Handbook of
Disruptive Behavior Disorders

Handbook of
Disruptive Behavior Disorders

Edited by

Herbert C. Quay and
Anne E. Hogan

University of Miami
Coral Gables, Florida

Kluwer Academic / Plenum Publishers
New York, Boston, Dordrecht, London, Moscow

ISBN 0-306-45974-4

© 1999 Kluwer Academic / Plenum Publishers, New York
233 Spring Street, New York, N.Y. 10013

10 9 8 7 6 5 4 3 2 1

A C.I.P. record for this book is available from the Library of Congress.

Printed in the United States of America

Contributors

Michael G. Aman, Ph.D. • The Nisonger Center for Mental Retardation and Developmental Disabilities, The Ohio State University, Columbus, Ohio 43210-1296

Russell A. Barkley, Ph.D. • Department of Psychiatry, University of Massachusetts Medical Center, Worcester, Massachusetts 01655

Betsey A. Benson, Ph.D. • The Nisonger Center for Mental Retardation and Developmental Disabilities, The Ohio State University, Columbus, Ohio 43210-1296

Dennis P. Cantwell[†], M.D. • Neuropsychiatric Institute, University of California, Los Angeles, Los Angeles, California 90095

Caryn L. Carlson, Ph.D. • Department of Psychology, University of Texas at Austin, Austin, Texas 78712-1189

F. Xavier Castellanos, M.D. • Child Psychiatry Branch, National Institute of Mental Health, Bethesda, Maryland 20892-1251

Patricia Chamberlain, Ph.D. • Oregon Social Learning Center, Eugene, Oregon 97401

Virginia I. Douglas, Ph.D. • Department of Psychology, McGill University and Montreal Children's Hospital, Montreal, Quebec, Canada H3A 1B1

Celia B. Fisher, Ph.D. • Department of Psychology, Fordham University, New York, New York 10458

Steven R. Forness, Ph.D. • Department of Special Education, University of California, Los Angeles, Los Angeles, California 90095-1759

Susan Frauenglass, Ph.D. • La Rabida Children's Hospital and Research Center, University of Chicago, Chicago, Illinois 60649

Paul J. Frick, Ph.D. • Department of Psychology, University of Alabama, Tuscaloosa, Alabama 35487

Rachel A. Gordon, Ph.D. • Department of Psychiatry, University of Chicago, Chicago, Illinois 60637

Laurence L. Greenhill, M.D. • Division of Child Psychiatry, New York State Psychiatric Institute/Columbia University, New York, New York 10032

Scott W. Henggeler, Ph.D. • Department of Psychiatry and Behavioral Sciences, Medical University of South Carolina, Charleston, South Carolina 29425-0742

Barbara Henker, Ph.D. • Department of Psychology, University of California, Los Angeles, Los Angeles, California 90095-1563

Stephen P. Hinshaw, Ph.D. • Department of Psychology, University of California, Berkeley, Berkeley, California 94720-1650

[†]Deceased.

97817

Kimberly Hoagwood, Ph.D. • Division of Mental Disorders, Behavioral Research, and AIDS, National Institute of Mental Health, Rockville, Maryland 20857-8030

Anne E. Hogan, Ph.D. • Department of Psychology, University of Miami, Coral Gables, Florida 33124-0721

Abel Ickowicz, M.D. • Department of Psychiatry, The Hospital for Sick Children, Toronto, Ontario, Canada M5G 1X8

Peter S. Jensen, M.D. • Division of Mental Disorders, Behavioral Research, and AIDS, National Institute of Mental Health, Rockville, Maryland 20857-8030

Kenneth A. Kavale, Ph.D. • Department of Special Education, The University of Iowa, Iowa City, Iowa 52242-1529

Rachel G. Klein, Ph.D. • Department of Clinical Psychology, Columbia University, and New York State Psychiatric Institute, New York, New York 10032

Benjamin B. Lahey, Ph.D. • Department of Psychiatry, University of Chicago, Chicago, Illinois 60637

Jane E. Ledingham, Ph.D. • School of Psychology, University of Ottawa, Ottawa, Ontario, Canada K1N 6N5

David LeMarquand, Ph.D. • Research Unit on Children's Psychosocial Maladjustment, University of Montreal, Montreal, Quebec, Canada H3T 1J7

Bryan R. Loney • Department of Psychology, University of Alabama, Tuscaloosa, Alabama 35487

Salvatore Mannuzza, Ph.D. • Department of Clinical Psychology, Columbia University, and New York State Psychiatric Institute, New York, New York 10032

Rob McGee, Ph.D. • Department of Preventive and Social Medicine, University of Otago Medical School, Dunedin, New Zealand

Jaap van der Meere, Ph.D. • Department of Experimental Clinical Psychology, University of Groningen, 9712 TS Groningen, The Netherlands

Terri L. Miller, Ph.D. • Department of Psychiatry, University of Chicago, Chicago, Illinois 60637

Jaap Oosterlaan, Ph.D. • Department of Clinical Psychology, University of Amsterdam, 1018 WB Amsterdam, The Netherlands

Teron Park, M.A. • Department of Psychology, University of California, Berkeley, Berkeley, California 94720-1650

William E. Pelham, Jr., Ph.D. • Department of Psychology, State University of New York at Buffalo, Buffalo, New York 14260-4110

Steven R. Pliszka, Ph.D. • Department of Psychiatry, The University of Texas Health Science Center at San Antonio, San Antonio, Texas 78284-7792

Margot Prior, Ph.D. • Department of Psychology, University of Melbourne, Parkville, Victoria 3052, Australia

Herbert C. Quay, Ph.D. • Department of Psychology, University of Miami, Coral Gables, Florida 33124-0721

Anne W. Riley, Ph.D. • School of Public Health, Johns Hopkins University, Baltimore, Maryland 21205

Donald K. Routh, Ph.D. • Department of Psychology, University of Miami, Coral Gables, Florida 33124-0721

Kalyani Samudra, M.D. • Department of Psychiatry, University of Colorado Health Sciences Center and Children's Hospital, Denver, Colorado 80218

Ann Sanson, Ph.D. • Department of Psychology, University of Melbourne, Parkville, Victoria 3052, Australia

Russell Schachar, M.D. • Department of Psychiatry, The Hospital for Sick Children, Toronto, Ontario, Canada M5G 1X8

Sonja K. Schoenwald, Ph.D. • Department of Psychiatry and Behavioral Sciences, Medical University of South Carolina, Charleston, South Carolina 29425-0742

Joseph A. Sergeant, Ph.D. • Department of Clinical Psychology, University of Amsterdam, 1018 WB Amsterdam, The Netherlands

Leanne Tamm, M.A. • Department of Psychology, University of Texas at Austin, Austin, Texas 78712-1189

Richard E. Tremblay, Ph.D. • Research Unit on Children's Psychosocial Maladjustment, University of Montreal, Montreal, Quebec, Canada H3T 1J7

Frank Vitaro, Ph.D. • Research Unit on Children's Psychosocial Maladjustment, University of Montreal, Montreal, Quebec, Canada H3T 1J7

Hill M. Walker, Ph.D. • Department of Special Education, University of Oregon, Eugene, Oregon 97403-1215

Daniel A. Waschbusch, Ph.D. • Department of Psychology, Dalhousie University, Halifax, Nova Scotia, Canada B3H 4J1

Bruce Waslick, M.D. • Division of Child Psychiatry, New York State Psychiatric Institute/ Columbia University, New York, New York 10032

John S. Werry, M.S. • Department of Psychiatry, University of Auckland, Auckland, New Zealand

Carol K. Whalen, Ph.D. • Department of Psychology and Social Behavior, University of California, Irvine, Irvine, California 92697-7085

Sheila Williams, Ph.D. • Department of Preventive and Social Medicine, University of Otago Medical School, Dunedin, New Zealand

Preface

The purpose of this *Handbook* is to provide the researcher, clinician, teacher, and student in all mental health fields with as up-to-date information as possible about what have come to be called the Disruptive Behavior Disorders of children and adolescents. To accomplish our purpose we have called upon 51 researchers and theorists in psychology, child and adolescent psychiatry, and education to provide comprehensive reviews of research in their areas of expertise. That this *Handbook* has more than 2600 references attests to both the amount of research interest in these disorders and the coverage provided by our authors.

The Disruptive Behavior Disorders, as labeled in the current taxonomy (DSM-IV), are Attention-Deficit/Hyperactivity Disorder (three subtypes), Conduct Disorder (two subtypes), and Oppositional Defiant Disorder.

Taken together, these disruptive disorders account for at least three fourths of the combined prevalence of all psychopathological disorders of childhood and adolescence. In particular, the two subtypes of Conduct Disorder—with their links to school failure and dropout, juvenile delinquency, criminality, and other indices of dysfunction in adulthood—are extremely costly both to society and to the individuals afflicted.

An understanding of the biological and psychosocial etiologies of these disorders, the settings that engender and maintain them, their natural history, and what may be the most effective intervention and prevention strategies for them are of prime importance to all professionals who must deal with these troubled and troublesome youth.

Part I covers the classification, epidemiology, and assessment of all three categories of the Disruptive Behavior Disorders.

Part II provides reviews of the research on Attention-Deficit/Hyperactivity Disorder, covering information processing, cognitive functioning, the child with this disorder in the family, school, and peer group, as well as reviews of the psychobiology, risk factors, pharmacotherapy, behavioral interventions, adolescent and adult outcomes, and theories of the disorder.

Part III provides reviews of the research on Conduct Disorder and Oppositional Defiant Disorder. Topics include cognitive functioning; problems posed by children with these disorders in the family, community, and school; and the psychobiological, temperament, and behavioral precursors and associated environmental risk factors for these disorders. Additional topics include pharmacotherapy and interventions in the home, community, school, and residential settings, as well as outcomes and prevention.

Part IV deals with special problems and issues, including the Disruptive Behavior Disorders in the mentally retarded, ethical and legal issues in research, and issues related to gender and ethnicity, as well as research problems encountered in studying these disorders.

The editors wish to acknowledge the special contributions of John S. Werry, M.D. Beyond his co-authorship of Chapter 21, he reviewed all of the biologically oriented chapters, providing us with the benefit of his expertise.

We also want to note, with sorrow, the untimely passing of Dennis P. Cantwell, M.D.

Denny will be missed by all of us in the field but especially by his residents and fellows. It is most unfortunate that many young psychiatrists will no longer have the opportunity to train with him and to benefit from his wit and wisdom.

Herbert C. Quay
Anne E. Hogan

Contents

III. Oppositional Defiant Disorder and Conduct Disorder

IV: Special Problems and Issues

I

Overview of the Disruptive Behavior Disorders

1

Classification of the Disruptive Behavior Disorders

HERBERT C. QUAY

INTRODUCTION

As is now well known, the development of a taxonomy of the phenomenon to be studied is a necessary first step in scientific inquiry. In psychopathology, the measurement or assessment of the constituent elements (most often referred to as symptoms) is the next step, leading to the classification (diagnosis) of individuals for intervention, research study, or both.

The bases and purposes of, and requisites for, a classification system for psychopathological behavior have been discussed elsewhere (see Blashfield, 1984; Blashfield & Livesley, 1991; Millon, 1991; Morey, 1991; Quay, 1986a) and need not be enumerated here.

Since the *Diagnostic and Statistical Manual of Mental Disorders* (4th edition [DSM-IV]; American Psychiatric Association, 1994) is now the most widely used classification system for clinical purposes in the United States and is becoming extremely influential in research in child and adolescent psychopathology, this chapter is organized around the DSM-IV Disruptive Behavior Disorders (DBD): Attention-Deficit/Hyperactivity Disorder (ADHD), Conduct Disorder (CD), and Oppositional-Defiant Disorder (ODD).* Alternatives to, and suggested expansions upon, the DSM-IV for classification are discussed later in this chapter.

OVERVIEW OF THE DEVELOPMENT OF DSM-IV

The DSM-IV section on the DBD is part of a larger section "Disorders Usually Diagnosed in Infancy, Childhood or Adolescence" that is itself a relatively small section of the overall DSM-IV. The development of the DBD section was undertaken with the same guidelines as was the entire DSM-IV. These guidelines included (1) basing proposed changes from DSM-III-R (American Psychiatric Association, 1987) on empirical reviews and reports rather than solely on expert opinion or committee consensus and (2) new criteria maximizing as much as possible the correspondence with other diagnostic systems (see Shaffer *et al.*, 1989).

In the case of each of the DBD, changes from DSM-III-R were instituted after initial literature reviews and small group sessions. Subsequently, the results of field trials were used to finalize the operational criteria (symptom lists),

HERBERT C. QUAY • Department of Psychology, University of Miami, Coral Gables, Florida 33124-0721.

Handbook of Disruptive Behavior Disorders, edited by Quay and Hogan. Kluwer Academic/Plenum Publishers, New York, 1999.

*These disorders are grouped under the heading of Attention-Deficit and Disruptive Behavior Disorders. However, all three disorders have come to be referred to as disruptive. That usage is carried on in this chapter and subsequent chapters in this Handbook.

to set thresholds for the number of symptoms required to make a diagnosis, to establish criteria for duration of symptoms, to include situational pervasiveness and age of onset of symptoms in ADHD, and to choose the method of subtyping CD.

Empirical research into the classification of behavior disorders in children and adolescents goes back at least 50 years. These studies became increasingly sophisticated when the development of electronic computers made factor analysis and other types of multivariate statistical analyses of large numbers of variables and large numbers of cases practicable. A number of comprehensive reviews of these studies were published from 1978 to about 1988 (Achenbach & Edelbrock, 1978; Quay, 1972, 1979, 1986a).

It is also important to recognize that preceding DSM-IV, there was DSM-III-R (American Psychiatric Association, 1987), DSM-III (American Psychiatric Association, 1980), and DSM-II (American Psychiatric Association, 1968); the latter, however, provided very little with regard to disorders of childhood and adolescence. Since there have been a multitude of research studies on the DBD that have used DSM-III and DSM-III-R criteria, I briefly review, for each diagnostic category, the changes that have occurred in the thinking about the DBD culminating in DSM-IV.

DSM-IV ADHD

Comparisons with DSM-III and DSM-III-R

DSM-III permitted the diagnosis of two subtypes: Attention-Deficit Disorder with Hyperactivity (ADDH) and without Hyperactivity, based on lists of three different clusters of symptoms: Inattention, Impulsivity, and Hyperactivity.

Despite a much lower prevalence of ADD without Hyperactivity, evidence began to accumulate suggesting that the subtype distinction had both validity and utility (see Carlson, 1986; Lahey & Carlson, 1991; Lahey, Carlson, & Frick, 1997, for reviews). However, DSM-III-R did away with the "without" subtype but let it in the back door by way of the "Undifferentiated" subtype.

The DSM-III-R operational criteria were collapsed into a list of 14 symptoms, of which 9 were reworded from DSM-III and 4 were new. Despite the requirement that 8 of the 14 symptoms be present, it became possible to meet criteria for ADDH with *no* symptoms of inattention, at least as these had been considered in DSM-III. As McBurnett (1997) has pointed out, two children could each exhibit 8 symptoms, yet only share 2 in common. It is clear that the DSM-III-R approach could, and no doubt did, lead to considerable heterogeneity among diagnosed cases.

DSM-IV provides lists for two types of symptoms, Inattention and Hyperactivity-Impulsivity (see Table 1), permits diagnosis based on meeting criteria of six or more symptoms from either list, and provides for three subtypes: Predominantly Inattentive, Predominantly Hyperactive-Impulsive, and Combined. In addition to meeting criteria for number of symptoms, there are criteria for duration, maladaptiveness, age of onset, and impairment in two or more settings.

TABLE 1.   Operational Criteria (Abridged) for Attention-Deficit/Hyperactivity Disorder in the DSM-IV

Inattention
   Fails to give close attention to detail; careless mistakes
   Difficulty sustaining attention
   Does not seem to listen when spoken to
   Does not follow through; fails to finish
   Difficulty organizing
   Avoids, dislikes tasks requiring sustained mental effort
   Often loses things
   Easily distracted
   Forgetful
Hyperactivity
   Fidgets, squirms
   Leaves seat
   Runs about or climbs excessively
   Difficulty playing quietly
   Often "on the go"
Impulsivity
   Blurts out answers
   Difficulty awaiting turn
   Interrupts or intrudes on others

The Field Trials

As is the case for CD and ODD, the ADHD symptom lists, threshold score, and other criteria were heavily influenced by the results of field trials. Table 2 provides an outline of the methodology for the field trials for all three of the DBD.

Symptom Selection

Frick and colleagues (1994) have provided data on the chance-corrected positive predictive power (PPP) and negative predictive power (NPP) of each symptom in predicting a score at or above the interview schedule diagnostic threshold for both Inattention (six symptoms) and Hyperactivity-Impulsivity (five symptoms) with that symptom removed. PPP is the pro-

TABLE 2.   Subjects and Assessments Utilized in the DSM-IV Field Trials for ADHD, CD, and ODD

Subjects

440 clinic-referred cases from 7 different outpatient and inpatient settings: 336 males, 104 females; ages 4–17 (mean age 9.5)

Ethnicity: 61% European American, 20% African American, 15.2% Hispanic American, 1.6% Asian American, 2.1% Other

Assessments

Diagnostic Interview Schedule for Children (DISC-2), slightly modified
    Child (DISC-2C)
    Parent (DISC-2P)
    Teacher (DISC2-T)
    (not all informants interviewed for all subjects)

Children's Global Assessment Scale (CGAS)
    Completed by both parent and interviewer with Impairment defined as a score of 60 or worse

Parent ratings of child's problems in completing homework

Teacher ratings of accuracy and quality of academic work completed in the classroom

Teacher estimation of extent of child's social impairment

Parent report of school suspensions and police contacts

Official records of police contact (subsample of 86 cases)

Clinician's (validation) diagnosis based on all available information and on the criteria for any version of the DSM or ICD or their own criteria

Note. From Lahey, Applegate, Barkley, *et al.*(1994) and Lahey, Applegate, McBurnett, *et al.* (1994). Reprinted with permission.

portion of individuals with the symptom who have the disorder, and NPP is the proportion of individuals without the symptom who do not have the disorder. Each symptom had moderate to high PPP (mean of .69) and NPP (mean of .76) at or above the threshold for Inattention, as well as for Hyperactivity-Impulsivity (.73 and .65).

Diagnostic Threshold

In setting the diagnostic threshold as reported by Lahey, Applegate, McBurnett, and colleagues (1994), initial analyses determined that the number of Hyperactivity-Impulsivity symptoms was strongly related to scores on both the interviewer and parent versions of the Children's Global Assessment Scale (CGAS; Shaffer *et al.*, 1983) but the number of Inattention symptoms was not. Therefore, CGAS scores were used as external criteria for selection of the threshold score for the Hyperactivity-Impulsivity symptoms. Since the number of Inattention symptoms was related to both teacher and parent measures of impairment in academic functioning, these two measures were used to select the threshold for Inattention symptoms.

As reported by Lahey, Applegate, McBurnett, and colleagues (1994) a score of five Hyperactivity-Impulsivity symptoms predicted CGAS impairment for both parent and interviewer and optimized agreement with the validation diagnosis. The kappa for test–retest agreement was .66. Although these analyses indicated that a threshold of five symptoms provided the best identification of impaired cases and agreement with clinicians, Lahey, Applegate, McBurnett, and colleagues stated that "In order to minimize the identification of normally active children as exhibiting attention deficit hyperactivity disorder, however, the DSM-IV Child Disorder Work Group chose the more conservative threshold of six symptoms of hyperactivity-impulsivity for DSM-IV" (pp. 1676–1677).

Similar analyses were conducted to set the threshold for Inattention symptoms. For the identification of cases with academic impairment as rated by either teacher or parent, both six and seven symptoms produced a similar result. Test–retest agreement peaked at seven symptoms. The association of the number of Inattention symptoms and validation diagnosis was best at six symptoms, although the kappa was a moderate .42. More detailed analyses revealed that the clinicians diagnosed ADHD when six Hyperactivity-Impulsivity symptoms were present *regardless* of the number of Inattention symptoms present. Because the model of ADHD adopted for the field trials was based on the assumption that the diagnosis of ADHD would be defined as the presence of clinically significant numbers of symptoms of *both* Inattention and Hyperactivity-Impulsivity, this finding related to the diagnosis of ADHD indicated that DSM-IV ADHD would maximize agreement with clinicians only if a subtype diagnosis could be made on the basis of significant levels of Hyperactivity-Impulsivity alone.

In the end, a definition was adopted in which a diagnosis could be made on the basis of either six or more Inattention symptoms, six or more Hyperactivity-Impulsivity symptoms, or both. Thus, the three subtypes were identified by this definition. Additional analyses revealed that the predominantly hyperactive-impulsive cases were younger than either the combined type or the predominantly inattentive type, whereas those with the combined type were younger than those with the predominantly inattentive type.

Age of Onset

Applegate and colleagues (1997) have addressed the validity of the DSM-IV age-of-onset criterion of impairment due to symptoms before age 7. They compared cases who met symptom criteria and who either did or did not meet the DSM-IV age-of-onset-of-impairment criterion to determine whether they differed on variables that addressed the validity of the ADHD diagnosis. They compared the (age-of-onset) groups on the rate of validation diagnoses of ADHD, on two types of impairment (CGAS and Academic) characteristic of ADHD, and on rates of other disorders that might have better accounted for the ADHD symptoms.

Their results first indicated that the great majority of cases who met symptom criteria for one of the three subtypes were reported by parents to have an age of onset of the *first symptom* before age 7; the median age of onset of the first symptom was 1 year of age. However, the median age of onset of *impairment* due to symptoms was 3.5 years.

For the combined subtype, 82% of cases had an age of onset of impairment of less than 7 years and 96% had at least one symptom prior to age 7. Ninety-eight percent of the Predominantly Hyperactive-Impulsive type exhibited impairment before age 7, and 100% had at least one symptom before age 7. In contrast, only 57% of the Predominantly Inattentive were impaired by age 7 although 85% had at least one symptom prior to age 7.

The difference in age of onset of impairment among the three groups was statistically significant. With regard to age of onset of the first symptom, the Predominantly Inattentive group had a significantly later age of onset than the other two groups who did not differ.

Applegate and colleagues (1997) then compared cases in the combined type who had earlier versus later age of onset of impairment. The hypothesis was that those 18% with a later age of onset of impairment would be less impaired at the time of assessment, less likely to receive a validation diagnosis of ADHD, and more likely to meet criteria for other diagnoses. Although those cases with both earlier and later onset of impairment differed significantly from those individuals who did *not* meet ADHD symptom criteria on all variables, there were no differences between the earlier and later onset subgroups of the combined type on any of the criterion variables. Thus, once symptom criteria for the combined subtype were met, the age of onset of impairment did not matter.

A similar result was obtained for cases who met criteria for the Predominantly Inattentive type: Age of onset of impairment was not related to degree of impairment at assessment, validation diagnosis, or comorbidity.

Only the Predominantly Inattentive subtype contained cases (43%) in which the age of onset of the first symptom was *later* than 7 years; therefore, only this group could be studied with respect to earlier (less than 7 years) versus later (7 to 8 years) age of onset of the first symptom. While both groups differed from the non-ADHD cases, they did not differ from each other. Since only two cases had an onset later than 8 years, "later" onset essentially means after age 7 but before age 8.

It would appear that the DSM-IV criteria with respect to age of onset of impairment prior to 7 years is problematic. Applegate and colleagues (1997) noted that a considerable number of youth who met symptom criteria for ADHD did not have a reported age of onset of impairment before 7 years of age. This is more the case for the combined and Predominantly Inattentive subtypes; almost all (98%) of the Hyperactive-Impulsive subtype were impaired prior to age 7. Later onset of impairment was not associated with either less impairment, more comorbid diagnoses, or fewer validation diagnoses at assessment; therefore, the DSM-IV age-of-onset-of-impairment criterion may result in the failure to diagnose cases who meet symptom criteria and are impaired.

Critique of the Field Trials and DSM-IV ADHD

It is obvious that there is some lack of independence of the ADHD symptoms and both the parent and teacher reports of global and academic impairment, and especially the validation diagnosis. It is difficult to see how parents, particularly, could report large numbers of symptoms without reporting impairment. Of necessity, the clinicians had access to the symptom reports in making their validation diagnoses.

At the same time, the finding that Inattentive symptoms were not related to CGAS impairment but were related to academic impairment, while the reverse was true for the Hyperactive-Impulsive symptoms, argues for the differential validity of the two types of symptoms.

Based on the research cited earlier indicating both different background factors and corre-lates of Attention-Deficit Disorder with and without Hyperactivity, the DSM-IV subtypes seem well justified. The fact that DSM-IV permits the diagnosis of ADHD without the presence of *any* symptoms of Inattention seems paradoxical. However, it may be that younger children diagnosable as the Hyperactive-Impulsive subtype have not yet developed or manifested the attentional symptoms that will occur when their attentional capacity is challenged.

Wolraich, Hannah, Pinnock, Baumgaertel, and Brown (1996) obtained teacher ratings on all DSM-IV items for the DBD on a countywide sample of 8258 children in grades K–5. A factor analysis resulted in separate factors for Inattention and Hyperactivity-Impulsivity.

Given the research referred to earlier and the occasional finding of independent dimensions of attention problems and excess motor behavior in multivariate statistical studies (see Quay, 1986a), the question arises as to whether there are two *separate* disorders with different underlying pathologies in terms of disinhibition-impulsivity and "true" attentional deficits (see Quay, 1997; Chapters 4 and 5, this volume). DSM-IV now permits the diagnosis of both conditions as well as the combined subtype, thus facilitating research that can explore basic differences among all three subtypes. In fact, such research has already begun to appear (e.g., Faraone, Biederman, Weber, & Russell, 1998; Gaub & Carlson, 1997; Morgan, Hynd, Riccio, & Hall, 1996).

DSM-IV CD

Comparison with DSM-III and DSM-III-R

DSM-III provided separate diagnostic criteria for four subtypes of CD: Undersocialized Aggressive, Undersocialized Nonaggressive, Socialized Aggressive, and Socialized Nonaggressive. Diagnoses required a duration of at least 6 months. Criteria for each category contained the same set of five behaviors indicating social attachment or lack thereof. The separate symptom criteria required that only one of either two symptoms (for Undersocialized

Aggressive and Socialized Aggressive) or four symptoms (for Undersocialized Nonaggressive and Socialized Nonaggressive) be present.

DSM-III-R provided a list of 13 symptoms, with at least 3 present for at least 6 months to meet criteria. Three subtypes were briefly described. In the Group Type, conduct problems occurring mainly as a group activity with peers predominated. In the Solitary Aggressive subtype, aggressive physical behavior toward both adults and peers was predominant. An Undifferentiated subtype with a mixture of clinical features that could not be classified as either of the other subtypes was also listed. In contrast to DSM-III there were no separate operational criteria, either inclusionary or exclusionary, for making subtype diagnoses.

DSM-IV provides a list of 15 symptoms grouped, for mnemonic purposes, under the rubrics of Aggression to People and Animals, Destruction of Property, Deceitfulness or Theft, and Serious Violations of the Rules (see Table 3). Diagnosis requires the presence of three or more symptoms in the past 12 months with at least one symptom present in the past 6 months. In addition, there must be present clinically significant impairment in social, academic, or occupational functioning. Two subtypes are provided based on age of onset of at least one symptom: childhood onset (prior to age 10 years) and adolescent onset (no symptoms prior to age 10 years).

The Field Trials

Symptom Selection

As was the case for ADHD, Frick and colleagues (1994) have provided data on the chance-corrected PPP and NPP for predicting a score at or above the diagnostic threshold for the 15 symptoms used for the provisional diagnosis of CD, as well as 3 alternate symptoms. The PPPs for all of the symptoms were moderate to high, while the NPPs (proportion without symptoms but with CD) were much lower. As Frick and colleagues (1991) noted earlier, the high PPP–low NPP pattern is typical for symptoms with low base rates, which in this study ranged from 3% for fire-setting to 34% for stealing. As these authors stated, "the low NPP suggests that the absence of symptoms should not be considered highly indicative of the absence of the disorder" (Frick et al., 1994, p. 537). What the authors mean is that the absence of any *particular* symptom does not mean that the disorder is absent.

Diagnostic Threshold

As reported by Lahey, Applegate, Barkley, and colleagues (1994), the analyses of the association of the number of CD symptoms with both parent and interviewer CGAS ratings were not helpful in choosing a diagnostic threshold. Even a single CD symptom resulted in the CGAS score selected as indicating clinically significant impairment. Number of school suspensions was also not helpful as there was a linear relationship between symptoms and suspensions with no optimal cutting point.

However, number of lifetime police contacts (when the delinquent subsample was eliminated) showed the greatest upward inflection at three symptoms. Furthermore, a threshold of three symptoms using the past year—one

TABLE 3. Operational Criteria (Abridged) for Conduct Disorder in DSM-IV

Aggression to people and animals
  Bullies, threatens or intimidates
  Initiates physical fights
  Has used a weapon
  Physically cruel to people
  Physically cruel to animals
  Has stolen while confronting victim
  Forced sexual activity
Destruction to property
  Fire-setting with intent to damage
  Destroys others' property
Deceitfulness or theft
  Breaking into house, building, or car
  "Cons" others
  Stealing without confrontation
Serious violations of rules
  Stays out at night beginning before age 13
  Runs away from home overnight at least twice
  Truant from school before age 13

symptom past 6 months best predicted the validation diagnoses (kappa about .60) and test–retest reliability (kappa of .64).

In light of the discussion on subtyping of CD to follow, it would be of interest to know whether certain subsets of three symptoms predicted police contacts while others did not. Given that some of the 15 symptoms are violations of the law almost certain to attract official attention (e.g., fire-setting, breaking and entering, stealing, truancy, forced sex) while others are much less likely to result in official intervention (e.g., bullying, "conning" others, initiating fights), meeting CD criteria on the basis of three of the former would seem more likely to result in police contacts than meeting criteria with three symptoms of the latter.

Subtyping of CD

The subtyping of CD on the basis of an informant's report of the onset of a single symptom prior to or after age 10 years represents a radical departure from earlier DSMs, from the DSM-IV subtyping of ADHD on the basis of differing clusters of symptoms, from ICD-10 (World Health Organization, 1992; discussed later in this chapter), and from the symptom-based subtypes found throughout the multivariate statistical literature. This departure seems to be the result of a convergence of factors. Of the four subtypes of DSM-III the two nonaggressive subtypes had very little empirical underpinning and were rarely diagnosed. Although DSM-III-R essentially retained the undersocialized versus socialized subtypes (solitary vs. group), the criteria for making a subtype diagnosis were sketchy at best. These factors resulted in considerable dissatisfaction with behaviorally based subtypes, at least as found in DSM-III and DSM-III-R.

Lahey and colleagues (1998) have noted research suggesting early onset as predictive of adverse consequences into adulthood, the prior lack of established criteria in the DSMs for the amount or type of aggression required to exhibit the aggressive subtype of CD, and the finding that boys who meet criteria for CD show fluctuating levels of aggression over time.*

It is obvious that many of the DSM-IV symptoms of CD are age-related and are more likely to occur at an earlier or later age (this issue will be discussed in more detail later in this chapter). What follows is that age of onset is likely to be related to clusters of symptoms that, in themselves, may define behavioral subtypes. In fact, in the narrative descriptions of the CD subtypes, DSM-IV states "Individuals with the childhood-onset type are usually male, frequently display physical aggression toward others, [and] have disturbed peer relationships . . ." (American Psychiatric Association, 1994, p. 86). In contrast, the adolescent-onset type "are less likely to display aggressive behaviors and tend to have more normative peer relationships (although they often display conduct problems in the company of others)" (p. 87).

Lahey and colleagues (1998) have reported on the development of age of onset as the basis for subtyping CD in DSM-IV. Using data from the field trials, these authors first determined that 28.6% of the clinical sample met DSM-IV criteria for CD and 5.8% of a household sample met DSM-III-R criteria for CD. The youngest age of onset of any symptom of CD reported by either parent or youth defined the age of onset. Cases of childhood onset (first symptom before age 10) and adolescent onset (first symptom at age 10 or older) were then compared on a number of other measures.

In the clinic sample there was a significantly greater proportion of females in the adolescent-onset group than in the childhood-onset group, but in the household sample this was not the case. In both samples, earlier age of onset was related to the presence of more aggressive symptoms. Data provided by Lahey (personal communication, April 1997) revealed that in the clinic sample, 84% of early-onset cases had *two* or more aggressive symptoms as opposed to 40% of the adolescent-onset youths. In the household sample the proportions were almost exactly the same for having

*With respect to these issues, however, I note that dimensional measures do provide criteria to distinguish aggressive subtypes. It is also true that individuals also fluctuate in terms of meeting criteria for CD over time (Lahey *et al.*, 1995).

one or more aggressive symptoms: 84% early onset versus 39% late onset.

The number of nonaggressive symptoms was not related to age of onset in either the clinic or household samples. As might be expected, the number of nonaggressive symptoms was related to the youth's being older at the time of assessment.

Given the association of age of onset and greater number of aggressive symptoms, it is surprising that no significant associations of age of onset were found for either parent or interviewer ratings of impairment, police contacts, school expulsions, or school suspensions. In the clinic sample, but not in the household sample, childhood onset was significantly related to a higher number of maternal and paternal antisocial behaviors.

In their discussion, Lahey and colleagues (1998) noted that because age of onset is strongly related to level of aggression, it appears that subtyping on one dimension would have the effect of subtyping on the other as well. However, as noted earlier, they argued that because level of aggression fluctuates over time (see Lahey *et al.,* 1995), subtyping on the basis of age of onset is more straightforward. At the same time, they pointed out that the DSM-IV subtyping scheme classifies essentially the same cases as does earlier subtyping based on aggression.

Fluctuating levels of aggression over time clearly present a problem in subtyping CD on the basis of aggressive versus nonaggressive (or delinquent) symptoms, but if subtyping by age of onset of the first symptom is to be valid the ascertainment of that age of onset must be accurate and reliable. Angold, Erkanli, Costello, and Rutter (1996) have pointed out that the accuracy of either child or parent recall and report is unlikely to be determinable. One can conceive of the rare situation in which the onset of a first symptom was so sudden and dramatic as to be "marked on the calendar," such as might be the case in posttraumatic stress disorder. The time of first onset of a CD symptom, however, is unlikely to be so dramatic and memorable.

Reliability, in terms of the onset date for a symptom as reported on two different occasions, can be much more easily determined. Angold and colleagues (1996) studied the reliability of symptom onsets in both child and parent reports on a structured interview schedule obtained at two different times an average of 5 days apart. For the child self-reports, they found that only 42.4% of 161 symptoms reported on both occasions had reported onsets even within 1 year of one another. For parent reports, 60.2% of onset reports were within 1 year of one another. Furthermore, when these researchers looked at the precision, that is, the extent to which children or parents could pinpoint onset (e.g., "sometime last year" vs. "in March of last year"), they found that for both children and parents CD and ODD symptoms were less precisely reported than symptoms of other types of disorders.

These findings are disquieting even given the relatively low degree of precision required for CD subtyping (i.e., onset before or after age 10). On the other hand, the high degree of overlap between age of onset and aggressive versus nonaggressive (delinquent) symptoms in the field trial data (Lahey *et al.,* 1998) suggests that reports of onset as prior to or after age 10 will identify aggressive versus nonaggressive cases.

Critique of DSM-IV CD

The field trial results (Lahey, Applegate, Barkley, *et al.,* 1994) clearly indicated that each of the 15 symptoms had a positive relationship in predicting a CD diagnosis, but there are a number of troublesome problems with such a large and varied list of symptoms combined with a low threshold for meeting diagnostic criteria. As was pointed out earlier, at least 7 of the 15 symptoms consist of unlawful acts. Thus, it is likely that most youth who have been adjudicated delinquent will meet CD criteria. However, many youth who are legally delinquent do not obtain high scores on dimensional measures of either undersocialized or socialized aggression but on dimensions of disorder not considered disruptive or do not have high scores on *any* dimension of disorder (see Quay, 1987, for a review).

Finally, if age of onset subtyping does not produce subgroups similar to the earlier categories undersocialized versus socialized, then a considerable amount of research demonstrating meaningful differences in these subtypes (see Quay, 1986b, 1987) will be ignored.

DSM-IV ODD

Comparisons with DSM-III and DSM-III-R

DSM-III described Oppositional Disorder as a pattern of disobedient, negativistic, and provocative opposition to authority figures. Diagnostic criteria provided for an onset after age 3 and before age 18, a 6-month duration, and a threshold of at least two of five symptoms, but with no violation of the basic rights of others or of major age-appropriate societal norms or rules as in CD.

"Defiant" was added to the title of the disorder in DSM-III-R, where it was described as a pattern of negativistic, hostile, and defiant behavior without the more serious violations of the basic rights of others in CD. It was also noted that because cases diagnosed as CD were likely to have all the symptoms of ODD as well, a CD diagnosis preempted a diagnosis of ODD. DSM-III-R provided a list of nine symptoms, requiring that at least five be present for at least 6 months. Furthermore, a criterion was considered to be met "only if the behavior is considerably more frequent than that of most people of the same mental age" (American Psychiatric Association, 1987, p. 57).

In DSM-IV, ODD is a pattern of negativistic, hostile, and defiant behavior lasting at least 6 months in which at least four of eight criteria are present. The symptom list is the same as that in DSM-III-R but with the deletion of "often swears and uses obscene language" (see Table 4). As in DSM-III-R, a criterion is considered to be met "only if the behavior occurs more frequently than is typically observed in individuals of comparable age and developmental level" (American Psychiatric Association, 1994, p. 94) and "the distur-

bance in behavior causes clinically significant impairment in social, academic or occupational functioning" (p. 94). A CD diagnosis remains preemptive of an ODD diagnosis.

The Field Trials

Symptom Selection

Frick and colleagues (1994) have reported chance-corrected PPP and NPP for the eight ODD symptoms in predicting the interview schedule diagnosis of ODD. PPP values ranged from .88 to .51 (mean approximately .70); the NPP values ranged from .76 to .34 (mean = .62). Although the ODD symptoms have poor utility in the prediction of a diagnosis of CD, a number of CD symptoms had utility in predicting ODD. In fact, six CD symptoms had higher PPP values (.73–1.00) than the average of the ODD symptoms: use of a weapon, firesetting, cruelty to people, cruelty to animals, staying out late at night, and initiating fights.

Diagnostic Threshold

Lahey, Applegate, Barkley, and colleagues (1994) reported that for both parent and interviewers the CGAS impairment criterion was reached at four symptoms. For the validation diagnosis, three symptoms resulted in a kappa of .59 and four symptoms produced a kappa of .55. For test–retest reliability, both three, four, and six symptoms resulted in essentially equal kappas (.54). The more conservative threshold of four symptoms was chosen to minimize the

TABLE 4. Operational Criteria (Abridged) for Oppositional-Defiant Disorder in DSM-IV

Often loses temper
Often argues with adults
Often actively defies or refuses to comply
Often deliberately annoys people
Often blames others
Often touchy or easily annoyed
Often angry and resentful
Often spiteful or vindictive

number of false positives although more cases would be missed than if the threshold were set at three symptoms.

In a general population sample of 1071 children, ages 9, 11, and 13 (screened so as to oversample for disorder), Angold and Costello (1996) found the prevalence of DSM-IV ODD to be 2.4% when both impairment and a preemptive diagnosis of CD were considered, but without consideration of the 6-month duration criterion. The subsequent use of this criterion, however, made no change in the prevalence rate. However, the youngest children were already age 9 when first studied.

Because the results of the field trials (Lahey, Applegate, Barkley, *et al.*, 1994) indicated that the presence of only two or three ODD symptoms produced as good agreement with validation diagnoses and test–retest reliability as did the chosen threshold of four symptoms, Angold and Costello (1996) also compared cases with two or three ODD symptoms plus parent- or child-rated impairment with those who had four symptoms. These cases were, by definition, impaired, by the measures used by Angold and Costello (see Angold *et al.*, 1995, for a description), in that they had one or more of five other measures of diminished function (e.g., receiving treatment) and that 22% met criteria for another diagnosis (vs. 27% meeting full DSM-IV criteria); these authors suggested reducing the number of symptoms required for ODD to two or three, but maintaining the requirement for impairment.

Angold and Costello's (1996) Table 2 (p. 1210) notes, however, that 54 cases met full DSM-IV criteria while an additional 45 cases had three symptoms plus impairment, and an added 53 cases had two symptoms plus impairment. Thus, a three-symptom threshold adds 83% more cases and a two-symptom cutoff almost triples the original number of cases by adding a total of 98 cases to the original 54. According to Angold (personal communication, 1998), at three-plus symptoms, the weighted population prevalence rate is 4.4%, while at two-plus symptoms, it is 8%.

Are ODD and CD Independent Syndromes?

The addition of OD (later ODD) to the DSM was controversial from the beginning, in part because of the lack of a firm empirical foundation for the disorder as separate from CD. One apparent reason for the addition of ODD (although to this writer's knowledge, nowhere documented) was the reluctance of clinicians to give a child, particularly a younger one, a diagnosis of CD because of the connotation of this diagnosis as regards treatability and prognosis.

In an early discussion of CD and ODD in light of preparations for DSM-IV, Loeber, Lahey, and Thomas (1991) suggested that a possible distinction between ODD and CD could be conceptualized in at least three ways: as distinct entities, as more or less severe expressions of the same etiology "wherein some youths progress over time from the less severe symptoms (ODD) to the more severe symptoms (CD)" (p. 379), or as largely distinct disorders with one or more etiological factors in common. There is, of course, at least one additional possibility: that ODD and CD may be distinct disorders but are so highly associated that they most often occur simultaneously.

It is clear that CD and ODD are related, both empirically, as will be discussed later, and conceptually, as they are both considered in DSM-IV as DBD. From a developmental perspective, many of the operational criteria of both ODD and CD are age-related. The symptoms of ODD are all within the physical and mental capacity of a 4-year-old to perform. In contrast, some of the symptoms of CD, for example, use of weapons, stealing with confrontation, forced sexual activity, breaking and entering, and school truancy, are simply not in the behavioral repertoire of the overwhelming majority of preschoolers or early-elementary-age children.

Also relevant is the developmental course of the symptoms. Loeber and colleagues (1991) have reviewed much of the literature (on nonclinical samples), which indicates that in most children such symptoms as threatening, cruelty to animals, attention-demanding, physical attacks, temper tantrums, and disobedience at home decline with age; these are symptoms considered by Loeber and colleagues to be "oppositional." In contrast, behaviors characterized by Loeber and colleagues as "covert" CD, such as truancy from school, alcohol or marijuana use, stealing, and stealing at school, increase with age. As I noted earlier, these "nonaggressive" delinquent symptoms are associated with adolescent-onset CD.

Thus, younger children could meet criteria for ODD without meeting criteria for CD, while most older children who meet childhood-onset CD criteria would likely meet ODD criteria as well, giving rise to the DSM-IV rule that excludes a diagnosis of ODD if CD criteria (of either subtype) are met.

If, as these developmental considerations suggest, ODD is a less severe disorder, but is a precursor of CD (at least to the childhood-onset subtype) then we need to know the probability of progression from ODD to CD. Studies relevant to this issue are described in Chapter 19, this volume.

The case for considering ODD and CD as independent disorders can be bolstered if (1) the two can be shown to be independent syndromes by statistical analysis and (2) they have differential relationships with other relevant variables, including differences in etiology and response to treatment.

Although the question of the independence of CD and ODD had not arisen at the time, my 1986 review (Quay, 1986a) of the multivariate statistical studies indicated consistent findings of two independent "conduct disorder" dimensions often labeled Undersocialized Aggressive and Socialized Aggressive. Of the 8 DSM-IV symptoms of ODD, 3 (loses temper, defies, is touchy) have their counterparts among the 15 symptoms most often found in the Undersocialized Aggressive syndrome. Of the 15 symptoms of DSM-IV CD, 4 (bullying, fighting, destroying property, lying) appear in the Undersocialized Aggressive cluster and 3 (running away from home,

staying out at night, truant from school) appear in the Socialized Aggressive dimension (see Quay, 1986a, Tables 1.4 and 1.5).

These comparisons, however, leave five DSM-IV ODD symptoms and eight CD symptoms unaccounted for in these multivariate studies. This does not mean that these symptoms *never* appeared in *any* multivariate study in a CD (or other) factor, but these five ODD and eight CD symptoms were not found frequently in the two CD factors.

In their study of parent ratings of 8194 6- to 16-year-olds referred to American and Dutch mental health services, Achenbach, Conners, Quay, Verhulst, and Howell (1989) found two CD dimensions in both younger (6–11) and older (12–16) boys and girls. These were labeled "Aggressive" and "Delinquent." Abbreviated item descriptions for the two dimensions are provided in Table 5.

The Aggressive factor (which contains 19 items) includes some form of 5 of the 8 DSM-IV ODD symptoms: has a strong temper, argues, defies, is touchy (irritable), angry, and

TABLE 5. Parent-Rated Items (Abridged) for the Aggressive and Delinquent Syndromes

Aggressive	Delinquent
Argues	Alcohol, drugs
Brags, boasts	Bad companions
Bullies	Cheats, lies
Demands attention	Destroys others' things
Disobedient at home	Disobedient at school
Doesn't feel guilty	Runs away from home
Easily jealous	Sets fires
Impulsive	Steals at home
Loud	Steals outside home
Screams	Truancy
Shows off	Vandalism
Starts fights	
Stubborn, irritable	
Sudden mood changes	
Sulks	
Swearing, obscenity	
Talks too much	
Teases	
Temper tantrums	

Note. From Achenbach *et al.* (1989).

resentful (sulks); and 2 of the 15 DSM-IV CD symptoms: bullies and physically fights.

None of the DSM-IV ODD symptoms appear on the Delinquent factor. However, 6 of the 15 DSM-IV CD symptoms appear on this factor: fire-setting, property destruction, stealing (stealing outside the home), running away from home, and truancy.

On the basis of this large sample of parent ratings on 215 items of behavioral-emotional deviance, it is difficult to argue for a dimension of ODD that is independent of the aggressive CD dimension. There is obviously very convincing evidence for two dimensions of CD, one of which subsumes symptoms most of which are not only norm-violating but clearly illegal.

In a study of 2600 4- to 16-year-olds assessed at intake into mental health services and 2600 demographically matched nonreferred children, Achenbach, Howell, Quay, and Conners (1991) found an increase with age of scores on the Delinquent dimension along with a decrease with age in scores on the Aggressive dimension. Given the nature of the items on those dimensions, this finding was to be expected and parallels the findings of Loeber and colleagues (1991) noted earlier.

More recently, Frick and colleagues (1993) attacked the problem by the use of multidimensional scaling of the extent to which CD and ODD symptoms appeared on the same factors in studies published between 1980 and 1990. Two solutions were considered. The first was a single bipolar dimension (the conceptual equivalent of two orthogonal factors) with the more overtly aggressive CD and ODD symptoms at one pole and the more covertly aggressive (or, in my terms, socialized aggressive) items at the other. This solution was much like the earlier findings of Loeber and Schmaling (1985) who coined the terms "overt" and "covert" CD.

The second solution provided for two bipolar dimensions, the conceptual equivalent of four factors. The second bipolar dimension was labeled destructive versus nondestructive. The destructive-covert quadrant contained vandalism, stealing, fire-setting, and lying and was labeled "property violations." The destructive-overt quadrant contained assault, spitefulness, cruelty, fighting, bullying, and blaming others and received the designation of "aggression." The nondestructive-covert quadrant contained running away, truancy, substance abuse, breaking rules, and swearing and was called "status violations." Finally, the overt-nondestructive quadrant covered high temper, defiance, arguing, stubbornness, annoying others, and touchiness and was labeled "oppositional."

It is the appearance of this pole that provides evidence for the independence of an oppositional syndrome. This pattern does contain six of the eight DSM-IV symptoms of ODD (high temper, arguing, defiance, annoying others, touchiness, anger). It is of interest that nine DSM-IV CD symptoms are spread over the remaining three quadrants, suggesting the possibility of three behavioral subtypes of CD.

When considering the two solutions it should be noted that multidimensional scaling and exploratory factor analysis have a common issue: when to stop factoring. In this instance the two-pole solution clearly allows us to have hopes for the independence of ODD from CD as a syndrome of DBD.

Frick and colleagues (1991) directly tested the factorial independence of CD and ODD by factor analyzing teacher and parent responses to a structured interview inquiring about all DSM-III and DSM-III-R symptoms of ODD and CD in a sample of 177 clinic-attending boys ages 7–12 years. For the parent reports a two-factor solution was obtained wherein all ODD symptoms and four CD symptoms (bullying, breaking major rules, lying, and fighting) loaded on the first factor. The second factor encompassed lying, stealing without confrontation, truancy, breaking and entering, and vandalism.

For the teacher reports a similar pattern appeared. For the two sources combined, considered by the authors to produce the most important results, the first factor loaded ODD symptoms plus bullying and fighting. The second factor was composed of CD items (of both socialized and undersocialized types, but predominantly of the socialized type).

A cluster analysis resulted in the authors' distinguishing three clusters of subjects: (1)

high on ODD/Aggression but low on CD, (2) high on both ODD and CD, and (3) high on neither. Of interest was the failure to find a cluster of cases high on CD *only.*

Rey and Morris-Yates's (1993) checklist ratings from the parents of 528 consecutive clinic referrals divided into three groups: those with DSM-III-R CD diagnoses (*n* = 189), those with ODD diagnoses (*n* = 75), and those with other diagnoses (*n* = 264). An analysis of all 528 cases resulted in the acceptance of an oblique four-factor solution. These correlated factors were labeled "aggression," "delinquency," "oppositionality," and "escapism." The factors of aggression and oppositionality correlated .54, aggression and delinquency correlated .25, and oppositionality and delinquency correlated only .06.

Subjects in the ODD and CD groups were then clustered on the basis of their scores on the four factors. Two clusters were extracted. A cross-tabulation of clinical diagnosis with cluster membership indicated that 17% of the ODD cases and 69% of those in the CD group were in the first cluster; 83% of the OD group and 31% of the CD group were in the second cluster. The association of group and cluster membership was highly significant but the kappa was a moderate .44.

The interpretation of the results of this study in support of independent ODD and CD dimensions must be tempered by the fact that the two factors were correlated .54; the correlations of the factor scores, which would likely have been higher, were not reported. It is also troublesome to note that although the second cluster contained 81% of the diagnosed ODD cases, it also contained 31% of the CD group.

In fact, the results of this study can be used to argue for the existence of the undersocialized aggressive and socialized aggressive subtypes of CD (factor correlation .25). Among the CD cases, those with the highest factor score on delinquency were the 128 cases in cluster one. The next highest scores were obtained by the 12 ODD cases in cluster one.

Fergusson, Horwood, and Lynskey (1994) have also looked at whether CD and ODD are factorially distinct. They studied a birth cohort

sample of 739 15-year-olds using data provided by official reports of police contact and parental and self-reports with respect to DSM-III-R criteria for DBD. Item-level analysis was not possible as many item frequencies in this normal sample were too low to permit factor analysis. Instead, items were, a priori, formed into scales of ODD, covert CD, and overt CD for both parent and self-reports.

Confirmatory factor analysis revealed that the best solution was one of correlated, but distinct, factors of ODD, overt CD, and covert CD. The correlations among the three factors were, however, quite high: ODD correlated .70 with overt CD and .76 with covert CD; the two CD factors correlated .76.

A further analysis, which included ADHD symptom scales, revealed a distinct ADHD factor that was, however, correlated .68 with both CD factors and .89 with ODD. A higher-order analysis revealed two factors. The first was labeled "Behavior Problems" and subsumed the lower-order ODD and ADHD factors. The second higher-order factor was labeled "Antisocial Behaviors" and subsumed both overt and covert CD factors. The two factors were, however, correlated .85, "suggesting strong association between tendencies to disruptive behaviors and tendencies to delinquency" (Ferguson *et al.,* 1994, p. 1152).

The results of this study provide evidence for ODD as distinct from either of the two CD dimensions, but it is obvious that the high degree of association and with both dimensions of CD will make it more difficult to find differential correlates of ODD and CD than if the two dimensions, and their measurement, were more truly independent.

It seems most consistent with the evidence to consider ODD and the two subtypes of CD to be conceptually separate but closely related disorders. It also is likely that ODD is a precursor of childhood-onset CD, but that ODD is not likely to be a precursor to adolescent-onset CD (see Hinshaw, Lahey, & Hart, 1993). If the progression from ODD to CD is highly predictable, this would be evidence for considering the symptoms of ODD as the less severe, but earlier, manifestations of aggressive CD. Similarly, findings that cases of aggressive

CD also meet, or retrospectively would have met, criteria for ODD at an earlier age would be evidence for a single ODD-CD dimension with different manifestations at different ages. These developmental pathways are considered in detail in Chapter 19, this volume.

ALTERNATIVE APPROACHES TO CLASSIFICATION

DBD in ICD-10

Outside North America the most widely used taxonomic system is the *International Classification of Diseases,* tenth edition (ICD-10; World Health Organization, 1992). Table 6

lists the ICD-10 DBD with brief descriptions of their characteristics. As can be seen, DSM-IV ADHD, CD, and ODD have their counterparts in ICD-10 with similar symptoms and criteria for age of onset, duration, and situational pervasiveness. However, impairment as a criterion does not formally appear in ICD-10 but is implied in the narrative. In ICD-10 the number of symptoms required for a diagnosis (threshold) is not dealt with formally as it is in DSM-IV.

The major differences between the DBD categories of the two systems clearly lies in the subtyping of both ADHD–Hyperkinetic disorder and CD. ICD-10 melds the three ADHD subtypes into a single subtype: Disturbance of Activity and Attention. The ICD-10 Hyper-

TABLE 6.   Major Categories of DBD in ICD-10 (Descriptions Abridged)

Hyperkinetic Disorder

Combination of overactive, poorly modulated behavior with marked inattention and lack of persistence
> Pervasive over situations and time
> Both impaired attention and overactivity necessary for diagnosis
> Onset before age 6

Subtypes
> Disturbance of activity and attention
>> Criteria for hyperkinetic disorder met
> Hyperkinetic conduct disorder
>> Criteria for both hyperkinetic disorder and conduct disorder met

Conduct Disorder

Repetitive and persistent pattern of dissocial, aggressive, and defiant conduct. Major violations of age-appropriate social expectations. Behaviors on which diagnosis is based include excessive fighting and bullying, cruelty to animals or other people, severe destructiveness to property, fire-setting, repeated lying, truancy from school and running away from home, unusually frequent and severe temper tantrums, defiant and provocative behavior, and persistent and severe disobedience

Duration of 6 months or longer
Subtypes
> Conduct disorder confined to the family context
>> Overall criteria are met but abnormal behavior confined to home and/or to interactions with members of nuclear family or immediate household
>> Social relationships outside the family within normal range
> Unsocialized conduct disorder
>> Overall criteria are met but not merely oppositional, defiant or disruptive behavior. Significant, pervasive abnormality in relationships with other children.
> Socialized conduct disorder
>> Meets overall criteria but involves persistent dissocial or aggressive behavior occurring in individuals well integrated into their peer group

Oppositional Defiant Disorder

Essential feature is a pattern of persistently negativistic, hostile, defiant, provocative, and disruptive behavior outside the normal range but not including the more serious violations of rights of others as in conduct disorder.
If conduct disorder criteria are met, that diagnosis takes precedence.

kinetic–Conduct Disorder subtype is, in DSM-IV, seen as two separate disorders occurring together (ADHD and CD) rather than as a subtype of ADHD. In ICD-10 a diagnosis of Hyperkinetic Disorder takes precedence over a diagnosis of CD so as to permit this subtype diagnosis to be made.

The CD subtypes of ICD-10 are based on behavioral differences rather than age of onset and the unsocialized and socialized subtypes are very close to those of DSM-III-R. There has never been a DSM counterpart of the ICD-10 "confined to the family context" subtype. Such a circumscribed form of CD has never, to my knowledge, been found in the multivariate statistical literature, but it is not likely that variables describing limitations of CD behavior to the family have been entered into such analyses.

If, as we have already discussed, cases of childhood-onset CD show a preponderance of undersocialized-aggressive type symptoms, while adolescent onset cases show a preponderance of socialized (or "delinquent") symptoms, the DSM-IV and ICD-10 approaches to subtyping will likely identify most of the same cases.

ICD-10 also permits diagnosis of "Mixed Disorders of Conduct and Emotion" wherein CD criteria as well as criteria for a chidhood or adult internalizing disorder are met.

Alternatives from a Behavioral Perspective

An extensive critique of the entire DSM-IV and alternative proposals have been offered from a behaviorist perspective in a series of papers (see Follette, 1996, for introductory comments). A critique of the disorders of childhood and adolescence with particular reference to the DBD has been offered by Scotti, Morris, McNeil, and Hawkins (1996). These authors explicitly recognize that both traditional or structural (i.e., syndromic) assessment and functional (i.e., behavioral) assessment have their strengths and weaknesses. They also recognize that behaviorists overdid the earlier denial of the value of symptoms-based structural classification.

Employing a treatment perspective, Scotti and colleagues (1996) correctly noted that DSM-IV categories have little to say about either skills or behavioral assets that may covary with the symptoms of any disorder and that may also be very important in developing interventions. At the same time, they recognize the utility of syndromes made up of intercorrelated behaviors at two levels of analysis: descriptive, and causal in the sense of a common etiology, mechanism, and function.

Although they argued for the incorporation of functional analysis into any diagnostic system, Scotti and colleagues (1996) also raised a troubling issue. That is, an 8-year-old child who initiates fights, bullies others, and hurts animals and a 16-year-old adolescent who sets fires, steals from others' homes and is truant from school would both receive a diagnosis of CD (although I add here, very likely different subtypes). In this instance, as the authors pointed out, the treatment plan, its duration, and the most likely outcomes would be very different.

The need for the clinician to have a great deal of other information is recognized in DSM-IV by the uses of Axis III (General Medical Conditions), Axis IV (Psychosocial and Environmental Problems), and Axis V (Global Assessment of Functioning). Scotti and colleagues (1996) suggested that Axis III be revamped to include psychosocial and environmental *resources* as well as deficits and that a "new" Axis IV be developed to be labeled "Idiographic case analysis." This axis would cover biological factors, general medical conditions, and other factors in terms of their roles as antecedents, repertoires, and consequences.

In essence, the Scotti and colleagues (1996) critique is not aimed at the reliability and validity of the DSM-IV categories of DBD per se, but at their limitations as providing adequate information for a plan of *behavioral* intervention.

It seems doubtful that these "add ons" are likely to become a part of the DSM in the near future. There is, of course, nothing to prevent clinicians (and researchers) from using the basic DSM-IV categories while collecting the added information necessary for whatever purposes the diagnostic process has been undertaken.

Proactive and Reactive Aggression as a Basis for Subtyping CD

A very different alternative conception has been offered by Dodge, Lochman, Harnish, Bates, and Petit (1997). In considering the subtyping of CD, these authors state: "We hypothesize that a new distinction should be made based on the topography of the child's aggressive behavior itself" (p. 37). "We posit a distinction between *reactively aggressive* (RA) and *proactively aggressive* (PA) [italics in original] children" (p. 38). Dodge and colleagues argued that the distinction between the two types of aggression can be made phenomonologically and on the basis that they have different antecedents and different physiological-biological concomitants.

In Study I (Dodge *et al.,* 1997), 504 third-grade children were assessed by teacher ratings for PA and RA behavior. Fifty-seven children received high scores on both scales and were labeled pervasively aggressive, 34 were classified as RA, and 17 were classified as PA. Thus, a total of 108 of the 504 children (21%) received one of the three aggressive "diagnoses" producing a prevalence rate for the three subtypes combined considerably above that of a DSM-IV diagnosis of CD (see Chapter 2, this volume). Furthermore, 53% of those classified were in the combined subtype, so that less than half the cases maintained the distinction between RA and PA.

When the three aggressive groups were compared along with the nonaggressive group (NA), a number of differences emerged. In general, the pervasively aggressive group and the RA group had experienced the most deleterious early life influences and were concurrently more impaired. The PA group more often did not differ from the NA group.

It remains for future research to determine the relationship of the Dodge and colleagues (1997) three subtypes and DSM-IV CD diagnoses. Future longitudinal research will also be necessary to determine which taxonomy predicts persistence, response to treatment, and both biological and social etiological variables.

Categorical versus Dimensional Classification

Space limitations do not permit an extensive discussion of categorical as opposed to dimensional assessment of the DBD. Both approaches permit the determination of "caseness" versus not by meeting the established threshold as in the DSM-IV, or by exceeding a statistical threshold (e.g., above the 70th percentile) in the case of standardized dimensional measures. In the absence of a nonfallible external criterion, either type of cutoff to determine "caseness" is at least somewhat arbitrary.

However, dimensional measures permit the use of more information as the entire range of symptoms or scores is available for analysis of the relationship of the dimension to any other variable. In categorical diagnosis, the number of subthreshold symptoms is ignored in the "noncases" as is the number of suprathreshold symptoms in the "cases," although ratings of severity can be made as in DSM-IV.

Fergusson and Horwood (1995) have shown, for example, that dimensional scores based on DSM-III-R criteria for ADHD, ODD, and CD taken at age 15 were better predictors of substance abuse, juvenile offending, and school dropout at age 16 than were DSM-III-R categorical diagnoses.

However, it is possible that one or more of the DBD, or some subtypes of the DBD, may be truly categorical (type or disease entity or taxon) rather than dimensional (see Meehl, 1995). Most psychopathological disorders are most likely dimensions (Grove, 1991), but recent work has indicated that adult psychopaths are a discrete class (Harris, Rice, & Quinsey, 1994). It is important to note that a taxon does not need to derive from a single causative agent. One can speculate that those cases of childhood-onset CD who graduate to Adult Antisocial Personality Disorder might be determined by appropriate research (see Meehl, 1995) to comprise a discrete class. Determination of taxonicity with respect to the Primarily Inattentive and Primarily Hyperactive-Impulsive subtypes of ADHD would be a crucial step forward in determining whether these two subtypes are actually separate disorders. However, using DSM-III-R criteria in a large-scale study of twins, Levy, Hay, McStephen, Wood, and Waldman (1997) concluded that ADHD was best viewed as an extreme of behavior varying genetically throughout the population rather than as a discrete disorder.

Despite the emphasis in this chapter on categorical classification as exemplified in the DSM-IV, the reader will find that much of the research reported in subsequent chapters in this volume is based on dimensional measures for subject selection. Many of these measures are discussed in Chapter 3 (this volume) or are briefly described in the chapters that follow.

REFERENCES

Achenbach, T. M., & Edelbrock, C. S. (1978). The classification of child psychopathology: A review and analysis of empirical efforts. *Psychological Bulletin, 85,* 1275–1301.

Achenbach, T. M., Conners, C. K., Quay, H. C., Verhulst, F. C., & Howell, C. T. (1989). Replication of empirically derived syndromes as a basis for taxonomy of child/adolescent psychopathology. *Journal of Abnormal Child Psychology, 17,* 299–323.

Achenbach, T. M., Howell, C. T., Quay, H. C., & Conners, C. K. (1991). National survey of problems and competencies among four- to sixteen-year-olds. *Monographs of the Society for Research in Child Development, 36* (3, Serial No. 225).

American Psychiatric Association. (1968). *Diagnostic and statistical manual of mental disorders* (2nd ed.). Washington, DC: Author.

American Psychiatric Association. (1980). *Diagnostic and statistical manual of mental disorders* (3rd ed.). Washington, DC: Author.

American Psychiatric Association. (1987). *Diagnostic and statistical manual of mental disorders* (3rd ed., rev.). Washington, DC: Author.

American Psychiatric Association. (1994). *Diagnostic and statistical manual of mental disorders* (4th ed.). Washington, DC: Author.

Angold, A., & Costello, E. J. (1996). Toward establishing an empirical basis for the diagnosis of Oppositional Defiant Disorder. *Journal of the American Academy of Child and Adolescent Psychiatry, 35,* 1205–1212.

Angold, A., Prendergast, M., Cox, A., Harrington, R., Simonoff, E., & Rutter, M. (1995). The Child and Adolescent Psychiatric Assessment (CAPA). *Psychological Medicine, 25,* 739–753.

Angold, A., Erkanli, A., Costello, E. J., & Rutter, M. (1996). Precision, reliability and accuracy in dating symptom onsets in child and adolescent psychopathology. *Journal of Child Psychology and Psychiatry, 37,* 657–664.

Applegate, B., Lahey, B. B., Hart, E. L., Biederman, J., Hynd, G. W., Barkley, R. A., Ollendick, T., Frick, P. J., Greenhill, L., McBurnett, K., Newcorn, J. H., Kerdyk, L., Garfinkel, B., Waldman, I., & Shaffer, D. (1997). Validity of the age of onset criterion for attention-deficit/hyperactivity disorder: A report from the DSM-IV field trials. *Journal of the American Academy of Child and Adolescent Psychiatry, 36,* 1211–1221.

Blashfield, R. K. (1984). *The classification of psychopathology.* New York: Plenum.

Blashfield, R. K., & Livesley, W. J. (1991). Metaphorical analysis of psychiatric classification as a psychological test. *Journal of Abnormal Psychology, 100,* 262–270.

Carlson, C. L. (1986). Attention deficit disorder without hyperactivity: A review of preliminary experimental evidence. In B. B. Lahey & A. E. Kazdin (Eds.), *Advances in clinical child psychology* (Vol. 9, pp. 153–175). New York: Plenum.

Dodge, K. A., Lochman, J. E., Harnish, J. D., Bates, J. E., & Petit, G. S. (1997). Reactive and proactive aggression in school children and psychiatrically impaired, chronically assaultive youth. *Journal of Abnormal Psychology, 106,* 37–51.

Faraone, S. V., Biederman, J., Weber, W., & Russell, R. L. (1998). Psychiatric, neuropsychological, and psychosocial features of DSM-IV subtypes of Attention-Deficit/Hyperactivity Disorder: Results from a clinically referred sample. *Journal of the American Academy of Child and Adolescent Psychiatry, 37,* 185–193.

Fergusson, D. M., & Horwood, L. J. (1995). Predictive validity of categorically and dimensionally scored measures of disruptive childhood behaviors. *Journal of the American Academy of Child and Adolescent Psychiatry, 34,* 477–485.

Fergusson, D. M., Horwood, L. J, & Lynskey, M. T. (1994). Structure of DSM-III-R criteria for disruptive childhood behaviors: Confirmatory factor models. *Journal of the American Academy of Child and Adolescent Psychiatry, 33,* 1145–1155.

Follette, W. C. (1996). Introduction to the special section on the development of theoretically coherent alternatives to the DSM system. *Journal of Consulting and Clinical Psychology, 64,* 1117–1119.

Frick, P. J., Lahey, B. B., Loeber, R., Stouthamer-Loeber, M., Green, S., Hart, E. L., & Christ, M. A. G. (1991). Oppositional defiant disorder and conduct disorder in boys: Patterns of behavioral covariation. *Journal of Clinical Child Psychology, 20,* 202–208.

Frick, P. J., Lahey, B. B., Loeber, R., Tannenbaum, L., Van Horn, Y., Christ, M. A. G., Hart, E. L., & Hanson, K. (1993). Oppositional defiant disorder and conduct disorder: A meta-analytic review of factor analyses and cross-validation in a clinic sample. *Clinical Psychology Review, 13,* 319–340.

Frick, P. J., Lahey, B. B., Applegate, B., Kerdyck, L., Ollendick, T., Hynd, G. W., Garfinkel, B., Greenhill, L., Biederman, J., Barkley, R. A., McBurnett, K., Newcorn, J., & Waldman, I. (1994). DSM-IV field trials for the disruptive behavior disorders: Symptom utility estimates. *Journal of the American Academy of Child and Adolescent Psychiatry, 33,* 529–539.

Gaub, M., & Carlson, C. L. (1997). Behavioral characteristics of DSM-IV subtypes on a school-based population. *Journal of Abnormal Child Psychology, 25,* 103–111.

Grove, W. M. (1991). When is a diagnosis worth making? A comparison of two statistical prediction strategies. *Psychological Reports, 68,* 3–17.

Harris, G. T., Rice, M. E., & Quinsey, V. L. (1994). Psychopathy as a taxon: Evidence that psychopaths are a discrete class. *Journal of Consulting and Clinical Psychology, 62,* 387–397.

Hinshaw, S. P., Lahey, B. B., & Hart. E. L. (1993). Issues of taxonomy and comorbidity in the development of conduct disorder. *Development and Psychopathology, 5,* 31–49.

Lahey, B. B., & Carlson, C. L. (1991). Validity of the diagnostic category of Attention Deficit without Hyperactivity: A review of the literature. *Journal of Learning Disabilities, 24,* 110–120.

Lahey, B. B., Applegate, B., Barkley, R. A., Garfinkel, B., McBurnett, K., Kerdyk, L., Greenhill, L., Hynd, G. W., Frick, P. J., Newcorn, J., Biederman, J., Ollendick, T., Hart, E. L., Perez, D., Waldman, I., & Shaffer, D. (1994). DSM-IV field trials for oppositional defiant disorder and conduct disorder in children and adolescents. *American Journal of Psychiatry, 151,* 1163–1171.

Lahey, B. B., Applegate, B., McBurnett, K., Biederman, J., Greenhill, L., Hynd, G. W., Barkley, R. A., Newcorn, J., Jensen, P., Richters, J., Garfinkel, B., Kerdyk, L., Frick, P. J., Ollendick, T., Perez, D., Hart, E. L., Waldman, I., & Shaffer, D. (1994). DSM-IV field trials for attention deficit hyperactivity disorder in children and adolescents. *American Journal of Psychiatry, 151,* 1673–1685.

Lahey, B. B., Loeber, R., Hart, E. L., Frick, P. J., Applegate, B., Zhang, Q., Green, S. M., & Russo, M. F. (1995). Four-year longitudinal study of conduct disorder in boys: Patterns and predictors of persistence. *Journal of Abnormal Psychology, 104,* 83–93.

Lahey, B. B., Carlson, C. L., & Frick, P. J. (1997). Attention deficit disorder without hyperactivity. In T. A. Widiger, A. J. Francis, H. A. Pincus, R. Ross, M. B. First, & W. Davis (Eds.), *DSM-IV Sourcebook* (Vol 3., pp. 163–188). Washington, DC: American Psychiatric Association.

Lahey, B. B., Loeber, R., Quay, H. C., Applegate, B., Shaffer, D., Waldman, I., Hart, E. L., McBurnett, K., Frick, P. J., Jensen, P., Duncan, M., Canino, G., & Bird, H. (1998). Validity of DSM-IV subtypes of conduct disorder based on age on onset. *Journal of the American Academy of Child and Adolescent Psychiatry, 37,* 435–442.

Levy, F., Hay, D. A., McStephen, M., Wood, C., & Waldman, I. (1997). Attention-deficit hyperactivity disorder: A category or a continuum? Genetic analysis of a large-scale twin study. *Journal of the American Academy of Child and Adolescent Psychiatry, 36,* 737–744.

Loeber, R., & Schmaling, K. B. (1985). Empirical evidence for overt and covert patterns of antisocial conduct problems: A meta-analysis. *Journal of Abnormal Child Psychology, 13,* 337–352.

Loeber, R., Lahey, B. B., & Thomas, C. (1991). Diagnostic conundrum of oppositional defiant disorder and conduct disorder. *Journal of Abnormal Psychology, 100,* 379–390.

McBurnett, K. (1997). Attention-deficit hyperactivity disorder: A review of diagnostic issues. In T. A. Widiger, A. J. Francis, H. A. Pincus, R. Ross, M. B. First, & W. Davis (Eds.), *DSM-IV Sourcebook* (Vol 3., pp. 111–143). Washington, DC: American Psychiatric Association.

Meehl, P. E. (1995). Bootstraps taxometrics solving the classification problems in psychopathology. *American Psychologist, 50,* 266–275.

Millon, T. (1991). Classification in psychopathology: Rationale, alternatives and standards. *Journal of Abnormal Psychology, 100,* 245–261.

Morey, L. C. (1991). Classification of mental disorders as a collection of hypothetical constructs. *Journal of Abnormal Psychology, 100,* 289–293.

Morgan, A. E., Hynd, G. W., Riccio, C. A., & Hall, J. (1996). Validity of the DSM-IV ADHD Predominantly Inattentive and Combined types: Relationship to previous DSM diagnoses/subtypes. *Journal of the American Academy of Child and Adolescent Psychiatry, 35,* 325–333.

Quay, H. C. (1972). Patterns of aggression, withdrawal, and immaturity. In H. C. Quay & J. S. Werry (Eds.), *Psychopathological disorders of childhood* (pp. 1–29). New York: Wiley.

Quay, H. C. (1979). Classification. In H. C. Quay & J. S. Werry (Eds.), *Psychopathological disorders of childhood* (2nd ed., pp. 1–42). New York: Wiley.

Quay, H. C. (1986a). Classification. In H. C. Quay & J. S. Werry (Eds.), *Psychopathological disorders of childhood* (3rd ed., pp. 1–34). New York: Wiley.

Quay, H. C. (1986b). Conduct disorders. In H. C. Quay & J. S. Werry (Eds.), *Psychopathological disorders of childhood* (3rd ed., pp. 35–72). New York: Wiley.

Quay, H. C. (1987). Patterns of delinquent behavior. In H. C. Quay (Ed.), *Handbook of juvenile delinquency* (pp. 118–183). New York: Wiley.

Quay, H. C. (1997). Inhibition and attention deficit hyperactivity disorder. *Journal of Abnormal Child Psychology, 25,* 7–14.

Rey, J. M., & Morris-Yates, A. (1993). Are oppositional and conduct disorders of adolescents separate conditions? *Australian and New Zealand Journal of Psychiatry, 27,* 281–287.

Scotti, J. R., Morris, T. L., McNeil, C. B., & Hawkins, R. P. (1996). DSM-IV and disorders of childhood and adolescence: Can structural criteria be functional? *Journal of Consulting and Clinical Psychology, 64,* 1177–1191.

Shaffer, D., Gould, M. S., Brasic, J., Ambrosini, P., Fisher, P., Bird, H., & Aluwahlia, S. (1983). A Children's Global Assessment Scale (CGAS). *Archives of General Psychiatry, 40,* 1228–1231.

Shaffer, D., Campbell, M., Cantwell, D., Bradley, S., Carlson, G., Cohen, D., Denckla, M., Frances, A., Garfinkel, B., Klein, R., Pincus, H., Spitzer, R., Volkmar, F., & Widiger, T. (1989). Child and adolescent psychiatric disorders in DSM-IV: Issues facing the Work Group. *Journal of the American Academy of Child and Adolescent Psychiatry, 28,* 830–835.

Wolraich, M. L., Hannah, J. N., Pinnock, T. Y., Baumgaertel, A., & Brown, J. (1996). Comparison of diagnostic criteria for attention deficit hyperactivity disorder in a county-wide sample. *Journal of the American Academy of Child and Adolescent Psychiatry, 35,* 319–324.

World Health Organization. (1992). *International classification of diseases* (10th ed.). Geneva, Switzerland: Author.

2

Developmental Epidemiology of the Disruptive Behavior Disorders

BENJAMIN B. LAHEY, TERRI L. MILLER,
RACHEL A. GORDON, and ANNE W. RILEY

Epidemiology is both a scientific discipline and a powerful set of investigative methods that have been adopted by other fields, including the fields that study the behavior problems of children and adolescents. The discipline of epidemiology was developed to study the etiology of diseases, and the methods of epidemiology evolved in service of that aim. Because the mental health disciplines also seek to understand the origins of disorders, it has been to our advantage to adopt many of the methods of epidemiology.

In this chapter we attempt to accomplish five things: (1) briefly describe the methods that define epidemiology as they have been applied to the Disruptive Behavior Disorders (DBD); (2) explain the unique role played by population-based studies in identifying risk and protective factors; (3) provide a review and annotated bibliography of existing epidemiologic studies of DBD (the data sets of many of these are available for public use); (4) summarize major findings to date on prevalence, comorbidity, and selected risk and protective factors; and (5) highlight areas in which information is sparse to suggest directions for future research. This chapter might best be viewed as a progress report on a field of mental health research that is still emerging, despite the many studies that have been conducted over the past 20 years.

BASIC CONCEPTS OF EPIDEMIOLOGY

Epidemiology's focus on the origins and proliferation of diseases in the general population required the development of the methods and statistics of *sampling.* To describe the parameters of a disease in a population, one must either gather data on all members of that population or draw a sample that is *representative* of the population. The goal of representative sampling is the limitation of *bias.* Samples selected using nonrepresentative methods can be biased in ways that lead to invalid conclusions when results are generalized to the general population.

BENJAMIN B. LAHEY, TERRI L. MILLER, and RACHEL A. GORDON • Department of Psychiatry, University of Chicago, Chicago, Illinois 60637. ANNE W. RILEY • School of Public Health, Johns Hopkins University, Baltimore, Maryland 21205.

Handbook of Disruptive Behavior Disorders, edited by Quay and Hogan. Kluwer Academic/Plenum Publishers, New York, 1999.

An example of the kinds of errors that can be made using nonrepresentative samples comes from research on human sexual behavior. The first large-scale surveys of sexual behavior did not use representative samples. For example, subjects in the Kinsey studies (Kinsey, Pomeroy, & Martin, 1948; Kinsey, Pomeroy, Martin, & Gebhard, 1953) either were members of easily recruited groups (e.g., college fraternities and sororities) or were friends of already-interviewed subjects recruited through networking. Other early studies were based on the readership of magazines such as *Playboy* or *Redbook*. When a large survey of sexual behavior was conducted more recently using a representative household sample (Michael, Gagnon, Laumann, & Kolata, 1994), it was found that the earlier surveys had overestimated by double or triple the rates of sexual behaviors believed to be relevant to the spread of HIV (homosexual behavior, extramarital sexual behavior, and specific high-risk sexual practices). Had scientists and policy makers relied only on findings from the earlier studies, they would have been seriously misinformed about the expected rate of the spread of HIV and would not have formulated optimal prevention strategies.

Perhaps the best known sampling bias was described over 50 years ago by Berkson (1946) and is known today as "Berkson's Bias." For a number of reasons, samples drawn from medical clinics tend to overestimate the degree of comorbidity among medical conditions relative to representative samples of the general population. True to the principle of Berkson's Bias, samples of children and adolescents with emotional and behavioral disorders drawn from specialty mental health clinics have higher rates of comorbidity than youths in the general population (Goodman *et al.*, 1997; McConaughy & Achenbach, 1994). Children in mental health clinic samples also are more impaired, are less likely to be prepubertal girls, are less likely to belong to racial or ethnic groups of color, and are more likely to have parents who have received mental health services than are youths with the same disorders in the general population who have not received mental health services (Goodman *et al.*, 1997). Thus, clinic

samples are biased in important ways and their use can lead to erroneous conclusions regarding psychopathology in the general population. In subtler but equally important ways, community samples that are not representative ("convenience samples") also can be biased in ways that lead to invalid conclusions.

Although psychologists and psychiatrists are becoming increasingly aware of the dangers of generalizing from nonrepresentative samples, most published studies of DBD have used such samples. Most of our knowledge of DBD is based on studies of samples drawn solely from clinics or juvenile detention facilities and of nonrepresentative community samples, which are subject to biases that can distort findings. It is essential that we move toward studies of representative samples using state-of-the-art measurement strategies to avoid a science based on misinformation. Psychology and psychiatry owe an important debt to epidemiology for its contributions in the area of sampling. The size of that debt should grow as our understanding of the importance of representative sampling spreads.

Epidemiology and the Study of Risk and Protective Factors

Epidemiology assumes that disorders are not randomly distributed in the population, but are more likely to occur under some conditions than under others (Hennekens, Buring, & Mayrent, 1987; Rutter, 1981). Sampling theory allows us to "map" the nonrandom distribution of disorders, and this map can point toward causes. For example, the association between cigarette smoking and lung cancer was identified long before the role of altered DNA in cancer and the role of cigarette smoke in altering DNA were understood. The mental health fields have every reason to expect that the same kinds of clues to causal factors will come from the study of risk and protective factors for behavior problems in population-based samples. However, such benefits require the adoption of sophisticated methods of sampling. Conclusive studies of risk and protective factors can be conducted only by using representative samples that yield unbiased estimates of relationships between risk factors and psychopathology.

It has become conventional to speak of variables that are statistically associated with disorders as *correlates,* and to restrict the term *risk factor* to variables that precede (temporally and logically) disorders and might eventually be shown to be *causes* of that disorder (Offord, 1995). Similarly, the term *protective factor* is typically restricted to variables that precede the disorder and might reduce the likelihood of that disorder.

In the child and adolescent mental health field, one important reason for restricting the terms risk and protective factors to variables that temporally and logically precede disorders is to avoid mistakenly identifying variables influenced by "child effects" as risk factors. For example, many studies that have identified a correlation between Conduct Disorder (CD) and parenting variables have not ruled out the possibility that atypical parenting could be the *result* of the child's CD behaviors (and other disruptive behaviors that may have antedated them developmentally). That is, there is evidence that the behavior of children can causally influence the parenting behaviors of adults (Bell & Harper, 1977; Lytton, 1990; see also Chapter 15, this volume, for a discussion of this issue). Only studies that rule out child effects and other confounding factors can confirm the status of correlates as risk or protective factors. Longitudinal studies, twin studies, and randomized interventions focused on putative risk factors are among the types of designs that can accomplish this.

Demographic factors that are associated with the prevalence of disorders are a special case. Age, gender, racial or ethnic background, socioeconomic status (SES), family structure, and other demographic factors may confer increased or decreased risk for some disorders, but would not ordinarily be considered to be "causes" of disorders (Offord, 1995). Demographic factors might be better conceptualized as distal variables that work indirectly through a variety of proximal variables (e.g., biological maturation, acculturation, parental supervision) to exert their influences. For the sake of simplicity, however, we refer to demographic factors as potential risk factors in this chapter.

It is important to distinguish between risk factors for the *onset* of a disorder and risk factors for the *persistence* of the disorder, as they often are not the same (Costello & Angold, 1995). Both types of risk factors are important, as understanding risk factors for onset may lead to advances in prevention, whereas knowledge of risk factors for persistence may lead to improvements in treatments. It is important to point out, however, that few studies reviewed in this chapter made this distinction. That is, they present correlations between potential risk factors and the youth's meeting criteria for a disorder (or receiving elevated ratings on a dimension of psychopathology) at a given time. Variables that increase the likelihood of the onset of that disorder and variables that increase its likelihood of persisting over time both might be correlated with meeting criteria for the disorder at a single point. Thus, in these studies it is not possible to distinguish among factors that increase risk for onset, for persistence, or for both. That distinction requires (1) prospective longitudinal studies that begin before the risk period for the disorder for at least a large part of the sample, and (2) the use of data analytic techniques that distinguish between risk for onset and persistence. To date, this important distinction has been made in few studies.

Caseness, Prevalence, and Incidence

Among the key concepts of epidemiology are *prevalence* (the proportion of individuals who meet criteria for a disorder during a defined period) and *incidence* (the proportion of individuals who meet criteria for a disorder for the first time during a defined time). Knowledge of the prevalence and incidence rates of disorders is useful for many scientific and administrative purposes, such as estimating the rate of spread of epidemics and planning health services.

The value of the concepts of prevalence and incidence depends on the concept of *caseness.* Before one can count cases of disorder to estimate prevalence and incidence, one must be able to distinguish reliably between cases and noncases.

The issue of caseness is a particularly complex one for child and adolescent psychopathology, as the identification of defensible boundaries between "normality" and "disorder" presents many difficulties (Boyle et al., 1996; Lahey, Applegate, Barkley, et al., 1994; Lahey, Applegate, McBurnett, et al., 1994; Zarin & Earls, 1993). Boyle and colleagues (1996) recently illustrated the problems of case definition. Using data from a population-based study in Ontario, they examined several plausible operational definitions of mental disorder. Using the same basic data on symptoms and impairment, the investigators found that these definitions produced markedly different prevalence rates, levels of test–retest reliability, and associations with potential risk factors in the same sample.

Even seemingly minor changes in diagnostic criteria can produce large differences in the prevalence of mental disorders (Boyle et al., 1996; Lahey et al., 1990). By the same token, different studies using the same diagnostic criteria but employing different methods of assessment (interviews by clinicians, behavior checklists, or diagnostic interviews) can be expected to yield different prevalence estimates. One might even expect different versions of the same general approach to assessment, such as different checklists (or different structured interviews or clinicians trained in different ways), to yield different prevalence rates. That is, one should assume that prevalence estimates and other epidemiologic findings are method-specific until shown to be otherwise (Lahey, Applegate, Barkley, et al., 1994; Lahey, Applegate, McBurnett, et al., 1994). This should not be surprising, as it is a truism of psychometrics that different methods of assessment should be assumed to yield different results until correspondence between the methods has been established empirically. Still, in the field of child and adolescent mental health we have proceeded as if diagnostic constructs were independent of the operations of measurement.

Toward Defensible Definitions of Caseness

Boyle and colleagues (1996) suggested that differences in definitions of caseness are one of the key reasons that wide ranges of prevalence estimates have been published for mental disorders among children. Moreover, they suggested that there is currently no defensible way to choose one definition over another. A number of key issues that must be addressed before the field can agree on standard definitions of caseness for child and adolescent psychopathology are discussed in the following sections (Boyle et al., 1996; Lahey, Applegate, Barkley, et al., 1994; Lahey, Applegate, McBurnett, et al., 1994; Zarin & Earls, 1993).

Are There Natural Thresholds between Normality and Abnormality?

Decisions about caseness are straightforward when clear discontinuities in nature can be identified. For example, the qualitative difference between the minerals gold and copper is one that trained observers can identify readily. At present, however, there is scant evidence that such natural discontinuities exist in child and adolescent psychopathology. Like many other theorists, we believe that the most reasonable assumption at this time is that most (if not all) types of psychopathology are inherently continuous and that diagnoses represent dichotomized dimensions of psychopathology. Boyle and colleagues (1996) put it this way:

> For the most prevalent categories of childhood psychiatric disorder (i.e., conduct disorder, oppositional defiant disorder, attention-deficit hyperactivity disorder, separation anxiety disorder, and overanxious disorder), DSM provides a symptom list and, from the count of symptoms, identifies the number at or above which a child is to be classified as exhibiting a disorder. This approach to classification explicitly acknowledges that these disorders are dimensional phenomena in which symptoms can be substituted for one another to achieve a threshold. If our approach to classification acknowledges a dimensional component, then we must show that our categorical representations (i.e., disorder as present or absent) are both sensible and nonarbitrary. (pp. 1440–1441)

There are a number of ways in which one can search for evidence of natural dichotomies in psychopathology. Distributions of numbers of symptoms can be examined for evidence of bimodality, which may indicate separate, if overlapping, distributions of numbers of symptoms for those with or without the putative disorder. Alternatively, one could examine plots of numbers of symptoms against indices of functional impairment for indications of curvilinearity. Curvilinearity in these functions may indicate reasonable points of distinguishing "normal" from "abnormal" numbers of symptoms in terms of degree of impairment. Similarly, one could use behavior-genetic methods to determine whether one potential diagnostic threshold is associated with greater heritability or shared environmental influence than other potential thresholds. Each of these methods has been used, however, with no indication of natural dichotomies for DBD to date (Lahey, Applegate, Barkley, et al., 1994; Lahey, Applegate, McBurnett, et al., 1994; Levy, Hay, McStephen, Wood, & Waldman, 1997; see also Chapter 1, this volume, for a discussion of this topic).

It should be noted that the problem of how to dichotomize what appear to be natural continua is not unique to the mental health fields. In medicine, the definition of hypertension provides a good analogy to psychopathology. There is a continuum of diastolic blood pressure on which all individuals can be given a score. The widely accepted dichotomization of this continuum into "normal blood pressure" and "hypertension" was made possible only by the discovery of the curvilinear relationship between diastolic pressure and death from cardiovascular event. Unfortunately, no data are currently available to support such dichotomizations in the mental health fields. The lack of evidence supporting the existence of natural dichotomies should not be taken as a reason not to continue to search for it, however. Indeed, much more research on this topic is needed before firm conclusions are reached. For the purposes of this chapter, however, we take the position that diagnoses represent dichotomizations of continuous dimensions of psychopathology in the absence of adequate data to support those dichotomizations.

Is It Necessary or Advantageous to Dichotomize Dimensions of Psychopathology?

It should be emphasized that epidemiology does not require the use of dichotomous diagnoses for many purposes. For example, one could relate potential risk and protective factors for onset or persistence to dimensions of psychopathology instead of diagnoses. Indeed, many of the epidemiologic studies summarized in this chapter treated behavior problems as continuous dimensions.

Epidemiologists often point to the potential advantages of dichotomizing both continuous risk factor variables and continuous measures of dysfunction, however. First, clinicians face the need to make dichotomous decisions regarding psychopathology on a daily basis; they must decide to treat or not to treat. Because most forms of treatment are associated with some degree of iatrogenic risk, it is not always in the patient's best interest to provide treatment. Because epidemiologic data can contribute importantly to the definition of caseness, finding the most reasonable point of demarcation between disorder and nondisorder could be of great benefit to clinical decision making. By the same token, it would be valuable to know the number of youths in a population who need services and how they are distributed in that population. Such knowledge would assist in planning services, budgeting for those services, and studying barriers to the receipt of mental health services.

There also are statistical advantages to dichotomizing dimensional measures under some circumstances. Pearson correlations (and other statistical procedures that are based on them) reflect the degree of covariation across the entire range of scores on both variables. Often risk variables and disorders are, in fact, related across the full range of both continua and such statistics are appropriate. On the other hand, treating all risk variables and measures of psychopathology as continua may hide potent risk relationships at the ends of those continua when only variation at the extremes are relevant. For example, the Pearson correlation between birth weight and intelligence in children is $r = .20$, accounting for only 4% of the variance in intelligence (Scott, Shaw, & Urbano, 1994). When birth weight (<2500 g) and intelligence are dichotomized, however, the relative risk for severe mental retardation among low versus normal birth weight children is over 5.0 (Scott et al., 1994). Birth weight is not an important predictor of intelligence for most children (those within the normal ranges of birth weight and intelligence), but low birth weight is an important predictor of very low intelligence. It is possible that some important risk relationships for child and adolescent psychopathology similarly reflect variation only at the extremes of the continua of the risk factor and the dimension of psychopathology. Reliance solely on continuous measures of risk and psychopathology might easily lead to an underestimate of the importance of these relationships.

Role of Functional Impairment in Diagnostic Caseness

DSM-IV (American Psychiatric Association, 1994) definitions of mental disorder require two key conditions to be met to make diagnoses: (1) the requisite number of symptomatic behaviors or emotions must be present, and (2) those symptoms must be judged to have created significant functional impairment or distress. Similarly, the Center for Mental Health Services (CMHS) definition of "serious emotional disturbance" requires the presence of "functional impairment which substantially interferes with or limits the child's role or functioning in family, school, or community activities" (Definition of children with serious emotional disturbance, *Federal Register,* 1993, p. 29425).

Although an emphasis on functional impairment and distress seems essential, two key questions must be answered before measures of impairment can play a role in the assessment of psychopathology in childhood and adolescents. First, what kinds of functional impairment and distress should be measured and how should we measure them? Second, how much functional impairment is necessary and sufficient to conclude that a set of symptoms constitutes a disorder? Most measures of functional impairment are themselves continua (e.g., scores on a measure of classroom academic problems or numbers of "dislike most" votes in a classroom sociometric exercise). One could easily use functional impairment to set nonarbitrary

thresholds for diagnoses if functional impairment itself were dichotomous, but generally that is not the case. Alternatively, one could use continuous measures of impairment to set nonarbitrary diagnostic thresholds if the relationships between numbers of symptoms and measures of impairment were curvilinear, revealing natural points of demarcation between "normal" and "abnormal" numbers of symptoms. To date, however, the available evidence suggests that the relationships between continuous numbers of symptoms and continuous measures of impairment are linear (e.g., Lahey, Applegate, Barkley, *et al.,* 1994; Lahey, Applegate, McBurnett, *et al.,* 1994).

Paradoxically, the researchers involved in establishing empirical diagnostic thresholds for DSM-IV (American Psychiatric Association, 1994) definitions of DBD found that they had to arbitrarily dichotomize continuous measures of impairment (based on distributions in a normative sample) before using them to reduce somewhat the arbitrariness of diagnostic thresholds (Lahey, Applegate, Barkley, *et al.,* 1994; Lahey, Applegate, McBurnett, *et al.,* 1994). Clearly, we must go beyond such practices in the future. If natural dichotomies cannot be identified, the field should acknowledge that fact and work toward widely endorsed conventions for dichotomizing dimensions of psychopathology when categorical treatments of psychopathology are in the best interests of children.

How Should Information from Different Informants Be Used?

The field of mental health epidemiology also has been slow to integrate another obvious fact about the assessment of psychopathology into our thinking: Different informants (e.g., children, parents, teachers) provide different information on child and adolescent psychopathology (Achenbach, McConaughy, & Howell, 1987). It should not be surprising, therefore, that different informants and different combinations of informants yield different prevalence levels for diagnoses and that those diagnoses show different patterns of correlations with potential risk factors and impairment variables (Boyle *et al.,* 1996; Hart, Lahey, Loeber, & Hanson, 1994). It will be of great importance to take differences between informants into consideration in the future and to attempt to identify the optimal informants (and perhaps combinations of informants) for each dimension of psychopathology.

DEVELOPMENTAL PSYCHOPATHOLOGY AND DEVELOPMENTAL EPIDEMIOLOGY

The interdisciplinary subfield of developmental psychopathology combines the methods and assumptions of developmental psychology with those of abnormal child psychology and psychiatry (Achenbach, 1974; Sroufe & Rutter, 1984). Thus, the focus of developmental psychopathology is on both individual differences *among* individuals in adaptive functioning and developmental changes and continuities over time *within* individuals. Developmental epidemiology weds the concepts of epidemiology with developmental psychopathology (Costello & Angold, 1995; Rutter, 1988; Scott *et al.,* 1994). Therefore, the perspective of developmental epidemiology favors designs that allow the analysis of developmental change, preferably in prospective longitudinal studies that allow the strongest causal inferences about risk and protective factors.

Like epidemiology in general, developmental epidemiology studies risk factors for both the onset and persistence of disorders, but it encourages a focus on the role of developmental factors in risk–disorder relationships. For example, it is possible that childhood-onset CD is more strongly associated with parental antisocial behavior than is adolescent-onset CD (Lahey, Loeber, Quay, Frick, & Grimm, 1997). In addition, developmental transitions from one form of disorder to another (such as from Oppositional Defiant Disorder [ODD] to CD) that are sometimes referred to as "precursor" relationships and sometimes discussed under the rubric of "heterotypic continuity" are of particular interest to developmental epidemiologists.

The broader fields of epidemiology and biostatistics have developed a number of techniques for examining developmental effects, such as event history analysis, but many of the statistical methods and experimental designs of developmental epidemiology are derived from developmental and educational psychology (i.e., longitudinal analyses of change).

REVIEW OF POPULATION-BASED STUDIES OF THE DISRUPTIVE BEHAVIOR DISORDERS

In this chapter, we review the published literature on the epidemiology of DBD. Studies of national samples are described in Table A1 in the Appendix and studies of more local samples are described in Table A2, also in the Appendix. Although epidemiologic studies can be conducted using samples that are representative of clinics or other institutions, we limit this review to birth cohort samples, household samples, and school-based samples to reduce overlap with other chapters in this volume. Even with these limitations, the literature on the epidemiology of DBD is quite large. Using a combination of searches of electronic databases and other methods, a total of 39 population-based studies of DBD were identified that met the inclusion criteria described in the following sections. Of these studies, 11 used nationally representative samples (7 of these studies were conducted in the United States) and 28 used samples representative of smaller geopolitical units (15 of these studies were conducted in the United States).

It is important to note that the primary goal of many of these studies was not to study DBD, even though relevant data were collected in studies with other primary goals (e.g., a description of the adolescent labor force for the purpose of economic planning). Even among studies with a mental health focus, however, there was a notable lack of shared agendas across studies. Each study seems to have been designed with different questions in mind and the published data have been treated in many different ways. As a result, it is difficult to collate data on even the most basic topics. Future progress in developmental epidemiology would be aided greatly by the emergence of a coherent research agenda for developmental epidemiology.

Inclusion Criteria for This Review

Dependent Variables

Studies are included if they employed either dimensional ratings of disruptive and antisocial behavior or structured diagnostic interviews of Attention-Deficit/Hyperactivity Disorder (ADHD), ODD, or CD. Studies are included only if they reported on data at the individual level (e.g., delinquent acts committed by individuals as opposed to overall crime rates of different neighborhoods). Studies employing diagnostic measures had to allow participants to receive multiple diagnoses where criteria for more than one disorder were met.

If one accepts the fact that apparently minor differences in methods of measuring dependent variables (e.g., diagnostic criteria, instruments, informants) can make considerable differences in findings, the difficulties inherent in summarizing findings from methodologically diverse studies are obvious. Mindful of this concern, we have presented the salient methodologic features of each study to allow readers to come to their own conclusions. Because conventions for the measurement of mental disorders have not been agreed on by the field, one can do little more at present than highlight methodologic differences.

Perhaps the most serious limitation of these studies stems from the wide range of instruments used to measure disruptive behaviors, ranging from rating scales to structured diagnostic interviews. Moreover, because many of the studies were not designed to focus on DBD, the range of disruptive behaviors covered varies widely. For example, the frequently used Behavior Problem Index (Zill, 1985) includes an "antisocial" subscale, but that scale does not include items referring to such hallmarks of CD as fighting, stealing, or running away from home. Such variations in measures undoubtedly contribute to the lack of consistent findings across studies.

Informants

Only studies using parents, teachers, peers, the youths themselves, or some combination as informants are included. "Official records" of delinquent or antisocial behavior (e.g., rates of detention or arrest, adjudication or conviction, commitment or incarceration) confound rates of behavior with responses to that behavior by the criminal and juvenile justice systems, either of which may vary systematically across sociodemographic groups. Due to the biases inherent in these types of measures, studies employing them as the sole indices of disruptive behavior are not included.

Age Range

Only studies of youths 4–18 years of age are included, although some longitudinal studies followed youths into early adulthood.

Sampling Strategies

Studies are included only if they employed household-based, school-based, or birth-cohort-based sampling strategies, selecting either entire target populations or probability samples of those populations. Some leeway is given on the representativeness of sampling (e.g., studies of only one gender or one racial or ethnic group are included), but studies that, for example, selected only schools or neighborhoods with high crime rates are excluded. Similarly, samples drawn from institutions other than schools or obstetric hospitals (e.g., mental health clinics, pediatric clinics, perinatal intensive care units, juvenile detention centers) are not included.

Sample Size

Studies are included only if their sample sizes were at least 500. In the case of longitudinal studies, only the sample sizes at the first wave of data collection are required to meet this criterion. For studies using a two-stage design (in which a total population or large sample was first screened for disruptive behavior problems, and a subsample was then selected for intensive assessment), only the first-stage samples have to meet this requirement.

Population of Reference

Samples must be representative of youths in a school district, city, county, or larger geographical unit.

Independent Variables

Studies must have reported findings on the relationship between the DBDs and basic demographic factors (e.g., age, gender, SES), family variables (e.g., family constitution, parenting), or residential factors (e.g., neighborhood characteristics).

Results

Studies are included only if the results of significance tests were reported or if specific references were made to the significance of the findings. An exception is made for findings regarding gender differences, which often were reported in the form of gender ratios without tests of significance.

Limitations of Studies Reviewed

Dependent Variables

In the studies reviewed in this chapter, there is an unfortunate inverse relationship between the comprehensiveness of the evaluation of the dependent variables and the size of the population of reference. In particular, most studies of national samples used brief measures of psychopathology that obtained useful information on common conduct problems, but obtained less information on more serious antisocial behaviors and other types of psychopathology. Only the Achenbach national study (Achenbach, Howell, Quay, & Conners, 1991) used a comprehensive psychopathology rating scale. No U.S. national study obtained sufficient information to make diagnostic classifications. In the United States, some local-site studies conducted diagnostic assessments, but

small sample sizes often necessitated combining some lower-rate disorders, such as ODD and CD, into a single category. This practice makes sense if the two disorders have the same correlates, but combining them precludes determining whether they do. Outside the United States, studies of both local and national samples have been conducted using diagnostic assessments, but it is not clear that the results can be generalized to U.S. youths.

Informants

There also is a regrettable inverse association between sample size and the number of informants on the youth's behavior problems. Most U.S. national studies used a single informant on the youth's psychopathology. Only the Achenbach U.S. national study (Achenbach *et al.*, 1991) used parent, youth, and teacher informants to provide multiple perspectives. Generally, studies conducted outside the United States are more likely to include all three key informants.

Functional Impairment

This database is also seriously limited in that few U.S. national studies obtained information on the youth's functional impairment and distress. Because many children exhibit behaviors and emotions that are considered to be symptoms of psychopathology, but do not exhibit a significant degree of impairment or distress, DSM-IV (American Psychiatric Association, 1994) and other diagnostic systems require the presence of both the requisite symptoms and significant functional impairment or distress associated with those symptoms before a diagnosis can be made. Most of the studies reviewed, however, did not use any measure of functional impairment.

Independent Variables

In the national studies reviewed, the independent variables do not begin to cover the full range of potential risk and protective factors for child and adolescent psychopathology. For example, parental psychopathology is an important risk factor for child and adolescent psychopathology. The National Longitudinal Survey of Youth Child Data (NLSY; Baker, Keck, Mott, & Quinlan, 1993) was exceptional in obtaining information on delinquent behavior and substance use by the mother, but even the NLSY did not obtain information on other types of maternal psychopathology or on any type of psychopathology in the biological father or other caretakers. Other national studies obtained even less information on the family history of psychopathology. Omission of key risk factors such as parental psychopathology and other potential risk and protective factors seriously limits efforts to model risk for psychopathology in children and adolescents and can lead to erroneous conclusions. For example, if parental psychopathology is a strong risk factor for a disorder in children, but parental psychopathology is not measured, variables that are correlated with parental psychopathology may be incorrectly identified as risk factors for childhood disorder because parental psychopathology was not controlled in the model.

Sampling Strategies

All of the studies reviewed employed strategies designed to yield representative samples of some subset of the general population, but these strategies may have biased conclusions. In particular, most studies excluded some proportion of the population from the study (e.g., youths who were hospitalized or incarcerated, youths with chronic physical illness or disability, youths not attending public schools, youths who were not native speakers of the language in which the interview was written). If any of these excluded groups exhibit different prevalences of DBD than the included groups, estimates of prevalence and risk based on the study samples could be biased if generalized to the general population. For example, most studies did not include youths who were residents of correctional facilities. The most recent available 1-day census data indicate that 0.5% of black youths ages 7–21 years were being held in custody on any given day compared

with 0.1% of white youths (Austin, Krisberg, DeComo, Rudenstine, & Del Rosario, 1995; *U.S. Population Estimates,* 1997). If most of these incarcerated youths met criteria for CD, the exclusion of this proportion of youths from each racial group would not have a large impact on the prevalence rates for CD in the two groups, but the difference could be large enough to bias tests of statistical significance.

Sample Sizes and Statistical Power

The sample sizes of these studies vary widely. Many studies provided excellent statistical power for testing main effects for moderate or larger effect sizes, but only a few studies had the larger sample sizes necessary to test interactions with age, gender, racial or ethnic background, or other key demographic variables. Interactions between these variables and risk factors would not be surprising and would be of great scientific and policy interest. For example, a statistically significant interaction between a risk factor and gender would indicate that the risk factor operates differently for girls and boys. In such a case, the main effect for that risk factor would not accurately represent the risk–disorder relationship for either girls or boys. Knowledge of such interactions would be of profound importance to theories of the origins of DBD. Therefore, having adequate statistical power to test at least two-way interactions is of the utmost importance for future population-based studies of child and adolescent psychopathology.

Testing for these interactions requires sufficient sample sizes for each demographic group. Most of the studies reviewed in this chapter sampled girls and boys equally. If the overall sample size supported testing two-way interactions, sampling the two genders with equal probability would an appropriate strategy. Similar strategies may be appropriate for testing interactions with age. Testing interactions with other variables, such as racial or ethnic background, may require different strategies, however. Typically, it would be necessary to oversample youths from less populous racial or ethnic groups to have sufficient statistical power to examine interactions. For example, the total sample size and oversampling strategy used in the NLSY study (Baker *et al.*, 1993) provide adequate statistical power for assessing relationships *within* subsamples of black, Hispanic, and white youths, but other U.S. national studies did not select adequate samples of children from racial or ethnic groups of color to examine interactions.

Treatment of Race and Ethnicity

In a broader sense, the studies reviewed generally do not promote our understanding of similarities and differences among different racial and ethnic groups because of the ways in which race and ethnicity were conceptualized and assessed. Many of these studies treated "race" and "ethnicity" as interchangeable terms rather than as distinct though related concepts. Moreover, all of the studies treated these variables as simple categorical designations rather than as multidimensional constructs encompassing culture and identity that potentially could be causally related to disorder. In addition, the categories employed frequently confounded the two variables (e.g., reporting sample proportions of whites, blacks, and Hispanics). Consequently, we regretfully have chosen to use the hybrid term "race/ethnicity" in discussing these studies, as the variables were not sufficiently differentiated.

Many of these studies were so unconcerned with the issue of sociodemographic variation that they did not even report the racial/ethnic (or gender) composition of their samples. Among those that did, many did not describe the methods by which participants were assigned to racial/ethnic categories. When the methods were described, they were often problematic. For example, in the National Survey of Youth (NSY; Elliott, Ageton, Huizinga, Knowles, & Canter, 1983), participants usually were assigned to racial/ethnic categories by the interviewers based on their visual appearance rather than by self-identification. As noted previously, a few studies oversampled smaller racial/ethnic groups to allow comparisons across groups. This strategy may have created more confusion than information, however. For example, oversampling Hispanic families as a single group may have obscured differences between groups of Hispanic origin that have different histories of immigration and acculturation. It may be more informative to oversample one or more specific Hispanic groups (e.g., Mexican Americans) in future studies. The problem of potentially obscuring meaningful differences among racial and ethnic subgroups by distinguishing only the broadest groupings is also relevant to blacks, Asians, Native Americans, and whites (see also Chapter 28, this volume).

SUMMARY OF KEY FINDINGS

In Tables A3 through A7 (Appendix, this volume), each reference includes a number indicating the study on which the publication is based (from Appendix Tables A1 and A2). These numbers are given to help the reader determine when multiple papers are based on the same sample.

Prevalence of the Disruptive Behavior Disorders

It is important to keep in mind that the calculation of prevalence rates of behavior disorders is simple arithmetically, but fraught with the many problems of definition and measurement discussed earlier. Variations in time frames (e.g., 3-month vs. 12-month prevalence), informants, diagnostic definitions, and algorithms for determining whether diagnostic criteria have been met (e.g., the type and amount of functional impairment required) also can make considerable differences in estimates of prevalence (Boyle *et al.*, 1996; Lahey *et al.*, 1990).

For the sake of simplicity, we use the terms ADHD, ODD, and CD in the next sections to refer to all of the various definitions of each disorder, which include DSM-III, DSM-III-R, and DSM-IV (American Psychiatric Association, 1980, 1987, 1994); ICD-9 and ICD-10 (World Health Organization, 1977,

1992); and Rutter's suggested scheme for classification (Rutter, 1965). The reader may refer to the description of each study in the Appendix, Tables A1 and A2, for the more detailed information. One must keep in mind that many factors make any summary of prevalence estimates of questionable value.

Prevalence Estimates of ADHD

Ranges of prevalence estimates for DBD are presented in the Appendix, Table A3. Ignoring age and variations in methodology, estimates of the prevalence of various definitions of ADHD among girls and boys combined ranged from 0.0% to 16.6%, with a median of about 2.0%.

Prevalence Estimates of CD

As presented in Table A3 (Appendix), a wide range of estimates of the prevalence of various definitions of CD have been reported, ranging from 0.0% to 11.9% for girls and boys combined. The median of the percentages presented in Table A3 was about 2.0%.

Prevalence Estimates of ODD

The range of estimates of the prevalence of ODD for girls and boys shown in Table A3 (Appendix) ranged from 0.3% to 22.5%, with the median of all estimates being about 3.2%.

Comorbidity among the Disruptive Behavior Disorders

A great deal has been written about comorbidity among mental disorders during childhood and adolescence (Biederman, Newcorn, & Sprich, 1991; Caron & Rutter, 1991; Jensen, Martin, & Cantwell, 1997; Nottleman & Jensen, 1995). As the term *comorbidity* has been used in a number of different ways, an explicit definition is necessary. In this chapter, we use the term to refer simply to meeting criteria for two or more disorders during the same period (e.g., the past 12 months). Consequently, all of the difficulties associated with the concept of prevalence discussed previously necessarily also apply to the concept of comorbidity.

Among clinic-based samples, findings consistently suggest high rates of comorbidity among DBD (Biederman et al., 1991). A number of general-population studies also provide information on the comorbidity of ADHD with CD and ODD. As shown in Table A4 (Appendix), tests of significance were calculated (or enough data were presented to allow us to calculate them) to determine whether ADHD and CD (or CD and/or ODD as a combined category) overlapped at greater than chance levels in five reports from four studies (Anderson, Williams, McGee, & Silva, 1987; Bird et al., 1988; Bird, Gould, & Staghezza, 1993; Fergusson, Horwood, & Lynskey, 1993; Wolraich, Hannah, Pinnock, Baumgaertel, & Brown, 1996). In each case, the degree of overlap between the two disorders was statistically significant. In a report from the Dunedin study, however, McGee and colleagues (1990) did not find a statistically significant degree of overlap when the two disorders were assessed at an older age and using different informants than in the analyses reported by Anderson and colleagues (1987). Several other studies reported the degree of overlap among DBD, but not enough information was provided to calculate tests of significance.

When considered together, these data suggest that ADHD and CD (or CD and/or ODD combined) co-occur at higher than chance rates. Unfortunately, only one of these studies provided data on the overlap of ADHD with ODD, findings that suggest that ADHD and ODD also co-occur at higher than chance rates. None of the studies provided data on the overlap of CD with ODD. These studies generally either did not measure both ODD and CD or combined them into a single category because sample sizes were too small to consider the disorders separately. Because some theories of the development of DBD are based on the presumed overlap between ODD and CD (e.g., Lahey & Loeber, 1994; Loeber, Lahey, & Thomas, 1991), the inability to draw conclusions regarding comorbidity between ODD and CD represents an important gap in knowledge.

If DBD co-occur at higher than chance levels, that fact would have important methodologic implications for the study of risk factors for DBD. If, for example, ADHD and CD tend to co-occur, it would be easy to conclude incorrectly that a risk factor for one of those disorders was a risk factor for both disorders. Similarly, it would be easy to confuse a risk factor specific to the comorbid form of the disorder with a factor related to risk for each disorder separately. To avoid these kinds of errors, it is necessary to separate comorbid cases from cases that occur separately. This has been done in almost none of the studies reviewed in this chapter, perhaps because of the large sample sizes that such a strategy would require. Regardless of the difficulties in doing so, however, if DBD do tend to co-occur at greater than chance levels, we will not understand the risk factors for DBD until they are studied both separately and together.

POTENTIAL INDIVIDUAL-LEVEL RISK FACTORS FOR THE DISRUPTIVE BEHAVIOR DISORDERS

Associations of DBD with demographic and other potential individual-level risk factors are summarized in Table A5 (Appendix). When both bivariate and multivariate models were reported, we table only the bivariate statistics. The results of multivariate analyses are tabled only when bivariate correlations were not reported. We take this approach for two reasons. First, our intent is to broadly summarize simple associations among potential risk factors and DBD. Second, the marked differences in multivariate models across studies make them very difficult to compare.

For many potential risk factors, a lack of consistent findings across studies means that only tentative conclusions can be reached. In some cases, however, clear associations with potential risk factors can be seen in the current database. Apparently, some associations are strong enough to be detected in spite of methodologic differences among the studies.

Age

Few of the studies reviewed were designed explicitly to provide information about age-related changes in DBD, either through cross-sectional comparisons across a broad age range or through the longitudinal study of age-related change over time. In addition, even when statistical analyses of age-related changes could have been made, many published reports did not provide them. Unfortunately, those studies that did test for age effects often had sample sizes that provided little power for detecting differences. It is quite remarkable that the fundamentally important developmental variable of age has received so little attention to date in population-based research. Clearly, much work remains to be done to foster a developmental perspective on the epidemiology of psychopathology in children and adolescents.

ADHD

Longitudinal studies of clinic-referred children consistently show age-related declines in ADHD behaviors (e.g., Barkley, Fisher, Edelbrock, & Smallish, 1990; Gittelman, Mannuzza, Shenker, & Bonagura, 1985; Hart et al., 1995), but the few population-based studies that report on potential age differences in ADHD provided inconsistent findings. Five reports from three studies (Cohen et al., 1993; McDermott, 1993, 1996; Offord, Boyle, & Racine, 1989; Velez, Johnson, & Cohen, 1989) showed significant age-related decreases in the prevalence of ADHD across childhood and adolescence, but another report from one of these studies found no age differences (Offord et al., 1987), perhaps because of differences in the informants used in the analyses. In contrast, two studies reported age-related increases in ADHD from preschool to elementary school ages, with little or no age-related changes after entry to elementary school (Achenbach et al., 1991; Bird, Gould, Yager, Staghezza, & Canino, 1989). Two other studies (Costello et al., 1996; Lewinsohn, Hops, Robert, Seeley, & Andrews, 1993) reported no significant age differences, but these studies covered relatively narrow age ranges.

Thus, it is not clear whether ADHD behaviors change with age in the general population. At this point, the most reasonable hypothesis is that reports of ADHD symptoms increase from preschool ages to elementary ages (perhaps due to increased demands on the child in elementary school to pay attention and stay still), with relatively small age-related declines from elementary school entry through adolescence. It should be noted, however, that Hart and colleagues (1995) found that the age-related decline in the prevalence of ADHD from childhood through adolescence in a clinic sample was due to declines in hyperactive-impulsive behaviors only, with no age-related changes found for inattentive behaviors. The distinction between these two dimensions of ADHD behaviors in DSM-IV (American Psychiatric Association, 1994) may lead to clearer findings on potential developmental changes in ADHD behaviors in future population-based studies.

CD

Data on potential age-related changes in CD also are inconsistent across the studies reviewed. Reports from the Ontario Child Health Study (Offord et al., 1987; Offord, Boyle, & Racine, 1989) indicated significantly higher rates of the diagnosis of CD among 12- to 16-year-olds than among 4- to 11-year-olds, but a comparison of 6- to 11-year-olds and 12- to 16-year-olds in a second Ontario sample revealed no significant age differences in CD (Offord et al., 1996). One study reported age-related declines in the diagnosis of CD in males, with females showing increases in the CD until age 16 and then decreases (Cohen et al., 1993; Velez et al., 1989). Two other studies (Costello et al., 1996; Lewinsohn et al., 1993) found no significant age-related differences in the diagnosis of CD, but these studies covered relatively narrow age ranges. Thus, these data on age-related changes in the diagnosis of CD support no conclusions.

Two studies that used dimensional measures of aggression found age-related declines (Achenbach et al., 1991; McDermott, 1993, 1996), although one study found that the declines were limited to males (McDermott, 1996) and a third study that used a less comprehensive measure of aggression found no age-related declines (Roberts & Baird, 1972). In contrast, four studies found age-related increases in mostly nonaggressive delinquent behavior from middle childhood into adolescence (Achenbach et al., 1991; Aneshensel & Sucoff, 1996; Elliott et al., 1983; Pedersen & Wichstrøm, 1995), with some evidence of a peak in delinquency at 16–17 years and a decline afterward (Pedersen & Wichstrøm, 1995). One study that used a broad measure of conduct problems including both aggressive and nonaggressive behaviors found no age-related differences (Wichstrøm, Skogen, & Øia, 1996).

The discrepant results for CD might be explained by two factors. First, findings from studies that distinguished between aggressive and nonaggressive CD behaviors were consistent enough to suggest that inconsistent results among many studies could be the result of a failure to distinguish between these two dimensions. That is, it appears likely that aggressive CD behaviors become less common with increasing age, whereas nonagressive CD behaviors become more common with age (Achenbach et al., 1991). If this proves to be the case, grouping aggressive and nonaggressive CD behaviors together could easily produce inconsistent findings on age-related change. Second, it is possible that there are gender differences in age-related changes in CD behaviors (e.g., McDermott, 1996). Studies that used all male or mixed male and female samples might have yielded inconsistent results for this reason as well.

ODD

Most of the studies reviewed reported no age-related differences in ODD, but one study reported age-related declines (Velez et al., 1989), whereas Aneshensel and Sucoff (1996) reported age-related increases in ODD. As a result, it is not clear at this point whether rates of ODD behavior change with age.

Comment on Age Differences

The unclear pattern of results on potential age-related changes in DBD may be partly the result of methodologic differences that are confounded with age. Differences in instruments, designs, and statistical power all may contribute to the inconsistent findings. In addition, the age of the youths often was confounded with the identity of the informants in some studies. Teachers were sometimes interviewed only for younger children, whereas the youths were interviewed only when they were older. Although this pattern of changing informants makes good developmental sense, it confounds age-related changes with changes in informants. Disentangling changes in informants from changes in age should be a priority for future research to clarify possible developmental changes in DBD.

Gender

ADHD

Many of the studies reviewed reported significantly higher rates of ADHD among boys than girls (Al-Kuwaiti, Hossain, & Absood, 1995; Bird *et al.*, 1989; Cohen *et al.*, 1993; Fergusson *et al.*, 1993; McDermott, 1993, 1996; Offord *et al.*, 1987; Williams, McGee, Anderson, & Silva, 1989). On the other hand, many other studies reported no gender difference for ADHD (e.g., Graham & Rutter, 1973; Lewinsohn *et al.*, 1993; McGee *et al.*, 1990; Verhulst, van der Ende, Ferdinand, & Kasius, 1997; Vikan, 1985), including two studies that used the ICD construct of hyperkinesis rather than the DSM construct of ADHD (Graham & Rutter, 1973; Vikan, 1985). On the other hand, no study reported significantly higher rates of ADHD among girls than boys.

Reported gender ratios tended to be larger and more consistent among younger than older children. For example, Offord and colleagues (1987) found a 3:1 male to female ratio among 4- to 11-year-olds, and a 2.1:1 male to female ratio among 12- to 16-year-olds. Similarly, Co-

hen and colleagues (1993) reported a 2:1 male to female ratio among 10- to 13-year-olds, a 1.8:1 ratio among 14- to 16-year-olds, and a nearly equal male to female ratio among 17- to 20-year-olds. The patterns of differences in other studies were generally similar.

These findings suggest the tentative hypothesis that, except when the restrictive hyperkinesis definition is used, ADHD is more common among males at early ages, but that the male:female gender ratio declines with increasing age. An inspection of age-related changes in mean numbers of ADHD symptoms across studies suggests that this may result from a steeper decline in ADHD symptoms with increasing age among boys than girls. These generalizations can only be considered to be hypotheses, however, and not even well-supported hypotheses at this stage. Again, the confounding of age with informant in some studies creates difficulties in interpretation that must be addressed in future studies.

CD

Numerous studies reviewed have found that CD is significantly more common in boys than girls using a variety of categorical and dimensional measures (Achenbach *et al.*, 1991; Al-Kuwaiti *et al.*, 1995; Anastas & Reinherz, 1984; Barbarin & Soler, 1993; Butler & Golding, 1986; Davie, Butler, & Goldstein, 1972; Elliott *et al.*, 1983; McDermott, 1996; Offord *et al.*, 1987; Pedersen & Wichstrøm, 1995; Roberts & Baird, 1972; Verhulst *et al.*, 1997; Wichstrøm *et al.*, 1996). No study found that CD was significantly more common in girls than boys. The longitudinal Dunedin study (Anderson *et al.*, 1987; Feehan, McGee, Raja, & Williams, 1994; McGee *et al.*, 1985; McGee *et al.*, 1990) and the New York Child Longitudinal Study (Cohen *et al.*, 1993; Velez *et al.*, 1989; Williams *et al.*, 1989) reported inconsistent patterns of higher rates for boys during some but not all assessments. These inconsistencies may be related to differences in informants at different ages in the Dunedin study, but the same informants were used at all ages in the New York study. Reports from the two Ontario studies indicated that males were significantly more likely to meet criteria for CD than females when the teacher was the informant (and when parent and teacher reports were combined), but not when only the parent's report of symptoms was considered (Offord, Boyle, & Racine, 1996), and that the gender difference was found only among the offspring of parents with mental disorders (Offord et al., 1989).

One study reported no gender difference for the diagnosis of CD (Lewinsohn et al., 1993), but only the youth informant was interviewed and rates of CD were very low for both genders. Two studies using dimensional measures found no gender differences (Aneshensel & Sucoff, 1996; Luster & McAdoo, 1994). Other studies reported gender ratios, but did not provide a statistical test of the difference. In most of these studies, however, the rate of CD was considerably higher in boys than girls.

These findings suggest that CD is more common in boys than girls in the general population. This appears to be true for both aggressive and nonaggressive aspects of CD behaviors (Achenbach et al., 1991). It is not possible to estimate the overall gender ratio for the diagnosis of CD meaningfully, however, because of the marked methodologic differences across studies. There is some evidence that the male:female ratio may be higher for CD that emerges before puberty and is marked by higher levels of aggression than for CD that emerges during adolescence and is characterized by lower levels of aggression (McGee et al., 1990), but these data are confounded by differences in informants. In addition, the male:female gender ratio may be higher when CD is not comorbid with emotional disorders (Graham & Rutter, 1973).

ODD

Evidence regarding gender differences for ODD in the reviewed studies is quite inconsistent. Two studies found significantly more ODD among boys (Aneshensel & Sucoff, 1996; Offord et al., 1996). One longitudinal study of adolescents (Lewinsohn et al., 1993) found significantly higher rates at the first assessment, but not at the follow-up assessment a year later. McDermott (1996) found higher rates of ODD behaviors in boys than girls among 5- to 8-year-old children, but not in older children or adolescents, and four studies found no significant gender difference in rates of ODD (Bird et al., 1989; Cohen et al., 1993; Velez et al., 1989; Verhulst et al., 1997; Williams et al., 1989). No study found significantly higher rates of ODD among girls than boys, however. Future studies with adequate statistical power will be needed to determine whether there are gender differences in ODD.

Race and Ethnicity

The studies reviewed provide weak and inconsistent evidence on potential racial and ethnic differences in the prevalence of DBD. Velez and colleagues (1989) found lower rates of the diagnosis of CD among White youths than all other racial or ethnic groups combined during one longitudinal assessment, but not another, and found no differences for ADHD and ODD. All other reviewed studies that used diagnostic measures as the dependent variable did not find racial or ethnic differences for any DBD diagnosis.

Among studies using dimensional measures, Achenbach and colleagues (1991) found higher rates among white youths than nonwhite youths on aggression and attention problems, but not delinquency. In contrast, Elliott and colleagues (1983) and Loeber, Farrington, Stouthamer-Loeber, and van Kammen (1998) found higher rates of delinquency among black than white youths, and Aneshensel and Sucoff (1996) and Fridrich and Flannery (1995) found higher rates of conduct problems among Hispanic than non-Hispanic youths. Most studies, however, found no differences on dimensional measures of the DBD.

It would be of great importance to obtain information on possible racial and ethnic differences in prevalence in studies that employ more sophisticated conceptualizations of these variables and that are designed to have sufficient statistical power to examine the potential roles of race and ethnicity while controlling for SES and other confounds. This would require either very large sample sizes or oversamples of selected racial or ethnic groups. Such samples also would allow the examination of potential racial and ethnic differences in the relationship between potential risk factors and disorders.

POTENTIAL FAMILY-LEVEL RISK FACTORS FOR THE DISRUPTIVE BEHAVIOR DISORDERS

Findings on potential risk factors at the level of the family are summarized in Table A6 (Appendix). Because many variables were measured within each construct, it is difficult to reach firm conclusions in many cases. However, these data strongly suggest that further study of family factors would be worthwhile.

Family Structure and Family Size

The majority of the studies reviewed indicate that children from two-biological-parent families have lower rates of DBD than children from families containing one biological parent. Not all studies found one-parent families to have higher rates of child disorders, but none found lower rates among one-parent families. There appears to be something about two-parent families that is associated with lower risk for DBD. At this point, however, it is not possible to generate well-supported hypotheses as to why children from two-parent families are at lower risk. Intact families may have fewer children with DBD because they provide better supervision, because they are less likely to contain a parent with serious psychopathology, or for many other reasons.

A clue that may lead to an eventual understanding of the causal connection between family structure and DBD in the children is that *change* in family structure has been linked to risk for behavior problems in the child in two longitudinal studies (Achenbach, Howell, McConaughy, & Stanger, 1995; Stanger, McConaughy, & Achenbach, 1992) and that the

total number of changes in parenting figures during childhood has been correlated with the prevalence of DBD in another longitudinal study (Fergusson & Lynskey, 1993a). That is, both stable one-parent and two-parent families are less likely to have children with behavior problems than families in which the custodial parent (usually the biological mother) has had more than one partner (Najman et al., 1997). Interestingly, Barbarin and Soler (1993) found the risk of CD among black families to be higher among families headed by a single biological mother than among three-generation families, suggesting that the number of parent figures, per se, is not the key variable. The causal variable related to family structure is likely to be either some aspect of changes in parenting or some characteristic of parents who frequently change partners (e.g., psychopathy), or both, but it seems unlikely to be an inherent characteristic of single-parent families.

Maternal Age

Several studies reviewed suggest that young age of the mother at the birth of the child (defined as her age at the birth of her first child or of the study child in different studies) is linked to the risk for CD in her offspring. Because this variable could reflect a number of different potential causal processes (e.g., differences in reproductive processes, differences in parenting behavior, limiting effects of earlier childbearing on maternal education, greater tendency for antisocial women to give birth at younger ages), it would be valuable to give attention to this variable in future studies. That is, maternal age seems likely to be correlated with one or more causal risk factors for CD, and as such, it is an important scientific clue.

Parental Psychopathology and Substance Abuse

Many studies of clinic-referred children and adolescents have linked child and adolescent CD to antisocial behavior in their biological parents (e.g., Lahey et al., 1988), but these studies could be influenced by referral biases because children with disorders who are referred to clinics are more likely to have parents who have sought treatment for their own psychopathology than children with the same disorders who are not referred to clinics (Goodman et al., 1997). Relatively few population-based studies have assessed parental psychopathology, but findings from the majority of the studies reviewed, as summarized in Appendix Table A6, show a significant association between depression, antisocial behavior, and substance abuse in parents and DBD in their children. Although these results are not completely consistent across studies or informants, they suggest the hypothesis that psychopathology is familial in the general population and not an artifact of clinic referral.

Furthermore, the data suggest that the familial patterns are general rather than specific (i.e., several parental disorders are linked to several child disorders). The data from these studies have not been analyzed to disentangle comorbid diagnoses in the parent and child to directly assess the degree of specificity, however. When this has been done in clinic studies, a much greater degree of specificity has been demonstrated (Faraone, Biederman, Keenan, & Tsuang, 1991; Lahey et al., 1988). Additional research is clearly needed to test the hypothesis of familiality in DBD, to determine whether familiality is general or specific, and to explore the potential genetic and environmental mechanisms of familial transmission (see also Chapters 9 and 18, this volume, for more on these issues).

Family Functioning

As shown in Table A6 (Appendix), a number of studies reviewed found that DBD are more common among children from families that are broadly dysfunctional and whose parents' marital relationship is not harmonious, but there is some evidence from two longitudinal studies that this correlation may weaken as the age of the children increases (Fergusson & Lynskey, 1993a; Loeber et al., 1998). It will be important in future longitudinal studies to determine whether family problems antedate

child problems and, therefore, may play a causal role, or whether family problems result from having a child with problems. In particular, longitudinal studies of population-based samples could determine whether changes in family functioning precede changes in child behavior. If family problems are found to precede child problems, it will be possible for future studies to test hypotheses regarding the causal mechanisms underlying this association. For example, it is equally possible that family dysfunction directly increases the risk of DBD by causing distress in children, that it has indirect effects through disrupted parenting, or that it is not causally related to DBD at all, but is a noncausal reflection of parental psychopathology that may be shown in the future to be causally related to DBD. Any of these possibilities could be true for different children, of course.

Parenting

Despite the central importance of parenting in theories of the origins of DBD and in the treatment of DBD (e.g., Patterson, Reid, & Dishion, 1992), relatively few of the studies reviewed assessed the relationship between parenting and DBD. The studies that did measure parenting, however, usually found associations between a broad range of aspects of parenting and DBD (Table A6, Appendix). The inclusion of valid measures of parental monitoring, supervision, physical punishment, and other aspects of parenting in future population-based studies would allow the testing of hypotheses that are of enormous importance to the field's conceptualization of DBD. These studies must be longitudinal in design, however, to rule out child effects.

POTENTIAL SOCIOECONOMIC AND RESIDENTIAL RISK FACTORS FOR THE DISRUPTIVE BEHAVIOR DISORDERS

Findings on the relationship of DBD to several aspects of SES, including family income, parental education, and occupational status, and to residential risk factors, such as living in urban environments or high-crime neighborhoods, are summarized in Table A7 in the Appendix.

SES

There is rather consistent evidence across many of the studies reviewed, summarized in Table A7 (Appendix), that risk for ADHD, ODD, and CD is higher among children from families with lower incomes, but that receipt of public financial aid is not a consistent correlate of DBD. There is also reasonably consistent evidence that DBD are related to a variety of other measures of family SES, including parental education, parental employment, parental occupational status, and composite indices of SES. These findings strongly suggest that the prevalence of DBD is inversely related to SES. No attempt has been made, however, to determine whether SES is more strongly associated with one DBD than with others (such as thorough analyses that disentangle comorbid cases) and the causal mechanisms underlying this association have rarely been explored.

Neighborhood Characteristics and Urbanization

As shown in Table A7 (Appendix), several studies reviewed have shown that neighborhood characteristics are consistently associated with CD behaviors, but not with other DBD. Neighborhoods that are associated with higher rates of CD behaviors have been characterized using both composite indices derived from census data (e.g., neighborhood crime rates, mean income of neighbors, use of public assistance) and parental perceptions of their neighborhoods (e.g., crime rates, quality of housing, safety, rates of unemployment), lending weight to these findings. Such findings are potentially of importance to theories of the origins of CD because of the specific relationship between neighborhood characteristics and CD behaviors. Again, however, the field has only begun to explore the causal mechanisms involved in the association between neighborhood characteristics

and rates of CD behavior. Notably, Sampson, Raudenbush, and Earls (1997) have suggested that neighborhood effects on crime rates are mediated by a willingness of neighbors to supervise youths from other families and otherwise work together for the common good, for example, by lobbying for more street lights.

In 1975, Rutter, Cox, Tupling, Berger, and Yule published a striking comparison between rates of psychopathology in the Isle of Wight sample and a similar sample drawn from an inner borough of London. Their findings suggested markedly higher rates of both conduct problems and emotional disorders in the urban environment. Since that time, two population-based studies have confirmed the finding of increased risk for conduct problems in urban environments in mixed-gender samples (Osborn, Butler, & Morris, 1984; Wichstrøm et al., 1996) and two studies have found higher rates of conduct problems in urban environments among girls (Ageton, 1983; Zahner, Jacobs, Freeman, & Trainor, 1993). A number of other studies have failed to replicate urbanization effects, however. Because the studies of urban– rural differences had limited statistical power and their sampling frames often did not include large cities, no conclusions can be reached at present on urbanization. This is unfortunate, as it is a variable of potential scientific and public policy importance.

SUMMARY AND FUTURE DIRECTIONS

Developmental epidemiology is an emerging field that has only begun to tap its potential. In time, it may have an increasingly important impact on the child and adolescent mental health fields. It is hoped that the field at large will be influenced to consider both sampling and developmental issues in the design and interpretation of future studies. In particular, longitudinal population-based studies could shed light on a number of key issues in developmental psychopathology that can only be studied when sampling bias is limited (e.g., risk and protective factors). Such designs should become a routine part of the array of methodologies used by researchers.

At this point in the early history of developmental epidemiology, we are in the unusual position of having far more data than findings. There are two primary reasons for this state of affairs. First, population-based studies of youth have not had a coherent agenda that organizes research. To a great extent, these studies have not been designed around specific questions (other than simple prevalence), and when they were driven by specific questions, these were not mental health questions. If we are to advance our understanding of the development of psychopathology in children and adolescents, we must conduct studies that are designed specifically to answer the most pressing empirical questions and end our reliance on studies that are designed for other purposes.

Although a number of nationally representative studies with strong statistical power have been conducted, they were funded primarily by sources other than mental health agencies. As a result, the largest national studies did not use the best or most comprehensive measures of DBD. In particular, these larger national studies often assessed high-rate, mild behavior problems, but did not assess the lower-rate, serious antisocial behaviors (e.g., theft, mugging, running away from home, rape) that have the greatest theoretical and policy importance.

Unfortunately, well-designed population-based studies are expensive, and when money is spent on one kind of research, less money is available for other kinds of research. This makes it difficult to fund the field of developmental epidemiology. It is our firm belief, however, that advances in the field of developmental psychopathology will be unacceptably slow, and often misguided, until adequate longitudinal population-based studies have been conducted that (1) definitively describe the development of the syndromes of psychopathology (the phenotypes), and (2) definitively confirm or rule out potential risk factors. Until the field of developmental psychopathology has this broad empirical framework, we will be working in the dark created by inadequate sample sizes, biased samples, and other very real limitations.

Second, mental health researchers have only begun to take seriously the notion that methodologic differences, such as differences in definitions of disorders or differences in informants, often produce differences in findings. If we are going to make the most of future population-based studies, we must reach greater agreement on definitions of caseness, fully understand the implications of differences in informants (and the advantages and disadvantages of combining discrepant information from multiple informants), and resolve other methodologic questions.

Relatively little can be concluded about the prevalence of DBD at this time. A wide range of diagnostic definitions, assessment instruments, informants (and combinations of informants), and adjustments for functional impairment have resulted in a range of prevalence estimates that is too broad to summarize. Clearly, the field needs to reach greater consensus on the definition of "caseness" for psychopathology in children and adolescents before tackling the issues of prevalence and incidence. In spite of the difficulties in defining prevalence, there is evidence across several studies that DBD tend to co-occur at higher than chance levels. Unfortunately, no evidence is available on the key question of the co-occurrence of ODD and CD at this time, largely because the studies that assessed these two disorders had insufficient sample sizes to assess their degree of comorbidity.

On a more positive note, enough is known at this point to advance several potentially important hypotheses about the development of DBD. First, it appears that ADHD and CD are more common among boys than girls. The evidence on gender differences for ODD is less clear, but is in the direction of greater prevalence among boys. Second, the population-based studies suggest that ADHD may decrease somewhat with advancing age from childhood through adolescence, replicating findings from clinic-based samples (Barkley *et al.,* 1990; Gittelman *et al.,* 1985; Hart *et al.,* 1995). In addition, the reviewed population-based studies suggest the hypothesis that the rate of developmental decline in the prevalence of ADHD behaviors is greater in boys than girls, reducing the gender difference in adolescence. In the case of CD, it is unfortunate that little is known about potentially important shifts in gender ratios across age, pubertal stage, and other developmental indices, but some studies suggest the important hypothesis that aggressive behaviors decline with age, whereas nonaggressive CD behaviors increase during late childhood and early-to-mid adolescence.

Current findings indicate that there is an inverse relationship between SES and DBD. Indeed, there is less need for future studies to confirm the inverse association between SES and DBD than to begin to *explain* this robust association. SES is a complex variable that subsumes many potentially important factors and processes. These include both directly related variables such as level of parental education and economic resources, and correlated variables such as neighborhood crime, school climates, and racial or ethnic background. It may be possible to identify the variables that underlie the link between SES and DBD by using statistical modeling, but we will not fully understand the processes underlying SES–DBD correlations until longitudinal studies have been conducted that examine the relationship between changes in the components of SES over time and changes in DBD over time. Because of the strength of the association between SES and DBD, efforts to decompose its active elements in the future should be a high research priority.

Similarly, current findings suggest that parental psychopathology, family and marital dysfunction, and atypical parenting are all likely correlates of DBD. It will be important for future studies to confirm these findings using longitudinal designs that can rule out child effects and other alternative interpretations. Moreover, such longitudinal studies would allow informative tests of hypotheses regarding the causal mechanisms involved in these correlations.

In light of methodological limitations regarding the measurement of race and ethnicity and the adequacy of sample sizes, little can be concluded about racial or ethnic differences in the prevalence of DBD or in risk–disorder relationships. Our lack of knowledge of potential associations of race and ethnicity with DBD and interactions with other demographic factors represents an important gap that must be addressed in future studies. Eliminating such gaps, however, requires large sample sizes and strategic oversampling, both of which are expensive. Answering such key questions will require a strong commitment from the mental health research community, and such a commitment can flow only from a full understanding of the issues and the stakes.

We must be very careful in interpreting the findings relevant to potential risk factors for DBD summarized in this chapter. In particular, these studies did not distinguish between risk factors for onset and risk for persistence of behavior problems. Because risk factors for onset and persistence may be different, the failure to distinguish between the onset and the persistence of behavior problems may result not only in conceptual confusion but also in a weakening of statistical power for the identification of either type of risk factor.

It is perhaps disheartening to see the small number of generalizations about risk that can be drawn with confidence from the large number of expensive studies that have been conducted to date. On the other hand, this review of existing studies does provide some potentially important hypotheses and clearly points to areas of gaps in knowledge. It is hoped that the future will bring population-based longitudinal studies with clear goals, strong measures of psychopathology and functional impairment obtained from multiple informants, adequate statistical power for testing interactions, and a more explanatory approach focusing on the causal mechanisms underlying sociodemographic patterns.

References

Achenbach, T. M. (1974). *Developmental psychopathology.* New York: Ronald.

Achenbach, T. M., McConaughy, S. H., & Howell, C. T. (1987). Child/adolescent behavioral and emotional problems: Implications of cross-informant correlations for situation specificity. *Psychological Bulletin, 101,* 213–232.

Achenbach, T. M, Howell, C. T., Quay, H. C., & Conners, C. K. (1991). National survey of problems and competencies among four- to sixteen-year-olds: Parents' reports for normative and clinical samples. *Monographs of the Society for Research in Child Development, 56*(3, Serial No. 225).

Achenbach, T. M., Howell, C. T., McConaughy, S. M., & Stanger, C. (1995). Six-year predictors of problems in a national sample of children and youth: I. Cross-informant syndromes. *Journal of the American Academy of Child and Adolescent Psychiatry, 34,* 336–347.

Ageton, S. S. (1983). The dynamics of female delinquency, 1976–1980. *Criminology, 21,* 555–584.

Al-Kuwaiti, M. A., Hossain, M. M., & Absood, G. H. (1995). Behaviour disorders in primary school children in Al Ain, United Arab Emirates. *Annals of Tropical Paediatrics, 15,* 97–104.

American Psychiatric Association. (1980). *Diagnostic and statistical manual of mental disorders* (3rd ed.). Washington, DC: Author.

American Psychiatric Association. (1987). *Diagnostic and statistical manual of mental disorders* (3rd ed., rev.). Washington, DC: Author.

American Psychiatric Association. (1994). *Diagnostic and statistical manual of mental disorders* (4th ed.). Washington, DC: Author.

Anastas, J. W., & Reinherz, H. (1984). Gender differences in learning and adjustment problems in school: Results of a longitudinal study. *American Journal of Orthopsychiatry, 54,* 110–122.

Anderson, J. C., Williams, S., McGee, R., & Silva, P. A. (1987). DSM-III disorders in preadolescent children: Prevalence in a large sample from the general population. *Archives of General Psychiatry, 44,* 69–76.

Andrews, V. C., Garrison, C. Z., Jackson, K. L., Addy, C. L., & McKeown, R. E. (1993). Mother–adolescent agreement on the symptoms and diagnoses of adolescent depression and conduct disorders. *Journal of the American Academy of Child and Adolescent Psychiatry, 32,* 731–738.

Aneshensel, C. S., & Sucoff, C. A. (1996). The neighborhood context of adolescent mental health. *Journal of Health and Social Behaviour, 37,* 293–310.

Angold, A., & Costello, E. J. (1996). Toward establishing an empirical basis for the diagnosis of oppositional defiant disorder. *Journal of the American Academy of Child and Adolescent Psychiatry, 35,* 1205–1212.

Austin, J., Krisberg, B., DeComo, R., Rudenstine, S., & Del Rosario, D. (1995). *Juveniles taken into custody: Fiscal year 1993* (NCJ No. 150422). Washington, DC: Office of Juvenile Justice and Delinquency Prevention.

Baker, P. C., Keck, C. K., Mott, F. L., & Quinlan, S. V. (1993). *NLSY Child Handbook: A guide to the 1986–1990 National Longitudinal Survey of Youth Child Data* (rev. ed.). Columbus, OH: Center for Human Resource Research.

Barbarin, O. A., & Soler, R. E. (1993). Behavioral, emotional, and academic adjustment in a national proba-

bility sample of African American children. *Journal of Black Psychology, 19,* 423–446.

Barkley, R. A., Fisher, M., Edelbrock, C. S., & Smallish, L. (1990). The adolescent outcome of hyperactive children diagnosed by research criteria: I. An 8-year prospective follow-up study. *Journal of the American Academy of Child and Adolescent Psychiatry, 29,* 546–557.

Bell, R. Q., & Harper, L. (1977). *Child effects on adults.* New York: John Wiley.

Berkson, J. (1946). Limitations of the application of fourfold table analysis to hospital data. *Biometrics, 2,* 47–53.

Biederman, J., Newcorn, J., & Sprich, S. (1991). Comorbidity of attention deficit hyperactivity disorder with conduct, depressive, anxiety, and other disorders. *American Journal of Psychiatry, 148,* 564–577.

Bird, H. R., Canino, G., Rubio-Stipec, M., Gould, M. S., Ribera, J., Sesman, M., Woodbury, M., Huertas-Goldman, S., Pagan, A., Sanchez-Lacay, A., & Moscoso, M. (1988). Estimates of the prevalence of childhood maladjustment in a community in Puerto Rico. *Archives of General Psychiatry, 45,* 1120–1126.

Bird, H. R., Gould, M., Yager, T., Staghezza, B., & Canino, G. (1989). Risk factors for maladjustment in Puerto Rican children. *Journal of the American Academy of Child and Adolescent Psychiatry, 28,* 847–850.

Bird, H. R., Gould, M. S., & Staghezza, B. M. (1992). Aggregating data from multiple informants in child psychiatry epidemiological research. *Journal of the American Academy of Child and Adolescent Psychiatry, 318,* 78–85.

Bird, H. R., Gould, M. S., & Staghezza, B. M. (1993). Patterns of diagnostic comorbidity in a community sample of children aged 9 through 16 years. *Journal of the American Academy of Child and Adolescent Psychiatry, 32,* 361–368.

Blum, H. M., Boyle, M. H., & Offord, D. R. (1988). Single-parent families: Child psychiatric disorder and school performance. *Journal of the American Academy of Child and Adolescent Psychiatry, 27,* 214–219.

Boyle, M. H., Offord, D. R., Hofman, H. G., Catlin, G. P., Byles, J. A., Cadman, D. T., Crawford, J. W., Links, P. S., Rae-Grant, N., & Szatmari, P. (1987). Ontario Child Health Study: I. Methodology. *Archives of General Psychiatry, 44,* 826–831.

Boyle, M. H., Offord, D. R., Racine, Y., Fleming, J. E., Szatmari, P., & Sanford, M. (1993). Evaluation of the revised Ontario Child Health Study Scales. *Journal of Child Psychology and Psychiatry, 34,* 189–213.

Boyle, M. H., Offord, D. R., Racine, Y., Sanford, M., Szatmari, P., Fleming, J. E., & Price-Munn, N. (1993). Evaluation of the Diagnostic Interview for Children and Adolescents for use in a general population sample. *Journal of Abnormal Child Psychology, 21,* 663–681.

Boyle, M. H., Offord, D. R., Racine, Y., Szatmari, P., Fleming, J., & Sanford, M. (1996). Identifying thresholds for classifying childhood psychiatric disorder: Issues and prospects. *Journal of the American Academy of Child and Adolescent Psychiatry, 35*, 1440–1448.

Butler, N. R., & Golding, J. (1986). *From birth to five: A study of the health and behaviour of Britain's 5-year-olds.* Oxford, England: Pergamon.

Caron, C., & Rutter, M. (1991). Comorbidity in child psychopathology: Concepts, issues, and research strategies. *Journal of Child Psychology and Psychiatry, 32*, 1063–1080.

Cohen, P., Cohen, J., Kasen, S., Velez, C. N., Hartmark, C., Johnson, J., Rojas, M., Brook, J., & Streuning, E. L. (1993). An epidemiological study of disorders in late childhood and adolescence: I. Age- and gender-specific prevalence. *Journal of Child Psychology and Psychiatry, 34*, 851–867.

Costello, E. J., & Angold, A. (1995). Developmental epidemiology. In D. Cicchetti & D. Cohen (Eds.), *Developmental psychopathology: Volume 1. Theory and methods* (pp. 23–56). New York: Wiley.

Costello, E. J., Angold, A., Burns, B. J., Stangl, D. K., Tweed, D. L., Erkanli, A., & Worthman, C. M. (1996). The Great Smoky Mountains Study of Youth: Goals, design, methods, and the prevalence of DSM-III-R disorders. *Archives of General Psychiatry, 53*, 1129–1136.

Costello, E. J., Farmer, E. M. Z., Angold, A., Burns, B. J., & Erkanli, A. (1997). Psychiatric disorders among American Indian and white youth in Appalachia: The Great Smoky Mountains Study. *American Journal of Public Health, 87*, 827–832.

Davie, R., Butler, N., & Goldstein, H. (1972). *From birth to seven: The second report of the National Child Development Study.* London: Longman.

Dawson, D. A. (1991). Family structure and children's health: United States, 1988. *Vital and Health Statistics* (DHHS Publication No. PHS 91-1506). Washington, DC: U.S. Government Printing Office.

Definition of children with a serious emotional disturbance. (1993). *Federal Register, 58*, 29422.

Dubow, E. F., & Ippolito, M. F. (1994). Effects of poverty and quality of the home environment on changes in the academic and behavioral adjustment of elementary school-age children. *Journal of Clinical Child Psychology, 23*, 401–412.

Elliott, D. S., & Huizinga, D. (1983). Social class and delinquent behavior in a national youth panel. *Criminology, 21*, 149–177.

Elliott, D. S., Ageton, S. S., Huizinga, D., Knowles, B. A., & Canter, R. J. (1983). *The prevalence and incidence of delinquent behavior, 1976–1980: National estimates of delinquent behavior by sex, race, social class, and other selected variables* (National Youth Survey Report No. 26). Boulder, CO: Behavioral Research Institute.

Esser, G., Schmidt, M. H., & Woerner, W. (1990). Epidemiology and course of psychiatric disorders in school-age children: Results of a longitudinal study. *Journal of Child Psychology and Psychiatry, 31*, 243–263.

Faraone, S. V., Biederman, J., Keenan, K., & Tsuang, M. T. (1991). Separation of DSM-III attention deficit disorder and conduct disorder: Evidence from a family-genetic study of American child psychiatric patients. *Psychological Medicine, 21*, 109–121.

Feehan, M., McGee, R., Raja, S. N., & Williams, S. (1994). DSM-III-R disorders in New Zealand 18-year-olds. *Australian and New Zealand Journal of Psychiatry, 28*, 87–99.

Fergusson, D. M., & Lynskey, M. T. (1993a). The effects of maternal depression on child conduct disorder and attention deficit behaviors. *Social Psychiatry and Psychiatric Epidemiology, 28*, 116–123.

Fergusson, D. M., & Lynskey, M. T. (1993b). Maternal age and behavioural outcomes in middle childhood. *Paediatric and Perinatal Epidemiology, 7*, 77–91.

Fergusson, D. M., Horwood, L. J., Shannon, F. T., & Lawton, J. M. (1989). The Christchurch Child Development Study: A review of epidemiological findings. *Paediatric and Perinatal Epidemiology, 3*, 302–325.

Fergusson, D. M., Horwood, L. J., & Lawton, J. M. (1990). Vulnerability to childhood problems and family social background. *Journal of Child Psychology and Psychiatry, 31*, 1145–1160.

Fergusson, D. M., Horwood, L. J., & Lynskey, M. T. (1993). Prevalence and comorbidity of DSM-III-R diagnoses in a birth cohort of 15 year olds. *Journal of American Academy of Child and Adolescent Psychiatry, 32*, 1127–1134.

Fergusson, D. M., Horwood, L. J., & Lynskey, M. T. (1994). Parental separation, adolescent psychopathology, and problem behaviors. *Journal of the American Academy of Child and Adolescent Psychiatry, 33*, 1122–1131.

Fridrich, A. H., & Flannery, D. J. (1995). The effects of ethnicity and acculturation on early adolescent delinquency. *Journal of Child and Family Studies, 4*, 69–87.

Garrison, C. Z., Addy, C. L., Jackson, K. L., McKeown, R. E., & Waller, J. L. (1992). Major depressive disorder and dysthymia in young adolescents. *American Journal of Epidemiology, 135*, 792–802.

Gittelman, R., Mannuzza, S., Shenker, R., & Bonagura, N. (1985). Hyperactive boys almost grown up. I. Psychiatric status. *Archives of General Psychiatry, 42*, 937–947.

Goodman, S. H., Lahey, B. B., Fielding, B., Dulcan, M., Narrow, W., & Regier, D. (1997). Representativeness of clinical samples of youth with mental disorders: A preliminary population-based study. *Journal of Abnormal Psychology, 106*, 3–14.

Graham, P., & Rutter, M. (1973). Psychiatric disorder in the young adolescent: A follow-up study. *Proceedings of the Royal Society of Medicine, 66*, 1226–1229.

Hart, E. L., Lahey, B. B., Loeber, R., & Hanson, K. S. (1994). Criterion validity of informants in the diagnosis of disruptive behavior disorders in children: A preliminary study. *Journal of Consulting and Clinical Psychology, 62*, 410–414.

Hart, E. L., Lahey, B. B., Loeber, R., Applegate, B., Green, S. M., & Frick, P. J. (1995). Developmental change in attention-deficit hyperactivity disorder in boys: A four-year longitudinal study. *Journal of Abnormal Child Psychology, 23,* 729–749.

Havighurst, R. J., Bowman, P. H., Liddle, G. P., Matthews, C. V., & Pierce, J. V. (1962). *Growing Up in River City.* New York: Wiley.

Hennekens, C. H., Buring, J. E., & Mayrent, S. L. (1987). *Epidemiology in medicine.* Boston: Little, Brown.

Huizinga, D., & Elliott, D. S. (1987). Juvenile offenders: Prevalence, offender incidence, and arrest rates by race. *Crime and Delinquency, 33,* 206–223.

Inter-university Consortium for Political and Social Research. (1985). *National Health Interview Survey, 1981* (ICPSR 8319). Ann Arbor, MI: Author.

Inter-university Consortium for Political and Social Research. (1994). *National Health Interview Survey, 1988* (ICPSR 9375). Ann Arbor, MI: Author.

Jensen, P. S., Martin, D., & Cantwell, D. P. (1997). Comorbidity in ADHD: Implications for research, practice, and DSM-IV. *Journal of the American Academy of Child and Adolescent Psychiatry, 36,* 1065–1079.

Kingery, P. M., Biafora, F. A., & Zimmerman, R. S. (1996). Risk factors for violent behaviors among ethnically diverse urban adolescents: Beyond race/ethnicity. *School Psychology International, 17,* 171–188.

Kinsey, A. C., Pomeroy, W. B., & Martin, C. E. (1948). *Sexual behavior in the human male.* Philadelphia: Saunders.

Kinsey, A. C., Pomeroy, W. B., Martin, C. E., & Gebhard, P. H. (1953). *Sexual behavior in the human female.* Philadelphia: Saunders.

Lahey, B. B., & Loeber, R. (1994). Framework for a developmental model of oppositional defiant disorder and conduct disorder. In D. K. Routh (Ed.), *Disruptive behavior disorders in childhood* (pp. 139–180). New York: Plenum.

Lahey, B. B., Piacentini, J. C., McBurnett, K., Stone, P. A., Hartdagen, S., & Hynd, G. W. (1988). Psychopathology in the parents of children with conduct disorder and hyperactivity. *Journal of the American Academy of Child and Adolescent Psychiatry, 27,* 163–170.

Lahey, B. B., Loeber, R., Stouthamer-Loeber, M., Christ, M. A. G., Green, S., Russo, M. F., Frick, P. J., & Dulcan, M. (1990). Comparison of DSM-III and DSM-III-R diagnoses for prepubertal children: Changes in prevalence and validity. *Journal of the American Academy of Child and Adolescent Psychiatry, 29,* 620–626.

Lahey, B. B., Applegate, B., Barkley, R. A., Garfinkel, B., McBurnett, K., Kerdyk, L., Greenhill, L., Hynd, G. W., Frick, P. J., Newcorn, J., Biederman, J., Ollendick, T., Hart, E. L., Perez, D., Waldman, I., & Shaffer, D. (1994). DSM-IV field trials for oppositional defiant disorder and conduct disorder in children and adolescents. *American Journal of Psychiatry, 151,* 1163–1171.

Lahey, B. B., Applegate, B., McBurnett, K., Biederman, J., Greenhill, L., Hynd, G. W., Barkley, R. A., Newcorn, J., Jensen, P., Richters, J., Garfinkel, B., Kerdyk, L., Frick, P. J., Ollendick, T., Perez, D., Hart, E. L., Waldman, I., & Shaffer, D. (1994). DSM-IV field trials for attention deficit/hyperactivity disorder in chil-

dren and adolescents. *American Journal of Psychiatry, 151,* 1673–1685.

Lahey, B. B., Flagg, E. W., Bird, H. R., Schwab-Stone, M. E., Canino, G., Dulcan, M. K., Leaf, P. J., Davies, M., Brogan, D., Bourdon, K., Horowitz, S. M., Rubio-Stipec, M., Freeman, D. H., Lichtman, J. H., Shaffer, D., Goodman, S. H., Narrow, W. E., Weissman, M. M., Kandel, D. B., Jensen, P. S., Richters, J. E., & Regier, D. A. (1996). The NIMH Methods for the Epidemiology of Child and Adolescent Mental Disorders (MECA) study: Background and methodology. *Journal of the American Academy of Child and Adolescent Psychiatry, 35,* 855–864.

Lahey, B. B., Loeber, R., Quay, H. C., Frick, P. J., & Grimm, J. (1997). Oppositional defiant disorder and conduct disorder. In A. Frances, T. Widiger, H. Pincus, R. Ross, M. B. First, & W. Davis (Eds.), *DSM-IV Source Book* (Vol. 3, pp. 189–210). Washington, DC: American Psychiatric Press.

Leslie, S. A. (1974). Psychiatric disorder in the young adolescents of an industrial town. *British Journal of Psychiatry, 125,* 113–124.

Leung, P. W. L., Luk, S. L., Ho, T. P., Taylor, E., Mak, F. L., & Bacon-Shone, J. (1996). The diagnosis and prevalence of hyperactivity in Chinese schoolboys. *British Journal of Psychiatry, 168,* 486–496.

Levy, F., Hay, D. A., McStephen, M., Wood, C., & Waldman, I. (1997). Attention-deficit disorder: A category or a continuum? Genetic analysis of a large-scale twin study. *Journal of the American Academy of Child and Adolescent Psychiatry, 36,* 737–744.

Lewinsohn, P. M., Hops, H., Robert, R. E., Seeley, J. R., & Andrews, J. A. (1993). Adolescent psychopathology: I. Prevalence and incidence of depression and other DSM-III-R disorders in high school students. *Journal of Abnormal Psychology, 102,* 133–144.

Loeber, R., Lahey, B. B., & Thomas, C. (1991). The diagnostic conundrum of oppositional defiant disorder and conduct disorder. *Journal of Abnormal Psychology, 100,* 379–390.

Loeber, R., Farrington, D. P., Stouthamer-Loeber, M., & van Kammen, W. (1998). *Antisocial behavior and mental health problems: Risk factors in childhood and adolescence.* Hillsdale, NJ: Erlbaum.

Luster, T., & McAdoo, H. P. (1994). Factors related to the achievement and adjustment of young African American children. *Child Development, 65,* 1080–1094.

Lynskey, M. T., Fergusson, D. M., & Horwood, L. J. (1994). The effect of parental alcohol problems on rates of adolescent psychiatric disorders. *Addiction, 89,* 1277–1286.

Lytton, H. (1990). Child and parent effects in boys' conduct disorder: A reinterpretation. *Developmental Psychology, 26,* 683–697.

McConaughy, S. H., & Achenbach, T. M. (1994). Comorbidity of empirically based syndromes in matched general population and clinical samples. *Journal of Child Psychology and Psychiatry, 35,* 1141–1157.

McDermott, P. A. (1993). National standardization of uniform multisituational measures of child and adolescent behavior pathology. *Psychological Assessment, 5,* 413–424.

McDermott, P. A. (1996). A nationwide study of developmental and gender prevalence for psychopathology in childhood and adolescence. *Journal of Abnormal Child Psychology, 24,* 53–66.

McGee, R., Silva, P. A., & Williams, S. (1984). Behaviour problems in a population of seven-year-old children: Prevalence, stability, and types of disorder. *Journal of Child Psychology and Psychiatry, 25,* 251–259.

McGee, R., Williams, S., Bradshaw, J., Chapel, J. L., Robins, A., & Silva, P. A. (1985). The Rutter scale for completion by teachers: Factor structure and relationships with cognitive abilities and family adversity for a sample of New Zealand children. *Journal of Child Psychology and Psychiatry, 26,* 727–739.

McGee, R., Feehan, M., Williams, S., Partridge, F., Silva, P. A., & Kelly, J. (1990). DSM-III disorders in a large sample of adolescents. *Journal of the American Academy of Child and Adolescent Psychiatry, 29,* 611–619.

Michael, R. T., Gagnon, J. H., Laumann, E. O., & Kolata, G. (1994). *Sex in America.* Boston: Little, Brown.

Najman, J. M., Behrens, B. C., Andersen, M., Bor, W., O'Callaghan, M., & Williams, G. M. (1997). Impact of family type and family quality on child behavior problems: A longitudinal study. *Journal of the American Academy of Child and Adolescent Psychiatry, 36,* 1357–1365.

National Center for Health Statistics. (1967). Plan, operation, and response results of a program of children's examinations. *Vital and Health Statistics* (PHS Publication No. 1000). Washington, DC: U.S. Government Printing Office.

Nottleman, E. D., & Jensen, P. S. (1995). Comorbidity of disorders in children and adolescents: Developmental perspectives. In T. H. Ollendick & R. J. Prinz (Eds.), *Advances in clinical child psychology* (Vol. 17, pp. 109–155). New York: Plenum.

Offord, D. R. (1995). Child psychiatric epidemiology: Current status and future prospects. *Canadian Journal of Psychiatry, 40,* 284–288.

Offord, D. R., Alder, R. J., & Boyle, M. H. (1986). Prevalence and sociodemographic correlates of conduct disorder. *American Journal of Social Psychiatry, 6,* 272–278.

Offord, D. R., Boyle, M. H., Szatmari, P., Rae-Grant, N., Links, P. S., Cadman, D. T., Byles, J. A., Crawford, J. W., Blum, H. M., Byrne, C., Thomas, H., & Woodward, C. A. (1987). Ontario Child Health Study: II. Six-month prevalence of disorder and rates of service utilization. *Archives of General Psychiatry, 44,* 832–836.

Offord, D. R., Boyle, M. H., & Racine, Y. (1989). Ontario Child Health Study: Correlates of disorder. *Journal of the American Academy of Child and Adolescent Psychiatry, 28,* 856–860.

Offord, D. R., Boyle, M. H., Fleming, J. E., Blum, H. M., & Grant, N. R. (1989). Ontario Child Health Study: Summary of selected results. *Canadian Journal of Psychiatry, 34,* 483–491.

Offord, D. R., Boyle, M. H., & Racine, Y. A. (1991). The epidemiology of antisocial behavior in childhood and adolescence. In D. J. Pepler & K. H. Rubin (Eds.), *The development and treatment of childhood aggression* (pp. 31–54). Hillsdale, NJ: Erlbaum.

Offord, D. R., Boyle, M. H., Racine, Y., Szatmari, P., Fleming, J. E., Sanford, M., & Lipman, E. L. (1996). Integrating assessment data from multiple informants. *Journal of the American Academy of Child and Adolescent Psychiatry, 35,* 1078–1085.

Osborn, A. F., Butler, N. R., & Morris, A. C. (1984). *The social life of Britain's five-year-olds: A report of the Child Health and Education Study.* London: Routledge & Kegan Paul.

Patterson, G. R., Reid, J. B., & Dishion, T. J. (1992). *Antisocial boys.* Eugene, OR: Castalia.

Pedersen, W., & Wichstrøm, L. (1995). Patterns of delinquency in Norwegian adolescents. *British Journal of Criminology, 35,* 543–562.

Pringle, M. L. K., Butler, N. R., & Davie, R. (1966). *11,000 seven-year-olds: First report of the National Child Development Study.* London: Longman.

Reinherz, H. Z., Fowler, P. C., Farkas, M. S., Raymundo, C. M., O'Regan, M., & Park, R. M. (1984). An epidemiological study of the behavior problems of young children. In S. A. Mednick, M. Harway, & K. M. Finello (Eds.), *Handbook of longitudinal research: Volume 1. Birth and childhood cohorts* (pp. 251–266). New York: Praeger.

Roberts, J., & Baird, J. T. (1972). Behavior patterns of children in school. *Vital and Health Statistics* (DHEW Publication No. HSM 72-1042). Washington, DC: U.S. Government Printing Office.

Rutter, M. (1965). Classification and categorization in child psychiatry. *Journal of Child Psychology and Psychiatry, 6,* 71–83.

Rutter, M. (1981). Epidemiological/longitudinal strategies and causal research in child psychiatry. *Journal of the American Academy of Child and Adolescent Psychiatry, 20,* 513–544.

Rutter, M. (1988). Epidemiological approaches to developmental psychopathology. *Archives of General Psychiatry, 45,* 486–495.

Rutter, M., Tizard, J., & Whitmore, K. (1970). *Education, health, and behaviour.* London: Longman.

Rutter, M., Cox, A., Tupling, C., Berger, M., & Yule, W. (1975). Attainment and adjustment in two geographical areas: I. The prevalence of psychiatric disorder. *British Journal of Psychiatry, 126,* 493–509.

Sampson, R. J., Raudenbush, S. W., & Earls, F. (1997). Neighborhoods and violent crime: A multilevel study of collective efficacy. *Science, 277,* 918–924.

Scott, K. G., Shaw, K. H., & Urbano, J. C. (1994). Developmental epidemiology. In S. L. Friedman & H. C. Haywood (Eds.), *Developmental follow-up: Concepts, domains, and methods* (pp. 351–374). San Diego: Academic Press.

Shaffer, D., Fisher, P., Dulcan, M. K., Davies, M., Piacentini, J., Schwab-Stone, M. E., Lahey, B. B., Bourdon, K., Jensen, P. S., Bird, H. R., Canino, G., & Regier, D. A. (1996). The NIMH Diagnostic Interview Schedule for Children Version 2.3 (DISC-2.3): Description, acceptability, prevalence rates, and performance in the MECA study. *Journal of the American Academy of Child and Adolescent Psychiatry, 35,* 865–877.

Silva, P. A. (1990). The Dunedin Multidisciplinary Health and Development Study: A 15 year longitudinal study. *Paediatric and Perinatal Epidemiology, 4,* 76–107.

Silva, P. A., McGee, R., Thomas, J., & Williams, S. (1982). A descriptive study of socio-economic status and child development in Dunedin five year olds. *New Zealand Journal of Educational Studies, 17,* 21–32.

Sroufe, L. A., & Rutter, M. (1984). The domain of developmental psychopathology. *Child Development, 55,* 17–29.

Stanger, C., McConaughy, S. H., & Achenbach, T. M. (1992). Three-year course of behavioral-emotional problems in a national sample of 4- to 16-year-olds: II. Predictors of syndromes. *Journal of the American Academy of Child and Adolescent Psychiatry, 31,* 941–950.

Szatmari, P., Boyle, M. H., & Offord, D. R. (1989). ADDH and conduct disorder: Degree of diagnostic overlap and differences among correlates. *Journal of the American Academy of Child and Adolescent Psychiatry, 28,* 865–872.

Szatmari, P., Offord, D. R., & Boyle, M. H. (1989). Ontario Child Health Study: Prevalence of attention deficit disorder with hyperactivity. *Journal of Child Psychiatry and Psychology, 30,* 219–230.

Trites, R. L., Dugas, E., Lynch, G., & Ferguson, B. (1979). Prevalence of hyperactivity. *Journal of Pediatric Psychology, 4,* 179–188.

U.S. population estimates by age, sex, race, and Hispanic origin: 1980 to 1996 (with extension to January 1, 1997) [machine-readable data files]. (1997). Washington, DC: U.S. Bureau of the Census.

Velez, C. M., Johnson, J., & Cohen, P. (1989). A longitudinal analysis of selected risk factors for childhood psychopathology. *Journal of the American Academy of Child and Adolescent Psychiatry, 28,* 861–864.

Verhulst, F. C., van der Ende, J., Ferdinand, R. F., & Kasius, M. C. (1997). The prevalence of DSM-III-R diagnoses in a national sample of Dutch adolescents. *Archives of General Psychiatry, 54,* 329–336.

Vikan, A. (1985). Psychiatric epidemiology in a sample of 1510 ten-year-old children. *Journal of Child Psychology and Psychiatry, 26,* 55–75.

Wadsworth, J., Burnell, I., Taylor, B., & Butler, N. (1985). The influence of family type on children's behaviour and development at five years. *Journal of Child Psychology and Psychiatry, 26,* 245–254.

Wang, Y., Chong, M., Chou, W., & Yang, J. O. (1993). Prevalence of attention deficit hyperactivity disorder in primary school children in Taiwan. *Journal of the Formosan Medical Association, 92,* 133–138.

Warheit, G. J., Zimmerman, R. S., Khoury, E. L., Vega, W. A., & Gil, A. G. (1996). Disaster related stresses, depressive signs and symptoms, and suicidal ideation among a multi-racial/ethnic sample of adolescents: A longitudinal analysis. *Journal of Child Psychology and Psychiatry, 37,* 435–444.

Wichstrøm, L. Skogen, K., & Øia, T. (1996). Increased rate of conduct problems in urban areas: What is the mechanism? *Journal of the American Academy of Child and Adolescent Psychiatry, 35,* 471–479.

Williams, S., McGee, R., Anderson, J., & Silva, P. A. (1989). The structure and correlates of self-reported symptoms in 11-year-old children. *Journal of Abnormal Child Psychology, 17,* 55–71.

Wolraich, M. L., Hannah, J. N., Pinnock, T. Y., Baumgaertel, A., & Brown, J. (1996). Comparison of diagnostic criteria for attention-deficit hyperactivity disorder in a countywide sample. *Journal of the American Academy of Child and Adolescent Psychiatry, 35,* 319–324.

World Health Organization. (1977). *International classification of disease* (9th ed.). Geneva, Switzerland: Author.

World Health Organization. (1992). *International classification of disease* (10th ed.). Geneva, Switzerland: Author.

Zahner, G. E. P., Jacobs, J. H., Freeman, D. H., & Trainor, K. F. (1993). Rural–urban child psychopathology in a northeastern U.S. state: 1986–1989. *Journal of the American Academy of Child and Adolescent Psychiatry, 32,* 378–387.

Zarin, D. A., & Earls, F. (1993). Diagnostic decision making in psychiatry. *American Journal of Psychiatry, 150,* 197–206.

Zill, N. (1985). *Behavior Problem Scales developed from the 1981 Child Health Supplement to the National Health Interview Survey.* Washington, DC: Child Trends.

3

Assessment of the Disruptive Behavior Disorders

Dimensional and Categorical Approaches

SUSAN FRAUENGLASS and DONALD K. ROUTH

INTRODUCTION

Disruptive Behavior Disorders (DBD) are those most commonly referred by parents and teachers for professional help (Kazdin, Siegel, & Bass, 1990; Wells & Forehand, 1985) and also the most common mental health problems presented in pediatricians' offices.* The assessment, differential diagnosis, and treatment of DBD thus require careful consideration. The foundation for any such assessment includes the definition of the disorder and the specific criteria to be used in its diagnosis. Any child may display DBD to some degree at specific times or in certain settings, but in order to be consid-

ered clinically significant, they must exceed the range of normal for the child's age group in terms of frequency, pervasiveness, severity, and interference with the child's ability to function adaptively (see Chapter 1, this volume). At older ages, these DBD and maladaptive interactions tend to have greater chronicity and severity.

"Caseness" is usually approximated somewhat arbitrarily by the number of standard deviations from the mean of a normal distribution or by meeting the formal criteria of a categorical classification system (see Chapter 1, this volume). DBD have been divided into Attention-Deficit/Hyperactivity Disorder (ADHD), Oppositional Defiant Disorder (ODD), and Conduct Disorder (CD) by the *Diagnostic and Statistical Manual of Mental Disorders* (DSM-IV; American Psychiatric Association, 1994), with diagnostic criteria established for each category. The way DBD are assessed depends on one's preference for defining them as either dimensional or categorical constructs. It also depends on whether the assessment is for clinical or for research purposes. Further, the fact that both assessment and treatment cost money may affect the threshold used in identifying these disorders.

This chapter presents assessment procedures that use dimensional and categorical perspectives to direct treatment. We begin by

*We use the term *disruptive behavior disorder* (DBD) to include the behaviors associated with Conduct Disorder, Oppositional Defiant Disorder, and Attention-Deficit/ Hyperactivity Disorder, whether these are conceptualized categorically or dimensionally and whether or not a formal diagnosis is warranted. Other terms in the literature that are also subsumed by our term DBD are "externalizing," "acting-out," and "disruptive behavior problems."

SUSAN FRAUENGLASS • La Rabida Children's Hospital and Research Center, University of Chicago, Chicago, Illinois 60649.   DONALD K. ROUTH • Department of Psychology, University of Miami, Coral Gables, Florida 33124-0721.

Handbook of Disruptive Behavior Disorders, edited by Quay and Hogan. Kluwer Academic/Plenum Publishers, New York, 1999.

examining these two theoretical perspectives. Then we present a comprehensive approach to assessment, followed by a description of selected assessment procedures available.

DIMENSIONAL APPROACH

Attention problems, noncompliant behavior, and aggressive behavior form a set of correlated dimensions of DBD behavior. The dimensional view first of all distinguishes DBD from internalizing disorders such as depression, anxiety, and social withdrawal (Achenbach & Edelbrock, 1978; Quay, 1979). The problem behavior theory of Jessor and Jessor (1977) suggests that the constellations of DBD occur in part because they fulfill developmental needs, such as peer bonding and independence from parents.

The dimensional view of DBD has several practical advantages. There are also research findings demonstrating correlated dimensions of behavior that change with age (McGee & Newcomb, 1992). Definitions of problem behavior syndromes are based on multivariate statistical analyses of standardized assessment data from large samples. Thus, the covariance structure of these checklist items is well established. The dimensional approach readily accepts adjustments for developmental levels. The youngest children studied seem to present a general group of problem behaviors not yet meriting the label of "disorder." These may resolve with age or continue as a clinically significant failure to develop self-regulation. Thus, the DSM-IV (American Psychiatric Association, 1994) criteria may overdiagnose preschool children, for whom a garden variety sample of disruptive behaviors is common (Campbell, 1990).

The pattern of responses describing a child's behavior corresponds to a position within a distribution, the mean of which is defined by reference to groups of children the same age and gender. From this perspective, the dimensional approach provides a clinically relevant means of interpreting the frequency, type, and intensity of DBD with respect to developmental changes. Dimensional evaluations are easily linked to treatment, since children can be allocated to interventions tailored to their particular profile. Children whose DBD interfere with their development and social interactions may be identified for treatment, even though they may not meet a categorical, criteria-based clinical diagnosis.

Unfortunately, this clinical flexibility has not yet led to a consensus as to what cutoff point marks a clinically significant level of DBD, whether that be 1, 1.5, or 2 standard deviations from the mean. Particular normative distributions must be carefully constructed because of differing environmental influences on development. The question as to what defines a "normal" population raises numerous issues. If an elevated level of DBD is characteristic of children in high-risk, stressful environments, is it therefore appropriate to define their clinical levels relative to their own population? Rather than reducing services by such a comparison, a definition of the prevalence of DBD relative to general norms is more appropriate to describe the problems of high-risk children. The identified prevalence could then highlight a community in crisis and intensify the services provided.

CATEGORICAL APPROACH

The absolute determination of the presence or absence of a disorder is more characteristic of the categorical approach. As noted earlier, numerous studies have identified the three specific disorders of ADHD, ODD, and CD. The characteristics and subtypes of these disorders are discussed in detail in Chapter 1, this volume.

The categorical approach has diagnostic utility for both clinical and research purposes. Clinically, meeting diagnostic criteria can be a prerequisite for receiving services, such as specialized school placement, or having treatment costs covered by insurance or managed care providers. The categorical approach incorporates an absolute criterion level to determine the presence of a disorder with the requirement that these criteria be applied relative to what is age appropriate, and that the behaviors are sufficiently distressing to self or others as to impair the child's ability to function adaptively. Impairment is necessary for the diagnosis to be made. These considerations suggest a "harmful dysfunction" or defective cognitive mechanism (Wakefield, 1992) corresponding to a specific intervention, similar to the medical model of diagnosis and treatment. Once a child is diagnosed with a behavior disorder in this categorical manner, treatment effects can be monitored with respect to reduced distress and impairment in the child's functioning (e.g., improved grades at school) and increasingly appropriate conduct.

Standardized diagnostic criteria (or dimensional measures) are essential for the dissemination of meaningful research information. Categorical definitions of dysfunction enable comparisons and synthesis of findings across studies. The initial diagnostic classification creates a comparison point for longitudinal studies of a disorder with or without treatment. Norms for assessment instruments are developed for both clinical or general populations. These groups must be defined by criteria which can be agreed on and applied in a uniform manner to specific individuals. Thus the categorical approach is often considered essential to the very process of assessment. In addition, understanding specific disorders directs research into examination of the premorbid risk factors, which may aid in prevention.

Criticisms of the categorical approach have been advanced both generally and specifically regarding the DBD, however. The number of criteria necessary for diagnosis creates an abrupt ledge between clinical populations that may be somewhat arbitrary. The criteria and definition of the disorders overlap among the DBD (Hinshaw, Lahey, & Hart, 1993), leading to debate about the utility of the categorical distinctions rather than the dimensional spectrum approach (see also Chapter 1, this volume). The application of DSM-lV (American Psychiatric Association, 1994) diagnostic criteria requires that the behavior be developmentally inappropriate, but operational criteria and normative information for each developmental level often are not provided, and the same criteria are meant to apply to children and adolescents. The behavioral

symptoms of young children typically lack specificity. Thus, labeling behavior as disordered at an early age constrains the flexibility needed when behavior changes with age (Campbell, 1990). Also, there can be extensive within-group variation since the several criteria met by one child to invoke a diagnosis may not overlap at all with the symptoms presented by another child diagnosed with the same disorder (Kasdin, 1995). Further, there continues to be opposition to labeling children with a diagnosis of a mental disorder because the labeling itself may negatively affect the environment's reaction to the child, and the child's self-esteem.

OBSERVER AND CONTEXT

In both the dimensional and categorical definitions of DBD, there is a certain arbitrariness in the cutoff used for clinical significance, whether that is in meeting enough criteria to rule in the presence of a disorder, or in reaching a psychometrically significant level of deviance from the norm. Norms can be biased because they represent a particular population. Symptom criteria presume a medical model in which a disorder exists or does not exist, as indicated at times by the difference of a single symptom that may be developmentally inappropriate. The criteria have been defined by empirical data over countless observations of children's behavior, but the context for these observations and characteristics of the observers also play a role in assessing behavior. Beyond accepting the relativistic constraints of our clinical formulations for a particular culture, this is also a practical matter for each new assessment. Observers judge both children's behavior and the world in which they live. Whether they have adapted well or poorly, children are reacting to their social ecology and expressing their biological and psychological inheritance. A critical component of assessment is recognizing the importance of both the context of the behavior and the characteristics of the person reporting the behavior. For example, increased parent stress and dysfunction have been linked to rating the child as more deviant (Kazdin, 1995).

The influence of genetic, family, social-ecological, and peer factors in the development and maintenance of DBD are described in detail in subsequent chapters in this handbook.

In addition to data from parents, the assessment needs to include information from the teacher. Any such information reported is of necessity filtered through the teacher's perspective and experience in interactions with the child. Teachers are often the motivating source for referrals, either directly or by drawing the parents' attention to the severity of the DBD. Children rarely refer themselves for treatment, particularly for their DBD. Others in the environment may suffer more from the DBD than do the children who manifest them. Thus, some awareness of how the child's behavior affects the teacher is important in both clinical assessment and treatment planning, and in research, in order to detect the presence of source bias in the data.

The individual characteristics of any observer become filters to the information provided about the child and must be considered in the assessment process. What individual, family, or environmental factors may be influencing parents' reports? Why have the parents chosen this time to seek services, or, if the DBD are identified only in research sampling, why have the parents not chosen to seek assistance? The point is emphasized because the assessment of DBD relies so heavily on parent and teacher report that source bias is endemic to the process. However, the more severe the DBD, the less of an effect this source of error will generate. Clinically, understanding the systemic influences is critical both in comprehensive assessment and in evaluating viable resources to be involved in treatment with the child.

Standardized direct observations of behavior are the most empirical response to this view of how experiences and interactions influence assessment. Thus, trained clinicians or technicians may be used to observe the child. Clinicians often make such observations of the child in the clinic, but home and school visits are generally impractical except for research purposes.

The coding of behavioral observations can yield information relevant to both clinical and research activities. The purpose of assessment as a clinical or research activity can affect the way DBD are operationalized. Ecological validity in clinical assessment is important for diagnosis and treatment planning. The process is malleable to systemic influence. The referral question directs assessment toward testing a range of hypotheses, leading to case conceptualization based on various sources of information. On the other hand, research assessments seek to control for the effects of various systemic influences and typically apply the same assessment protocol to each child in an effort to obtain uniform information. The way a sample is selected may vary across studies, with differing degrees of attention paid to the identification of comorbid disorders (see Chapter 2, this volume). There is a need for a consistent definition and approach to assessment so that research findings are comparable between studies. The debate regarding categorical versus dimensional approaches notwithstanding, the DSM-IV (American Psychiatric Association, 1994) definitions of ODD, CD, and ADHD provide a working consensus for much research and clinical assessment. Whichever approach is followed, the challenge is to conduct sufficiently comprehensive, developmentally sensitive, and multisystemic assessments of the child's behavior.

OVERVIEW OF COMPREHENSIVE ASSESSMENT

The strategies discussed in this chapter can be used to carry out a systematic assessment that is appropriate to the age of the child. It can lead to either a categorical diagnosis or a dimensional description of the child's behavior. Diagnosis is only one portion of an assessment, which should integrate information from the multiple contexts in which a child's behavior occurs. In the clinical setting, assessment must suggest treatment and evaluate its effectiveness. In terms of research, assessment must yield ecologically valid, empirically sound data on which to base investigations.

It is an implicit assumption in working with young children that they often cannot describe their internal experience and history reliably. They cannot pinpoint critical experiences, or attribute their behavior to their feelings or to external influences in a clear cause-and-effect relationship. Nevertheless, all children communicate something about their internal difficulties through their observable behavior and interactions with their social environment. Most young children will present disruptive behaviors at some point. The classification of these as having clinical significance presumes that the behaviors no longer fulfill a useful developmental role. They have become sufficiently intense to impair the child's ability to meet further developmental goals including appropriate social interaction (Patterson, DeBaryshe, & Ramsey, 1989). Thus the assessment presumes a clear understanding of normal development and behavior for children and families.

The three phases of the comprehensive behavioral assessment approach presented in the following sections are (1) initial diagnostic assessment, (2) treatment planning, and (3) evaluation of treatment effectiveness (or at least of clinical status at follow-up). An overview of these three phases is presented first, followed by more detailed discussion.

The diagnostic portion of the assessment may begin with screening via broad-band behavioral checklists, informal clinical interviews, or background information forms. It may then move to more specific checklists or standardized interviews and testing to detect learning or cognitive difficulties. When feasible, assessment may also include other procedures, such as peer ratings or nominations or direct observations in multiple settings. Functional analysis using single-subject experimental procedures is a useful though sometimes impractical ideal in treatment planning. Parents can complete paper-and-pencil measures while the child is being evaluated. The diagnostic assessment may be concluded with a session to assess family interaction patterns.

In this age of managed care, both treatment planning and evaluation are often based only on brief, informal interviews with parent and child and include no psychoeducational testing or information from school personnel. Such an approach cannot be expected to lead to reliable diagnostic information or treatment evaluation. Though this practice is common, it is difficult to defend either clinically or scientifically. Consumers should perhaps take a lesson from the editors of peer-reviewed scholarly journals and refuse to accept such an inadequate substitute for a proper assessment. Research-based practice guidelines need to be developed in order to ensure that mental health providers make adequate assessment an ordinary part of their services.

A careful diagnostic assessment is essential to differentiate DBD from anxiety disorders, pervasive developmental disorders, posttraumatic stress following abuse experiences, reactive attachment disorders, and disturbed behavior associated with histories of neglect. The symptoms of each of these disorders can mimic those of DBD. Assessment also assumes that a medical evaluation has been completed to rule out vision or hearing problems, lead poisoning, or other health problems that may affect behavior.

The focus questions and targets for information obtained for the diagnostic assessment fit into four main groups:

1. What are the current DBD being displayed? Clarify the referral question. For whom are they most distressing? Where and when do they occur? Define them in each area of the child's life. Are they developmentally appropriate or inappropriate?
2. What happened prior to the current assessment that might be relevant to the child's DBD? Obtain the biopsychosocial history to chart the onset, course, and contributing risk factors. Note, however, that many details of retrospectively obtained histories may prove to be inaccurate when compared with prospective information.
3. What strengths and weaknesses does the child present that might account for or contribute to the DBD? Complete a psychoeducational assessment to detect any cognitive processing deficits or academic achievement problems. What other diagnoses might account for the DBD?

4. How has the child's behavior affected the social environment and vice versa? What systematic factors contribute to or maintain the DBD? Why has the child been referred, and by whom? Evaluate the reliability of referral and informant sources as reporters of the child's DBD.

Once a diagnostic assessment is completed, the information is integrated for treatment planning. Two main issues are the focus of the comprehensive behavioral assessment at this stage: (1) What are the resources for intervention with the child and family? Which treatment approach is indicated, given the multisystemic profile? In which areas will intervention be necessary to support behavioral change in the child? (2) What is the child's developmental level in comparison with normative information? Where has development been delayed?

Finally, treatment effectiveness is assessed by readministering selected measures relevant to the areas in which intervention was conducted. The primary indicator of treatment effectiveness (or at least of relevant change) is decreased impairment due to the DBD. Improvements in the child's school performance, family functioning, and parenting stress are also common markers.

Initial Diagnostic Assessment

Assessment of Behavior

The core of comprehensive behavioral assessment is measuring the specific disruptive behaviors as they are currently presented by the child in various settings, either through independent actions, or during interactions with others. To establish test–retest reliability, the behaviors ideally should be measured multiple times in multiple settings. Since direct observations of this type are impractical for most clinical assessments, multiple informants provide information through interview, checklist measures, or both. A structured interview provides the most direct information regarding current symptoms for a categorical diagnosis using the DSM-IV (American Psychiatric Association, 1994) criteria. The structured format

requires strict adherence, so when a standardized interview measure is used for clinical purposes, background information must be obtained separately. For most clinical settings, completing both standardized and clinical or semistructured interviews is impractical, so the latter are typically used.

Information on previous DBD is collected to determine onset, course, and predisposing factors for the child's DBD. Whether current or past, each of the DBD is assessed along the following dimensions: (1) frequency and intensity of the behavior for a determination of clinical impairment (Kazdin, 1995), (2) repetitiveness and chronicity to indicate the onset and stability over time, and (3) developmental inappropriateness.

DBD may be acute or chronic. An abrupt onset of DBD at any age, without a pattern of prior difficulties, excludes a diagnosis of ADHD. Different precipitants may lead to ODD or CD symptoms, but their identification can point treatment in very different directions. The range of profiles may include maladjustment to stressful life events; reactions to a trauma such as sexual abuse or domestic violence; disrupted attachment related to factors such as neglect, abuse, multiple foster placements, maternal depression, or parental substance abuse; or difficulties transitioning from one developmental level to the next if required to do so prior to readiness. Thus information regarding onset, duration, and identifiable difficulties across developmental levels is requisite to differential diagnosis given the range of factors that may underlie the presentation of DBD.

The determination of developmental inappropriateness relies on an understanding of both the normal developmental patterns and the patterns presented in youth with DBD. As has been noted, young children tend to present nonspecific disruptive behavior that can lead to more DBD over the course of development.

Once the severity, course, and developmental inappropriateness of the DBD have been evaluated, the assessment considers the interaction between the child's behavior and the environment. The goal is to evaluate the level of impairment in adaptive functioning at home, in school, and with peers. The assessment of adaptive functioning addresses several diagnostic concerns. First, it delivers evidence of consistency in the DBD across settings, thus reducing the likelihood of missing system-specific etiological factors. Second, because multiple settings are assessed, multiple informants are likely to be used, thus reducing the likelihood of source bias. Personal perspectives and the interpersonal influence of the child's relationship to the informant must still be considered. There may be little correlation between the different reports of the child's behavior (Achenbach, McConaughy, & Howell, 1987). To assess the child's adaptive functioning with peers, direct reports through peer rating or nomination measures are ideal, but are impractical for clinical applications. Thus, parent, teacher, or self-reports of peer relationships are typically utilized instead.

History and Predisposing Risk Factors

Extensive research has been conducted to identify some of the predisposing risk factors for the DBD. Taking a careful history is necessary to utilize such research findings for differential diagnosis. Often a combination of clinical interview and forms for demographic information, developmental milestones, and medical history information is used. Any information presented on the intake paperwork should be queried directly to clarify or discuss it further.

Evaluation of predisposing risk factors provides both a general picture of high risk for negative developmental outcomes and a specific profile of risk factors for a particular type of psychopathology. These risk factors are considered in detail in Chapters 9, 18, and 19 (this volume). Also worth consideration is the developmental status of the family as a whole, including the family composition and the child's place in the family system. For example, when the primary caregiver is a grandparent, the resources for managing a problem behavior child may be diminished due to the large developmental gap, or the caregiver may be viewing developmentally normal behaviors as excessive and problematic.

Collateral Assessment for Differential Diagnosis

The next portion of the initial assessment is a basic psychoeducational assessment to determine the child's cognitive ability, language skills, perceptual processing, and motor skills development. For school age and older children, achievement is tested to determine whether a comorbid learning disability exists and what the areas of strength and weakness are as risk factors or targets for intervention. While this basic assessment is crucial for an accurate, informed diagnosis, in practice, resource issues and theoretical orientation often preclude psychoeducational testing. Its importance needs to be stressed, however, since DBD can arise from or be exacerbated by numerous cognitive factors. For example, a child with language difficulties might appear noncompliant when requests have not been understood, initiating a coercive interaction pattern with parents and teachers. Both low and high cognitive ability may contribute to DBD. A child with above average or gifted intellectual ability might display DBD because of boredom. The public schools are legally obliged to carry out such evaluations for children with suspected disabilities, and thus it may be possible to rely on school evaluations for part or all of this information. Liaison with the school system is important in any case, in terms of intervention as well as assessment.

Differential diagnosis of ADHD, ODD, or CD versus other types of psychopathology with similar symptoms may require further assessment of the child's emotional functioning and personality by interview or other methods. Children who are extremely anxious or depressed, who have experienced abuse or trauma, or who have a pervasive developmental disorder may present with behavior problems, poor attention and concentration, and irritability and anger. Further, children with ADHD, ODD, or CD often experience comorbid internalizing symptoms (see Chapter 2, this volume). Determining the cause-and-effect relationship between DBD and other difficulties may not be feasible; a differential or comorbid diagnosis is the goal to direct treatment appropriately.

Mood disorders, anxiety disorders, adjustment disorders, behavior problems associated with mental retardation, pervasive developmental disorders (learning and communication disorders), and Tourette's disorder should all be considered as possible diagnoses to be ruled out in the comprehensive behavioral assessment (Breen & Altepeter, 1990).

Contextual Assessment

DBD are multidetermined with a high probability of coexisting family and peer problems (Mandel, 1997). Thus, a comprehensive behavioral assessment must also consider the context in which the child's behavior occurs. This step in the diagnostic assessment phase has three main purposes: (1) to determine the interactive influences between systemic factors and the DBD, (2) to evaluate the reliability of the data provided by the referral source and other informants, and (3) to identify resources and readiness for intervention.

Various systemic conditions may also operate to sustain or exacerbate a child's DBD. The relationship is not unidirectional, however. The child's DBD clearly affect the environment and either give rise to or maintain problems such as parenting stress (Anastopoulos, Guevremont, Shelton, & DuPaul, 1992; Mash & Johnston, 1990), parent conflict about child rearing (Dadds & Powell, 1991; Jouriles *et al.*, 1991), and coercive parenting practices (Mann & MacKenzie, 1996). The primary contextual areas to be evaluated in terms of sustaining or exacerbating risk are parenting, family environment, peer interactions, and neighborhood risk. Aspects of parenting that are associated with DBD are discussed in Chapters 6, 15, and 19, this volume.

Given the amount of assessment information collected from various informants, determining the reliability of those sources is essential for a valid diagnosis. A parent profile of personal adjustment, psychological well-being, and medical history is developed to detect areas of bias in reporting child behavior in an overly negative or positive light. Also, clarification of the referral source sheds light on the parents' perceptions of the problem and motivation for treatment. Since the DBD have likely been occurring for some time, it is also useful to ask why the child was referred at this time. Teachers have often brought the problem to the parents' attention. Teacher report is also subject to bias; however, assessing the teacher's reliability as an informant is typically not done through standardized assessment measures, but through qualitative evaluation during a brief teacher interview, often over the telephone. Another way to do this is to obtain ratings from more than one of a child's teachers, if possible.

Finally, throughout the assessment of contextual factors, the examiner must be considering what systemic resources exist to support intervention. The parent profile, evaluation of family functioning, and teacher interview all provide information about the capacity of people to participate in the child's treatment, such as assimilating and utilizing parenting skills training, attending therapy sessions to modify interaction patterns, or enforcing a consistent behavior management program. Parents of children with DBD may have immature, impulsive, inattentive, depressed, hostile, or rejecting dispositions themselves (Frick *et al.*, 1992; Patterson, 1982); thus, their willingness to participate in treatment may be diminished. Often more information about their readiness to join in treatment efforts is provided during the first feedback session.

Conceptualization and Treatment Planning

Case conceptualization is a process which begins at the point of referral and continues throughout the diagnostic assessment phase. A working diagnosis and a list of possible disorders to be ruled out are used to guide the assessment process efficiently. Yet the potential exists that early conceptualizations preclude investigation of alternative explanations and increase the risk for misdiagnosis. Thus, case formulation should be viewed as a distinct activity in which all the assessment data are reviewed objectively in a comprehensive format. Table 1 presents the information that should be available about the child, compiled into an overview format. Using

TABLE 1.   Case Conceptualization Summary Form

I. Child profile
   Development levels
      Cognitive
      Emotional
      Physical
   Cognitive ability and achievement
      Intellectual level
      Strengths/weaknesses
      School performance
   Predisposing risk factors
      Prenatal/perinatal
      Medical history
      Vision and hearing
      Family history
         Maternal age
         Medical
         Psychopathology
      Socioeconomic status
      Abuse/neglect/trauma history
   Contextual risk factors
      Family composition
      Parent–Child interactions
      Parenting style/discipline
      Family interactions
      Marital satisfaction
      Peer interactions
      Child–Teacher interactions
II. Behavioral presentations
   Positive symptoms
      Frequency
      Intensity
      Duration
   Onset
   Course
   Level of impairment
III. Diagnostic impression

the child profile data and behavioral presentation summary, a diagnosis is made. Each area listed may contribute to, exacerbate, or maintain the DBD. Thus, each is a possible target for intervention. The case summary also provides a reference point for follow-up in the ongoing assessment process.

Treatment planning involves identifying the areas to be targeted for change and establishing specific, realistic goals for change in a given period. How areas of strength and competency can support improvements should be specified. Not only the child but also contextual factors may be targets for interventions, particularly those situational factors that exacerbate or maintain the behavior problems. As a treatment plan is formulated, consideration must be given to the contextual resources to support change. The more systemic involvement mobilized, the greater the likelihood of sustaining behavioral change, particularly in targeting coercive parent–child interaction patterns. All of the contextual information gathered comes into play in developing the treatment plan. Treatments and the resources necessary to implement them are discussed in Chapters 10, 11, 20, 21, 22, and 23 (this volume), as are evaluation criteria or methods.

Some Practical Implications

Current behavioral assessment procedures are becoming increasingly constrained by demands for brevity and cost-effectiveness. Clinicians and researchers must define and empirically justify the standards for appropriate assessment. Children are referred for mental health services because their symptoms are considered by someone to be developmentally inappropriate and sufficiently extreme to be interfering with their social or school functioning. A brief inquiry into the types of behaviors exhibited is sufficient to suggest that the child may fit within the spectrum of DBD. Next, a parent rating scale or standardized interview, a teacher checklist, and informal observations of the child provide sufficient information to make a diagnosis of a particular one of the DBD. This cursory approach to assessment may overlook certain comorbid problems or etiological factors, however, which would aim treatment in different directions or be greatly informative for research purposes.

A behavior management or pharmacological intervention for a child diagnosed with one of the DBD frequently provides symptom relief that is rewarding to the parents and teacher. But if the child shows irritability, acting out, and difficulty concentrating, representing Posttraumatic Stress Disorder (PTSD) following undisclosed sexual abuse, the effectiveness of such treatments may be only palliative in the short term. Certain core difficulties may thus be left unaddressed so that they become internalized. Depression and anxiety in children may also present as irritability, distractibility, short attention span, academic difficulties, and DBD manifested in a variety of ways, such as substance abuse. Learning disabilities or speech and language disorders can also lead to numerous problems, and not only in the school setting, because children may have difficulty understanding and following instructions at home also, making them appear oppositional. Further, learning disabled children often respond negatively to parental pressure to improve their academic performance and school behavior.

Although each of these examples seems self-evident given sufficient evaluation of the child and his or her interactive influences, today's clinician is necessarily aware of economic pressures to conduct brief assessments. This can result in diagnosis on the basis of overt presenting symptoms only rather than comprehensive assessment and etiological understanding on which to base treatment. This is not to say that detecting a learning disability, an internalizing disorder, or a traumatic history precludes diagnosis of DBD or necessarily provides answers about causes. Rather, the ongoing assessment process serves to focus treatment efforts and inform research. The assessment functions to deliver a diagnosis or establish inclusion and exclusion criteria; it also imparts findings relevant to service delivery and research. The assessment process should be viewed as ongoing, with new hypotheses and conceptualizations being generated as the child progresses developmentally and as the child's interactions with the social environment are further revealed over the course of treatment.

Clinically, the diagnostic assessment is geared toward treatment planning. Over the course of time as behavior management, parent training, or other intervention is started, subsequent assessments provide comparison points for evaluating treatment effectiveness or modifying the case conceptualization as necessary. The effects of pharmacologic intervention can also be informative, but comorbid difficulties in children with ADHD may require ongoing

evaluation. Over the course of treatment, the child may become more able to express feelings and to provide reliable self-reports.

Differential diagnosis through an ongoing assessment process is more problematic for research work, where inclusion and exclusion criteria must be met based on the initial assessment. Flexible, extended diagnostic assessments are usually impractical. However, such findings may be important in understanding changes over time or interpreting contradictory findings in longitudinal studies.

Particular Assessment Procedures

The following section provides an overview of selected assessment procedures available for use in a comprehensive assessment of DBD in children. Table 2 indicates the application of the various approaches to match the assessment approach just discussed. The measures listed in the following section are primarily for clinical purposes and comprise the core of a comprehensive integrated behavioral assessment approach. Further, when particular areas of difficulty are identified as primary targets of intervention, additional assessment may be required using more specific measures than those reviewed here to clarify the contributing factors.

Interviews

The most current standardized interview for the assessment of child and adolescent psychopathology is the Diagnostic Interview Schedule for Children, which has a parent version (DISC-P) and a child version (DISC-C) (Fisher et al., 1991; Schwab-Stone et al., 1993; Shaffer et al., 1993). These have the advantage of being keyed directly to the DSM and permit one to make an accurate diagnosis of ODD, CD, or ADHD. These interviews have received extensive field testing and are presently the ones most commonly used to make these diagnoses in funded research projects. They have the disadvantage that they are lengthy and somewhat cumbersome. In addition, the question of the construct validity of the categories of descriptive psychopathology is perennial.

TABLE 2.   Comprehensive Behavioral Assessment Goals and Procedures

Assessment goal	Procedure	
Measure the current behaviors across settings using multiple informants	Ratings:	Parent and teacher checklists
		Child self-report
		Peer nomination
	Interviews:	Parent
		Child
	Observations:	Child behavior
		Family interaction
		Peer interaction
Obtain biopsychosocial history and information about predisposing risk factors	Interview:	Parent
	Records:	Medical
		Psychological
		School
		Court and police
		Child protective services
Assess intellectual factors to determine cognitive strengths and weaknesses for differential or comorbid diagnosis, and to measure attention. impulsivity, distractibility, etc.	Psychoeducational assessment battery, including standardized intellectual, achievement, and executive processing measures	
Assess personality and emotional factors for differential diagnosis of other psychopathology (such as PDD, anxiety, depression, etc.)	Ratings:	Parent and teacher checklists
		Child self-report
	Interviews:	Parent
		Child
	Diagnostic play sessions with child	
Evaluate systemic factors to determine their influence on child's behavior, possible source bias in interview and checklist data, and availability of resources for treatment	Interviews:	Parent
		Child
	Other procedures:	Family problem solving
		Interaction
		Parent psychopathology measures
		Parenting stress measures
		Marital assessment measures
		Social support measures

Also, test–retest attenuation effects have been identified in structured diagnostic interviews, with fewer symptoms reported and thus significantly fewer diagnoses made in repeated interviews of children, particularly for those 6 to 9 years old (Edelbrock, Costello, Dulcan, Conover, & Kala, 1986). Reliability appears best for youth 11 years and older (Schwab-Stone et al., 1993; Shaffer et al., 1993). The time it takes to give these full interviews may not be reimbursed under managed care plans.

The Diagnostic Interview for Children and Adolescents (DICA; Boyle et al., 1993; Herjanic & Reich, 1982; Reich & Welner, 1988) is a structured interview that provides categorical information on 185 symptoms reflecting the DSM-IV (American Psychiatric Association, 1994) diagnostic criteria. In addition, the frequency, intensity, onset, and duration of symptoms are compiled into six areas (Relationship Problems, School Behavior, School Learning, Neurotic Symptoms, Somatic Symptoms, and Psychotic Symptoms). Versions are provided for parent and child (for children 6–12 years old) and for adolescents (13–17 years old).

Parent, Teacher, and Self-Report Checklists

Several broad-band checklists are available for general screening of behavior problems and for identifying comorbidity. They have the advantage of being brief, inexpensive, and easily administered. Parent and teacher measures can be sent before the first appointment for a more informed intake interview. Also, they can be used to measure treatment effects. As with any informant-based measure, there can be source bias. It is advisable to assess the informant's motivation to evaluate the child's behavior unduly positively or negatively. For the most part these measures are dimensional ones and are not keyed to the DSM. Thus, they do not lend themselves to making categorical diagnoses. In fact, the dimensions assessed are generally somewhat incommensurable with categories used by the DSM, even though they cover the same broad territory. The items and the formats for numerically rating them do not match precisely the criteria of any of the DSMs (see Chapter 1, this volume).

The widely used Child Behavior Checklist (CBCL; Achenbach & Edelbrock, 1983) is a parent-completed checklist that covers a wide range of children's behavior problems (118 items) and social competencies in and out of the home (20 items). Parents are asked to rate their child on each behavior as "not true" (0), "somewhat or sometimes true" (1), or "very true" (2). The responses yield scores on eight separate factors (Withdrawn, Somatic Complaints, Anxious/Depressed, Social Problems, Thought Problems, Attention Problems, Delinquent Behavior, Aggressive Behavior) and two composite factors for Internalizing and Externalizing behavior, as well as Total Problem Behaviors. The Internalizing factor represents overcontrolled, inhibited behaviors characterized as anxious or withdrawn. The Externalizing factor corresponds to undercontrolled, impulsive, and disruptive behaviors. Norms are provided for children aged 4–18 years, stratified by gender and age (4–11 years and 12–18 years). The CBCL is written at the fifth-grade reading level and requires approximately 20 min to complete. A shorter version is also available for 2- to 3-year-old children and a parallel one for young adults.

The psychometric properties of the CBCL have been demonstrated in many studies in the United States and abroad; these properties include internal consistency, test–retest reliabil-

ity, and criterion-related validity (clinic-referred children vs. a general community sample). The dimensions are based on extensive factor-analytic research. In addition, the CBCL is sensitive to the effects of treatments such as parent training, child behavior management, and pharmacological interventions. Moderate interrater reliability has been reported between parents, although several studies have indicated significant discrepancies between maternal and paternal ratings of child behavior.

The Teacher Report Form (TRF; Achenbach & Edelbrock, 1986) is a teacher-completed checklist that covers a wide range of children's behavior problems (118 items) and social competencies in the school setting (20 items). Teachers are asked to rate the child on each behavior as "not true" (0), "somewhat or sometimes true" (1), or "very true" (2). The responses yield scores on the same eight factors and two composite factors (plus Total Deviant Behavior) obtained from the parent-completed CBCL. Norms are provided for children ages 4–18, stratified by gender and age (4–11 years and 12–18 years). The TRF requires approximately 20 min to complete.

The established psychometric properties of the TRF include internal consistency, test–retest reliability, and criterion-related validity (clinic-referred vs. community samples). As with the CBCL, the dimensions emerged from extensive factor-analytic research. Interrater reliability has been reported between teachers, with correlation coefficients ranging from .30 to .84 and a median of .57.

The Youth Self Report (YSR; Achenbach & Edelbrock, 1987) is a 103-item adolescent-completed measure that assesses problem behaviors and social adjustment in a format similar to those for parent- and teacher-completed measures. Youths 11 to 18 years old are asked to rate whether each item is "not true" (0), "somewhat or sometimes true" (1), or "very true" (2) of their own behavior. The responses yield scores on the same factors obtained from the CBCL and the TRF and the composite factors of Internalizing and Externalizing, plus Total Deviant Behavior. Norms are provided separately by gender and are based on a sample from the northeastern United States with an adequate distribution in terms of socioeconomic status and race. The YSR is written at a fifth-grade reading level and requires approximately 20 min to complete.

The test–retest reliability of the YSR differs by gender, with girls displaying greater stability coefficients. Criterion-related validity has been established for clinic-referred versus nonreferred samples. Significant but moderate correlations have been reported between youth and adult reports for similar factors from the CBCL and the TRF (mean .45 for girls and .41 for boys). The YSR remains the primary self-report checklist used in screening for general behavior problems and identifying comorbidity. It is brief, inexpensive, and easily administered.

It is possible to combine data from the three types of informants on the Achenbach and Edelbrock scales to generate eight Cross-Informants Syndromes (Withdrawn, Somatic Complaints, Anxious/Depressed, Social Problems, Thought Problems, Attention Problems, Delinquent Behavior, and Aggressive Behavior; Achenbach & McConaughy, 1997). The cross-informant syndromes combine the scores of the items that are common across all three informants, and those obtained from only two informants, but statistically loaded on a particular syndrome. The three profiles are laid out similarly for quick visual comparisons, and a cross-informant computer program is available for more systematic comparison of scores (J. Arnold & Jacobowitz, 1993).

The Revised Behavior Problem Checklist (RBPC; Quay & Peterson, 1987) measures a broad range of child behavior problems and can be completed by parents, teachers, or other adults who have extensive contact with the child. Eighty-nine items are rated as "not a problem" (0), "a mild problem" (1), or "a severe problem" (2). The responses yield six factors: Conduct Disorder, Socialized Aggression, Attention Problems–Immaturity, Anxiety-Withdrawal, Psychotic Behavior, and Motor Excess. Norms are provided for children 5–17 years of age in two age groups, stratified by gender. The RBPC requires approximately 20 min to complete.

The psychometric properties of the RBPC have been acceptably demonstrated, although the specificity of the normative sample demands caution in using the norms provided in the manual. For research use, it is advisable to develop local norms.

Several specific checklists are available for DBD, including the Conners checklists, Barkley Home and School Situations Questionnaire, and the Eyberg Child Behavior Inventory.

The Revised Conners' Parent Rating Scale (CPRS-R; Conners, Sitarenios, Parker, & Epstein, 1998) is a 57-item parent-completed measure for the assessment of Cognitive Problems, Oppositional behavior, Hyperactivity-Impulsivity, Anxious-Shy behaviors, Perfectionism, Social Problems, and Psychosomatic behaviors in children ages 3–17 years. Parents indicate whether the child displays each of a number of behaviors, with the severity of each of the behaviors ranging from "not at all true" (0), to "very much true" (3). Norms are provided with stratification for gender and age. The CRPS-R requires less than 20 min to complete.

Limited psychometric data are available for the new version of the CPRS-R. Coefficient alphas for the seven scales ranged from .75 to .94 for males and .75 to .93 for females. Six-week test–retest correlations ranged from .13 to .78, with all but one being higher than .40. Using a discriminant function, the scales correctly classified over 90% of samples of children with ADHD and non-ADHD controls correctly. The previous version of this parent rating scale showed sensitivity to behavioral and pharmacological treatment effects (e.g., Barkley, 1988; Pelham et al., 1988). Ullmann and Sleator (1985) noted that the previous version of the CPRS-R assessed conduct problems and parent–child conflict as well as ADHD.

The Conners Teacher Rating Scale–Revised (CTRS-R; Goyette, Conners, & Ulrich, 1978) is a 28-item teacher-completed measure for the assessment of ADHD in children ages 3–17. As is the case for the other Conners scales, its items are not precisely related to those of any of the DSMs for this disorder. Teachers indicate whether the child displays each of a series of disruptive behaviors, with the severity of each behavior ranging from "not at all" (0) to "very much" (3). The responses yield three factors: Conduct Problems, Hyperactive, and Inattention-Passivity. Norms are provided with stratification for gender and age. The CTRS-R requires approximately 10 min to complete.

The CTRS-R has demonstrated good internal consistency, test–retest reliability, and convergent validity for children with disruptive behavior disorders versus normal children. Sensitivity to treatment effects including stimulant medication and behavior therapy has often been demonstrated (e.g., Barkley, 1988; Pelham et al., 1988).

Three additional forms of the Conners Teacher Rating Scale are available: the original longer version of 39 items, which includes internalizing behaviors; the 10-item Abbreviated Symptom Questionnaire of items most often endorsed by teachers for hyperactive children; and the 10-item IOWA CTRS, which yields two factors for Hyperactivity and Aggression (with the latter better labeled as oppositional behavior). The longer version has demonstrated validity in distinguishing hyperactive children from controls and in monitoring treatment effects.

Conners and his colleagues (1997) have also recently developed a 64-item self-report measure for the assessment of adolescent psychopathology, the Conners/Wells Adolescent Self-Report of Symptoms (CASS). Factor analysis suggests that it measures six factors: family problems, emotional problems, conduct problems, cognitive problems, anger control problems, and hyperactivity. The coefficient alphas for these scales range from .83 to .92, and their median test–retest reliability is .86. The CASS has some criterion-related validity (a correct classification rate over 80%) in distinguishing subjects with ADHD from controls.

The Home Situations Questionnaire (HSQ; Barkley, 1981) is a parent-completed measure designed to assess the severity and types of disruptive behavior problems observed in the home setting. Parents rate each of 16 problem behaviors for presence and severity on a scale ranging from mild (1) to severe (9). The items are not keyed to DSM criteria. The responses yield two scores, for Number of Problems and

Mean Severity. Breen and Altepeter (1990) analyzed the normative data and obtained four factors: Custodial Transactions, Non-Family Transactions, Task-Performance Transactions, and Isolate Play. When compared to the School Situations Questionnaire, the HSQ establishes the situational variability of a child's problem behavior. Such situational similarities and differences are essential to know in diagnosing Disruptive Behavior Disorders.

The School Situations Questionnaire (SSQ; Barkley, 1981) is a teacher-completed measure designed to assess the severity and types of disruptive behavior problems observed in the school setting. Teachers indicate whether each of 16 problems occur and, if so, how severe they are on a scale from mild (1) to severe (9). The responses yield two scores, for Number of Problems and Mean Severity. When compared to the Home Situations Questionnaire, the SSQ establishes the situational variability in a child's problem behavior.

The Eyberg Child Behavior Inventory (ECBI; Eyberg, 1980; Eyberg & Ross, 1978; Robinson, Eyberg, & Ross, 1980) is a 36-item parent-completed measure that assesses oppositional behavior and conduct problems. The items are not specifically keyed to the criteria of any of the DSMs. Parents first respond (yes or no) whether each disruptive behavior item is a problem with the child. Then the frequency of each behavior is rated from never (1) to always (7). The yes–no responses are scored for a total Problem Scale, and the frequencies are scored for the Intensity Scale. The ECBI requires only 10 min to complete.

The psychometric properties of the scale indicate good internal consistency, test–retest reliability, and interrater reliability between parents. Social desirability responding has not been problematic with this scale. The ECBI distinguishes nonreferred children from clinic-referred children with conduct problems. However, the normative data provided are not adequate for general clinical use.

The ADHD Comprehensive Teacher Rating Scale (ACTeRS; Ullmann, Sleator, & Sprague, 1984, 1985, 1988) is a 24-item teacher-completed measure that assesses disruptive behavior problems in four factors, including Attention, Hyperactivity, Oppositional, and Social Skills. It is not keyed to criteria of any of the DSMs. Teachers rate the frequency of each behavior from "almost never" (1) to "almost always" (5). Norms are provided for children in kindergarten through fifth grade, with separate data for boys and girls, but not stratified by age. Good psychometric properties have been demonstrated, though concurrent validity data have not been reported. The primary advantage of the ACTeRS may be its brevity.

Self-report measures specific to DBD are less commonly available than parent- or teacher-report ones, because the symptoms are most easily identified by those who experience their effects and are often not identified as problems by the child displaying them. The Self-Report Delinquency Scale (Elliott, Dunford, & Huizinga, 1987) is a 47-item measure for 11- to 21-year-olds. It was developed as part of the National Youth Survey to assess the frequency with which delinquent behaviors occurred in the past year. The Children's Hostility Inventory devised by Kazdin and his colleagues (Kazdin, Rodgers, Colbus, & Siegel, 1987) is a 38-item instrument for 6- to 13-year-olds that measures aspects of hostility and aggression with true–false responses to each statement. Although both of these measures have been used primarily for research purposes, they can provide essential information for differential diagnosis of ODD and CD.

For clinical purposes, the child is more likely to report not the behaviors themselves but social consequences of the behaviors as "the problems" causing emotional distress. Self-report checklists are more useful for measuring symptoms of depression and anxiety and provide information regarding the child's level of unhappiness. The Children's Depression Inventory (CDI; Kovacs, 1981, 1985) and the Reynolds Adolescent Depression Scale (RADS; Reynolds, 1987) are the most commonly used self-report measures for depressive symptoms.

Behavioral Observations

Formal coding systems for direct observations have been developed, though primarily for research purposes. In clinical practice, behavioral observations are typically used to obtain qualitative information about the child's behavior in order to specify the content of the reported behaviors, clarify discrepancies in informant reports, and detect behaviors not reported on checklists or in interviews. Table 3 details a range of observations. The examiner also considers how the child enters a novel environment; how the child interacts with parents, other family members, peers, or other adults; how well the child self-regulates emotions and behavior; and how quickly the child recovers when distressed. Specific observations may suggest the need for referral to another discipline. For example, an atypical gait or inability to walk in a straight line might suggest organic involvement, particularly with any history of traumatic brain injury, and such observations would indicate the need for neurological or neuropsychological consultation.

Direct observation of the child's behavior can also provide quantitative information, using standardized rating systems. Use of an observational coding system has the advantage of consistency in measuring the same set of behaviors at multiple times, yielding reliable information for diagnosis and for evaluation of treatment effectiveness. Direct observation may be particularly necessary to reconcile discrepant or unreliable informant reports and clarify interactional processes of which participants may not be aware. Despite the wealth of data obtained, observational methods have had little use outside of research settings because they are time intensive, require travel to natural settings, or if done in the clinic require observation rooms and equipment.

Currently, one of the most straightforward, practical coding systems available for direct observation in the school is the Direct Observation Form (DOF; Achenbach, 1991). The group setting provides information about both the child's behavior and the behaviors of others who may be influencing the child. Observations over a 10-min period are scored on 96 problem items with ratings of 0 for nonoccurrence, 1 for slight or ambiguous occurrence, 2 for definite occurrence of mild to moderate

TABLE 3. Behavioral Observation Form

Behavioral Observations

Child's name
Date of birth
Test date
Examiner

A. Physical appearance/motor skills
    1. Size: Large   Average   Small
    2. Unusual features/physical handicaps:
    3. Gait: On tiptoes   On heels   On whole feet
              Able to walk in straight line for 30 feet+
              Yes   No
              Stairs: Single foot   Alternating feet
    4. Gross motor:
    5. Fine motor:
    6. Dominance: Hand: Right   Left
                  Foot: Right   Left
    7. Other:
B. Affective/emotional state
    1. Rapport with examiner
        a. Eye contact: Often   Sometimes   Never
        b. Response to praise:
    2. Mood: Active   Passive   Anxious   Tense
              Calm   Confident
    3. Affect: Appropriate   Heightened   Flat
    4. Behavioral control: Independent   Need for cues
    5. Compliance:
    6. Reaction to success:
    7. Reaction to failure:
    8. Tolerance for frustration:
    9. Social behavior: Agreeable   Hostile
                  Passive
   10. Other:
C. Level of activity and attention
    1. Activity: High   Moderate   Low
    2. Adjustment to test situation
        a. Interest level: High   Fair   Low
        b. Level of cooperation: Excellent   Fair   Poor
    3. Level of self-confidence
        Self-confident and assured
        Moderate self-confidence
        Lacks self-confidence
        Distrusts ability
        Unaware of errors
    4. Attention span
        Long periods of concentration
        Average
        Distractible: Visual   Auditory

5. Perseverative, self-stimulating, or other interfering behaviors
6. Other
D. Work skills
    1. Motivation: Strong   Moderate   Poor
    2. Problem solving strategies
        a. Trial and error   Imitation   Random
        b. Ability to recognize errors and self-correct:
            Yes   Sometimes   No
        c. Ability to learn from demonstration:
            Yes   Sometimes   No
    3. Degree of organization
        a. Methodical   Haphazard   Disorganized
        b. Anticipates next step: Yes   No
        c. Identifies causal relationships: Yes   No
        d. Classification skills: Yes   No
    4. Effort: Tries hard   Fair   Minimal effort
    5. Work behavior
        Eager to make good impression
        Alert
        Impulsive
        Erratic
        Timid
        Responds very slowly
        Careless
        Requires firmness
        Creative
        Playful
        Tries to please
        Inhibited
        Perfectionist
    6. Other
E. Communication skills
    1. Spontaneous   Responsive   Requires prompting
    2. Expressive skills Yes   Sometimes   No
        Intelligible verbal responses
        Fluent speech
        Uses one-word responses
        Uses sentences
        Uses echolalic speech
        Perseverative speech
        Absence of speech
    3. Receptive skills:
        Follows verbal directions
        Responds to gestures
    4. Other
Additional comments:

intensity or for less than 3 min, and up to 4 for a definite occurrence of severe intensity or 3 or more min duration. On-task behavior is recorded as yes–no at the end of each min. The scores yield clinical cutoffs for six syndromes: Withdrawn-Inattentive, Nervous-Obsessive, Depressed, Hyperactive, Attention Demanding, and Aggressive. T-scores and percentile scores are provided for Internalizing and Externalizing dimensions.

Impairment

The child's level of impairment must be established for a DSM-IV (American Psychiatric Association, 1994) diagnosis to be made. In doing this, one can follow the same procedure by which the cutting scores were established for DSM-IV symptoms in field trials, via comparisons with the Children's Global Assessment Scale (CGAS) (e.g., Green, Shirk, Hanze, & Wanstrath, 1994). This is a standardized rating procedure that can be used by clinicians or by others who are knowledgeable about a child.

Clinical Interview and Background Information

The primary areas of information to be obtained from the interviews of parents, teachers, and the child include (1) details of the symptom presentation, onset, and course of the problem behaviors and (2) background information on predisposing risk factors, including medical, developmental, family history, family composition, socioeconomic status, and maternal age; the results of the most recent vision and hearing tests; any psychological evaluations; school records of grades, attendance, detention, and suspensions; and involvement with the law or child protective services agency. Other areas include (3) exacerbating or comorbid risk factors, including all aspects of family function, family stressors, parenting and discipline approaches used, educational achievement, the child's internalizing symptoms, and stressful or traumatic life events. Finally, there is (4) multisystemic impact of the DBD on parent–child interaction, other interpersonal relationships, and how the informant has attempted to adjust cognitively and emotionally to the problem behaviors.

The interview process is central to assessing all these areas but must do so with sensitivity to the informant's affective responses to delivering the information. Parents may feel guilt, defensiveness, or relief as they describe negative parenting experiences or their own difficulties such as substance abuse or antisocial behavior. Further, family conflict and the informant's negative attributions about the child can impede the interview process. Demographic forms that parents can complete while the child is being evaluated individually complement the interview process.

During the clinical interview of the child, information is gathered retrospectively and concurrently through interactions between the child and examiner, and behavioral observations of how the child enters the assessment situation. McConaughy and Achenbach (1994) have developed the Semistructured Clinical Interview for Children and Adolescents (SCICA) for ages 6–18 years. Areas of inquiry include activities, school, job, friends, family relations, fantasies, self-perceptions and feelings, parent- and teacher-reported problems, and achievement tests. Children 6–12 years old can be screened for fine or gross motor problems, and adolescents can be interviewed about somatic complaints, alcohol and drug use, and trouble with the law. Youth are encouraged to respond in a conversational format. The SCICA is scored in a format similar to that of the CBCL and TRF with ratings for the observed behavior on five scales (Anxious, Attention Problems, Resistant, Strange, and Withdrawn) and the child's self-report of difficulties on three scales (Aggressive Behavior, Anxious/Depressed, and Family Problems).

Greenspan (1981) has provided guidelines for conducting an unstructured child clinical interview, assessing levels of function in the following areas: physical, speech and language, mood, relationship capacity, affect, use of the environment, thematic development in play, and the examiner's subjective experience of the child. The child's play is viewed diagnostically to help determine developmental level and the child's internal dynamics.

At least two individual diagnostic sessions are necessary to engage a child and appropriately assess the behavior. Children may present as well-mannered and compliant in the initial session because of fear or shyness. Once engaged, the child can report information that reveals traumatic experiences of abuse or neglect, a comorbid internalizing disorder, or depression. At some point the examiner may want to use a query such as, "Sometimes when something bad happens to children, they get angry and act in ways that get them in trouble. Has anything happened to you like that?" The child's awareness of peer problems, any remorse about problem behaviors, and sense of inability to inhibit impulses are all areas to investigate through such interviews and through diagnostic play.

Parent and Family Measures

The multisystemic assessment of parent and family factors includes evaluation of parent psychological adjustment (particularly depression), marital adjustment, parenting stress, social support, parenting practices, and dyadic and family interactions. A great deal of the parent information, such as personal characteristics, parenting skills, behavior management techniques, disciplinary methods, monitoring of child activities, developmental expectations, and utilization of community resources, is obtained during the parent interview and through observation of the parent–child interaction. Demographic information about the family composition, parents' educational level, occupation, employment status, and medical history can be first collected on intake forms, then further queried during the parent interview. Much of the information collected on parent and family measures may also be addressed in subsequent interviews with the parent over the course of the assessment process as rapport increases and the interference of social desirability responding decreases. Numerous instruments to assess specific variables have been developed for research purposes, and many of these hold promise of clinical applications (see Barkley, 1997a, 1997b for recent reviews).

Parent Psychological Adjustment

The Symptom Checklist 90-R (SCL-90-R; Derogatis, 1983) and Beck Depression Inventory (BDI; Beck & Beck, 1972; Beck, Ward, Mendelson, Mock, & Erbaugh, 1961; Beck, Steer, & Garbin, 1988) are brief, cost-effective questionnaires to assess general parent

personality characteristics and the level of depressive symptomatology specifically.

The SCL-90-R is a 90-item checklist on which adults self-report the amount of distress experienced from psychological symptoms on a 5-point scale. The responses yield scores on nine dimensions (Somatization, Obsessive-Compulsive, Interpersonal Sensitivity, Depression, Anxiety, Hostility, Phobic Anxiety, Paranoid Ideation, and Psychoticism). Scores are also totaled for three distress indices (Global Severity Index, Positive Symptom Total, and Positive Symptom Distress Index). Profiles are available using clinical and nonclinical norms. Psychometric properties are strong. The SCL-R-90 has the advantage of providing general assessment of the parent's psychological status, which may either be associated with the child's behavior disorder (Barkley, Fisher, Edelbrock, & Smallish, 1991; Barkley, Anastopoulos, Guevremont, & Fletcher, 1992) or compromise treatment response (Forehand & MacMahon, 1981).

The BDI is a 21-item measure of symptoms of depression including cognitive, emotional, and somatic aspects. The adult respondent selects one of four statements in each item that best describes how he or she has felt in the past 7 days. A total score is obtained with clinical cutoffs. It requires a sixth-grade reading level and takes 5–10 min to complete. Its psychometric properties have been demonstrated in numerous studies and reviewed by Beck and colleagues (1988). It should be noted that faking either good or bad is relatively easy because of the obviousness of the content (Beck & Beamesderfer, 1974).

Marital Adjustment

One of two measures is typically used to assess marital adjustment: the Dyadic Adjustment Scale (DAS; Spanier, 1976; Spanier & Thompson, 1982) or the Locke–Wallace Marital Adjustment Test (LWMAT; Locke & Wallace, 1959). The DAS is a 32-item measure of marital adjustment that yields four factors (Dyadic Satisfaction, Dyadic Cohesion, Dyadic Consensus, and Affectional Expression). The

DAS provides no overall impression of the marital relationship. It does identify specific problem areas and permits comparison of the partners' reports with each other. The LWMAT uses a 7-point scale to rate eight areas of the marital relationship (Financial matters, Recreation, Demonstration of affection, Friends, Sexual relations, Conventionality, Philosophy of life, and Dealing with in-laws). The degree of concordance in each area and overall satisfaction are scored. Both of these measures are supported by extensive research and demonstrate reliability and validity in assessing marital discord (Carey, Spector, Lantinga, & Krauss, 1993). Early assessment of the marital adjustment can assist in treatment planning by identifying areas that can be separately targeted for intervention and thus improve the family's level of functioning in order to support behavior change in the disruptive child.

Parenting Stress and Social Support

The Parenting Stress Index (PSI; Abidin, 1995) is a 101-item measure that assesses the amount of stress in the parent–child relationship (for children up to 12 years old). Parents rate items on a 5-point scale, yielding 13 subscale scores which form two domain scores: stress due to characteristics of the parent (Depression, Attachment to Child, Restriction of Role, Sense of Competence, Social Isolation, Relationship with Spouse, and Parental Health), and stress due to characteristics of the child (Adaptability, Demandingness, Mood, Distractibility/Hyperactivity, and the degree to which the child is Acceptable to the parent and Reinforces the parent). Nineteen additional items can be included for a measure of Situational/Demographic Life Stress. An overall Stress Index score is also obtained. It requires a fifth-grade reading level and takes 15–20 min to complete. Research has demonstrated strong psychometric properties (Abidin, 1995) including the capacity to distinguish clinical from nonclinical samples (Breen & Barkley, 1978; Mash & Johnston, 1983), and longitudinal predictions of behavior problems from PSI scores obtained when the child was in infancy (Abidin,

Jenkins, & McGaughey, 1992). Maternal reports tend to indicate higher levels of parenting stress than do paternal reports (Webster-Stratton, 1984).

Parenting Practices

Many aspects of parenting, such as how the parent makes demands and obtains compliance from the child, and affective responsiveness to the child, can be readily observed in the clinic; other facets, such as monitoring of child activities, disciplinary techniques, or daily structuring of household routines, are difficult to observe outside the home. Several measures to screen parenting practices have been developed out of research studies, such as the Parenting Scale (D. S. Arnold, O'Leary, Wolff, & Acker, 1993). This instrument is a 30-item parent-report measure of the parents' attempts to discipline the misbehavior of their toddler. Sets of opposing statements about parenting behaviors are rated on a 7-point scale to obtain a total score and three domain scores (Laxness, Overreactivity, and Verbosity). The Parenting Scale displayed good reliability and validity, but its small age range limits its clinical applications.

Dyadic and Family Interactions

The Conflict Behavior Questionnaire (CBQ) and Issues Checklist (IC) were developed to measure the amount of conflict, negative communication, and anger regarding conflictual issues in the family system (Prinz, Foster, Kent, & O'Leary, 1979; Robin & Foster, 1984). Parallel versions of the CBQ are completed by parents (75 items) and adolescents (73 items) independently to identify the number of conflictual issues and the intensity of the anger. The CBQ and IC have the advantage of being easy and brief to administer (they require 10–15 min to complete) and sensitive to treatment effects (Foster, Prinz, & O'Leary, 1983). However, only comparison data are available.

Although not generally feasible for clinical applications, a variety of coding systems have been developed for direct observations of parent–child and family interactions (see Foster & Robin, 1997, for review).

CONCLUSION

The present scientific and professional consensus seems to favor the use of categorical diagnosis of ODD, ADHD, and CD. However, carrying out such categorical diagnosis reliably and validly requires the use of standardized interviews of some kind with the parent and child and of standardized ratings by teachers. We know of very few clinicians who actually use such procedures in their routine practice or treatment evaluation, for the obvious reason that they are cumbersome and expensive.

Thus, our recommendation for routine clinical assessment where cost is an important factor is to use informal interviews mainly for rapport building and contextual information. For formal assessment, we recommend the use of standardized behavioral checklists from the parent and teacher (and from the child also, if sufficiently mature to respond meaningfully). Given that such checklists are rarely keyed to the DSM categories, the recommended approach is a dimensional one. In addition, clinicians should depend on the public school system to meet its responsibilities in providing appropriate psychoeducational assessment. Making sure that the schools do what they are supposed to do in terms of assessment would have the additional benefit of cementing the liaison between the clinic and the school system, which is often a crucial part of intervention.

The comprehensive assessment procedures discussed at length in this chapter can be considered to represent an ideal approach to clinical assessment, to be followed if time and resources permit. Assessment for research purposes cannot be prescribed except to mention some of the possibilities. What is adequate for a scientific investigation depends on the particular hypotheses to be evaluated and, of course, the financial resources available. Granting agencies usually require a clear scientific ratio-

nale and justification for the particular procedures to be employed in a study.

REFERENCES

Abidin, R. R. (1995). *Parenting Stress Index—Professional manual* (3rd ed.). Odessa, FL; Psychological Assessment Resources.

Abidin, R. R., Jenkins, C. L., & McGaughey, M. C. (1992). The relationship of early family variables to children's subsequent behavioral adjustment. *Journal of Clinical Psychology, 21*, 60–69.

Achenbach, T. M. (1991). *Integrative guide for the 1991 CBCL/4–18, YSR, and TRF Profiles.* Burlington: University of Vermont, Department of Psychiatry.

Achenbach, T. M., & Edelbrock, C. S. (1978). The classification of child psychopathology: A review and analysis of empirical efforts. *Psychological Bulletin, 55*, 1275–1301.

Achenbach, T. M., & Edelbrock, C. S. (1983). *Manual for the Child Behavior Checklist and Revised Child Behavior Profile.* Burlington: University of Vermont, Department of Psychiatry.

Achenbach, T. M., & Edelbrock, C. S. (1986). *Manual for the Teacher Report Form and Child Behavior Profile.* Burlington: University of Vermont, Department of Psychiatry.

Achenbach, T. M., & Edelbrock, C. S. (1987). *Manual for the Child Behavior Checklist and Youth Self Report.* Burlington: University of Vermont, Department of Psychiatry.

Achenbach, T. M., & McConaughy, S. H. (1997). *Empirically based assessment of child and adolescent psychopathology: Practical applications* (2nd ed.).Thousand Oaks, CA: Sage.

Achenbach, T. M., McConaughy, S. H., & Howell, C. T. (1987). Child-adolescent behavioral and emotional problems: Implications of cross-informant correlations for situational specificity. *Psychological Bulletin, 101*, 213–232.

American Psychiatric Association. (1994). *Diagnostic and statistical manual of mental disorders* (4th ed.). Washington, DC: Author.

Anastopoulos, A. D., Guevremont, D. C., Shelton, T. L., & DuPaul, G. J. (1992). Parenting stress among families of children with Attention Deficit Hyperactivity Disorder. *Journal of Abnormal Child Psychology, 20*, 503–520.

Arnold, D. S., O'Leary, S. G., Wolff, L. S., & Acker, M. M. (1993). The Parenting Scale: A measure of dysfunctional parenting in discipline situations. *Psychological Assessment, 5*, 137–144.

Arnold, J., & Jacobowitz, D. (1993). *The Cross-Informant Program for the CBCL/4–18, YSR, & TRF.* Burlington: University of Vermont, Department of Psychiatry.

Barkley, R. A. (1981). *Hyperactive children: A handbook for diagnosis and treatment.* New York: Guilford.

Barkley, R. A. (1988). Child behavior rating scales and checklists. In M. Rutter, A. H. Tuma, & I. S. Lann (Eds.), *Assessment and diagnosis in child psychopathology* (pp. 113–155). New York: Guilford.

Barkley, R. A. (1997a). Attention-Deficit/Hyperactivity Disorder. In E. J. Mash & L. G. Terdal (Eds.), *Assessment in childhood disorders* (pp. 71–129). New York: Guilford.

Barkley, R. A. (1997b). *Defiant children: A clinician's manual for assessment and training* (2nd ed.). New York: Guilford.

Barkley, R. A., Fisher, M., Edelbrock, C. S., & Smallish, L. (1991). The adolescent outcome of hyperactive children diagnosed by research criteria: III. Mother–child interactions, family conflicts, and maternal psychopathology. *Journal of Child Psychology and Psychiatry, 32,* 233–256.

Barkley, R. A., Anastopoulos, A. D., Guevremont, D. C., & Fletcher, K. F. (1992). Adolescents with Attention Deficit Hyperactivity Disorder: Mother–adolescent interactions, family beliefs and conflicts, and maternal psychopathology. *Journal of Abnormal Child Psychology, 20,* 263–288.

Beck, A. T., & Beamesderfer, A. (1974). Assessment of depression. The Depression Inventory. In P. Pichot (Ed.), *Modern problems in pharmacopsychiatry* (pp. 151–169). Basel, Switzerland: Karger.

Beck, A. T., & Beck, R. W. (1972). Screening depressed patients in family practice: A rapid technique. *Postgraduate Medicine, 52,* 81–85.

Beck, A. T., Ward, C. H., Mendelson, M., Mock, J., & Erbaugh, J. (1961). An inventory for measuring depression. *Archives of General Psychiatry, 4,* 561–571.

Beck, A. T., Steer, R. A., & Garbin, M. G. (1988). Psychometric properties of the Beck Depression Inventory: Twenty-five years of evaluation. *Clinical Psychology Review, 8,* 77–100.

Boyle, M. H., Offord, D. R., Racine, Y., Sanford, M., Szatmari, P., Fleming, J. E., & Price-Munn, N. (1993). Evaluation of the Diagnostic Interview for Children and Adolescents for use in general population samples. *Journal of Abnormal Child Psychology, 21,* 663–681.

Breen, M. J., & Altepeter, T. S. (1990). *Disruptive behavior disorders in children: Treatment-focused assessment.* New York: Guilford.

Breen, M. J., & Barkley, R. A. (1978). Child psychopathology and parenting stress in girls and boys having Attention Deficit Disorder with Hyperactivity. *Journal of Pediatric Psychology, 2,* 265–280.

Campbell, S. B. (1990). *Behavior problems in preschool children.* New York: Guilford.

Carey, M. P., Spector, I. P., Lantinga, L. J., & Krauss, D. J. (1993). Reliability of the Dyadic Adjustment Scale. *Psychological Assessment, 5,* 238–240.

Conners, C. K., Wells, K. C., Parker, J. D. A., Sitarenios, G., Diamond, J. M., & Powell, J. W. (1997). A new self-report scale for assessment of adolescent psychopathology: Factor structure, reliability, validity, and diagnostic sensitivity. *Journal of Abnormal Child Psychology, 25,* 487–497.

Conners, C. K., Sitarenios, G., Parker, J. D. A., & Epstein, J. N. (1998). The Revised Conners' Parent Rating Scale (CPRS-R): Factor structure, reliability, and criterion validity. *Journal of Abnormal Child Psychology, 26,* 257–268.

Dadds, M. R., & Powell, M. B. (1991). The relationship of interpersonal conflict and global marital adjustment to aggression, anxiety, and immaturity in aggressive and nonclinic children. *Journal of Abnormal Child Psychology, 19,* 553–567.

Derogatis, L. R. (1983). *SCL-90-R administration, scoring, and procedures manual–II.* Towson, MD: Clinical Psychometric Research.

Edelbrock, C., Costello, A., Dulcan, M., Conover, N., & Kala, R. (1986). Parent–child agreement on child psychiatric symptoms assessed via structured interview. *Journal of Child Psychology and Psychiatry, 27,* 181–190.

Elliott, D. S., Dunford, F. W., & Huizinga, D. (1987). The identification and prediction of career offenders utilizing self-reported and official data. In J. D. Burchard & S. N. Burchard (Eds.), *Preventing delinquent behavior* (pp. 90–121). Newbury Park, CA: Sage.

Eyberg, S. M. (1980). Eyberg Child Behavior Inventory. *Journal of Clinical Child Psychology, 9,* 29.

Eyberg, S. M., & Ross, A. W. (1978). Assessment of child behavior problems: The validation of a new inventory. *Journal of Clinical Child Psychology, 7,* 113–116.

Fisher, P., Shaffer, D., Piacentini, J., Lapkin, J., Wicks, J., & Rojas, M. (1991). *Completion of the revisions of the NIMH Diagnostic Interview Schedule for Children (DISC-2).* Washington, DC: Epidemiology and Psychopathology Research Branch, National Institute of Mental Health.

Forehand, R., & McMahon, R. (1981). *Helping the noncompliant child: A clinician's guide to parent training.* New York: Guilford.

Foster, S. L., & Robin, A. L. (1997). Family conflict and communication in adolescence. In E. J. Mash & L. G. Terdal (Eds.), *Assessment of childhood disorders* (pp. 627–682). New York: Guilford.

Foster, S. L., Prinz, R. J., & O'Leary, K. D. (1983). Impact of problem-solving communication training and generalization procedures on family conflict. *Child and Family Behavior Therapy, 5,* 1–23.

Frick, P. J., Lahey, B. B., Loeber, R., Stouthamer-Loeber, M., Christ, M. A., & Hanson, K. (1992). Familial risk factors to oppositional defiant disorder and conduct disorder: Parental psychopathology and maternal parenting. *Journal of Consulting Clinical Psychology, 60,* 49–55.

Goyette, C. H., Conners, C. K., & Ulrich, R. F. (1978). Normative data on revised Conners Parent and Teacher Rating Scales. *Journal of Abnormal Child Psychology, 6,* 221–236.

Green, B., Shirk, S., Hanze, D., & Wanstrath, J. (1994). The Children's Global Assessment Scale in clinical practice: An empirical evaluation. *Journal of the*

American Academy of Child and Adolescent Psychiatry, 33, 1158–1164.

Greenspan, S. (1981). *The clinical interview of the child.* New York: McGraw-Hill.

Herjanic, B., & Reich, W. (1982). Development of a structured psychiatric interview for children: Agreement between child and parent on individual symptoms. *Journal of Abnormal Child Psychology, 10,* 307–324.

Hinshaw, S. P., Lahey, B. B., & Hart, E. L. (1993). Issues of taxonomy and comorbidity in the development of conduct disorder. *Development and Psychopathology, 5,* 31–49.

Jessor, R., & Jessor, S. L. (1977). *Problem behavior and psychological development: A longitudinal study of youth.* New York: Academic Press.

Jouriles, E. N., Murphy, C. M., Farris, A.M., Smith, D. A., Richters, J. E., & Waters, E. (1991). Marital adjustment, parental disagreements about child rearing, and behavior problems in boys: Increasing the specificity of the marital assessment. *Child Development, 62,* 1424–1433.

Kazdin, A. E. (1995). *Conduct disorders in childhood and adolescence.* Thousand Oaks, CA: Sage.

Kazdin, A. E., Rodgers, A., Colbus, D., & Siegel, T. (1987). Children's Hostility Inventory: Measurement of aggression and hostility in psychiatric inpatient children. *Journal of Clinical Child Psychology, 16,* 320–328.

Kazdin, A. E., Siegel, T. C., & Bass, D. (1990). Drawing upon clinical practice to inform research on child and adolescent psychotherapy: A survey of practitioners. *Professional Psychology: Research and Practice, 21,* 189–198.

Kovacs, M. (1981). Rating scales to assess depression in school-aged children. *Acta Paedopsychiatrica, 46,* 305–315.

Kovacs, M. (1985). The Children's Depression Inventory. *Psychopharmacology Bulletin, 21,* 995–998.

Locke, H., & Wallace, K. (1959). Short marital-adjustment and prediction tests: Their reliability and validity. *Marriage and Family Living, 21,* 251–255.

Mandel, H. P. (1997). *Conduct Disorder and underachievement: Risk factors, treatment, and prevention.* New York: Wiley.

Mann, B. J., & MacKenzie, E. P. (1996). Pathways among marital functioning, parental behaviors, and child behavior problems in school-age boys. *Journal of Clinical Child Psychology, 25,* 183–191.

Mash, E. J., & Johnston, C. (1983). Parental perceptions of child behavior problems, parenting self-esteem, and mothers' reported stress in younger and older hyperactive and normal children. *Journal of Consulting and Clinical Psychology, 51,* 86–99.

Mash, E. J., & Johnston, C. (1990). Determinants of parenting stress: Illustrations from families of hyperactive children and families of physically abused children. *Journal of Clinical and Child Psychology, 19,* 313–328.

McConaughy, S. H., & Achenbach, T. M. (1994). *Manual for the Semistructured Clinical Interview for Children and Adolescents.* Burlington: University of Vermont, Department of Psychiatry.

McGee, L., & Newcomb, M. D. (1992). General deviance syndrome: Expanded hierarchical evaluations at four ages from early adolescence to adulthood. *Journal of Consulting and Clinical Psychology, 60,* 766–776.

Patterson, G. R. (1982). *Coercive family processes.* Eugene, OR: Castalia.

Patterson, G. R., DeBaryshe, B. D., & Ramsey, E. (1989). A developmental perspective on antisocial behavior. *American Psychologist, 44,* 329–335.

Pelham, W. E., Schnedler, R. W., Nender, M. E., Nilsson, D. E., Miller, L., Budrow, M. S., Ronnei, M., Paluchowski, C., & Marks, D. A. (1988). The combination of behavior therapy and methylphenidate in the treatment of Attention Deficit Disorders: A therapy outcome study. In L. M. Bloomingdale (Ed.), *Attention Deficit Disorder: Vol. 3. New research in attention, treatment, and psychopharmacology* (pp. 29–48). New York: Pergamon.

Prinz, R. J., Foster, S. L., Kent, R. N., & O'Leary, K. D. (1979). Multivariate assessment of conflict in distressed and nondistressed mother–adolescent dyads. *Journal of Applied Behavioral Analysis, 12,* 691–700.

Quay, H. C. (1979). Classification. In H. C. Quay & J. S. Werry (Eds.), *Psychopathological disorders of childhood* (2nd ed., pp. 1–42). New York: Wiley.

Quay, H. C., & Peterson, D. R. (1987). *Manual for the Revised Behavior Problem Checklist.* Odessa, FL: Psychological Assessment Resources.

Reich, W., & Welner, Z. (1988). *Revised version of the Diagnostic Interview for Children and Adolescents (DICA-R).* St. Louis, MO: Washington University School of Medicine, Department of Psychiatry.

Reynolds, W. M. (1987). *Reynolds Adolescent Depression Scale: Professional manual.* Odessa, FL: Psychological Assessment Resources.

Robin, A. L., & Foster, S. L. (1984). Problem-solving communication training: A behavioral-family systems approach to parent–adolescent training. *Advances in Child Behavioral Analysis and Therapy, 3,* 195–240.

Robinson, E. A., Eyberg, S. M., & Ross, A. W. (1980). The standardization of an inventory of child conduct problem behavior. *Journal of Clinical Child Psychology, 48,* 117–118.

Schwab-Stone, M., Fisher, P., Piacentini, J., Shaffer, D., Davies, M., & Briggs, M. (1993). The Diagnostic Interview Schedule for Children—Revised version (DISC-R): II. Test–retest reliability. *Journal of the American Academy of Child and Adolescent Psychiatry, 32,* 658–665.

Shaffer, D., Schwab-Stone, M., Fisher, P., Cohen, P., Piacentini, J., Davies, M., Conners, C. K., & Regier, D. (1993). The Diagnostic Interview Schedule for Children—Revised version (DISC-R): I. Preparation, field testing, interrater reliability, and acceptability. *Journal of the American Academy of Child and Adolescent Psychiatry, 32,* 643–650.

Spanier, G. B. (1976). Measuring dyadic adjustment: New scales for assessing the quality of marriage and similar dyads. *Journal of Marriage and the Family, 38,* 15–38.

Spanier, G. B., & Thompson, L. (1982). A confirmatory analysis of the Dyadic Adjustment Scale. *Journal of Marriage and the Family, 44,* 731–738.

Ullmann, R., & Sleator, E. (1985). Attention deficit disorder children with or without hyperactivity: Which behaviors are helped by stimulants? *Clinical Pediatrics, 24,* 547–551.

Ullmann, R., Sleator, E., & Sprague, R. (1984). A new rating scale for diagnosis and monitoring of ADD children. *Psychopharmacology Bulletin, 20,* 106–164.

Ullmann, R., Sleator, E., & Sprague, R. (1985). A change of mind: Conners' Abbreviated Rating Scales reconsidered. *Journal of Abnormal Child Psychology, 13,* 553–566.

Ullmann, R., Sleator, E., & Sprague, R. (1988). *Manual for the ADD-H Comprehensive Teachers' Rating Scale.* Champaign, IL: MeriTech.

Wakefield, J. C. (1992). Disorder as harmful dysfunction: A conceptual critique of DSM-III-R's definition of mental disorder. *Psychological Review, 99,* 232–247.

Webster-Stratton, C. (1984). Mothers' and fathers' perceptions of child deviance: Roles of parent and child behaviors and parent adjustment. *Journal of Consulting and Clinical Psychology, 56,* 909–915.

Wells, K. C., & Forehand, R. (1985). Conduct and oppositional disorders. In P. H. Bornstein & A. E. Kazdin (Eds.), *Handbook of clinical behavior therapy with children* (pp. 218–265). Homewood, IL: Dorsey.

II

Attention-Deficit/Hyperactivity Disorder

4

Information Processing and Energetic Factors in Attention-Deficit/Hyperactivity Disorder

JOSEPH A. SERGEANT, JAAP OOSTERLAAN, and JAAP van der MEERE

BACKGROUND

Currently, children and adolescents with an excess of hyperactive, inattentive, and impulsive behavior are diagnosed as Attention-Deficit/Hyperactivity Disorder (ADHD; see the *Diagnostic and Statistical Manual of Mental Disorders* [DSM-IV], American Psychiatric Association, 1994, and chapter 1, this volume).*

Each of the three facets of the disorder—hyperactivity, inattention, and, most recently, impulsivity—has been the focus of experimental study. Objective measurement of overactivity using actometers has proven to be less than

*Children now diagnosed as ADHD have, in past research, been categorized under a number of labels. In this chapter, we uniformly use the term ADHD to describe all "hyperactive" and "attention-deficit" research subjects.

JOSEPH A. SERGEANT and JAAP OOSTERLAAN • Department of Clinical Psychology, University of Amsterdam, 1018 WB Amsterdam, The Netherlands. JAAP van der MEERE • Department of Experimental Clinical Psychology, University of Groningen, 9712 TS, Groningen, The Netherlands.

Handbook of Disruptive Behavior Disorders, edited by Quay and Hogan. Kluwer Academic/Plenum Publishers, New York, 1999.

straightforward. For example, position on ligaments and situations in which measurement occurs have been shown to affect results (Taylor, 1983). Nevertheless, ADHD children are more likely to be overactive in highly structured task conditions than in more informal settings (Goyette, Conners, & Ulrich, 1978; Porrino *et al.,* 1983; Zentall & Zentall, 1983) and even in their sleep (Porrino *et al.,* 1983). This suggests that overactivity is crucial to two of the three subtypes: the primarily hyperactive-impulsive and the combined subtype, distinguished in DSM-IV.

The second area of inquiry, "attention deficits," may be traced to work published in the early 1970s in which a series of studies from the Montreal group reported that ADHD children had poorer vigilance performance than controls (Sykes, Douglas, Weiss, & Minde, 1971; Sykes, Douglas, & Morgenstern, 1973). It was also found that the response strategy in ADHD children tended to be more often impulsive (fast, inaccurate performance) rather than reflective (slow, accurate performance) (Campbell, Douglas, & Morgenstern, 1971; Campbell, Endman, & Bernfeld 1977; Cohen, Weiss, & Minde,

1972; Hopkins, Perlman, Hechtman, & Weiss, 1979). Research also showed that ADHD children were less physiologically aroused and faster habituators than normals (Satterfield & Dawson, 1971). These findings suggested that ADHD children might have a deficit associated with vigilance, problem-solving strategy, or energetic state. In essence, these findings were interpreted at the end of the 1970s as evidence for the position that ADHD children were characterized by an attention deficit.

In the 1980s a series of publications appeared that questioned whether an attention deficit adequately explained the information-processing problems of ADHD children. When attention tasks of short duration were used and when the children were tested under supervision, ADHD children were able to divide their attentional resources among simultaneously presented stimuli with varying complexity (Klorman *et al.*, 1988; van der Meere & Sergeant, 1987; Sergeant & Scholten, 1983, 1985a, 1985b). ADHD children were also able

to focus their attention, that is, to ignore irrelevant stimuli in favor of processing relevant stimuli (van der Meere & Sergeant, 1988c). In addition, ADHD children were able to acquire automatic processing at the same rate as controls (van der Meere & Sergeant, 1988a). When tasks were attractive (activating), ADHD children were able to sustain attention for more than 36 min in paced tasks (van der Meere & Sergeant, 1988b), or for more than two hr in blocked-paced tasks (Sergeant, 1988) and in self-paced conditions (van der Meere, Wekking, & Sergeant, 1991). Thus, an attentional deficit hypothesis did not seem to explain the nature of the deficit in ADHD.

Recently, the third facet of ADHD, impulsivity, has been the focus of research attention. It has been strongly argued that impulsivity, or, more precisely, disinhibition, is the key to distinguishing this disorder from others (Barkley, 1994, 1997; Quay, 1988, 1997). This approach suggests that ADHD is the result of a failure to delay responding asso-

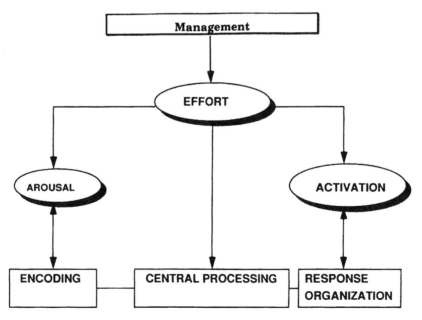

FIGURE 1.   A simplified representation of the cognitive-energetic model. The top box, "Management," contains typical executive functions. The three ellipses represent the three energetic pools, arousal, activation, and effort. Effort influences both arousal and activation. The three lower boxes represent the stages of information processing, encoding, central processing (search and decision), and motor organization with which these pools are associated.

ciated with inhibitory deficits (see Chapter 13, this volume, for a more complete exposition).

As yet, research has not conclusively indicated exactly what the primary defect in ADHD is. As noted in Chapter 1 (this volume), there is a strong possibility that the two subgroups of ADHD are two distinct disorders: one in which attentional defects are the core and one in which hyperactivity-impulsivity is the core.

We have advocated a research strategy in which a model of information processing is used to identify the locus of the ADHD deficit (Sergeant & van der Meere, 1994). Our approach utilizes the cognitive-energetic model (see Figure 1) described by Sanders (1983) and elaborated in ADHD by Sergeant & van der Meere (1990a, 1990b; 1994). We acknowledge that earlier work proposed that the ADHD deficit could be described as a dysfunction of both arousal and inhibition (Satterfield, Cantwell, & Satterfield, 1974).

OBJECTIVES

The aim of this chapter is to address critically the issue as to whether ADHD children are unable to inhibit, when appropriate, ongoing activity and if so, what the processes underlying the apparent inhibitory dysfunction are. The cognitive-energetic model guiding our research is briefly presented and we review some of the traditional clinical tests and tasks used to study inhibition. We suggest that clinical tests are insufficiently specific to conclude that the core of ADHD is an inhibition deficit. We argue that the claim of an inhibitory deficit in ADHD fails to take account of the fact that poor inhibitory performance is not specific to ADHD. We argue that energetic factors are critical to the performance deficits of ADHD children. We review electrophysiological and neural imaging studies to support the energetic position and argue that the evident problems of inhibitory control in ADHD children need to be studied with methods that can determine whether this apparent disinhibitory problem is modulated by energetic factors.

THE COGNITIVE-ENERGETIC MODEL

From the results of vigilance and human performance research the effects of factors such as sleep loss, noise, heat, and drugs on information processing are evident (see Warm, 1984). These factors later became known as *state factors* in contrast to *process (computational) factors*. The overall efficiency of processing in the cognitive-energetic model is said to be determined by process *and* state factors.

Process, or computational, mechanisms of attention include four general stages: encoding, search, decision, and motor organization (Sternberg, 1969). These stages of information processing are associated with experimental task variables. The processing of unbroken (physically intact) versus broken (physically degraded) stimuli is localized at encoding; the number of items to be searched in memory or on a visual display with search; deciding target present/absent with decision; and stimulus–response compatibility with motor organization. This linkage of stages with task variables made possible a search for the locus of the information-processing deficit in ADHD (van der Meere, 1988; Oosterlaan, 1996; Sergeant, 1981).

State factors include three energetic pools. The first is *effort* (Kahneman, 1973). Effort was conceived of as the necessary energy to meet the demands of a task. Factors that affected effort were variables such as cognitive load, which could be manipulated to increase task demands. Specifically, effort was said to be required when the current state of the organism did not meet the state required to perform a task. The effort pool was identified with the hippocampus (Pribram & McGuiness, 1975). Kahneman (1973) originally proposed that effort was best measured by pupil dilation; the greater the dilation, the more effort was being applied to the task. This prediction has been found to be generally correct; pupil dilation occurs when processing load is below seven to-be-recalled digits, but constriction occurs when load is increased beyond this point (Granholm, Asarnow, Sarkin, & Dykes, 1996). Other work has suggested that heart rate (HR) deceleration, respiratory sinus arrhythmia (van der Molen, Bashore, Halliday, & Callaway, 1991), and Event-Related Desynchronization (ERD) may reflect the operation of this pool (Boiten, Sergeant, & Geuze, 1992; van Winsum, Sergeant, & Geuze, 1984). Sanders (1983) assigned to effort the function of both exciting and inhibiting two other energetic pools: arousal and activation.

Arousal was defined as phasic responding that is time locked to stimulus processing (Pribram & McGuiness, 1975). Typical variables identified by Sanders (1983) as influencing arousal are signal intensity and novelty. The arousal pool was associated with the mesencephalic, reticular formation, and the amygdala. Arousal was said to be monitored by measures of time-locked physiological responding, such as electrodermal response (EDR) and HR acceleration–deceleration (Pribram & McGuiness, 1975). Sanders (1983) considered perceptual sensitivity (the ability to discriminate signal plus noise from noise only), measured by d′, to be a direct index of the arousal pool.

Tonic changes of physiological activity were thought to represent the operation of the *activation* pool (Pribram & McGuiness, 1975). The activation pool was identified with the basal ganglia and corpus striatum (Pribram & McGuiness, 1975). Sanders (1983) concluded that activation was affected by task variables such as preparation, manipulated by the period of time between a warning signal and the signal requiring a response (called the foreperiod); alertness (detrimentally influenced by sleep loss); time of day (performance after breakfast being better than at night) and time on task (maximum performance decrement being observed at around 30 min on a task). Activation is associated with tonic physiological readiness to respond. It was proposed that within vigilance tasks, response bias (the tendency to opt systematically for one response, for example, "yes," which would lead to many true positives but also to a high false positive rate), measured by β, was the appropriate performance measure of the activation pool.

As reviewed by Sergeant and van der Meere (1990a), drugs are considered to influence state factors; the locus of effect of drugs should be determined by those task variables with which they interact. As noted in that review, barbiturates interact with encoding variables and are said to have their locus at the encoding stage and the associated arousal pool. Amphetamines were shown to interact with motor output variables and the associated activation pool (Frowein, 1981).

Of importance for the review of the ADHD deficit is the relationship between effort and the activation pool. Sanders (1983) suggested a direct pathway between effort and response choice based on research by Gaillard (1978). Later research has shown that when long periods of motor preparation are required, subjects will wait until the application of effort will have maximum payoff for minimum allocation of energy (Hackley & Miller, 1995). These findings suggest that the effort and activation pools are tightly connected and have considerable effect on motor output.

The cognitive-energetic model also includes an overriding, management, or evaluation mechanism (see Figure 1). This mechanism is associated with planning, monitoring, detection of errors, and their correction. Task variables that affect this mechanism are knowledge of results and cost-benefits (Sanders, 1983). Thus the complete model has three levels: a lower stratum with four stages of processing, a middle level with three energetic pools, and a higher level mechanism of management or control. This latter mechanism shows considerable similarities to the executive functions associated with the prefrontal cortex (Barkley, 1996; Pennington, Bennetto, McAleer, & Roberts, 1996; see also Chapter 5, this volume). The place of management in the model is depicted in Figure 1.

We use this model in organizing the research that we review with respect to the inhibition-deficit hypothesis of ADHD.

OPERATIONALIZATIONS OF RESPONSE INHIBITION

The terms inhibition and disinhibition have had a variety of meanings and experimental operationalizations. *Disinhibition* has been conceptualized as, or defined by (1) fast but inaccurate responding, (2) response perseveration, and (3) a failure to respond appropriately in a response conflict task. These conceptualizations are linked to performance on clinical tests designed to measure each of them and are discussed in the next section of this chapter.

Disinhibition has been further operationalized as (1) a failure to inhibit a response to "distracting," task-irrelevant stimuli; (2) a failure of appropriate oculomotor delay in looking to a remembered spatial location; (3) a failure of prepulse inhibition of the startle eyeblink; (4) a failure to inhibit a response to a misleading cue in a spatial location task; (5) a failure to inhibit to-be-ignored stimuli in a dichotic listening task; (6) a failure to inhibit an earlier appropriate, but now inappropriate, response in an S–R compatibility–incompatibility task; (7) a failure to show latent inhibition; (8) a failure to suppress inappropriate responding in Go/No-Go tasks; (9) failure to suppress inappropriate responding in the stop-signal task; (10) failure to suppress inappropriate responding in the change task; (11) a failure to inhibit an experimenter-induced prepotent response when it is no longer appropriate; and (12) a failure to slow or inhibit responding as a result of the detection of an error.*

These operationalizations of disinhibition are related to information-processing tasks that are reviewed in sections following the review of clinical tests.

Clinical Tests

Fast Inaccurate Responses: MFFT

The Matching Familiar Figures Test (MFFT) was devised to measure disinhibition as fast but inaccurate responding (Kagan, Rosman, Day, Albert, & Phillips, 1964). The test involves choosing, out of six to eight possible designs, the one that is most like the standard. Scores consist of the mean time in making a response and the number of errors (mismatches). Fast but inaccurate performance has been found consistently in ADHD children (Barkley, 1991; Campbell et al., 1971; Campbell et al., 1977; Cohen et al., 1972; DuPaul, Anastopoulos, Shelton, Guevremont, & Metevia, 1992; Hopkins et al., 1979; Milich & Kramer, 1984; Sergeant, van Velthoven, & Virginia, 1979).

Milich, Hartung, Martin, and Haigler (1994) observed that a portion of the validity of the MFFT was derived from the fact that it differentiated ADHD children known to have problems in impulse control from those who did not. However, as they noted, there are other psychological processes besides disinhibition (e.g., attentional or motivational difficulties) that could account for this differentiation. Furthermore, performance on the MFFT poorly correlates with teacher ratings or observations of impulsivity in the classroom (Sergeant et al., 1979). Schachar and Logan (1990) summarized findings that MFFT performance varies with IQ, search strategy, and awareness of appropriateness of inhibiting a response until all variants have been compared.

In contrast to the fast, inaccurate responding reported with the MFFT, reaction time (RT) studies consistently show that ADHD children are slow, inaccurate performers rather than fast, inaccurate performers (Klorman et al., 1988; van der Meere & Sergeant, 1987; 1988a, 1988b, 1988c; van der Meere, van Baal, & Sergeant, 1989; van der Meere et al., 1991). More puzzling for the inhibition-deficit hypothesis is the consistent finding that ADHD children slow down even more when they are asked to perform as quickly as possible (Kalverboer & Brouwer, 1983; Milich & Kramer, 1984; Sergeant & Scholten, 1985b; Stevens, Stover, & Backus, 1970). If disinhibition is defined as fast, inaccurate responding, these studies do not support the claim of an inhibition deficit in ADHD children. (See Chapter 5, this volume, for a somewhat different conclusion with respect to MFFT findings.)

---

*It can be argued that all of these conceptualizations or operationalizations, with the exception of latent inhibition, can be subsumed under failure of passive avoidance, that is, the failure to withhold responding that will lead to punishment, punishment being broadly defined so as to include "being incorrect" with or without actual aversive consequences.

Response Perseveration: Wisconsin Card Sorting Test

The Wisconsin Card Sorting Test (WCST), developed by Berg (1948) and Grant and Berg (1948), is purported to be a measure of frontal lobe functioning (Milner, 1963). The subject is required to detect a change in a "target set." Perseveration of responses for an earlier set (the measure of disinhibition), categories reached, and set maintenance are dependent variables. The WCST can differentiate between ADHD children and controls (Boucagnani & Jones, 1989; Carter, Krener, Chaderjian, Northcutt, & Wolfe, 1995; Chelune, Fergusson, Koon, & Dickey, 1986; Shue & Douglas, 1992). The results suggest that ADHD dysfunction is associated with lateral frontal areas related to functions such as conceptualization of the problem, planning, and organization.

However, Reader, Harris, Scherholz, and Denckla (1994) found no indication of extreme perseverative errors in an ADHD sample. A review of the WCST studies suggests that the comparisons in which ADHD and controls differed were confined to a younger age group (Barkley, Grodzinsky, & DuPaul, 1992). In addition, the WCST does not discriminate patients with and without focal frontal damage (Anderson, Damasio, Jones, & Tranel, 1991). Mountain and Snow (1993) reviewed the literature on the WCST and concluded that a variety of processes and brain structures are responsible for performance on this test, making it difficult to conclude specifically that ADHD children have a disinhibitory defect due to impaired frontal functioning.

Response Conflict: Stroop

The Stroop test (Stroop, 1935) contains words denoting colors printed in an incongruent color (e.g., the word *red* printed in blue). According to Posner (1978), the Stroop effect produces response conflict in which an overlearned response (word reading) has to be inhibited for the benefit of another (color naming). Pardo, Pardo, Janer, and Raichle (1990) using positron emission tomography reported that

performance on the Stroop was mediated by the anterior cingulate gyrus.

Barkley and colleagues (1992) found five studies in which the Stroop interference measure distinguished ADHD children from controls. Two later studies also reported significant differences between ADHD and control children (Leung & Connolly, 1996; Pennington, Grossier, & Welsh, 1993). Earlier Cohen and colleagues (1972) had used the Stroop in a study with ADHD children and controls but found no difference in performance between the two groups. Seidman, Biederman, Faraone, Weber, and Oullette (1997) reported that the critical interference score of the Stroop failed to differentiate ADHD children and adolescents, when scores were adjusted for socioeconomic status (SES), family history, comorbidity, and "all confounds."

These findings from the three clinical measures suggest, in general, that the Stroop may be the best test of inhibition in ADHD, although it is highly sensitive to other variables correlated with ADHD. Hence, without control for these confounds, it is uncertain whether the Stroop is measuring disinhibition that is uniquely due to ADHD.

Information-Processing Tasks and Measures

A shortcoming of the clinical tests is that they produce common outputs such as errors or response latency that may be the result of a web of underlying cognitive processes. In contrast, information-processing tasks are purported to differentiate the cognitive process involved in inhibition.

Inhibition to Distracting Stimuli

An inability of the subject to inhibit responses to distractors (irrelevant stimuli) provides another operationalization of disinhibition. With some exceptions (Ceci & Tishman, 1984; McIntyre, Blackwell, & Denton, 1978; Radosh & Gittelman, 1981; Rosenthal & Allen, 1980; Zentall & Shaw, 1980), the majority of studies using external distractors (e.g., radio music, noise, color discrepancy, peripheral pictures) have failed to show that ADHD children are more easily distracted than normals (see for reviews, Douglas, 1983; Douglas & Peters, 1979; van der Meere & Sergeant, 1988c). In contrast to what the distractor hypothesis predicts, task performance of ADHD children may even *improve* in the presence of a distractor (Abikoff, Szeibel, & Courtney, 1990; Zentall & Meyer, 1987; Zentall, Zentall, & Barack, 1978). Consequently, the disinhibition hypothesis of ADHD defined in terms of inability to resist distraction has been only partially supported.

Oculomotor Inhibition

The oculomotor delayed-response task requires that the subject look at a fixation point and observe (but not gaze at) a briefly presented cue whose presentation point varies in degree of arc from the fixation point. On command, the subject directs his or her gaze to the to-be-remembered locus of the cue. A greater number of premature saccades have been found in an ADHD group than controls (Ross, Hommer, Breiger, Varley, & Radant, 1994). No significant differences were found between ADHD and controls for the speed of responding on signal or accuracy of locating the cue. Methylphenidate (MPH) had no effect on the dependent variables. As noted by these authors, it is possible that this task measures a different sort of inhibition than that measured by the stop-signal task (discussed later in this chapter).

Prepulse Inhibition

Prepulse inhibition of the startle eyeblink is induced by evoking a startle eyeblink response preceded by a stimulus, called the prepulse. The prepulse inhibits (reduces) the amplitude and latency of the eyeblink (Graham, 1975). The startle reflex is evoked by a second stimulus, usually a loud noise. The inhibition of the startle eyeblink is thought to be modulated at the basal ganglia and to reflect early phases of stimulus encoding (Graham, 1975). Ornitz,

Hanna, and De Traversay (1992) found no difference between ADHD and control children in prepulse inhibition of the startle eyeblink.

Goldstein and Blumenthal (1995) in a small sample of ADHD children found no difference in the amplitude of inhibition of the prepulse effect. They also reported that the point of maximum reduction of the startle response was reached *faster* in ADHD than control subjects.

If disinhibition is equated with a failure of prepulse inhibition, these two reports are inconsistent with a disinhibition explanation for ADHD. Further, the fast automatic response of the ADHD children suggests that the automatic allocation of arousal is *more* efficient in ADHD children than controls. Should this finding be replicated, it would argue strongly against an arousal pool explanation of the ADHD deficit.

Spatial Location Tasks

In the Posner spatial location task (Posner & Raichle, 1994), cues can be informative (valid), noninformative (invalid), or neutral. Several versions of this paradigm exist, but only one is discussed here. Two boxes are presented on a screen in the left and right visual fields. One of the boxes is illuminated and is called the cue. A valid cue occurs when, for example, a box is illuminated and the target (an asterisk) appears in the box. The cue is invalid when the box is illuminated and the target does not appear in the box. A neutral condition is when the target appears in a box but *neither* box is illuminated. The typical finding is that RT for detection of a target is faster on valid trials than on neutral trials, and slower on invalid trials than neutral trials. This finding has been variously interpreted. One hypothesis is that the processing of the invalid cue requires the subject to reallocate attention; this reallocation involves a switch of attention and requires response inhibition.

A study by Swanson and colleagues (1991) found no main effect for group on RT or errors in this task. ADHD children exhibited slower RTs to the right visual field targets than to the left visual field targets in the noncued and invalid cued conditions but only when the delay between the appearance of the cue and the appearance of the target was long (800 ms) and not when it was short (100 ms). However, there were no visual field differences in the valid cue condition. Controls did not show any visual field differences under any of the three conditions.

The right visual field disadvantage for ADHD subjects was not replicated by Nigg, Swanson, and Hinshaw (1997), who found a left rather than a right field disadvantage. However, they reported a group main effect in which the ADHD subjects had slower RTs bilaterally over all conditions.

Novak, Solanto, and Abikoff (1995) reported no differences between ADHD and control children, despite the fact that the valid–invalid effect was clearly present in the task. Tomporowski, Tinsley, and Hager (1994) likewise found that ADHD children performed less well than controls and college students but did not find any visual field interaction with group.

Carter and colleagues (1995) reported that ADHD subjects were slower than controls and that there was a validity (valid cue) effect, slower RTs to right visual field targets, and notably at the slower 800-ms interval.

Pearson, Yaffee, Loveland, and Norton (1995) reported for RT no significant group main effect or interaction with the validity effect, although errors did distinguish ADHD children from controls.

The absence of a main effect for group in three (of five) studies suggest that this task is not robust in revealing either an inhibition or attention switch deficit in ADHD. The findings of a right hemisphere disadvantage are compromised by the failure of a left hemisphere disadvantage as well.

Van der Meere and Sergeant (1988b) used a task in which children were instructed to pay attention to the top-left to bottom-right (relevant) diagonal of a display but to ignore the other (irrelevant) diagonal. In half of the trials, a target appeared on the relevant diagonal and a "yes" response was required. A "no" response was required if the target was not presented on

the relevant diagonal. Targets in incorrect loci (foils) were presented on less than 10% of the target trials. ADHD children did not respond to foils more frequently than controls.

Dichotic Listening

Another type of interference occurs when subjects are required to process information presented to one ear rather than the other. Dichotic listening requires division of attention to simultaneous input to both ears. Errors of detection of signals to the designated ear and intrusion of signals from the to-be-ignored ear are used as dependent variables in this task. ADHD subjects have performed more poorly than controls in a dichotic vigilance task but not in a dichotic listening task (Loiselle, Stamn, Matinsky, & Whipple, 1980). However, in a dichotic listening task Prior, Sanson, Freethy, and Geffen (1985) reported higher d' in controls than ADHD children. Analysis of commissions and their RTs revealed that ADHD children were faster to the right than left ear, *irrespective* of shadowing instructions (Prior *et al.*, 1985). MPH does not improve ADHD performance on dichotic listening (Hiscock, Kinsbourne, Caplan, & Swanson, 1979). Given the uncertainty of the locus of the dichotic listening effect (Broadbent, 1971), we regard these studies as neutral with respect to the ADHD disinhibition hypothesis.

Stimulus–Response (S–R) Compatibility–Incompatibility

S–R compatibility–incompatibility requires that the subject first map stimulus location symmetrically to response side (target right, response right hand) and then reverse the pattern. During the reversal phase the previous dominant response requires suppression. ADHD children compared with controls and LD non-ADHD children were slower in the incompatible condition (van der Meere *et al.*, 1989). This finding implicated a deficiency in motor selection for the ADHD group. Brandeis and colleagues (1998) reported a partial replication of the S–R compatibility interaction with ADHD (inattentive subtype). A second study, using separate groups of pure ADHD without reading disability (RD), a RD group without ADHD, and a control group reported a full replication of the original differential ADHD interaction with S–R compatibility (Hall, Halperin, Schwartz, & Newcorn, 1997).

However, Zahn, Kruesi, and Rapoport (1991) did not find an S–R incompatibility interaction in boys with disruptive behavior disorders. Oosterlaan and Sergeant (1995) failed to replicate the interaction of S–R incompatibility with ADHD and argued that this was due to the event rate used. Indeed, van der Meere, Vreeling, and Sergeant (1992) demonstrated that event rate interacted with ADHD, with ADHD children becoming *slower* in this task in the slow event rate. The role of event rate and its place in the energetic system is discussed later in this chapter.

S–R incompatibility is moderately robust in differentiating ADHD children without LD from both controls and LD children without ADHD. Thus ADHD children may have a motor output deficit which may be dependent on the event rate of the task. As discussed later, this finding implicates an energetic dysfunction in ADHD.

Inhibition of Prepotent Responses

In this section we consider the role of inhibition in three different tasks and the inhibition of responses following an error. Inhibition of prepotent responses is considered a crucial test of the inhibition hypothesis (Barkley, 1997; see also Chapter 13, this volume).

Latent Inhibition. Latent inhibition is produced when a stimulus is passively pre-exposed for a number of trials and there is a subsequent decrease in the ability to form a new association of the pre-exposed stimulus with a new event (Lubow, 1989). The passive stimulus exposure presumably builds up an inhibitory effect in establishing a new conditioned relationship at the encoding stage. Lubow and Josman (1993) compared ADHD and control children. No latent inhibition effect was found in the ADHD

group. This finding is consonant with the hypothesis that ADHD children have a weak behavioral inhibition system (BIS) (Gray, 1982) that does not react to the "novelty" of the pre-exposed stimulus, and thus no habituation has occurred when it is presented later as a conditioning stimulus. Alternatively, this result can be interpreted as suggesting that disinhibitory deficits in ADHD are not due to stimulus factors, that is, input side effects, since in normals the inhibitory effect is caused by passive pre-exposure to stimuli. This finding is consonant with studies showing that external distractors do not have detrimental effects on information processing in ADHD children (see, for review, Douglas & Peters, 1979).

Go/No-Go Task. Several studies have shown that, when ADHD children are instructed to respond Go on signal trials and refrain from responding on No-Go trials, they commit more No-Go responses or errors of commission (Iaboni, Douglas, & Baker, 1995; Milich *et al.*, 1994; Shue & Douglas, 1992). Higher proportions of No-Go responses have also been reported in children with attentional problems (Grünewald-Züberbier, Grünewald, Rasche, & Netz, 1978). These data support the inhibitory deficit hypothesis in ADHD. Unclear, however, is the mechanism involved in this deficit, for example, motor selection or preparation.

Stop-Signal Task. The stop-signal task is currently the most direct measure of the processes required in inhibiting a response (Logan & Cowan, 1984; Logan, Cowan, & Davis, 1984). In this task, subjects are instructed to respond when a signal is presented and to inhibit their intended response to the signal when a stop signal (usually a tone) is presented. Stop signals are presented at different intervals before the subject's expected response. The closer the stop signal is presented to the "point of no return," the more difficult it becomes to inhibit the response. This task, in contrast to the Go/No-Go paradigm, requires suppression of a response which is already being executed.

Recently, Oosterlaan, Logan, and Sergeant (1998) conducted a meta-analysis of eight studies employing the stop-signal task studies. For the first dependent variable, the inhibition function, consistent and robust differences were found between ADHD and control children; ADHD children were less able to inhibit inappropriate responses than controls.

ADHD children also had slower stop-signal reaction times (SSRTs) than controls. Thus, poor response inhibition was attributed to slow inhibitory processing. For the third dependent variable, ZRFT-slope, no group differences were found; ADHD children did not differ from controls in their ability to trigger an inhibitory response or in variability in the latency of the inhibitory process. However, Conduct Disordered (CD) children showed impairments similar to ADHD children. Therefore, the meta-analytic findings do not support the notion that response inhibition deficits are *specifically* related to ADHD. Rather, the results suggest that poor response inhibition characterizes children with behavior characterized as disruptive (see Chapter 1, this volume).

Another issue raised by the finding that ADHD children have slower inhibitory processes (SSRT) is whether this reflects a generally slow mode of information processing characteristic of ADHD children, since ADHD children also have slower RT to the target the non–stop-signal trials.

The stop-signal task contains a third measure, ZRFT, which is the probability of triggering or inhibitory process. Oosterlaan and colleagues (1998) in their meta-analysis found no difference for this measure between ADHD children and controls or between ADHD and CD subjects or CD and control children. ZRFT is unable to explain the observed lack of inhibition to the stop signal.

The Change Task. For purposes of studying controlled adaptive functioning, the ability to suppress a response and subsequently initiate an alternative response (response reengagement) has been studied in an extension of the stop-signal task: the change task. Results of studies using this task (Oosterlaan & Sergeant, 1998; Schachar & Tannock, 1995; Schachar, Tannock, Marriott, & Logan, 1995) confirm earlier reports using the stop-signal task that

ADHD children are less able to inhibit a response compared to controls. Furthermore, these studies replicated the finding of slower inhibitory processing in ADHD children than controls. ADHD children were also observed in two of these studies (Schachar & Tannock, 1995; Schachar et al., 1995) to have slower response reengagement than controls. However, Oosterlaan and Sergeant (1998b) failed to replicate this finding.

In summary, the stop-signal studies indicate that ADHD children are less likely to inhibit a response than controls. However, measures of inhibition do not differentiate ADHD children from CD children; the stop-signal findings are not specific with respect to ADHD.

Sternberg's Response Bias Task. Another means of generating prepotent responses is to bias the responding of the subject to one response rather than another. In a study by Sternberg (1969), subjects were instructed to remember a memory set and compare this with sets of items presented on a display. A target was a match between a memory set item and one of the display set items. If a match occurred, a "yes" response was required; otherwise a "no" response was required. Sternberg varied both set size and target probability, with the more frequent targets biasing subjects toward "yes" responses; increasing the set size led to an increase of both "yes" and "no" RTs. Subjects responded faster to the most frequent response type ("yes" or "no") *independent* of the set size. This finding was interpreted to demonstrate independence of search and decision as well as a bias in the motor decision process toward faster processing of the more frequent response. This finding was replicated by Brookhuis and colleagues (1983).

Using the response bias task, one can test whether disinhibition is related to overly fast stimulus identification, a difficulty in stopping and changing the response (van der Meere, Gunning, & Stemerdink, 1996). The baseline condition had a 50% target–nontarget probability. In the response bias condition, target probability was 30%, requiring 30% "yes" responses and 70% "no" responses. Although ADHD children had slower correct "yes" *and* "no" responses than controls irrespective of condition, they were able to stop and change their intended response to the same extent as controls. There was no evidence of impulsive scanning or decision making. Consequently, these findings indicate that ADHD children are able to inhibit and change an intended response, even in conditions with high cognitive load. Errors were equally fast for ADHD and control children. Thus, a "fast guess" or impulsive strategy was absent in ADHD children.

Inhibitory Effect of Error Detection

As noted earlier in this chapter, the cognitive-energetic model was designed to include a superordinate, management, or evaluation mechanism. Vigilance researchers had shown that knowledge of results enabled the subject to adjust and improve performance. Rabbitt and Rodgers (1977) showed that subjects can correct errors faster than they can make correct responses. Presumably, this means that the subject detects the error and error correction is actually initiated before completion of the incorrect response. However, on the trial following an error, the subject takes more time to respond, apparently to ensure that a correct response is made. This is known as RT after an error (RTE+1), the "1" indicating first *correct* trial after an error. Active control of processing or allocation of attentional resources on RTE+1 trials requires inhibition of responding.

Sergeant and van der Meere (1988) found that as cognitive load increased in a search task, controls slowed RTE+1 in a linear fashion. ADHD children did not perform in this manner. When processing load was low, ADHD children had a much slower RTE+1 than controls. In contrast, when processing load was high and one would expect a slow RTE+1, ADHD children were faster than controls.

Recently, RTE+1 has been shown to become slowed by MPH (Krusch *et al.,* 1996). Drugs are considered as influencing energetic but not computational factors in the cognitive-energetic model. Krusch and colleagues' finding indicates the influence of an energetic factor on inhibitory processing.

Since both overly slow and overly fast RTE+1 latencies were observed in ADHD children, and since poor inhibition would have predicted only fast RTE+1, these findings argue against a disinhibition hypothesis. A failure to adjust to task demands, referred to as attentional allocation (Sergeant & Scholten, 1985b), offers a better account of these findings.

Summary of Studies of Response Inhibition

To recapitulate the findings with traditional clinical measures, it is unclear whether these are pure measures of response inhibition, since a variety of processes are involved.

This issue is illustrated in a study using the WCST. Fristoe, Salthouse, and Woodard, (1997) used measures of speed of performance, working memory, feedback usage, and card sorting performance (perseverative errors, categories achieved, conceptual level responses) on the WCST to predict age-related differences. They showed that speed of performance was independent of feedback and working memory in predicting the age effect. Importantly, the classical measures of card-sorting performance were independent of the so-called executive functions, working memory, and feedback use in predicting age-effects. Speed of processing (an energetic variable) accounted for the major part of the variance. Thus age-related effects on the WCST are only in part determined by measures of executive functioning and may be better explained by speed of processing. This type of fine-grained analysis is needed for clinical tests and could be facilitated by using the additive factor method (Sergeant & van der Meere, 1990b).

Twelve information-processing tasks have been reviewed to determine support for the disinhibition hypothesis in ADHD; these are summarized in Table 1.

Three tasks, the Go/No-Go, stop-signal and change task provide clear support for this hypothesis. The stop-signal and change tasks indicate that a slow inhibitory process underlies poor response inhibition in ADHD children, but this is not specific to this group; inhibitory

TABLE 1.   Performance Evidence and the Inhibition Hypothesis

None	Some	Clear
Distractor	Oculomotor delay	Go/no-go
Prepulse inhibition	Spatial location	Stop-signal
Latent inhibition	Dichotic listening	Change task
Sternberg response bias	S–R compatibility	
RTE+1		

performance measures do not differentiate ADHD from CD children. Four tasks provide some support for the inhibition hypothesis and five tasks do not. Few reports are available to determine whether claims of an inhibition deficit are specific to ADHD or apply to other externalizing disorders.

ENERGETICS

We now argue that what has been considered as evidence of an inhibition deficit in ADHD may, at least in part, be explained in terms of an energetical dysfunction. We bolster this claim by reviewing research using vigilance measures, and the variables of event rate, contingent rewards, and MPH, all of which are thought to influence the energetic state of the subject. Research is reviewed in which electrophysiological indices of energetic functioning and neuroimaging have been used. These measures complement performance measures as indices of arousal, activation, and effort. We argue against the claim that ADHD is an inhibition dysfunction the locus of which is in the frontal cortex (Barkley, 1997) and favor the position that inhibition has its locus in a circuit involving the septo-hippocampal system and its connections to the frontal cortex (Gray, 1982), a circuit involving the basal ganglia (Le Moal, 1995),* or both. These circuits are important, because they necessarily require that energetics be implicated in a comprehensive account of ADHD.

*The first author gratefully acknowledges this point made by J. Swanson.

Tasks and Energetics

Earlier in this chapter (see also Figure 1), we noted that performance deficits in ADHD children could be linked to the three energetic pools and the superordinate management mechanism of the cognitive-energetic model. Two of these pools, activation and effort, are especially relevant to the inhibition hypothesis in ADHD. Activation is directly related to the motor organization (output) side of the cognitive-energetic model, which has been implicated in ADHD (van der Meere et al., 1992). Effort in this model encompasses terms such as motivation and response to contingencies, which are also thought to be disrupted in ADHD children. We reconsider and discuss the role of the arousal pool with respect to an alternative hypothesis that ADHD is an input deficit that is reflected in poor vigilance performance, particularly in diminished d'.

Vigilance Energetics and Response Inhibition

Two important measures derived from the Continuous Performance Task (CPT; Rosvold, Mirsky, Sarason, Bransome, & Beck, 1956) are d' and β. As noted earlier, d' is a measure of perceptual sensitivity (the ability to distinguish signal and noise from noise only) and is directly modulated by the arousal pool. β is considered an index of response bias, whereby subjects may be overcautious and commit more errors of omission or may be less conservative and make a high number of errors of commission. As noted earlier, fast commission errors are considered to be a measure of impulsiveness or disinhibition. Vigilance research has shown that *reduced readiness to respond* is associated with a more conservative response strategy (high β); thus, β in the cognitive-energetic model is considered a measure of activation.

Halperin and colleagues (1988) analyzed different types of commission errors on an A-X (an X following an A is the target) CPT. A-not-X errors (responding to another letter following an A) had faster RTs than correct responses and were considered as *impulsive* errors. X-only errors (responses to an X not preceded by an A) had longer RTs than correct responses and were considered to reflect *inattention* to the letter before the X. A-only errors (a response to an A prior to the presentation of the next letter) had RTs not different from correct responses. However, A-only errors with slow RTs were considered to reflect the inability of the child to wait for the next letter and were thus also considered *impulsive*.

Impulsive (A-not-X) errors correlated significantly with teacher ratings of conduct problems, hyperactivity, and impulsivity. Inattention errors (X-only) were significantly correlated only with a rating of inattention-passivity. A-only errors were not related to any of the teacher behavior ratings.

Halperin and colleagues (1990) subsequently reported that a combination of A-not-X and slow A-only errors were significantly greater in a group of nonreferred children subtyped by behavior ratings as hyperactivity/aggressive than in a group subtyped as hyperactive, aggressive, or controls. Inattention (X-only) errors were greater in the hyperactive subgroup as compared to the other subgroups.

Halperin, Matier, Bedi, Sharma, and Newcorn (1992) reported that both impulsivity and inattention errors differentiated an ADHD group from a normal control group but not from a group with other psychiatric diagnoses. The non-ADHD psychiatric group did not differ from the normal group on impulsive errors but made more inattentive errors.

Halperin and colleagues' (1988) operationalization of impulsivity is partly based on the assumption that *both* fast and inaccurate responding (A not X errors) and slow and inaccurate responding (slow A-only errors) are valid indices of the inability to suppress responding to inappropriate stimuli. When a subject can respond "yes" (target) or "no" (not a target) a fast RT "no" response to a target may also be considered to be impulsive. What processes cause the fast RT errors? These errors may reflect any combination of process(es), such as short inspection time, rapid decision making, adjusting performance to test one's limits, or lack of planning. To sustain the claim that fast commission errors reflect only impulsivity, convergent evidence is required to show that fast commission errors *specifically* reflect an impulsive strategy and not a failure in one of the information-processing stages. Such a failure cannot be determined by the classical CPT, since it, for example, does not vary cognitive load, stimulus clarity, or response complexity (Sergeant & van der Meere, 1990b).

Response bias (β) has been considered a measure of impulsivity (Corkum, Schachar, & Siegel, 1996). The rationale is that β reflects the subject's confidence or conservativeness in responding. Conservative responding means that the subject is less likely to indicate that a stimulus is a target. Risky or impulsive responding is indicated by a low β, when the subject requires less evidence (fast responding) to decide that a stimulus is a target. One would expect that, if impulsivity characterizes ADHD children, the majority of studies would have shown that β differentiated ADHD children from controls. In a meta-analysis by Losier, McGrath, and Klein (1996), β did not distinguish ADHD children from controls. However, two studies showed that ADHD children had a lower β than controls (Nuechterlein, 1983; Satterfield, Schell, & Nicholas, 1994), as would be predicted from a "fast guess" or impulsive strategy of responding. Further, van Leeuwen and colleagues (1998) found that β differentiated ADHD from control subjects and β became *stricter* (reflecting less disinhibition) with time on task in ADHD subjects. Whether β changes with time on task and reflects changes in strategy or activation is an open question, since previous studies have not systematically used task variables that modify β.

In summary, in contrast to the proposal of Halperin and colleagues (1988), that fast A-not-X errors are equivalent to slow A-only errors, slow errors need not reflect impulsivity, but may be merely slow errors. A process or stage explanation of slow commission errors is that they reflect continued processing of stimuli the quality of which has begun to decline past an optimal point of processing. Thus they are long and still inaccurate (Ollman, 1977). This type of error has been reported by Sergeant and Scholten (1985b) and Sergeant (1988).

An energetic explanation of commission errors is that when they occur early in the task they reflect overarousal. Errors that occur later in the task, *omission* errors, reflect low activation (Sanders, 1983). Study of when in the task errors occur and what type of errors they are is needed before slow errors can be considered a valid measure of disinhibition. Similarly, the vigilance measure most appropriate for measuring impulsivity (β), has not been shown to differentiate consistently between ADHD and control children. The task variables of, for example, knowledge of results and response contingencies need to be manipulated in information-processing tasks in order to determine the role of β in ADHD.

Event Rate and Response Inhibition

Event rate, the speed with which stimuli are presented, has been shown to be an important determinant of performance and to have its locus in the activation pool (Sanders, 1983). Detection deficits in patients with right frontal lesions occur more often in a slow event rate (1 stimulus every s) than with a fast event rate (1 every 0.14 s) (Wilkins, Shallice, & McCarthy, 1987). This suggests that performance is dependent on the event rate of the task. Event rate alters the energetic state of the subject; that is, compared with the medium condition, the fast condition may induce either overarousal or overactivation, resulting in fast, inaccurate responding. A slow event rate may induce underarousal or underactivation, resulting in slow, inaccurate responding (Sanders, 1983).

Event rate differentiates controls from ADHD children in a wide variety of tasks (Chee, Logan, Schachar, Lindsay, & Wachsmuth, 1989; Conte, Kinsbourne, Swanson, Zirk, & Samuels, 1986; Dalby, Kinsbourne, Swanson, & Sobel, 1977; van der Meere *et al.,* 1992). In general, ADHD children have been found to perform more poorly in conditions of relatively slow event rates as compared with fast and moderate event rates.

Van der Meere, Stemerdink, and Gunning (1995) compared ADHD children with and without a Tic Disorder (TD) and a normal control group, using a Go/No-Go task. Stimuli were presented at three rates: a fast presentation rate (1 s), a medium presentation rate (4 s) and a slow presentation rate (8 s). Results indicated that ADHD children with and without comorbid TD made more errors of commission (i.e., responses to the No-Go stimuli) than controls. Of interest was the finding that the inefficient task behavior of ADHD-only children was related to the event rate. These children made more errors of commission in the fast and slow conditions, but not in the medium condition, thus substantially replicating the findings of van der Meere and colleagues (1992). These results suggest that ADHD children's lack of response inhibition is modulated by their inability to adjust their state.

Another type of experimental manipulation is an experimenter-paced versus a subject-self-paced task. Long self-paced tasks place demands on the effort pool of the subject (Broadbent, 1971), whereas long experimenter-paced tasks are thought to place demands primarily on the activation pool (Sanders, 1983). Sonuga-Barke, Taylor, Sembi, and Smith (1992) found that, when given a choice between a small, immediate reward and a large, delayed reward, ADHD children chose immediate reward but only when this led to shorter total task duration irrespective of the amount of reward available. When trial length was paced by the experimenter, ADHD children waited for the larger, delayed reward.

In contrast, Schweitzer and Sulzer-Azaroff (1995) reported that in a task with a choice between a large, delayed reward and a small, immediate reward in which trial length was held constant, control children chose delayed, large rewards but ADHD children more often chose the immediate, small reward. In the ensuing discussion between Sonuga-Barke (1996) and Schweitzer (1996) of the interpretation of these results, Schweitzer (1996) reported further data supporting the claim that ADHD children prefer immediate rather than delayed reward with overall duration of the task being held constant.

Sonuga-Barke, Houlberg, and Hall (1994) using the MFFT found that ADHD children in a self-paced task responded quickly only when by doing so they could reduce the total task duration. In contrast, when trial length was paced by the experimenter, ADHD children had equal RTs but remained more inaccurate than controls. On the basis of these results (and others), Sonuga-Barke (1996) argued that ADHD children are "delay aversive" and do not have a failure of inhibition.

Studies using different event rates indicate that performance in ADHD children is dependent on this variable, suggesting that the activation pool of ADHD children is in a nonoptimal state, particularly in a slow-event-rate condition. Results of tasks in which delay is controlled by the experimenter have, in general, been interpreted as evidence of delay aversion in ADHD children. The usefulness of the concept of delay aversion (Sonuga-Barke, 1996) in comparison with disinhibition, however, is not clear. If an ADHD child finds waiting aversive, a logical strategy is to shorten the waiting period by selecting a smaller reward. This would seem to be disinhibition, by most definitions, as it is inefficient performance for obtaining the greatest reward.

Performance on paced tasks appear to be dependent on event rate that can either normalize (fast event rate) or detrimentally influence performance (slow event rate in all studies and, in some instances, fast event rate). An inhibition-deficit explanation of the information-processing performance of ADHD needs to show that disinhibitory responding occurs *independently* of event rate. Currently, no evidence exists that this is the case.

Contingencies

In the cognitive-energetic model, contingent reward operates on the management part of the system. The effect of reward has been conceived of as central to ADHD (Douglas, 1983, 1989). Several tasks have been used to assess response inhibition and the effects of reward on performance in ADHD children.

Daugherty and Quay (1991) reported a study using a task in which the probability of a reward decreased by 10% with each succeeding 10 trials (i.e., from 90% to 0%). Both the comorbid ADHD+CD group and CD group tended to persist in responding despite increasingly unfavorable odds. It is not clear whether the poor performance of ADHD+CD children points to a deficit in response inhibition or is due to an unusual sensitivity to reward, or both.

Gordon (1979) used a delay task (DRL; differential reinforcement for low-rate responding) in which the child was told, if he "waits first" before pressing the button, he can earn a point. The task is programmed to dispense "points" on a fixed-interval basis (usually 6 s) The child is not told the interval. If the child responds before this time, the timer resets and another 6 s must elapse before a point is dispensed after a key press. Premature responses and earned points are recorded to compute an "efficiency ratio" (points earned divided by total responses). Gordon (1979) and McClure and Gordon (1984) showed that ADHD children were unable to withhold their responses as evidenced by their large number of nonrewarded responses. Solanto (1990) compared the performance of ADHD children to controls under conditions of baseline, reward, and response cost. Although ADHD children had lower efficiency ratio under all three conditions they improved their performance equally under both reward and response cost.

Daugherty and Quay (1991), however, reported that ADHD, ADHD+CD, anxious-withdrawn children, and controls did not differ on this task. Similarly, Loge, Staton, and Beatty (1990) reported no difference between ADHD subjects and normals on a DRL.

Other studies have failed to find differences between ADHD and control groups in the effect of reward or response cost on measures of RT and of inhibitory control (Douglas & Parry, 1994; Iaboni et al., 1995). Iaboni and colleagues (1995) found that ADHD children responded faster in response cost than in reward. The number of commission errors made by ADHD children was greater than controls but there was no differential effect between the groups due to reward or response cost.

Oosterlaan and Sergeant (1998a), using the stop-signal task, compared the impact of reward and response cost on response inhibition in ADHD children, normal control children, and two psychopathological groups: a group of disruptive children and a group of anxious children. Response contingencies were used to enhance children's effort. The aim was to determine whether inhibition effects would be similar for reward and response cost. It was reasoned that, if contingencies are ineffective in ameliorating poor response inhibition, this would render an effort explanation unlikely and provide support for the primacy of an inhibition deficit in ADHD. In contrast, it was argued that, if effort underlies impaired response inhibition, this impairment would be remedied by response contingencies. Compared with normal controls, ADHD children showed a lower probability of inhibition and slower inhibitory processes under both reward and response cost. This finding does not support Douglas's earlier suggestion (1989) that response cost is particularly effective with ADHD children and strengthens their inhibitory control. This finding also does not support an effort hypothesis of ADHD.

Solanto, Wender, and Bartell (1997), using an A-X CPT, reported a tendency ($p = .07$) for a combination of reward for correct responses and response cost for errors to improve d' but to have no effect on deterioration of performance over time. β decreased over time on task irrespective of condition (contingencies or MPH). This diminished tendency to respond over time would not be predicted by the disinhibition hypothesis.

Van der Meere, Hughes, Börger, and Sallee (1995), who used the CPT with a reward

and nonreward condition, reported that ADHD children not comorbid for CD did not differ from controls in the effect of reward. However, ADHD+CD children differed from both controls and ADHD children in being more sensitive to the effect of reward (improvement in performance) with time on task, in contrast to Solanto and colleagues (1997).

The studies just mentioned suggest that response contingencies have subtle interactions with task structure and with group membership. Further, there is evidence that inhibition deficits can be observed in both ADHD and CD children, independent of response contingencies. From an energetic point of view, this suggests that lack of effort cannot explain the inhibitory deficit observed in the ADHD or ADHD+CD group. One possibility is that the effort pool is more involved in the CD group. Differences between studies for the ADHD+CD group may reflect a difference in the number and type of the ADHD and CD symptoms in the comorbid groups.

Methylphenidate and Energetics

MPH clearly enhances the ability to sustain attention in ADHD children. Losier and colleagues (1996; see also Chapter 10, this volume, for an extensive discussion) conducted a meta-analysis of 15 studies using the CPT and MPH with ADHD children. Their analysis indicated that MPH decreased errors of both commission and omission. They further analyzed the relationship between d' and β and, for example, shorter target duration, fewer trials, higher target probabilities, and type of stimuli. They concluded that MPH operated on the input side of the system and, in particular, on the arousal pool. If this argument is proved to be correct, it would imply that inhibitory deficits have a locus very different from our postulated activation deficit in the cognitive-energetic model.

We question Losier and colleagues' (1996) conclusion for two reasons. In the 15 studies the two CPT task variables of shorter target duration (exposure time) and fewer trials result in a short time on task (varying from 5 to 17 min with a modal time of 9 min). It is, therefore, open to question whether the time-on-task effect measured in these tasks reflects only arousal or activation as well. Since time on task was relatively short and arousal effects were measured early in the CPT, some studies might reflect only arousal effects, others a combination of arousal and early activation effects. Critical for the arousal hypothesis is that the greatest difference between groups be found *early* in time on task, as for example, in the study by Sykes and colleagues (1973).

In contrast, Corkum and colleagues (1996) and van der Meere, Shalev, Börger, and Gross-Tsur (1995) showed that the greatest time-on-task effect was found in the last phase of the task, implicating the activation pool. Further, they used a relatively long event rate, thus placing extra activation demands on their ADHD group. Consequently, one CPT study (Sykes *et al.,* 1973) indicates that arousal may be involved and two other CPT studies implicate the activation pool. It is conceivable that both findings validly reflect an ADHD energetic deficiency, measured in tasks with different time on task.

A second reason that we question Losier and colleagues' (1996) conclusion that ADHD is an input deficit is that the input stage is, in the cognitive-energetic model, the encoding stage. Sergeant and van der Meere (1990b) reviewed the eight available encoding studies in ADHD subjects. No evidence was found for an encoding stage deficiency. Hence, these studies suggest that ADHD does not involve an input dysfunction.

When motor demands and MPH have been manipulated, for example, using the stop-signal task, MPH has been shown to improve the probability of inhibition and SSRT (Tannock, Schachar, & Logan, 1995). However, MPH in one study did not show an interaction with S–R incompatibility (de Sonneville, Njiokik-tjien, & Hilhorst, 1991). Two studies failed to find a response bias interaction with MPH (van der Meere *et al.,* 1996; Fobel-Smithee, Klorman, Brumaghim, & Borgstedt, 1998). Which motor process or processes interact with MPH have not yet been conclusively identified, with the excep-

tion of motor inhibition in the stop-signal task. The contrast in studies suggests that the inhibition processes in these two types of tasks may be different or that MPH targets a motor process not measured by response bias tasks.

In this section we have reviewed the relationship between tasks and energetic factors. Using vigilance measures d′ and β, there is clear-cut evidence that d′ is lower in ADHD children than controls. In general β has not differentiated between the groups but, it can be argued, it has not been optimally studied. From the point of view of an inhibition hypothesis, this is disconcerting, since β should differentiate ADHD from controls. At the same time, a high β can be achieved by *fast* omission errors (subject is quick to respond that the stimulus is *not* a target), which could also reflect disinhibition.

In summary, we favor the interpretation that limitations in energetic maintenance, allocation, or both occur in ADHD children, and these limitations lead to apparent disinhibitory behavior. Further clarity on this issue may be gained by coupling psychophysiological measures that tap the energetic pools to tasks that measure performance. For example, reward has been shown to be associated with less alpha power in the left mid and left frontal regions, whereas punishment is associated with less alpha power in the right frontal region (Sobotka, Davidson, & Senulis, 1992). These investigators also reported that these effects were independent of preparation as measured by the contingent negative variation (CNV). CNV amplitude was larger during fast than slow trials, suggesting that the energetic factor associated with preparation may be independent of the energetic effects of reward and punishment.

State Regulation and Energetics

General

We have argued that the disinhibition in ADHD is related to the energetics of the psychophysiological system. Energetics and the concept of state have a long history with regard to functioning of the nervous system. Hebb

(1949) wrote that neuropsychological functioning and organization was dependent on "a very delicate timing which might be disturbed by metabolic changes as well as by sensory events that do not accord with the pre-existent central processes" (p. xix). Thus, performance deficiencies may reflect mismatches between the actual state of the organism and the state required to perform a particular task. As noted earlier, the concept of state refers to the overall level of alertness of the subject (Posner, 1978). State regulation, in turn, refers to "energy mobilization," which is necessary to change the state of the organism in the direction that is optimal for a task or situation, referred to as the "required or target state" (Hockey, 1979). State regulation has a strong resemblance to terms such as mental effort and motivation, and may be considered to be the energetic part of frontal lobe functioning (Mulder, 1986).

Electrophysiology, Energetics, and Inhibition

Research into the relationship between energetics and inhibition in ADHD began in the 1970s. The then provocative finding was that ADHD children were, contrary to expectation, underaroused (Satterfield & Dawson, 1971). Satterfield and colleagues (1974) followed up this report by a review that suggested that a subgroup of ADHD children had a predominance of slow EEG activity, increased energy in the low-frequency bands, and large amplitude of evoked responses. They interpreted these results as indicating that an ADHD subgroup had low central nervous system (CNS) arousal. This, they hypothesized, was due to "insufficient CNS inhibition" (p. 841) and the fact that low CNS inhibition and low arousal covary. It was then found that ADHD boys under 7.5 years had smaller event-related potentials (P2–N2), suggestive of being underaroused. In contrast, older ADHD children had larger event-related potentials, suggesting overarousal (Satterfield & Braley, 1977). Satterfield, Schell, Backs, and Hidaka (1984) reported that in normal children but not ADHD children power spectral intensities decreased with increasing age, which was inter-preted as evidence of slower maturation of the CNS in ADHD children. Grünewald-Züberbier and colleagues (1978) showed that, in the period immediately prior to a motor response, alpha attenuation and CNV amplitude (reflecting the activation pool) were lower in ADHD children. Grünewald, Grünewald-Züberbier, and Netz (1978) found in a Go/No-Go task that alpha attenuation was related to No-Go responses. This work supported the hypothesis that energetic failures underlie the inhibitory dysfunction of ADHD children.

Klorman (1995) concluded that lower autonomic nervous system (ANS) responsiveness was characteristic of ADHD, which, like event-related potentials, could be improved by using MPH (Klorman, Salzman, Pass, Borgstedt, & Dainer, 1979; Michael, Klorman, Saltzman, Borgstedt, & Dainer, 1981). The influence of MPH on ANS responsiveness has been found for both younger (Klorman, Brumaghim, Fitzpatrick, Borgstedt, & Strauss, 1994) and adolescent children with ADHD (Klorman, Brumaghim, Fitzpatrick, & Borgstedt, 1992). Tannock, Ickowicz, and Schachar (1995) demonstrated that in a working memory task high doses of MPH (0.9 mg/kg) improved performance in a fast but not a slow event rate. These findings suggests that MPH has, on the one hand, normalizing effects on ANS and CNS arousal-activation and, on the other hand, that the MPH effect on performance measures is dependent on the event rate used in a task.

A slow event rate induces underactivation in ADHD children compared with controls (van der Meere *et al.,* 1992). Succeeding research (van der Meere, Hughes, *et al.,* 1995) indicated that ADHD children showed a rapid performance decrement when stimuli were presented slowly (no manipulation of event rate) and when children had to perform without supervision. In terms of state regulation, the data suggest that ADHD children are not able, or are unwilling, to allocate extra energy in order to adjust their underactive state during the later course of the CPT.

This hypothesis has been recently tested using the 0.10 Hz component of HR variability, which is considered to be a psychophysiological index of mental effort (Mulder, 1992). The more effort the subject allocates, the smaller the variability of the 0.10 Hz component. The variability of the 0.10 Hz component was found to be related to on- and off-task behavior of ADHD children: the smaller the variance of the 0.10 Hz, the less on-task behavior; the larger variance in 0.10 Hz, the more off-task behavior while performing a CPT without supervision and using a slow presentation rate (Börger, van der Meere, Ronner, Alberts, & Geuze, 1997). Because only one stimulus presentation rate was used with only an unsupervised condition, interactions between event rate and supervision could not be determined. The investigators also could not determine whether the 0.10 Hz component, which increased with time on task was due to the activation or the effort pool.

Using a stop-signal task, Jennings, van der Molen, Pelham, Brock-Debski, and Hoza, (1997) concluded that ADHD children have an appropriate capability for inhibition, but that the regulation of response processes requires greater control in ADHD relative to controls. Based on Gray's model (Gray, 1982) and the predictions derived from this model by Fowles (1988), Iaboni, Douglas, and Ditto (1997) hypothesized that HR reactivity during reward reflects activity in the behavioral activation system (BAS), and skin conductance level (SCL) during extinction reflects activity in the BIS. Compared with controls, ADHD children failed to show increased skin conductance level (SCL) during extinction, suggesting a weak BIS, as predicted by Quay (1997). ADHD children also displayed faster HR habituation to reward, which is consistent with the prediction that ADHD children have a less dominant BAS (Quay, 1988, 1997). These results clearly implicate a weak BIS and a possible energetic dysfunction in that system in ADHD children.

Neuroimaging Studies

Because the inhibition hypothesis of ADHD has, for some researchers, been tightly linked with the "frontal" metaphor (Barkley, 1997; Pennington & Ozonoff, 1996), the ob-

jective of this section is to address the evidence favoring a frontal deficit or an energetic deficit hypothesis. Considerable interest has been generated in reports using a variety of neuroimaging modalities: anatomical magnetic resonance imaging (MRI), functional MRI (fMRI), positron emission tomography (PET), and Single Positron Emission Computerized Tomography (SPECT). PET methodology reflects use of brain glucose and fMRI the flow of blood in the brain. These methods differ in their temporal resolution; fMRI has temporal resolution superior to that of PET and SPECT.

Lou, Henriksen, and Bruhn (1984) and Lou, Henriksen, Bruhn, Borner, and Nielsen (1989) used SPECT measures of blood flow and reported that ADHD subjects had hypoperfusion of striatal and frontal brain areas (about 10% lower than normal) and hyperperfusion of occipital brain areas. Importantly, when MPH was administered, perfusion increased in the left but not right striatum (Lou et al., 1989). Castellanos and colleagues (1994) reported that ADHD males had smaller *right* caudate volumes while controls exhibited a right larger than left asymmetry which was not the case with the ADHD subjects. In contrast, Filipek, Semrud-Clikeman, Steingard, Kennedy, and Biederman (1997) reported smaller *left* caudate areas in ADHD children, who also differed from controls by having larger left than right frontal lobes.

Zametkin and colleagues (1990) used PET and reported that adults with a history of ADHD in childhood had about 10% lower global glucose metabolism than the control subjects in many brain areas. However, subsequent study of ADHD adolescents and controls (Zametkin et al., 1993) found decreased glucose metabolism in only 6 out of 60 brain imaged areas.

Casey, Castellanos, and colleagues (1997) correlated MRI scans of ADHD children and age-matched normal controls with three tasks: a forced-choice discrimination, S–R compatibility, and Go/No-Go. Significant differences in RT were observed between ADHD and normals on all three tasks. Correlations were performed between RT and accuracy with MRI scans in the three tasks.

The results of this study are complex and are often inconsistent with respect to the ADHD control comparison. For example, in the control condition of the discrimination task, accuracy for the ADHD subjects was positively correlated with right caudate volume, while for the control subjects accuracy is negatively correlated with caudate volume. In the inhibition trials on this task, accuracy was positively correlated with right prefrontal volume for the controls but there was no such correlation for the ADHD subjects. In the inhibition condition of the Go/No-Go task, accuracy was *negatively* correlated with right prefrontal volume in the ADHD group while there was no correlation between prefrontal volume and accuracy in the control group. Direct comparisons of the ADHD and control groups with respect to inhibition and MRI results are limited by the small number of correlations for either group between the two types of variables, that is, inhibition performance and MRI. There were no systematic correlates across the groups between inhibitory performance and brain regions imaged in this study.

Filipek and colleagues (1997) reported that right anterior-superior hemisphere regions (right posterior prefrontal cortex, motor association area, and midanterior cingulate) are reduced in ADHD children. These areas are implicated in the arousal and executive networks proposed by Posner and Raichle (1994). If replicated, the results could suggest that *both* an energetic and a control mechanism would explain the ADHD deficit. This argument is strengthened by the finding that both speed and accuracy in a forced-choice discrimination task was greater in normal children with larger anterior cingulate volumes (Casey, Trainor, *et al.*, 1997).

In view of the involvement of the basal ganglia in the arousal pool (Robbins & Everitt, 1995) and the volumetric deficiencies mentioned in the preceding paragraph, the performance deficiencies of ADHD children implicate the right frontal cortex, the cerebellum, and the basal ganglia (Houk & Wise, 1995). In addition, volumetric studies suggest a smaller anterior corpus callosum in ADHD adolescents

(Giedd *et al.*, 1994). This is of interest, since there is evidence that callosal efficiency is related to sustained attention (Rueckert, Sorensen, & Levy, 1994) and that patients with right frontal lesions involving the corpus callosum show a clear decline in performance with time on task (Rueckert & Grafman, 1996). Using intact children who were subgrouped into those with a prior high and low information-processing efficiency of the corpus callosum, Rueckert and Levy (1996) reported that the poorest sustained-attention performance was found in the inefficient group, especially when a slow event rate was used. These combined findings suggest that energetic differences between ADHD and control children may be related to a circuit that involves the basal ganglia, anterior corpus callosum, and right frontal structures.

Evidence for such a failure in circuitry using PET imaging in a vigilance task recently has been reported (Paus *et al.*, 1997). These researchers showed that in normal subjects decline in RT with time on task was related to lower cerebral blood flow in the medial thalamus, midbrain brain reticular formation, and substantia innominata (structures involved in the regulation of arousal and activation). When subjects began the vigilance task, in which arousal is required, large increases in cerebral blood flow were observed in the right frontal lobe. As time on task progressed and the activation pool was required, cerebral blood flow in the right ventro-lateral frontal cortex decreased.

These results are consonant with the two-component energetic allocation (arousal and activation) as discussed earlier. Further, the reported asymmetries are consonant with models of lateralized energetic specialization of the brain (Kinsbourne, 1973; Kinsbourne & Hicks, 1978; Posner & Raichle, 1994; Tucker & Williamson, 1984). Of interest is the finding that ADHD children (especially those with LD) improve lateralized performance when right hemispheric inhibition is increased by MPH (Malone, Kershner, & Siegal, 1988). It should be noted that a succeeding study demonstrated that this effect was accounted for by those children with comorbid LD and may, therefore, reflect reading ability rather than ADHD itself (Malone, Couitis, Kershner, & Logan, 1994). Hence, while normal controls may show the predicted pattern of energetic allocation in a vigilance task (Paus *et al.*, 1997), it remains to be demonstrated whether the double energetic allocation in vigilance will discriminate ADHD from control children.

Some remarks concerning imaging methodology seem appropriate. The very large number of independent tests conducted without adjustment of alpha level reported in neuroimaging studies makes it possible that false positive results have been reported. Further, the majority of neuroimaging studies employ the subtractive methodology, which makes the assumption that the difference between rest and task measured by a difference image is a valid index of functioning.

A more convincing methodology is the additive factor method (Jonides *et al.*, 1997). This method requires that the task demands be linearly increased and that the neuroimaging effect be monitored over a range of these demands. Correlations between anatomical MRI and task performance (not measured with MRI) cannot prove that the *processes* required for cognitive tasks are the same ones measured in a resting condition. It has been further shown in PET research that event rate has considerable effect on which structures of the brain are activated (Bench *et al.*, 1993).

On the basis of imaging studies, the locus of the ADHD deficit seems to involve a circuit that includes (right) frontal structures, corpus callosum, the caudate, and the basal ganglia. How far these structures reflect performance deficits on particular tasks or generalize between tasks is currently undetermined. Neuroimaging studies, at this point, remain suggestive but not conclusive concerning the role of energetic factors. Imaging studies suggest that complex circuits spreading throughout the brain, not just the frontal cortex, are involved in some of the classical measures of behavioral inhibition.

CONCLUSIONS

We have argued that it is an oversimplification to conclude that ADHD children uniquely suffer from an inhibition deficit that accounts for all of the experimental findings of impaired performance on a myriad of tasks (Barkley, 1997, see also Chapter 13, this volume). Without doubt, the results of a wide variety of tests and tasks can be interpreted as showing disinhibition in ADHD. However, alternative explanations for many of the findings have not yet been ruled out. We have drawn attention to the role of state or energetic factors that may generate responses that suggest an inhibitory defect. Furthermore, reward, response cost, and event rate influence findings to such a degree that the usefulness of disinhibition as an overall explanatory concept can be called into question.

A second line of difficulty with an inhibition deficit explanation of ADHD is that various tasks purported to measure inhibition have failed to distinguish ADHD from controls. More seriously, tasks designed to measure a specific aspect of inhibition either find no evidence of an inhibition defect or find evidence that can be only partially dovetailed into an inhibition explanation. For example, Sergeant and van der Meere (1988) demonstrated that error detection and correction can occur normally in ADHD children; only at the highest level of cognitive load do ADHD children respond without due reflection.

A third point is that tasks considered as relatively pure measures of inhibition, for example, the stop-signal task, when used to discriminate between ADHD, CD, and comorbid ADHD+CD children are unable to find a deficit specific to ADHD (see Oosterlaan *et al.*, 1998). This finding could be interpreted to mean that all three groups are representative of a common disinhibitory psychopathology (Quay, 1988, 1997). Alternatively, these groups may exhibit a common deficit on the stop-signal task but this deficit may be produced by (as yet unknown) different mechanisms. Whichever interpretation is later found to be correct, it does not appear that ADHD children are the only psychopathological subgroup who have inhibitory difficulties.

We do not know whether the hypothesized inhibitory deficit in ADHD reflects a central (cortical) or a peripheral (motor) deficit. For example, in the stop-signal task it has been shown with ERPs and the electromyogram that two classes of failures to stop can be distinguished: central and peripheral (De Jong, Coles, & Logan, 1995). The central mechanism operates by inhibiting response activation processes in cortical motor structures to prevent central outflow of motor commands. The peripheral mechanism operates by preventing the actual execution of central motor commands by blocking transmission of such commands. This latter mechanism can inhibit responses even when the central mechanism has passed the point of no return. Apparent failures of response suppression need not always reflect impulsivity but may reflect deficits in either central or peripheral control mechanisms. It is of interest that the central mechanism described here is similar to Gray's (1982) suggestion that central BIS enervation leads to peripheral inhibition of ongoing motor programs.

Response inhibition is part of what has been referred to as an executive function (Barkley, 1996; Denckla, 1994; Pennington & Ozonoff, 1996). Executive function is believed to be a prefrontal function. Pennington and Ozonoff (1996) concluded: "Since an underlying inhibition deficit provides a straightforward explanation of ADHD, we can make a fairly strong case for a primary EF deficit" (p. 80). This is, in our opinion, an oversimplification. First, it does not take account of what *produces* the apparent disinhibitory behavior. Second, the strong version of the "frontal hypothesis" fails to take into account the many circuits required in neuropsychological tests of frontal functioning. There are a variety of alternatives other than the prefrontal lobes. The (pre)frontal lobe is the end station of a limbic and midbrain system. State regulation and inhibition are, we suggest, interwoven to such a degree that we wonder whether it is possible to develop tasks that measure purely the one or the other concept. The available imaging research suggests that circuits rather than specific loci are implicated in ADHD.

In the brief review of neuroimaging studies, the heterogeneity of findings and their dependence on event rate was noted. At this point we draw attention to a commonality among these studies. Authors have reported not only frontal functioning differences but also midbrain and basal ganglia differences between ADHD and control children. The frontal results have been emphasized without due attention to the midbrain and basal ganglia circuits. Animal research has shown that dopaminergic innervation of the nucleus accumbens septi mediates activation on the overall probability of responding but not its speed (Cole & Robbins, 1989). Modulation of activity in both the dorsal and ventral striatum influences the preparation of responses in anticipation of a signal to respond. We emphasize that the reciprocal relation between these circuits and frontal circuits has yet to be clarified before identifying impulsive responding as being evidence of a frontal dysfunction.

We have noted that both imaging and information-processing studies have produced results suggesting a greater right hemisphere dysfunction in ADHD. However, some studies indicate that this apparent right hemisphere effect may be due to comorbid LD (Malone *et al.*, 1994). Hence, prior to acceptance of a right hemisphere dysfunction, imaging studies need to take account of and control for LD.

We have argued that the hypothesized inhibition deficit in ADHD is dependent on the state of the subject and the allocation of energy to the tasks at hand. We acknowledge that the cognitive-energetic model is not without its limitations. For example, specificity of the relationship of measures to pools is not, at present, satisfactory. Second, in animal studies it is known that there is not always a direct relationship between performance and energetics (Brener, 1987).

The considerable evidence that ADHD children manifest problems in inhibition (passive avoidance), means that a deficit in *behavioral* inhibition is difficult to deny. The question becomes that of what lies behind the observed deficit. Quay (1988, 1997) has argued that the underlying problem is an underresponsive BIS (Gray, 1984). According to Gray, the BIS involves the septo-hippocampal area and its connections to the frontal cortex.

Why does the BIS not work as well in ADHD as it does in controls and anxious children? It is highly unlikely that the problem is anatomical; no evidence exists that parts of the BIS are missing in ADHD children. What is more likely is that the BIS is *underaroused*, possibly due to diminished norepinephrine inputs from the locus coeruleus. Why does MPH enhance performance in ADHD children? One possibility is that it increases *arousal/activation* in the BIS.

We can also entertain the possibility that the BIS of the ADHD child responds adequately to cues of punishment or nonreward but that the output of the BIS, whereby go-behavior is suppressed, is faulty. In terms of the cognitive-energetic model, there is inadequate *activation* of the actual inhibitory mechanism. It seems that effort is a less attractive explanation for the ADHD deficit, since inhibitory differences can be observed, despite reward and response cost. The evidence suggests that the activation pool is necessary for inhibition of a motor response to occur and is crucial in explaining disinhibition in ADHD.

References

Abikoff, H., Szeibel, P. J., & Courtney, M. E. (1990). *The effects of auditory distractors on the academic performance of ADHD and normal boys.* Poster presented at the annual meeting of the American Academy of Child and Adolescent Psychiatry, Chicago.

American Psychiatric Association. (1994). *Diagnostic and statistical manual of mental disorders* (4th ed.). Washington, DC: Author.

Anderson, S. W., Damasio, H., Jones, R. D., & Tranel, D. (1991). Wisconsin card sorting test performance as a measure of frontal lobe damage. *Journal of Clinical and Experimental Neuropsychology, 13,* 909–992.

Barkley, R. A. (1991). The ecological validity of laboratory and analogue assessment methods of ADHD symptoms. *Journal of Abnormal Child Psychology, 19,* 149–178.

Barkley, R. A. (1994). Impaired delayed responding: A unified theory of Attention-Deficit Hyperactivity Disorder. In D. K. Routh (Ed.), *Disruptive behavior disorders in childhood: Essays honoring Herbert C. Quay* (pp. 11–57). New York: Plenum.

Barkley, R. A. (1996). Linkages between attention and executive functions. In G. R. Lyon & N. A. Krasnegor (Eds.), *Attention, memory, and executive function* (pp. 307–326). Baltimore: Brookes.

Barkley, R. A. (1997). Behavioral inhibition, sustained attention, and executive functions: Constructing a unifying theory of ADHD. *Psychological Bulletin, 121,* 65–94.

Barkley, R. A., Grodzinsky, G., & DuPaul, G. (1992). Frontal lobe functions in attention deficit disorder with and without hyperactivity: A review and research report. *Journal of Abnormal Child Psychology, 20,* 163–188.

Bench, C. J., Frith, C. D., Grasby, P. M., Friston, K. J., Paulesu, E., Frackowiak, R. S. J., & Dolan, R. J. (1993). Investigations of the functional anatomy of attention using the Stroop test. *Neuropsychologia, 31,* 907–922.

Berg, E. A. (1948). A simple objective test for measuring flexibility in thinking. *Journal of General Psychology, 39,* 15–22.

Boiten, F., Sergeant, J. A., & Geuze., R. (1992). Event-related desynchronization: The effects of energetic and computational demands. *Electroencephalography and Clinical Neurophysiology, 82,* 302–309.

Börger, N., Meere, J. J. van der, Ronner, A., Alberts, A., & Geuze, R. (1997). *Heart rate variability and sustained attention in ADHD* (Manuscript in preparation).

Boucagnani, L. L., & Jones, R. W. (1989). Behaviors analogous to frontal dysfunction in children with attention deficit hyperactivity disorder. *Archives of Clinical Neuropsychology, 4,* 161–173.

Brandeis, D., Leeuwen, T. van, Rubia, K., Vitacco, D., Steger, J., Pascual-Marqui, R. D., & Steinhausen, H.-Ch. (1998). Neuroelectric mapping reveals precursor of stop failures in children with attention deficits. *Behavioural Brain Research, 94,* 111–125.

Brener, J. (1987). Behavioral energetics: Some effects of uncertainty on the mobilization and distribution of energy. *Psychophysiology, 24,* 499–512.

Broadbent, D. E. (1971). *Decision and stress.* New York: Academic Press.

Brookhuis, K. A., Mulder, G., Mulder, L. J. J., Gloerich, A. B. M., Dellen, H. J. van, Meere, J. J. van der, & Ellerman, H. H. (1983). Late positive components and stimulus evaluation time. *Biological Psychology, 13,* 107–123.

Campbell, S. B., Douglas, V. I., & Morgenstern, G. (1971). Cognitive styles in hyperactive children and the effect of methylphenidate. *Journal of Child Psychology and Psychiatry, 12,* 55–67.

Campbell, S. B., Endman, M. W., & Bernfeld, G. (1977). A three-year follow-up of hyperactive preschoolers into elementary school. *Journal of Child Psychology and Psychiatry, 18,* 239–250.

Carter, C. S., Krener, P., Chaderjian, M., Northcutt, C., & Wolfe, V. (1995). Asymmetrical visual-spatial attentional performance in ADHD: Evidence for a right hemispheric deficit. *Biological Psychiatry, 37,* 788–797.

Casey, B. J., Castellanos, F. X., Giedd, J. N., Marsh, W. L., Hamburger, S. D., Schubert, A. B., Vauss, Y. C., Vaituzis, C. K., Dickstein, D. P., Sarfatti, S. E., & Rapoport, J. L. (1997). Implication of right frontostriatal circuitry in response inhibition and attention deficit/hyperactivity disorder. *Journal of the American Academy of Child and Adolescent Psychiatry, 36,* 374–383.

Casey, B. J., Trainor, R., Giedd, J., Vauss, Y., Vaituzis, C. K., Dickstein, D. P., Sarfatti, S. E., Hamburger, S., Kozuch, P., & Rapoport, J. L. (1997). The role of the anterior cingulate in automatic and controlled processes: A developmental neuroanatomical study. *Developmental Psychobiology, 30,* 61–69.

Castellanos, F. X., Giedd, J. N., Eckburg, P., Marsh, W. L., Vaituzis, C., Kaysen, D., Hamburger, S., Hamburger, S., & Rapoport, J. L. (1994). Quantitative morphology of the caudate nucleus in attention deficit hyperactivity disorder. *American Journal of Psychiatry, 151,* 1791–1796.

Ceci, S. J., & Tishman, J. (1984). Hyperactivity and incidental memory: Evidence for attentional diffusion. *Child Development, 55,* 192–203.

Chee, P., Logan, G., Schachar, R., Lindsay, P., Wachsmuth, R. (1989). Effects of event rate and display time on sustained attention in hyperactive, normal and control children. *Journal of Abnormal Child Psychology, 17,* 371–391.

Chelune, G. J., Fergusson, W., Koon, R., & Dickey, T. O. (1986). Frontal lobe disinhibition in attention deficit disorder. *Child Psychiatry and Human Development, 16,* 221–234.

Cohen, N. J., Weiss, G., & Minde, K. (1972). Cognitive styles in adolescents previously diagnosed as hyperactives. *Journal of Child Psychology and Psychiatry, 13,* 203–209.

Cole, B. J., & Robbins, T. A. W. (1989). Effects of 6-hydroxydopamine lesions of the nucleus accumbens septi on performance of a 5-choice serial reaction time task in rats: Implications for theories of selective attention and arousal. *Behavioural Brain Research, 33,* 165–179.

Conte, R., Kinsbourne, M., Swanson, J., Zirk, H., & Samuels, M. (1986). Presentation rate effects on paired associate learning by attention deficit disordered children. *Child Development, 57,* 681–687.

Corkum, P. V., Schachar, R. J., & Siegel, L. S. (1996). Performance on the continuous performance task and the impact of reward. *Journal of Attention Disorders, 1,* 114–121.

Dalby, J. I., Kinsbourne, M., Swanson, J. M., & Sobel, M. P. (1977). Hyperactive children's underuse of learning time: Correction by stimulant treatment. *Child Development, 48,* 1448–1453.

Daugherty, T. K., & Quay, H. C. (1991). Response perseveration and delayed responding in childhood behavior disorders. *Journal of Child Psychology and Psychiatry, 32,* 453–461.

De Jong, R., Coles, M. G. H., & Logan, G. D. (1995). Strategies and mechanisms in nonselective and selective inhibitory motor control. *Journal of Experimental Psychology, 21,* 498–511.

Denckla, M. B. (1994). Measurement of executive function. In G. R. Lyon (Ed.), *Frames of reference for the assessment of learning disabilities: New views on measurement issues* (pp. 117–142). Baltimore: Brookes.

Douglas, V. I. (1983). Attentional and cognitive problems. In M. Rutter (Ed.), *Developmental neuropsychiatry* (pp. 280–328). New York: Guilford.

Douglas, V. I. (1989). Can Skinnerian theory explain attention deficit disorder? A reply to Barkley. In L. M. Bloomingdale & J. Swanson (Eds.), *Attention deficit disorder: Current concepts and emerging trends in attentional and behavioral disorders of childhood* (pp. 235–254). Elmsford, NY: Pergamon.

Douglas, V. I., & Parry, P. A. (1994). Effects of reward and nonreward on frustration and attention in attention deficit disorder. *Journal of Abnormal Child Psychology, 22,* 281–302.

Douglas, V. I., & Peters, K. G. (1979). Towards a clearer definition of the attentional cognitive deficit of hyperactive children. In G. A. Hale & M. Lewis (Eds), *Attention and cognitive development* (pp. 173–247). New York: Plenum.

DuPaul, G. J., Anastopoulos, A. D., Shelton, T. L., Guevremont, D. C., & Metevia, L. (1992). Multimethod assessment of attention deficit hyperactivity disorder: The diagnostic utility of clinic-based tests. *Journal of Clinical Child Psychology, 21,* 394–402.

Filipek, P. A., Semrud-Clikeman, M., Steingard, R. J., Kennedy, D. N., & Biederman, J. (1997). Volumetric MRI analysis comparing attention-deficit hyperactivity disorder and normal controls. *Journal of Child Neurology, 48,* 589–601.

Fobel-Smithee, J. A., Klorman, R., Brumaghim, J. T., & Borgstedt, A. D. (1998). Methylphenidate does not modify the impact of response frequency or stimulus sequence on performance and event-related potentials of children with Attention Deficit Hyperactivity Disorder. *Journal of Abnormal Child Psychology, 26,* 233–245.

Fowles, D. C. (1988). Psychophysiology and psychopathology: A motivational approach. *Psychophysiology, 25,* 373–391.

Fristoe, N. M., Salthouse, T. A., & Woodard, J. L. (1997). Examination of aged-related deficits on the Wisconsin Card Sorting Test. *Neuropsychology, 11,* 428–436.

Frowein, H. W. (1981). *Selective drug effects on information processing.* Doctoral thesis, University of Tilburg, Tilburg, The Netherlands.

Gaillard, A. W. K. (1978). *Slow brain potentials preceding task performance.* Amsterdam: Academische Pers.

Giedd, J. N., Castellanos, F. X., Casey, B. J., Kozuch, P., King, A. C., Hamburger, S. D., & Rapoport, J. L. (1994). Quantitative morphology of the corpus callosum in Attention Deficit Hyperactivity Disorder. *American Journal of Psychiatry, 151,* 665–669.

Goldstein, D. J., & Blumenthal, T. D. (1995). Startle eyeblink elicitation in Attention Deficit Disordered children using low-intensity acoustic stimuli. *Perceptual and Motor Skills, 80,* 227–231.

Gordon, M. A. (1979). The assessment of impulsivity and mediating behavior in hyperactive and nonhyperactive boys. *Journal of Abnormal Child Psychology, 7,* 317–326.

Goyette, C. H., Conners, C. K., & Ulrich, R. F. (1978). Normative date on revised Conners parent and teacher rating scales. *Journal of Abnormal Child Psychology, 6,* 221–236.

Graham, F. K. (1975). The more or less startling effects of weak prestimulation. *Psychophysiology, 12,* 238–248.

Granholm, E., Asarnow, R. F., Sarkin, A. J., & Dykes, K. L. (1996). Papillary responses index cognitive resource limitations. *Psychophysiology, 33,* 457–461.

Grant, D. A., & Berg, E. A. (1948). A behavioral analysis of degree of reinforcement and ease of shifting to new responses in a Weigel-type card-sorting problem. *Journal of Experimental Psychology, 38,* 404–411.

Gray, J. A. (1982). *The neuropsychology of anxiety: An enquiry into the functions of the septo-hippocampal system.* New York: Oxford University Press.

Gray, J. A. (1984). *The psychology of fear and stress.* Cambridge, England: Cambridge University Press.

Grünewald, G., Grünewald-Züberbier, E., & Netz, J. (1978). Late components of average evoked potentials in children with different abilities to concentrate. *Electroencephalography and Clinical Neurophysiology, 44,* 617–625.

Grünewald-Züberbier, E., Grünewald, G., Rasche, A., & Netz, J. (1978). Contingent negative variation and alpha attenuation responses in children with different abilities to concentrate. *Electroencephalography and Clinical Neurophysiology, 44,* 37–47.

Hackley, S., & Miller, J. (1995). Response complexity and precue interval effects on the lateralized readiness potential. *Psychophysiology, 32,* 230–241.

Hall, S. J., Halperin, J. M., Schwartz, S. T., & Newcorn, J. H. (1997). Behavioral and executive functions in children with Attention-Deficit Hyperactivity Disorder. *Journal of Attention Disorders, 1,* 235–244.

Halperin, J. M., Wolf, L. E., Pascualvaca, D. M., Newcorn, J. H., Healey, J. M., O'Brien, J. D., Morganstein, A., & Young, J. G. (1988). Differential assessment of attention and impulsivity in children. *Journal of the American Academy of Child and Adolescent Psychiatry, 27,* 326–329.

Halperin, J. M., O'Brien, J. D., Newcorn, J. H., Healey, J. M., Pascualvaca, D. M., Wolf, L. E., & Young, J. G. (1990). Validation of hyperactive, aggressive, and mixed hyperactive/aggressive childhood disorders: A research note. *Journal of Child Psychology and Psychiatry, 31,* 455–459.

Halperin, J. M., Matier, K., Bedi, G., Sharma, V., & Newcorn, J. H. (1992). Specificity of inattention, impulsivity, and hyperactivity to the diagnosis of attention-deficit hyperactivity disorder. *Journal of the American Academy of Child and Adolescent Psychiatry, 31,* 190–196.

Hebb, D. O. (1949). *Organization of behavior.* New York: Wiley.

Hiscock, M., Kinsbourne, M., Caplan, G., & Swanson, J. M. (1979). Auditory attention in hyperactive children: Effects of stimulant medication on dichotic listening performance. *Journal of Abnormal Psychology, 88,* 27–32.

Hockey, R. (1979). Stress and cognitive components of skilled performance. In V. Hamilton & D. M. Warburton (Eds.), *Human stress and cognition* (pp. 141–177). Chichester, England: Wiley.

Hopkins, J., Perlman, T., Hechtman, L., & Weiss, G. (1979). Cognitive style in adults originally diagnosed as hyperactives. *Journal of Child Psychology and Psychiatry, 20,* 209–216.

Houk, J. C., & Wise, S. P. (1995). Distributed modular architectures linking basal ganglia, cerebellum, and cerebral cortex: Their role in planning and controlling action. *Cerebral Cortex, 5,* 95–110.

Iaboni, F., Douglas, V. I., & Baker, A. G. (1995). Effects of reward and response costs on inhibition in ADHD children. *Journal of Abnormal Psychology, 104,* 232–240.

Iaboni, F., Douglas, V. I., & Ditto, B. (1997). Psychophysiological response of ADHD children to reward and extinction. *Psychophysiology, 34,* 116–123.

Jennings, J. R., Molen, M. W. van der, Pelham, W., Brock-Debski, K., & Hoza, B. (1997). Psychophysiology of inhibition in boys with attention deficit disorder. *Developmental Psychology, 33,* 308–318.

Jonides, J., Schumacher, E. H., Smith, E. E., Lauber, E. J., Awh, E., Minoshima, S., & Koeppe, R. A. (1997). Verbal working memory load affects regional brain activation as measured by PET. *Journal of Cognitive Neuroscience, 9,* 462–475.

Kagan, J., Rosman, B. L., Day, D., Albert, J., & Phillips, W. (1964). Information processing in the child, significance of analytic and reflective attitudes. *Psychological Monographs, 1* (Whole No. 578).

Kahneman, D. (1973). *Attention and effort.* Englewood Cliffs, NJ: Prentice-Hall.

Kalverboer, A. F., & Brouwer, W. H. (1983). Visuomotor behaviour in preschool children in relation to sex and neurological status. *Journal of Child Psychology and Psychiatry, 24,* 65–88.

Kinsbourne, M. (1973). The control of attention by interaction between the cerebral hemispheres. In S. Kornblum (Ed.), *Attention and performance* (Vol. 4, pp. 239–256). New York: Academic Press.

Kinsbourne, M., & Hicks, R. E. (1978). Functional cerebral space: A model for overflow, transfer and interference effects in human performance. A tutorial review. In J. Requin (Ed.), *Attention and performance* (Vol. VII, pp. 345–362). Hillsdale, NJ: Erlbaum.

Klorman, R. (1995). Psychophysiological determinants. In M. Hersen & R. T. Ammerman (Eds.), *Advanced abnormal child psychology* (pp. 59–85). Hillsdale, NJ: Erlbaum.

Klorman, R., Salzman, L. F., Pass, H. L., Borgstedt, A. D., & Dainer, K. B. (1979). Effects of methylphenidate on hyperactive children's evoked response during passive and active attention. *Psychophysiology, 16*, 23–29.

Klorman, R., Brumaghim, J. L., Coons, H. W., Peloquin, L.-J., Strauss, J., Lewine, J. D., Borgstedt, A. D., & Goldstein, M. (1988). The contributions of event-related potentials to understanding the effects of stimulants on information processing in attention deficit disorder. In L. F. Bloomingdale & J. A. Sergeant (Eds.), *Attention deficit disorder* (Vol. 5, pp. 199–218). Oxford, England: Pergamon.

Klorman, R., Brumaghim, J. L., Fitzpatrick, P. A., Borgstedt, A. D. (1992). Methylphenidate reduces abnormalities of stimulus classification in adolescents with attention deficit disorder. *Journal of Abnormal Psychology, 101*, 130–138.

Klorman, R., Brumaghim, J. L., Fitzpatrick, P. A., Borgstedt, A. D., & Strauss, J. (1994). Clinical and cognitive effects of methylphenidate on attention deficit disorders as a function of aggression/oppositionality and age. *Journal of Abnormal Psychology, 103*, 206–221.

Krusch, D. A., Klorman, R., Brumaghim, J. T., Fitzpatrick, P. A., Borgstedt, A. D., & Strauss, J. (1996). Slowing during and after errors in ADD: Methylphenidate slows reactions of children with Attention Deficit Disorder during and after an error. *Journal of Abnormal Child Psychology, 24*, 633–650.

Le Moal, M. (1995). Mescocorticolimbic dopaminergic neurons: Functional and regulatory roles. In F. E. Bloom & D. J. Kupfer (Eds.), *Psychopharmacology: The fourth generation of progress* (pp. 283–294). New York: Raven.

Leeuwen, T. H. van, Steinhausen, H.-Ch., Overtoom, C. C. E., Pasqual-Marqui, R. D., Klooster, B. van't, Rothemberger, A., Sergeant, J. A., & Brandeis, D. (1998). The continuous performance test revisited with neuroelectric mapping: Impaired orienting in children with attention deficits. *Behavioural Brain Research, 94*, 97–110.

Leung, P. W. L., & Connolly, K. J. (1996). Distractibility in hyperactive and conduct-disordered children. *Journal of Child Psychology and Psychiatry, 37*, 305–312.

Logan, G. D., & Cowan, W. B. (1984). On the ability to inhibit thought and action: A theory of an act of control. *Psychological Review, 91*, 295–327.

Logan, G. D., Cowan, W. B., & Davis, K. A. (1984). On the ability to inhibit thought and action: A model and a method. *Journal of Experimental Psychology, 10*, 276–291.

Loge, D. V., Staton, D. V., & Beatty, W. W. (1990). Performance of children with ADHD on tests sensitive to frontal lobe dysfunction. *Journal of the American Academy of Child and Adolescent Psychiatry, 29*, 540–545.

Loiselle, D. L., Stamn, J. S., Matinsky, S., & Whipple, S. (1980). Evoked potential and behavioral signs of attentive dysfunctions in hyperactive boys. *Psychophysiology, 17*, 193–201.

Losier, B. J., McGrath, P. J., & Klein, R. M. (1996). Error patterns on the continuous performance test in non-medicated and medicated samples of children with and without ADHD: A meta-analytic review. *Journal of Child Psychology and Psychiatry, 37*, 971–988.

Lou, H. C., Henriksen, L., & Bruhn, P. (1984). Focal cerebral hypoperfusion in children with dysphasia and/or attention deficit disorder. *Archives of Neurology, 41*, 825–829.

Lou, H. C., Henriksen, L., Bruhn, P., Borner, H., & Nielsen, J. B. (1989). Striatal dysfunction in attention deficit and hyperkinetic disorder. *Archives of Neurology, 46*, 48–52.

Lubow, R. E. (1989). *Latent inhibition and conditioned attention theory.* Cambridge, England: Cambridge University Press.

Lubow, R. E., & Josman, Z. E. (1993). Latent inhibition deficits in hyperactive children. *Journal of Child Psychology and Psychiatry, 34*, 959–973.

Malone, M., Kershner, J. R., & Siegal, L. (1988). The effects of methylphenidate on levels of processing and laterality in children with Attention Deficit Disorder. *Journal of Abnormal Child Psychology, 16*, 379–395.

Malone, M., Couitis, J., Kershner, J. R., & Logan, W. J. (1994). Right hemisphere dysfunction and methylphenidate effects in children with Attention-Deficit/Hyperactivity Disorder. *Journal of Child and Adolescent Psychopharmacology, 4*, 245–253.

McClure, F. D., & Gordon, M. (1984). Performance of disturbed hyperactive and nonhyperactive children on an objective measure of hyperactivity. *Journal of Abnormal Child Psychology, 12*, 561–571.

McIntyre, C. W., Blackwell, S. L., & Denton, C. L. (1978). Background characteristics of aggressive, hyperactive and aggressive-hyperactive boys. *Journal of Abnormal Child Psychology, 6*, 483–494.

Meere, J. J. van der. (1988). *Attention deficit disorder with hyperactivity: A misconception.* Doctoral thesis, University of Groningen, Groningan, The Netherlands.

Meere, J. J. van der, & Sergeant, J. A. (1987). A divided attention experiment in pervasively hyperactive children. *Journal of Abnormal Child Psychology, 16*, 379–391.

Meere, J. J. van der, & Sergeant, J. A. (1988a). Acquisition of attentional skill in pervasively hyperactive children. *Journal of Child Psychology and Psychiatry, 29*, 301–310.

Meere, J. J. van der, & Sergeant, J. A. (1988b). Controlled processing and vigilance in hyperactivity: Time will tell. *Journal of Abnormal Child Psychology, 16*, 641–655.

Meere, J. J. van der, & Sergeant, J. A. (1988c). A focused attention experiment in pervasively hyperactive children. *Journal of Abnormal Child Psychology, 16*, 627–639.

Meere, J. J. van der, Baal, M. van, & Sergeant, J. A. (1989). The additive factor method: A differential diagnostic tool in hyperactivity and learning disablement. *Journal of Abnormal Child Psychology, 17,* 409–422.

Meere, J. J. van der, Wekking, E., & Sergeant, J. A. (1991). Sustained attention and pervasive hyperactivity. *Journal of Child Psychology and Psychiatry, 32,* 275–284.

Meere, J. J. van der, Vreeling, H. J., & Sergeant, J. A. (1992). A motor presetting study in hyperactives, learning disabled and control children. *Journal of Child Psychology and Psychiatry, 34,* 1347–1354.

Meere, J. J. van der, Hughes, K. A., Börger, N., & Sallee, F. R. (1995). The effect of reward on sustained attention in ADHD children with and without CD. In J. Sergeant (Ed.), *European approaches to hyperkinetic disorder: Eunethydis* (pp. 241–253). Zurich, Switzerland: Fotorator.

Meere, J. J. van der, Shalev, R., Börger, N., & Gross-Tsur, V. (1995). Sustained attention, activation and MPH in ADHD. *Journal of Child Psychology and Psychiatry, 36,* 697–703.

Meere, J. J. van der, Stemerdink, N., & Gunning, B. (1995). Effects of presentation rate of stimuli on response inhibition in ADHD children with and without tics. *Perceptual and Motor Skills, 81,* 259–262.

Meere, J. J. van der, Gunning, B., & Stemerdink, N. (1996). Changing a response set in normal development and in ADHD children with and without tics. *Journal of Abnormal Child Psychology, 24,* 767–786.

Michael, R. L., Klorman, R., Salzman, L. F., Borgstedt, A. D., & Dainer, K. B. (1981). Normalizing effects of methylphenidate on hyperactive children's vigilance performance and evoked potentials. *Psychophysiology, 18,* 665–677.

Milich, R., & Kramer, J. (1984). Reflections on impulsivity: An empirical investigation of impulsivity as a construct. In K. D. Gadow (Ed.), *Advances in learning and behavioral disabilities* (Vol. 3, pp. 57–94). Greenwich, CT: JAI.

Milich, R., Hartung, C. M., Martin, C. M., & Haigler, E. D. (1994). Behavioral disinhibition and underlying processes in adolescents with disruptive behavior disorders. In D. K. Routh (Ed.), *Disruptive behavior disorders in childhood: Essays honoring Herbert C. Quay* (pp. 109–138). New York: Plenum.

Milner, B. (1963). Effects of different brain lesions on card sorting. *Archives of Neurology, 9,* 90–100.

Molen, M. W. van der, Bashore, T. R., Halliday, R., & Callaway, E. (1991). Chronophysiology: Mental chronometry augmented by physiological time markers. In J. R. Jennings & M. G. H. Coles (Eds.), *Handbook of cognitive psychophysiology: Central and autonomic nervous system approaches* (pp. 9–178). Chichester, England: Wiley.

Mountain, M. A., & Snow, W. G. (1993). Wisconsin card sorting test as a measure of frontal pathology: A review. *Clinical Neuropsychology, 7,* 108–118.

Mulder, G. (1986). The concept and measurement of mental effort. In G. R. J. Hockey, A. W. K. Gaillard, &

M. G. H. Coles (Eds.), *Energetics and human information processing* (pp. 178–198). Dordrecht, The Netherlands: Martinus Nijhoff.

Mulder, L. J. (1992). Measurement and analysis methods of heart rate and respiration for use in applied environments. *Biological Psychology, 34,* 205–236

Nigg, J. T., Swanson, J. M., & Hinshaw, S. P. (1997). Covert visual spatial attention in boys with attention deficit hyperactivity disorder: Lateral effects, methylphenidate response and results for parents. *Neuropsychologia, 35,* 165–176.

Novak, G. P., Solanto, M., & Abikoff, H. (1995). Spatial orienting and focused attention in attention deficit hyperactivity disorder. *Psychophysiology, 32,* 546–559.

Nuechterlein, K. (1983). Signal detection in vigilance tasks and behavioral attributes among offspring of schizophrenic mothers and among hyperactive children. *Journal of Abnormal Psychology, 92,* 4–28.

Ollman, R. (1977). Choice reaction time and the problem of distinguishing task effects from strategy effects. In S. Dornic (Ed.), *Attention and performance* (Vol. 7, pp. 99–113). Hillsdale, NJ: Erlbaum.

Oosterlaan, J. (1996). *Response inhibition in children with Attention Deficit Hyperactivity and related disorders.* Doctoral thesis, University of Amsterdam, Amsterdam, The Netherlands.

Oosterlaan, J., & Sergeant, J. A. (1995). Response choice and inhibition in ADHD, anxious and aggressive children: The relationship between S–R compatibility and stop signal task. In J. A. Sergeant (Ed.), *European approaches to hyperkinetic disorder: Eunethydis* (pp. 225–240). Zurich, Switzerland: Fotorotar.

Oosterlaan, J., & Sergeant, J. A. (1998a). Response inhibition and the effects of reward and response cost: A comparison between ADHD, disruptive, anxious and normal children. *Journal of Abnormal Child Psychology, 26,* 161–174.

Oosterlaan, J., & Sergeant, J. A. (1998b). Response inhibition and response re-engagement in attention-deficit/hyperactivity disorder, disruptive, anxious and normal children. *Behavioural Brain Research, 94,* 33–44.

Oosterlaan, J., Logan, G. D., & Sergeant, J. A. (1998). Response inhibition in ADHD, CD, comorbid ADHD+CD, anxious and normal children: A meta-analysis of studies with the stop task. *Journal of Child Psychology and Psychiatry, 39,* 411–426.

Ornitz, E. M., Hanna, G. L., & De Traversay, J. (1992). Prestimulation-induced startle modulation in Attention-Deficit Hyperactivity Disorder and Nocturnal Enuresis. *Psychophysiology, 29,* 437–451.

Pardo, J. V., Pardo, P. J., Janer, K. W., & Raichle, M. E. (1990). The anterior cingulate cortex mediates processing selection in the Stroop attentional conflict paradigm. *Proceedings of the National Academy of Sciences, 87,* 256–259.

Paus, T., Zatorre, R. J., Hofle, N., Caramanos, Z., Gotman, J., Petrides, M., & Evans, A. C. (1997). Time-related changes in neural systems underlying attention and arousal during the performance of an auditory vigilance task. *Journal of Cognitive Neuroscience, 9,* 392–408.

Pearson, D. A., Yaffee, L. S., Loveland, K. A., & Norton, A. M. (1995). Covert visual attention in children with attention deficit hyperactivity disorder: Evidence for developmental immaturity. *Development and Psychopathology, 7,* 351–367.

Pennington, B. F., & Ozonoff, S. (1996). Executive functions and developmental psychopathology. *Journal of Child Psychology and Psychiatry, 37,* 51–87.

Pennington, B. F., Grossier, D., & Welsh, M. C. (1993). Contrasting cognitive deficits in Attention Deficit Hyperactivity Disorder versus Reading Disability. *Developmental Psychology, 29,* 511–523.

Pennington, B. F., Bennetto, L., McAleer, O. K., & Roberts, R. J., Jr. (1996). Executive functions and working memory: Theoretical and measurement issues. In G. R. Lyon & N. A. Krasnegor (Eds.), *Attention, memory and executive function* (pp. 327–348). Baltimore: Brookes.

Porrino, L. J., Rapoport, J. L., Behar, D., Sceery, W., Ismond, D. R., & Bunney, W. E. (1983). A naturalistic assessment of the motor activity of hyperactive boys: I. Comparison with normal controls. *Archives of General Psychiatry, 40,* 681–687.

Posner, M. I. (1978). *Chronometric explorations of mind.* Hillsdale, NJ: Erlbaum.

Posner, M. I., & Raichle, M. E. (1994). *Images of mind.* New York: Scientific American Library.

Pribram, K. H., & McGuiness, D. (1975). Arousal, activation and effort in the control of attention. *Psychological Review, 82,* 116–149.

Prior, M., Sanson, A., Freethy, C., & Geffen, G. (1985). Auditory attentional abilities in hyperactive children. *Journal of Child Psychology and Psychiatry, 26,* 289–304.

Quay, H. C. (1988). Attention deficit disorder and the behavioral inhibition system: The relevance of the neuropsychological theory of Jeffrey A. Gray. In L. M. Bloomingdale & J. Sergeant (Eds.), *Attention deficit disorder: Criteria, cognition, intervention* (pp. 117–125). Oxford, England: Pergamon.

Quay, H. C. (1997). Inhibition and attention deficit hyperactivity disorder. *Journal of Abnormal Child Psychology, 25,* 7–13.

Rabbitt, P., & Rodgers, B. (1977). What does a man do after he makes an error: An analysis of response programming. *Quarterly Journal of Experimental Psychology, 29,* 727–743.

Radosh, A., & Gittelman, R. (1981). The effects of appealing distractors on the performance of hyperactive children. *Journal of Abnormal Child Psychology, 9,* 179–189.

Reader, M. J., Harris, E. L., Scherholz, L. J., & Denckla, M. B. (1994). Attention Deficit Hyperactivity Disorder and executive functioning. *Developmental Neuropsychology, 10,* 493–512.

Robbins, T. W., & Everritt, B. (1995). Arousal systems and attention. In M. S. Gazzaniga (Ed.), *The cognitive neuroscience* (pp. 615–624). Cambridge, MA: MIT Press.

Rosenthal, H. R., & Allen, T. W. (1980). Intratask distractibility in hyperkinetic and nonhyperkinetic children. *Journal of Abnormal Child Psychology, 8,* 175–187.

Ross, R. G., Hommer, D., Breiger, D., Varley, C., & Radant, A. (1994). Eye movement task related to frontal lobe functioning in children with Attention deficit Disorder. *Journal of the American Academy of Child and Adolescent Psychiatry, 33,* 869–874.

Rosvold, H. E., Mirsky, A. F., Sarason. I., Bransome, E. D., & Beck. L. H. (1956). A continuous performance test of brain damage. *Journal of Consulting Psychology, 20,* 343–350.

Rueckert, L., & Grafman, J. (1996). Sustained attention deficits in patients with right frontal lesions. *Neuropsychologia, 34,* 953–963.

Rueckert, L., & Levy, J. (1996). Further evidence that the callosum is involved in sustaining attention. *Neuropsychologia, 34,* 927–935.

Rueckert, L., Sorensen, L., & Levy, J. (1994). Callosal efficiency is related to sustained attention. *Neuropsychologia, 32,* 159–173.

Sanders, A. F. (1983). Towards a model of stress and performance. *Acta Psychologica, 53,* 61–97.

Satterfield, J. H., & Braley, B. W. (1977). Evoked potentials and brain maturation in hyperactive and normal children. *Electroencephalography and Clinical Neurophysiology, 43,* 43–51.

Satterfield, J. H., & Dawson, M. E. (1971). Electrodermal correlates of hyperactivity in children. *Psychophysiology, 8,* 191–197.

Satterfield, J. H., Cantwell, D. P., & Satterfield, B. T. (1974). Pathophysiology of the hyperactive child syndrome. *Archives of General Psychiatry, 31,* 839–844.

Satterfield, J. H., Schell, A. M., Backs, R. W., & Hidaka, K. C. (1984). A cross-sectional and longitudinal study of age effects of electrophysiological measures in hyperactive and normal children. *Biological Psychiatry, 19,* 973–990.

Satterfield, J. H., Schell, A. M., & Nicholas, T. (1994). Preferential neural processing of attended stimuli in attention-deficit hyperactivity disorder and normal boys. *Psychophysiology, 31,* 1–10.

Schachar, R., & Logan, G. (1990). Impulsivity and inhibitory control in normal development and childhood psychopathology. *Developmental Psychology, 26,* 710–720.

Schachar, R., & Tannock, R. (1995). Test of four hypotheses for the comorbidity of attention-deficit hyperactivity disorder. *Journal of the American Academy of Child and Adolescent Psychiatry, 34,* 639–648.

Schachar, R., Tannock, R., Marriott, M., & Logan, G. (1995). Deficient inhibitory control in attention deficit hyperactivity disorder. *Journal of Abnormal Child Psychology, 23,* 411–438.

Schweitzer, J. B. (1996). Debate and argument: Delay aversion versus impulsivity: Testing for dysfunction in ADHD. *Journal of Child Psychology and Psychiatry, 37,* 1027–1028.

Schweitzer, J. B., & Sulzer-Azaroff, B. (1995). Self-control in boys with attention deficit hyperactivity disorder: Effects of added stimulation and time. *Journal of Child Psychology and Psychiatry, 36,* 671–686.

Seidman, L. L., Biederman, J., Faraone, S. V., Weber, W., & Oullette, C. (1997). Towards defining a neuropsychology of Attention Deficit-Hyperactivity Disorder: Performance of children and adolescents from a large clinically referred sample. *Journal of Consulting and Clinical Psychology, 65,* 150–160.

Sergeant, J. A. (1981). *Attentional studies in hyperactivity.* Doctoral thesis, University of Groningen, Groningen, The Netherlands.

Sergeant, J. A. (1988). From DSM-III Attention Deficit Disorder to functional defects. In L. M. Bloomingdale & J. A. Sergeant (Eds.), *Attention deficit disorder: Criteria, cognition, intervention* (Vol. 5, pp. 183–198). Oxford, England: Pergamon.

Sergeant, J. A., & Meere, J. J. van der. (1988). What happens after a hyperactive commits an error? *Psychiatry Research, 28,* 157–164.

Sergeant, J. A., & Meere, J. J. van der. (1990a). Additive factor methodology applied to psychopathology with special reference to hyperactivity. *Acta Psychologica, 74,* 277–295.

Sergeant, J. A., & Meere, J. J. van der. (1990b). Convergence of approaches in localizing the hyperactivity deficit. In B. B. Lahey & A. E. Kazdin (Eds.), *Advancements in clinical child psychology* (Vol. 13, pp. 207–245). New York: Plenum.

Sergeant, J. A., & Meere, J. J. van der. (1994). Towards an empirical child psychopathology. In D. K. Routh (Ed.), *Disruptive behavior disorders in childhood: Essays honoring Herbert C. Quay* (pp. 59–85). New York: Plenum.

Sergeant, J. A., & Scholten, C. A. (1983). A stages-of-information processing approach to hyperactivity. *Journal of Child Psychology and Psychiatry, 22,* 49–60.

Sergeant, J. A., & Scholten, C. A. (1985a). On data limitations in hyperactivity. *Journal of Child Psychology and Psychiatry, 26,* 111–124.

Sergeant, J. A., & Scholten, C. A. (1985b). On resource strategy limitations in hyperactivity: Cognitive impulsivity reconsidered. *Journal of Child Psychology and Psychiatry, 26,* 97–109.

Sergeant, J. A., Velthoven, R. van, & Virginia, A. (1979). Hyperactivity, impulsivity and reflectivity: An examination of their relationship and implications for clinical child psychology. *Journal of Child Psychology and Psychiatry, 20,* 47–60.

Shue, K. L., & Douglas, V. I. (1992). Attention Deficit Hyperactivity Disorder and the frontal lobe syndrome. *Brain and Cognition, 20,* 104–124.

Sobotka, S. S., Davidson, R. J., & Senulis, J. A. (1992). Anterior brain electrical asymmetries in response to reward and punishment. *Electroencephalography and Clinical Neurophysiology, 83,* 236–247.

Solanto, M. V. (1990). The effects of reinforcement and response-cost on a delayed response task in children with attention deficit hyperactivity disorder: A research note. *Journal of Child Psychology and Psychiatry, 31,* 803–808.

Solanto, M. V., Wender, E. H., & Bartell, S. S. (1997). Effects of methylphenidate and behavioral contingencies on vigilance in AD/HD: A test of the reward dysfunction hypothesis. *Journal of Child and Adolescent Psychopharmacology, 7,* 123–136.

Sonneville, L. M. J. de, Njiokiktjien, C., & Hilhorst, R. C. (1991). Methylphenidate induced changes in ADDH information processors. *Journal of Child Psychology and Psychiatry, 32,* 285–296.

Sonuga-Barke, E. J. S. (1996). Debate and argument: When "impulsiveness" is delay aversion: A reply to Schweitzer and Sulzer-Azaroff. *Journal of Child Psychology and Psychiatry, 33,* 1023–1025.

Sonuga-Barke, E. J. S., Taylor, E., Sembi, S., & Smith, J. (1992). Hyperactivity and delay aversion—II: The effect of delay on choice. *Journal of Child Psychology and Psychiatry, 33,* 387–398.

Sonuga-Barke, E. J. S., Houlberg, K., & Hall, M. (1994). When is "impulsiveness" not impulsive: The case of hyperactive children's cognitive style. *Journal of Child Psychology and Psychiatry, 35,* 1247–1253.

Sternberg, S. (1969). Discovery of processing stages: Extensions of Donders' method. In W. G. Koster (Ed.), *Attention and performance* (Vol. 2, pp. 276–315). Amsterdam: North Holland.

Stevens, D. A., Stover, C. F., & Backus, J. T. (1970). The hyperkinetic child: Effects of incentives on the speed of rapid tapping. *Journal of Consulting and Clinical Psychology 34,* 56–59.

Stroop, J. R. (1935). Studies of inference in serial verbal reactions. *Journal of Experimental Psychology, 18,* 643–662.

Swanson, J. M., Posner, M. I., Potkin, S., Bonforte, S., Youpa, D., Cantwell, D., & Crinella, F. (1991). Activating tasks for the study of visual-spatial attention in ADHD children: A cognitive anatomical approach. *Journal of Child Neurology, 6* (Suppl.), S119–S127.

Sykes, D. H., Douglas, V. I., Weiss, G., & Minde, K. K. (1971). Attention in hyperactive children and the effect of methylphenidate (Ritalin). *Journal of Child Psychology and Psychiatry, 12,* 129–139.

Sykes, D. H., Douglas, V. I., & Morgenstern, G. (1973). Sustained attention in hyperactive children. *Journal of Child Psychology and Psychiatry, 14,* 213–220.

Tannock, R., Ickowicz, A., & Schachar, R. (1995). Differential effects of methylphenidate on working memory in ADHD children with and without comorbid anxiety. *Journal of the American Academy of Child and Adolescent Psychiatry, 34,* 886–896.

Tannock, R., Schachar, R., & Logan, G. (1995). Methylphenidate and cognitive flexibility: Dissociated dose effects in hyperactive children. *Journal of Abnormal Child Psychology, 23,* 235–266.

Taylor, E. (1983). Drug response and diagnostic validation. In M. Rutter (Ed.), *Developmental neuropsychiatry* (pp. 348–368). New York: Guilford.

Tomporowski, P. D., Tinsley, V., & Hager, L. D. (1994). Visuospatial attentional shifts and choice responses of adults and ADHD and non-ADHD children. *Perceptual and Motor Skills, 79,* 1479–1490.

Tucker, D. M., & Williamson, P. A. (1984). Asymmetric neural control systems in human self-regulation. *Psychological Review, 91,* 185–215.

Warm, J. S. (1984). *Sustained attention in human performance.* New York: Wiley.

Wilkins, A. J., Shallice, T., & McCarthy, R. (1987). Frontal lesions and sustained attention. *Neuropsychologia, 25,* 359–365.

Winsum, W. van, Sergeant, J. A., & Geuze, R. (1984). The functional significance of event-related desynchronization of alpha rhythm in attentional and activating tasks. *Electroencephalography and Clinical Neurophysiology, 58,* 519–524.

Zahn, T., Kruesi, M. J. P., & Rapoport. J. L. (1991). Reaction time indices of attention deficits in boys with disruptive behavior disorders. *Journal of Abnormal Child Psychology, 19,* 233–252.

Zametkin, A. J., Nordahl, T. E., Gross, M., King, A. C., Semple, W. E., Rumsey, J., Hamburger, S., & Cohen, R. M. (1990). Cerebral glucose metabolism in adults with hyperactivity of childhood onset. *New England Journal of Medicine, 323,* 1361–1366.

Zametkin, A. J., Liebenauer, L. L., Fitzgerald, G. A., King, A. C., Minkunas, D. V., Herscovitch, P., Yamada, E. M., & Cohen, R. M. (1993). Brain metabolism in teenagers with attention deficit hyperactivity disorder. *Archives of General Psychiatry, 50,* 333–340.

Zentall, S. S., & Meyer, M. J. (1987). Self-regulation of stimulation for ADD-H children during reading and vigilance task performance. *Journal of Abnormal Child Psychology, 15,* 519–536.

Zentall, S. S., & Shaw, J. H. (1980). Effects of classroom noise on performance and activity of second-grade hyperactives and control children. *Journal of Educational Psychology, 71,* 830–840.

Zentall, S. S., & Zentall, T. R. (1983). Optimal stimulation: A model of disordered activity and performance in normal and deviant children. *Psychological Bulletin, 94,* 446–471.

Zentall, S. S., Zentall, T. R., & Barack, R. B. (1978). Distraction as a function of within-task stimulation for hyperactive and normal children. *Journal of Learning Disabilities, 11,* 13–21.

5

Cognitive Control Processes in Attention-Deficit/Hyperactivity Disorder

VIRGINIA I. DOUGLAS

For many years investigators have worked toward achieving a better understanding of the causes of the impaired performance of children with Attention-Deficit/Hyperactivity Disorder (ADHD) on cognitive, information-processing, and neuropsychological tasks. These efforts have led to a recent emphasis on identifying the "core" or "primary" dysfunction responsible for ADHD children's cognitive problems. In this chapter, I attempt an overview of the extensive and often confusing literature in this area, emphasizing findings that I believe must be encompassed in a working conceptualization of the cognitive deficits associated with ADHD. I also point to conceptual and statistical problems that I believe are impeding research progress on ADHD.

DEFINING REGULATORY CONTROL PROBLEMS: PERVASIVE VERSUS SPECIFIC REGULATORY DEFICITS

Over the past several years, I have emphasized the role of dysfunctional regulatory or control processes in ADHD (Douglas, 1983,

1988, 1989). Recognizing the difficulties involved in dealing empirically with this complex and potentially vague concept, I recommended an approach that involves defining different aspects of regulatory control that appear to be problematic for ADHD children, proposing environmental or task manipulations that would be expected to increase or minimize demands on each aspect, and comparing the effects of these manipulations on the performance of ADHD and control groups.

Pervasive Control Problems

Some of the regulatory difficulties of ADHD children have pervasive, generalized effects on their cognitive performance, thus influencing performance at a macro level. These pervasive problems are of considerable interest in their own right. In addition, however, they must be taken into account when attempting to study more specific regulatory processes. Stated differently, experimental manipulations thought to affect specific aspects of regulation must be studied *against the background* of these more pervasive regulatory problems.

The noncompliant behaviors of ADHD children provide readily observable evidence of pervasive control problems. They include, for example, engaging in irrelevant conversation,

VIRGINIA I. DOUGLAS • Department of Psychology, McGill University and Montreal Children's Hospital, Montreal, Quebec, Canada H3A 1B1.

Handbook of Disruptive Behavior Disorders, edited by Quay and Hogan. Kluwer Academic/Plenum Publishers, New York, 1999.

playing with the equipment, or failing to follow instructions. Investigators wishing to study more specific regulatory processes may attempt, explicitly or implicitly, to minimize the confounding effects of these behaviors by such strategies as adopting a firm, authoritative approach or rewarding compliance.

Several investigators have pointed to a more subtle manifestation of defective regulation. Although difficult to define, it has serious effects on cognitive performance. I have referred to the problem as a failure to allocate adequate attention or effort to meet task demands (Douglas, 1983, 1988). Sergeant and van der Meere (1991; see also Chapter 4, this volume) recognized the problem by emphasizing deficiencies in the mechanisms supplying the energetic resources for information processing. I also spoke of an apparent lack of "intrinsic motivation," and of the difficulty observers experience in judging whether an ADHD child "can't" or "won't" improve his performance (Douglas, 1983, 1989, 1990). Levy and Hobbes (1996) used the term "incentive motivation" to differentiate between an involuntary failure to marshal adequate effort, and deliberate noncompliance or laziness. These concerns reflect the peculiar *blending of motivational and cognitive difficulties* that seems to typify the performance of ADHD children. There is some evidence that manipulations such as the amount of stimulation provided by the task or testing situation and the speeding or slowing of event rates can influence this aspect of regulatory control.

Another important, but less studied, pervasive manifestation of regulatory problems in ADDH children is the high degree of variability or inconsistency in their performance (see Chapter 4, this volume). Later in the chapter, I discuss a recent attempt by my colleagues and me to apply a new method of statistical analysis to gain a better understanding of this phenomenon.

Finally, working from a different theoretical perspective, several investigators have pointed to "stylistic" differences in the approach of ADHD children to problem-solving tasks. Concepts such as "impulsive (or nonreflective) cognitive style," "delay aversion," and

"delay of gratification" are used to refer to pervasive differences of this kind.

More Specific Control Problems

Regulatory problems that have been revealed by specific manipulations typically involve demands for *sustained effort, response preparation, adaptation to changing demands,* and *maintaining focus* despite distracting or conflicting events. The problems include the ability to maintain performance across time, to maintain and adjust readiness to respond to designated stimuli, to shift responses flexibly to meet task demands, to adapt response speed on demand or following an error, and to inhibit responding to inappropriate stimuli.

Examples of task manipulations and measures to assess these aspects of regulatory control include assessing performance across repeated trials or repeated administrations of a task, varying the length of preparatory intervals, manipulating the predictability (uncertainty) of response demands, assessing response times following an error, and introducing task-irrelevant stimuli.

Stimulant and Reinforcement Effects

I have argued that stimulant medication and some reinforcement contingencies improve performance by acting on regulatory processes (Douglas, 1989; Douglas, Barr, O'Neill, & Britton, 1986; Douglas, Barr, Amin, O'Neill, & Britton, 1988; Douglas, Barr, Desilets, & Sherman, 1995). An important question is whether the effects of these interventions are confined to the more pervasive aspects of regulation, or whether effects can also be shown on the specific manipulations of regulatory demands just described.

Criteria for an Adequate Conceptualization of the Cognitive Deficits Associated with ADHD

My move toward a regulatory deficiency hypothesis was not made easily. Like other investigators, I would prefer to trace the cause of the cognitive deficiencies in ADHD to a more simple explanatory mechanism. I believe, however, that recent attempts to achieve this goal have failed to account for some key findings and may have caused unnecessary confusion. In previous papers (Douglas, 1983, 1984, 1985, 1988, 1989), I argued that an adequate conceptualization of the cognitive problems of children with ADHD must account for (1) evidence of *both* attentional and inhibitory deficits; (2) findings pointing to difficulties in *both* maintaining preparatory set and in adjusting set flexibly to meet changing demands; (3) evidence suggesting defective regulation of arousal–activation levels to meet situational demands; (4) an inclination to seek immediate reinforcement; and (5) impaired performance on tasks requiring such executive functions as planning, organization, and self-monitoring. In this chapter, I argue, further, that a working conceptualization of the disorder must account for (6) the dramatic and pervasive improvement produced by stimulant medication; (7) the effects of rewards and stimulating events on performance, including apparent early habituation of these effects; (8) evidence that ADHD children respond *too quickly* on some tasks and *too slowly* on others, together with evidence that stimulants can improve their performance while *either slowing or speeding* responding, depending on the nature of task demands; and (9) findings of slow, variable reaction times and high error rates on a variety of laboratory tasks. These pervasive deficits may well constitute the most consistent finding in the ADHD literature, yet we remain unable to explain them adequately, and investigators frequently fail to recognize their confounding effects when studying more specific task manipulations.

COMPARING THEORETICAL APPROACHES

In my early attempts to conceptualize the cognitive deficits of ADHD children, I emphasized both attentional and inhibitory problems (Douglas, 1972, 1980, 1984). However, when the name of the disorder was changed to reflect evidence showing that high activity levels were typically accompanied by cognitive deficits, the new label, Attention Deficit Disorder, referred only to attentional problems (see Chapter 1, this volume). Although impulsive symptoms were included in the diagnostic criteria, the new label probably resulted in insufficient emphasis on inhibitory deficits.

More recently, however, some investigators, most notably Barkley (1994, 1996, 1997a, 1997b; see also Chapter 13, this volume) and Sergeant and van der Meere (Sergeant, 1995, 1996; Sergeant & van der Meere, 1990b, 1994; see also Chapter 4, this volume), have questioned the role of defective attention in ADHD. Barkley's conceptualization relies heavily on defective inhibitory and delayed response processes; Sergeant and van der Meere emphasize the inadequate allocation of cognitive-energetic resources during the motor output stage of information processing. It should be noted that Barkley's emphasis on inhibition has similarities to Quay's (1988a, 1988b, 1997) earlier attempt to explain ADHD symptoms within Gray's (1985, 1987) psychobiological theory of instrumental learning and emotion as resulting from underresponsivity of the behavioral inhibition system (BIS). Precursors to Sergeant and van der Meere's emphasis on cognitive-energetic processes include hypothesized differences in arousal, arousability, or control of arousal levels (Douglas, 1980; Kinsbourne, 1983; Satterfield, Schell, Backs, & Hidaka, 1984; Zahn, Abate, Little, & Wender, 1975); suggestions that ADHD children respond in unique ways to reinforcement contingencies (Barkley, 1989; Douglas, 1985, 1989; Douglas & Parry, 1994; Haenlein & Caul, 1987); and the "stimulation seeking" hypothesis of Zentall and Zentall (1983).

Although I accept arguments that ADHD children show problems implicating inhibition and motor output, I believe that ignoring or underestimating the importance of attentional and regulatory problems is likely to have negative effects on both theory building and the development of effective diagnostic and treatment procedures. Thus, I argue that the defective regulatory control hypothesis provides a more inclusive conceptual framework within which attentional, inhibitory, and motor processing problems can be integrated.

Barkley's Inhibition or Delayed-Response Model

Strongly influenced by the thinking of Bronowski (1977), Barkley (1994; see also Chapter 13, this volume) argued that the multiple deficits observed in ADHD, including apparent attentional problems, can be traced to a single cardinal feature: an impairment in the development of delayed responding or response inhibition. As I discuss later, there has been recurring debate about whether attentional or inhibitory deficits are primary in ADHD, or whether they should be viewed as two intricately interdependent, interacting processes. Some theorists argue that concentration deficits result from an inability to inhibit responding to extraneous stimuli. Others argue that the processing of irrelevant stimuli is caused by a more basic failure to allocate adequate, focused attention to critical task demands. Consequently, several of the tasks used with ADHD children have been described as assessing either attention or inhibition, depending on the investigator's theoretical preference.

Barkley's (1994) attempt to establish the primacy of disinhibition differs from my own conceptualization, in which attentional and inhibitory deficits are viewed as different manifestations of an underlying *regulatory control problem*. As I have emphasized previously (Douglas, 1980, 1984), there is convincing evidence to support *both* facilitating (activating) *and* inhibitory problems in ADHD. It should be noted, however, that in his more recent writing, Barkley appears to be shifting toward a greater emphasis on control processes (Barkley, 1997a, 1997b). Thus, the major source of my current disagreement with Barkley centers on his continuing reliance on inhibition as the central explanatory concept in his attempt to construct a model of ADHD (see Chapter 13, this volume).

Sergeant and van der Meere's Cognitive-Energetic Approach

In a recent review article, Sergeant and van der Meere (1994) reiterated their conclusion that "children with attention deficit with hyperactivity are not attentionally deficient" (p. 60). They argued, instead, for a deficit involving the allocation of energetic resources. However, they limited this problem to the *motor output* stage of processing. In reaching this conclusion, they drew on Sternberg's (1969, 1975) additive-factors model and Sanders's (1977, 1983) cognitive-energetic model of information processing. Both models posit independent (though somewhat different) stages at the basic, functional level of information processing. In addition, Sanders's model (described in Chapter 4, this volume) includes other levels supplying the energetic resources for information processing. Sanders's model has particular appeal for ADHD researchers because of a long-standing belief that defective allocation of attention and effort plays an important role in the disorder.

However, caution is necessary when applying the Sternberg and Sanders models to ADHD children. The assumption of independent information-processing stages has not been universally accepted. In addition, both models are based on findings from carefully controlled experiments with highly practiced, well-motivated adult subjects, factors that may limit their application to abnormal samples, particularly children whose approach to information processing is typically disorganized and poorly regulated.

Sergeant and van der Meere's (1990a, 1990b, 1994; see also Chapter 4, this volume) rejection of attentional problems is based on studies in which they were unable to show that ADHD children's performance was more impaired than that of controls by manipulations known to increase processing demands at the encoding and search stages of Sternberg's model. More specifically, they found no evidence of abnormalities in attentional *structural* processes in any of the stimulus-processing stages. Because an "arousal" pool provides energetic resources for stimulus-processing in Sanders's (1977, 1983) model, however, their failure to find stimulus-processing difficulties also appeared to rule out deficiencies in arousal, as well as in those functions of Sanders's "effort mechanism" that are responsible for controlling arousal. Sergeant and van der Meere concluded that the deficit associated with ADHD must be located *following* the stimulus-processing stages; that is, at the motor output (response) stage. Interestingly, they do not mention the possibility of motor output problems involving structural deficits. They emphasize, rather, an energy-related dysfunction implicating Sanders's effort mechanism, and possibly the "activation" pool, which provides energetic resources for the motor output stage.

In disagreement with Sergeant and van der Meere (1990a, 1990b, 1994), I argue that there is considerable evidence to implicate deficits in the stimulus-processing stages of information processing. If this conclusion is accepted, it becomes necessary to reconsider Sergeant and van der Meere's application of Sanders's model to ADHD. It should be stressed, first, that the presence of deficits in one or more stimulus-processing stages would not necessarily imply a *structural* cause. Using the same reasoning that Sergeant and van der Meere used to account for motor output problems, the cause could be located at the *effort* or *arousal* levels of Sanders's model. This raises the possibility that a defective effort-control mechanism could be responsible for inadequate allocation of energetic resources during *both* stimulus processing and response output.

Acceptance of this position would narrow the difference between my emphasis on regulatory processes as controlling attention and effort and Sergeant and van der Meere's emphasis on a defective effort mechanism. It should be noted that effort is described in Sanders's model as a *management system* that modifies arousal and activation to meet task demands. In addition, Sanders attributes *both* activating and inhibitory functions to the effort mechanism. Thus, within the domain of energy allocation,

Sanders's effort concept clearly has a regulatory or control function.

It is also noteworthy that, although Sergeant and van der Meere (1990a, 1990b, 1994) place most emphasis on the allocation of energetic resources, as I discuss shortly, several of their papers deal with the failure of ADHD children to cope with more specific regulatory requirements involving preparation and flexible adaptation to task demands. In addition, Oosterlaan and Sergeant (1995) recently suggested that it may be necessary to posit a general impairment in executive functioning to account for the different types of cognitive deficit they observed in their study. Finally, as Sergeant, van der Meere, and Oosterlaan point out in Chapter 4 (this volume), Sanders's model includes a higher-level "evaluation mechanism" which evaluates the adequacy of performance and the appropriate functioning of arousal and activation, thus sharing essential characteristics with executive and regulatory concepts. Although these authors did not invoke Sanders's evaluation mechanism in their earlier theorizing about ADHD, it may be necessary to rethink this question.

SCOPE AND LIMITATIONS OF THE REVIEW

In reviewing evidence of ADHD deficits on a wide variety of cognitive tasks, I address the theoretical issues just discussed, keeping in mind the criteria outlined earlier that I believe must be met in order to arrive at an adequate conceptualization of the underlying cognitive dysfunction in ADHD. This chapter is organized around a number of cognitive domains, including attention, inhibition, motor control, preparation and adjustment, cognitive style, complex memory and visual-memory search processes, and executive functions. It focuses on studies using children (usually males) who meet either earlier criteria for ADD with Hyperactivity or current criteria for ADHD, Combined Type, and for whom ADHD appears to be the *primary* diagnosis. I emphasize findings comparing ADHD and normal control children, touching only briefly on comparisons with other clinical groups. This decision is based on space limitations and on my belief that a clear understanding of ADHD–normal control differences constitutes the first step toward delineating the cognitive dysfunctions associated with ADHD. Although it would be gratifying to discover measures that identify deficits unique to ADHD, it is probably more realistic to work toward identifying *constellations* of measures that differentiate ADHD from other diagnostic groups. A similar position was advanced by Pennington and Ozonoff (1996), who spoke of the possibility of establishing *profile differences* between the childhood disorders.

Finally, although I agree that neurological and neurochemical processes play an essential role in ADHD, I limit my discussion to the nature of the defective *cognitive* functions that neurological theories must explain, and to the need for sound experimental methods and manipulations to assess these functions.

In the earlier parts of the chapter, I concentrate on findings from laboratory-based measures from the information-processing and cognitive psychology literature. In later sections, I emphasize findings from studies that used more complex tasks, including measures of stylistic differences in the approach to problem solving, and neuropsychological tasks originally developed to assess executive processes in patients with frontal lobe injuries.

Because of the importance of the relationship between the deficits shown by ADHD children and the effects of stimulant medication and reinforcement contingencies on them, I touch briefly on the implications of evidence from these interventions.

FINDINGS FROM COGNITIVE AND INFORMATION-PROCESSING TASKS

Deficits in Sustained Attention

Vigilance or Continuous Performance tasks (CPT) are among the most frequently used measures to assess cognitive processes in ADHD.

The value of this research has been seriously compromised, however, by variations in the paradigms used and in differences in such task parameters as event rates, task duration, and stimulus presentation times.

All of the versions reviewed here share the basic requirement that subjects must critically monitor the appearance of a series of continually changing stimuli, while *maintaining preparation* to respond to relatively infrequent, unpredictably occurring, correct "target" stimuli and *inhibiting* responding to more frequently appearing incorrect stimuli.

A series of articles highly critical of vigilance research (Corkum & Siegel, 1993; Sergeant & van der Meere, 1990b; Trommer, Hoeppner, Lorber, & Armstrong, 1988b) no doubt contributed to current disenchantment with the explanatory role of attention in ADHD. Confusion also developed from the use of the term "sustained" to refer to both overall performance levels and the decrement that typically occurs as subjects are required to maintain vigilance over an extended time period (e.g., 10 or 20 min).

Measures of Overall CPT Performance

A review by Corkum and Siegel (1993) focused mainly on measures reflecting overall performance. They reported that significant ADHD–control differences were found on both omission errors and commission errors in approximately 50% of the studies they reviewed. In reply to criticisms from Koelega (1995), they argued that an updated analysis (Corkum & Siegel, 1995) yielded similar figures. They emphasized the disappointing inconsistencies in the findings and pointed to the pitfalls in using CPT tasks for diagnostic purposes. Nevertheless, since their 50% figures hardly represent chance findings, their conclusion that "there is no compelling evidence for a sustained deficit in ADHD children" (Corkum & Siegel, 1993, p. 1217) probably caused more pessimism than the results merited.

More recently, Losier, McGrath, and Klein (1996) carried out a meta-analysis of ADHD vigilance studies. They also reviewed studies comparing methylphenidate (MPH) and placebo effects on performance. Perhaps because of their more demanding criteria for inclusion of studies in their analyses, their conclusions were considerably more supportive of the discriminative validity of vigilance measures. A "vote counting" procedure showed that 82% of the studies reported significantly more errors of omission and commission in ADHD than in control groups. Calculation of effect sizes revealed significant group effects on both types of errors. ADHD children missed twice as many targets as normal children and made more than twice as many commission errors. MPH significantly reduced omission errors in the 14 studies reviewed; 8 of the studies reported significant improvement on commission errors. On average, ADHD children made 39% fewer omission errors and 29% fewer commission errors on MPH than on placebo; both findings reached statistical significance.

Losier and colleagues (1996) also used results from a signal-detection analysis to argue against a response bias explanation of either the ADHD–control differences or the MPH effects. The mean discriminability score (d') of ADHD children was significantly lower than that of normal children, whereas the difference on response bias (Beta) (see Chapter 4, this volume, for a definition of these terms) did not reach significance. They also reported a significant drug effect on the d' measure, but not on Beta.

Although many of the early CPT studies failed to assess reaction times (RTs), there is now evidence confirming that ADHD subjects typically show slower and more variable RTs than controls (Klorman, Salzman, Pass, Borgstedt, & Dainer, 1979). There is also evidence that the improvement in accuracy observed on MPH is sometimes accompanied by faster RTs and decreased RT variability (Coons, Klorman, & Borgstedt, 1987; Klorman et al., 1979; Peloquin & Klorman, 1986).

Evidence from Studies of Event-Related Potentials

Several investigators have attempted to obtain additional information about the processing stages implicated in ADHD and the ac-

tion of MPH by monitoring event-related potentials (ERPs) during CPT performance. The most consistent findings have been obtained from the measure of P3 (or P3b) *amplitude,* which is thought to reflect capacity allocation during stimulus evaluation processes (Jonkman, 1997; Klorman, 1991). In a recent review of ERP studies, Jonkman (1997) reported that smaller P3 amplitudes were found in ADHD than control samples in 6 out of 8 studies. Although some investigators found differences only for target stimuli, others reported smaller amplitudes to both targets and nontargets, possibly implicating a *generalized* deficiency in attention allocation. In a review of MPH effects, Jonkman (1997) reported that MPH increased P3 amplitude in 9 out of 14 studies. As in the ADHD–control comparisons, changes in amplitude were sometimes found for both targets and nontargets.

Reports on measures of P3 (or P3b) *latency* on the CPT have been less consistent. Earlier studies in Klorman's laboratory did not find either ADHD–control differences or stimulant effects on P3b latency (Klorman *et al.,* 1979; Michael, Klorman, Salzman, Borgstedt, & Dainer, 1981; Peloquin & Klorman, 1986). These findings seemed to suggest that both the processing deficit in ADHD and the effects of MPH occurred following stimulus evaluation; that is, following identification of the stimulus as a target or nontarget. However, later studies (Brumaghim, Klorman, Strauss, Lewine, & Goldstein, 1987; Coons *et al.,* 1987; Klorman, Brumaghim, Fitzpatrick, & Borgstedt, 1991) showed that MPH both shortened P3b latencies and reduced their variability. These investigators suggested that the changes observed on MPH reflected a reduction and stabilization in the time taken to evaluate task stimuli. They attributed this improvement to increased capacity allocation *during stimulus evaluation.* Based on a measure reflecting the difference between RT and P3b latency, Klorman and colleagues (1991) also concluded that MPH enabled ADHD adolescents to undertake response processing with the benefit of earlier completion of stimulus evaluation processes.

Sustained Attention over Time on Task

Sergeant and van der Meere's (1990b; see Chapter 4, this volume) criticism of the sustained-attention hypothesis centered on a failure of several studies to meet classical criteria for a sustained-attention deficit. They argued that it is necessary to demonstrate, first, that both ADHD and control groups show the expected performance decrement over time and, second, that the decrement is more pronounced in the ADHD group. This would be demonstrated by a significant *interaction* between subject groups and time on task.

Some investigators have argued that these criteria are too stringent (Seidel & Joschko, 1990). Interestingly, however, two recent studies (Hooks, Milich, & Lorch, 1994; van der Meere, Shalev, Borger, & Gross-Tsur, 1995) showed differential deterioration in ADHD and control children. Hooks and colleagues (1994) reported that both omission errors and the d' measure showed a sharper decline in ADHD than in control boys. Using extremely slow and variable intertrial intervals (10 to 35 s), van der Meere and colleagues (1995) found a greater increase in RTs in their ADHD group. This effect was maximized in an "experimenter-absent" condition (see Draeger, Prior, & Sanson, 1986).

In keeping with their emphasis on energetic factors, van der Meere and colleagues (1995) favored a "suboptimal activation" hypothesis to explain their findings. This interpretation is based on the assumption that slow presentation rates produce less stimulation than fast rates. Evidence that ADHD children are particularly affected by event rates was also reported by Chee, Logan, Schachar, Lindsay, and Wachsmuth (1989). In another study, Alberts and van der Meere (1992) suggested a "self-stimulation" hypothesis to explain findings in which ADHD children appeared to prevent a deterioration over time by "looking away," presumably at other objects in the room, during blank periods between stimuli. It is not clear, however, that slow event rates were responsible for the steeper decline in the van der Meere and colleagues (1995) study. Hooks and colleagues (1994), unlike van der Meere and

colleagues (1995), obtained their findings using a relatively typical event rate.

Effects of Stimulants and Reinforcement

Van der Meere and colleagues (1995) reported that MPH "literally erased" (p. 701) both the overall difference and the decrement across trials in the ADHD group. Several other recent studies support the conclusion that MPH acts both to speed RTs and to counteract the decrement in performance of ADHD subjects (De Sonneville, Njiokiktjien, & Hilhorst, 1991; Klorman et al., 1991; Klorman, Brumaghim, Fitzpatrick, Borgstedt, & Strauss, 1994; Levy & Hobbes, 1996). These results suggest stimulant action on the processes regulating *both* overall attentional allocation and the maintenance of attention on later trials.

Citing opinions from the treatment literature that stimulants and behavioral contingencies act similarly to compensate for an elevated reward threshold in ADHD, Solanto, Wender, and Bartell (1997) designed a study to compare the effects of the two interventions on the maintenance of attention across trials. ADHD children were assessed in four treatment conditions (placebo + feedback, placebo + response contingencies, MPH + feedback, and MPH + response contingencies). MPH improved overall performance levels and reduced deterioration in d' over time. In contrast, the response contingencies improved d' but did not affect the slope of deterioration. Solanto and colleagues used Sanders's (1977, 1983) model to interpret their results. Because MPH affected the slope of deterioration, they argued that it acted on Sanders's effort component, which supplies both the arousal and the activation pools. Since the contingencies affected only overall d', these investigators suggested that their effect was confined to increasing arousal.

An alternative interpretation of the findings could also be considered. In a recent study, in which we used heart rate (HR) changes to monitor the response of ADHD and control children to the repeated introduction and removal of rewards (Iaboni, Douglas, & Ditto, 1996), we found that the ADHD group habituated more quickly than controls to the reward contingencies. It could be argued, therefore, that MPH and the response contingencies improved effort allocation in the Solanto and colleagues (1997) study, but that the effects of reward habituated too early to prevent the decline on later trials. As I discuss later, there is other evidence suggesting that ADHD children habituate to the effects of reward and other stimulating events more quickly than controls.

Summary of CPT Findings

Extensive research with vigilance tasks strongly supports the hypothesis that ADHD children show attentional deficits during stimulus processing. The findings on commission errors also support an inhibition problem. In addition, there is clear evidence that MPH reduces these deficits and combats a decline in performance across trials, probably by activating effort and capacity allocation.

Although there is some debate about the use of signal detection methods with CPT data (Koelega, 1995), findings on the d' measure suggest a deficit in the arousal component of Sanders's (1977, 1983) model. It is interesting to note that, in one of their papers, Sergeant and van der Meere (1990b) referred to the "remarkable consistency" in findings of d' deficits in ADHD. These investigators themselves found an overall deficit in d' in the same study in which they failed to show a steeper decline in performance in their ADHD group (Sergeant & van der Meere, 1988). In their discussion of this finding, they referred to the possibility that children with ADHD have a *constant arousal deficit*. They apparently abandoned this hypothesis, however, probably because of other findings from their laboratory (to be discussed next).

Selective or Focused Attention

Memory Search Paradigm

Sergeant and van der Meere's position (see Chapter 4, this volume) that ADHD children do not show attentional deficits was influenced

by several failures to locate information-processing deficits within the stimulus-processing stages of the Sternberg (1969, 1975) model. Most of their studies used variations of Sternberg's (1969) memory scanning task (described in Chapter 4, this volume). In several studies, they assessed the effects of manipulating processing loads which, in the Sternberg model, affects memory search. Drawing on the attentional model of Shiffrin and Schneider (1977), van der Meere, van Baal, and Sergeant (1989) defined Sternberg's search stage as assessing divided attention, which Shiffrin and Schneider consider to be one aspect of controlled selective attention.

Their studies using the manipulation of processing load (reviewed in Sergeant & van der Meere, 1990b) frequently yielded *overall* group differences on error rates, RT, or RT variability. However, the load manipulations failed to show *differential* effects on ADHD samples, thus leading them to conclude that ADHD children do not have a selective attention deficit. In another study, van der Meere and Sergeant (1988) failed to show that ADHD children were differentially vulnerable to distractors. Considered together, these findings led them to conclude that ADHD children do not have a selective, divided, or focused attention deficit (Sergeant & van der Meere, 1990b).

Early stimulant medication studies by Klorman and his colleagues (reviewed in Klorman, 1991), in which they compared MPH effects on high versus low loads on the memory search task, provided indirect support for Sergeant and van der Meere's position. As in studies using the CPT, they have generally found that MPH can reduce errors, speed RT, and decrease RT variability (Brumaghim *et al.*, 1987; Fitzpatrick, Klorman, Brumaghim, & Keefover, 1988; Klorman, Brumaghim, Fitzpatrick, & Borgstedt, 1992; Klorman *et al.*, 1994). However, speeding effects in two of the earlier studies (Brumaghim *et al.*, 1987; Fitzpatrick *et al.*, 1988) were comparable for small and large memory loads. In addition, P3b latency, which marks the time of completion of stimulus evaluation (identification of the stimulus as a target or nontarget) was not changed by MPH. These findings from the earlier studies in Klorman's laboratory suggested that the improvement in RT occurred following stimulus evaluation; that is, during the motor output stage.

Critique and Contrary Findings

It is important to keep in mind that Sergeant and van der Meere's (1990b) conclusions regarding the absence of selective, divided, and focused attention deficits, as well as their criticism of the sustained-attention hypothesis, were based on failures to obtain significant *interactions* between subject groups and the various within-task manipulations used in their studies (early vs. late trials, low vs. high loads, presence or absence of distractors). Within-task manipulations represent a sound approach for studying the differential effects of critical task variables in experimental and control groups. As clinical researchers have long recognized, however, this approach is also very exacting (Chapman & Chapman, 1978; Cohen & Cohen, 1983; Pennington & Ozonoff, 1996; Zahn, Kruesi, & Rapoport, 1991). Interactions are difficult to obtain because they depend on demonstrating differences between differences. The problem is further exacerbated when subject samples are small or when there is high variability in the data; both of these conditions frequently apply to these studies. Thus, the usual cautions about drawing conclusions from negative results are particularly relevant.

In the case of the processing load manipulation, there is another reason for caution in interpreting the failures to find subject group interactions. Developmental studies have also frequently failed to show interactions between age and processing load (Klorman et al., 1994; van der Meere, Gunning, & Stemerdink, 1996; Sergeant, 1996). Stated differently, speed of scanning items on Sternberg-like tasks appears to level off at an early age. Enns and Cameron (1987), for example, found no slope differences between 4- and 7-year-olds. The early development of this skill would be expected to make it relatively insensitive to subject group differences, particularly in children older than 6 or 7 years.

It is also necessary to consider the fact that effects of these task manipulations must be assessed against the background of large overall group differences. Indeed, as mentioned previously, ADHD children often have inferior scores on accuracy, RT, and RT variability, even in baseline conditions. Klorman and colleagues (1992, 1994) also expressed concern that group differences in baseline conditions can make the application of Sternberg's additive-factors logic to findings from load manipulations problematic.

Evidence from Other Selective Attention Studies

An early review from our laboratory (Douglas & Peters, 1979) helped influence Sergeant and van der Meere (1990b) to conclude that ADHD children do not show selective attention problems. Our review was partially motivated by the then prevalent belief that ADHD children are "stimulus driven" and, consequently, must be protected from extraneous distractors by such extreme methods as isolating them in special cubicles in the classroom. We were also dubious about the attribution of all of the children's attentional problems to distractibility. We had observed serious attentional difficulties in relatively distraction-free laboratory environments, and we were unwilling to ascribe their poor performance to poorly defined external or internal distractors. Thus, we felt that at least equal emphasis should be placed on the inability of ADHD children to *focus* or to *invest attention* on task-relevant stimuli. We were impressed, as well, by the number of studies, including some of our own, that had failed to show distraction effects in ADHD groups. In addition, we were intrigued by occasional hints that some kinds of extraneous stimuli improved, rather than impaired, the children's performance.

These questions continue to concern ADHD researchers. Zentall and her colleagues followed up the observation that external stimulation may have positive effects on ADHD children. Emphasizing the role of optimal arousal levels on performance, Zentall and Zentall

(1983) reviewed evidence to support their hypothesis that ADHD children engage in stimulation-seeking behavior in order to increase chronically low arousal levels. This position raises the possibility that stimulation-seeking behaviors or the presence of extraneous stimuli may have either positive or negative effects on ADHD children's performance, depending on a variety of poorly understood factors.

In a later review of selective attention and distractibility studies (Douglas, 1983), I pointed to increasing evidence demonstrating that ADHD children are particularly vulnerable to novel or salient distractors and that they are most likely to show distractibility on difficult (effort-demanding) or boring (unstimulating) tasks. Although there have also been some negative reports, particularly from speeded classification tasks (Hooks *et al.*, 1994; Tarnowski, Prinz, & Nay, 1986), evidence that ADHD children show distractibility or selective attention deficits on some tasks and under some conditions continues to accumulate.

Incidental Memory Paradigm

In the Douglas and Peters (1979) review, we reported Peters's (1977) failure to demonstrate that the presence of extraneous stimuli impaired the ability of ADHD children to recall central stimuli on an incidental learning task. This task involves presenting subjects with a series of cards containing pictures of central stimuli, which they are directed to remember, and incidental stimuli, which they are told to ignore. The children are tested for recall of both the central and incidental stimuli; the underlying assumption is that processing of extraneous stimuli interferes with processing of central stimuli.

In a later study, using ingenious modifications of the incidental learning paradigm and sensitive recognition measures, Ceci and Tishman (1984) found that when encoding demands are low, as in the Peters (1977) study, ADHD children are able to pay more attention than control children to incidental stimuli without sacrificing processing of the central information. Indeed, on a measure that allowed them to benefit from processing both central and incidental stimuli, their recognition performance was *better* than that of the comparison group. Ceci and Tishman also found, however, that when demands were increased by limiting the time available for encoding, or by using difficult-to-encode central stimuli, the recognition accuracy of the ADHD group dropped below that of control children. In interpreting their findings, Ceci and Tishman described the attentional approach of ADHD children as "diffuse." This description appears to emphasize a failure to focus adequately on the central stimuli.

Two-Channel Selective Attention Paradigms

Two-channel paradigms, including dichotic listening tasks (described in Chapter 4, this volume) and tasks employing the visual and auditory modalities, have also yielded evidence of selective attention problems. In addition to assessing errors, several investigators have monitored the early ERP negative wave called processing negativity (PN). This measure reflects the amount of responsivity to relevant (designated) stimuli, as compared to responsivity to irrelevant stimuli. Normal subjects show larger amplitudes for the designated stimuli.

ADHD children typically make fewer correct detections on these tasks. Although findings from the negativity measure have been rather inconsistent, there is some agreement that ADHD children fail to show the expected pattern of preferential (selective) attention to designated stimuli, particularly on auditory tasks (Jonkman, 1997; Jonkman *et al.*, 1997b; Klorman, 1991, 1995; Satterfield, Schell, & Nicholas, 1994). There is also some evidence that MPH enhances the negativity measure (Jonkman *et al.*, 1997a).

Satterfield and colleagues (1994) also found evidence of deficient preferential processing using a two-channel auditory-visual paradigm and monitoring P3 amplitude and latency measures. They argued that their findings pointed to impaired responding to target stimuli, rather than difficulty in ignoring nontarget stimuli.

More Recent Findings from Sternberg Task

Although the findings from Klorman's laboratory reviewed earlier suggested that ADHD–control differences and MPH effects did not occur during Sternberg's stimulus-processing stages, more recent studies comparing P3b latencies to targets versus nontargets suggest that ADHD children show a selective attention deficit, which is ameliorated by MPH. Klorman and colleagues (1992) reported that ADHD adolescents failed to show the normal pattern of faster P3b latencies to targets than to nontargets. MPH reduced errors and speeded P3b latency to target stimuli. In a second study with young ADHD children, Klorman and colleagues (1994) again found that MPH produced differentially faster P3b latencies for targets. In reviewing these findings, Klorman (1995) argued that faster P3b latencies to targets reflect greater ease in identifying significant stimuli. He concluded, therefore, that ADHD is associated with a deficit in the *stimulus evaluation* processes which precede preparation and execution of a motor response. Klorman also emphasized that this evidence of a specific selective attention deficit to target stimuli demonstrates that the processing deficiencies of ADHD children are not entirely attributable to nonspecific arousal or motivation problems. Moreover, MPH appears to have a specific effect on selective attention that can be differentiated from more generalized effects on energetic processes.

Evidence for Inhibitory Problems in ADHD

Sonuga-Barke (1995) drew a distinction between "ongoing" and "momentary" inhibition. He defines *ongoing inhibition* as the ability to suppress responding *over a period* of delay. He restricts the term *momentary inhibition* to situations in which a dominant or prepotent response must be withheld *following a signal* that the response is inappropriate. Sonuga-Barke's definition of ongoing inhibition resembles my emphasis on pervasive stylistic differences in ADHD children, which are discussed later.

Sonuga-Barke (1995) also reminded us that Quay's (1988a, 1988b, 1997) approach to momentary disinhibition is *motivational.* In this approach, inhibition errors result from the failure of an underactive BIS to respond to conditioned cues for punishment or nonreward. Sonuga-Barke contrasted this with the *cognitive* approach adopted by Logan and Cowan (1984) in developing the Stop task to assess inhibitory processes during information processing.

Because the role of inhibition in ADHD is covered extensively in Chapters 4 and 13 (this volume), I limit my comments to some concerns about the methods currently available to assess momentary inhibitory processes in ADHD. Perhaps because of the belated interest in inhibition, these methods have received much less critical attention than methods for assessing attentional deficits. An exception is the measure of commission errors on the CPT although, as discussed earlier, the diagnostic usefulness of this measure will depend on adequate standardization studies.

Most of the other tasks currently in use to assess inhibition in ADHD are subject to several criticisms, including insufficient evidence of replicability of findings, confounding effects resulting from the inclusion of reinforcers within the inhibition tasks, and the use of research designs employing within-task manipulations without the necessary statistical controls.

Go/No-Go Tasks

The Shue and Douglas (1992) findings from a manually administered and scored Go/No-Go task (described in Chapter 4, this volume) are cited to support an inhibitory defect in ADHD children. However, our attempts to replicate our findings using a more reliable computerized version of the task have yielded inconsistent findings. A more concerted effort, with greater emphasis on the effects of presentation rates and age differences, might yield more positive results. However, another study by Trommer, Hoeppner, Lorber, and Armstrong (1988a), using a brief, hand-scored version, yielded confusing results. Although their *nonhyperactive* ADD group made more commission errors than normal controls, their ADD group with hyperactive symptoms showed more evidence of *attentional* problems, as reflected in more errors of omission and a failure to improve across trials.

Turning to the more complex Go/No-Go learning task used by Iaboni, Douglas, and Baker (1995), we must recognize that this task was designed to study the effects of different reinforcement contingencies on inhibition. Although the results clearly demonstrated a higher incidence of commission (inhibitory) errors in our ADHD group across the combinations of contingencies studied, we would not recommend the task as an inhibition measure because of the confounding effects of the reinforcement contingencies. In addition, the task taps relatively complex learning processes.

Differential Reinforcement for Low-Rate Responding

This task, in which subjects must repeatedly withhold responding for designated time intervals in order to receive rewards (Gordon, 1979; McClure & Gordon, 1984), also has the disadvantage of involving reinforcers. In addition, I was unable to find replication studies showing ADHD–control differences from other laboratories. My concern about this was increased by our failure to demonstrate differences between ADHD and control children in two (unpublished) attempts.

"Door Opening Task"

This task, developed by Daugherty and Quay (1991), assesses a child's willingness to continue to respond for reward in the face of diminishing payoffs. Although the task provides a novel way to assess an important aspect of ADHD behavior, it is not possible to separate the effects of the children's response to the reward contingencies from their inhibitory problems.

Designs Using Within-Task Manipulations of Inhibitory Demands

A recent study by Casey and colleagues (1997) used the within-task manipulation design discussed earlier to investigate the effects

of the presence or absence of inhibitory demands on the performance of ADHD and control children. Their inhibitory manipulations are somewhat questionable. Also of concern, however, is their use of the within-task design without appropriate statistical controls. These investigators used three control tasks and three experimental tasks, which included increased inhibitory demands. In analyzing their results, however, they did not test for the significant group interactions that would be necessary to establish that their manipulations of inhibitory demands had a *differential* effect on the ADHD group. Instead, they reported separate results for the two subject groups on the control and inhibition tasks. This is particularly problematic because their results showed large ADHD–control group differences on the control tasks. Although Casey and colleagues went on to report correlations between their cognitive task measures and magnetic resonance imaging (MRI) measures, their failure to assess the specific effects of the inhibitory manipulations makes it impossible to interpret these findings. In future studies using brain imaging techniques to study ADHD, it will be important to ensure that the growing sophistication of these techniques is matched by equally sophisticated cognitive assessment procedures.

Stroop Color–Word Interference Test

Research with the Stroop task (Stroop, 1935) reflects a similar problem. Most of the Stroop studies reviewed by Barkley, Grodinzsky, and DuPaul (1992), for example, failed to control for group differences on the Stroop cards that do not contain interfering stimuli (color naming and word reading). I feel reasonably confident, however, that the hypothesis that ADHD children are particularly vulnerable to interference effects on the Stroop will hold up. We recently replicated the early positive findings using a computerized version of the Stroop task and the necessary statistical controls (Berman, Douglas, & Dunbar, 1994).

In considering these findings from the Stroop task, it is also important to note that, although I have included it here with measures of inhibition, some investigators describe the Stroop as assessing *voluntary attentional control* (Dunbar & Sussman, 1995; MacLeod, 1991).

Stop-Signal Task

The Stop-Signal task, described in Chapter 4 (this volume), was developed by Logan and Cowan (1984) to provide a "pure" and reliable measure of defective inhibition during information processing. In a recent meta-analysis, Oosterlaan, Logan, and Sergeant (1998) reviewed findings from eight studies employing this task. The findings confirmed that the ADHD–control differences reported by Schachar and his colleagues (Schachar & Logan, 1990; Schachar & Tannock, 1995; Schachar, Tannock, & Logan, 1993; Schachar, Tannock, Marriott & Logan, 1995) are being replicated fairly consistently in other laboratories. (See Chapter 4, this volume, for a more detailed report of this review.) The impaired performance of ADHD children appears to be associated with *slow, variable inhibitory processes.*

There is some disagreement, however, about whether defective inhibition is specific to ADHD. Schachar and Tannock (1995) appeared to confirm an earlier finding that *pure* Conduct Disordered (CD) children do not show the deficit. However, their study included only five pure CD cases. In addition, evidence reported by Oosterlaan and Sergeant (1995, 1996a, 1996b) strongly supports the presence of inhibitory deficits in groups labeled "aggressive" or "disruptive," which they selected using different (non-DSM) criteria.

It is important to note that the Stop task shares some characteristics with the CPT, although the response required clearly differs. In both tasks, subjects must monitor stimuli carefully while maintaining preparation to make the appropriate response (either inhibit or respond) to rare and unpredictable stimuli. Also in both tasks, ADHD children are differentiated from normal controls by their slow, variable RTs. Thus, it appears that the tasks share common regulatory demands associated with remaining *vigilant,* maintaining *preparation* to respond, and coping with *unpredictability.* It

should be noted that Oosterlaan and Sergeant (1995) also suggested that the Stop task assesses preparation, as well as inhibition.

Stimulant Effects on Inhibitory Tasks

The limited available evidence supports the argument that MPH acts on inhibitory processes. Evidence on the effects of MPH on errors of commission on vigilance tasks was discussed earlier. Berman and colleagues (1994) found that MPH reduced errors on the computerized version of the Stroop task. Another study just completed in our laboratory showed that MPH reduced errors of commission on the complex Go/No-Go learning task used in the study by Iaboni and colleagues (1995). Trommer, Hoeppner, and Zecker (1991) also reported a reduction in commission errors on their simple Go/No-Go task in ADD children *without* hyperactive symptoms. Finally, MPH has been shown to improve performance on the Stop task (Tannock, Schachar, Carr, Chajczyk, & Logan, 1989; Tannock, Schachar, & Logan, 1995).

Psychophysiological Evidence of an Inhibitory Deficiency

A recent study in our laboratory (Iaboni *et al.,* 1996) used psychophysiological measures to test Quay's (1988a, 1988b, 1997) hypothesis that ADHD children show an inhibitory problem, as defined in Gray's (1982, 1987) model. Our study was based on findings by Fowles and his colleagues (Fowles, 1980, 1988) demonstrating that skin conductance reflects activity of Gray's BIS, whereas HR reflects activity of the Behavioral Activation System (BAS). Iaboni and colleagues recorded skin conductance levels during a repetitive motor task in which rewards were repeatedly introduced and removed. Extinction trials were expected to elicit activity in the BIS because the BIS acts to inhibit behavior in order to facilitate a more careful analysis of factors that may be responsible for the termination of rewards. In agreement with Quay's hypothesis, while control children showed the expected pattern, ADHD children showed a striking lack of electrodermal responsivity on the extinction trials.

At first glance, these results appear to disagree with those reported by Pliszka, Hatch, Borcherding, and Rogeness (1993). However, that study dealt with classical conditioning, whereas ours employed conditioned stimuli. As Quay (1997) has emphasized, Gray's formulations of the BIS and BAS refer exclusively to responding to conditioned stimuli, and the BIS is not involved in the formation of classically conditioned responses.

Motor Output, Motor Coordination, and Motor Control

Having failed to find deficits in ADHD children during stimulus processing, Sergeant and van der Meere (1990b) hypothesized that the cause of their slow RTs on information-processing tasks must be located at the motor output or response-processing stage. As noted earlier, these investigators did not discuss the possibility of basic motor control deficits. Rather, they attributed the hypothesized motor output dysfunction to inadequate allocation of energetic resources to processing at the motor stage. That is, they saw the deficits as originating at the effort mechanism, or possibly the activation pool of Sanders's model (Sergeant & van der Meere, 1990b; see also Chapter 4, this volume).

Do ADHD Children Have Basic Motor Control Deficits?

Before considering Sergeant and van der Meere's (1990b) attempts to demonstrate impaired processing at the motor output stage, it is important to recognize the long history of concern about possible motor control problems in ADHD children (see also Chapter 13, this volume).

Motor Control and Coordination

In an early paper (Douglas, 1972), I reported ADHD deficits on a number of tasks thought to assess fine and gross motor coordi-

nation. I was puzzled at that time, and remain puzzled, about the relationship between these motor control and coordination deficits and more generalized regulatory control problems. Denckla (Denckla & Rudel, 1978; Denckla, Rudel, Chapman, & Krieger, 1985), a pioneer in this area, reported deficiencies in motor proficiency in hyperactive boys using tasks assessing speed, rhythm, and "motor overflow." In a recent paper, Denckla (1996) spoke of motor control as a "neighbor/fellow traveller" (p. 264) of executive control functions. Thus, she also is impressed by the apparent relationship between control of motor movement and other aspects of regulatory control.

Continuing interest in these deficits is reflected in several recent studies. Mariani and Barkley (1997) compared ADHD boys (ages 4 and 5) with control boys on a large battery of academic and neuropsychological tasks. One of two factor scores that differentiated ADHD boys from controls reflected motor control problems. The second factor reflected problems with working memory and persistence. The emergence of these factors prompted Mariani and Barkley to conclude that ADHD must be conceptualized in a manner that recognizes both "the neuromaturational nature of the children's symptoms" and "the involvement of executive functions beyond the core problems in behavioral inhibition and sustained attention" (p. 111).

Oculomotor Control

Other studies have focused on abnormalities in oculomotor functioning in ADHD children, particularly those reflecting impaired smooth-pursuit eye movements (Bala et al., 1981; Bylsma & Pivik, 1989). In addition, Ross, Hommer, Breiger, Varley, and Radant (1994) recently reported that children with ADHD had difficulty delaying responding on an oculomotor delayed-response task. Since the ADHD children did not differ from controls on measures of latency or accuracy of the delayed response, Ross and colleagues concluded that the primary deficit in ADHD concerns inhibition of motor responding. However, the extremely short delay period (800 ms) used in this study makes it impossible to rule out additional problems with working memory, the ability to maintain response preparation, or both, since subjects were required to remember the position of the stimulus and maintain readiness to respond for only a brief period.

Findings from Neuroimaging

A recent neuroimaging study by Berquin and colleagues (1997) used MRI techniques to study possible differences in brain volume in the areas controlling movement. Their findings led them to speculate that "a cerebello-thalamo-prefrontal circuit dysfunction may subserve the motor control and inhibition and/or executive function deficits encountered in ADHD" (p. 1087). This is another example of research findings suggesting the need to consider a possible relationship between impaired motor control and more general regulatory control problems.

Motor Problems as Defined by Sanders's Motor Output Stage

Stimulus–Response Spatial Compatibility Paradigm. The S–R compatibility paradigm has been used to study possible deficits in *response choice* in ADHD children. In Sanders's model, response choice represents a substage of motor output, and is affected by compatibility manipulations. RTs have been shown to be shorter for compatible than for incompatible responses (Verfaellie, Bowers, & Heilman, 1990). This is attributed to an automatic tendency to respond in a compatible manner (on the same side as the stimulus), thus making it necessary to *inhibit* the prepotent compatible response before executing the incompatible response.

Van der Meere and colleagues (1989) reported a significant interaction on mean RTs between subject groups (ADHD vs. controls) and a compatible–incompatible manipulation, with the RTs of ADHD children showing more slowing in the incompatible condition. They interpreted this finding as supporting a motor ouput deficit involving response choice.

However, in a later study in which they investigated the effects of both event rate and compatibility demands, van der Meere, Vreeling, and Sergeant (1992) failed to show differential group effects on the compatibility manipulation. The event rate manipulation yielded a significant interaction in this study; therefore, they suggested that the slow event rates used in the earlier study may have been responsible for the group differences they obtained on the compatibility manipulation. Consequently, they suggested that ADHD children have a problem involving *response preparation,* another substage of motor output. This interpretation is based on the assumption in Sanders's model that event rates affect motor preparation.

Oosterlaan and Sergeant (1995) also failed a find a differential group effect using a compatibility manipulation. Noting the importance of event rates in the previous studies, they speculated that their failure to obtain group differences on the compatibility manipulation was due to the use of relatively fast event rates in their study.

Regulatory Demands for Adaptation, Preparation, and Flexible Responding

S–R Compatibility Task with Changing Response Requirements

We recently used a four-choice S–R compatibility paradigm to assess the response of ADHD children to heavier incompatibility demands and also to investigate the effects of predictability of response demands on the performance of ADHD and control children (Elbaz, Douglas, & Ditto, 1997). We predicted that the need to adapt flexibly to changing, unpredictable demands for compatible or incompatible responding would overtax the regulatory capabilities of ADHD children. The design included a fixed (predictable) compatible condition, a fixed incompatible condition, and a third mixed condition in which compatible and incompatible trials were randomly mixed. In the mixed condition, children were informed prior to each trial whether a compatible or incompatible response was required on that trial. The order of presentation of the three conditions, fixed compatible, fixed incompatible, and mixed compatible–incompatible, was counterbalanced across subjects. In order to increase processing demands, we used a four-choice S–R task rather than the two-choice tasks used in the previous studies.

Overall RTs of the ADHD children were slower than those of control children. The two groups also showed similar increases in RT in the fixed incompatible as compared with the fixed compatible condition, suggesting that the ADHD group did not experience differential difficulty with incompatible demands even on our four-choice task. However, analyses following a significant predictability X group interaction revealed that RTs of the ADHD group were more slowed than those of controls in the mixed condition. Thus, the ADHD group had more difficulty adjusting to unpredictable response demands.

Stroop Task with Unpredictable Response Requirements

We also pursued the hypothesis that ADHD children have particular difficulty adjusting to unpredictable demands using two computerized versions of the Stroop Color Word Interference task (Berman *et al.*, 1994). The two versions were presented to ADHD and control children in a counterbalanced order. In the "predictable" version, as in the traditional Stroop paradigm, instructions to read the word (or to name the color) were announced prior to a block of trials requiring the same response (either word reading or color naming) throughout all trials in the block. In the "unpredictable" version, children were informed by a high or low tone *prior to each stimulus* whether they were to read the word or name the color on that particular trial.

As we found with the mixed compatibility–incompatibility manipulation, children with ADHD were differentially affected by the unpredictable response demands. This was demonstrated by a dramatic increase in the tendency to make the more automatic word reading response.

Tasks Requiring Adaptation of Response Speeds

The ability to adapt to changing demands has also been investigated in several studies in which subjects were required to adapt their response speeds to changing conditions. Van der Meere and colleagues (1989) used the term "poor control adjustment" to refer to these findings. In an early study, Stevens, Stover, and Backus (1970) reported that, although ADHD children's spontaneous tapping speeds were faster than those of controls, they failed to respond to incentives to increase tapping speeds. Sergeant and Scholten (1985) also found that their ADHD group was unable to adjust to instructions for fast responding. Since speed instructions place heavy demands on the rapid deployment of processing resources, they concluded that ADHD children show deficient resource allocation. Sergeant and van der Meere (1988) found that ADHD children failed to slow their response speeds as a function of processing load after making an error, which was also seen as a failure in response adjustment.

The Change Task

Some studies using the Stop task have added a "reengagement" or "change" requirement. Following the successful completion of the stop response, subjects are required to execute a different response. Thus, the Change task assesses the ability to shift flexibly and rapidly from one response to another (De Jong, Coles, & Logan, 1995). Schachar and his colleagues (Schachar & Tannock, 1995; Schachar *et al.*, 1995) reported that ADHD children had difficulty with *both* the stop and change requirements on the new task. Oosterlaan and Sergeant (1996b) found greater variability in the latency of response reengagement, as well as reduced accuracy in their ADHD group. As with the Stop task, they found that a group of "disruptive" children showed a similar pattern.

In a discussion of ADHD findings on the Stop and Change tasks, Schachar and colleagues (1993) argued that these tasks assess two different aspects of regulation. De Jong and colleagues (1995) recently reported evidence from lateralized readiness potentials to argue that the tasks tap functionally distinct mechanisms and strategies, with the Change task more clearly associated with a centrally operating mechanism that selectively inhibits the "go" response, without impeding the execution of alternative movements.

Warned Reaction-Time Tasks

Warned reaction-time (WRT) tasks have also been used to assess preparatory and adaptive processes in ADHD. The simple WRT consists of a series of trials in which there is a warning signal, followed by a preparatory interval (PI), and a signal to respond. The warning signal helps prepare the subject to respond as quickly as possible to the response signal. In an early study (Cohen & Douglas, 1972) with the WRT task, we found that ADHD children had slower and more variable RTs than controls. Monitoring of skin conductance revealed that the warning signal failed to elicit normal orienting responses in the ADHD group, suggesting that it did not have the intended effect of facilitating preparation to receive and respond to the imperative signal. Zahn and colleagues (1991) replicated and extended these findings. They compared the effects of two manipulations, length (duration) and predictability (uncertainty) of PI on the RTs of normal boys and boys with diagnoses of Disruptive Behavior Disorders (DBD), many of whom met criteria for ADHD. In the duration manipulation they compared the effects of fixed (blocked) PIs of 2, 4, or 8 s on RT. The predictability manipulation involved presenting the same PIs (2, 4, or 8 s) in a variable, random order.

As in several ADHD studies previously discussed, Zahn and colleagues (1991) found slower and more variable *overall* RTs in boys with DBD than in control boys. Indeed, they mention that these were their strongest findings. Over and above these differences, however, they reported that the performance of boys with DBD was more sensitive to the PI duration and predictability manipulations.

The clearest group differences resulting from the manipulations were found on the longest (8-s) PI. In the fixed condition, longer PIs produced disproportionate slowing of RTs in the boys with DBD. Zahn and colleagues (1991) attributed this to impaired sustained attention, in the sense of impaired ability to maintain preparation as the PIs became longer. They stressed that the PIs on the WRT task lasted for only several seconds, as opposed to the CPT, where attention must be sustained over several minutes. In addition, however, unlike controls, boys with DBD achieved considerably faster RTs at the longest (8-s) PI when it occurred in the varied interval condition than when it occurred in the fixed interval condition. Thus, their particular difficulty with the long PI was most evident when it occurred within the context of other long PIs.

Several other investigators have obtained findings demonstrating that ADHD children have particular difficulty with long PIs (Elbaz *et al.*, 1997), long delays between cue presentation and target onset (Swanson, Posner, *et al.*, 1991; Tomporowski, Tinsley, & Hager, 1994), long preresponse delays (Sonuga-Barke & Taylor, 1991), and long intertrial intervals or slow event rates (Chee *et al.*, 1989; Conte, Kinsbourne, Swanson, Zirk, & Samuels, 1986; van der Meere *et al.*, 1992). These difficulties have been variously attributed to lapses of attention (Zahn *et al.*, 1991), aversion to delay (Sonuga-Barke & Taylor, 1991), or the lack of stimulation associated with overall slow event rates (van der Meere *et al.*, 1992).

There is also evidence to support the Zahn and colleagues (1991) finding showing that these difficulties are most apparent when long delays occur within a context of other long delays. We recently replicated the Zahn and colleagues (1991) results using a four-choice WRT task (Elbaz *et al.*, 1997). Analyses subsequent to obtaining a three-way interaction between groups, length of PI, and predictability of PI, revealed that, unlike controls, ADHD children showed considerably less slowing on long (8-s) PIs in the variable PI condition than in the fixed PI condition. Conte and colleagues (1986) obtained similar results from manipulations of presentation rates on a paired associates task. They found that slow rates had a debilitating effect on the performance of ADD children when presentation rates were fixed, but not in a condition in which slow and fast presentation rates were mixed.

These findings suggest that the appearance of sustained-attention or response-preparation deficits in ADHD is highly dependent on contextual factors, most notably slower average event rates and, possibly, the presence of monotonous repetition. Investigators have appealed to concepts such as underarousal (Conte et al., 1986) and impaired energetic mechanisms (Sanders, 1986, 1990; van der Meere et al., 1992) to explain these results. If these explanations are accepted, the findings provide some support for the previously discussed hypothesis that ADHD children have an abnormal need for stimulation and reinforcement (Douglas, 1985; Douglas & Peters, 1979; Haenlein & Caul, 1987; Kinsbourne, 1983; van der Meere et al., 1995; Zentall & Zentall, 1983).

Stimulant Effects on Preparation, Adaptation, and Flexible Responding

MPH has been shown to reduce inappropriate responses on WRT tasks while speeding RTs and decreasing RT variability (Cohen, Douglas, & Morgenstern, 1971; Douglas et al., 1988). In addition, Zahn, Rapoport, and Thompson (1980) found that amphetamine improved performance and increased HR rate deceleration to task stimuli on the WRT task in both ADHD and normal individuals. Tannock and colleagues (1995) reported that MPH improved the RTs of ADHD children on the Change task. Krusch and colleagues (1996) found that MPH affected the response of ADHD children to their own errors on the Sternberg task. MPH slowed their RTs both on trials on which they made an error and on trials following an error, suggesting that it heightened caution and effort when the children were experiencing uncertainty about their performance. Preliminary findings from our WRT and S–R compatibility tasks suggest that, besides speeding overall RTs and reducing RT variability, MPH eradicates evidence of the more specific vulnerability of ADHD children to long PIs in the fixed PI condition of the WRT and to unpredictability in the mixed condition of the S–R compatibility task.

Implications of MPH Findings

Findings from the tasks discussed thus far suggest that, besides having generalized energizing effects on arousal and activation, MPH helps ADHD children meet more specific demands for preparation, adaptation, inhibition, flexible responding, and selective and sustained attention. Thus, appropriately controlled allocation of energetic resources across multiple aspects of information processing is clearly implicated in the action of MPH.

The evidence that rewards and other stimulating factors have some of the same effects as MPH further supports the importance of arousal and activation in the disorder. It is possible, however, that rewards do not have the fine-tuned regulating effects that have been demonstrated with MPH. Douglas (1985, 1989) argued that it is particularly important to use contingent rewards with ADHD children in order to obtain these specific effects.

Investigators sometimes point to the fact that stimulants also improve the performance of normal individuals to argue that the effects in ADHD do not indicate pathological neurological or neurochemical processes. However, as I have argued previously (Douglas et al., 1988), even normal individuals seldom perform at their optimal levels, presumably because regulatory processes governing the allocation of attention and effort do not always function at full capacity. However, the discrepancy between optimal and typical performance is considerably larger and more pervasive in ADHD children, suggesting that these regulatory processes are chronically underactive in ADHD. Consequently, stimulant action on these processes would be expected to produce more dramatic effects in ADHD children.

Interpreting the Repeated Findings of Slow, Variable Reaction Times

As we have seen repeatedly, investigators studying the effects of specific task manipulations typically find overall slower and more variable RTs in their ADHD samples. Moreover, these differences frequently appear in control conditions, before the manipulations are introduced. I have presented evidence of the presence of this pattern in studies manipulating processing loads on the Sternberg task, compatibility–incompatibility demands on the S–R compatibility task, and length of preparatory intervals on WRT tasks. I have also reviewed evidence of slow, variable RTs on the CPT, Stop, and Change tasks.

Most researchers take care to rule out obvious causes for these patterns, such as group differences in IQ or failure of ADHD children to comply with task instructions. In my earlier discussion of pervasive regulatory deficits in ADHD, I mentioned two other possible causes that our laboratory decided to pursue. These are a general failure to allocate adequate effort to cognitive processing, a failure to allocate effort consistently across task trials, or both.

In a recent study (Leth-Steensen, Douglas, & Elbaz, 1997), we carried out a detailed investigation of the distributions of RTs in ADHD and control children using data from our study of the effects of manipulations of PIs on the choice reaction-time task. We were interested in assessing the relative contribution of a general inability to respond quickly, as opposed to inconsistent responding, which would produce a mixture of fast and slow responses. In addition, because we wanted to know whether the RT distributions from our ADHD sample reflected an immature response pattern typical of younger children, we collected parallel data from a group of normal children several years younger than our ADHD and control samples.

There is a growing recognition that new methods of statistical analysis are required to deal more adequately with RT data. More specifically, it has been demonstrated that studying the shapes of RT distributions can provide more information than the standard statistical measures of mean and variance (Heathcote, Popiel, & Mewhort, 1991; Hockley, 1984; Ratcliff & Murdock, 1976). Distributions of RTs are often not normal in form, but are typically positively skewed. Statistically, this positive skew results in a small number of extreme values having a disproportionate influence on the calculation of the RT mean (as well as increasing the variance). Standard methods for dealing with extreme RT values involve using statistical transformations to reduce the skew.

Observation of the RT distributions of ADHD children has frequently made me wonder, however, whether the positive skewing of their distributions could be regarded as an important phenomenon in its own right. Preliminary distributional analyses of data from our WRT task indicated that much of the observed difference in the RT means and variances between our age-matched ADHD and control children could be accounted for by differences in positive skew. In other words, the responding of the ADHD group was distinguished from that of the control group by the presence of a substantially larger number of abnormally slow responses rather than by an overall pattern of slow responses.

To pursue this observation, we obtained statistical summary measures of the distributional properties of our WRT data by fitting the ex-Gaussian distribution (Heathcote, 1996) to the RT distributions of three groups: ADHD boys, control boys, and a group of younger normal boys. These groups were matched on IQ and socioeconomic status with our ADHDs and controls. The ex-Gaussian is a theoretical distributional model which assumes that each response time can be represented as the sum of a normally distributed and an independent exponentially distributed random variable. The ex-Gaussian distribution has three parameters: mu and sigma, which respectively describe the mean and the standard deviation of the normal component; and tau, which describes both the mean and the standard deviation of the exponential component. In practice, mu and tau reflect the location of the leading edge (or mode) of the distribution and the size of its tail.

Traditional analyses of mean RT and RT variances from the WRT data confirmed that the overall RTs of the ADHD children and the younger controls were significantly slower than those of the control group. RTs of the ADHD children were also significantly more variable than those of the younger controls which, in turn, were significantly more variable than those of the older controls. However, analyses involving the three ex-Gaussian parameters revealed that the differences in RT means and variability between the ADHD and control groups were not due to significant differences in either mu or sigma, but to substantial differences in tau. In contrast, the differences in RT means and variability between the older and younger control groups were due to significant difference in all of the ex-Gaussian parameters. Thus, only findings from the ex-Gaussian analysis were able to clarify that the slower and more variable responding of the ADHD children cannot be attributed to developmental delay (which appears to be marked by overall slowing and spreading out of RTs) but, rather, to a tendency to respond abnormally slowly on a greater number of trials. These findings strongly suggest that inconsistent or erratic allocation of attention and effort plays a major role in the deficits shown by ADHD children on information-processing tasks.

Van der Molen (1996) argued that RT variability is the "dynamometer of attention" (p. 232), with high variability reflecting fluctuations and lapses in attentional allocation. Sanders (1983) argued that difficulties with basic cognitive processing result in consistently slow performance, whereas energetic deficiencies are reflected in high RT variability. Thus, in Sanders's model, our findings support a deficit at the energetic, rather than the functional level.

The observation that ADHD children show erratic RTs is not new. After carrying out detailed analyses of RT distributions for both correct and incorrect responses, Sergeant (1988) emphasized the importance of fluctuations in the children's processing times, which he attributed to poorly understood "inefficient control processes" (p. 196). Hicks, Mayo, and Clayton (1989) argued that ADHD children

can be best characterized by their excessive variability. They further hypothesized that stimulants act on the neural substrate responsible for the abnormal oscillations, which they consider to be the regulatory functions of the frontal lobes.

Besides having far-reaching theoretical and clinical implications, RT variability has important implications for the statistical approaches used to analyze RT data from ADHD samples. In particular, it raises serious doubts about applying statistical transformations in order to normalize RT distributions. It appears that these methods effectively eliminate the information that most clearly characterizes ADHD samples.

Stylistic Differences in the Approach of ADHD Children to Cognitive Tasks

Impulsive–Reflective Cognitive Style

General. The "cognitive style" concept has caused heated debate among psychologists over many years. In a recent review, Sternberg and Grigorenko (1997) remarked that, despite the disagreement the concept has engendered, the question of whether individuals show personal preferences in the way they use their cognitive abilities is still being debated. This question is particularly relevant for ADHD children, who often do not use their cognitive abilities, or use them in a manner not acceptable to adults.

The cognitive style of *reflection–impulsivity* was introduced by Kagan (1965a, 1965b) to refer to individual differences in the tendency to invest time and effort reflecting on alternative possibilities before making a decision in situations involving high response uncertainty. Kagan assessed this style using the Matching Familiar Figures test (MFFT) (described in Chapter 4, this volume), in which impulsivity is reflected in fast, inaccurate responses.

Because the term *impulsivity* has caused unnecessary confusion in ADHD research, it is important to distinguish between Kagan's definition and the use of the term in the information-processing literature to refer to the sacrifice of accuracy for speed on tasks involving relatively unambiguously correct responses and relatively fast processing times. Differences in the demands of fast versus slow processing tasks have also been emphasized by Rapport and Kelly (1991).

Although findings from the MFFT have been somewhat inconsistent, the available evidence suggests that ADHD children do not take sufficient time to search carefully through the alternatives and, consequently, make more errors than control groups (Douglas et al., 1988; Pennington & Ozonoff, 1996; Sonuga-Barke, 1995). Because of criticisms of the MFFT, it should be noted that some of these studies used ADHD and control groups adequately matched on IQ, and also employed more reliable, extended versions of the MFFT (see Douglas et al., 1988; Milich & Kramer, 1984; Salkind, 1978; Walker, 1986). The need to avoid including "time off task" in the calculation of response times (Douglas, 1983) continues to receive insufficient attention, and may account for the greater inconsistency in findings from the response-time measure.

Stimulant Effects on the MFFT. There is good evidence that MPH both *slows* response times and reduces errors on the MFFT. In addition, the slowing effects are more pronounced on higher MPH doses (Douglas et al., 1988; Rapport et al., 1988). At first glance, these results appear to disagree with the findings discussed earlier showing that MPH reduces errors and *speeds* RTs on the CPT, WRT, and Sternberg tasks. To reconcile these findings, it is necessary to consider the differences emphasized earlier between the MFFT and these fast processing tasks. It is also necessary to remember that response times of unmedicated ADHD children are *slower* than those of controls on the CPT, WRT, and Sternberg tasks, but *faster* on the MFFT. The slow-inaccurate pattern on fast-paced information-processing tasks clearly does not fit the fast-inaccurate criteria for impulsive responding. Nevertheless, as I argued earlier, the findings suggest that the slow RTs on these tasks *also* result from impaired regulation of attention and effort. Consequently, it should not

be surprising that activating effects of MPH on regulatory processes result in speeding of RTs on one type of task and slowing on the other.

Delay Aversion

Sonuga-Barke (1995) pointed to the need to differentiate between such hypothesized deficits as impaired inhibition, impulsivity, or inability to delay gratification and his concept of *delay aversion,* which he defines as reduced tolerance for delay. Sonuga-Barke carried out a series of studies in which ADHD and control children had to choose between small, immediate and large, delayed rewards (Mischel, 1983). By using ingenious manipulations, such as varying the amount of delay *after* the delivery of rewards, they were able to show that, at least under some conditions, ADHD children seemed more concerned with reducing overall delay times (delay aversion) than with maximizing either the amount or immediacy of rewards (Sonuga-Barke, Taylor, Sembi, & Smith, 1992). Sonuga-Barke, Houlberg, and Hall (1994) also demonstrated that ADHD children no longer showed an impulsive cognitive style on the MFFT when responding quickly did not reduce the total length of the session. On a more traditional version of the MFFT, in which trial length was determined by the children's response speeds, the ADHD group showed the expected impulsive pattern. In a second condition, in which a fixed delay was imposed, the response latencies of the ADHD and control groups were similar. It should also be noted, however, that this artificially induced reflective style did not reduce errors in the ADHD group to the level of the controls, suggesting that the ADHD children did not make efficient use of the additional time to search the response alternatives carefully.

Delay of Gratification

Schweitzer and Sulzer-Azaroff (1995) also used the delay of gratification paradigm with ADHD and control boys. Their study differed from those of Sonuga-Barke, in that children's choices were investigated over repeated exposure to the task. Overall, the controls showed a stronger tendency to choose the larger, delayed rewards. Of particular interest, this preference *increased* as they gained more experience with the task, whereas ADHD boys chose *fewer* large, delayed rewards on the second than on the first testing day.

Equally interesting, the ADHD boys showed increased motor activity with increasing exposure to the task. The authors suggested that they were providing their own immediate rewards by indulging in such activities as diving under the table and twirling in their chairs.

There are a number of other studies reporting that task performance and gross motor activity of ADHD children are particularly affected by novelty and task repetition (Alberts & van der Meere, 1992; Sykes, Douglas, Weiss, & Minde, 1971; Zentall & Zentall, 1976). There is also evidence suggesting that ADHD children satiate more quickly than controls to rewards, novelty, and stimulating task qualities, such as color (Barkley, 1989, 1990; Iaboni *et al.*, 1996; Zentall, 1975; Zentall & Meyer, 1987).

Complex Memory and Visual-Memory Search Tasks

Whether one chooses to emphasize stimulation seeking, cognitive impulsivity, delay aversion, or inability to delay gratification, the stylistic differences just described would be expected to have particularly deleterious effects on tasks requiring self-organized and persistent effort. These qualities typify complex memory tasks in which children must rehearse material for later recall. In some tasks it is also possible to observe their rehearsal strategies and the amount of time and effort they devote to rehearsal and retrieval. In addition, the children's attitudes about their own abilities and their metacognitive knowledge about effective strategies can be investigated.

Study Strategies on a Story Recall Task. O'Neill and Douglas (1991) assessed the study strategies used by ADHD and control boys when they were asked to study folktales in order to remember them. We scored accuracy of

recall and assessed the boys' metacognitive knowledge about effective strategies for remembering the tales, the amount of time and effort spent studying them, the quality of study strategies, the boys' predictions about how well they would be able to remember the tales, and their estimates of how well they had actually remembered them.

Interestingly, in spite of spending less time studying, expending less effort, and employing more superficial strategies, the ADHD boys did not differ from controls on gist recall. Thus, in the case of the simple, interesting, and well-structured folktales used in this study, their fast, cavalier approach paid off. Their metacognitive knowledge about effective memory strategies also did not appear to be deficient. However, in comparisons with controls, the ADHD boys evaluated their own performance more highly and made more optimistic predictions about their future performance.

Self-Paced Overt Rehearsal Task. In a second study, O'Neill and Douglas (1996) used a self-paced, multitrial free recall task in which ADHD and control boys were asked to rehearse the names of 24 pictures aloud. The examiner provided minimal external control or support. The boys were allowed to rehearse the pictures in their own style, at their own speed, and received no feedback about their performance. On each trial they were given a booklet containing the 24 cards and were asked to try to study them so that they would be able to remember them. This procedure made it possible to observe their rehearsal strategies as well as the amount of time and effort they devoted to rehearsal and retrieval.

The ADHD boys adopted a slapdash approach from the first trial, spending less time than the controls on both rehearsal and retrieval. Unlike the controls, who showed some evidence of using the more effective grouping or cumulative rehearsal strategy, the ADHD boys relied almost exclusively on simple repetition of single items. In a metacognitive evaluation of their knowledge about the effectiveness of the strategies, however, they showed that they were aware of the superiority of the grouping strategy. On this task, the ADHD boys' fast, perfunctory approach resulted in significantly poorer recall performance.

Other Evidence of Stylistic Differences

Several other investigators have reported that ADHD children use less effortful, less mature, or less organized perceptual, memory, or problem-solving strategies (Amin, Douglas, Mendelson, & Dufresne, 1993; August, 1987; Borcherding et al., 1988; Douglas & Benezra, 1990; Hamlett, Pelegrini, & Conners, 1987; Reid & Borkowski, 1987; Tant & Douglas, 1982; Weingartner et al., 1980); that they fail to apply these strategies even when they demonstrate knowledge about their superior effectiveness (August, 1987; Voelker, Carter, Sprague, Gdowski, & Lachar, 1989); that they seem to have an unrealistically positive view of their own competence (Barber, Milich, & Welsh, 1996; Hoza, Pelham, Milich, Pillow, & McBride, 1993); and that they fail to adopt an active, "mastery orientation" to tasks (Barber et al., 1996; Milich & Okazaki, 1991).

Stimulant Effects on Complex Cognitive Tasks

General

There is convincing evidence that MPH improves the performance of ADHD children on a number of complex cognitive tasks. There has been continuing concern, however, resulting from early reports of possible negative effects at high doses, particularly when the tasks require acquisition of new learning or flexible thinking (Sprague & Sleator, 1977; Swanson, Cantwell, Lerner, McBurnett, & Hanna, 1991). However, in a review of studies of dosage effects, Rapport and Kelly (1991) reported that all studies providing statistics on between-dose effects found higher dosages to be more effective. In addition, using an acute dosage, crossover design, Douglas and colleagues (1995) found linear improvements in performance on measures assessing cognitive flexibility on MPH doses up to 0.9 mg/kg.

It is important to note that the improvements observed on complex tasks are typically accompanied by stylistic changes in the children's approach. There are now several reports of MPH effects on effort ratings (Douglas et al., 1988, 1995), on persistence over repeated task administrations, or following a failure experience (Carlson, Pelham, Milich, & Hoza, 1993; Douglas et al., 1988; Milich, 1994; Milich, Carlson, Pelham, & Licht, 1991; Pelham, Kipp, Gnagy, & Hoza, 1997; Solanto & Wender, 1989).

Dosage Effects and Processing Demands

Our laboratory has also investigated possible interactions between MPH dosage and strength of processing demands. We have used different operational definitions of processing load, including the number of items to be processed and demands to continue processing across trials on multitrial learning tasks (Berman, Douglas, & Barr, in press; Douglas, Barr, O'Neill, & Desilets, 1997). If high doses interfere with complex processing, the negative effects should be most evident under high processing demands. However, if MPH acts on effort and persistence, higher doses would be expected to be most helpful in the most demanding conditions.

Paired Associates Learning. Douglas and colleagues (1997) studied the effects of MPH dosages of 0.3, 0.6, and 0.9 mg/kg on a paired associates learning (PAL) task in which children had to develop associations between lists of arbitrarily paired words and improve their mastery of the lists across repeated learning trials. To increase demands for effort, persistence, and self-organized learning, we modified the PAL used in our earlier studies (Douglas et al., 1986, 1988) by increasing the number of word pairs and extending the number of learning trials. In addition, subjects were required to monitor and organize their own progress in mastering the lists. They were not informed when they made an error; rather, the entire list of correct pairs was reread to them before each trial, thus making them responsible for identifying pairs they had not yet mastered and concentrating their effort on rehearsing them.

We found a significant trial-by-dosage interaction on number of pairs recalled, with *higher* dosages producing most improvement on *later* learning trials. In an earlier study comparing ADHD and control groups on the PAL (Douglas & Benezra, 1990), we found that the ADHD group fell further behind the controls on later trials. Later trials place heavier demands on self-regulation and persistence because the child must identify and rehearse the pairs not yet mastered, while retaining pairs learned on previous trials. Thus, our findings show that higher dosages were most effective when these demands were at a maximum.

Self-Paced Overt Rehearsal Task. Douglas and colleagues (1997) obtained similar results using the self-paced overt rehearsal task described earlier (O'Neill & Douglas, 1996). Despite the lack of examiner pacing or feedback, ADHD children adopted a more active and effortful style when they were receiving MPH. They spent more time rehearsing, received higher effort ratings, and recalled more items. As on the PAL, we found a significant trial-by-dosage interaction, with higher doses producing most improvement on later trials.

Visual-Memory Search Task. Berman and colleagues (in press) investigated the relationship between MPH dosage and processing demands using a visual-memory search (VMS) task. The VMS followed the basic format of the Sternberg task but was modified in several ways to increase processing demands. Although the number of items in the memory load varied from 1 to 4 as in the Sternberg, search loads were greatly extended, varying from 4 to 16 items. Consequently, the VMS required an organized, protracted, and integrated visual-memory search throughout the combined items in the memory and search sets. In addition, both the memory and search items changed on each trial.

On the error measure, we found a linear dose–response effect, with fewer errors at the higher dosages. There was no interaction between dosage and processing load. The RT measure, however, yielded several two- and three-way interactions involving dosage level and processing load. These interactions implicated three different operational definitions of processing load: number of items in the memory set, number of items in the search set, and the target-present versus target-absent condition. This last factor is associated with load because, on average, subjects must search through only half as many items when the target is present in order to reach a decision. All of the interactions revealed that higher doses caused the greatest slowing of RTs at the highest loads.

The amount of slowing in the high-dose–high-load conditions was extremely large. In addition, effort ratings were very high on the high doses. These findings suggest that the ADHD children were expending considerable time and effort to achieve relatively small additional gains in accuracy. Thus, MPH induced a cognitive style that appeared to be the opposite of impulsivity, adversity to delay, or overoptimism.

It is important to emphasize one further point regarding the MPH effects on the VMS task. The high doses did *not* slow RTs when ADHD children were dealing with low processing loads. Moreover, the evidence discussed earlier showed that MPH can *speed* RTs on the lower load Sternberg task, which has a format similar to the VMS. These findings demonstrate that stimulants do not simply speed or slow responding in ADHD children, but enable them to adapt their response times to specific task demands. Again, the evidence points to specific, well-modulated stimulant effects on regulatory control processes.

Executive Functions in ADHD

Researchers have long been aware of parallels between the cognitive deficits found in ADHD and those observed in patients with prefrontal lobe injuries. I made this observation in one of my earliest papers (Douglas, 1972). Since that time, there have been numerous studies investigating ADHD performance on tasks designed to assess executive functions thought to be mediated by the prefrontal cortex (for reviews, see Barkley *et al.*, 1992; Pennington & Ozonoff, 1996; Pennington, Groisser, & Welsh, 1993).

The "frontal lobe analogy" (Pennington & Ozonoff, 1996) helped increase interest in regulatory control processes in ADHD and their possible neural substrates (Castellanos *et al.,* 1994, 1996; Hynd *et al.,* 1993; Lou, Henriksen, Bruhn, Borner, & Nielsen, 1989; Zametkin *et al.,* 1990). However, there are limitations to the analogy. The causes of impaired functioning are probably present from birth in most ADHD children, with subsequent effects on cognitive development. In contrast, cognitive abilities typically develop normally in frontal patients up to the time they experience brain trauma. In addition, frontal patients sustain loss or serious damage to brain tissue, whereas in ADHD, the affected neural networks can probably be best described as "dysfunctional."

In addition, there has been growing dissatisfaction with tests such as the Wisconsin Card Sorting test (described in Chapter 4, this volume) and the Tower of Hanoi that purport to measure "higher level" executive functions such as planning, organization, and cognitive flexibility. These tests tap many different cognitive processes, both executive and nonexecutive (Goel & Grafman, 1995; Pennington, Bennetto, McAleer, & Roberts, 1996). Cohen and Servan-Schreiber (1992) recently called for simpler tasks that lend themselves to the analysis of specific cognitive processing mechanisms. Denckla (1996) recommended setting aside vague "supraordinate" or "higher-order" concepts and concentrating, instead, on such constructs as "maintenance of anticipatory set/preparedness to act" and "inhibition/freedom from interference." She also endorsed Heilman's (1994) emphasis on *intentionality,* which he breaks down into "initiate," "sustain," "inhibit/stop," and "shift" (Denckla, 1996, pp. 265–266).

There is considerable similarity between the specifications just described and the characteristics of several of the tasks reviewed in this chapter. Interestingly, many of the tasks discussed in the chapter have been included in recent reviews of measures assessing executive functions. Yet, many were in use by ADHD researchers before the frontal lobe hypothesis of ADHD became popular, and most were devel-oped for the purpose of studying basic cognitive and information-processing functions.

SUMMARY AND CONCLUSIONS

The evidence reviewed suggests that, in attempting to understand the cognitive deficits of ADHD children, we should concentrate on processes regulating consistent and sustained allocation of effort and attention, inhibition of inappropriate responding, preparation to process and respond to task stimuli, and flexible adaptation to changing task demands. At least for the present, it may be more profitable to choose measures capable of assessing these processes as simply and directly as possible.

Examples of potentially useful tasks reviewed in this chapter include the WRT, CPT, Stop, Change, and Stroop tasks. In addition, task manipulations, such as duration of preparatory intervals, event rates, predictability of task demands, and the presence or absence of extraneous stimuli, may sharpen the discriminability of such measures, provided there is clear evidence that the manipulations have a *differential* effect on ADHD children. The use of such measures for diagnostic purposes, however, will require the development of standardized versions with adequate age norms. It will also be necessary to use improved statistical techniques that take into account the high variability usually found in ADHD data.

The patterns of improvement produced by MPH implicate stimulant effects on regulatory processes responsible for the controlled, well-modulated allocation of cognitive resources. As cognitive assessment and brain imaging techniques become more sophisticated, investigation of the concomitant cognitive and neural changes produced by the stimulants should provide an additional "window" for exploring the neural substrates of ADHD.

This interpretation of the action of the stimulants also helps explain why they are effective only so long as ADHD children continue to take them and blood levels remain sufficiently high. It appears that the cognitive impairments associated with ADHD stem largely from a failure to activate neural processes that are considerably more intact than the childrens' typical performance would suggest.

Although rewards and other stimulating interventions, such as increased event rates, novelty, and colorful stimuli also appear to activate cognitive processing in ADHD, it appears that their effects may be more diffuse than that of the stimulants, unless considerable care is taken to deliver them contingently. It also appears that the effectiveness of some of these interventions may habituate quickly.

This conceptualization of the nature of the regulatory disorder in ADHD may also help explain why results from cognitive training focusing on teaching higher level problem-solving strategies have been somewhat disappointing. Evidence that ADHD children frequently fail to apply strategies with which they are familiar and which they understand are more effective underlines the central role of basic control processes. It must be stressed, however, that this observation should not discourage attempts to provide training and attractive opportunities for practicing skills and strategic approaches that the fast, careless style of ADHD children has prevented them from acquiring.

Finally, the vexing question remains as to whether cognitive interventions aimed at strengthening the basic kinds of control processes described in this chapter could have beneficial effects. Certainly, the nature of these processes suggests that environmental factors, such as failure to monitor ADHD children's performance or to provide consistent feedback are likely to exacerbate their problems. Perhaps it is not too optimistic also to speculate that early training using gamelike versions of the information-processing tasks and manipulations recommended earlier could facilitate the development of these regulatory control processes in ADHD children.

REFERENCES

Alberts, E., & Meere, J. J. van der. (1992). Observations of hyperactive behaviour during vigilance. *Journal of Child Psychology and Psychiatry, 33*, 1355–1364.

Amin, K., Douglas, V. I., Mendelson, M. J., & Dufresne, J. (1993). Separable/integral classification by hyperactive and normal children. *Development and Psychopathology, 5*, 415–431.

August, C. J. (1987). Production deficiencies in free recall: A comparison of hyperactive, learning disabled and normal children. *Journal of Abnormal Child Psychology, 15*, 429–440.

Bala, S. P., Cohen, B., Morris, A. G., Atkin, A., Gittelman, R., & Kates, W. (1981). Saccades of hyperactive and normal boys during ocular pursuit. *Developmental Medicine and Child Neurology, 23*, 323–336.

Barber, M. A., Milich, R., & Welsh, R. (1996). Effect of reinforcement schedule and task difficulty on the performance of attention deficit hyperactivity disordered and control boys. *Journal of Clinical Child Psychology, 25*, 66–76.

Barkley, R. A. (1989). The problem of stimulus control and rule-governed behavior in children with attention deficit disorder with hyperactivity. In J. Swanson & L. Bloomingdale (Eds.), *Attention deficit disorders* (pp. 39–72). New York: Pergamon.

Barkley, R. A. (1990). The problem of stimulus control and rule governed behavior in Attention Deficit Disorder with Hyperactivity. In J. Swanson & L. M. Bloomingdale (Eds.), *Attention deficit disorder: Current concepts and emerging trends in attentional and behavioral disorders of children* (Vol. 3, pp. 203–228). New York: Spectrum.

Barkley, R. A. (1994). Impaired delayed responding. A unified theory of attention-deficit hyperactivity disorder. In D. K. Routh (Ed.), *Disruptive behavior disorders: Essays in honor of Herbert Quay* (pp. 11–57). New York: Plenum.

Barkley, R. A. (1996). Linkages between attention and executive functions. In G. R. Lyon & N. A. Krasnegor (Eds.), *Attention, memory and executive function* (pp. 307–326). Baltimore: Brookes.

Barkley, R. A. (1997a). *ADHD and the nature of self control.* New York: Guilford.

Barkley, R. A. (1997b). Inhibition, sustained attention, and executive functions: Constructing a unifying theory of ADHD. *Psychological Bulletin, 121*, 65–94.

Barkley, R. A., Grodzinsky, G., & DuPaul, G. J. (1992). Frontal lobe functions in attention deficit disorder with and without hyperactivity: A review and research report. *Journal of Abnormal Child Psychology, 20*, 163–188.

Berman, T., Douglas, V. I., & Dunbar, K. (1994). *Flexibility of Attention in ADHD Children.* Poster presentation at the annual meeting of the American Psychological Association, Los Angeles.

Berman, T., Douglas, V. I., & Barr, R. G. (in press). *Does methylphenidate improve high level cognitive processing in children with attention-deficit hyperactivity disorder? Journal of Abnormal Psychology.*

Berquin, P. C., Giedd, J. N., Jacobsen, L. K., Hamburger, S. D., Krain, A. L., Rapoport, J. L., & Castellanos, F. X. (1997). *The cerebellum in attention-deficit/hyperactivity disorder: A morphometric MRI study. Neurology, 50*(4), 1087–93.

Borcherding, B., Thompson, K., Kruesi, M., Bartko, J., Rapoport, J. L., & Weingartner, H. (1988). Automatic and effortful processing in attention deficit/hyperactivity disorder. *Journal of Abnormal Child Psychology, 16,* 333–345.

Bronowski, J. (1977). *Human and animal languages: A sense of the future.* Cambridge, MA: MIT Press.

Brumaghim, J., Klorman, R., Strauss, J., Lewine, J., & Goldstein, G. (1987). Does methylphenidate affect information processing? Findings from two studies on performance and P3b latency. *Psychophysiology, 24,* 361–373.

Bylsma, F. W., & Pivik, R. T. (1989). The effects of background illumination and stimulant medication on smooth pursuit eye movements of hyperactive children. *Journal of Abnormal Child Psychology, 17,* 73–90.

Carlson, C. L., Pelham, W. E., Milich, R., & Hoza, R. (1993). ADHD boys' performance and attributions following success and failure: Drug effects and individual differences. *Cognitive Therapy and Research, 17,* 269–287.

Casey, B. J., Castellanos, F. X., Giedd, J. N., Marsh, W. L., Hamburger, S. D., Schubert, A. B., Vauss, Y. C., Vaituzis, A. C., Dickstein, D. P., Sarfatti, S. E., & Rapoport, J. L. (1997). Implications of right frontostriatal circuitry in response inhibition and attention deficit/hyperactivity disorder. *Journal of the American Academy of Child and Adolescent Psychiatry, 36,* 374–383.

Castellanos, F., Giedd, J., Eckburg, P., Marsh, W., Vaituzis, C., Kaysen, D., Hamburger, S., & Rapoport, J. (1994). Quantitative morphology of the caudate nucleus in attention deficit hyperactivity disorder. *American Journal of Psychiatry, 151,* 1791–1796.

Castellanos, F., Giedd, J., Eckburg, P., Marsh, W., Vaituzis, C., Kaysen, D., Hamburger, S., & Rapoport, J. (1996). Quantitative brain magnetic resonance imaging in Attention-Deficit Hyperactivity Disorder. *Archives of General Psychiatry, 53,* 607–616.

Ceci, S. J., & Tishman, J. (1984). Hyperactivity and incidental memory: Evidence for attentional diffusion. *Child Development, 55,* 192–203.

Chapman, L. J., & Chapman, J. P. (1978). The measurement of differential deficit. *Journal of Pediatric Research, 14,* 303–311.

Chee, P., Logan, G., Schachar, R., Lindsay, P., & Wachsmuth, R. (1989). Effects of event rate and display time on sustained attention in hyperactive, normal, and control children. *Journal of Abnormal Child Psychology, 17,* 371–391.

Cohen, J., & Cohen, P. (1983). *Applied multiple regression/correlation analysis for the behavioral sciences* (2nd ed.). Hillsdale, NJ: Erlbaum.

Cohen, J. D., & Servan-Schreiber, D. (1992). Context, cortex, and dopamine: A connectionist approach to behavior and biology in schizophrenia. *Psychological Review, 99,* 45–77.

Cohen, N., Douglas, V., & Morgenstern, G. (1971). The effect of methylphenidate on attentive behavior and autonomic activity in hyperactive children. *Psychopharmacology, 22,* 282–294.

Cohen, N. J., & Douglas, V. I. (1972). Characteristics of the orienting response in hyperactive and normal children. *Psychophysiology, 9,* 238–245.

Coons, H., Klorman, R., & Borgstedt, A. (1987). Effects of methylphenidate on adolescents with a childhood history of attention deficit disorder: II. Information processing. *Journal of the American Academy of Child and Adolescent Psychiatry, 26,* 368–374.

Conte, R., Kinsbourne, M., Swanson, J., Zirk, H., & Samuels, M. (1986). Presentation rate effects on paired associate learning by attention deficit disorder children. *Child Development, 57,* 681–687.

Corkum, P., & Siegel, L. (1993). Is the continuous performance task a valuable research tool for use with children with attention-deficit hyperactivity disorder? *Journal of Child Psychology and Psychiatry, 34,* 1217–1239.

Corkum, P., & Siegel, L. (1995). Debate and argument: Reply to Dr. Koelega: Is the Continuous Performance Task useful in research with ADHD children? Comments on a review. *Journal of Child Psychology and Psychiatry, 36,* 1487–1493.

Daugherty, T. K., & Quay, H. C. (1991). Response perseveration and delayed responding in childhood behavior disorders. *Journal of Child Psychology and Psychiatry, 32,* 453–461.

De Jong, R., Coles, M. G. H., & Logan, G. D. (1995). Strategies and mechanisms in nonselective and selective inhibitory motor control. *Journal of Experimental Psychology, 21,* 498–511.

De Sonneville, L. M. J., Njiokiktjien, C., & Hilhorst, R. C. (1991). Methylphenidate-induced changes in ADHD information processors. *Journal of Child Psychology and Psychiatry, 32,* 285–295.

Denckla, M. B. (1996). A theory and model of executive function: A neuropsychological persepective. In G. R. Lyon & A. Krasnegor (Eds.), *Attention, memory and executive function* (pp. 263–278). Baltimore: Brookes.

Denckla, M. B., & Rudel, R. G. (1978). Anomalies of motor development in hyperactive boys. *Annals of Neurology, 3,* 231–233.

Denckla, M. B., Rudel, R. G., Chapman, C., & Krieger, J. (1985). Motor proficiency in dyslexic children with and without attentional disorders. *Archives of Neurology, 42,* 228–231.

Douglas, V. I. (1972). Stop, look and listen: The problem of sustained attention and impulse control in hyperactive and normal children. *Canadian Journal of Behavioural Science, 4,* 259–282.

Douglas, V. I. (1980). Treatment and training approaches to hyperactivity: Establishing internal or external control? In C. K. Whalen & B. Henker (Eds.), *Hyperactive children: The social ecology of identification and treatment* (pp. 238–317). New York: Academic Press.

Douglas, V. I. (1983). Attentional and cognitive problems. In M. Rutter (Ed.), *Developmental neuropsychiatry* (pp. 280–329). New York: Guilford.

Douglas, V. I. (1984). The psychological processes implicated in ADD. In L. M. Bloomingdale (Ed.), *Attention deficit disorder: Diagnostic, cognitive, and therapeutic understanding* (pp. 147–162). New York: Spectrum.

Douglas, V. I. (1985). The response of ADD children to reinforcement. In L. M. Bloomingdale (Ed.), *Attention deficit disorder: Identification, course and rationale* (pp. 49–66). Jamaica, NY: Spectrum.

Douglas, V. I. (1988). Cognitive deficits in children with Attention Deficit Disorder with Hyperactivity. *Journal of Child Psychology and Psychiatry* (Monograph Suppl.), 65–81.

Douglas, V. I. (1989). Can Skinnerian theory explain attention deficit disorder? A reply to Barkley. In L. M. Bloomingdale & J. A. Sergeant (Eds.), *Attention deficit disorder: Current concepts and emerging trends in attentional and behavioral disorders of childhood* (pp. 235–254). Elmsford, NY: Pergamon.

Douglas, V. I. (1990, August). *Diagnosis and treatment of attention deficit hyperactivity disorder: Has research helped?* Invited address presented at the annual meeting of the American Psychological Association, Boston.

Douglas, V. I., & Benezra, E. (1990). Supraspan verbal memory in attention deficit disorder with hyperactivity, normal and reading-disabled boys. *Journal of Abnormal Child Psychology, 18,* 617–638.

Douglas, V. I., & Parry, P. A. (1994). Effects of reward and non-reward on frustration and attention in attention deficit disorder. *Journal of Abnormal Child Psychology, 22,* 281–302.

Douglas, V. I., & Peters, K. G. (1979). Toward a clearer definition of the attention deficit of hyperactive children. In G. A. Hale & M. Lewis (Eds.), *Attention and cognitive development* (pp. 173–247). New York: Plenum.

Douglas, V. I., Barr, R. G., O'Neill, M. E., & Britton, B. G. (1986). Short term effects of methylphenidate on the cognitive, learning and academic performance of children with attention deficit disorder in the laboratory and in the classroom. *Journal of Child Psychology and Psychiatry, 27,* 191–211.

Douglas, V. I., Barr, R. G., Amin, K., O'Neill, M. E., & Britton, B. G. (1988). Dosage effects and individual responsivity to methylphenidate in attention deficit disorder. *Journal of Child Psychology and Psychiatry, 29,* 453–475.

Douglas, V. I., Barr, R. G., Desilets, J., & Sherman, E. (1995). Do high doses of stimulants impair flexible thinking in attention deficit hyperactivity disorder? *Journal of the American Academy of Child and Adolescent Psychiatry, 34,* 877–885.

Douglas, V. I., Barr, R. G., O'Neill, M. E., & Desilets, J. (1997). *Effects of methylphenidate on the allocation of time and effort.* Manuscript in preparation.

Draeger, S., Prior, M., & Sanson, A. (1986). Visual and auditory attention performance in hyperactive children:

Competence or compliance. *Journal of Abnormal Child Psychology, 14,* 411–424.

Dunbar, K., & Sussman, D. (1995). Toward a cognitive account of frontal lobe function: Simulating frontal lobe deficits in normal subjects. In J. Grafman, K. Holyoak, & F. Boller (Eds.), *Annals of the New York Academy of Sciences* (Vol. 769, pp. 289–304). New York: New York Academy of Sciences.

Elbaz, Z., Douglas, V. I., & Ditto, B. (1997). *Effects of preparatory intervals on reaction times of children with attention deficit hyperactivity disorder.* Manuscript in preparation.

Enns, J. T., & Cameron, S. (1987). Selective attention in young children: The relations between visual search, filtering, and priming. *Journal of Experimental Child Psychology, 44,* 38–63.

Fitzpatrick, P., Klorman, R., Brumaghim, J. T., & Keefover, R. W. (1988). Effects of methylphenidate on stimulus evaluation and response processes: Evidence from performance and event-related potentials. *Psychophysiology, 25,* 292–304.

Fowles, D. C. (1980). The three arousal model: Implications of Gray's two-factor learning theory for heart rate, electrodermal activity, and psychopathy. *Psychophysiology, 17,* 87–104.

Fowles, D. C. (1988). Psychophysiology and psychopathology: A motivational approach. *Psychophysiology, 25,* 373–391.

Goel, V., & Grafman, J. (1995). Are the frontal lobes implicated in "planning" functions? Interpreting data from the Tower of Hanoi. *Neuropsychologica, 33,* 623–642.

Gordon, M. A. (1979). The assessment of impulsivity and mediating behavior in hyperactive and nonhyperactive boys. *Journal of Abnormal Psychology, 6,* 317–326.

Gray, J. A. (1982). *The neuropsychology of anxiety.* New York: Oxford University Press.

Gray, J. A.(1985). A whole and its parts: Behavior, the brain, cognition and emotion. *Bulletin of the British Psychological Society, 38,* 99–112.

Gray, J. A. (1987). *The psychology of fear and stress* (2nd ed.). Cambridge, England: Cambridge University Press.

Haenlein, M., & Caul, W. F. (1987). Attention deficit disorder with hyperactivity: A specific hypothesis of reward dysfunction. *Journal of the American Academy of Child and Adolescent Psychiatry, 26,* 356–362.

Hamlett, K. W., Pelegrini, D. S., & Conners, C. K. (1987). An investigation of executive processes in the problem-solving of Attention Deficit Hyperactivity Disorder–hyperactive children. *Journal of Pediatric Psychology, 12,* 227–239.

Heathcote, A. (1996). RTSYS: A DO application for the analysis of reaction time data. *Behavior Research Methods, Instruments and Computers, 28,* 427–445.

Heathcote, A., Popiel, S. J., & Mewhort, D. J., (1991). Analysis of response time distributions: An example using the Stroop task. *Psychological Bulletin, 109,* 340–347.

Heilman, K. (1994, January). Intention. Paper presented at the NICHD conference on Attention, Memory, and Executive Function. Bethesda, MD.

Hicks, R. E., Mayo, J., Jr., & Clayton, C. (1989). Differential psychopharmacology of methylphenidate and the neuropsychology of childhood hyperactivity. *International Journal of Neuroscience, 45,* 7–32.

Hockley, W. E. (1984). Analysis of response time distributions in the study of cognitive processes. *Journal of Experimental Psychology: Learning, Memory, and Cognition, 6,* 598–615.

Hooks, K., Milich, R., & Lorch, E. P. (1994). Sustained and selective attention in boys with attention deficit hyperactivity disorder. *Journal of Clinical Child Psychology, 23,* 69–77.

Hoza, B., Pelham, W. E., Milich, R., Pillow, D., & McBride, K. (1993). The self perceptions and attributions of attention deficit hyperactivity disordered and nonreferred boys. *Journal of Abnormal Child Psychology, 21,* 271–286.

Hynd, G. W., Hern, K. L., Novey, E. S., Eliopulos, D., Marshall, R., Gonzalez, J. J., & Voeller, K. K. (1993). Attention deficit-hyperactivity disorder and asymmetry of the caudate nucleus. *Journal of Child Neurology, 8,* 339–347.

Iaboni, F., Douglas, V. I., & Baker, A. G. (1995). Effects of reward and response costs on inhibition in Attention Deficit Hyperactivity Disorder children. *Journal of Abnormal Psychology, 104,* 232–240.

Iaboni, F., Douglas, V. I., & Ditto, B. (1996). Psychophysiological response of ADHD children to reward and extinction. *Psychophysiology, 34,* 116–123.

Jonkman, L. (1997). *Effects of methylphenidate on brain activity and behavior of children with attention-deficit hyperactivity disorder.* Unpublished doctoral dissertation, Universiteit Utrecht, Utrecht, The Netherlands.

Jonkman, L. M., Kemner, C., Verbaten, M. N., Koelega, H. S., Camfferman, G., van der Gaag, R. J., Buitelaar, J. K., & van Engeland, H. (1997a). Effects of methylphenidate on event-related potentials and performance of attention-deficit hyperactivity disorder children in auditory and visual selective attention tasks. *Biological Psychiatry, 41,* 595–611.

Jonkman, L. M., Kemner, C., Verbaten, M. N., Koelega, H. S., Camfferman, G., van der Gaag, R. J., Buitelaar, J. K., & van Engeland, H. (1997b). Event related potentials and performance of ADHD children and normal controls in auditory and visual selective attention tasks. *Biological Psychiatry, 41,* 690–702.

Kagan, J. (1965a). Individual differences in the resolution of response uncertainty. *Journal of Personality and Social Psychology, 2,* 154–160.

Kagan, J. (1965b). Reflection–impulsivity and reading ability in primary grade children. *Child Development, 36,* 609–628.

Kinsbourne, M. (1983). Toward a model of the attention deficit disorder. In M. Perlmutter (Ed.), *The Minnesota Symposia on Child Psychology. Development and policy concerning children with special needs* (Vol. 16, pp. 137–166). Hillsdale, NJ: Erlbaum.

Klorman, R. (1991). Cognitive event-related potentials in attention deficit disorder. *Journal of Learning Disabilities, 24,* 130–140.

Klorman, R. (1995). Psychophysiological determinants. In M. Hersen & R. T. Ammerman (Eds.), *Advanced abnormal child psychology* (pp.59–85). Hillsdale, NJ: Erlbaum.

Klorman, R., Salzman, L. F., Pass, H. L., Borgstedt, A. D., & Dainer, K. B. (1979). Effects of methylphenidate on hyperactive children's evoked responses during passive and active attention. *Psychophysiology, 16,* 23–29.

Klorman, R., Brumaghim, J., Fitzpatrick, P., & Borgstedt, A. (1991). Methylphenidate speeds evaluation processes of attention deficit disorder adolescents during a continuous performance test. *Journal of Abnormal Child Psychology, 19,* 263–283.

Klorman, R., Brumaghim, J., Fitzpatrick, P., & Borgstedt, A. (1992). Methylphenidate reduces abnormalities of stimulus classification in adolescents with attention deficit disorder. *Journal of Abnormal Psychology. 101,* 130–138.

Klorman, R., Brumaghim, J., Fitzpatrick, P., Borgstedt, A., & Strauss, J. (1994). Clinical and cognitive effects of methylphenidate on children with attention deficit disorder as a function of aggression/oppositionality and age. *Journal of Abnormal Psychology, 103,* 206–221.

Koelega, H. (1995). Is the continuous performance task useful in research with ADHD children? Comments on a review. *Journal of Child Psychology and Psychiatry, 36,* 1477–1485.

Krusch, D. A., Klorman, R., Brumaghim, J. T., Fitzpatrick, P. A., Borgstedt, A. D., & Strauss, J. (1996). Methylphenidate slows reactions of children with attention deficit disorder during and after an error. *Journal of Abnormal Child Psychology, 24,* 633–650.

Leth-Steensen, C., Douglas, V., & Elbaz, Z. (1997). *Variability and skew in the responding of children with attention deficit hyperactivity disorder: A response time distributional approach.* Manuscript in preparation.

Levy, F., & Hobbes, G. (1996). Does haloperidol block methylphenidate? Motivation or attention? *Psychopharmacology, 126,* 70–74.

Logan, G. D., & Cowan, W. B. (1984). On the ability to inhibit thought and action: A theory of an act of control. *Psychological Review, 91,* 295–327.

Losier, B., McGrath, P., & Klein, R. (1996). Error patterns on the continuous performance test in non-medicated and medicated samples of children with and without ADHD: A meta-analytic review. *Journal of Child Psychology and Psychiatry, 37,* 971–987.

Lou, H. C., Henriksen, L., Bruhn, P., Borner, H., & Nielsen, J. B. (1989). Striatal dysfunction in attention deficit and hyperkinetic disorder. *Archives of Neurology, 46,* 48–52.

MacLeod, C. M. (1991). Half a century of research on the Stroop effect: An integrative review. *Psychological Bulletin, 109,* 163–203.

Mariani, M. A., & Barkley, R. A. (1997). Neuropsychological and academic functioning in preschool boys with attention deficit hyperactivity disorder. *Developmental Neuropsychology, 13,* 111–129.

McClure, F. D., & Gordon, M. (1984). Performance of disturbed hyperactive and nonhyperactive children on an objective measure of hyperactivity. *Journal of Abnormal Child Psychology, 12,* 561–572.

Meere, J. J. van der, & Sergeant, J. A. (1988). Focused attention in pervasively hyperactive children. *Journal of Abnormal Child Psychology, 16,* 627–639.

Meere, J. J. van der, Baal, M. van, & Sergeant, J. A. (1989). The additive factor method: A differential diagnostic tool in hyperactivity and learning disability. *Journal of Abnormal Child Psychology, 17,* 409–422.

Meere, J. J. van der, Vreeling, H. J., & Sergeant, J. A. (1992). A motor presetting study in hyperactive, learning disabled and control children. *Journal of Child Psychology and Psychiatry, 33,* 1347–1354.

Meere, J. J. van der, Shalev, R., Borger, N., & Gross-Tsur, V. (1995). Sustained attention, activation and MPH in ADHD: A research note. *Journal of Child Psychology and Psychiatry, 36,* 697–703.

Meere, J. J. van der, Gunning, W., & Stemerdink, N. (1996). Changing a response set in normal development and in ADHD children with and without tics. *Journal of Abnormal Child Psychology, 24,* 767–786.

Michael, R. L., Klorman, R., Salzman, L. F., Borgstedt, A. D., & Dainer, K. B. (1981). Normalizing effects of methylphenidate on hyperactive children's vigilance performance and evoked potentials. *Psychophysiology, 18,* 655–677.

Milich, R. (1994). The response of children with ADHD to failure: If at first you don't succeed, do you try, try again? *School Psychology Review, 23,* 11–28.

Milich, R., & Kramer, J. (1984). Reflections on impulsivity: An empirical investigation of impulsivity as a construct. In K. D. Gadow & I. Bialer (Eds.), *Advances in learning and behavioral disabilities* (pp. 57–94). Greenwich, CT: JAI.

Milich, R., & Okazaki, M. (1991). An examination of learned helplessness among attention-deficit hyperactivity disordered boys. *Journal of Abnormal Child Psychology, 19,* 607–623.

Milich, R., Carlson, C., Pelham, W. E., & Licht, B. (1991). Effects of methylphenidate on the persistence of ADHD boys following failure experiences. *Journal of Abnormal Child Psychology, 19,* 519–536.

Mischel, W. (1983). Delay of gratification as process and as person variable in development. In D. Magnusson & U. L. Allen (Eds.), *Human development: An interactional perspective* (pp. 149–166). New York: Academic Press.

O'Neill, M., & Douglas, V. I. (1991). Study strategies and story recall in Attention Deficit Disorder and Reading Disability. *Journal of Abnormal Child Psychology, 19,* 671–692.

O'Neill, M., & Douglas, V. I. (1996). Rehearsal strategies and recall performance in boys with and without Attention Deficit Hyperactivity Disorder. *Journal of Pediatric Psychology, 21,* 73–88.

Oosterlaan, J., & Sergeant, J. A. (1995). Response choice and inhibition in ADHD, anxious and aggressive children: The relationship between S–R compatibility and stop signal task. In J. A. Sergeant (Ed.), *European approaches to hyperkinetic disorder* (pp. 225–240). Zurich, Switzerland: Fotorotar.

Oosterlaan, J., & Sergeant, J. A. (1996a). Inhibition in ADHD, aggressive, and anxious children: A biologically based model of child psychopathology. *Journal of Abnormal Child Psychology, 24,* 19–36.

Oosterlaan, J., & Sergeant, J. A. (1996b). *Response inhibition and response re-engagment in ADHD, disruptive, anxious and normal children.* Manuscript submitted for publication.

Oosterlaan, J., Logan, G. D., & Sergeant, J. A. (1998). Response inhibition in ADHD, CD, comorbid ADHD+CD, anxious and normal children: A meta-analysis of studies with the stop task. *Journal of Child Psychology and Psychiatry, 39,* 411–425.

Pelham, W. E., Kipp, H. L., Gnagy, E. M., & Hoza, B. (1997). Effects of methylphenidate and expectancy on ADHD children's performance, self-evaluations, persistence, and attributions on a cognitive task. *Experimental and Clinical Psychopharmacology, 5,* 3–13.

Peloquin, L., & Klorman, R. (1986). Effects of methylphenidate on normal children's mood, event-related potentials, and performance in memory scanning and vigilance. *Journal of Abnormal Psychology, 95,* 88–98.

Pennington, B. F., & Ozonoff, S. (1996). Executive functions and developmental psychopathology. *Journal of Child Psychology and Psychiatry, 37,* 511–587.

Pennington, B. F., Groisser, L., & Welsh, R. (1993). Contrasting cognition deficits in ADHD versus reading disabilities. *Developmental Psychology, 29,* 511–523.

Pennington, B. F., Bennetto, L., McAleer, O., & Roberts, R. J., Jr. (1996). Executive functions and working memory: Theoretical and measurement issues. In G. R. Lyon & A. Krasnegor (Eds.), *Attention, memory and executive function* (pp. 327–348). Baltimore: Brookes.

Peters, K. G. (1977). *Selective attention and distractibility in hyperactive and normal children.* Unpublished doctoral dissertation, McGill University, Montreal, Quebec, Canada.

Pliszka, S. R., Hatch, J. P., Borcherding, S., & Rogeness, G. A. (1993). Classical conditioning with attention deficit hyperactivity disorder and anxiety disorder: A test of Quay's model. *Journal of Abnormal Psychology, 21,* 411–424.

Quay, H. (1997). Inhibition and Attention Deficit Hyperactivity Disorder. *Journal of Abnormal Child Psychology, 25,* 7–13.

Quay, H. C. (1988a). Attention deficit disorder and the behavioral inhibition system: The relevance of the neuropsychological theory of Jeffrey A. Gray. In L. M. Bloomingdale & J. A. Sergeant (Eds.), *Attention deficit disorder: Criteria, cognition, intervention* (pp. 117–125). Oxford, England: Pergamon.

Quay, H. C. (1988b). The behavioral reward and inhibition systems in childhood behavior disorders. In L. M. Bloomingdale (Ed.), *Attention deficit disorder. New research in attention, treatment and psychopharmacology* (Vol. 3, pp. 176–186). Oxford, England: Pergamon.

Rapport, M. D., & Kelly, K. L. (1991). Psychostimulant effects on learning and cognitive function: Findings and implications for children with attention deficit hyperactivity disorder. *Clinical Psychology Review, 11*, 61–92.

Rapport, M. D., Stoner, G., DuPaul, G. J., Kelly, K. L., Tucker, S. B., & Schoeler, T. (1988). Attention deficit disorder and methylphenidate: A multilevel analysis of dose–response effects on children's impulsivity across settings. *Journal of the American Academy of Child and Adolescent Psychiatry, 27*, 60–69.

Ratcliff, R., & Murdock, B. B. (1976). Retrieval processes in recognition memory. *Psychological Review, 83*, 190–214.

Reid, M. K., & Borkowski, J. G. (1987). Causal attributions of hyperactive children: Implications for teaching strategies and self-control. *Journal of Educational Psychology, 79*, 296–307.

Ross, R. G., Hommer, D., Breiger, D., Varley, C., & Radant, A. (1994). Eye movement task related to frontal lobe functioning in children with attention deficit disorder. *Journal of the American Academy of Child and Adolescent Psychiatry, 33*, 869–874.

Salkind, N. J. (1978). The development of norms for the Matching Familiar Figures Test. *Journal Supplement Abstract Service, 8*, 1718.

Sanders, A. F. (1977). Structural and functional aspects of the reaction process. In S. Dornic (Ed.), *Attention and performance* (Vol. 6, pp. 3–25). New York: Wiley.

Sanders, A. F. (1983). Towards a model of stress and human performance. *Acta Psychologica, 53*, 61–97.

Sanders, A. F. (1986). Energetical states underlying task performance. In G. R. Hockey, A. W. K. Gaillard, & M. G. H. Coles (Eds.), *Energetics and human information processing* (pp. 139–154). Dordrecht, The Netherlands: Nijhoff.

Sanders, A. F. (1990). Issues and trends in the debate on discrete vs. continuous processing of information. *Acta Psychologica, 74*, 123–167.

Satterfield, J. H., Schell, A. M., Backs, R. W., & Hidaka, K. C. (1984). A cross-sectional and longitudinal study of age effects of electrophysiological measures in hyperactive and normal children. *Electroencephalography and Clinical Neurophysiology, 57*, 199–207.

Satterfield, J. H., Schell, A. M., & Nicholas, T. (1994). Preferential neural processing of attention stimuli in attention-deficit hyperactivity disorder and normal boys. *Psychophysiology, 31*, 1–10.

Schachar, R., & Tannock, R. (1995). Test of four hypotheses for the comorbidity of ADHD and conduct disorder. *Journal of the American Academy of Child and Adolescent Psychiatry, 34*, 639–648.

Schachar, R., Tannock, R., & Logan, G. (1993). Inhibitory control, impulsiveness, and Attention Deficit Hyperactivity Disorder. *Clinical Psychology Review, 13*, 721–739.

Schachar, R., Tannock, R., Marriott, M., & Logan, G. (1995). Deficient inhibitory control in attention deficit hyperactivity disorder. *Journal of Abnormal Child Psychology, 23*, 411–437.

Schachar, R. J., & Logan, G. D. (1990). Impulsivity and inhibitory control in normal development and childhood psychopathology. *Developmental Psychology, 26*, 710–720.

Schweitzer, J. B., & Sulzer-Azaroff, B. (1995). Self-control in boys with attention deficit hyperactivity disorder: Effects of added stimulation and time. *Journal of Child Psychology and Psychiatry, 36*, 671–686.

Seidel, W. T., & Joschko, M. (1990). Evidence of difficulties in sustained attention in children with ADHD. *Journal of Abnormal Child Psychology, 18*, 217–229.

Sergeant, J. A. (1988). From DSM-III Attentional Deficit Disorder to Functional Defects. In L. M. Bloomingdale & J. A. Sergeant (Eds.), *Attention deficit disorder* (Vol. 5, pp. 183–198). Oxford, England: Pergamon.

Sergeant, J. A. (1995). Hyperkinetic disorder revisited. In J. A. Sergeant (Ed.), *European approaches to hyperkinetic disorder* (pp. 7–17). Zurich, Switzerland: Fotorotar.

Sergeant, J. A. (1996). A theory of attention: An information processing perspective. In G. R. Lyon & A. Krasnegor (Eds.), *Attention, memory and executive function* (pp. 57–70). Baltimore: Brookes.

Sergeant, J. A., & Meere, J. van der. (1988). What happens after a hyperactive child commits an error? *Psychiatry Research, 24*, 157–164.

Sergeant, J. A., & Meere, J. van der. (1990a). Additive factor method applied to psychopathology with special reference to childhood hyperactivity. *Acta Psychologica, 74*, 277–295.

Sergeant, J. A., & Meere, J. van der. (1990b). Convergence of approaches in localizing the hyperactivity deficit. In B. B. Lahey & A. E. Kazdin (Eds.), *Advances in clinical child psychology* (Vol. 13, pp. 207–245). New York: Plenum.

Sergeant, J. A., & Meere, J. van der. (1991). Ritalin effects and information processing in hyperactivity. In L. L. Greenhill & B. B. Osman (Eds.), *Ritalin: Theory and patient management* (pp. 1–13). New York: Mary Ann Liebert.

Sergeant, J. A., & Meere, J. van der. (1994). Toward an empirical child psychopathology. In D. K. Routh (Ed.), *Disruptive behavior disorders in childhood* (pp. 59–85). New York: Plenum.

Sergeant, J. A., & Scholten, C. A. (1985). On resource strategy limitations in hyperactivity: Cognitive impulsivity reconsidered. *Journal of Child Psychology and Psychiatry, 26*, 97–109.

Shiffrin, R. M., & Schneider, W. (1977). Controlled and automatic human information processing: 1. Detection, search and attention. *Psychological Review, 84*, 1–66.

Shue, K. L., & Douglas, V. I. (1992). Attention deficit hyperactivity disorder and the frontal lobe syndrome. *Brain and Cognition, 20*, 104–124.

Solanto, M. V., & Wender, E. H. (1989). Does methylphenidate constrict cognitive functioning? *Journal of the American Academy of Child and Adolescent Psychiatry, 26*, 879–902.

Solanto, M., Wender, E., & Bartell, S. (1997). Effects of methylphenidate and behavioral contingencies on vigilance in AD/HD: A test of the reward dysfunction hypothesis. *Journal of Child and Adolescent Psychopharmacology, 7*, 123–136.

Sonuga-Barke, E. J. S. (1995). Disambiguating inhibitory dyfunction in childhood hyperactivity. In J. Sergeant (Ed.), *Eunethydis: European approaches to hyperkinetic disorder* (pp. 209–223). Zurich, Switzerland: Fotorotar.

Sougua-Barke, E. J. S., & Taylor, E. (1991). The effect of delay on hyperactive and non-hyperactive children's response times: A research note. *Journal of Child Psychology and Psychiatry, 33*, 1091–1096.

Sonuga-Barke, E. J. S., Taylor, E., Sembi, S., & Smith, J. (1992). Hyperactivity and delay aversion: I. The effect of delay on choice. *Journal of Child Psychology and Psychiatry, 33*, 399–410.

Sonuga-Barke, E. J. S., Houlberg, K., & Hall, M. (1994). When is "impulsiveness" not impulsive? The case of hyperactive children's cognitive style. *Journal of Child Psychology and Psychiatry, 35*, 1247–1253.

Sprague, R. I., & Sleator, E. K. (1977). Methylphenidate in hyperkinetic children: Differences in dose effects on learning and social behavior. *Science, 198*, 1274–1276.

Sternberg, S. (1969). Discovery of processing stages: Extensions of Donder's method. In W. G. Koster (Ed.), *Attention and performance* (Vol. 2, pp. 276–315). Amsterdam: Noord-Holland.

Sternberg, S. (1975). Memory scanning: New findings and currentcontroversies. *Quarterly Journal of Experimental Psychology, 27*, 281–285.

Sternberg, R., & Grigorenko, E. (1997). Are cognitive styles still in style? *American Psychologist, 52*, 700–712.

Stevens, D. A., Stover, C. F., & Backus, J. T. (1970). The hyperkinetic child: Effects of incentives to the speed of rapid tapping. *Journal of Consulting and Clinical Psychology, 4*, 56–59.

Stroop, J. R. (1935). Studies of interference in serial verbal reactions. *Journal of Experimental Psychology, 18*, 643–662.

Swanson, J. M., Cantwell, D., Lerner, M., McBurnett, K., & Hanna, G. (1991). Effects of stimulant medication on learning in children with ADHD. *Journal of Learning Disabilities, 24*, 219–230.

Swanson, J. M., Posner, S., Bonforte, S., Youpa, D., Fiore, C., Cantwell, D., & Crinella, F. (1991). Activating tasks for the study of visual-spatial attention in ADHD children: A cognitive anatomical approach. *Journal of Child Neurology, 6*, 119–127.

Sykes, D. H., Douglas, V. I., Weiss, G., & Minde, K. K. (1971). Attention in hyperactive children and the effect of methylphenidate (Ritalin). *Journal of Child Psychology and Psychiatry, 12*, 129–139.

Tannock, R., Schachar, R., Carr, R. P., Chajczyk, D., & Logan, G. D. (1989). Effects of methylphenidate on inhibitory control in hyperactive children. *Journal of Child Psychology and Psychiatry, 17*, 473–491.

Tannock, R., Schachar, R. J., & Logan, G. (1995). Methylphenidate and cognitive flexibility: Dissociated dose effects in hyperactive children. *Journal of Abnormal Child Psychology, 23*, 235–266.

Tant, J. L., & Douglas, V. I. (1982). Problem solving in hyperactive, normal, and reading disabled boys. *Journal of Abnormal Child Psychology, 10*, 285–306.

Tarnowski, K. J., Prinz, R. J., & Nay, S. M. (1986). Comparative analysis of attentional deficits in hyperactive and learning disabled children. *Journal of Abnormal Psychology, 95*, 341–345.

Tomporowski, P., Tinsley, Y., & Hager, L. (1994). Visuospatial attentional shifts and choice responses of adults and ADHD and non-ADHD children. *Perceptual and Motor Skills, 79*, 1479–1490.

Trommer, B., Hoeppner, J. A., Lorber, R., & Armstrong, K. (1988a). The Go-No Go paradigm in Attention Deficit Disorder. *Annals of Neurology, 24*, 610–614.

Trommer, B., Hoeppner, J. A., Lorber, R., & Armstrong, K. (1988b). Pitfalls in the use of a continuous performance test as a diagnostic tool in Attention Deficit Disorder. *Developmental and Behavioral Pediatrics, 9*, 339–345.

Trommer, B., Hoeppner, J. A., & Zecker, S. G. (1991). The Go-No Go Test in Attention Deficit Disorder is sensitive to methylphenidate. *Journal of Child Neurology, 6*, s128–s131.

Van der Molen, M. W. (1996). Energetics and the reaction process: Running threads through experimental psychology. In O. Neumann & A. F. Sanders (Eds.), *Handbook of perception and action* (Vol. III, pp. 229–275). London: Academic Press.

Verfaellie, M., Bowers, D., & Heilman, K. M. (1990). Attentional processes in spatial stimulus–response compatibility. In R.W. Proctor & T. G. Reeve (Eds.), *Stimulus–response compatibility* (pp. 261–275). Amsterdam: Elsevier.

Voelker, S. L., Carter, R. A., Sprague, D. J., Gdowski, C. L., & Lachar, D. (1989). Developmental trends in memory and metamemory in children with Attention Deficit Hyperactivity Disorder. *Journal of Pediatric Psychology, 14*, 75–88.

Walker, N. W. (1986). What ever happened to the norms for the matching familiar figures test? *Perceptual and Motor Skills, 63*, 1234–1242.

Weingartner, H., Rapoport, J. L., Buchsbaum, M. S., Bunney, W. E., Ebert, M. H., Mikkelsen, E. J., & Caine, E. D. (1980). Cognitive processes in normal and hyperactive children and their response to amphetamine treatment. *Journal of Abnormal Psychology, 89*, 25–37.

Zahn, T. P., Abate, F., Little, B., & Wender, P. (1975). MBD, stimulant drugs and ANS activity. *Archives of General Psychiatry, 32*, 381–387.

Zahn, T. P., Rapoport, J. L., & Thompson, C. L. (1980). Autonomic and behavioral effects of dextroamphetamine and placebo in normal and hyperactive prepubertal boys. *Journal of Abnormal Child Psychology, 8*, 145–160.

Zahn, T. P., Kruesi, M. J. P., & Rapoport, J. L. (1991). Reaction time indices of attention deficits in boys with disruptive behavior disorders. *Journal of Abnormal Child Psychology, 19,* 233–252.

Zametkin, A. J., Nordahl, T. E., Gross, M., King, C., Semple, W. E., Rumsey, J., Hamburger, S., & Cohen, R. M. (1990). Cerebral glucose metabolism in adults with hyperactivity of childhood onset. *New England Journal of Medicine, 323,* 1361–1366.

Zentall, S. S. (1975). Optimal stimulation as a theoretical basis of hyperactivity. *American Journal of Orthopsychiatry, 45,* 549–563.

Zentall, S. S., & Meyer, M. J. (1987). Self-regulation of stimulation for ADD-H children during reading and vigilance task performance. *Journal of Abnormal Child Psychology, 15,* 519–536.

Zentall, S. S., & Zentall, T. R. (1976). Activity and task performance of hyperactive children as a function of environmental stimulation. *Journal of Consulting and Clinical Psychology, 44,* 693–697.

Zentall, S. S., & Zentall, T. R. (1983). Optimal stimulation: A model of disordered activity and performance in normal and deviant children. *Psychological Bulletin, 94,* 446–471.

6

The Child with Attention-Deficit/ Hyperactivity Disorder in Family Contexts

CAROL K. WHALEN and BARBARA HENKER

Attention Deficit/Hyperactivity Disorder (AD-HD) is a family affair. There is robust evidence of the family's role in both nature and nurture. Twin and family pedigree studies provide compelling evidence of high heritability of the syndrome itself as well as of more specific behavioral domains such as impulsivity and inattentiveness (Edelbrock, Rende, Plomin, & Thompson, 1995; Gillis, Gilger, Pennington, & DeFries, 1992; Gjone, Stevenson, & Sundet, 1996; Goodman & Stevenson, 1989; Zahn-Waxler, Schmitz, Fulker, Robinson, & Emde, 1996; see also Chapter 9, this volume). Psychosocial studies demonstrate that ADHD is also a transactional disorder. Family factors function as causes, correlates, and consequences, as children with ADHD influence and react to their social and physical environments. Although such bidirectional processes of influence define any parent–child relationship, ADHD can be considered a special case in that this disorder imposes more than the usual slate

of challenges and demands on caregivers. Moreover, children with ADHD may be particularly vulnerable to adverse or even less than optimal environmental influences. The challenges presented by a child with ADHD can easily overwhelm the family system, especially when (1) available resources are limited, perhaps by family adversity, single parenthood, or parental psychopathology; (2) the child's deficits and problems are so severe that even skillful and persistent attempts at accommodation and amelioration are ineffective; or (3) there is a poor fit between the personalities and behavioral styles of parent and child. In this chapter we discuss current thinking and research on the family contexts, cognitions, and interpersonal exchanges that characterize ADHD. But first, as an aid to interpretation and integration, we highlight some methodological issues fundamental to research on ADHD families.

APPROACHES TO THE STUDY OF FAMILY FACTORS

The diversity of approaches to the study of family factors compels caution when integrating and drawing conclusions from the clinical and empirical literatures. Despite this caveat, we attempt such an integration in the

CAROL K. WHALEN • Department of Psychology and Social Behavior, University of California, Irvine, Irvine, California 92697-7085. BARBARA HENKER • Department of Psychology, University of California, Los Angeles, Los Angeles, California 90095-1563.

Handbook of Disruptive Behavior Disorders, edited by Quay and Hogan. Kluwer Academic/Plenum Publishers, New York, 1999.

following pages. Thus, it seems appropriate to begin with a brief review of some methodological issues that must be considered when interpreting and integrating research findings.

Causal Directions

Families share many genes as well as many aspects of their everyday environments. Thus, it is not surprising that links between child ADHD and family factors have been documented repeatedly. The usual tendency is to interpret such links as demonstrating family-to-child influences. The hazards of such ready assumptions are cast into sharp relief by Stormont-Spurgin and Zentall's (1995) finding that mothers' reports of greater amounts of family support predicted higher ratings of child aggression 6 months later. Although it is conceivable that social support exacerbated the child's difficulties, it is more reasonable to speculate that parents of difficult children are especially likely to seek needed social support. Despite recent advances in behavioral genetics and statistical methodologies, the direction or degree of causality remains difficult to discern. The associations that are emerging from the research literature provide promising hypotheses about causal arrows, but their primary value is in elucidating developmental pathways, guiding treatment, and predicting long-term outcomes.

Assessment Modes

The vast majority of studies use questionnaires or rating scales; direct observations of child behaviors and parent–child interactions are relatively rare. Questionnaires have the advantages of economy, standardization, and portability. These instruments also suffer from well-known limitations, including subjectivity, variability across informants, and vulnerability to bias. Behavioral assessments provide relatively objective and unbiased glimpses of relationship qualities and interaction styles. However, these assessments are often conducted under artificial laboratory conditions in order to facilitate precision, objectivity, and stan-

dardization. The unfamiliar setting, the structured nature of activities, and the proximity of observers and recording equipment all influence and perhaps contaminate behaviors in unknown ways. Moreover, behavioral assessments are relatively narrow, given the impracticality of aggregating information across a broad sample of settings, intervals, and activities.

The potential role of source factors is also an important consideration when evaluating and comparing research investigations. Because of their availability to research staff and their centrality to the family, mothers are often the single source of information not only about their own characteristics and actions, but also about family climate, paternal characteristics, and child behaviors. Stronger inferences can usually be drawn from studies that include independent sources of information, such as parent reports of family history, directly observed parent–child interactions, and teacher evaluations of child behaviors. But because of the numerous logistic hurdles endemic to such multisource approaches, they are rarely used.

Diagnostic Heterogeneity

Until recently, children with ADHD and those with oppositional-defiant (ODD) or conduct disorders (CD) were grouped into a single externalizing category, with few studies distinguishing "pure" and comorbid subgroups. Comorbidity is very common, with more than half of children diagnosed with ADHD typically showing CD or ODD as well (Bauermeister, Canino, & Bird, 1994; see also Chapters 22 and 28, this volume). The result is that many of the conclusions drawn about ADHD may in fact apply specifically to ODD or CD, whether or not accompanied by ADHD. In other cases, the link between child problems and family dimensions seems strongest in children showing both types of problems, perhaps because such comorbidity is often an index of severity. The importance of differentiating between children with ADHD-only versus those with ADHD+ ODD/CD is underscored by intriguing evidence of distinctive developmental pathways for such subtypes, pathways that may be distinguished on the basis of symptomatology as well as age of onset, biological substrates, and family factors (Loeber & Hay, 1997; Moffitt, 1990).

Methodological Heterogeneity

When one reviews ADHD studies, one finds wide divergence in the samples, family dimensions, assessment modalities, and outcome factors examined. Studies may focus on preschool, school-age, or adolescent youngsters. Samples may be obtained from clinics or communities. Children may show earlier or later onset of problems, higher or lower symptom severity, and several or no comorbid disorders. The family factors and stressors identified may occur earlier or later in the child's development, be mild or severe, be brief or protracted, have narrow or widespread impact, and occur singly or in conjunction with other adverse influences. In brief, there is a host of potentially important and largely unexamined factors that vary across studies. These variations may underlie many of the conflicting results that appear in the literature, and they also impede our ability to unravel the complexities and reach definitive conclusions about the multiple roles of the family. Even so, there is a substantial body of informative research that has both heuristic and clinical implications, as illustrated in the following pages.

FAMILY CONTEXTS, CONCEPTS, AND CONTACTS

It has long been known that adverse environmental conditions, such as family dysfunction and low socioeconomic status (SES), are associated with greater risk of developing childhood behavior disorders. As an organizing scheme, we divide the diverse family factors that have been examined into three overlapping clusters: contexts, concepts, and contacts. *Contexts* are background or setting factors, including global dimensions such as SES and more proximal dimensions such as marital status, social support resources, and parental psy-

chopathology. *Concepts* are attitudes, perceptions, and attributions. Included in this category are parents' perceptions of their child's problems; their self-perceived parenting stress, competence, and satisfaction; and their causal reasoning about problem sources and solutions. *Contacts* are the most proximal of the variables, including observed parent-child interaction patterns as well as parenting styles, socialization practices, and emotional climate in the home.

This tripartite scheme is presented for ease of communication. The distinctions are somewhat arbitrary and the boundaries quite fluid. For example, maternal depression and maternal perceptions of parenting stress and satisfaction are inextricably enmeshed, and both are associated with day-by-day transactions between mother and child. Another example can be found in a structural equation analysis of multiple parent-related factors that illustrated the intricate direct and indirect influences of economic pressure, spousal and social network support, parental depression, and positive parenting (Simons, Lorenz, Wu, & Conger, 1993). One finding regarding mothers, for example, was that spousal support moderated the impact of economic strain by reducing the disruptive effects of depression on parenting behavior. Thus, rather than functioning as discrete characteristics or occurrences that can simply be aggregated or studied in isolation, these clusters interact in a complex web of multidirectional influences.

Family Contexts

Diverse facets of family environments have been linked to child externalizing disorders. Some studies examine the influence of individual risk factors; others use a composite index as a cumulative measure of overall adversity. A typical example is that used in the seminal Dunedin Multidisciplinary Health and Development Study in New Zealand: A 6-point index of family disadvantage was constructed based on low SES, solo parenting, large family size, parental separations, perceived family support, and maternal depression (Feehan, McGee, &

Williams, 1993; McGee *et al.,* 1990; see also Chapter 19, this volume). In this section we focus first on a few key family contextual variables: parental psychopathology, personality, and marital discord. Then, studies that used composite adversity indexes are examined.

Parental Psychopathology: Antisocial Behavior, Depression, and ADHD

Numerous studies have linked child ADHD to parental psychopathology. Compared with the general population, parents and other first-degree relatives of children with ADHD show elevated rates of psychiatric disorders and also are more likely to have problems with drug and alcohol use, criminal activity, job performance, and marital discord (Barkley, Fischer, Edelbrock, & Smallish, 1991; Biederman *et al.,* 1992; Cunningham, Benness, & Siegel, 1988; Hechtman, 1996).

Several early studies reported disproportionate rates of parental (and especially paternal) antisocial behavior in children with ADHD. With the recent efforts to distinguish between ADHD-only and ADHD+ODD/CD subtypes, it is becoming apparent that the link with parental antisocial behavior is relatively specific to the latter subgroup; in fact, parental antisocial behavior is associated with childhood ODD/CD whether or not accompanied by ADHD (Faraone *et al.,* 1995; Frick, Lahey, Christ, Loeber, & Green, 1991; Lahey *et al.,* 1988; see also Chapter 15, this volume). The only parental disorder that has been associated specifically and consistently with ADHD is maternal or paternal history of childhood ADHD (Frick *et al.,* 1991).

Maternal depression has also been associated with childhood ADHD, although the literature reveals some inconsistencies (Faraone *et al.,* 1995; Frick, 1994). As with paternal antisocial behavior, both clinical and epidemiological findings suggest that rates of maternal depression are higher in the comorbid ADHD+ODD/CD subgroup (Barkley *et al.,* 1991; Lahey *et al.,* 1988). Living with, and being responsible for a child with ADHD poses daily challenges, and success experiences are far fewer

than would be expected on the basis of parental actions and efforts. Because mothers typically take on a greater proportion of child management burdens than do fathers, and because depression occurs much more frequently in women than in men, one would expect higher rates of depression in mothers. The child-to-parent direction of effect is further buttressed by Hechtman's (1996) observation that the mental health of family members tends to improve with time, and that the change is most marked when the child with ADHD moves out of the family home. The possibility of reciprocal mother–father effects is suggested by Brown and Pacini's (1989) intriguing report that, in a sample of parents of children with ADHD, the depression scores of mothers and fathers were inversely associated. In summary, there are sound reasons to assume child-to-parent directionality, but there are also good reasons to consider biological bases as well as third variables such as marital discord that may contribute to the development of both disorders.

Parental Personality

One set of family factors that has not been well studied is parental personality, individual differences in modes of thinking and behaving that are within the "normal" range. Nigg and Hinshaw (1998) not only examined such nonclinical individual differences, but they also distinguished between overt and covert antisocial behaviors in children with ADHD. Higher rates of *overt* antisocial behavior were linked primarily to maternal characteristics such as depression. In contrast, higher rates of *covert* antisocial acts (stealing) were related to paternal characteristics, including greater openness and a history of substance abuse. These links to parental traits and disorders emerged over and above SES, a contextual variable that has been associated with child conduct problems in a number of studies (Coie & Dodge, 1998; Offord *et al.,* 1992).

A link between maternal anxiety and low levels of overt antisocial behavior also emerged, suggesting that maternal anxiety may serve a protective function for this behavioral domain.

As Nigg and Hinshaw (1998) note, there are several alternative explanations of this pattern. Boys with ADHD who have anxious mothers may themselves be more inhibited and thus less likely to transgress. Or, these boys may limit noncompliant and aggressive acts in an attempt to help ameliorate their mothers' anxiety. A third possibility is that anxious mothers may be more likely than their nonanxious counterparts to anticipate and attempt to control problem behaviors in their sons, for example, through limit-setting and careful monitoring. These alternative interpretations lend themselves nicely to empirical tests. The findings from this study were complex and at times puzzling. For example, the predictive association between maternal neuroticism and overt aggression was positive, whereas that between maternal anxiety disorder and overt aggression was negative. Needed now are attempts at systematic replication of this exploratory study as well as extension to other samples, behavioral domains, and personality characteristics.

Marital Discord and Divorce

Marital discord or divorce surfaces frequently in the families of children with ADHD. Although there are some exceptions to this pattern (Johnston, 1996; Prinz, Myers, Holden, Tarnowski, & Roberts, 1983), the bulk of the evidence suggests, once again, that this dimension is related more strongly to ODD/CD than to ADHD per se and is thus most evident among children with ADHD when there are also aggression or conduct problems (Loeber, Brinthaupt, & Green, 1990). There is suggestive evidence that the unsalutary effects of separation or divorce stem not so much from the attendant stress and disruption, but rather from the intense conflict and discord that often precede divorce (see Frick, 1994). This conclusion is buttressed by Amato and Keith's (1991) report that children in high-conflict, intact homes have poorer adjustment than children from divorced homes. Many questions about links between marital and child problems remain, including whether the

effects are due specifically to discord or more generally to an aggregate of risk factors that typically accompany marital problems (Rutter, 1989). Other key questions relate to the pathogenic aspects of discord. For example, do negative effects on the child result from the lack of a secure parent–child relationship, a climate of tension and emotional distress, or impairment of parenting (Erel & Burman, 1995)? Questions also remain about direction of causality. Not only can marital discord exert harmful effects on children, but difficult-to-manage children can undermine the spousal relationship. Such reciprocal effects may evolve into self-perpetuating vicious cycles, with marital discord exacerbating child behavior problems and the behavior problems in turn placing additional stress on troubled spousal relations.

Cumulative Family Adversity

Psychosocial risk factors tend to cluster. To illustrate from one epidemiological study, Sandberg, Wieselberg, and Shaffer (1980) found that 47% of children from low SES backgrounds came from broken homes and 46% had mentally distressed mothers, compared to 15% and 24% at other SES levels. For the most part, investigators have been unsuccessful in their attempts to link isolated risk factors with specific disorders. When groups of children are assessed, it does not seem that marital conflict, low SES, parental psychopathology, or any single risk factor is associated specifically with ADHD. The aggregate of adverse experiences seems to be more critical than any single stressor or set of stressors. As signaled by Rutter's (1979) seminal research, there may in fact be a dose–response relationship, with the decisive factor being the overall level or degree of adversity (Biederman, Milberger, Faraone, Kiely, Guite, Mick, Ablon, Warburton, & Reed, 1995).

When children with ADHD are compared with their nondiagnosed peers on these types of indicators, it is often found that the ADHD group has experienced higher levels of both family and environmental adversity. Longitudinal studies also indicate that family stress and adversity predict continuing problems over the years of development (Campbell, 1994, 1997). In a 4-year prospective study, Biederman and colleagues (1996) divided an ADHD sample into three subgroups: those whose problems abated during childhood (early remitters), those who improved during adolescence (late remitters), and those who continued to experience serious difficulties (persistent ADHD). Indicators of psychosocial adversity, along with family history of ADHD, were markedly elevated among those in the persistent group and moderately elevated among the late remitters. In contrast, there were no differences in these indexes between normal controls and the early remitters. Another important finding was that the early remitters did not differ from the other children with ADHD in terms of initial symptom picture, age of onset, or problem duration. Family adversity seemed to be the best discriminator.

The literature is not entirely consistent, however, on the pervasiveness of links between ADHD and family adversity. Some studies failed to find such links after relevant variables such as comorbidity were controlled (Frick, 1994; Szatmari, Offord, & Boyle, 1989). There is evidence that adverse family environments may be associated more strongly with conduct problems or other comorbid disorders than with ADHD per se (August, MacDonald, Realmuto, & Skare, 1996; Bauermeister et al., 1994; Loeber et al., 1990), and that family adversity may play the largest role in children who have combined ADHD+ODD/CD problems (Moffitt, 1990). Still other studies suggest a global vulnerability that applies to any child experiencing adverse family environments rather than a specific link between family risk and ADHD (Biederman, Milberger, Faraone, Kiely, Guite, Mick, Ablon, Warburton, Reed, & Davis, 1995; Offord, Boyle, & Racine, 1989). The most valid conclusion at this point seems to be that psychosocial adversity may lower the threshold for problem development in general; there is no evidence of a profile of environmental risk factors specific to ADHD (Schachar, 1991).

Concepts: Perceived Competence, Support, and Causal Attributions

Within the realm of family cognitions, we focus on two main domains: parental perceptions of internal and external resources, and parental attributions about child behaviors. In the resource domain we include parent-perceived competence and self-efficacy, stress, and social support, as well as parenting satisfaction. In the attribution domain we include underlying theories about initial problem sources and probable solutions as well as day-to-day causal reasoning about why their child behaves or fails to behave in certain ways.

Parental Perceptions of Internal and External Resources

Mothers of children with ADHD, compared with mothers of nondiagnosed children, report higher levels of stress and social isolation and lower levels of social support, self-perceived competence, and parenting self-esteem (Beck, Young, & Tarnowski, 1990; Brown & Pacini, 1989; Campbell, 1994; Edwards, Schulz, & Long, 1995; Fischer, 1990; Mash & Johnston, 1983a, 1983b; Sandberg et al., 1980). The most compelling links emerge, once again, in the families of those children who show a combination of ADHD and oppositional or conduct problems. Anastopoulos, Guevremont, Shelton, and DuPaul (1992) found that, in families with a child with ADHD, it was the child's oppositional-defiant behavior that predicted parenting stress. Johnston (1996) examined parent characteristics and parent–child interactions in three family groups: those with nonproblem children, and those with children with ADHD who exhibited either higher (HOD) or lower (LOD) levels of oppositional-defiant behavior. By their own report, parents in both ADHD groups used more negative-reactive and fewer positive parenting strategies than did those in the nonproblem group. Whereas the two ADHD groups did not differ significantly in reported parenting behaviors, parenting self-esteem was lowest in the HOD group. The relevance of these parental perceptions to child outcomes is suggested by the findings from a longitudinal study of preschoolers with problems that high parenting stress predicted poorer child adjustment over time (Heller, Baker, Henker, & Hinshaw, 1996).

When considering maternal parenting stress and satisfaction, it is important to focus not only on the child with ADHD, but also on other family members, especially fathers and siblings. Mash and Johnston (1983a) found that, compared to mothers, fathers view the problem behaviors of children with ADHD as less severe. This finding highlights the important role that fathers can play as a source of validation and support for mothers who typically put in much longer shifts than do fathers on the firing line with a difficult child. In a companion study, Mash and Johnston (1983b) found that mothers' reports of parenting competence, stress, and satisfaction were correlated with the quality of sibling interactions. Despite the difficulties of including fathers and siblings in research studies, these findings point to the need to look beyond the mother–child relationship and learn more about the family as a transactional system, both to further our understanding of ADHD and to guide intervention efforts.

Causal Attributions

For many years, attributional theorists have been describing how people generate theories to understand the events they observe, and causal ascriptions are key ingredients of these lay theories (Jones & Davis, 1965). Studies of parental attributions have demonstrated links between the causal explanations that parents use when explaining their child's behavior and parental perceptions of, and affective reactions to, child (mis)behaviors (Gretarsson & Gelfand, 1988). Moreover, these cognitive appraisals mediate behavioral responses and parenting practices (Bugental, Blue, & Cruzcosa, 1989; Dix, Ruble, Grusec, & Nixon, 1986; Geller & Johnston, 1995; Johnston & Patensude, 1994).

Parental attributions regarding children with ADHD may be especially consequential, given the chronicity of this disorder and the fact that these parents confront demands and burdens that far exceed those of most parents. The ways in which parents explain problem sources and solutions can have important implications not only for child outcomes, but also for the mental health and well-being of parents and their willingness to persist in time-consuming intervention efforts.

A study by our own research team contrasted the causal attributions of parents with older versus younger ADHD and non-ADHD school-age boys (Henker, Whalen, Carter, Garland, & Heller, 1996). Parents participated in a structured interview designed to assess their causal attributions for their own child's behaviors and misbehaviors. Following these interviews, the boys participated in a 5-week research summer program, after which behavioral ratings were obtained from the staff who had become well acquainted with these youngsters over the course of the program. One immediately apparent difference between parents of children with ADHD and those with non-problem children was that the former generated a larger number of causal attributions to explain their sons' behaviors, and those parents who offered the largest number of causal explanations had sons who were perceived most negatively by the summer school staff. Parents of boys with ADHD also gave their children less credit for positive behaviors than did parents of non-ADHD children, and they were more likely to attribute their sons' good behaviors to themselves than to their sons. Consistent with these findings are those reported by Johnston and Freeman (1997) indicating that parents of a child with ADHD, in contrast to parents of normal controls, perceive the prosocial behaviors of their own child as less internal and less stable. In a related study, these investigators found that parents of children with ADHD responded less positively to prosocial behaviors presented in the context of inattentive-overactive or oppositional-defiant behaviors than they did to prosocial behaviors that accompanied other prosocial behaviors (Freeman, Johnston, & Barth, 1997). Given their cumulative experiences with child misbehavior, it is not difficult to see how parents of children with ADHD begin to diverge from parents of normal children in their perceptions and causal analyses.

Henker and colleagues (1996) examined not only who received the credit or blame, but also whether the acts were perceived as volitional. One major developmental task during childhood is the acquisition of intentional control over one's own behavior, and most parents view their child's behaviors as increasingly volitional as the child matures (Dix *et al.,* 1986). Parents of older (in contrast to younger) non-ADHD children displayed this pattern, whereas those of older ADHD children did not. In other words, parents of older ADHD boys were less likely than parents of older control boys to view their son's misbehaviors as volitional. The importance of this difference is suggested by the fact that parents who gave *fewer* child volitional attributions had sons who received more negative staff evaluations.

The association between nonvolitional attributions on the part of the parent and troublesome behavior on the part of the child is particularly compelling when one recalls that the child's behaviors were evaluated by independent judges (i.e., summer-school staff) and occurred when the parents were not present. Parental perceptions of low volitional control in boys with ADHD may be a joint function of cumulative failure experiences with these children and increasing acknowledgment or acceptance of a physiological basis for the problems. A diagnosis may in itself lead parents to relieve a child of a certain amount of responsibility for misbehavior (Walker, Garber, & Van Slyke, 1995; Whalen & Henker, 1976).

Studies of attributional reasoning in parents of nonreferred children indicate that parents typically become more upset by and respond more intensely to children's transgressions when they view these acts as intentional rather than beyond the child's control (Geller & Johnston, 1995; see Miller, 1995, for a review). Perhaps nonvolitional attributions help parents

with difficult children regulate their own emotions and prevent or contain negative affectivity. Parental perceptions of physiological causation and child nonvolition may be strengthened over time in children who are participating in long-term stimulant treatment regimens, given the tendency to reason backward from treatment to etiology (Whalen & Henker, 1997).

These findings have implications for understanding parenting practices, treatment adherence, and child outcomes. When parents view their child as not accountable, even if such perceptions are accurate, they may be less likely to raise their expectations progressively and provide age-appropriate challenges as their child matures. Parents who do not view their child as capable of intentional self-regulation may also be less willing to endorse or apply appropriate behavior change strategies and more likely to rely on medication as the sole treatment modality.

There is also suggestive evidence from previous studies that parents can overattribute volitionality to their child. Volitional attributions regarding child misbehavior have been linked to abusive and dysfunctional parenting and to parental perceptions of helplessness and incompetence (e.g., Baden & Howe, 1992; Bugental, Blue, & Lewis, 1990; Smith & O'Leary, 1995). The delineation of optimal levels of parent-perceived volitionality is an important topic for future research. These levels can be expected to vary not only across individuals and situations, but also across developmental stages, types of behavior problems, and phases of treatment.

Parental perceptions and attributions may also be important during the adolescent years. Barkley, Anastopoulos, Guevremont, and Fletcher (1992) examined causal attributions of mothers of three groups of adolescents: those with ADHD+ODD, those with ADHD-only, and a normal control group. Once again, the role of conduct problems appeared to be paramount. Mothers in the ADHD+ODD group attributed more malicious intent to the conduct of their teens than did mothers in the other two groups, who did not differ from each other. These mothers were also more likely than mothers in the control group to communicate negatively when discussing a putatively neutral topic with their teenager, to express extreme and unreasonable beliefs about their parent–teen relations, and to report greater personal distress and less marital satisfaction. These maternal differences did not occur in a vacuum, of course. As would be expected, teens in the ADHD+ODD displayed more negative perceptions and behaviors than their counterparts in the other two groups, once again attesting to the transactional nature of family influences.

As suggested earlier, parental attributions may mediate several facets of treatment response, including acceptance of specific modalities, compliance with the regimen, and interpretation of results. Borden and Brown (1989) examined attributions during an intervention program in which one of three medication conditions (stimulants, placebos, or no pills) was combined with cognitive behavioral treatment. Parents in the no-pill group expressed the strongest beliefs that their children were capable of solving their own problems, whereas those in the placebo group were more likely to believe that solutions would result from external and uncontrollable factors. These findings suggest that there may be inadvertent attributional effects of medication for children with ADHD, and that these effects may be most probable when the treatment is ineffective (e.g., when placebos are given).

A final illustration of the potential significance of parental attributional styles is provided by a recent study of attributional reasoning in boys with externalizing disorders and their mothers (Bickett, Milich, & Brown, 1996). As would be expected from the findings just reported, mothers of the externalizing boys showed a generalized tendency to infer negative motives or dispositions when accounting for their son's misbehavior. And, as has been shown in previous studies (e.g., Crick & Dodge, 1994), boys with externalizing problems failed to distinguish between hostile and ambiguous situations, tending to infer hostile intentions in both instances. What was particularly intriguing about these findings was that

mothers' responses were similar to those of their sons in that mothers also made indiscriminate inferences about hostile intentions. Parental tendencies toward hostile attributional reasoning may not only maintain abrasive and coercive patterns of interaction, but may also serve to encourage, through modeling and reinforcement, similar dysfunctional cognitions in their children.

Contacts: Parenting Practices, Parent–Child Interactions, and Sibling Relations

The contact dimension can be considered the most proximal level of empirical analysis, involving what parents and children actually do for, to, and with each other. To illustrate major concepts and findings, we take examples from the literatures on parent negativity and depression.

Parenting Negativity

Mother–child interactions are qualitatively and quantitatively distinctive when the child has ADHD (Campbell, Breaux, Ewing, Szumowski, & Pierce, 1986; Cunningham & Barkley, 1979; Humphries, Kinsbourne, & Swanson, 1978). Mash and Johnston (1982) reported that during both free play and structured task activities, mothers of children with ADHD were more directive and negative than were mothers of normal children. Although the children with ADHD were more negative and noncompliant than their peers, the mother's negativity emerged even when the child was behaving appropriately. Mothers of children with ADHD also tended to be less responsive when their children initiated interaction. Observed negativity on the part of mothers has been linked directly to child noncompliance and stealing (Anderson, Hinshaw, & Simmel, 1994). Interestingly, in this latter study there was no association between maternal negativity and child displays of overt aggression, a reminder of the multidimensionality of externalizing behavior problems discussed in Chapter 1 (this volume).

Studies of adolescents with ADHD indicate that parent–child transactions continue to be problematic. When mothers interacted with their ADHD teenagers, especially teenagers who show both ADHD and ODD problems, there were higher rates of negative, controlling, and conflictful behaviors, and fewer instances of positive and facilitating behaviors, than in mother–adolescent dyads without ADHD (Barkley *et al.*, 1991, 1992; Fletcher, Fischer, Barkley, & Smallish, 1996). Particularly noteworthy was the fact that this negative interaction style distinguished ADHD from normal groups only during discussions of putatively neutral, nonproblematic topics. There were no group differences during discussions of conflict-laden topics, most likely because this situation elicited high rates of negative behaviors in the control group as well. Thus, the family problems experienced during the adolescent years may be concerned not so much with the negativity displayed but rather with the range of situations that elicit this negativity and the intensity of the reaction.

The prognostic significance of negative parent–child interaction styles during early development has also been demonstrated. Fagot and Leve (1998) reported that parent negativity (critical, coercive, aggressive behavior) when children were ages 18–24 months predicted teacher ratings of externalizing behavior problems at school entry (age 5). The continuation of such associations into the school-age years has been documented in a longitudinal study of difficult-to-manage boys: Observed negative maternal affect and intrusive control when children were age 4 predicted externalizing problems at age 9 (Campbell, Pierce, Moore, Marakovitz, & Newby, 1996). It is quite likely that a substantial component of this less than optimal parenting is the result of atypically high rates of noncompliant and disruptive behavior on the child's part. But the associations tend to hold even when the child's symptomatology is controlled statistically (Campbell, March, Pierce, Ewing, & Szumowski, 1991; Campbell *et al.*, 1996). Whatever the initial causes, it is clear that negative interaction patterns can be established early in the child's life,

often by or before preschool age, and that a bidirectional, self-perpetuating cycle of unsalutary interactions may result (Campbell, 1995; Cunningham & Barkley, 1979). Frick (1994) suggested that ADHD may develop independently of parenting practices, but that the child's behavior problems may disrupt the parenting process, and the resultant ineffective or coercive parenting may place the child at risk for the development of conduct problems.

Maternal Depression

Intriguing patterns of mother–child interaction are also emerging from fine-grained observational studies of depressed mothers interacting with their children. Comparing mother–infant interactions of depressed and nondepressed first-time mothers, Campbell, Cohn, and Meyers (1995) found that mothers who showed transient depression did not differ from nondepressed mothers, but when the depression lasted at least 6 months, both the mothers and their infants showed decreased levels of positive affect and engagement during feeding, toy play, and face-to-face interaction. There were no differences in rates of negative, rejecting, or intrusive behaviors, all of which occurred rarely in this relatively low-risk sample.

This pattern changes, however, when the focus is on older children and families who are at greater risk because of environmental adversity. These studies have demonstrated that depressed mothers can be distinguished from nondepressed mothers by their higher rates of disapproval and criticism, irritability, negative affective tone, unresponsiveness, disengagement, and lower levels of sensitivity (Gelfand & Teti, 1990; Nolen-Hoeksema, Wolfson, Mumme, & Guskin, 1995; Tarullo, DeMulder, Ronsaville, Brown, & Radke-Yarrow, 1995). Conrad and Hammen (1989) found an intriguing interaction between maternal depression and child misbehavior. There were no differences between depressed and nondepressed mothers in rates of either positive or negative interactions toward nondisturbed children. But when they had children with behavior problems, depressed mothers were more negative and critical in their interactions than were non-depressed mothers. Depressed mothers also seemed to be more accurate in their ratings of disturbed children. There was no general tendency to exaggerate the problems of their youngsters but rather a specific tendency to perceive symptomatic behaviors in those children who had been independently identified as having problems. Taken together, these findings suggest that depressed mothers may be more attuned to or less tolerant of child dysfunction. It has also been suggested that, rather than being more accurate and realistic in their perceptions, depressed mothers may actually distort their observations in a negative direction, but there has been little empirical support for this hypothesis (Richters, 1992).

Gelfand and Teti (1990) suggested that children vary temperamentally, situationally, and developmentally in their susceptibility to deficient parenting. Some youngsters will cope better than others with maternal depressive episodes, because of their personal resources as well as various protective factors such as marital harmony or a strong relationship with the father. Although these studies of maternal depression were not specific to children with ADHD, they suggest that the combination of a depressed mother and a child with ADHD may be especially pernicious, resulting in high levels of conflict, negative or ineffective socialization practices, disengagement and withdrawal, and demoralization of both mother and child.

Sibling Interactions

As noted previously, sibling relationships have not been examined extensively. In an early study of interaction patterns, Mash and Johnston (1983b) observed that school-age sibling dyads that included a child with ADHD interacted more negatively than dyads with non-problem children, and in fact few behavioral differences were noted between the hyperactive boys and their nondiagnosed sibs. Stormont-Spurgin and Zentall (1995) reported that preschool children who exhibited both hyperactivity and aggression experienced dispropor-

tionately high rates of counteraggression from their siblings, according to maternal reports. Thus, there are emerging indications of problematic behavior patterns in (as yet) nondiagnosed siblings, although the data are sparse. These behavioral findings are consistent with family pedigree studies indicating that siblings of children with ADHD have higher than average rates of behavioral, mood, and anxiety disorders, school failure, and other signs of psychosocial dysfunction (Faraone *et al.*, 1993, 1995; see also Chapter 9, this volume).

The fact that many siblings of children with ADHD do not function as well as their peers is not surprising, given the commonalities in genetic makeup and environmental influences. Even without being able to disentangle cause from effect or nature from nurture, the fact that some siblings display relatively high rates of dysfunctional behavior has consequences for children with ADHD, to the extent that the siblings' actions help maintain abrasive interaction patterns and almost certainly have a negative impact on the quality of family life. The findings are also consistent with the notion that children with ADHD serve as negative social catalysts (Whalen & Henker, 1992). The factors associated with adaptive versus maladaptive sibling outcomes are especially worthy of empirical examination.

FAMILY INFLUENCES: CAUSES, MODULATORS, AND CONSEQUENCES

Thus far the discussion has focused primarily on the contents of family influences. By way of summarizing these large and diverse literatures, we now turn to a brief examination of potential processes or mechanisms that may help explain and predict links between family factors and child behaviors.

The Family as Source

Findings from several empirical strands, including those from family and twin studies, are converging on the conclusion that genetic and other biological contributions are paramount in the etiology of ADHD (see Chapter 8, this volume). In a subgroup of children diagnosed with ADHD, however, psychosocial variables may play an etiological role above and beyond their influence on severity, course, and treatment responsiveness. Biederman, Faraone, Keenan, Knee, and Tsuang (1990) found that the risk of ADHD among relatives of ADHD probands was high whether there was psychosocial advantage or adversity, indicating that environmental advantage did not protect against familial risk for ADHD. In contrast, lower SES and separation or divorce did increase the risk of ADHD among relatives of the control group. Findings such as these have led to speculation that there may be a nonfamilial or psychogenic form of ADHD that is seen in youngsters from low-SES backgrounds who experience substantial family adversity (e.g., Bauermeister, Alegria, Bird, Rubio-Stipec, & Canino, 1992; Biederman *et al.*, 1990).

Consistent with this psychogenic subgroup hypothesis are the findings from a prospective longitudinal study of inattentiveness and hyperactivity in children from low-SES backgrounds (Carlson, Jacobvitz, & Sroufe, 1995). Children were assessed during the preschool (age $3\frac{1}{2}$) and early elementary years (ages 6–8), and again during middle childhood (age 11). Measures included not only a comprehensive set of ratings and history variables, but also directly observed behaviors of parent and child while engaged in structured teaching tasks. A combination of maternal personality dimensions (anxiety and aggression), caregiving behaviors, and contextual factors predicted the development and stability of ADHD during childhood. The ADHD group differed from controls in terms of intrusive and overstimulating caregiving. These parent behaviors, such as teasing or provoking a child who is already aroused, or physically stimulating a child in the absence of expressed need, are thought to interfere with the child's development of arousal regulation and self-control. Also associated with ADHD were two contextual variables, relationship status at the child's birth (married or long-term relationship versus

single, divorced, or long-term separation) and quality of emotional support available to mother. These investigators suggest that one of the multiple routes to the development of ADHD may be overstimulating caregiving by a mother who is isolated in the caregiving relationship and lacking in external social support. Although cause-and-effect questions cannot be answered definitively, these findings illustrate how family dimensions may play influential roles in the development of early problem behaviors. Interestingly, family contextual variables did not improve the prediction of hyperactivity in the later elementary years beyond the influence of hyperactivity in the early elementary years. Over the years, these family factors may combine with child disruptiveness in a self-stabilizing cycle of dysfunctional behavior (Carlson *et al.*, 1995).

The Family as Modulator

There is little disagreement that the family context affects problem extensiveness and severity, response to treatment, and long-term outcomes. Family influences such as marital conflict and coercive parenting may be especially important in the development of aggression and conduct problems in children with ADHD, as discussed in the preceding sections. Because of its diagnostic intent, much of the literature on family factors examines negative influences, focusing on unsalutary practices and conditions. An alternate view of ADHD that may have heuristic as well as clinical value is that the constellation of problem behaviors and their malleability over the course of development provide a natural laboratory for parent and child to engage in mutual problem solving aimed at developing the cognitive perspectives, adaptive skills, and external resources needed to confront the ADHD challenge. Developmental transitions (e.g., entry into preschool) and family stressors (e.g., separation, illness) ineluctably provide critical teaching moments for mastering or succumbing to such challenges. The ways in which parents guide their children through such events may facilitate adaptive coping and positive relationships. Alternatively, eventful and even everyday challenges can overwhelm resources, increase interpersonal conflict, and cement dysfunctional action patterns (Campbell, 1995). Some support for this view emerged from an observational study of mother–father–child triads in a nonclinic sample. Westerman and Schonholtz (1993) found that joint parental support of the child's problem-solving efforts was associated directly with marital adjustment (as reported by fathers) and inversely with child behavior problems (as reported by teachers as well as by fathers). The link between observed family interaction and teacher reports, an independent source of information about the child, makes these findings particularly compelling.

The protective or buffering role that fathers may play has been largely overlooked, despite recent recognition of the need to study paternal contributions to child development (Parke, 1995; Phares & Compas, 1992). In a study of the impact of maternal depression, Tannenbaum and Forehand (1994) found that adolescents whose mothers reported depressive mood were more likely to have both internalizing and externalizing problems. The subgroup who had good (low-conflict) relationships with their fathers, however, showed fewer problems and seemed to be functioning as well as their peers whose mothers were not depressed. The literature is laced with suggestions that those children with ADHD who fare best enjoy a positive relationship with a special, caring family member (Weiss & Hechtman, 1993). The empirical literature on protective factors is still quite sketchy, and studies are needed that compare the profiles of personal and interpersonal resources of children with ADHD who show good versus poor long-term outcomes (Whalen & Henker, 1998).

The Family as Outcome

Families are ineluctably changed through their experiences with a child with ADHD. Although the usual caveats about inferring direction of causality obtain, there is suggestive empirical evidence of child-to-parent effects. Perhaps the most compelling examples are studies in which parents are observed interacting with their children or adolescents when the child is on stimulant medication versus placebo. These studies have demonstrated marked differences in the behaviors of the parent that are linked to the medication-related changes in child behaviors. Mothers and fathers tend to be more negative and controlling when the child is on placebo and more positive and supportive when the child is on medication (Barkley, 1989; Barkley & Cunningham, 1979; Humphries et al., 1978). The degree and rapidity of change in parental behaviors in response to the medication condition of the child weighs against the interpretation that negative parental behavior initially caused the child's problematic behavior. These studies demonstrate, instead, that parents of children and adolescents with ADHD can modulate their interactive style in accordance with the child's actions.

Over the long term, however, the effects on family members may be more pernicious and enduring. Pervasive child problems demand considerable parental resources, often resulting in failure, fatigue, and demoralization; isolated and circumscribed living; strained marital relationships; and neglect or overindulgence of siblings. Despite these chronic, high-demand conditions, many parents marshal the resources needed to cope adaptively with the multiple challenges they confront. And many children with ADHD improve to the point of being indistinguishable as adults (see Chapter 12, this volume). Perhaps the greatest research need is for multifactorial studies that help us locate and make the connections between pervasive and persistent ADHD problems, on the one hand, and successful long-term outcomes, on the other. The challenge for the future is to track the corrective and compensatory experiences that divert the trajectories for some children into more benign and beneficial pathways.

REFERENCES

Amato, P. R., & Keith, B. (1991). Parental divorce and the well-being of children: A meta-analysis. *Psychological Bulletin, 110,* 26–46.

Anastopoulos, A. D., Guevremont, D. C., Shelton, T. L., & DuPaul, G. J. (1992). Parenting stress among families of children with attention deficit hyperactivity disorder. *Journal of Abnormal Child Psychology, 20,* 503–520.

Anderson, C. A., Hinshaw, S. P., & Simmel, C. (1994). Mother–child interactions in ADHD and comparison boys: Relationships with overt and covert externalizing behavior. *Journal of Abnormal Child Psychology, 22,* 247–265.

August, G. J., MacDonald, A. W., Realmuto, G. M., & Skare, S. S. (1996). Hyperactive and aggressive pathways: Effects of demographic, family, and child characteristics on children's adaptive functioning. *Journal of Clinical Child Psychology, 25,* 341–351.

Baden, A. D., & Howe, G. W. (1992). Mothers' attributions and expectancies regarding their conduct-disordered children. *Journal of Abnormal Child Psychology, 20,* 467–485.

Barkley, R. A. (1989). Hyperactive girls and boys: Stimulant drug effects on mother–child interactions. *Journal of Child Psychology and Psychiatry, 30,* 379–390.

Barkley, R. A., & Cunningham, C. E. (1979). The effects of methylphenidate on the mother–child interactions of hyperactive children. *Archives of General Psychiatry, 36,* 201–208.

Barkley, R. A., Fischer, M., Edelbrock, C., & Smallish, L. (1991). The adolescent outcome of hyperactive children diagnosed by research criteria—III. Mother–child interactions, family conflicts and maternal psychopathology. *Journal of Child Psychology and Psychiatry, 32,* 233–255.

Barkley, R. A., Anastopoulos, A. D., Guevremont, D. C., & Fletcher, K. E. (1992). Adolescents with attention deficit hyperactivity disorder: Mother–adolescent interactions, family beliefs and conflicts, and maternal psychopathology. *Journal of Abnormal Child Psychology, 20,* 263–288.

Bauermeister, J. J., Alegria, M., Bird, H. R., Rubio-Stipec, M., & Canino, G. (1992). Are attentional-hyperactivity deficits unidimensional or multidimensional syndromes? Empirical findings from a community survey. *Journal of the American Academy of Child and Adolescent Psychiatry, 31,* 423–431.

Bauermeister, J. J., Canino, G., & Bird, H. (1994). Epidemiology of disruptive behavior disorders. *Child and Adolescent Psychiatric Clinics of North America, 3,* 177–194.

Beck, S. J., Young, G. H., & Tarnowski, K. J. (1990). Maternal characteristics and perceptions of pervasive and situational hyperactives and normal controls. *Journal of the American Academy of Child and Adolescent Psychiatry, 29,* 558–565.

Bickett, L. R., Milich, R., & Brown, R. T. (1996). Attributional styles of aggressive boys and their mothers. *Journal of Abnormal Child Psychology, 24,* 457–472.

Biederman, J., Faraone, S. V., Keenan, K., Knee, D., & Tsuang, M. T. (1990). Family-genetic and psychosocial risk factors in DSM-III attention deficit disorder. *Journal of the American Academy of Child and Adolescent Psychiatry, 29,* 526–533.

Biederman, J., Faraone, S. V., Keenan, K., Benjamin, J., Krifcher, B., Moore, C., Sprich-Buckminster, S., Ugaglia, K., Jellinek, M. S., Steingard, R., Spencer, T., Norman, D., Kolodny, R., Kraus, I., Perrin, J., Keller, M. B., & Tsuang, M. T. (1992). Further evidence for family-genetic risk factors in attention deficit hyperactivity disorder: Patterns of comorbidity in probands and relatives in psychiatrically and pediatrically referred samples. *Archives of General Psychiatry, 49,* 728–738.

Biederman, J., Milberger, S., Faraone, S. V., Kiely, K., Guite, J., Mick, E., Ablon, S., Warburton, R., & Reed, E. (1995). Family-environment risk factors for attention-deficit hyperactivity disorder: A test of Rutter's indicators of adversity. *Archives of General Psychiatry, 52,* 464–470.

Biederman, J., Milberger, S., Faraone, S. V., Kiely, K., Guite, J., Mick, E., Ablon, J. S., Warburton, R., Reed, E., & Davis, S. G. (1995). Impact of adversity on functioning and comorbidity in children with Attention-Deficit Hyperactivity Disorder. *Journal of the American Academy of Child and Adolescent Psychiatry, 34,* 1495–1503.

Biederman, J., Faraone, S., Milberger, S., Guite, J., Mick, J., Chen, L., Mennin, D., Marrs, A., Ouellette, C., Moore, P., Spencer, T., Norman, D., Wilens, T., Kraus, I., & Perrin, J. (1996). A prospective 4-year follow-up study of Attention-Deficit Hyperactivity and related disorders. *Archives of General Psychiatry, 53,* 437–446.

Borden, K. A., & Brown, R. T. (1989). Attributional outcomes: The subtle messages of treatments for attention deficit disorder. *Cognitive Therapy and Research, 13,* 147–160.

Brown, R. T., & Pacini, J. N. (1989). Perceived family functioning, marital status, and depression in parents of boys with attention deficit disorder. *Journal of Learning Disabilities, 22,* 581–587.

Bugental, D. B., Blue, J., & Cruzcosa, M. (1989). Perceived control over caregiving outcomes: Implications for child abuse. *Developmental Psychology, 25,* 532–539.

Bugental, D. B., Blue, J., & Lewis, J. (1990). Caregiver beliefs and dysphoric affect directed to difficult children. *Developmental Psychology, 26,* 631–638.

Campbell, S. B. (1994). Hard-to-manage preschool boys: Externalizing behavior, social competence, and family context at two-year followup. *Journal of Abnormal Child Psychology, 22,* 147–166.

Campbell, S. B. (1995). Behavior problems in preschool children: A review of recent research. *Journal of Child Psychology and Psychiatry, 36,* 113–149.

Campbell, S. B. (1997). Behavior problems in preschool children: Developmental and family issues. In T. H. Ollendick & R. J. Prinz (Eds.), *Advances in clinical child psychology* (Vol. 19, pp. 1–26). New York: Plenum.

Campbell, S. B., Breaux, A. M., Ewing, L. J., Szumowski, E. K., & Pierce, E. W. (1986). Parent-identified problem preschoolers: Mother–child interaction during play at intake and 1-year follow-up. *Journal of Abnormal Child Psychology, 14,* 425–440.

Campbell, S. B., March, C., Pierce, E., Ewing, L. J., & Szumowski, E. K. (1991). Hard-to-manage preschool boys: Family context and stability of externalizing behavior. *Journal of Abnormal Child Psychology, 19,* 301–318.

Campbell, S. B., Cohn, J. F., & Meyers, T. (1995). Depression in first-time mothers: Mother–infant interaction and depression chronicity. *Developmental Psychology, 31,* 349–357.

Campbell, S. B., Pierce, E. W., Moore, G., Marakovitz, S., & Newby, K. (1996). Boys' externalizing problems at elementary school age: Pathways from early behavior problems, maternal control, and family stress. *Development and Psychopathology, 8,* 701–719.

Carlson, E. A., Jacobvitz, D., & Sroufe, L. A. (1995). A developmental investigation of inattentiveness and hyperactivity. *Child Development, 66,* 37–54.

Coie, J. D., & Dodge, K. A. (1998). The development of aggression and antisocial behavior. In W. Damon & N. Eisenberg (Eds.), *Handbook of child psychology* (5th ed.): *Vol. 3. Social, emotional and personality development* (pp. 779–861). New York: Wiley.

Conrad, M., & Hammen, C. (1989). Role of maternal depression in perceptions of child maladjustment. *Journal of Consulting and Clinical Psychology, 57,* 663–667.

Crick, N. R., & Dodge, K. A. (1994). A review and reformation of social information-processing mechanisms in children's social adjustment. *Psychological Bulletin, 115,* 74–101.

Cunningham, C. E., & Barkley, R. A. (1979). The interactions of normal and hyperactive children with their mothers in free play and structured tasks. *Child Development, 50,* 217–224.

Cunningham, C. E., Benness, B. B., & Siegel, L. S. (1988). Family functioning, time allocation, and parental depression in the families of normal and ADDH children. *Journal of Clinical Child Psychology, 17,* 169–177.

Dix, T. H., Ruble, D. N., Grusec, J. E., & Nixon, S. (1986). Social cognition in parents: Inferential and affective reactions to children of three age levels. *Child Development, 57,* 879–894.

Edelbrock, C., Rende, R., Plomin, R., & Thompson, L. A. (1995). A twin study of competence and problem behavior in childhood and early adolescence. *Journal of Child Psychology and Psychiatry, 36,* 775–785.

Edwards, M. C., Schulz, E. G., & Long, N. (1995). The role of the family in the assessment of attention deficit hyperactivity disorder. *Clinical Psychology Review, 15,* 375–394.

Erel, O., & Burman, B. (1995). Interrelatedness of marital relations and parent–child relations: A meta-analytic review. *Psychological Bulletin, 118,* 108–132.

Fagot, B., & Leve, L. (1998). Teacher ratings of externalizing behavior at school entry for boys and girls: Similar early predictors and different correlates. *Journal of Child Psychology and Psychiatry, 39,* 555–566.

Faraone, S. V., Biederman, J., Lehman, B. K., Spencer, T., Norman, D., Seidman, L. J., Kraus, I., Perrin, J.,

Chen, W. J., & Tsuang, M. T. (1993). Intellectual performance and school failure in children with attention deficit hyperactivity disorder and in their siblings. *Journal of Abnormal Psychology, 102,* 616–623.

Faraone, S. V., Biederman, J., Chen, W. J., Milberger, S., Warburton, R., & Tsuang, M. T. (1995). Genetic heterogeneity in Attention-Deficit Hyperactivity Disorder (ADHD): Gender, psychiatric comorbidity, and maternal ADHD. *Journal of Abnormal Psychology, 104,* 334–345.

Feehan, M., McGee, R., & Williams, S. M. (1993). Mental health disorders from age 15 to age 18 years. *Journal of the American Academy of Child and Adolescent Psychiatry, 32,* 1118–1126.

Fischer, M. (1990). Parenting stress and the child with attention deficit hyperactivity disorder. *Journal of Clinical Child Psychology, 19,* 337–346.

Fletcher, K. E., Fischer, M., Barkley, R. A., & Smallish, L. (1996). A sequential analysis of the mother–adolescent interactions of ADHD, ADHD/ODD, and normal teenagers during neutral and conflict discussions. *Journal of Abnormal Child Psychology, 24,* 271–297.

Freeman, W. S., Johnston, C., & Barth, F. M. (1997). Parent attributions for inattentive-overactive, oppositional-defiant, and prosocial behaviours in children with attention deficit hyperactivity disorder. *Canadian Journal of Behavioural Science, 29,* 239–248.

Frick, P. J. (1994). Family dysfunction and the disruptive disorders: A review of recent empirical findings. In T. H. Ollendick & R. J. Prinz (Eds.), *Advances in clinical child psychology* (Vol. 16, pp. 203–226). New York: Plenum.

Frick, P. J., Lahey, B. B., Christ, M. A. G., Loeber, R., & Green, S. (1991). History of childhood behavior problems in biological relatives of boys with attention-deficit hyperactivity disorder and conduct disorder. *Journal of Clinical Child Psychology, 20,* 445–451.

Gelfand, D. M., & Teti, D. M. (1990). The effects of maternal depression on children. *Clinical Psychology Review, 10,* 329–353.

Geller, J., & Johnston, C. (1995). Predictors of mothers' responses to child noncompliance: Attributions and attitudes. *Journal of Clinical Child Psychology, 24,* 272–278.

Gillis, J. J., Gilger, J. W., Pennington, B. F., & DeFries, J. C. (1992). Attention deficit disorder in reading-disabled twins: Evidence for a genetic etiology. *Journal of Abnormal Child Psychology, 20,* 303–315.

Gjone, H., Stevenson, J., & Sundet, J. M. (1996). Genetic influence on parent-reported attention-related problems in a Norwegian general population twin sample. *Journal of the American Academy of Child and Adolescent Psychiatry, 35,* 588–596.

Goodman, R., & Stevenson, J. (1989). A twin study of hyperactivity—II. The aetiological role of genes, family relationships and perinatal adversity. *Journal of Child Psychology and Psychiatry, 30,* 691–709.

Gretarsson, S. J., & Gelfand, D. M. (1988). Mothers' attributions regarding their children's social behavior and personality characteristics. *Developmental Psychology, 24, 264–269.*

Hechtman, L. (1996). Families of children with attention deficit hyperactivity disorder: A review. *Canadian Journal of Psychiatry, 41, 350–360.*

Heller, T. L., Baker, B. L., Henker, B., & Hinshaw, S. P. (1996). Externalizing behavior and cognitive functioning from preschool to first grade: Stability and predictors. *Journal of Clinical Child Psychology, 25,* 376–387.

Henker, B., Whalen, C. K., Carter, M. J., Garland, K., & Heller, T. (1996, January). *Explaining positive and negative behaviors: Causal attributions generated by parents of ADHD vs nonADHD boys.* Poster presented at the meeting of the International Society for Research in Child and Adolescent Psychopathology, Santa Monica, CA.

Humphries, T., Kinsbourne, M., & Swanson, J. (1978). Stimulant effects on cooperation and social interaction between hyperactive children and their mothers. *Journal of Child Psychology and Psychiatry, 19,* 13–22.

Johnston, C. (1996). Parent characteristics and parent–child interactions in families of nonproblem children and ADHD children with higher and lower levels of oppositional-defiant behavior. *Journal of Abnormal Child Psychology, 24,* 85–104.

Johnston, C., & Freeman, W. (1997). Attributions for child behavior in parents of children without behavior disorders and children with attention deficit–hyperactivity disorder. *Journal of Consulting and Clinical Psychology, 65,* 636–645.

Johnston, C., & Patensude, R. (1994). Parent attributions for inattentive-overactive and oppositional-defiant child behaviors. *Cognitive Therapy and Research, 18,* 261–275.

Jones, E. E., & Davis, K. E. (1965). From acts to dispositions: The attribution process in person perception. In L. Berkowitz (Ed.), *Advances in experimental social psychology* (Vol. 2, pp. 219–226). New York: Academic Press.

Lahey, B. B., Piacentini, J. C., McBurnett, K., Stone, P., Hartdagen, S. E., & Hynd, G. (1988). Psychopathology and antisocial behavior in the parents of children with conduct disorder and hyperactivity. *Journal of the American Academy of Child and Adolescent Psychiatry, 27,* 163–170.

Loeber, R., & Hay, D. (1997). Key issues in the development of aggression and violence from childhood to early adulthood. *Annual Review of Psychology, 48,* 371–410.

Loeber, R., Brinthaupt, V. P., & Green, S. M. (1990). Attention deficits, impulsivity, and hyperactivity with or without conduct problems: Relationships to delinquency and unique contextual factors. In R. J. McMahon & R. DeV. Peters (Eds.), *Behavior disorders of adolescence: Research, intervention, and policy in clinical and school settings* (pp. 39–61). New York: Plenum.

Mash, E. J., & Johnston, C. (1982). A comparison of the mother–child interactions of younger and older hyperactive and normal children. *Child Development, 53,* 1371–1381.

Mash, E. J., & Johnston, C. (1983a). Parental perceptions of child behavior problems, parenting self-esteem, and mothers' reported stress in younger and older hyperactive and normal children. *Journal of Consulting and Clinical Psychology, 51,* 86–99.

Mash, E. J., & Johnston, C. (1983b). Sibling interactions of hyperactive and normal children and their relationship to reports of maternal stress and self-esteem. *Journal of Clinical Child Psychology, 12,* 91–99.

McGee, R., Feehan, M., Williams, S., Partridge, F., Silva, P. A., & Kelly, J. (1990). DSM-III disorders in a large sample of adolescents. *Journal of the American Academy of Child and Adolescent Psychiatry, 29,* 611–619.

Miller, S. A. (1995). Parents' attributions for their children's behavior. *Child Development, 66,* 1557–1584.

Moffitt, T. E. (1990). Juvenile delinquency and attention deficit disorder: Boys' developmental trajectories from age 3 to age 15. *Child Development, 61,* 893–910.

Nigg, J. T., & Hinshaw, S. P. (1998). Parent personality traits and psychopathology associated with antisocial behaviors in childhood attention-deficit hyperactivity disorder. *Journal of Child Psychology and Psychiatry, 39,* 145–159.

Nolen-Hoeksema, S., Wolfson, A., Mumme, D., & Guskin, K. (1995). Helplessness in children of depressed and nondepressed mothers. *Developmental Psychology, 31,* 377–387.

Offord, D. R., Boyle, M. H., & Racine, Y. (1989). Ontario Child Health Study: Correlates of disorder. *Journal of the American Academy of Child and Adolescent Psychiatry, 28,* 856–860.

Offord, D. R., Boyle, M. H., Racine, Y. A., Fleming, J. E., Cadman, D. T., Blum, H. M., Byrne, C., Links, P. S., Lipman, E. L., and Macmillan, H. L. (1992). Outcome, prognosis and risk in a longitudinal follow-up study. *Journal of the American Academy of Child and Adolescent Psychiatry, 31,* 916–923.

Parke, R. D. (1995). Fathers and families. In M. H. Bornstein (Ed.), *Handbook of parenting* (Vol. 3, pp. 27–63). Hillsdale, NJ: Erlbaum.

Phares, V., & Compas, B. E. (1992). The role of fathers in child and adolescent psychopathology: Make room for Daddy. *Psychological Bulletin, 111,* 387–412.

Prinz, R. J., Myers, deR., Holden, E. W., Tarnowski, K. J., & Roberts, W. A. (1983). Marital disturbance and child problems: A cautionary note regarding hyperactive children. *Journal of Abnormal Child Psychology, 11,* 393–399.

Richters, J. (1992). Depressed mothers as informants about their children: A critical review of the evidence for distortion. *Psychological Bulletin, 112,* 485–499.

Rutter, M. (1979). Protective factors in children's responses to stress and disadvantage. *Annals of the Academy of Medicine, 8,* 324–338.

Rutter, M. (1989). Isle of Wight revisited: Twenty-five years of child psychiatric epidemiology. *Journal of the American Academy of Child and Adolescent Psychiatry, 28,* 633–653.

Sandberg, S. T., Wieselberg, M., & Shaffer, D. (1980). Hyperkinetic and conduct problem children in a primary school population: Some epidemiological considerations. *Journal of Child Psychology and Psychiatry, 21,* 293–311.

Schachar, R. (1991). Childhood hyperactivity. *Journal of Child Psychology and Psychiatry, 32,* 155–191.

Simons, R. L., Lorenz, F. O., Wu, C., & Conger, R. D. (1993). Social network and marital support as mediators and moderators of the impact of stress and depression on parental behavior. *Developmental Psychology, 29,* 368–381.

Smith, A. M., & O'Leary, S. G. (1995). Attributions and arousal as predictors of maternal discipline. *Cognitive Therapy and Research, 19,* 459–471.

Stormont-Spurgin, M., & Zentall, S. S. (1995). Contributing factors in the manifestation of aggression in preschoolers with hyperactivity. *Journal of Child Psychology and Psychiatry, 36,* 491–509.

Szatmari, P., Offord, D. R., & Boyle, M. H. (1989). Correlates, associated impairments and patterns of service utilization of children with attention deficit disorder: Findings from the Ontario Child Health Study. *Journal of Child Psychology and Psychiatry, 30,* 205–217.

Tannenbaum, L., & Forehand, R. (1994). Maternal depressive mood: The role of the father in preventing adolescent problem behaviors. *Behavior Research and Therapy, 32,* 321–325.

Tarullo, L. B., DeMulder, E. K., Ronsaville, D. S., Brown, E., & Radke-Yarrow, M. (1995). Maternal depression and maternal treatment of siblings as predictors of child psychopathology. *Developmental Psychology, 31,* 395–405.

Walker, L. S., Garber, J., & Van Slyke, D. A. (1995). Do parents excuse the misbehavior of children with physical or emotional symptoms? An investigation of the pediatric sick role. *Journal of Pediatric Psychology, 20,* 329–345.

Weiss, G., & Hechtman, L. T. (1993). *Hyperactive children grown up. ADHD in children, adolescents, and adults* (2nd ed.). New York: Guilford.

Westerman, M. A., & Schonholtz, J. (1993). Marital adjustment, joint parental support in a triadic problem-solving task, and child behavior problems. *Journal of Clinical Child Psychology, 22,* 97–106.

Whalen, C. K., & Henker B. (1976). Psychostimulants and children: A review and analysis. *Psychological Bulletin, 83,* 1113–1130.

Whalen, C. K., & Henker, B. (1992). The social profile of attention-deficit hyperactivity disorder: Five fundamental facets. *Child and Adolescent Psychiatric Clinics of North America, 1,* 395–410.

Whalen, C. K., & Henker, B. (1997). Stimulant pharmacotherapy for attention deficit/hyperactivity disorders: An analysis of progress, problems, and prospects. In S. Fisher & R. Greenberg (Eds.), *From placebo to panacea: Putting psychiatric drugs to the test* (pp. 323–355). New York: Wiley.

Whalen, C. K., & Henker, B. (1998). Attention-deficit/hyperactivity disorders. In T. H. Ollendick & M. Hersen (Eds.), *Handbook of child psychopathology* (3rd ed., pp. 181–211). New York: Plenum.

Zahn-Waxler, C., Schmitz, S., Fulker, D., Robinson, J., & Emde, R. (1996). Behavior problems in 5-year-old monozygotic and dizygotic twins: Genetic and environmental influences, patterns of regulation, and internalization of control. *Development and Psychopathology, 8,* 103–122.

7

The Child with Attention-Deficit/ Hyperactivity Disorder in School and Peer Settings

BARBARA HENKER and CAROL K. WHALEN

INTRODUCTION

Many children with Attention-Deficit/Hyperactivity Disorder (ADHD) are salient stimuli on the social landscape. They engage in high rates of behaviors that are unexpected, inappropriate, immature, and generally devalued by others. Their intentions may be sound, but their implementations often clash with the setting, the social script, or other people's activities. Even though interpersonal dysfunction is rarely listed as a core symptom or defining characteristic of ADHD, there is no question that most of these youngsters experience serious problems negotiating their social worlds (Gaub & Carlson, 1997a; Whalen & Henker, 1992). It is almost as though they have failed to master a critical developmental task, one that involves synchronizing one's own actions and manner with the ongoing flow of social commerce. There is increasing recognition of the critical role of social dysfunction in children with ADHD and speculation that deficits

BARBARA HENKER • Department of Psychology, University of California, Los Angeles, Los Angeles, California 90095-1563. CAROL K. WHALEN • Department of Psychology and Social Behavior, University of California, Irvine, Irvine, California 92697-7085.

Handbook of Disruptive Behavior Disorders, edited by Quay and Hogan. Kluwer Academic/Plenum Publishers, New York, 1999.

in this domain may persist into adulthood, contributing in diverse ways to the continued interpersonal and occupational difficulties experienced by many individuals with ADHD (see Chapter 12, this volume).

In this chapter we consider how children with ADHD function in peer and school settings. As a reflection of the state of the field, this account may appear more speculative than other chapters in this handbook. There is an extensive theoretical and empirical literature on children's social development, but our understanding of the social worlds of children with ADHD remains sketchy. Symptoms of interpersonal dysfunction can be listed and counted, as they often are in teacher and parent rating scales. But the true nature of the social problems confronted by and with ADHD children continues to elude practitioners and researchers alike. Perhaps one reason for this circumscribed understanding is that these problems are transactional in nature, embedded in and influencing the social ecology. Contextual processes are not only difficult to study but also easily overlooked when the focus is on enumerating psychiatric symptoms that are viewed as residing in the child.

The literature on peer and school patterns that is sampled in this chapter is characterized by methodological heterogeneity. Most studies center on middle childhood, but others involve the preschool or adolescent years. A substantial proportion of the database stems from teacher or parent sources, but information has also been obtained from peers as well as from direct observations in natural and experimental settings. Some studies focus on clinically referred groups, whereas others examine epidemiological samples. Youngsters drawn from clinic referrals are likely to have more serious disturbances and higher rates of comorbid disorders than are those drawn from community studies. There is also a greater gender disparity (male preponderance) in referred samples, perhaps because males are more likely to exhibit disruptive behaviors that require intervention. Given these differences in diagnoses and severity, it can be expected that the quality and extent of social dysfunction differ as well. Referral biases, source factors, and developmental differences all influence research findings in largely unknown ways. Thus, integrating the diverse literatures is always somewhat hazardous, and the propositions presented in this chapter should be considered more heuristic than conclusive.

We begin with a look at profiles of social dysfunction in children with ADHD and then delineate some of the processes that might help account for these problems. The next section considers consequences of social dysfunction, immediate as well as longer term. Because of the relative neglect of girls with ADHD, we include a section on possible gender differences in development and characteristics. The final sections focus on school settings, learning environments, and academic achievement.

PROFILES OF SOCIAL DYSFUNCTION IN CHILDREN WITH ADHD

Clinical observation and systematic research demonstrate that the vast majority of children with ADHD show one of three social behavior patterns. Although not yet empirically validated, these categories serve a heuristic function and also provide a convenient rubric for illustrating the heterogeneity of so-

cial patterns within ADHD. For ease of communication, we label these subtypes aggressive/assertive, active/maladroit, and reluctant/avoidant. The aggressive/assertive children are oppositional with adults and contentious or disruptive with peers. They seem to be "doing their own thing" rather than what they are asked to do, what others are doing, or what the situation suggests. If they want something, they may take it without appearing to consider the context or consequences. Their needs and desires are prepotent and their energies directed toward satisfying them. In these pursuits, they often interfere with other people and violate social norms. These are the youngsters most likely to receive dual diagnoses of ADHD and either oppositional defiant disorder (ODD) or conduct disorder (CD).

The second subgroup, active/maladroit, are distinguished by their social busyness and their vigorous pursuit of interpersonal contact. Even though they seem to seek and enjoy other people, harmonious and mutually satisfying relations elude these youngsters. Often inadvertently, their acts interrupt ongoing activities, frustrate the goals of others, and impair the affective tone of social exchange. Their initiations may be ill timed, inept, or inappropriate to the situation. A socially competent child seeking to join a peer group activity is likely to observe the action for a while, select the opportune moment and mode of entry, and then approach somewhat tentatively, being careful to follow the flow and read the reactions of others. In contrast, a child with ADHD may barge right in and attempt to redirect the activity or rewrite the rules, apparently oblivious to the desires or behaviors of others. The short-term result is often conflict and confrontation. The longer-term result tends to be peer rejection and exclusion.

Even though the appearance and consequences of their behavior may be similar to those of the aggressive/assertive group, the flavor of their social encounters differs. These youngsters seem directed toward active social engagement rather than toward getting their way. An intensive, impulsive, and at times overzealous response style may prevent them from processing subtle social cues and enacting appropriate social scripts. They often seem puzzled and even saddened when their social efforts meet with disfavor.

The third subgroup, labeled reluctant/avoidant, shows a markedly different response profile. They are more likely to be outliers and onlookers than active participants, neither seeking nor seeming to enjoy peer contact. Many of these youngsters meet criteria for the *Diagnostic and Statistical Manual of Mental Disorders* (DSM-IV; American Psychiatric Association, 1994) predominantly inattentive (IA) subtype of ADHD and are likely to have internalizing problems as well, especially signs of social anxiety, shyness, and withdrawal. In the language of peer sociometrics, these youngsters are more likely to be neglected than actively rejected. There are some indications that girls diagnosed with ADHD may be especially likely to fit this profile.

These forms of social dysfunction merit research attention because they suggest distinctive developmental pathways and heterogeneous etiological influences. Perhaps most important, careful delineation of social behavior profiles should help guide therapeutic programs with the goal of matching treatments to individuals in order to optimize long-term outcomes. The goal of this chapter is not to validate subtypes or map comorbidities, but it is noteworthy that a recent review of ADHD patterns resulted in a recommendation that two of the three profiles delineated here be added as ADHD subtypes in DSM-V: ADHD, aggressive subtype, and ADHD, anxious subtype (Jensen, Martin, & Cantwell, 1997).

PROCESSES ASSOCIATED WITH SOCIAL DYSFUNCTION

The "what" of social dysfunction is much better understood than the "how" and the "why." The extent to which social problems result from limitations of ability versus application remains unknown. And within the application domain, questions continue about the degree of intentionality and the relative contributions of affect, motivation, and cognition to the social behavior of children with ADHD. In this section we discuss some mechanisms that may underlie social dysfunction in these youngsters.

Social Information-Processing Deficits

Even very young children have a wealth of knowledge about the social scene. They readily learn what they can and cannot, should and should not do; who is supposed to do what to whom; and how the rules of engagement vary across social contexts. Effective and harmonious social transactions require complex skills including cue utilization, situation–behavior matching, perspective taking, script mastery, response modulation, and outcome evaluation. Because children with ADHD have such serious problems getting along with others, it is often assumed that they have social information-processing deficiencies and perhaps, more generally, social learning disabilities that are analogous to reading or mathematical disabilities (Greene *et al.*, 1996). Social information-processing problems have been documented repeatedly in overly aggressive boys (Coie & Dodge, 1997), but the findings are far less compelling regarding ADHD per se. Boys with ADHD appear to be competent at identifying and evaluating social behaviors (Whalen, Henker, & Granger, 1990) and there is scattered evidence that, on occasion, they may even be more socially perspicacious than their peers (Whalen & Henker, 1985). Their knowledge of social scripts seems to be intact, but they often have difficulties enacting these scripts, perhaps because of lack of interest, overarousal, or heightened challenge.

One potentially important aspect of social information processing is causal reasoning—how children explain why things happen to and around them. In a study comparing causal attributions in boys with ADHD and their nondiagnosed peers, Hoza, Pelham, Milich, Pillow, and McBride (1993) found that the ADHD group were more likely to take responsibility for social successes and less likely to take responsibility for social failures. The clinical importance of this pattern is suggested by previous studies demonstrating links between perceived personal responsibility and helplessness versus mastery-oriented approaches to challenging tasks (Dweck & Leggett, 1988). Additional studies by Milich and colleagues, however, remind us of the pitfalls of drawing conclusions about ADHD from studies with nonproblem children. Milich (1994) reported that, whereas nondiagnosed children who attribute failure to a lack of effort are more likely than their peers to show a mastery orientation to problem solving, children with ADHD seem to show the opposite pattern, that is, more mastery behavior when they externalize rather than internalize their failures.

Differing Social Goals, Agendas, and Motivations

Research on children's social development points toward the importance of children's social goals and their abilities to balance conflicting agendas (Renshaw & Asher, 1983). We previously suggested that children with ADHD may have nonnormative social goals and agendas, as illustrated by a series of studies of sociometric choices made by boys with ADHD, nondiagnosed age-mates, and teachers (Whalen & Henker, 1985, 1992). When asked to identify children on the basis of specific characteristics such as "good student" or "causes trouble," the responses of children with ADHD were similar to those of their peers. But when asked to select classmates who were "fun to be with," the responses of these two groups diverged. Boys in the comparison group did not express liking for peers perceived as causing trouble; ratings of these two dimensions were inversely correlated. For the ADHD group, however, perceptions of troublemaking did not rule out liking; these two dimensions proved unrelated. Interestingly, teacher nominations were highly congruent with those of both the ADHD and the nondiagnosed groups for all categories except one: "fun to be with." In this instance teacher nominations more closely paralleled those of the control children than those of the ADHD group.

These peer preference patterns suggest that children with ADHD may be distinguished by differing social goals or agendas; they seem to have a greater tolerance or even enjoyment of deviant behavior. The hypothesis that children with ADHD are more oriented toward fun seeking and troublemaking, whereas nondiagnosed peers focus more on cooperation and rule following, was recently supported, for the aggressive subgroup, in an intriguing study of social goals by Melnick and Hinshaw (1996). Links were also demonstrated between these social goals and peer status, suggesting the potential value of including social agendas and goal hierarchies as treatment targets in behavior change programs, at least for children who show ADHD combined with aggression.

Modulation of Behavior and Affect

Although children with ADHD may have age-appropriate social knowledge and skills, many seem to have difficulty modulating their actions in accordance with changing settings and cues (Whalen & Henker, 1992). In some instances it may be their intense style of responding that annoys or interferes with other people; these youngsters may approach in a manner that is too intrusive, forceful, vigorous, or loud. In other instances, they fail to change roles when the situation requires such shifts. Two studies of structured interaction have demonstrated that role shifts are major challenges for many children with ADHD, whether the required shift is from leader to follower (Whalen, Henker, Collins, McAuliffe, & Vaux, 1979) or from talk show guest to host (Landau & Milich, 1988).

Whether glad, mad, or sad, many children with ADHD show high levels of affective arousal and expression. There are some indications from self-report measures that children with ADHD are more prone to anger, or perhaps more willing to acknowledge angry feelings (Whalen & Henker, 1991). Children who are emotionally reactive would be expected to have difficulties with self-regulation, and both dimensions have been linked to externalizing behavior problems (Eisenberg et al., 1996). In one recent observational study of response to frustration, high emotional reactivity and poor emotion regulation were strongly associated with each other and each also correlated with low peer standing in boys with ADHD (Hinshaw & Melnick, 1995). Sensation seeking has also been linked to ADHD, and there are suggestions that these children may have more difficulty than others their age maintaining optimal levels of arousal (MacDonald, 1988). Such difficulties regulating affect and arousal could result in both high rates of discord and in escalation rather than containment once conflict emerges. Despite the importance of these response domains for social development (see Crick & Dodge, 1994), affect expression and regulation remain understudied areas for children with ADHD. Of particular interest is the extent to which problems relate specifically to negative emotionality or more generally to the intensity, expressivity, and regulation of affect and arousal whether positive or negative.

CONSEQUENCES OF SOCIAL DYSFUNCTION

Peer Neglect and Rejection

Children with ADHD are generally less liked and more disliked than other youngsters, and they are more apt to be ignored or actively rejected by their peers (Gaub & Carlson, 1997a). Negative peer status is a critical dimension not only because of its associations with loneliness, low self-esteem, and restricted learning opportunities, but also because it predicts serious long-term difficulties with adjustment and achievement (Parker & Asher, 1987). There are multiple pathways to peer dislike and rejection. Aggression often plays a pivotal role, but it is neither a necessary nor a sufficient condition for social disapproval. In combination with ADHD, however, aggression appears to be a powerful predictor of peer rejection. Nonaggressive children with ADHD are also likely to suffer peer disfavor, perhaps as a function of social withdrawal and awkwardness (Hinshaw & Melnick, 1995).

The rapidity with which social disapproval can develop is remarkable; enduring negative appraisals often emerge after only a few minutes of observation or interaction (Buhrmester, Whalen, Henker, MacDonald, & Hinshaw, 1992; Erhardt & Hinshaw, 1994; Whalen, Henker, Castro, & Granger, 1987). Children with ADHD are often last to be selected as partners for school projects, seatmates for bus trips, or teammates for soccer games. Peers may worry that a child with ADHD will get them in trouble with parents or teachers by diverting them from assigned tasks or encouraging them to break rules and disobey instructions. As a group, children with ADHD have difficulty making friends and even more difficulty protecting and repairing friendships. Their parents often report, sadly, that the only friend their child has is a much younger child who lives down the block.

Despite a pervasive climate of neglect or rejection, some of the bold and illicit behavior of children with ADHD may capture the attention of their peers. Well-behaved children may be charmed by the misadventures of youngsters with ADHD. Inadvertently, such reactions can encourage misbehavior on the part of children with ADHD, who often find it difficult to obtain social approval through normative routes such as cooperative engagement, athletic pursuits, or academic achievement. The power of peer attention to maintain disruptive behavior in a child with ADHD was demonstrated recently by Northrup and colleagues (1997) in a classroom setting. Especially noteworthy in this study was that these reinforcing effects were found when the child was taking placebo but not when he was taking methylphenidate (MPH), which appeared to attenuate the reinforcing effects of peer attention.

Reputational Biases and Interpersonal Expectancy Effects

One of the most disappointing aspects of ADHD treatment programs is that changes in peer standing and friendship patterns lag far behind welcome improvements in externalizing behavior and task performance (Whalen &

Henker, 1997; Whalen *et al.,* 1989). There are many plausible reasons for this gap between behavior and peer appeal, including the strong possibility that subtle behavioral deficits or idiosyncrasies remain after the more obvious problems remit. Children with ADHD may learn to constrain their aggressive impulses; cooperate with others and wait their turn; respond in an age-appropriate rather than a silly, immature fashion; attend to the flow of social exchange; and shift behavior as they shift settings. But the fine points of social transactions may continue to elude them. They may acquire the appropriate phrases but say them in the wrong manner, with the wrong affect, or at the wrong time. They may learn not to intrude or interrupt but still be unable to engage in a reciprocal conversation. They may learn not to retaliate when provoked but remain unable to repair the breach left by a disagreement or confrontation. They may learn to enact basic social scripts but remain oblivious to more subtle cues that signal constraint or fine tuning. Social nuances are difficult to teach and also to measure, and thus there may be continuing but undetected difficulties in these elusive realms.

Another likely cause for the intractability of peer status problems is the potent influence of past experience and future expectation. School-age children can be unforgiving. Hymel (1986) demonstrated that children interpret identical actions in different ways, depending on their liking of the actor. They tend to credit liked peers for positive behavior and make excuses rather than blame them for negative behavior. In contrast, children tend not to give the benefit of the doubt to disliked peers who transgress, and they view positive behavior as stemming from unstable causes that are unlikely to recur. Thus, rather than change their evaluations and expectancies when they notice behavioral improvements, peers may reinterpret the causes of these behaviors in a direction consistent with a disliked child's prior reputation.

Such expectancy biases may extend beyond an individual's personal experience. People respond to strangers on the basis of preexisting beliefs; a diagnostic label or descriptive phrase can influence actual behavior as well as attitudes and attributions. Such interpersonal expectancies can result in self-fulfilling prophecies when a person responds to a labeled other in ways that encourage the other to engage in the behavior and misbehavior connoted by that label. Ever since Rosenthal and Jacobson's (1968) seminal (and controversial) study, "Pygmalion in the classroom," there has been active research interest in such interpersonal expectancy effects.

Most of the relevant work has focused on adult-to-child effects. Harris, Milich, and colleagues addressed the question of whether such effects occur when children are on both sides of the equation—the perceiver and the target (Harris, Milich, Johnston, & Hoover, 1990). When they led school-age boys who were randomly assigned to the perceiver role to think that an unfamiliar "target" boy with whom they were about to interact displayed the disruptive behavior associated with ADHD, there were salient effects on the behavior of perceivers as well as targets. The perceivers who received the ADHD expectancy were less friendly, less talkative, and less involved in the interaction than were perceivers who were given a neutral expectancy consisting only of their partner's name and grade. There was also substantially more reciprocity in the interactions of dyads who received the neutral versus the ADHD expectancy, as indexed by the strength of the associations between the behaviors of the two partners. When a similar study was conducted using boys with ADHD as well as nondiagnosed peers, these investigators found that both the perceivers' ADHD expectancy and the diagnostic status of the target had adverse affects on actual interactions (Harris, Milich, Corbitt, Hoover, & Brady, 1992). These findings remind us that including ADHD as a handicapping condition eligible for special educational services can be a double-edged sword to the extent that it stigmatizes those very children selected for assistance (Milich, McAninch, & Harris, 1992).

Isolation and Restricted Social Learning Opportunities

Lack of connectedness with the peer group and the attendant isolation severely circumscribe social learning experiences. Children who are rejected by peers are excluded from opportunities to observe socially competent exchanges, practice problem-solving routines, and hone social skills. They have restricted access to the natural classrooms provided by peer cultures, and the effects may be apparent in terms of both initial skill acquisition and corrective learning experiences. Truncated learning opportunities can be especially detrimental to children with ADHD, because many of these youngsters may have a deficit in social attention that is analogous to their task-attention problems in the classroom (Buitelaar, Swinkels, de Vries, van der Gaag, & van Hooff, 1994). They seem to spend less time watching other children than do their peers (Cunningham, Siegel, & Offord, 1985) and may be less likely to benefit from nonparticipant observation of social exchange.

Fragile Friendships and Lack of Intimacy

The bulk of the research evidence concerns negative social behaviors—those considered aggressive, disruptive, or noncompliant. These are the behaviors that demand attention and control if tasks are to be completed, learning is to be accomplished, and social harmony is to be maintained. These are also the behaviors that are most responsive to treatment, especially to stimulants (Whalen & Henker, 1991, 1997; see also Chapter 10, this volume). But there are important aspects of our social worlds that have not received sufficient empirical attention. How do children learn the meaning of friendship and master the stages of friendship building? How do they learn to adapt and to protect relationships while negotiating the unpredictable and often bumpy terrain of everyday life? How do they regulate affect and balance multiple performance and social goals? How do they learn empathy, caring, trust, and other intimacy skills?

The few studies of prosocial behavior in children with ADHD have not demonstrated distinctive deficits in these domains (Buhrmester et al., 1992). But the empirical literature is still sketchy, most likely because the positive aspects of social relationships are often subtle and difficult to measure. As discussed in preceding sections, when children with ADHD are treated successfully in the sense that disruption, noncompliance, and aggression diminish, their peer standing may not improve commensurately. We also know that adults with ADHD continue to have rocky relationships even after their most salient behavior problems have diminished (Weiss & Hechtman, 1993; Wender, 1995; see also Chapter 12, this volume). One possible reason for these residual problems is a deficiency in the acquisition or performance of complex and satisfying prosocial skills such as those involved in support, companionship, and intimacy.

Social Catalytic Effects

Several studies have demonstrated that the behavior of children with ADHD can have negative catalytic effects on the social environment. Whether in classrooms, playgrounds, or homes, the level of disharmony often rises in the presence of a child with ADHD. Other children engage in elevated rates of disruptive behavior when working or playing with a child with ADHD. Peers tend to show lower levels of responsivity, reciprocity, cooperation, and communicative efficiency and higher levels of control or disengagement when their partners are children with ADHD in contrast to nondiagnosed age-mates (Clark, Cheyne, Cunningham, & Siegel, 1988; Cunningham & Siegel, 1987; Landau & Milich, 1988; Madan-Swain & Zentall, 1990). Granger, Whalen, Henker, and Cantwell (1996) demonstrated that negative effects on the behavior of nondiagnosed peers may be most likely to occur when the setting requires mutual problem solving and interdependent goal attainment. Undesirable peer behaviors may result from modeling and disinhibition, or they may represent compensatory attempts on the part of nondiagnosed children to achieve their goals, regulate their affect, and maintain their status. Also noteworthy is the fact that teachers and parents tend to be more negative and controlling toward or in the presence of children with ADHD (Campbell, Breaux, Ewing, Szumowski, & Pierce, 1986; Cunningham & Barkley, 1979; Mash & Johnston, 1982; Whalen, Henker, & Dotemoto, 1980, 1981). These reactions from significant others, whether children or adults, can prompt a cycle of spiraling social cacophony.

There is also a positive side to this behavioral reciprocity. When children with ADHD receive stimulants and their behavior improves, the actions of others also change in positive directions. Teachers and parents make fewer controlling and corrective responses, mothers increase in warmth and engagement, and peers reduce their rates of negative and controlling acts (Barkley, 1989; Cunningham, Siegel, & Offord, 1991; Schachar, Taylor, Wieselberg, Thorley, & Rutter, 1987; Whalen *et al.,* 1980, 1981). Cunningham and colleagues (1991) reported that, despite the fact that medication-related reductions in negative and controlling behavior emerged in children with ADHD as well as in their nondiagnosed peers, these reductions did not seem to be linked directly. This dissociation suggests that peers may be responding to improvements in other domains such as task orientation or to more subtle changes such as enhanced attention to social cues and conventions. The positive effects that medication can have on task orientation and attention outside the classroom were demonstrated by a study of baseball performance conducted by Pelham and colleagues (1990). Medication had no significant effects on basic skills such as batting and throwing, but boys with ADHD were better able to attend to the game and follow the action when taking MPH versus placebo. Athletics is a critically important social arena for school-age boys. Peers may be unforgiving when a child with ADHD misses the ball not because of skill deficits, but rather because he is making faces at people in the stands or

throwing his glove in the air rather than focusing on the batter.

Even when children with ADHD are appropriately medicated, however, their social transactions can be distinguished from those of their peers. Using a peer pairing strategy, Hubbard and Newcomb (1991) assigned nondiagnosed boys to either another nondiagnosed boy or a medicated ADHD boy. The mixed dyads showed more solitary play and less associative interaction, less verbal reciprocity, lower levels of affective expression, and less ability to repair disruptions. Because the dyad was the unit of analysis, it is not possible to disentangle the contributions of each partner, but previous studies suggest bidirectional effects. The paramount point here is that, despite the dramatic methylphenidate-related improvements documented in numerous studies, medication does not normalize peer relations.

Long-Term Outcomes and Adult ADHD

In many children with ADHD, peer problems persist for years (see Chapter 12, this volume). The potential predictive utility of social dysfunction was demonstrated in a 4-year follow-up study by Greene, Biederman, Faraone, Sienna, and Garcia-Jetton (1997), who found that boys diagnosed with ADHD plus social disabilities had elevated rates of comorbid disorders, especially substance use and conduct disorders, after baseline mood, attention, and conduct problems were controlled. ADHD also appears to place children at risk for educational and vocational disadvantage. As a group, they complete fewer years of schooling and change jobs more frequently than other adults, outcomes that may be attributable, in part, to difficulties getting along (Mannuzza, Klein, Bessler, Malloy, & Hynes, 1997). Interestingly, Mannuzza, Klein, Bessler, Malloy, and LaPadula (1993) reported that a disproportionate number of their ADHD probands (approximately 20%, compared to 5% of controls) owned and operated their own business, perhaps a reflection of "niche-picking" (Scarr & McCartney, 1983) that allows these formerly ADHD individuals to function in settings that minimize external structure, constraint, and oversight. Caution is indicated, however, because this finding was not replicated in a new sample (Mannuzza et al., 1997).

GIRLS WITH ADHD: AN UNDERSTUDIED SUBGROUP

One of the most robust findings about ADHD is that boys outnumber girls, often by four or five to one (Wolraich, Hannah, Pinnock, Baumgaertel, & Brown, 1996; see also Chapter 2, this volume). Because of the preponderance of males in any group of youngsters with ADHD, it is difficult to recruit a sufficient number of girls for any single-site study, and the vast majority of ADHD studies focus predominantly or exclusively on boys. Thus, many questions remain about the degree to which the vast and developing knowledge base for ADHD applies to girls. Studies are beginning to demonstrate some similarities between boys and girls with ADHD with respect to familial psychopathology, treatment responsiveness, and long-term outcomes (Whalen & Henker, 1998). Evidence of gender differences is also building, however, especially with respect to severity of externalizing problems, associated cognitive impairments, and the course and severity of comorbid disorders. In particular, girls with ADHD are generally less aggressive, disruptive, and hyperactive, and prevalence rates for comorbid ADHD+ ODD/CD are lower for girls than for boys (Bird, Gould, & Staghezza, 1993; Carlson, Tamm, & Gaub, 1997; Gaub & Carlson, 1997b; Jensen, Martin, & Cantwell, 1997).

By contrast, girls diagnosed with ADHD appear to have high rates of developmental immaturity, cognitive impairment, and associated learning difficulties. Because they tend not to disturb other people, these girls may be underrecognized and undertreated (McGee & Feehan, 1991; Wolraich et al., 1996). With the expanding use of DSM-IV (American Psychiatric Association, 1994), however, more girls may be identified because of the decoupling of inattention and impulsivity and the delineation of the "predominantly inattentive" subtype that does not include externalizing symptoms (Lahey et al., 1994). Noteworthy in this context is the fact that the marked male preponderance during childhood does not seem to characterize samples of adults with ADHD, a pattern consistent with the hypothesis that girls with ADHD may be underrepresented during childhood because their behaviors are less likely to disturb other people (Spencer, Biederman, Wilens, & Faraone, 1994).

Other girls with ADHD have externalizing symptoms analogous to those seen in boys. Keenan and Shaw (1997) integrated a large body of research on normal and atypical development into an intriguing perspective on sex differences in early problem behaviors. These authors presented evidence congenial with their hypothesis that parents (and, later, teachers and peers) engage in differential socialization of boys and girls during the earliest years of life, channeling girls' problem behaviors into internalizing domains. They also suggested that girls' more rapid maturation—especially the development of language, emotion regulation, and self-control—leads to adaptive coping skills and the emergence of prosocial behaviors that buffer them from both genetic and environmental risks. Thus, girls who do experience problems are likely to grow out of them quickly or to have them shaped into an internalized form. The minority of girls who develop more slowly than expected, showing delays in the acquisition of empathy, emotion regulation, and social problem solving, may be at special risk of developing externalizing disorders. Whereas slow or erratic development of adaptive, self-regulatory skills is often tolerated in boys, such delays violate parental and societal expectancies for girls. These girls do not respond as expected to socialization efforts, and they create unexpected challenges and special frustrations for parents. The result is likely to be conflictful interactions, ineffective socialization, and escalation of problem behaviors.

It is interesting to speculate that there is a third subgroup of girls with ADHD, those who show neither cognitive impairments nor severely aggressive behavior, but rather engage in behavior viewed by many as gender-inappropriate. In their longitudinal study of predictors of externalizing behavior from age 18 months to 5 years, Fagot and Leve (1998) found intriguing gender differences. Boys who were rated high on externalizing behavior by teachers showed many problems at home and in school. Girls rated high by teachers tended not to show these problems. Rather, these girls showed high intellectual performance, although they rated themselves as low on cognitive competence. Fagot and Leve suggested that this may be a subgroup of particularly bright girls who are excited by school and active and assertive in the classroom in a way that is viewed by teachers as gender-inappropriate. The low self-perceived competence may be a sign that these girls are already beginning to internalize the critical reactions of other people. They may "earn" their externalizing ratings through high rates of verbalization, active engagement, and bids for attention in the classroom rather than from aggression and oppositionality. These and other findings raise interesting questions about whether a subgroup of girls may be falsely diagnosed as having externalizing problems in general and ADHD in particular.

In summary, there may be three subgroups of girls with ADHD: those who are developmentally immature and have marked problems with attention and cognition; those who show severe externalizing problems; and those who are especially bright, engaged, and assertive, qualities that conflict with society's gender norms. Because they tend to withdraw rather than disrupt, girls in the first subgroup may be underdiagnosed. Because their behaviors are considered gender-inappropriate and are therefore likely to disturb others, girls in the third subgroup may in fact be falsely diagnosed. These intriguing notions about differential ADHD profiles for girls are highly speculative and in need of empirical testing. Especially lacking thus far are studies of peer relations in girls. Compared to their male counterparts, girls with disruptive behavior disorders (DBD) are more disliked by peers even though they seem to show lower levels of many symptomatic behaviors (Carlson *et al.,*

1997). This apparent discrepancy raises questions about whether the social dysfunctions in girls are more subtle and difficult to document than those in boys, perhaps centering on prosocial facets and peer settings that do not lend themselves to observation by adults. Alternatively, as just discussed, similar disruptions or misbehavior may be judged as more severe or less acceptable in girls because they diverge more markedly from gender-based norms.

THE WORLD OF PEOPLE MEETS THE WORLD OF TASKS

Schools are unique environments. If children's settings were graded in terms of elasticity or flexibility, homes would be placed at one end of the continuum. Families are often able to adapt activities and routines to accommodate many of the behavioral differences of children with ADHD. At the middle of the gradient one might find most peer environments such as parties and playgroups. Peers are typically less accommodating than parents, but there is a certain amount of give in most peer cultures. Schools, and especially classrooms, are located near the opposite end of this gradient, characterized by high degrees of structure and constraint and relatively little capacity to adapt to individual differences. Schools come with sets of behavioral prescriptions and proscriptions. School means discoveries and new skills, but school also means work. Not only are there regimens and rules to follow but there are also performance expectations and multiple social cues that must be processed and negotiated while attempting to meet these expectations. Thus, in many ways the classroom is the crucible within which ADHD is most salient and meets its severest challenges.

The vast majority of children with ADHD have difficulty functioning under the constraints imposed by classrooms and demonstrate serious problems achieving in school. But this does not mean that a disproportionate number of children with ADHD have "learning disabilities" in the more technical sense. School problems run the gamut from troubles getting to school or not getting expelled to accomplishing a specific academic task, such as learning the difference between "threw" and "through" (and also proving that it was learned). Some school difficulties undoubtedly stem from the interpersonal realm; problems with teachers reflect not only transactions parallel to those with peers but the added challenge of working with someone in authority. School problems can also stem from the routines imposed by formal schooling: getting places on time, sitting when others sit, organizing one's desktop, doing what is asked, and, for the older ones, remembering to do and turn in your homework. School failure or underachievement can stem from any of several transactional difficulties in either the interpersonal realm, with teachers and peers, or the task realm—learning to read, spell, write, and calculate.

Conceptualizing Learning Disabilities

Next to ODD/CD, learning disability (LD) is probably the most common codiagnosis for ADHD. In the not too distant past, it was thought that perhaps 50% or more of the children with attentional-hyperactive-impulsive problems were also underachievers, meeting diagnostic criteria for LD (Lambert & Sandoval, 1980). In some sources, the figure goes as high as 92% (Silver, 1981). In the majority of these early studies, however, the overlap was assessed in heterogeneous samples of children who were receiving remedial educational services rather than in those who were carefully evaluated and diagnosed. This percentage has been dropping somewhat over the last two decades in conjunction with the development of better delimited assessment and research strategies. We return to this point in a later section.

Despite recent gains, classificatory and definitional problems continue to plague the study of LD. Illustrative definitions are presented in Table 1. In most arenas, the definition incorporated into the Education for All Handicapped Children Act (PL 94-142) is the one that guides clinical and educational practice (see Definition 1, Table 1). In 1990, under

Public Law 101-476, the Education for All Handicapped Children Act (PL 94-142) was retitled as the Individuals with Disabilities Education Act (IDEA). Current publications in the field of LD now refer to the federal definition as the IDEA definition. It is important to distinguish between the IDEA definition itself and the criteria required for identification of a child as having LD. There are two essential differences. First, the identification guidelines do not address either the psychological process component or the neurological components specified in the definition. Both of these are left as options, but not requirements, in operationalizing the criteria (Mercer, 1997) and, thus, in assessing individual children for the presence of LD. One result is widely varying practices in whether or how these components are incorporated into assessments. Second, the definition does not mention a discrepancy between intelligence and achievement, but the guidelines require a demonstrated discrepancy to identify academic and language problems.

Dissatisfaction with the IDEA definition was apparent almost from the outset, and at least a dozen major alternatives have been put forth by professional and advocacy groups over the last two decades. The sources of the dissatisfaction have centered on the fact that the definition is nonspecific, implying that LD is one general entity, and that it defines largely by exclusion rather than specification. It is of little help to either clinicians or researchers in identifying individuals (Lyon, 1996). The alternative that is most widely used is that proposed by the National Joint Committee on Learning Disabilities (Hammill, 1990). Although this definition does acknowledge both the heterogeneity and the likely comorbidity seen in LD, it remains a poor guide for identification. The DSM-IV (American Psychiatric Association, 1994) has taken a step in the desired direction by providing separate designations of disorder for the major academic domains of reading, written expression, and mathematics, as well as language disorders.

Virtually every definition of LD relies on the "surprise" or unexpected nature of the academic deficit or delay. Compared to expectations

TABLE 1.   Selected Definitions of Learning Disabilities and Dyslexia

1. Federal Register definition (IDEA)

   "Specific learning disability" means a disorder in one or more of the basic psychological processes involved in understanding or in using language, spoken or written, which may manifest itself in an imperfect ability to listen, think, speak, read, write, spell, or to do mathematical calculations. The term includes such conditions as perceptual handicaps, brain injury, minimal brain dysfunction, dyslexia, and developmental aphasia. The term does not include children who have learning problems which are primarily the result of visual, hearing, or motor handicaps, of mental retardation, of emotional disturbance, or of environmental, cultural, or economic disadvantage.

   Note: This definition was originally from the National Advisory Committee on Handicapped Children conference sponsored by the U.S. Office of Education, September, 1967, and was incorporated into the Education for All Handicapped Children Act (P.L. 94-142) and published by the U.S. Office of Education (1977, p. 65083). It was reissued under P.L. 101-476, the Individuals with Disabilities Education Act (IDEA).

2. NJCLD definition (revised)

   "Learning disabilities" is a general term that refers to a heterogeneous group of disorders manifested by significant difficulty in the acquisition and use of listening, speaking, reading, writing, reasoning, or mathematical abilities. These disorders are intrinsic to the individual, presumed to be due to central nervous system dysfunction, and may occur across the life span. Problems in self-regulatory behavior, social perception, and social interaction may exist with learning disabilities but do not by themselves constitute a learning disability. Al-

though learning disabilities may occur concomitantly with other handicapping conditions (for example, sensory impairment, mental retardation, social and emotional disturbance) or with extrinsic influences (such as cultural differences, insufficient or inappropriate instruction), they are not the result of these conditions or influences.

3. DSM-IV diagnostic criteria for reading disorder

   A. Reading achievement, as measured by individually administered standardized tests of reading accuracy or comprehension, is substantially below that expected given the person's chronological age, measured intelligence, and age-appropriate education.

   B. The disturbance in Criterion A significantly interferes with academic achievement or activities of daily living that require reading skills.

   C. If a sensory deficit is present, the reading difficulties are in excess of those usually associated with it (American Psychiatric Association, 1994).

4. Orton Dyslexia Society Research Definition

   "Dyslexia" is one of several distinct learning disabilities. It is a specific language-based disorder of constitutional origin characterized by difficulties in single-word decoding, usually reflecting insufficient phonological processing. These difficulties in single-word decoding are often unexpected in relation to age and other cognitive and academic abilities; they are not the result of generalized developmental disability or sensory impairment. Dyslexia is manifest by variable difficulty with different forms of language, often including, in addition to problems with reading, a conspicuous problem with acquiring proficiency in writing and spelling (Lyon, 1995).

for a given age or grade, this child is not doing well. The anchor or standard for what is expected is the child's intelligence. If the child is not bright or does not do well on a standardized IQ test, then poor school achievement is expected and not considered surprising. Implicit in this use of the intelligence construct is the assumption that IQ is an index of potential or capacity, that a child's intelligence somehow sets a ceiling or imposes limits on the rate or amount of school learning to be anticipated.

Despite its strong face validity, this discrepancy requirement poses a number of difficulties. Discrepancy formulas are applied in a similar fashion across the full range of skills and abilities, yet with disparate results. It is not rare to see a 15-point discrepancy between IQ and achievement when the IQ is 130 or

145, for example, yet it is extremely rare to find a discrepancy of this size when the IQ is 85 or even 100. In other words, it is easier for a child to qualify as having a LD if the child's IQ is higher, rather than lower. A student who earns a score of 110 on the Woodcock–Johnson reading measures and a score of 130 on the WISC III may still qualify as learning disabled in most states.

Another questionable assumption inherent in the discrepancy notion is that IQ and achievement tests differ in fundamental ways, the former tapping potential or capacity and the latter tapping learning. Both conceptions are in error, and the two types of tests have more similarities than differences. Their content domains do differ, with IQ tests sampling from a broad range of life experiences and achievement tests more restricted to school-based content. But both are actually achievement tests and both are good indicators of scholastic aptitude; both tap performance and both tap problem-solving skills. It is not necessary to embrace a capacity definition of intelligence to appreciate that IQ scores index stable characteristics and can serve as efficient predictors of school success.

In the United States, the required discrepancy is usually 1 to 2 standard deviation units or 15–30 score points, but this criterion varies from state to state, or even from school district to school district, an unsatisfactory practice. Moats and Lyon (1993) commented that this is a remarkable situation in which a child can incur a disorder or be cured of one simply by moving to another state.

The size of the required discrepancy, the formula used in calculating it, whether the component scores must be standard scores, whether to use a regression-based formula and if so which one—these are obvious problems in applying discrepancy criteria, but they are also soluble or at least potentially soluble. There are more serious difficulties, including the fact that IQ scores and achievement test results are not independent. The expected correlation of IQ and scholastic achievement is around .60 or slightly above. In clinically referred samples, this correlation typically runs higher, as high as .85 (Fletcher *et al.*, 1996). A severe reading problem that persists over time is likely to be linked with a decreasing IQ score, and detected discrepancies are unlikely to sustain. But the most telling criticism is that the diagnosis does not seem to be *valid*. Discrepancy criteria do not differentiate children with reading disability (RD) from simply slow or poor readers. These two groups perform similarly on many tasks related to reading, such as word recognition, and both seem to have core phonological deficits (Stanovich & Siegel, 1994). Thus, children who do and do not meet criteria for RD cannot be distinguished by their performance on academic tasks (Fletcher *et al.*, 1994; Shaywitz, Escobar, Shaywitz, Fletcher, & Makuch, 1992).

When one defines something by what it is not, that is, by exclusionary criteria, the definition lacks substance. One consequence is that research on the mechanisms or processes involved proceeds without specification of the characteristics of the population being studied, that is, without benefit of clear selection criteria. A related consequence is that the results of such studies are difficult to interpret and apply (Lyon, 1995). A new working definition has been constructed by the Orton Dyslexia Society Research Committee in collaboration with other scientists and clinicians. As can be seen in Table 1, Definition 4, this working definition goes beyond previous definitions in the sense that it is theory driven, it identifies candidate sources of difficulty for poor readers, and it specifies the criterial skills for becoming a competent reader. In other words, this definition specifies *inclusionary* as well as exclusionary criteria and, as such, should serve a heuristic function for clinical researchers as well as a means of facilitating communication among clinicians, teachers, and parents (Lyon, 1995).

The technical exactness of the discrepancy approach creates an illusion that a disorder or disability has been identified when, in fact, only its result has been detected. A larger than expected difference between two scores on two measures of attainment that are expected to be well correlated is indeed worthy of note, but it is the signal that something is amiss, not the identification of what is wrong. Discrepancies alone tell us nothing about why they are occurring. What are the reasons that Johnny can't read? Once we rule out environmental disadvantage, family adversity, detectable brain damage, poor teaching, and other obvious candidates, there remain a substantial number of children who have difficulty learning.

Conceptualizing the Overlap between ADHD and LD

Does ADHD confer an added risk for LD? Depending on conceptualization, sampling, and methodology, this question can be reasonably answered "yes," "no," or "it all depends." Epidemiological studies, which are useful because they control for ascertainment or referral bias, suggest that the two disorders are associated at chance or only slightly above chance levels (Shaywitz, Fletcher, & Shaywitz, 1994). Family genetic studies lead to similar conclusions. There is solid evidence that both LD and ADHD have strong genetic contributions, but the two disorders appear to be transmitted independently. One exception to the growing consensus of independent transmission is the report by Stevenson, Pennington, Gilger, DeFries, and Gillis (1993), who aggregated the results of two samples to estimate that 75% of the overlap between spelling disability and hyperactivity is heritable. Because this figure is often cited, it reminds us that this estimate refers to genetic influences on comorbidity and not on the characteristics, in this case spelling and hyperactivity, being compared. Of the 402 children in the London sample analyzed by Stevenson and colleagues, 17 children showed both conditions, for a comorbidity rate of 4.2%, a figure significantly higher than the 2.4% expected by chance. Faraone, Biederman, Lehman, Keenan, and colleagues (1993) concluded, after analyzing the comorbidity in their Massachusetts sample, that the overlap between ADHD and LD is not only smaller than previously thought, but may also be artifactual in nature, perhaps the result of nonrandom mating. (See also Chapter 9, this volume.)

In referred samples, there is no question that ADHD places a young person at risk for having serious problems of both school adjustment and achievement, so much so that there may be ample justification for considering ADHD itself as a major subtype of LD (Pennington & Welsh, 1995). As an example, Faraone, Biederman, Lehman, Spencer, and colleagues (1993) found that in a group of children with "pure" ADHD, 34% had repeated a grade and 63% had been judged in need of academic tutoring, even though only 17% of these youngsters met regression-based criteria for RD. In other words, despite average IQs and a relatively low rate of diagnosed RD, the evidence for underachievement and school problems was widespread. After reviewing more than two dozen studies of the overlap, DuPaul and Stoner (1994) concluded that a child with ADHD is three to four times more likely than a peer to display serious learning problems. As high as it is, this ratio is lower than the estimate by the same reviewers that children with LD are seven times more likely to have ADHD.

A superb, heuristic review of the bidirectional associations between poor school achievement and DBD is provided by Hinshaw (1992), who cautions that plausible developmental models for explaining the causes of these associations have received little systematic study. It is reasonable, for example, to hypothesize that early language difficulties, which are associated with both ADHD and underachievement at high rates, is one such causal candidate (Cantwell & Baker, 1991). Yet the developmental sequelae of early language problems, like those of subaverage IQ, are not at all specific to inhibition failures. In fact, according to Hinshaw, the most common behavioral outcome of early language delay is internalizing problems (see also Stevenson, Richman, & Graham, 1985).

Processes and Mechanisms

Another way to look at the overlap between ADHD and LD, rather than calculating comorbidities or tracing family pedigrees, is to examine the cognitive, neurodevelopmental, and behavioral processes that may or may not be shared. *Oo-day oo-yay oh-nay ig-pay attin-lay?* If you can comprehend this sentence when you hear it, and if you can produce an answer such as, "Atcherlee-nay, illy-say!" then you probably have intact phonemic awareness, as well as a working knowledge of both English orthography and Pig Latin. If you can do it rapidly, you probably also have good phonological recoding skills. These two skills, joined by verbal short-term memory, make up the trio of language processing abilities thought to underlie single-word decoding, the fundamental process in learning to read.

Consensus is building that phonemic or phonological awareness is most central to the task of reading, followed closely by phonological recoding. Phonological awareness is awareness of the sound structure of language. It is indexed by the ability to discriminate and replicate the 44 speech-sound constituents of words and associate them with our alphabet (e.g., knowing that *dot* rhymes with *pot* and that both have the same number of sounds; being able to say dog without the /d/ sound). Recoding phonemes from lexical store is often assessed by rapid naming of letters, colors, or objects (Lyon, 1995; Torgesen, 1996). The third element of phonological processing, verbal working memory, is tapped by measures of working memory span such as sentence repetition tasks or digits forward (Lyon, 1995).

The different elements of the phonological "processor" cohere well, often to the point where apparently different tasks such as memory span and phonological awareness correlate perfectly (Wagner, Torgesen, Laughon, Simmons, & Rashotte, 1993). The evidence that phonological difficulties underpin RD is strong, with 80% to 90% of the children in epidemiologic samples of poor readers showing such deficits (Fletcher *et al.*, 1994).

By contrast, contemporary reformulations and neuropsychological studies of ADHD are converging on executive function (EF) deficits as the core cognitive processes primary to this disorder. Almost two decades ago, Douglas (1983) described ADHD as a defect in self-regulation, a construct that comprises three major spheres: organization and planning, the mobilization and maintenance of effortful attention, and the inhibition of inappropriate responding. Through a systematic analysis of tasks on which hyperactive children performed well (phonemic processing, verbal memory) and less well (logical search, matrix solutions), Douglas (1988; Chapter 5, this volume) advanced a set of hypotheses implicating regulatory control mechanisms and investment of effort in contrast to attention, memory, or increased distractibility.

Other benchmarks in our theoretical understanding of basic executive and inhibitory processes in ADHD have come from the research program of Sergeant and his colleagues and students (see Sergeant, 1996, and Chapter 4, this volume) which validates the view that attention is a management process governing the allocation of resources, and from the support that has been accruing to Quay's hypothesis that ADHD may be a disorder of the behavioral inhibition system described by Gray (see Quay, 1997). In a well-articulated theoretical account, Barkley (1997; Chapter 13, this volume) garners considerable support for his alternative model, which also emphasizes inhibitory failure in ADHD and expands on the consequences of disinhibition.

One research design for exploring the separability and overlap of deficits in two disorders is the double dissociation design. As explained by Pennington, Groisser, and Welsh (1993), a design to compare ADHD and RD would require a pure RD group, a pure ADHD group, a comorbid group, and a control group using a $2 \times 2 \times 2$ research design in which the final factor is a within-subjects measure of the two cognitive processes of interest. If a double dissociation exists, the pure ADHD group should show evidence of EF deficits but not phonological deficits, and a pure RD group should show the converse pattern.

Several studies have supported the notion of a double dissociation between ADHD and IQ-discrepant language or RD; children with ADHD seem to have core deficits in EF while children with IQ-discrepant learning or language disorders demonstrate phonological deficits (Korkman & Pesonen, 1994; Pennington *et al.*,1993; Tarnowski, Prinz, & Nay, 1986). The profile of the comorbid group from Pennington and colleagues (1993) is of particular interest because these students did not differ from the RD-only group in either domain but did differ from the ADHD-only group on both an EF score and a composite phonological score; this cognitive profile held after controlling for IQ. Pennington and colleagues interpreted their findings as supporting a secondary phenocopy hypothesis in which a primary RD sometimes leads to the *symptoms* of ADHD. The primary–secondary question is even better addressed through longitudinal studies but, with a few notable exceptions (McGee, Williams, Share, Anderson, & Silva, 1986), little such research has been conducted to date. Earlier studies that have compared a pure ADHD sample with a comorbid group have found less clear differentiation between the two, but this is perhaps an effect of severity (August & Garfinkel, 1990; Halperin, Gittelman, Klein, & Rudel, 1984). The children in these studies were recruited from mental health clinic referrals, however, whereas the Pennington sample was school-based. In fact, according to Pennington and Ozonoff (1996), the one study in the literature that did not show EF deficits in children with ADHD is one that used a community sample, raising the remote possibility that EF deficits are a selection artifact (McGee, Williams, Moffitt, & Anderson, 1989).

In line with this double dissociation perspective, research findings are converging on the conclusion that children with reading and language disorders are impaired, compared to controls, on phonological tasks, whereas children with ADHD are the more impaired on EF tasks. Pennington and Welsh (1995) suggest that, "in their 'pure' forms, language-related disorders (e.g., dyslexia) are neuropsychologically independent from executive function disorders (e.g., ADHD) with regard to the core cognitive deficits and underlying brain mechanisms involved" (p. 269). The ADHD subtypes now recognized in DSM-IV (American Psychiatric Association, 1994) may reflect this distinction, to the extent that children who fit criteria for the ADHD-Inattentive subtype share characteristics with those considered LD, whereas children meeting criteria for the Hyperactive-Impulsive subtype may have more extensive problems with EF.

At the present time, the executive metaphor is a plausible one for framing the core deficits in ADHD, yet there are many reasons that it is far from satisfactory. The definitions of the construct are still quite fluid and are necessarily general and broad (see Chapter 4, this volume). In the measurement realm, the situation appears nearly chaotic, with long lists of EF tasks that vary greatly from one another, and many of the tasks are so multifaceted that it is nearly impossible to understand the meaning of a score. In the Wisconsin Card Sort Task (WCST), for example, a poor performance (few categories) could as easily be due to poor task attention as to excellent abstractive abilities, with the latter resulting in more incorrect trials because the child is trying out a complicated strategy.

Despite these severe difficulties, many EF batteries have proven useful in studies of children with ADHD, as noted in Chapter 4 (this volume). In a summary of 18 studies of EF in ADHD, Pennington and Ozonoff (1996) reported positive results in 15 of these 18 or a total of 40 of 60 measures. There was some specificity in the profiles, with ADHD children doing consistently well on both visuospatial measures and verbal memory tasks in the non-EF arena and less well on EF tasks and on tests of vigilance and perceptual speed.

Teachers as Prototypes for Executive Functions

There appear to be three essential features that typify most EF tasks:

1. The assessment target tends to be the doing of something rather than the knowing of something.
2. The goal is to act in a way that conflicts with automatic or well-practiced responses.
3. The conflict is initiated by a verbal instruction or arbitrary rule.

We have distilled this list from an analysis by Hayes, Gifford, and Ruckstuhl (1996), who point out that the conflict, in EF tasks, is often between verbal and nonverbal sources of behavior regulation, a competition between semantic meaning and primary stimulus properties. On the Stroop, for example, the child is to name the color, not the word, yielding an instruction-produced competition between a well-practiced response and a novel, contrasting response, whereas on Tower of Hanoi problems, the child must desist from the obvious strategy of moving one element with each hand or resting one on the table and, instead, hold a complex set of regulations in mind. What is at issue, in short, is the flexibility and effectiveness of verbal self-regulation or rule regulation and not the adequacy of the verbal knowledge base.

Given these basic requirements for a good test of EF, it could be argued that the best prototype or proxy for such a test is a classroom teacher. By virtue of curricular goals and classroom contexts, teachers pose EF tasks throughout each school day. Inevitably, we would argue, a good teacher is designing EF tasks, evaluating the results, and drawing inferences about the reasons for classroom harmony, student progress, or the lack thereof.

Perhaps this parallel can be taken an additional step. One difficulty in interpreting scores from neuropsychological EF tasks, as pointed out by Denckla (1996), is that their sensitivity and specificity depend on the individual's competence in the content domain of the task. On a Stroop inference paradigm, for example, a child who shows fast speed in naming the color of the ink rather than the word is credited with good inhibition of prepotent responses. Yet what about a child with this same facile performance who is also an incompetent reader and does not read color names automatically? For this latter child, the ink-color-naming task will not be a sensitive indicator of inhibitory EF.

Again, parallels can be seen to the tasks of classroom teaching. Neuropsychologists try to solve the problem of domain competence by pairing tasks that share a specific domain such as word knowledge, yet one task places a demand on EF while the other does not. Teachers can similarly present individualized tasks to children that allow the separation of content-specific competence and can do so across a vast array of contents and skills. In fact, content-controlled tasks are exactly what a good teacher can and does provide in the course of daily instruction. A competent teacher is often in a good position to know whether an incorrect arithmetic answer is due to inadequate calculation skills or impulsivity, or whether a missing homework item is better attributable to a skill problem or an EF problem. When the ideal teacher assigns a classroom task, the level of difficulty is adjusted to match the competencies of the students.

The ratings and judgments by teachers have long played a controversial role in the study of ADHD. The fact that the diagnosis itself is based, in large part, on these ratings is often the target of sharp criticism. There is little doubt that such ratings are imprecise or more global than measures obtained from either laboratory tasks or behavior observation systems. Whereas lab tasks can reliably distinguish three, four, or even more types of attentional functioning, teacher ratings of these same content domains often produce only one or at most two factors. Such ratings also show halo effects, in which the impact of salient negative behaviors seems to spread to other domains, particularly to ratings of attentiveness.

On the other hand, a sturdy case can be made for both the ecological and the predictive validity of teacher judgments. Teachers are trained in human development and acquire, over the years, an extensive normative base for comparison. They are more likely than behavioral observers to witness the rare but telling incident, and they do not have the personal involvement of parents that may impede objective assessment. Teachers are able to take contextual factors into account as they evaluate and compare. And their judgments are particularly valuable because of their implicit understanding of the importance of EF and their agility in tailoring academic tasks to make use of and enhance EF in their students. When it comes to ADHD, it may very well be that the kind of attention that makes the most difference in real life is the kind that these children do not pay. A second kind of attention deficit, as one of our young participants told us, is the kind that they can't get enough of. And teachers are the best detectors of both of these.

This consideration of teachers as EF assessors is an ideal. But conditions are rarely ideal, and teachers must teach within the constraints of imperfect knowledge, crowded classes, student heterogeneity, and other challenges. Thus another critical need is to assess settings and situations. We know that some children considered to have ADHD, even cross-situational ADHD, show remarkable contextual variation in their behavior (Granger *et al.,* 1996; Whalen *et al.,* 1978; Whalen, Henker, Collins, Finck, & Dotemoto, 1979). We know that many of them (at least enough to produce statistically significant effects) do better working one-on-one than in a group and that other classroom dimensions such as task structure or social context influence performance. Our current diagnostic models of developmental psychopathology, and of ADHD in particular, focus almost solely on symptom counts or clusters and provide no means of bringing these situational or transactional perspectives to bear on our understanding of a child's disorder.

Similarly, recognition of the importance of understanding developmental influences and trajectories is virtually universal. A responsible clinician always takes a developmental history and makes an attempt to understand the contexts that may have influenced or are influencing the current problem. Yet when that same clinician turns to the taxonomy, or when a researcher seeks to identify a case for inclusion in a study, these developmental and contextual factors are typically given only a cursory glance, enough perhaps to complete an impairment rating that will then play no further role. Important progress has been made in understanding the relationships of attentional and social dysfunctions, in understanding the transactions between children and reading. This progress has been made in spite of the nosology, diagnostic criteria, and notions of comorbidity, and not because of them.

The study of contextual variation lags far behind that of behavioral symptoms and traits. We need a much more extensive examination of context dependency and of the environmental triggers that can alter the expression and course of behavioral traits (Jensen, Mrazek, *et al.,* 1997). We need to understand the situational side of the person–situation interaction so that we can learn how adaptive niche-picking occurs and incorporate this knowledge into our intervention programs. The first need, however, is not for a taxonomy of situations that will parallel psychiatric nosologies, but rather for theoretical developments that will push our understanding of situational influences in the way that recent theories of ADHD have advanced our understanding of children with inhibitory dysfunctions.

CONCLUSION

Two decades ago, we described the consensus that the diagnostic term *hyperactivity* was a misnomer, but a relatively benevolent and harmless one (Whalen & Henker, 1976). We were reluctant to see it replaced by the ADD classification with its inclusion of both "deficit" and "disorder." Over these ensuing years, societal understanding and acceptance of behavioral and learning disorders has grown greatly. ADD and LD, and now ADHD, have become household terms and carry few apparent pejorative connotations. In fact, many video artists and Hollywood celebrities wear one of these diagnoses almost as a badge of distinction. Perhaps their visibility as successful role models has removed some of the stigma associated with having an acknowledged "deficit."

When we look to the future, we find ourselves again reluctant to relegate ADHD to the dustbin or wherever former categories are put, in spite of the fact that neither attention nor hyperactivity are entirely appropriate core descriptors for this pattern of developmental variation. Perhaps the American Psychiatric Association should be asked for a moratorium on further name changes until there is solid, validated consensus on the latent constructs or g factor equivalents for ADHD.

We yield to temptation and close using the metaphor of the transactional disorder we are seeking to understand. The diagnosis is clearly the combined type: We scientists have been hyperactive in gathering fragmented collections of symptoms and recombining them into shifting clusters; impulsive in seeking premature closures; and inattentive to the fundamental rules of construct validation. What the field needs now is to seek less attention for revisions to the nosology, pay more attention to validating its best theories, and planfully organize and implement ways to better integrate the enabling influences of both neurophysiology and situational context into its construct systems. To achieve this end will be an executive, self-regulatory, inhibitory task of some magnitude.

REFERENCES

American Psychiatric Association. (1994). *Diagnostic and statistical manual of mental disorders* (4th ed.). Washington, DC: Author.

August, G. J., & Garfinkel, B. D. (1990). Comorbidity of ADHD and reading disability among clinic-referred children. *Journal of Abnormal Child Psychology, 18,* 29–45.

Barkley, R. A. (1989). Hyperactive girls and boys: Stimulant drug effects on mother–child interactions. *Journal of Child Psychology and Psychiatry, 30,* 379–390.

Barkley, R. A. (1997). *ADHD and the nature of self-control.* New York: Guilford.

Bird, H. R., Gould, M. S., & Staghezza, B. M. (1993). Patterns of diagnostic comorbidity in a community sample of children aged 9 through 16 years. *Journal of the American Academy of Child and Adolescent Psychiatry, 32,* 361–368.

Buhrmester, D., Whalen, C. K., Henker, B., MacDonald, V., & Hinshaw, S. P. (1992). Prosocial behavior in hyperactive boys: Effects of stimulant medication and comparison with normal boys. *Journal of Abnormal Child Psychology, 20,* 103–121.

Buitelaar, J. K., Swinkels, S. H. N., de Vries, H., van der Gaag, R. J., & van Hooff, J. A. R. A. M. (1994). An ethological study on behavioural differences between hyperactive, aggressive, combined hyperactive/aggressive and control children. *Journal of Child Psychology and Psychiatry, 35,* 1437–1446.

Campbell, S. B., Breaux, A. M., Ewing, L. J., Szumowski, E. K., & Pierce, E. W. (1986). Parent-identified problem preschoolers: Mother–child interaction during play at intake and 1-year follow-up. *Journal of Abnormal Child Psychology, 14,* 425–440.

Cantwell, D. P., & Baker, L. (1991). Association between attention deficit–hyperactivity disorder and learning disorders. *Journal of Learning Disabilities, 24,* 88–95.

Carlson, C. L., Tamm, L., & Gaub, M. (1997). Gender differences in children with ADHD, ODD, and co-occurring ADHD/ODD identified in a school population. *Journal of the American Academy of Child and Adolescent Psychiatry, 36,* 1706–1714.

Clark, M. L., Cheyne, J. A., Cunningham, C. E., & Siegel, L. S. (1988). Dyadic peer interaction and task orientation in attention-deficit-disordered children. *Journal of Abnormal Child Psychology, 16,* 1–15.

Coie, J. D., & Dodge, K. A. (1998). The development of aggression and antisocial behavior. In W. Damon & N. Eisenberg (Eds.), *Handbook of child psychology* (5th ed.): Vol. 3. *Social, emotional, and personality development* (pp. 779–861). New York: Wiley.

Crick, N. R., & Dodge, K. A. (1994). A review and reformulation of social information-processing mechanisms in children's social adjustment. *Psychological Bulletin, 115,* 74–101.

Cunningham, C. E., & Barkley, R. A. (1979). The interactions of normal and hyperactive children with their mothers in free play and structured tasks. *Child Development, 50,* 217–224.

Cunningham, C. E., & Siegel, L. S. (1987). Peer interactions of normal and attention-deficit-disordered boys during free-play, cooperative task, and simulated classroom situations. *Journal of Abnormal Child Psychology, 15,* 247–268.

Cunningham, C. E., Siegel, L. S., & Offord, D. R. (1985). A developmental dose–response analysis of the effects of methylphenidate on the peer interactions of attention deficit disordered boys. *Journal of Child Psychology and Psychiatry, 26,* 955–971.

Cunningham, C. E., Siegel, L. S., & Offord, D. R. (1991). A dose–response analysis of the effects of methylphenidate on the peer interactions and simulated classroom performance of ADD children with and without conduct problems. *Journal of Child Psychology and Psychiatry, 32,* 439–452.

Denckla, M. B. (1996). Research on executive function in a neurodevelopmental context: Application of clinical measures. *Developmental Neuropsychology, 12,* 5–15.

Douglas, V. I. (1983). Attentional and cognitive problems. In M. Rutter (Ed.), *Developmental neuropsychiatry* (pp. 280–329). New York: Guilford.

Douglas, V. I. (1988). Cognitive deficits in children with attention deficit disorder with hyperactivity. In L. M. Bloomingdale & J. Sergeant (Eds.), *Attention deficit disorder: Criteria, cognition, intervention* (pp. 65–81). Elmsford, NY: Pergamon.

DuPaul, G. J., & Stoner, G. (1994). *ADHD in the schools: Assessment and intervention strategies.* New York: Guilford.

Dweck, C. S., & Leggett, E. L. (1988). A social-cognitive approach to motivation and personality. *Psychological Review, 95,* 256–273.

Eisenberg, N., Fabes, R. A., Guthrie, I. K., Murphy, B. C., Maszk, P., Holmgren, R., & Suh, K. (1996). The relations of regulation and emotionality to problem behavior in elementary school children. *Development and Psychopathology, 8,* 141–162.

Erhardt, D., & Hinshaw, S. P. (1994). Initial sociometric impressions of ADHD and comparison boys: Predictions from social behaviors and non-behavioral variables. *Journal of Consulting and Clinical Psychology, 62,* 833–842.

Fagot, B., & Leve, L. (1998). Teacher ratings of externalizing behavior at school entry for boys and girls: Similar early predictors and different correlates. *Journal of Child Psychology and Psychiatry, 39,* 555–566.

Faraone, S. V., Biederman, J., Lehman, B. K., Keenan, K., Norman, D., Seidman, L. J., Kolodny, R., Kraus, I., Perrin, J., & Chen, W. J. (1993). Evidence for the independent familial transmission of attention deficit hyperactivity disorder and learning disabilities: Results from a family genetic study. *American Journal of Psychiatry, 150,* 891–895.

Faraone, S. V., Biederman, J., Lehman, B. K., Spencer, T., Norman, D., Seidman, L. J., Kraus, I., Perrin, J., Chen, W. J., & Tsuang, M. T. (1993). Intellectual performance and school failure in children with attention deficit hyperactivity disorder and in their siblings. *Journal of Abnormal Psychology, 102,* 616–623.

Fletcher, J. M., Shaywitz, S. E., Shankweiler, D., Katz, L., Liberman, I. Y., Stuebing, K. K., Francis, D. J., Fowler, A. E., & Shaywitz, B. A. (1994). Cognitive profiles of reading disability: Comparisons of discrepancy and low achievement definitions. *Journal of Educational Psychology, 86,* 6–23.

Fletcher, J. M., Francis, D. J., Stuebing, K. K., Shaywitz, B. A., Shaywitz, S. E., Shankweiler, D. P., Katz, L., & Morris, R. D. (1996). Conceptual and methodological issues in construct definition. In G. R. Lyon & N. A. Krasnegor (Eds.), *Attention, memory, and executive function* (pp. 17–42). Baltimore: Brookes.

Gaub, M., & Carlson, C. L. (1997a). Behavioral characteristics of DSM-IV ADHD subtypes in a school-based population. *Journal of Abnormal Child Psychology, 43,* 103–111.

Gaub, M., & Carlson, C. L. (1997b). Gender differences in ADHD: A meta-analysis and critical review. *Journal of the American Academy of Child and Adolescent Psychiatry, 36,* 1036–1045.

Granger, D. A., Whalen, C. K., Henker, B., & Cantwell, C. (1996). ADHD boys' behavior during structured classroom social activities: Effects of social demands, teacher proximity, and methylphenidate. *Journal of Attention Disorders, 1,* 16–30.

Greene, R. W., Biederman, J., Faraone, S. V., Ouellette C. A., Penn, C., & Griffin, S. M. (1996). Toward a new psychometric definition of social disability in children with attention-deficit hyperactivity disorder. *Journal of the American Academy of Child & Adolescent Psychiatry, 35,* 571–578.

Greene, R. W., Biederman, J., Faraone, S. V., Sienna, M., & Garcia-Jetton, J. (1997). Adolescent outcome of boys with attention-deficit/hyperactivity disorder and social disability: Results from a 4-year longitudinal follow-up study. *Journal of Consulting and Clinical Psychology, 65,* 758–767.

Halperin, J. M., Gittelman, R., Klein, D. F., & Rudel, R. G. (1984). Reading-disabled hyperactive children: A distinct subgroup of attention deficit disorder with hyperactivity? *Journal of Abnormal Child Psychology, 12,* 1–14.

Hammill, D. (1990). On defining learning disabilities: An emerging consensus. *Journal of Learning Disabilities, 23,* 74–85.

Harris, M. J., Milich, R., Johnston, E. M., & Hoover, D. W. (1990). Effects of expectancies on children's social interactions. *Journal of Experimental Social Psychology, 26,* 1–12.

Harris, M. J., Milich, R., Corbitt, E. M., Hoover, D. W., & Brady, M. (1992). Self-fulfilling effects of stigmatizing information on children's social interactions. *Journal of Personality and Social Psychology, 63,* 41–50.

Hayes, S. C., Gifford, E. V., & Ruckstuhl, L. E., Jr. (1996). Relational frame theory and executive function: A behavioral approach. In G. R. Lyon & N. A. Krasnegor (Eds.), *Attention, memory, and executive function* (pp. 263–278). Baltimore: Brookes.

Hinshaw, S. P. (1992). Externalizing behavior problems and academic underachievement in childhood and adolescence: Causal relationships and underlying mechanisms. *Psychological Bulletin, 111,* 127–155.

Hinshaw, S. P., & Melnick, S. M. (1995). Peer relationships in boys with attention-deficit hyperactivity disorder with and without comorbid aggression. *Development and Psychopathology, 7,* 627–647.

Hoza, B., Pelham, W. E., Milich, R., Pillow, D., & McBride, K. (1993). The self-perceptions and attributions of attention deficit hyperactivity disordered and nonreferred boys. *Journal of Abnormal Child Psychology, 21,* 271–286.

Hubbard, J. A., & Newcomb, A. F. (1991). Initial dyadic peer interaction of attention deficit–hyperactivity disorder and normal boys. *Journal of Abnormal Child Psychology, 19,* 179–195.

Hymel, S. (1986). Interpretations of peer behavior: Affective bias in childhood and adolescence. *Child Development, 57,* 431–445.

Jensen, P. S., Martin, D., & Cantwell, D. P. (1997). Comorbidity in ADHD: Implications for research, practice, and DSM-V. *Journal of the American Academy of Child and Adolescent Psychiatry, 36,* 1065–1079.

Jensen, P. S., Mrazek, D., Knapp, P. K., Steinberg, L., Pfeffer, C., Schowalter, J., & Shapiro, T. (1997). Evolution and revolution in child psychiatry: ADHD as a disorder of adaptation. *Journal of the American Academy of Child and Adolescent Psychiatry, 36,* 1672–1679.

Keenan, K., & Shaw, D. (1997). Developmental and social influences on young girls' early problem behavior. *Psychological Bulletin, 121,* 95–113.

Korkman, M., & Pesonen, A. E. (1994). A comparison of neuropsychological test profiles of children with attention deficit hyperactivity disorder and/or learning disorder. *Journal of Learning Disabilities, 27,* 383–392.

Lahey, B. B., Applegate, B., McBurnett, K., Biederman, J., Greenhill, L., Hynd, G. W., Barkley, R. A., Newcorn, J., Jensen, P., Richters, J., Garfinkel, B., Kerdyk, L., Frick, P. J., Ollendick, T., Perez, D., Hart, E. L., Waldman, I., & Shaffer, D. (1994). DSM-IV field trials for attention-deficit/hyperactivity disorder in children and adolescents. *American Journal of Psychiatry, 151,* 1673–1685.

Lambert, N. M., & Sandoval, J. (1980). The prevalence of learning disabilities in a sample of children considered hyperactive. *Journal of Abnormal Child Psychology, 8,* 33–50.

Landau, S., & Milich, R. (1988). Social communication patterns of attention-deficit-disordered boys. *Journal of Abnormal Child Psychology, 16,* 69–81.

Lyon, G. R. (1995). Toward a definition of dyslexia. *Annals of Dyslexia, 45,* 3–27.

Lyon, G. R. (1996). Learning disabilities. In E. J. Mash & R. A. Barkley (Eds.), *Child psychopathology* (pp. 390–435). New York: Guilford.

MacDonald, K. B. (1988). *Social and personality development: An evolutionary synthesis.* New York: Plenum.

Madan-Swain, A., & Zentall, S. S. (1990). Behavioral comparisons of liked and disliked hyperactive children in play contexts and the behavioral accommodations by their classmates. *Journal of Consulting and Clinical Psychology, 58,* 197–209.

Mannuzza, S., Klein, R. G., Bessler, A., Malloy, P., & La-Padula, M. (1993). Adult outcome of hyperactive boys. *Archives of General Psychiatry, 50,* 565–576.

Mannuzza, S., Klein, R. G., Bessler, A., Malloy, P., & Hynes, M. E. (1997). Educational and occupational outcome of hyperactive boys grown up. *Journal of the American Academy of Child and Adolescent Psychiatry, 36,* 1222–1227.

Mash, E. J., & Johnston, C. (1982). A comparison of the mother–child interactions of younger and older hyperactive and normal children. *Child Development, 53,* 1371–1381.

McGee, R., & Feehan, M. (1991). Are girls with problems of attenton underrecognized? *Journal of Psychopathology and Behavioral Assessment, 13,* 187–198.

McGee, R., Williams, S., Share, D. L., Anderson, J., & Silva, P. A. (1986). The relationship between specific reading retardation, general reading backwardness, and behavioural problems in a large sample of Dunedin boys: A longitudinal study from five to eleven years. *Journal of Child Psychology and Psychiatry, 27,* 597–610.

McGee, R., Williams, S., Moffitt, T., & Anderson, J. (1989). A comparison of 13-year-old boys with attention deficit and/or reading disorder on neuropsychological measures. *Journal of Abnormal Child Psychology, 17,* 37–53.

Melnick, S. M., & Hinshaw, S. P. (1996). What they want and what they get: The social goals of boys with ADHD and comparison boys. *Journal of Abnormal Child Psychology, 24,* 169–185.

Mercer, C. D. (1997). *Students with learning disabilities* (5th ed.). Upper Saddle River, NJ: Merrill.

Milich, R. (1994). The response of children with ADHD to failure: If at first you don't succeed, do you try, try, again? *School Psychology Review, 23,* 11–18.

Milich, R., McAninch, C. B., & Harris, M. J. (1992). Effects of stigmatizing information on children's peer relations: Believing is seeing. *School Psychology Review, 21,* 400–409.

Moats, L. C., & Lyon, G. R. (1993). Learning disabilities in the United States: Advocacy, science, and the future of the field. *Journal of Learning Disabilities, 26,* 282–294.

Northup, J., Jones, K., Broussard, C., DiGiovanni, G., Herring, M., Fusilier, I., & Hanchey, A. (1997). A preliminary analysis of interactive effects between common classroom contingencies and methylphenidate. *Journal of Applied Behavior Analysis, 30,* 121–125.

Parker, J. G., & Asher, S. R. (1987). Peer relations and later personal adjustment: Are low-accepted children at risk? *Psychological Bulletin, 102,* 357–389.

Pelham, W. E., McBurnett, K., Harper, G. W., Milich, R., Murphy, D. A., Clinton, J., & Thiele, C. (1990). Methylphenidate and baseball playing in ADHD children: Who's on first? *Journal of Consulting and Clinical Psychology, 58,* 130–133.

Pennington, B. F., & Ozonoff, S. (1996). Executive functions and developmental psychopathology. *Journal of Child Psychology and Psychiatry, 37,* 51–87.

Pennington, B. F., & Welsh, M. (1995). Neuropsychology and developmental psychopathology. In D. Cicchetti & D. J. Cohen (Eds.), *Developmental psychopathology: Vol. 1. Theory and methods* (pp. 254–290). New York: Wiley.

Pennington, B. F., Groisser, D., & Welsh, M. C. (1993). Contrasting cognitive deficits in attention deficit hyperactivity disorder versus reading disability. *Developmental Psychology, 29,* 511–523.

Quay, H. C. (1997). Inhibition and attention deficit hyperactivity disorder. *Journal of Abnormal Child Psychology, 25,* 7–13.

Renshaw, P. D., & Asher, S. R. (1983). Children's goals and strategies for social interaction. *Merrill-Palmer Quarterly, 29,* 353–374.

Rosenthal, R., & Jacobson, L. (1968). *Pygmalion in the classroom.* New York: Holt, Rinehart, & Winston.

Scarr, S., & McCartney, K. (1983). How people make their own environments: A theory of genotype → environment effects. *Child Development, 54,* 424–435.

Schachar, R., Taylor, E., Wieselberg, J., Thorley, G., & Rutter, M. (1987). Changes in family function and relationships in children who respond to methylphenidate. *Journal of the Academy of Child and Adolescent Psychiatry, 26,* 728–732.

Sergeant, J. (1996). A theory of attention: An information processing perspective. In G. R. Lyon & N. A. Krasnegor (Eds.), *Attention, memory, and executive function* (pp. 45–56). Baltimore: Brookes.

Shaywitz, S. E., Escobar, M. D., Shaywitz, B. A., Fletcher, J. M., & Makuch, R. (1992). Evidence that dyslexia may represent the lower tail of a normal distribution of reading ability. *New England Journal of Medicine, 326,* 145–150.

Shaywitz, S. E., Fletcher, J. M., & Shaywitz, B. A. (1994). Issues in the definition and classification of attention deficit disorder. *Topics in Language Disorders, 14,* 1–25.

Silver, L. B. (1981). The relationship between learning disabilities, hyperactivity, distractibility, and behavioral problems: A clinical analysis. *Journal of the American Academy of Child Psychiatry, 20,* 385–397.

Spencer, T., Biederman, J., Wilens, T., & Faraone, S. V. (1994). Is attention-deficit hyperactivity disorder in adults a valid disorder? *Harvard Review of Psychiatry, 1*, 326–335.

Stanovich, K. E., & Siegel, L. S. (1994). Phenotypic performance profile of children with reading disabilities: A regression-based test of the phonological-core variable-difference model. *Journal of Educational Psychology, 86*, 24–53.

Stevenson, J., Richman, N., & Graham, P. (1985). Behaviour problems and language abilities at three years and behavioural deviance at eight years. *Journal of Child Psychology and Psychiatry, 26*, 215–230.

Stevenson, J., Pennington, B. F., Gilger, J. W., DeFries, J. C., & Gillis, J. J. (1993). Hyperactivity and spelling disability: Testing for shared genetic aetiology. *Journal of Child Psychology and Psychiatry, 34*, 1137–1152.

Tarnowski, K. J., Prinz, R. J., & Nay, S. M. (1986). Comparative analysis of attentional deficits in hyperactive and learning-disabled children. *Journal of Abnormal Psychology, 95*, 341–345.

Torgesen, J. K. (1996). A model of memory from an information processing perspective. The special case of phonological memory. In G. R. Lyon & N. A. Krasnegor (Eds), *Attention, memory, and executive function* (pp. 157–183). Baltimore: Brookes.

Wagner, R. K., Torgesen, J. K., Laughon, P., Simmons, K., & Rashotte, C. A. (1993). Development of young readers' phonological processing abilities. *Journal of Educational Psychology, 85*, 83–103.

Weiss, G., & Hechtman, L. T. (1993). *Hyperactive children grown up: ADHD in children, adolescents, and adults* (2nd ed.). New York: Guilford.

Wender, P. H. (1995). *Attention-deficit hyperactivity disorder in adults.* New York: Oxford University Press.

Whalen, C. K., & Henker B. (1976). Psychostimulants and children: A review and analysis. *Psychological Bulletin, 83*, 1113–1130.

Whalen, C. K., & Henker, B. (1985). The social worlds of hyperactive children. *Clinical Psychology Review, 5*, 1–32.

Whalen, C. K., & Henker, B. (1991). The social impact of stimulant treatment for hyperactive children. *Journal of Learning Disabilities, 24*, 231–241.

Whalen, C. K., & Henker, B. (1992). The social profile of attention-deficit hyperactivity disorder: Five fundamental facets. *Child and Adolescent Psychiatric Clinics of North America, 1*, 395–410.

Whalen, C. K., & Henker, B. (1997). Stimulant pharmacotherapy for attention deficit/hyperactivity disorders: An analysis of progress, problems, and prospects. In S. Fisher & R. Greenberg (Eds.), *From placebo to panacea: Putting psychiatric drugs to the test* (pp. 323–355). New York: Wiley.

Whalen, C. K., & Henker, B. (1998). Attention-deficit/hyperactivity disorders. In T. H. Ollendick & M. Hersen (Eds.), *Handbook of child psychopathology* (3rd ed., pp. 181–211). New York: Plenum.

Whalen, C. K., Collins, B. E., Henker, B., Alkus, S. R., Adams, D., & Stapp, J. (1978). Behavior observations of hyperactive children and methylphenidate (Ritalin) effects in systematically structured classroom environments: Now you see them, now you don't. *Journal of Pediatric Psychology, 3*, 177–187.

Whalen, C. K., Henker, B., Collins, B. E., Finck, D., & Dotemoto, S. (1979). A social ecology of hyperactive boys: Medication effects in structured classroom environments. *Journal of Applied Behavior Analysis, 12*, 65–81.

Whalen, C. K., Henker, B., Collins, B. E., McAuliffe, S., & Vaux, A. (1979). Peer interaction in a structured communication task: Comparisons of normal and hyperactive boys and of methylphenidate (Ritalin) and placebo effects. *Child Development, 50*, 388–401.

Whalen, C. K., Henker, B., & Dotemoto, S. (1980). Methylphenidate and hyperactivity: Effects on teacher behaviors. *Science, 208*, 1280–1282.

Whalen, C. K., Henker, B., & Dotemoto, S. (1981). Teacher response to the methylphenidate (Ritalin) versus placebo status of hyperactive boys in the classroom. *Child Development, 52*, 1005–1014.

Whalen, C. K., Henker, B., Castro, J., & Granger, D. (1987). Peer perceptions of hyperactivity and medication effects. *Child Development, 58*, 816–828.

Whalen, C. K., Henker, B., Buhrmester, D., Hinshaw, S. P., Huber, A., & Laski, K. (1989). Does stimulant medication improve the peer status of hyperactive children? *Journal of Consulting and Clinical Psychology, 57*, 545–549.

Whalen, C. K., Henker, B., & Granger, D. A. (1990). Social judgment processes in hyperactive boys: Effects of methylphenidate and comparisons with normal peers. *Journal of Abnormal Child Psychology, 18*, 297–316.

Wolraich, M. L., Hannah, J. N., Pinnock, T. Y., Baumgaertel, A., & Brown, J. (1996). Comparison of diagnostic criteria for attention-deficit hyperactivity disorder in a county-wide sample. *Journal of the American Academy of Child and Adolescent Psychiatry, 35*, 319–324.

8

The Psychobiology of Attention-Deficit/Hyperactivity Disorder

F. XAVIER CASTELLANOS

INTRODUCTION

The aim of this chapter is to link the advances in our understanding of Attention-Deficit/Hyperactivity Disorder (ADHD) delineated in this book to evolving models of brain function and dysfunction. The model presented here is a compendium and elaboration of others proposed over the past three decades. For economy, comprehensive reviews are cited rather than primary sources whenever possible, since the principal goal is to outline broad areas of previous work and directions for future studies, rather than to claim the status of a complete theory.

The thesis advanced is that ADHD is a disorder of deficient and delayed self-regulation, due largely to genetic differences in the rate of development and functional integrity of brain systems modulated by dopamine (DA), norepinephrine (NE), and possibly epinephrine (EPI), that encompass at least five anatomic components: the prefrontal cortex (PFC), basal ganglia, locus coeruleus (LC), cerebellum, and

amygdala–septo-hippocampal system. Finally, there is also evidence that the putative deviations in brain development interact with genetic control of lateralization of brain function such that right-sided circuits are those that are predominantly affected.

ADHD IS A DISORDER OF DEFICIENT SELF-REGULATION

Chapters 4, 5, and 13 in this volume advance the notion that ADHD is not merely a deficit of attention, an excess of locomotor activity, or their simple conjunction. The unifying abstraction that currently best encompasses the faculties principally affected in ADHD has been termed executive function (EF), which is an evolving concept (see, e.g., Lyon & Krasnegor, 1996). This concept and its limitations are dealt with in much more detail in the aforementioned chapters, but it is worth noting here that there is now impressive empirical support for its importance in ADHD. This evidence has been summarized in an excellent review of the neuropsychological literature by Pennington and Ozonoff (1996), who reported that 15 of 18 controlled studies found significant EF deficits in ADHD on one or more measures, with significant deficits on a total of 40 out of

F. XAVIER CASTELLANOS • Child Psychiatry Branch, National Institute of Mental Health, Bethesda, Maryland 20892-1251.

Handbook of Disruptive Behavior Disorders, edited by Quay and Hogan. Kluwer Academic/Plenum Publishers, New York, 1999.

60 EF measures. Consistent deficits were also found on tests of vigilance, which is one of the lower level faculties modulated by EF, but the most robust and consistent deficits were found on motor inhibition tasks (average effect size 0.85), whereas significant differences were found in only 19 of 54 non-EF measures. This relative specificity of EF in ADHD was particularly noted on verbal measures, on which ADHD children did not demonstrate any consistent deficits. However, EF deficits are not unique to ADHD, although the pattern of deficits is distinct from that found in autism. In general, the problem of discriminant validity has not been addressed satisfactorily up to now, but the conceptual and technical tools required are available. For example, although distractibility is accepted as one of the core symptoms of ADHD, children with ADHD do not differ from controls in electrophysiological responses to unattended stimuli. Instead, they are deficient in the preferential processing required for attended stimuli (Satterfield, Schell, & Nicholas, 1994). One mechanism through which such preferential processing is performed, known as "biased competition," is now being actively investigated in nonhuman primates and in humans undergoing functional brain imaging (Desimone, 1996). If Satterfield and colleagues' results are confirmed in "pure" ADHD (their sample was highly comorbid for Conduct Disorder [CD]), these results may represent an important clue to the nature of the central neurobiological deficits in ADHD.

ADHD IS A DISORDER OF DELAYED SELF-REGULATION

Kinsbourne (1973) proposed that minimal brain dysfunction could be understood as a neurodevelopmental lag. Evidence of neurodevelopmental delays in ADHD has been found in electrophysiological studies (Buchsbaum & Wender, 1973; Chabot & Serfontein, 1996; Klorman, Brumaghim, Fitzpatrick, Borgstedt, & Strauss, 1994; Satterfield & Braley, 1977), neuropsychological investigations (Chelune, Ferguson, Koon, & Dickey, 1986; Pontius &

Ruttiger, 1974), and in adaptive functioning (Roizen, Blondis, Irwin, & Stein, 1994; Stein, Szumowski, Blondis, & Roizen, 1995).

The lag hypothesis implies an ultimately favorable prognosis, as behavioral deviance diminishes with increasing age. Improvements with maturation have been consistently reported in a substantial proportion of individuals followed longitudinally (Gittelman, Mannuzza, Shenker, & Bonagura, 1985; Mannuzza, Klein, Bessler, Malloy, & LaPadula, 1993; Weiss, Hecthman, MIlroy, & Perlman, 1985). However, a favorable outcome is not always attained, whether the measures are electroencephalographic (Corning, Steffy, Anderson, & Bowers, 1986), neuropsychological (Fischer, Barkley, Edelbrock, & Smallish, 1990), or in psychiatric outcome (Mannuzza et al., 1993; see also Chapters 12 and 13, this volume). Delayed neurological maturation of frontal-striatal circuits has also been reported in Obsessive-Compulsive Disorder (OCD) (Rosenberg et al., 1997) and in Autism (Zilbovicius et al., 1995), demonstrating that delayed maturation may be a correlate of neuropsychiatric illness generally, and may not be specific to ADHD. Despite these limitations, the concept of a delay in self-regulation has clinical implications and is another important, albeit also nonspecific, component of the pathophysiology of ADHD.

BRAIN MATURATION AND ADHD

As noted previously, there is substantial neuropsychological, electrophysiological, and phenomenological evidence of delayed development in ADHD. What is lacking is clear evidence that brain development per se is delayed. The study of human brain development may be said to be still in its infancy, but the availability of neuroimaging techniques and rapid progress in developmental neuroscience is accelerating our understanding.

Interestingly, there is remarkably little change in total cerebral volume from ages 5 to 18, whether measured by magnetic resonance imaging (MRI) (Giedd et al., 1996; Reiss,

Abrams, Singer, Ross, & Denckla, 1996) or in postmortem specimens (Dobbing & Sands, 1973). This is surprising, because at the microscopic level, brain anatomy is changing qualitatively and quantitatively (Huttenlocher, 1984). The period between toddlerhood and adolescence is marked by widespread pruning of synapses at an astronomical rate (estimated in the rhesus monkey as 25,000 synapses lost per second for several years) (Bourgeois & Rakic, 1993). Because of electrophysiological and neuropsychological evidence that neurological maturation proceeds along a caudal–frontal gradient (Epstein, 1986; Thatcher, 1997), it was expected that the orderly progression of synaptic overgrowth and subsequent pruning would also begin in caudal regions. However, synaptogenesis, synaptic pruning, and neurotransmitter receptor production proceed in a synchronous manner throughout the cortex, "rather than as a system-by-system cascade" (Lidow, Goldman-Rakic, & Rakic, 1991, p. 10218). Thus, it appears unlikely that these tightly determined processes are the ones that account for relatively subtle maturational changes.

Since the time of Yakovlev and Lecours (1967), neurological maturation has been associated with differential regional myelination. For a variety of technical reasons, it has been difficult to study myelination in humans rigorously during development. Reiss and colleagues (1996) have taken the first step by confirming that the proportion of brain that is composed of white matter increases robustly in healthy children between the ages of 6 and 18 years. Giedd and colleagues (1996) at the National Institute of Mental Health (NIMH) obtained similar measures in a large cross-sectional sample of children with ADHD and matched healthy controls (> 100 subjects per group) with the goal of determining whether differential regional myelination patterns discriminate children with ADHD from controls. The corresponding analyses are just beginning at the time of the writing of this chapter.

Of course, even MRI measures of myelination are crude, and it would not be surprising if the pertinent processes that differentiate brain development in ADHD turn out to be subtler. Developmental neuroscientists and the Human Genome Project are likely to remain our (mainly inadvertent) collaborators in the years to come.

THE PRIMARY ETIOLOGY OF ADHD IS GENETIC

The family (Faraone et al., 1992), adoption (Cadoret & Stewart, 1991), and twin studies (Goodman & Stevenson, 1989; Levy, Hay, McStephen, Wood, & Waldman, 1997; Thapar, Hervas, & McGuffin, 1995) supporting a genetic etiology for most cases of ADHD are discussed in detail in Chapter 9 (this volume). Heritability estimates in twin studies range from 0.60 to 0.90 and there is at least a fivefold increase in relative risk to first-degree relatives of probands with ADHD compared to the risk in the general population (Smalley, 1997). By comparison, however, the relative risk in Autism is much higher (greater than 75:1).

Thus, despite its substantial heritability, the individual genes that are associated with an increased risk of ADHD are likely to have modest effects in isolation. For this reason, a consensus has emerged that progress in understanding the genetics of psychiatric disorders such as ADHD will require the recruitment of multiplex families (those with at least 2 full affected siblings) in order to conduct genome-wide scans for DNA markers that are shared more often than would be expected by chance (0.50 between full siblings). Once such markers are detected and replicated independently, it will be possible to apply positional cloning techniques to locate specific genetic variants that can be tested in independent data sets. This approach has been powerful in single-gene disorders, and it should also be useful in detecting genes of moderate effect in complex genetic disorders. The alternative is to pursue specific candidate genes that are hypothesized to have a role in the pathophysiology of a given disorder. In ADHD, several preliminary reports of such candidate genes have been published.

Immunologically Related Genes

One group has focused on the immunological complement cascade protein C4B, which was found to be decreased in 23 probands with ADHD, their mothers, or both (Warren et al., 1995). In a recent report extending their finding, 55% of 31 probands with ADHD (versus 8% of controls) had a C4B null gene together with a specific hypervariable sequence on the nearby gene encoding the leukocyte marker HLA-DR4 (Odell, Warren, Warren, Burger, & Maciulis, 1997). We conducted a small replication study in collaboration with Warren and colleagues that was inconclusive. The level of C4B in our 21 probands with ADHD (mean 177 µg/mL, SD 85) did not differ significantly from that of the 15 healthy age-matched controls (215 ± 125) (Castellanos, Warren, Marsh, & Rapoport, 1996). However, this small study was not limited to subjects of northern European extraction as were the Utah samples, and we did not analyze HLA-DR4 in our subjects. Pending replication by other groups, it is tempting to wonder whether subjects with low C4B who are positive for HLA-DR4 may also have a greater vulnerability for other neuropsychiatric symptoms linked to autoimmune dysfunction (Swedo et al., 1998). For example, in children with the proposed syndrome of Pediatric Autoimmune Neuropsychiatric Disorders Associated with Streptococcus (PANDAS), it has been hypothesized that immune responses to streptococcal antigens also injure basal ganglia regions, as has been demonstrated in Sydenham's chorea (Giedd et al., 1995; Husby, Van de Rijn, Zabriskie, Abdin, & Williams, 1976).

Dopaminergic Genes in ADHD

The remaining candidate genes studied to date in ADHD have been dopaminergic. An allelic* variation in the DA transporter gene (DAT1)[†] was significantly associated with ADHD in a study of 53 families (Cook et al.,

1995). This polymorphism[‡] is located in the untranscribed 3' portion of the DAT1 gene, so that its functional significance remains unclear. Nevertheless, this finding has now been replicated in two independent samples (Gill, Daly, Heron, Hawi, & Fitzgerald, 1997; Waldman et al., 1996).

The DA 4 receptor (DRD4) has a large number of allelic variations, many of which are determined by the number of 48 base pair repeats in exon 3. The second most common form of DRD4 contains 7 repeats (DRD4*7R) and has been associated with the psychological trait of Novelty Seeking in some samples (Benjamin et al., 1996; Ebstein et al., 1996) but not in others (Malhotra et al., 1996; Sullivan et al., 1998). DRD4*7R was significantly associated with ADHD in a sample of 39 California patients contrasted to Canadian controls (LaHoste et al., 1996). Again, our group was unable to confirm this finding in 41 probands with ADHD and 56 ethnically matched controls (Castellanos et al., 1998). However, the same group has reported a replication using within-family controls that eliminates potential confounds due to ethnic variations in allele frequencies (Swanson, Sunohara, et al., 1998).

DRD4*7R does not exist in the mouse, but transgenic mice lacking DRD4 have been found to be less active in open field tests, and to have *improved* locomotor coordination, along with increased DA synthesis and turnover in striatum (Rubinstein et al., 1997). The technique of "knocking out" specific genes has some

---

*Except for genes on the sex chromosomes, all genes are inherited as pairs, one from each parent. Alternative forms of a given gene are called *alleles*.

†The DAT1 gene has two main alleles. The most commonly found form contains a DNA segment that is repeated 10 times, and the alternate form contains 9 repetitions. Since the 10-repeat allele is longer than the 9-repeat version, they can be distinguished by gel electrophoresis.

‡Some genetic variants are extremely rare, but others are found in substantial proportions of a given population. Common allelic variations are termed *polymorphisms*. Some polymorphisms result in changes in the protein structure of the gene product and are said to have functional significance. The polymorphism in DAT1 is found outside the region that codes for the transporter protein structure so it is not clear how function of DAT would be affected. If DAT1 increases the vulnerability for ADHD, one possibility is that this variation may affect the quantity of DAT that is transcribed and produced.

value in revealing the role of a given gene and its products, but the caveats on interpreting results from such studies are similar to those that apply to brain lesion studies, since the procedure eliminates not only the particular gene product but also all its interactions with its molecular "partners" throughout life. Fortunately, there are now gene "knock-out" mice for all 5 DA receptors (see review by Swanson, Castellanos, Murias, LaHoste, & Kennedy, 1998) and techniques have been developed that will allow genes to be turned on or off at the experimenter's whim (Nestler & Aghajanian, 1997).

To date, studies that have found evidence supporting one DA candidate gene in ADHD have not found significant effects for the other. This pattern of inconsistent findings has been the rule in complex genetic disorders. The increasing momentum of the Human Genome Project suggests that progress in understanding the molecular nature of ADHD will be attainable in the near future by the application of improved genetic analysis technologies and sampling strategies that reduce genetic heterogeneity. Such progress is not likely to lead to gene therapy techniques, but rather to a more nuanced understanding of the variety of disorders that are currently subsumed under the diagnosis of ADHD, as is now taking place in Alzheimer's disease with regard to age of onset. The difficulty is that until we are better able to determine what the biologically meaningful subtypes of ADHD are, our statistical power to detect true genetic effects will remain limited.

Phenomenological studies have offered some tentative answers. For example, it has been suggested that ADHD combined with CD or Antisocial Personality Disorder may "signal a distinct subtype of ADHD" (Faraone et al., 1995, p. 344). Children who have ADHD combined with reading disorder (RD) are neuropsychologically (Pennington, Groisser, & Welsh, 1993) and neuropsychopharmacologically (Halperin et al., 1997) distinct from children who have ADHD without RD. To date, the genetic validity of these and other distinctions (e.g., Inattentive type versus Combined type) has not been tested.

ADHD REFLECTS DYSFUNCTION IN DOPAMINERGIC SYSTEMS

Operation of the Dopaminergic Systems

For over a decade, there has been a consensus that no single neurotransmitter hypothesis of ADHD is tenable (Zametkin & Rapoport, 1987). However, for convenience, this discussion focuses first on DA, before turning to NE and EPI.

After synaptic release, DA is primarily deactivated by reuptake into the presynaptic terminal via the specific DA transporter (DAT1) (Bannon, Granneman, & Kapatos, 1995). Once inside the nerve terminal, monoamines, whether DA, NE, or serotonin (5HT), are repackaged into synaptic vesicles by the same vesicular monoamine transporter (VMAT2) (Bonisch & Eiden, 1998). Methylphenidate (MPH) blocks DAT1 and the NE transporter (NET) (Sonders, Zhu, Sahniser, Kavanaugh, & Amara, 1997), whereas amphetamines produce efflux through DAT1, NET, and VMAT2, and thus affect not only DA and NE but also 5HT (Henry, Sagne, Botton, Isambert, & Gasnier, 1998). The nearly immediate effect of either type of stimulant is an increase in the synaptic concentration of monoamines, which produces an initially increased postsynaptic effect. However, most monoaminergic circuits are tightly regulated, both by long-distance and local feedback from inhibitory receptors located mostly in presynaptic nerve terminals (see review in Castellanos, 1997b). These *autoreceptors* and other feedback circuits rapidly regulate the level of synaptic neurotransmitter release. The net effect of a particular dose of a given stimulant is thus a complex function of multiple elements, including pharmacokinetic factors (Le Moal, 1995; Roth & Elsworth, 1995). Also relevant is the particular system being affected, that is, whether it is primarily limbic, cognitive, or sensorimotor.

Dopamine and Locomotor Activity

Evidence for a dopaminergic role in ADHD is extensive (Castellanos, 1997b; Levy, 1991) including animal models in which dopaminergic terminals were destroyed with 6-hydroxydopa in neonatal rats (Shaywitz, Klopper, & Gordon, 1978), or with low doses of the neurotoxin MPTP in primates (Roeltgen & Schneider, 1991), or in the DAT1 knock-out mouse with its dramatic hyperkinesis (Giros, Jaber, Jones, Wightman, & Caron, 1996). It has been more difficult to find clear evidence of dopaminergic dysfunction in children with ADHD. Markers of DA metabolism (chiefly levels of the metabolite homovanillic acid [HVA]) in blood, urine, or cerebrospinal fluid (CSF) do not consistently differ from controls (Pliszka, McCracken, & Maas, 1996; Rogeness, Javors, & Pliszka, 1992). In part, this reflects intrinsic methodological limitations (Rogeness et al., 1992). Thus, although blood and urine are obtained relatively easily, they reflect peripheral as well as central metabolism. Further, most studies of urinary metabolites have used samples collected over 24 hr, rather than timed specimens collected during the performance of particular tasks (Hanna, Ornitz, & Hariharan, 1996). CSF measures (at least for HVA and the 5HT metabolite, 5-hydroxyindoleacetic acid [HIAA]) primarily reflect CNS metabolism, but they still do so indirectly, and it is ethically impossible to obtain CSF from well-characterized pediatric controls under controlled conditions. Despite these limitations, our group was able to conduct a sizable study of CSF in 45 boys with ADHD. Though we were limited to within-group correlational analyses, we found significant positive correlations between CSF HVA (obtained during drug-free baseline) and ratings of hyperactivity in two independently collected samples (Castellanos et al., 1994; Castellanos, Elia, et al., 1996). Furthermore, after baseline severity, CSF HVA was the best predictor of improvements in hyperactivity in a double-blind crossover study of MPH, dextroamphetamine (DEX), and placebo (N = 45), and in a subsequent controlled trial of pemoline in a subset of patients (n = 16). CSF HVA did not correlate significantly with performance on attentional tests. These results were interpreted as supporting a mediating role of central DA activity in stimulant drug efficacy in ADHD and in motoric hyperactivity but not in vigilance (Castellanos, Elia, et al., 1996). A similar positive correlation between plasma HVA and objectively measured activity levels (r = .35, N = 45, p < .02) has been reported; plasma HVA did not correlate significantly with measures of vigilance or impulsivity on the Continuous Performance Task (CPT) (Halperin et al., 1997).

Dopamine and Development

When considering the monoamines, it is important to attend to age factors. Of the three monoamines, DA is the most developmentally dynamic. DA metabolite levels in CSF peak in infancy and decline rapidly over the next 12 years (Hedner, Lundell, Breese, Mueller, & Hedner, 1986). The rate of decrease slows by early adolescence, but continues inexorably, as demonstrated by decreases in DAT1 during healthy aging of 6.6% per decade (Volkow et al., 1996). Brain blood flow and metabolism also decline during the pediatric age range (Chugani, Phelps, & Mazziotta, 1987) and so does the overall level of locomotor activity in healthy children (Levy, 1980). Activity levels of normal children have not been compared to CSF DA metabolites, but the conclusion that the two are positively correlated is supported by studies carried out in adults (Banki, 1977; Post, Kotin, Goodwin, & Gordon, 1973) and in animals (Chaouloff, Laude, Guezennec, & Elghozi, 1986). In a 4-year longitudinal study of 106 boys with ADHD, the symptoms of hyperactivity-impulsivity, but not of inattention, declined linearly with increasing age (Hart, Lahey, Loeber, Applegate, & Frick, 1995), further supporting the hypothesis that central DA levels are positively correlated with symptoms of hyperactivity-impulsivity in ADHD.

Dopamine Agonists, Antagonists, and Autoreceptors

One possible explanation for the puzzling efficacy of both stimulants and neuroleptics in decreasing the behavioral symptoms of ADHD in children might be that the effects of stimulants, in clinical doses, are mediated primarily by inhibitory autoreceptors (Zametkin &

Rapoport, 1987). In the only clinical test of this hypothesis, Solanto (1986) administered a very low dose of MPH (0.1 mg/kg) and placebo to 12 children with DSM-III ADDH (see Chapter 1, this volume). In this carefully controlled study, she found a significant decrease in locomotor activity on drug, but no significant effects on an attentional measure, and concluded that her data provided more support for the notion that "stimulant drug effects are mediated by inhibitory autoreceptors rather than that they are due to effects at postsynaptic receptors sites" (p. 100). This small but potentially pivotal study has unfortunately been neither refuted nor replicated. It is also not possible to determine whether the apparent selectivity of the drug effect for locomotor activity rather than for attention reflected a true difference, or whether it reflected the small sample size. Still, it remains an excellent example of an elegant hypothesis-driven clinical study, and deserves greater attention than it has received. It is worth noting that DA neurons from the ventral tegmental area (VTA), which primarily innervate cortex and limbic regions, do not have inhibitory autoreceptors (Meador-Woodruff, Damask, & Watson, 1994). This intriguing absence may underlie the lack of long-term tolerance to the therapeutic effects of the stimulants in ADHD (Castellanos, 1997b).

Dopamine and Hyperactive Rats

Further evidence supporting a link between DA and hyperactivity comes from the study of genetically inbred rat strains derived from the Wistar–Kyoto (WKY) rat, the spontaneously hypertensive-hyperactive rat (SHR), and two derived strains, one of which is hypertensive and not hyperactive (WKHT), and another that is hyperactive but not hypertensive (WKHA) (Hendley & Fan, 1992). The latter strain differs from the remaining ones in having significantly increased DA uptake and the lowest rate of NE uptake in prefrontal cortex, though not in striatum. Recent work has focused on locating the genetic substrates of the hyperactivity in WKHA rats. A highly significant quantitative locus (lod score 9.5) has been identified in rat chromosome 8 that does not correspond to rat DAT1 but otherwise remains unidentified (Moisan et al., 1996).

Dopamine and Reward and Salience

Since the discovery that intracranial self-stimulation sites were principally populated by midbrain DA neurons, DA has been implicated in brain circuits mediating reward and reinforcement. Some "DA neurons and neurons in the ventral striatum only respond to reward when it is not entirely predictable, such as during the trial-and-error learning of tasks with specific constraints and during self-initiated movements without preceding reward-predicting stimuli. . . . It appears . . . that the response is due to the *salient,* alerting stimulus property of primary reward during learning" (Schultz, Apicella, Ljungberg, Romo, & Scarnati, 1993, p. 234; emphasis added). Salience and the hedonic elements of reward are often confounded, but when they are experimentally dissociated, it is salience that is dopaminergically based (Berridge, Vernier, & Robinson, 1989; Peciña, Berridge, & Parker, 1997; Robinson & Berridge, 1993; Schultz & Romo, 1990). The only brain region that was consistently activated by low doses of either MPH or dextroamphetamine (DEX) in rat (Porrino & Lucignani, 1987; Porrino, Lucignani, Dow-Edwards, & Sokoloff, 1984) is the nucleus accumbens, which is the brain region most closely linked to reward and salience.

Reward hypotheses of ADHD have been proposed (see Solanto, Wender, & Bartell, 1997) but the distinction between hedonic and salient components has not been attended to, which may explain in part why results have not always been consistent. In an explicit test of the reward dysfunction hypothesis, Solanto and colleagues (1997) found that while both MPH and behavioral contingencies improved performance on a CPT, only MPH "enhanced processes that mediate the regulation of effort over time" (p. 123). The processes that regulate effort over time are likely modulated, at least partly, by DA in the prefrontal cortex.

Dopamine and Executive Function

Whereas the DA cells arising in the substantia nigra pars compacta (SNpc) primarily innervate the striatum (i.e., caudate nucleus and putamen), the VTA contains DA cells that innervate the nucleus accumbens and the frontal cortex diffusely (Goldman-Rakic, Lidow, Smiley, & Williams, 1992). Work in primates has demonstrated that DA is involved in "direct gating of selective excitatory synaptic inputs to prefrontal neurons during cognition" (Williams & Goldman-Rakic, 1995, p. 572). The applicability of these effects in humans was demonstrated in a study in which volunteers underwent blood flow measurements with positron-emission tomography after double-blind placebo and DEX while performing two distinct cognitive tasks. In both types of tasks, DEX enhanced the signal-to-noise ratio of cortical activation by increasing activation in those regions previously found to be associated with the specific task and by decreasing nonspecific activation in uninvolved regions (Mattay *et al.,* 1996). Although this elegant experiment has not been conducted in subjects with ADHD, it offers an example of what is likely taking place in the cortex when individuals with ADHD benefit from stimulant medications. In the PFC the classic model of a hypofunctioning DA system is most likely to be correct in ADHD (Castellanos, 1997b).

ADHD REFLECTS DYSFUNCTION IN NORADRENERGIC AND ADRENERGIC NEUROTRANSMISSION

Although DA hypotheses of ADHD have their appeal, they do not account for the substantial efficacy of NE drugs for symptoms of hyperactivity-impulsivity, and for the poor efficacy of direct DA agonists (McCracken, 1991; Zametkin & Rapoport, 1987). However, the reverse is also true, because NE agents such as the tricyclic antidepressants, while unquestionably effective compared to placebo (see meta-analysis in Spencer *et al.,* 1996), have had modest effects when contrasted to MPH, particularly in cognitive testing (Garfinkel, Wender, Sloman, & O'Neill, 1983; Rapoport, Quinn, Bradbard, Riddle, & Brooks, 1974), with one exception (Kupietz & Balka, 1976).

In a review of the putative interaction between NE, DA, and possibly EPI, Pliszka and colleagues (1996) summarized the work of Posner and colleagues in delineating an NE posterior parietal network associated with vigilance (Posner & Dehaene, 1994) and DA prefrontal-striatal-thalamo-cortical circuits associated with executive functions. They proposed seven possible lesions in these distributed circuits: (1) a fundamental dysregulation in paragigantocellularis (the major excitatory input to the LC), (2) a deficit in central EPI, (3) dysfunction in peripheral EPI, (4) dysfunction "of brainstem mechanisms which effect a 'hand off' from the posterior NE-mediated system to more DA-mediated anterior executive system" (p. 270), (5) disruptions in PFC (either dorsolateral or medial-orbital), (6) excessive DA activity in nucleus accumbens, and (7) deficient dorsolateral PFC regulation of LC.

The last of these possibilities is supported by work on the modulating effects of both DA and NE in PFC functioning of primates and rodents (summarized in Arnsten, 1997; sell also Arnsten, Steere, & Hunt, 1996). Arnsten (1997) began by noting that DA, within a narrow range, is crucial for optimal PFC functioning. High levels of stress increase PFC DA beyond the optimal range, thus drastically impairing working memory performance. High levels of NE also "shut down" the PFC, via effects on $\alpha 1$ receptors (NE at physiological levels has greater affinity for $\alpha 2$ than for $\alpha 1$ receptors). The decrement in PFC function can be completely blocked by agonists for the $\alpha 2A$ receptor (such as the subtype-specific agonist guanfacine), which are densely distributed throughout PFC. Guanfacine improves PFC function in aged monkeys, and it produced improvements in CPT testing in children in an open trial (Chappell *et al.,* 1995). Arnsten (1997) provided substantial evidence that the LC influences PFC function, but she also noted "the PFC provides one of the few 'intelligent' inputs to the locus coeruleus" (p. 159) with evidence of both inhibitory and excitatory modulation. Clinical indirect evidence in support of an NE role in ADHD also comes from the replicated finding that children with ADHD and RD have significantly higher levels of the NE metabolite, 3-methoxy-4-hgdroxyphenylglycol (MHPG), in plasma than do children with ADHD without RD (Halperin *et al.*, 1997). Further interpretation of this finding awaits confirmation in a study that includes a healthy control group. Nevertheless, it is incontrovertible that DA and NE systems interact at multiple levels, including at the PFC. This complex relationship, implicated in ADHD, also appears to involve EPI.

EPI is a potent endogenous (α_2 agonist and has been implicated in ADHD as the potential source of "a defect in tonic adrenaline mediated inhibition of locus coeruleus stimulation" (Mefford & Potter, 1989, p. 33). A preliminary study in 12 boys with ADHD found decreased urinary EPI excretion during intelligence testing relative to controls (Hanna *et al.*, 1996), supporting the EPI hypothesis (as further elaborated by McCracken, 1991). However, enthusiasm for catecholamine studies of ADHD has diminished in proportion to increasing interest in molecular genetic and neuroimaging techniques. The latter are briefly reviewed in the remaining pages of this chapter, but greater detail is available elsewhere (Castellanos, 1997a). The reader should note that all ADHD pediatric neuroimaging samples to date have been characterized by considerable comorbidity, especially for Oppositional Defiant Disorder (ODD), with one exception (Filipek *et al.*, 1997; Semrud-Clikeman *et al.*, 1994).

THE BRAIN REGIONS IMPLICATED IN ADHD INCLUDE THE PREFRONTAL CORTEX, BASAL GANGLIA, LOCUS COERULEUS, CEREBELLUM, AND POSSIBLY AMYGDALA

The essential nature of PFC for the performance of EF (Denckla, 1996) is captured "by the metaphor of a symphony orchestra in which the conductor of the symphony is the frontal lobes and the nonfrontal regions of the cortex represent the various musical sections of the symphony" (Thatcher, 1991, p. 417). Rather than attempt to summarize the immense literature on the PFC (superbly condensed in Fuster, 1997), the following discussion is based on a pair of synthetic reviews that are strongly recommended (Houk & Wise, 1995; Wise, Murray, & Gerfen, 1996).

Wise and colleagues take as their starting point the fundamental nature of the key cells in PFC, the cortical pyramidal cells. They are the central integrators of multiple inputs, and they have the capability of firing in graded strengths rather than in all-or-none fashion (Houk & Wise, 1995). Because of this, pyramidal cells are well suited to carry out complex calculations, integrating higher order information from all brain regions, and carrying out top-down regulation of other lower order processes. Pyramidal cells are exquisitely sensitive to, among other factors, their DA and NE afferents, as discussed previously.

Alexander, DeLong, and Strick (1986) noted that several discrete circuits could be delineated connecting prefrontal pyramidal cell afferents to basal ganglia relay stations, which then synapse at thalamic nuclei, which in turn feed back to cortex. These cortical-striatal-thalamo-cortical circuits provide both positive and negative feedback to other cortical regions, and they serve as the anatomic substrate for EF. Since the Alexander and colleagues study, these circuits have been the object of intense study in rodents, nonhuman primates, and humans (Albin, Young, & Penney, 1995; DeLong, 1990; Gerfen, 1992; Yeterian & Van Hoesen, 1978). In Figure 1, PFC is schematized as a single rectangular box with excitatory outputs to other cortical regions (here limited to parietal cortex) (Halperin *et al.*, 1997), caudate nucleus and nucleus accumbens (referred to as striatum) (Mink & Thach, 1993; Parent, 1990), amygdala (Haber & Fudge, 1997), LC (Arnsten, 1997), and subthalamic nucleus (STN) (Smith & Grace, 1992; Wichmann, Bergman, & DeLong, 1994). Cortical, thalamic, and STN efferents

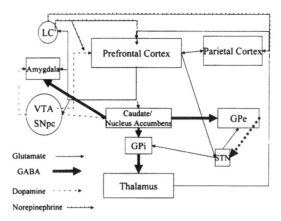

FIGURE 1. Schematic "circuit diagram" of brain regions putatively involved in ADHD. LC = locus coeruleus, VTA = ventral tegmental area, SNpc = substantia nigra pars compacta, GP$_i$ = globus pallidus internal segment, GP$_e$ = globus pallidus external segment, STN = subthalamic nucleus. The GABAergic projection from GP$_e$ is weaker than the other links of the circuit. Cerebellar circuits are not included in this diagram, but they may interact through the thalamus; the cerebellar vermis interacts with the amygdala.

are all glutamatergic and excitatory. All striatal and pallidal output neurons* are GABAergic and inhibitory. VTA and SNpc DA neurons can be excitatory or inhibitory depending on whether they activate D1 or D2 DA receptors, respectively. LC NE neurons also have complex effects depending on the balance of NE receptors activated and the state of the organism (Rajkowski, Kubiak, & Aston-Jones, 1994).

Signals that travel from the striatum *directly* to GP$_i$ disinhibit thalamic excitatory fibers, with the net result being positive feedback to the cortex. The *indirect pathway* includes the GP$_e$ and STN, with the latter receiving an important input directly from the PFC. Neuronal traffic through this pathway maintains the tonic level of inhibition produced by this system as its default state. Thus, the indirect pathway can be said to be the brain's braking mechanism (Wichman & DeLong, 1993). The identification of functionally segregated direct and indirect circuits that allow for complex regulation of inhibitory and excitatory influences at

*The *striatum* is composed of the caudate nucleus, putamen, and nucleus accumbens. The *pallidum* is composed of the lateral globus pallidus (or external GP (GP$_e$)) and the medial globus pallidus (also known as the internal segment of the globus pallidus (GP$_i$)). To further complicate matters, the putamen and globus pallidus are also sometimes described as the *lenticular nucleus*.

thalamic and cortical levels has been one of the principal achievements of the past decade (Gerfen, 1992). The tripartite classification of these circuits (association, limbic, and sensory-motor) parallels the disorders of EF, emotional regulation, and motor control such as ADHD, OCD, and Tourette's disorder, respectively (Baxter, 1990; Hallett, 1993; Modell, Mountz, Curtis, & Greden, 1989; Saint-Cyr, Taylor, & Nicholson, 1995).

Anatomic Studies of Brain Differences in ADHD

The schematic shown in Figure 1 represents regions that are known to be linked in functional circuits and that have also been hypothesized to be implicated in the pathophysiology of ADHD. However, most of the work underlying these insights has come from preclinical observations. One way of testing these hypotheses is to determine whether patients with ADHD differ from controls in these anatomic regions.

MRI is ideally suited for quantification of the corpus callosum, and all research groups have started there. Although total corpus callosum area in ADHD subjects has not differed from controls, smaller anterior regions have been found (Baumgardner *et al.*, 1996; Giedd *et* al., 1994; Hynd et al., 1991) and one study reported smaller posterior area (Semrud-Clikeman et al., 1994). The largest MRI study did not confirm these differences (Castellanos, Giedd, et al., 1996) although there were methodological differences which have not yet been resolved.

In healthy subjects, the right anterior brain is slightly but consistently larger than the left. Significant decreases of this asymmetry in ADHD have been reported using computed tomography (Shaywitz, Shaywitz, Byrne, Cohen, & Rothman, 1983), and MRI (Castellanos, Giedd, et al., 1996; Filipek et al., 1997; Hynd, Semrud-Clikeman, Lorys, Novey, & Eliopulos, 1990).

Abnormalities of caudate nucleus volume (Castellanos, Giedd, et al., 1996; Filipek et al., 1997), or asymmetry (Castellanos, Giedd, et al., 1996; Hynd et al., 1993; Mataró, García-Sánchez, Junqué, Estévez-González, & Pujol, 1997) have been reported although the studies differ in whether normal caudate is asymmetric, and whether this asymmetry normally favors the right or the left caudate. These inconsistencies may reflect differences in methodology and comorbidity.

The output nuclei of the basal ganglia are the internal segment of the globus pallidus and the substantia nigra pars reticulata, but the latter cannot be measured with MRI, and the globus pallidus can be measured only as a unit (lateral and medial segments together), and then only with difficulty. Still, this region has been found to be significantly smaller in ADHD (Aylward et al., 1996; Castellanos, Giedd, et al., 1996), although these two studies again differed in finding the larger difference on the left and right sides, respectively.

An early computed tomography study found a trend toward greater cerebellar atrophy in adults with a prior history of hyperkinetic minimal brain dysfunction (Nasrallah et al., 1986). We recently found that the cerebellar vermis is significantly smaller in ADHD (Berquin et al., 1998), although a similar observation was made in childhood-onset schizophrenia (Jacobsen et al., 1997). These findings are consistent with the more prominent role ascribed to the cerebellum in cognition and modulation of emotions (Schmahmann, 1996).

Functional Brain Imaging Studies of ADHD

The best-known functional study used [^{18}F]-fluoro-2-deoxy-D-glucose (FDG) positron emission tomography (PET) to demonstrate decreased frontal cerebral metabolism in adults with ADHD (Zametkin et al., 1990). Subsequent work also detected increases in right caudate metabolism after amphetamine under some conditions (Matochik et al., 1993), although inconsistent results in adolescents (Ernst et al., 1994; Zametkin et al., 1993) have led the authors to explore other techniques in ADHD. Other investigators of brain function have measured local cerebral blood flow, which closely approximates neuronal activity, with a variety of techniques including ^{133}Xenon inhalation and single positron emission computerized tomography (SPECT). Decreased blood flow has been found in ADHD subjects in the striatum (Lou, Henriksen, & Bruhn, 1990) and in prefrontal regions (Amen, Paldi, & Thisted, 1993). However, these results remain tentative because ethical constraints make it difficult to obtain truly independent observations from normal controls. A more promising technique may be blood oxygenation level dependent (BOLD) functional magnetic resonance imaging (fMRI), which obviates the need to use ionizing radiation. A preliminary report using this new technology has once again shown hypoperfusion in the right caudate, which reversed on optimal dose MPH treatment (Teicher et al., 1996). However, the exquisite sensitivity of this technique to motion artifact remains an obstacle.

ADHD MAY REFLECT DYSFUNCTION IN THE BEHAVIORAL INHIBITION SYSTEM MEDIATED BY THE AMYGDALA-SEPTO-HIPPOCAMPAL SYSTEM

Based on extensive work done primarily in rodents, Gray (1982) described three systems of behavioral regulation: a DA mediated reward or facilitation system, a fight-or-flight system that responds to unconditioned pain or punishment, and a behavioral inhibition system (BIS) that provides for "the cessation of ongoing behavior, an increase in nonspecific arousal, and a focusing of attention on relevant environmental cues" (Quay, 1997, p. 8). The anatomic substrates of BIS in rodents are the amygdala-septo-hippocampal system and its connections to the PFC, and its chemical bases are believed to be NE inputs from the LC and 5-HT inputs from the raphe nucleus. The influential role of the amygdala and its intricate interactions with limbic-related DA neurons in VTA and SNpc have drawn recent interest (Burns, Annett, Kelley, Everitt, & Robbins, 1996; Haber & Fudge, 1997; Han, McMahan, Holland, & Gallagher, 1997). Quay (1983, 1988, 1997) has been the most eloquent proponent of the view that ADHD can best be understood as the result of a hypofunctioning BIS, and that CD is associated with an overactive reward system.

There is both pharmacologic and neuropsychological evidence for an underactive BIS in ADHD. Because stimulants affect both NE and DA systems, their effects do not discriminate between the relative importance of the two systems. However, BIS functioning is impaired, whether in rodents or humans, by antianxiety drugs such as benzodiazepines or barbiturates, which are strikingly ineffective in ADHD. Iaboni, Douglas, and Ditto (1997) have presented the best evidence of the continuing relevance of the BIS theory. These authors examined heart rate (HR) and skin conductance levels (SCL) of 18 children with ADHD and 18 normal children performing a repetitive motor task during reward and extinction conditions. The authors predicted that increased HR in response to reward would reflect activation of the behavioral activation system, whereas increased SCL in response to extinction would reflect activation of the BIS. They found an impressive absence of SCL changes in the ADHD children during extinction trials, in contrast to the normal children, who exhibited robust evidence of autonomic responsivity. The only difficulty with this study is that 12 of the ADHD boys also met criteria for ODD and a further 4 met

criteria for CD. Thus, it is not clear whether their results can be ascribed solely to their primary disorder, ADHD, or whether comorbidity with CD and ODD played a major role. Neuroimaging studies are just now beginning to address the role of the amygdala-septal-hippocampal complex in substance abuse (Breiter et al., 1997); these techniques are likely to be useful in ADHD.

ADHD, BRAIN LATERALIZATION, AND RIGHT HEMISPHERE SYNDROMES

Extensive discussions of brain asymmetry can be found elsewhere (see Davidson & Hugdahl, 1995; Hellige, 1993). A credible argument cannot be made that ADHD represents dysfunction of exclusively right-sided structures, but a preponderance of the evidence from a variety of sources (Carter, Krener, Chaderjian, Northcutt, & Wolfe, 1995; Casey et al., 1997; Denckla, Rudel, Chapman, & Krieger, 1985; Duane, Clark, & Gottlob, 1996; García-Sánchez, Estévez-González, Suárez-Romero, & Junqué, 1997; Gross-Tsur, Shalev, Manor, & Amir, 1995; Malone, Kershner, & Siegel, 1988; Malone, Couitis, Kershner, & Logan, 1994; Malone, Kershner, & Swanson, 1994; Mann, Lubar, Zimmerman, Miller, & Muenchen, 1992; Nigg, Swanson, & Hinshaw, 1997; Voeller, 1995; Voeller & Heilman, 1988; Weinberg & Harper, 1993), including most of the neuroimaging studies just cited, suggests that brain dysfunction in ADHD is weighed toward the right hemisphere (Brumback & Staton, 1982; Heilman, Voeller, & Nadeau, 1991).

CONCLUSIONS AND FUTURE DIRECTIONS

Current models of the neurobiology of ADHD remain highly speculative in their details; even as the overall outline becomes clearer, unresolved questions remain at every level of analysis but provide a blueprint for systematic investigation in the middle term.

1. Although we have still not reached a consensus regarding the core neuropsychological-neurophysiological deficits in ADHD, there are broadly based candidates, such as EF, or more specific (but polymorphous) concepts, such as inhibition, delay aversion, or reward and salience. As we further refine our operational definitions and hypotheses, we need to attend more rigorously to the problem of discriminant validity, particularly with regard to other disruptive behavior disorders and learning disorders.

2. Most, though not all, neurobiological studies of ADHD have tended to preferentially include patients that would now be classified as DSM-IV (American Psychiatric Association, 1994) Combined type ADHD. Are there fundamental differences between ADHD subtypes? Are DSM-IV criteria stringent enough to allow comparison of studies across groups, or should ICD-10 (World Health Organization, 1992) criteria also be applied, as has recently been proposed (Swanson, Castellanos, *et al.,* 1998)?

3. As reflected by the dearth of neurobiological studies on ADHD in girls, this review has not discussed the male predominance. We need to determine whether the neurobiology of ADHD differs by sex, and whether there are specific or nonspecific protective and vulnerability factors.

4. We do not have neurobiological data relating to long-term outcome. How important will genetic factors be?

5. Genetic studies of multiplex families are proceeding in more than a dozen centers. At least in the United States., there has yet to be any coordination among centers. Based on the disappointing results of other such endeavors (e.g., in Tourette's syndrome), it is likely that a collaborative approach ultimately will be needed, if not in the first phase, then certainly for the replication phases that are now required by genetics journals before publication.

6. Candidate gene studies are "easier" than multiplex family studies, but it is highly likely that many pertinent candidates exist outside the DA system. Subtle genetic variants that influence (but do not prevent) normal brain development, especially those that affect lateralization should be given high priority when they are identified in nonhuman systems.

7. Pharmacological approaches to ADHD have been limited to monoaminergically active drugs. Will new drugs that modulate amino acid neurotransmitters, such as GABA and glutamate (Ferraro *et al.,* 1997), expand our options and our insights into ADHD?

8. In the burgeoning field of neuroimaging, much work needs to be done to resolve methodological issues, and the focus needs to be on understanding normal brain development and psychiatric disorders through longitudinal study. A workshop organized by several NIH institutes (Tools for Pediatric Neuroimaging, Reston, VA, 1997) has begun exploring a consortium approach for these purposes. While these technologies are not yet able to reliably provide diagnostic information, the proximal goal is that of developing anatomic and functional imaging phenotypes that can be used to improve the utility of genetic-molecular approaches. An iterative approach using both anatomic and functional techniques and incorporating state-of-the-art cognitive neuroscience paradigms will be needed.

Despite the cavernous gaps in our knowledge, we can anticipate an increasing tempo of research in the field of child and adolescent psychopathology, benefiting from the explosive growth of genetics, neuroscience, and neuroimaging. However, those exciting developments will not benefit our patients without the continuing efforts of the current and future generations of child psychiatrists and psychologists.

REFERENCES

Albin, R. L., Young, A. B., & Penney, J. B. (1995). The functional anatomy of disorders of the basal ganglia. *Trends in Neuroscience, 18,* 63–64.

Alexander, G. E., DeLong, M. R., & Strick, P. L. (1986). Parallel organization of functionally segregated circuits linking basal ganglia and cortex. *Annual Review of Neuroscience, 9,* 357–381.

Amen, D. G., Paldi, J. H., & Thisted, R. A. (1993). Brain SPECT imaging. *Journal of the American Academy of Child and Adolescent Psychiatry, 32,* 1080–1081.

American Psychiatric Association. (1994). *Diagnostic and statistical manual of mental disorders* (4th ed.). Washington, DC: Author.

Arnsten, A. F. (1997). Catecholamine regulation of the prefrontal cortex. *Journal of Psychopharmacology, 11*, 151–162.

Arnsten, A. F., Steere, J. C., & Hunt, R. D. (1996). The contribution of alpha 2-noradrenergic mechanisms of prefrontal cortical cognitive function. Potential significance for attention-deficit hyperactivity disorder. *Archives of General Psychiatry, 53*, 448–455.

Aylward, E. H., Reiss, A. L., Reader, M. J., Singer, H. S., Brown, J. E., & Denckla, M. B. (1996). Basal ganglia volumes in children with attention-deficit hyperactivity disorder. *Journal of Child Neurology, 11*, 112–115.

Banki, C. M. (1977). Correlation between cerebrospinal fluid amine metabolites and psychomotor activity in affective disorders. *Journal of Neurochemistry, 28*, 255–257.

Bannon, M. J., Granneman, J. G., & Kapatos, G. (1995). The dopamine transporter: Potential involvement in neuropsychiatric disorders. In F. E. Bloom & D. J. Kupfer (Eds.), *Psychopharmacology: The fourth generation of progress* (pp. 179–188). New York: Raven.

Baumgardner, T. L., Singer, H. S., Denckla, M. B., Rubin, M. A., Abrams, M. T., Colli, M. J., & Reiss, A. L. (1996). Corpus callosum morphology in children with Tourette syndrome and attention deficit hyperactivity disorder. *Neurology, 47*, 477–482.

Baxter, L. R. (1990). Brain imaging as a tool in establishing a theory of brain pathology in obsessive compulsive disorder. *Journal of Clinical Psychiatry, 51*(2 (Suppl.)), 22–25.

Benjamin, J., Li, L., Patterson, C., Greenberg, B. D., Murphy, D. L., & Hamer, D. H. (1996). Population and familial association between the D4 dopamine receptor gene and measures of Novelty Seeking. *Nature Genetics, 12*, 81–84.

Berquin, P. C., Giedd, J. N., Jacobsen, L. K., Hamburger, S. D., Krain, A. L., Rapoport, J. L., & Castellanos, F. X. (1998). The cerebellum in attention-deficit/hyperactivity disorder: A morphometric study. *Neurology, 50*, 1087–1093.

Berridge, K., Vernier, I. L., & Robinson, T. E. (1989). Taste reactivity analysis of 6-hydroxydopamine induced aphagia: Implications for arousal and anhedonia hypotheses of dopamine function. *Behavioral Neuroscience, 103*, 36–45.

Bonisch, H., & Eiden, L. (1998). Catecholamine reuptake and storage: Overview. *Advances in Pharmacology, 42*, 149–164.

Bourgeois, J. P., & Rakic, P. (1993). Changes of synaptic density in the primary visual cortex of the macaque monkey from fetal to adult stage. *Journal of Neuroscience, 13*, 2801–2820.

Breiter, H. C., Gollub, R. L., Weisskoff, R. M., Kennedy, D. N., Makris, N., Berke, J. D., Goodman, J. M., Kantor, H. L., Gastfriend, D. R., Riorden, J. P., Mathew, R. T., Rosen, B. R., & Hyman, S. E. (1997). Acute effects of cocaine on human brain activity and emotion. *Neuron, 19*, 591–611.

Brumback, R. A., & Staton, R. D. (1982). Right hemisphere involvement in learning disability, attention deficit disorder, and childhood major depressive disorder. *Medical Hypotheses, 8*, 505–514.

Buchsbaum, M., & Wender, P. (1973). Average evoked responses in normal and minimally brain dysfunctioned children treated with amphetamine. *Archives of General Psychiatry, 29*, 764–770.

Burns, L. H., Annett, L., Kelley, A. E., Everitt, B. J., & Robbins, T. W. (1996). Effects of lesions to amygdala, ventral subiculum, medial prefrontal cortex, and nucleus accumbens on the reaction to novelty: Implication for limbic–striatal interactions. *Behavioral Neuroscience, 110*, 60–73.

Cadoret, R. J., & Stewart, M. A. (1991). An adoption study of attention deficit/hyperactivity/aggression and their relationship to adult antisocial personality. *Comprehensive Psychiatry, 32*, 73–82.

Carter, C. S., Krener, P., Chaderjian, M., Northcutt, C., & Wolfe, V. (1995). Asymmetrical visual-spatial attentional performance in ADHD: Evidence for a right hemispheric deficit. *Biological Psychiatry, 37*, 789–797.

Casey, B. J., Castellanos, F. X., Giedd, J. N., Marsh, W. L., Hamburger, S. D., Schubert, A. B., Vauss, Y. C., Vaituzis, A. C., Dickstein, D. P., Sarfatti, S. E., & Rapoport, J. L. (1997). Implication of right frontostriatal circuitry in response inhibition and attention-deficit/hyperactivity disorder. *Journal of the American Academy of Child and Adolescent Psychiatry, 36*, 374–383.

Castellanos, F. X. (1997a). Neuroimaging of attention-deficit hyperactivity disorder. *Child and Adolescent Psychiatric Clinics of North America, 6*, 383–411.

Castellanos, F. X. (1997b). Toward a pathophysiology of attention-deficit/hyperactivity disorder. *Clinical Pediatrics, 36*, 381–393.

Castellanos, F. X., Elia, J., Kruesi, M. J. P., Gulotta, C. S., Mefford, I. N., Potter, W. Z., Ritchie, G. F., & Rapoport, J. L. (1994). Cerebrospinal fluid monoamine metabolites in boys with attention-deficit hyperactivity disorder. *Psychiatry Research, 52*, 305–316.

Castellanos, F. X., Elia, J., Kruesi, M. J. P., Marsh, W. L., Gulotta, C. S., Potter, W. Z., Ritchie, G. F., Hamburger, S. D., Rapoport, J. L., & Kruesi, M. J. (1996). Cerebrospinal homovanillic acid predicts behavioral response to stimulants in 45 boys with attention-deficit/hyperactivity disorder. *Neuropsychopharmacology, 14*, 125–137.

Castellanos, F. X., Giedd, J. N., Marsh, W. L., Hamburger, S. D., Vaituzis, A. C., Dickstein, D. P., Sarfatti, S. E., Vauss, Y. C., Snell, J. W., Lange, N., Kaysen, D., Krain, A. L., Ritchie, G. F., Rajapakse, J. C., & Rapoport, J. L. (1996). Quantitative brain magnetic resonance imaging in attention-deficit/hyperactivity disorder. *Archives of General Psychiatry, 53*, 607–616.

Castellanos, F. X., Lau, E., Tayebi, N., Lee, P., Long, R. E., Giedd, J. N., Sharp, W. S., Marsh, W. L., Walter, J. M., Hamburger, S.D., Ginns, E. I., Rapoport, J. L., & Sidransky, E. (1998). Lack of association between a dopamine-4 receptor polymorphism and attention-deficit/hyperactivity disorder: Genetic and brain morphometric analyses. *Molecular Psychiatry, 3,* 431–434.

Castellanos, F. X., Warren, R. P., Marsh, W. L., & Rapoport, J. L. (1996). [Complement 4B protein in ADHD: Attempted replication in an independent sample.] Unpublished raw data.

Chabot, R. J., & Serfontein, G. (1996). Quantitative electroencephalographic profiles of children with attention deficit disorder. *Biological Psychiatry, 40,* 951–963.

Chaouloff, F., Laude, D., Guezennec, Y., & Elghozi, J. L. (1986). Motor activity increases tryptophan, 5-hydroxyindoleacetic acid, and homovanillic acid in ventricular cerebrospinal fluid of the conscious rat. *Journal of Neurochemistry, 46,* 1313–1316.

Chappell, P. B., Riddle, M. A., Scahill, L., Lynch, K. A., Schultz, R., Arnsten, A., Leckman, J. F., & Cohen, D. J. (1995). Guanfacine treatment of comorbid attention-deficit hyperactivity disorder and Tourette's syndrome: Preliminary clinical experience. *Journal of the American Academy of Child and Adolescent Psychiatry, 34,* 1140–1146.

Chelune, G. J., Ferguson, W., Koon, R., & Dickey, T. O. (1986). Frontal lobe disinhibition in attention deficit disorder. *Child Psychiatry and Human Development, 16,* 221–234.

Chugani, H. T., Phelps, M. E., & Mazziotta, J. C. (1987). Positron emission tomography study of human brain functional development. *Annals of Neurology, 22,* 487–497.

Cook, E. H., Jr., Stein, M. A., Krasowski, M. D., Cox, N. J., Olkon, D. M., Kieffer, J. E., & Leventhal, B. L. (1995). Association of attention deficit disorder and the dopamine transporter gene. *American Journal of Human Genetics, 56,* 993–998.

Corning, W. C., Steffy, R. A., Anderson, E., & Bowers, P. (1986). EEG "maturational lag" profiles: Follow-up analyses. *Journal of Abnormal Child Psychology, 14,* 235–249.

Davidson, R. J., & Hugdahl, K. (Eds.). (1995). *Brain asymmetry.* Cambridge, MA: MIT Press.

DeLong, M. R. (1990). Primate models of movement disorders of basal ganglia origin. *Trends in Neuroscience, 13,* 281–285.

Denckla, M. B. (1996). A theory and model of executive function. A neuropsychological perspective. In G. R. Lyon & N. A. Krasnegor (Eds.), *Attention, memory, and executive function.* (pp. 263–278). Baltimore: Brookes.

Denckla, M. B., Rudel, R. G., Chapman, C., & Krieger, J. (1985). Motor proficiency in dyslexic children with and without attentional disorders. *Archives of Neurology, 42,* 228–231.

Desimone, R. (1996). Neural mechanisms for visual memory and their role in attention. *Proceedings of the Na-tional Academy of Sciences of the United States of America, 93,* 13494–13499.

Dobbing, J., & Sands, J. (1973). Quantitative growth and development of human brain. *Archives of Diseases of Children, 48,* 757–767.

Duane, D. D., Clark, M., & Gottlob, L. (1996). Right hemisphere dysfunction correlates with non-wakefulness in attention deficit disorder [Abstract]. *Neurology, 46* [Suppl], A125.

Ebstein, R. P., Novick, O., Umansky, R., Priel, B., Osher, Y., Blaine, D., Bennett, E. R., Nemanov, L., Katz, M., & Belmaker, R. H. (1996). Dopamine D4 receptor (D4DR) exon III polymorphism associated with the human personality trait of Novelty Seeking. *Nature Genetics, 12,* 78–80.

Epstein, H. T. (1986). Stages in human brain development. *Brain Research, 395,* 114–119.

Ernst, M., Liebenauer, L. L., King, A. C., Fitzgerald, G. A., Cohen, R. M., & Zametkin, A. J. (1994). Reduced brain metabolism in hyperactive girls. *Journal of the American Academy of Child and Adolescent Psychiatry, 33,* 858–868.

Faraone, S. V., Biederman, J., Chen, W. J., Krifcher, B., Keenan, K., Moore, C., Sprich, S., & Tsuang, M. T. (1992). Segregation analysis of attention deficit hyperactivity disorder. *Psychiatric Genetics, 2,* 257–275.

Faraone, S. V., Biederman, J., Chen, W. J., Milberger, S., Warburton, R., & Tsuang, M. T. (1995). Genetic heterogeneity in attention deficit hyperactivity disorder (ADHD): Gender, psychiatric comorbidity, and maternal ADHD. *Journal of Abnormal Psychology, 104,* 334–345.

Ferraro, L., Antonelli, T., O'Connor, W. T., Tanganelli, S., Rambert, F., & Fuxe, K. (1997). The antinarcoleptic drug modafinil increases glutamate release in thalamic areas and hippocampus. *NeuroReport, 8,* 2883–2887.

Filipek, P. A., Semrud-Clikeman, M., Steingard, R. J., Renshaw, P. F., Kennedy, D. N., & Biederman, J. (1997). Volumetric MRI analysis comparing attention-deficit hyperactivity disorder and normal controls. *Neurology, 48,* 589–601.

Fischer, M., Barkley, R. A., Edelbrock, C. S., & Smallish, L. (1990). The adolescent outcome of hyperactive children diagnosed by research criteria: II. Academic, attentional, and neuropsychological status. *Journal of Consulting and Clinical Psychology, 58,* 580–588.

Fuster, J. M. (1997). *The prefrontal cortex. Anatomy, physiology, and neuropsychology of the frontal lobe* (3rd ed.). Philadelphia: Lippincott-Raven.

García-Sánchez, C., Estévez-González, A., Suárez-Romero, E., & Junqué, C. (1997). Right hemisphere dysfunction in subjects with attention-deficit disorder with and without hyperactivity. *Journal of Child Neurology, 12,* 107–115.

Garfinkel, B. D., Wender, P. H., Sloman, L., & O'Neill, I. (1983). Tricyclic antidepressant and methylphenidate treatment of attention deficit disorder in children.

Journal of the American Academy of Child Psychiatry, 22, 343–348.

Gerfen, C. R. (1992). The neostriatal mosaic: Multiple levels of compartmental organization. *Trends in Neuroscience, 15,* 133–139.

Giedd, J. N., Castellanos, F. X., Casey, B. J., Kozuch, P., King, A. C., Hamburger, S. D., & Rapoport, J. L. (1994). Quantitative morphology of the corpus callosum in attention deficit hyperactivity disorder. *American Journal of Psychiatry, 151,* 665–669.

Giedd, J. N., Rapoport, J. L., Kruesi, M. J. P., Parker, C., Schapiro, M. B., Allen, A. J., Leonard, H. L., Richter, D., Kaysen, D., Dickstein, D. P., Marsh, W. L., Kozuch, P. L., Vaituzis, A. C., Hamburger, S. D., & Swedo, S. E. (1995). Sydenham's chorea: Magnetic resonance imaging of the basal ganglia. *Neurology, 45,* 2199–2202.

Giedd, J. N., Snell, J. W., Lange, N., Rajapakse, J. C., Casey, B. J., Kozuch, P. L., Vaituzis, A. C., Vauss, Y. C., Hamburger, S. D., Kaysen, D., & Rapoport, J. L. (1996). Quantitative magnetic resonance imaging of human brain development: Ages 4–18. *Cerebral Cortex, 6,* 551–560.

Gill, M., Daly, G., Heron, S., Hawi, Z., & Fitzgerald, M. (1997). Confirmation of association between attention deficit hyperactivity disorder and a dopamine transporter polymorphism. *Molecular Psychiatry, 2,* 311–313.

Giros, B., Jaber, M., Jones, S. R., Wightman, R. M., & Caron, M. G. (1996). Hyperlocomotion and indifference to cocaine and amphetamine in mice lacking the dopamine transporter. *Nature, 379,* 606–612.

Gittelman, R., Mannuzza, S., Shenker, R., & Bonagura, N. (1985). Hyperactive boys almost grown up: I. Psychiatric status. *Archives of General Psychiatry, 42,* 937–947.

Goldman-Rakic, P. S., Lidow, M. S., Smiley, J. F., & Williams, M. S. (1992). The anatomy of dopamine in monkey and human prefrontal cortex. *Journal of Neural Transmission Supplement, 36,* 163–177.

Goodman, R., & Stevenson, J. (1989). A twin study of hyperactivity: I. An examination of hyperactivity scores and categories derived from Rutter Teacher and Parent Questionnaires. *Journal of Child Psychology & Psychiatry and Allied Disciplines, 30,* 671–689.

Gray, J. A. (1982). *The neuropsychology of anxiety: An enquiry into the functions of the septo-hippocampal system.* Oxford, England: Oxford University Press.

Gross-Tsur, V., Shalev, R. S., Manor, O., & Amir, N. (1995). Developmental right-hemisphere syndrome: Clinical spectrum of the nonverbal learning disability. *Journal of Learning Disabilities, 28,* 80–86.

Haber, S. N., & Fudge, J. L. (1997). The interface between dopamine neurons and the amygdala: Implications for schizophrenia. *Schizophrenia Bulletin, 23,* 471–482.

Hallett, M. (1993). Physiology of basal ganglia disorders: An overview. *Canadian Journal of Neurologic Sciences, 20,* 177–183.

Halperin, J. M., Newcorn, J. H., Koda, V. H., Pick, L., McKay, K. E., & Knott, P. (1997). Noradrenergic

mechanisms in ADHD children with and without reading disabilities: A replication and extension. *Journal of the American Academy of Child and Adolescent Psychiatry, 36,* 1688–1697.

Han, J. S., McMahan, R. W., Holland, P., & Gallagher, M. (1997). The role of an amygdalo-nigrostriatal pathway in associative learning. *Journal of Neuroscience, 17,* 3913–3919.

Hanna, G. L., Ornitz, E. M., & Hariharan, M. (1996). Urinary epinephrine excretion during intelligence testing in attention-deficit hyperactivity disorder and normal boys. *Biological Psychiatry, 40,* 553–555.

Hart, E. L., Lahey, B. B., Loeber, R., Applegate, B., & Frick, P. J. (1995). Developmental change in attention-deficit/hyperactive disorder in boys: A four year longitudinal study. *Journal of Abnormal Child Psychology, 23,* 729–749.

Hedner, J., Lundell, K. H., Breese, G. R., Mueller, R. A., & Hedner, T. (1986). Developmental variations in CSF monoamine metabolites during childhood. *Biology of the Neonate, 49,* 190–197.

Heilman, K. M., Voeller, K. K. S., & Nadeau, S. E. (1991). A possible pathophysiologic substrate of attention deficit hyperactivity disorder. *Journal of Child Neurology, 6,* S76–S81.

Hellige, J. B. (1993). *Hemispheric asymmetry: What's right and what's left.* Cambridge, MA: Harvard University Press.

Hendley, E. D., & Fan, X. M. (1992). Regional differences in brain norepinephrine and dopamine uptake kinetics in inbred rat strains with hypertension and/or hyperactivity. *Brain Research, 586,* 44–52.

Henry, J. P., Sagne, C., Botton, D., Isambert, M. F., & Gasnier, B. (1998). Molecular pharmacology of the vesicular monoamine transporter. *Advances in Pharmacology, 42,* 236–239.

Houk, J. C., & Wise, S. P. (1995). Distributed modular architectures linking basal ganglia, cerebellum, and cerebral cortex: Their role in planning and controlling action. *Cerebral Cortex, 5,* 95–110.

Husby, G., Van de Rijn, I., Zabriskie, J. B., Abdin, Z. H., & Williams, R. C. (1976). Antibodies reacting with cytoplasm of subthalamic and caudate nuclei neurons in chorea and acute rheumatic fever. *Journal of Experimental Medicine, 144,* 1094–1110.

Huttenlocher, P. R. (1984). Synapse elimination and plasticity in developing human cerebral cortex. *American Journal of Mental Deficiency, 88,* 488–496.

Hynd, G. W., Semrud-Clikeman, M., Lorys, A. R., Novey, E. S., & Eliopulos, D. (1990). Brain morphology in developmental dyslexia and attention deficit disorder/hyperactivity. *Archives of Neurology, 47,* 919–926.

Hynd, G. W., Semrud-Clikeman, M., Lorys, A. R., Novey, E. S., Eliopulos, D., & Lyytinen, H. (1991). Corpus callosum morphology in attention-deficit hyperactivity disorder: Morphometric analysis of MRI. *Journal of Learning Disabilities, 24,* 141–146.

Hynd, G. W., Hern, K. L., Novey, E. S., Eliopulos, D., Marshall, R., Gonzalez, J. J., & Voeller, K. K. S.

(1993). Attention deficit hyperactivity disorder and asymmetry of the caudate nucleus. *Journal of Child Neurology, 8,* 339–347.

Iaboni, F., Douglas, V. I., & Ditto, B. (1997). Psychophysiological response of ADHD children to reward and extinction. *Psychophysiology, 34,* 116–123.

Jacobsen, L. K., Giedd, J. N., Berquin, P. C., Krain, A. L., Hamburger, S. D., Kumra, S., & Rapoport, J. L. (1997). Quantitative morphology of the cerebellum and fourth ventricle in childhood onset schizophrenia. *American Journal of Psychiatry, 154,* 1663–1669.

Kinsbourne, M. (1973). Minimal brain dysfunction as a neurodevelopmental lag. *Annals of the New York Academy of Sciences, 205,* 268–273.

Klorman, R., Brumaghim, J. T., Fitzpatrick, P. A., Borgstedt, A. D., & Strauss, J. (1994). Clinical and cognitive effects of methylphenidate on children with attention deficit disorder as a function of aggression/oppositionality and age. *Journal of Abnormal Psychology, 103,* 206–221.

Kupietz, S. S., & Balka, E. B. (1976). Alterations in the vigilance performance of children receiving amitriptyline and methylphenidate pharmacotherapy. *Psychopharmacology, 50,* 29–33.

LaHoste, G. J., Swanson, J. M., Wigal, S. B., Glabe, C., King, N., Kennedy, J. L., & Wigal, T. (1996). Dopamine D4 receptor gene polymorphism is associated with attention deficit hyperactivity disorder. *Molecular Psychiatry, 1,* 121–124.

Le Moal, M. (1995). Mesocorticolimbic dopaminergic neurons. Functional and regulatory roles. In F. E. Bloom & D. J. Kupfer (Eds.), *Psychopharmacology: The fourth generation of progress* (pp. 283–294). New York: Raven.

Levy, F. (1980). The development of sustained attention (vigilance) and inhibition in children: Some normative data. *Journal of Child Psychology and Psychiatry and Allied Disciplines, 21,* 77–84.

Levy, F. (1991). The dopamine theory of attention deficit hyperactivity disorder (ADHD). *Australian and New Zealand Journal of Psychiatry, 25,* 277–283.

Levy, F., Hay, D. A., McStephen, M., Wood, C., & Waldman, I. (1997). Attention-deficit hyperactivity disorder: A category or a continuum? Genetic analysis of a large-scale twin study. *Journal of the American Academy of Child and Adolescent Psychiatry, 36,* 737–744.

Lidow, M. S., Goldman-Rakic, P. S., & Rakic, P. (1991). Synchronized overproduction of neurotransmitter receptors in diverse regions of the primate cerebral cortex. *Proceedings of the National Academy of Sciences of the United States of America, 88,* 10218–10221.

Lou, H. C., Henriksen, L., & Bruhn, P. (1990). Focal cerebral dysfunction in developmental learning disabilities. *Lancet, 335,* 8–11.

Lyon, G.R., & Krasnegor, N.A. (Eds). (1996). *Attention, memory, and executive function.* Baltimore: Brookes.

Malhotra, A. K., Virkkunen, M., Rooney, W., Eggert, M., Linnoila, M., & Goldman, D. (1996). The association between the dopamine D$_4$ receptor (D4DR) 16 amino acid repeat polymorphism and Novelty Seeking. *Molecular Psychiatry, 1,* 388–391.

Malone, M. A., Kershner, J. R., & Siegel, L. (1988). The effects of methylphenidate on levels of processing and laterality in children with attention deficit disorder. *Journal of Abnormal Child Psychology, 16,* 379–395.

Malone, M. A., Couitis, J., Kershner, J. R., & Logan, W. J. (1994). Right hemisphere dysfunction and methylphenidate effects in children with attention-deficit/hyperactivity disorder. *Journal of Child and Adolescent Psychopharmacology, 4,* 245–253.

Malone, M. A., Kershner, J. R., & Swanson, J. M. (1994). Hemispheric processing and methylphenidate effects in attention-deficit hyperactivity disorder. *Journal of Child Neurology, 9,* 181–189.

Mann, C. A., Lubar, J. F., Zimmerman, A. W., Miller, C. A., & Muenchen, R. A. (1992). Quantitative analysis of EEG in boys with attention-deficit hyperactivity disorder: Controlled study with clinical implications. *Pediatric Neurology, 8,* 30–36.

Mannuzza, S., Klein, R. G., Bessler, A., Malloy, P., & LaPadula, M. (1993). Adult outcome of hyperactive boys: Educational achievement, occupational rank, and psychiatric status. *Archives of General Psychiatry, 50,* 565–576.

Mataró, M., García-Sánchez, C., Junqué, C., Estévez-González, A., & Pujol, J. (1997). Magnetic resonance imaging measurement of the caudate nucleus in adolescents with attention-deficit hyperactivity disorder and its relationship with neuropsychological and behavioral measures. *Archives of Neurology, 54,* 963–968.

Matochik, J. A., Nordahl, T. E., Gross, M., Semple, W. E., King, A. C., Cohen, R. M., & Zametkin, A. J. (1993). Effects of acute stimulant medication on cerebral metabolism in adults with hyperactivity. *Neuropsychopharmacology, 8,* 377–386.

Mattay, V. S., Berman, K. F., Ostrem, J. L., Esposito, G., Van Horn, J. D., Bigelow, L. B., & Weinberger, D. R. (1996). Dextroamphetamine enhances "neural network-specific" physiological signals: A positron-emission tomography rCBF study. *Journal of Neuroscience, 16,* 4816–4822.

McCracken, J. T. (1991). A two-part model of stimulant action on attention-deficit hyperactivity disorder in children. *Journal of Neuropsychiatry, 3,* 201–209.

Meador-Woodruff, J. H., Damask, S. P., & Watson, S. J., Jr. (1994). Differential expression of autoreceptors in the ascending dopamine systems of the human brain. *Proceedings of the National Academy of Sciences of the United States of America, 91,* 8297–8301.

Mefford, I. N., & Potter, W. Z. (1989). A neuroanatomical and biochemical basis for attention deficit disorder with hyperactivity in children: A defect in tonic adrenaline mediated inhibition of locus coeruleus stimulation. *Medical Hypotheses, 29,* 33–42.

Mink, J., & Thach, T. (1993). Basal ganglia intrinsic circuits and their role in behavior. *Current Opinion in Neurobiology, 3,* 950–957.

Modell, J. G., Mountz, J. M., Curtis, G. C., & Greden, J. F. (1989). Neurophysiologic dysfunction in basal ganglia/limbic striatal and thalamocortical circuits as a pathogenetic mechanism of obsessive-compulsive disorder. *Journal of Neuropsychiatry, 1,* 27–36.

Moisan, M. P., Courvoisier, H., Bihoreau, M. T., Gauguier, D., Hendley, E. D., Lathrop, M., James, M. R., & Mormède, P. (1996). A major quantitative trait locus influences hyperactivity in the WKHA rat. *Nature Genetics, 14,* 471–473.

Nasrallah, H. A., Loney, J., Olson, S. C., McCalley-Whitters, M., Kramer, J., & Jacoby, C. G. (1986). Cortical atrophy in young adults with a history of hyperactivity in childhood. *Psychiatry Research, 17,* 241–246.

Nestler, E. J., & Aghajanian, G. K. (1997). Molecular and cellular basis of addiction. *Science, 278,* 58–63.

Nigg, J. T., Swanson, J. M., & Hinshaw, S. P. (1997). Covert visual spatial attention in boys with attention deficit hyperactivity disorder: Lateral effects, methylphenidate response and results for parents. *Neuropsychologia, 35,* 165–176.

Odell, J. D., Warren, R. P., Warren, W. L., Burger, R. A., & Maciulis, A. (1997). Association of genes within the major histocompatibility complex with attention deficit hyperactivity disorder. *Neuropsychobiology, 35,* 181–186.

Parent, A. (1990). Extrinsic connections of the basal ganglia. *Trends in Neuroscience, 13,* 254–258.

Peciña, S., Berridge, K. C., & Parker, L. A. (1997). Pimozide does not shift palatability: Separation of anhedonia from sensorimotor suppression by taste reactivity. *Pharmacology, Biochemistry and Behavior, 58,* 801–811.

Pennington, B. F., & Ozonoff, S. (1996). Executive functions and developmental psychopathology. *Journal of Child Psychology and Psychiatry and Allied Disciplines, 37,* 51–87.

Pennington, B. F., Groisser, D., & Welsh, M. C. (1993). Contrasting cognitive deficits in attention deficit hyperactivity disorder versus reading disability. *Developmental Psychology, 29,* 511–523.

Pliszka, S. R., McCracken, J. T., & Maas, J. W. (1996). Catecholamines in attention-deficit hyperactivity disorder: Current perspectives. *Journal of the American Academy of Child and Adolescent Psychiatry, 35,* 264–272.

Pontius, A. A., & Ruttiger, K. F. (1974). Frontal lobe system maturational lag in juvenile delinquents shown in Narratives Test. *Adolescence, 11,* 509–518.

Porrino, L. J., & Lucignani, G. (1987). Different patterns of local brain energy metabolism associated with high and low doses of methylphenidate: Relevance to its action in hyperactive children. *Biological Psychiatry, 22,* 126–138.

Porrino, L. J., Lucignani, G., Dow-Edwards, D., & Sokoloff, L. (1984). Correlation of dose-dependent effects of acute amphetamine administration on behavior and local cerebral metabolism in rats. *Brain Research, 307,* 311–320.

Posner, M. I., & Dehaene, S. (1994). Attentional networks. *Trends in Neuroscience, 17,* 75–79.

Post, R. M., Kotin, J., Goodwin, F. K., & Gordon, E. K. (1973). Psychomotor activity and cerebrospinal fluid amine metabolites in affective illness. *American Journal of Psychiatry, 130,* 67–72.

Quay, H. C. (1983). The behavioral reward and inhibition system in childhood behavior disorder. In L. M. Bloomingdale (Ed.), *Attention deficit disorder: New research in attention, treatment, and psychopharmacology: Proceedings of the Third High Point Hospital Symposium on ADD* (pp. 176–186). Oxford, England: Pergamon.

Quay, H. C. (1988). Attention deficit disorder and the behavioral inhibition system: The relevance of the neuropsychological theory of Jeffrey A. Gray. In L. M. Bloomingdale & J. A. Sergeant (Eds.), *Attention deficit disorder: Criteria, cognition, intervention* (pp. 117–126). Oxford, England: Pergamon.

Quay, H. C. (1997). Inhibition and attention deficit hyperactivity disorder. *Journal of Abnormal Child Psychology, 25,* 7–13.

Rajkowski, J., Kubiak, P., & Aston-Jones, G. (1994). Locus coeruleus activity in monkey: Phasic and tonic changes are associated with altered vigilance. *Brain Research Bulletin, 35,* 607–616.

Rapoport, J. L., Quinn, P. O., Bradbard, G., Riddle, K. D., & Brooks, E. (1974). Imipramine and methylphenidate treatments of hyperactive boys: A double-blind comparison. *Archives of General Psychiatry, 30,* 789–793.

Reiss, A. L., Abrams, M. T., Singer, H. S., Ross, J. L., & Denckla, M. B. (1996). Brain development, gender and IQ in children: A volumetric imaging study. *Brain, 119,* 1763–1774.

Robinson, T. E., & Berridge, K. C. (1993). The neural basis of drug craving: An incentive-sensitization theory of addiction. *Brain Research Reviews, 18,* 247–291.

Roeltgen, D. P., & Schneider, J. S. (1991). Chronic low-dose MPTP in nonhuman primates: A possible model for attention deficit disorder. *Journal of Child Neurology, 6,* S82–S89

Rogeness, G. A., Javors, M. A., & Pliszka, S. R. (1992). Neurochemistry and child and adolescent psychiatry. *Journal of the American Academy of Child and Adolescent Psychiatry, 31,* 765–781.

Roizen, N. J., Blondis, T. A., Irwin, M., & Stein, M. A. (1994). Adaptive functioning in children with attention-deficit hyperactivity disorder. *Archives of Pediatric & Adolescent Medicine, 148,* 1137–1142.

Rosenberg, D. R., Averbach, D. H., O'Hearn, K. M., Seymour, A. B., Birmaher, B., & Sweeney, J. A. (1997). Response inhibition abnormalities in pediatric obsessive compulsive disorder: Implications for delayed developmental maturation of fronto-striatal circuitry. *Archives of General Psychiatry, 54,* 831–838.

Roth, R. H., & Elsworth, J. D. (1995). Biochemical pharmacology of midbrain dopamine neurons. In F. E. Bloom & D. J. Kupfer (Eds.), *Psychopharmacology: The fourth generation of progress* (pp. 227–243). New York: Raven.

Rubinstein, M., Phillips, T. J., Bunzow, J. R., Falzone, T. L., Dziewczapolski, G., Zhang, G., Fang, Y., Larson, J. L., McDougall, J. A., Chester, J. A., Saez, C., Pugsley, T. A., Gershanik, O., Low, M. J., & Grandy, D. K. (1997). Mice lacking dopamine D4 receptors are supersensitive to ethanol, cocaine, and methamphetamine. *Cell, 90,* 991–1001.

Saint-Cyr, J. A., Taylor, A. E., & Nicholson, K. (1995). Behavior and the basal ganglia. *Advances in Neurology, 65,* 1–28.

Satterfield, J. H., & Braley, B. W. (1977). Evoked potentials and brain maturation in hyperactive and normal children. *Electroencephalography and Clinical Neurophysiology, 43,* 43–51.

Satterfield, J. H., Schell, A. M., & Nicholas, T. (1994). Preferential neural processing of attended stimuli in attention-deficit hyperactivity disorder and normal boys. *Psychophysiology, 31,* 1–10.

Schmahmann, J. D. (1996). From movement to thought: Anatomic substrates of the cerebellar contribution to cognitive processing. *Human Brain Mapping, 4,* 174–198.

Schultz, W., & Romo, R. (1990). Dopamine neurons of the monkey midbrain: Contingencies of responses to stimuli eliciting immediate behavioral reactions. *Journal of Neurophysiology, 63,* 607–624.

Schultz, W., Apicella, P., Ljungberg, T., Romo, R., & Scarnati, E. (1993). Reward-related activity in the monkey striatum and substantia nigra. *Progress in Brain Research, 99,* 227–235.

Semrud-Clikeman, M., Filipek, P. A., Biederman, J., Steingard, R., Kennedy, D., Renshaw, P., & Bekken, K. (1994). Attention-deficit hyperactivity disorder: Magnetic resonance imaging morphometric analysis of the corpus callosum. *Journal of the American Academy of Child and Adolescent Psychiatry, 33,* 875–881.

Shaywitz, B. A., Klopper, J. H., & Gordon, J. W. (1978). Methylphenidate in 6-hydroxydopamine-treated developing rat pups. Effects on activity and maze performance. *Archives of Neurology, 35,* 463–469.

Shaywitz, B. A., Shaywitz, S. E., Byrne, T., Cohen, D. J., & Rothman, S. (1983). Attention deficit disorder: Quantitative analysis of CT. *Neurology, 33,* 1500–1503.

Smalley, S. L. (1997). Genetic influences in childhood-onset psychiatric disorders: Autism and attention-deficit/hyperactivity disorder. *American Journal of Human Genetics, 60,* 1276–1282.

Smith, I. D., & Grace, A. A. (1992). Role of the subthalamic nucleus in the regulation of nigral dopamine neuron activity. *Synapse, 12,* 287–303.

Solanto, M. V. (1986). Behavioral effects of low-dose methylphenidate in childhood attention deficit disorder: Implications for a mechanism of stimulant drug action. *Journal of the American Academy of Child Psychiatry, 25,* 96–101.

Solanto, M. V., Wender, E. H., & Bartell, S. S. (1997). Effects of methylphenidate and behavioral contingencies on sustained attention in attention-deficit hyperactivity disorder: A test of the reward dysfunction hypothesis. *Journal of Child and Adolescent Psychopharmacology, 7,* 123–136.

Sonders, M. S., Zhu, S. J., Zahniser, N. R., Kavanaugh, M. P., & Amara, S. G. (1997). Multiple ionic conductances of the human dopamine transporter: The actions of dopamine and psychostimulants. *Journal of Neuroscience, 17,* 960–974.

Spencer, T., Biederman, J., Wilens, T. E., Harding, M., O'Donnell, D., & Griffin, S. (1996). Pharmacotherapy of attention-deficit hyperactivity disorder across the life cycle. *Journal of the American Academy of Child and Adolescent Psychiatry, 35,* 409–432.

Stein, M. A., Szumowski, E., Blondis, T. A., & Roizen, N. J. (1995). Adaptive skills dysfunction in ADD and ADHD children. *Journal of Child Psychology and Psychiatry and Allied Disciplines, 36,* 663–670.

Sullivan, P. F., Fifield, W. J., Kennedy, M. A., Mulder, R. T., Sellman, J. D., & Joyce, P. R. (1998). No association between novelty seeking and the type 4 dopamine receptor gene (DRD4) in two New Zealand samples. *American Journal of Psychiatry, 155,* 98–101.

Swanson, J., Castellanos, F. X., Murias, M., LaHoste, G. S., & Kennedy, J. (1998). Cognitive neuroscience of attention deficit hyperactivity disorder (ADHD) and hyperkinetic disorder (HKD). *Current Opinion in Neurobiology, 8,* 263–271.

Swanson, J. M., Sergeant, J. A., Taylor, E., Sonuga-Barke, E. J. S., Jensen, P. S., & Cantwell, D. P. (1998). Seminar: Attention-deficit hyperactivity disorder and hyperkinetic disorder. *Lancet, 351,* 429–433.

Swanson, J. M., Sunohara, G. A., Kennedy, J. L., Regino, R., Fineberg, E., Wigal, T., Lerner, M., Williams, L., LaHoste, G. J., & Wigal, S. B. (1998). Association of the dopamine receptor D4 (DRD4) gene with a refined phenotype of attention deficit hyperactivity disorder (ADHD): A family-based approach. *Molecular Psychiatry, 3,* 38–41.

Swedo, S. E., Leonard, H. L., Mittleman, B., Allen, A. J., Garvey, M. A., Perlmutter, S. J., Lougee, L., Dow, S. P., Zamkoff, J., & Dubbert, B. K. (1998). Pediatric autoimmune neuropsychiatric disorders associated with streptococcal infections (PANDAS): A clinical description of the first fifty cases. *American Journal of Psychiatry, 155,* 264–271.

Teicher, M. H., Polcari, A., English, C. D., Anderson, C. M., Andersen, S. L., Glod, C. A., & Renshaw, P. (1996). Dose-dependent effects of methylphenidate on activity, attention, and magnetic resonance imaging measures in children with ADHD [Abstract]. *Society for Neuroscience Abstracts, 22,* 1191.

Thapar, A., Hervas, A., & McGuffin, P. (1995). Childhood hyperactivity scores are highly heritable and show sibling competition effects: Twin study evidence. *Behavioral Genetics, 25,* 537–544.

Thatcher, R. W. (1991). Maturation of the human frontal lobes: Physiological evidence for staging. *Developmental Neuropsychology, 7,* 397–419.

Thatcher, R. W. (1997). Human frontal lobe development: A theory of cyclical cortical reorganization. In N. A. Krasnegor, G. R. Lyon, & P. S. Goldman-Rakic (Eds.), *Development of the prefrontal cortex: Evolution, neurobiology, and behavior* (pp. 85–113). Baltimore: Brookes.

Voeller, K. K. (1995). Clinical neurologic aspects of the right-hemisphere deficit syndrome. *Journal of Child Neurology, 10* (Suppl. 1), S16–22.

Voeller, K. K. S., & Heilman, K. M. (1988). Motor impersistence in children with attention deficit hyperactivity disorder: Evidence for right-hemisphere dysfunction [Abstract]. *Annals of Neurology, 24,* 323–323.

Volkow, N. D., Ding, Y. S., Fowler, J. S., Wang, G. J., Logan, J., Gatley, S. J., Hitzemann, R., Smith, G., Fields, S. D., & Gur, R. (1996). Dopamine transporters decrease with age. *Journal of Nuclear Medicine, 37,* 554–559.

Waldman, I. D., Rowe, D. C., Abramowitz, A., Kozel, S., Mohr, J., Sherman, S. L., Cleveland, H. H., Sanders, M. L., & Stever, C. (1996). Association of the dopamine transporter gene (DAT1) and attention deficit hyperactivity disorder in children [Abstract]. *American Journal of Human Genetics, 59,* A25.

Warren, R. P., Odell, J. D., Warren, W. L., Burger, R. A., Maciulis, A., & Torres, A. R. (1995). Is decreased blood plasma concentration of the complement C4B protein associated with attention-deficit hyperactivity disorder? *Journal of the American Academy of Child and Adolescent Psychiatry, 34,* 1009–1014.

Weinberg, W. A., & Harper, C. R. (1993). Vigilance and its disorders. *Neurologic Clinics, 11,* 59–78.

Weiss, G., Hechtman, L., Milroy, T., & Perlman, T. (1985). Psychiatric status of hyperactives as adults: A controlled prospective 15-year follow-up of 63 hyperactive children. *Journal of the American Academy of Child Psychiatry, 24,* 211–220.

Wichmann, T., & DeLong, M. R. (1993). Pathophysiology of Parkinsonian motor abnormalities. In H. Narabayashi, T. Nagatsu, N. Yanagisawa, & Y. Mizuno (Eds.), *Advances in neurology* (Vol. 60, pp. 53–61). New York: Raven.

Wichmann, T., Bergman, H., & DeLong, M. R. (1994). The primate subthalamic nucleus: I. Functional properties in intact animals. *Journal of Neurophysiology, 72,* 494–506.

Williams, G. V., & Goldman-Rakic, P. S. (1995). Modulation of memory fields by dopamine D1 receptors in prefrontal cortex. *Nature, 376,* 572–575.

Wise, S. P., Murray, E. A., & Gerfen, C. R. (1996). The frontal cortex–basal ganglia system in primates. *Critical Reviews in Neurobiology, 10,* 317–356.

World Health Organization. (1992). *International classification of diseases* (10th ed.). Geneva, Switzerland: Author.

Yakovlev, P. I., & Lecours, A. R. (1967). The myelogenetic cycles of regional maturation of the brain. In A. Minkowski (Ed.), *Regional development of the brain in early life* (pp. 3–70). Oxford, England, & Edinburgh, Scotland: Blackwell.

Yeterian, E. H., & Van Hoesen, G. W. (1978). Cortico-striate projections in the rhesus monkey: The organization of certain cortico-caudate connections. *Brain Research, 139,* 43–63.

Zametkin, A. J., & Rapoport, J. L. (1987). Neurobiology of attention-deficit disorder with hyperactivity: Where have we come in 50 years? *Journal of the American Academy of Child and Adolescent Psychiatry, 26,* 676–686.

Zametkin, A. J., Nordahl, T. E., Gross, M., King, A. C., Semple, W. E., Rumsey, J., Hamburger, S. D., & Cohen, R. M. (1990). Cerebral glucose metabolism in adults with hyperactivity of childhood onset. *New England Journal of Medicine, 323,* 1361–1366.

Zametkin, A. J., Liebenauer, L. L., Fitzgerald, G. A., King, A. C., Minkunas, D. V., Herscovitch, P., Yamada, E. M., & Cohen, R. M. (1993). Brain metabolism in teenagers with attention-deficit hyperactivity disorder. *Archives of General Psychiatry, 50,* 333–340.

Zilbovicius, M., Garreau, B., Samson, Y., Remy, P., Barthelemy, C., Syrota, A., & Lelord, G. (1995). Delayed maturation of the frontal cortex in childhood autism. *American Journal of Psychiatry, 152,* 248–252.

9

Risk Factors for Attention-Deficit/Hyperactivity Disorder

KALYANI SAMUDRA and DENNIS P. CANTWELL*

INTRODUCTION

As discussed in Chapters 4, 5, and 13, a large body of evidence has accumulated about impairments in cognitive, social, and school functioning in children with Attention-Deficit/ Hyperactivity Disorder (ADHD)† (Cantwell, 1996), which has generated increased interest in research on risk factors for this disorder. Risk factors are defined as variables that increase the probability of any form of psychopathology. In contrast, protective factors modify an individual's response to risk factors and thus reduce the chance of disorder or of a maladaptive outcome. Resilience is defined as successful adaptation despite exposure to risk or adversity (Masten, 1994).

The following observations were noted by Coie and colleagues (1993) about risk and protective factors:

1. A specific area of dysfunction is usually associated with a number of different risk factors; further, a single risk factor may be associated with diverse areas of adaptive functioning and with diverse disorders.
2. Some risk factors may act only at certain points in development; others may predict poor functioning across the lifespan.
3. Risk factors can have additive or cumulative effects on an individual's susceptibility to dysfunction or disorder; this susceptibility can increase with the number, duration, or "toxicity" of risk factors involved.
4. Protective factors may act in a number of ways. They can reduce dysfunction directly, buffer the effects of a risk factor, interfere with the pathway through which the risk factor leads to dysfunction, or prevent the occurrence of a risk factor.

Protective factors for ADHD can be divided into two categories: (1) characteristics of the individual, such as temperament, disposition, and behavioral and cognitive skills; and (2) characteristics of the individual's environment such as social support, parental warmth, appropriate discipline, family cohesion, and adult supervision (Coie et al., 1993).

Rutter (1985) pointed out that protective factors need not be positive experiences or desirable traits. In fact, a stressful event can have what he called a steeling effect if an individual copes with it successfully. In addition, protective factors may have no noticeable effect in the

*Deceased.
†In this chapter we use the current term, ADHD, which subsumes the earlier labels of hyperactivity and attention-deficit disorder.

KALYANI SAMUDRA • Department of Psychiatry, University of Colorado, Health Sciences Center and Children's Hospital, Denver, Colorado 80218.   DENNIS P. CANTWELL • Neuropsychiatric Institute, University of California, Los Angeles, Los Angeles, California 90095.

Handbook of Disruptive Behavior Disorders, edited by Quay and Hogan. Kluwer Academic/Plenum Publishers, New York, 1999.

absence of a relevant risk factor with which they can interact. Finally, the same characteristic in a child can be protective in one situation but may place the child at risk in another. For example, compliance can be protective in a normal school or home environment, but it can put the child at risk in an abusive environment (Masten & Wright, 1998).

There are two common research designs in studies of risk factors. One compares levels of risk factors in two populations: A group of children with specific behavioral or emotional problems is compared with a matched control group of children without such problems. Another design assesses the prevalence of psychopathology and potentially associated risk factors in a large community population. This can be done cross-sectionally or longitudinally. In the longitudinal design, risk factors are assessed at one point; at a later point, psychopathology and functioning are measured. Unlike cross-sectional designs, the longitudinal design can suggest causal relationships between risk factors and psychopathology or other maladaptive outcomes.

Potential risk factors for ADHD that have been studied can be divided roughly into five categories: (1) family-genetic, (2) family-environmental, (3) pre- and perinatal, (4) temperament and developmental, and (5) nutrition and diet. Studies of risk factors help us understand the etiology of disorders and develop effective intervention strategies to counteract them.

GENETIC RISK FACTORS

Family Studies

Pedigree Studies

ADHD appears to be a highly familial disorder. In an early study, Morrison and Stewart (1971) interviewed the parents of 59 ADHD and 41 control children; they found that 20% of the parents in the ADHD group, compared to 5% of the parents of controls, had a retrospective diagnosis of ADHD. Cantwell (1972) compared the parents of 50 ADHD children and 50 matched control children and found that 20% of ADHD children had an ADHD parent compared to only 2% of normal controls. In both studies the authors noted that parents of ADHD children had a higher prevalence of alcoholism, hysteria, and sociopathy than did parents of normal controls. One concern about these earlier studies is the extent to which the ADHD subjects were comorbid for conduct disorder (CD) or oppositional defiant disorder (ODD) without the researchers being aware of it. For example, in the studies just cited, the greater prevalence of sociopathy in parents of ADHD children could be a function of the unidentified presence of ODD/CD in the ADHD probands. In fact, there is some evidence that parental Antisocial Personality Disorder and alcoholism are associated with comorbid CD in probands rather than with the presence of ADHD (Stewart, DeBlois, & Cummings, 1980).

Biederman, Faraone, Keenan, Knee, and Tsuang (1990) have found significantly greater morbidity risks for ADHD in first-degree relatives (parents and siblings) of ADHD children when compared with relatives of psychiatric controls and those of pediatric clinic controls. They compared 457 first-degree family members of 73 clinically referred ADHD children and adolescents with those of 26 psychiatric and 26 normal controls. They used structured diagnostic interviews in a blinded manner and controlled for gender, generation of the relative, age of proband, socioeconomic status (SES) and family intactness. The relatives of ADHD probands had a significantly higher morbidity risk for ADHD (25.1% vs. 5.3% vs. 4.6%).

Faraone, Biederman, and Milberger (1994) expanded this work to include the extended family by collecting parent-elicited information about second-degree relatives (aunts, uncles, and grandparents) of 140 ADHD children and those of 120 normal controls. They found that these second-degree relatives of ADHD children were at higher risk for ADHD than were second-degree relatives of controls and that the highest risk occurred in those related to an ADHD parent of an ADHD child. One can draw limited conclusions from these results given the lack of a direct clinical assessment of ADHD in the relatives. However, the investigators suggested that further work assessing ADHD prevalence in second-degree relatives using blinded structured interviews may help delineate patterns of familial transmission in ADHD.

Sibling studies have been designed with two purposes. First, siblings of ADHD probands have been used as a comparison group to control for SES, parental education and psychopathology, and family adversity. Such studies have suggested that ADHD children and adults usually have poorer outcomes than their siblings (Hechtman, 1996).

Siblings of ADHD probands have also been compared to siblings of non-ADHD individuals with the hypothesis that if the disorder is familial, rates of ADHD should be higher in siblings of ADHD probands than in siblings of normal controls. Welner, Welner, Stewart, Palkes, and Wish (1977) studied siblings of 53 clinic-referred ADHD subjects and siblings of 38 controls. The groups were matched for gender (male), ethnicity (white), age (mean 11 years), and SES (middle class). The probands met Stewart's modified research criteria (Stewart, Pitts, Craig, & Dieruf, 1966) for ADHD and had siblings at least 6 years of age. No individuals had evidence of psychosis, organic brain disorder, or neurologic illness; all lived with their mothers and attended school. ADHD was more common in brothers of ADHD probands (26%) than in brothers of controls (9%), ($p = 0.054$). No significant differences were found in ADHD in the sisters of the two groups. Non-ADHD brothers of probands were significantly more likely to have symptoms of depression and anxiety than were non-ADHD brothers of controls, though no such differences were noted in sisters. The authors suggested that this finding may relate to the stress of living with a brother with ADHD. Moreover, the authors found no difference in antisocial symptoms in siblings of probands compared to siblings of controls. ADHD brothers of probands did not have more antisocial symptoms than brothers of controls, but the ADHD probands themselves had more an-

tisocial symptoms compared to non-ADHD controls. However, this finding may reflect an increased likelihood of referral in ADHD boys with antisocial symptoms.

Faraone, Biederman, Lehman, Spencer, and colleagues (1993) examined academic and intellectual functioning in 140 children with ADHD, 120 normal control children, and their 303 siblings. The probands were predominantly Caucasian boys. As expected, the ADHD probands had more school failure and lower IQs than did controls. However, the siblings of ADHD probands also showed significantly higher rates of school problems and intellectual impairments, a finding that further supports the hypothesis that ADHD is familial. It should be noted that IQ and school failure are not necessarily independent. Lower IQ may lead to school failure, and IQ has a strong genetic component. Furthermore, the authors commented that achievement and IQ are often discrepant in children with ADHD; when such a discrepancy is absent, it may be because the disorder has impaired both.

One study of concordance rates in full and half siblings also supports the heritability of ADHD. Safer (1973) published the concordance rates of minimal brain dysfunction (the diagnostic predecessor of ADHD) based on his study of 19 full and 22 half-sibling pairs. Within each pair, the children had been reared by the same mother. Full siblings had significantly higher concordance (10 pairs) than half siblings (2 pairs), adding more support to the hypothesis that genetic factors as opposed to shared environment are extremely important in the development of this disorder.

In summary, ADHD is more likely to occur in first-degree relatives (and possibly even in second-degree relatives) of ADHD children than in those of non-ADHD children. Siblings of ADHD individuals generally have a better functional outcome than the ADHD probands but do more poorly than siblings of controls. They have more ADHD, depression, and anxiety symptoms than siblings of controls, although not more antisocial behavior. Concordance for ADHD symptoms is higher in full siblings than half siblings. Thus, pedigree studies provide strong evidence for the role of familial factors in the development of ADHD.

Twin and Adoption Studies

Is the familiality of ADHD based on shared genes or on a common environment within families? Twin and adoption studies have provided evidence for the role of genetics in the expression of ADHD. Twin studies have been based on the premise that if ADHD is genetically influenced, it should occur with greater concordance among monozygotic (MZ) twins, who share 100% of their genes, than among dizygotic (DZ) twins, who share only half of their genetic material.

Goodman and Stevenson (1989) studied 13-year-old twins (29 MZ pairs and 45 same-sex DZ pairs) in which at least one twin met criteria for pervasive ADHD. MZ twins were more alike than were DZ twins on parent and teacher ratings of hyperactivity and on objective attentional measures. The investigators also examined adverse family factors and perinatal adversity, and concluded that genetic risk factors accounted for approximately 30%–50% of the interindividual variation in childhood hyperactivity and inattentiveness, or about half of the explainable variance.

Gillis, Gilger, Pennington, and DeFries (1992) examined reading-disabled twin pairs participating in the Colorado Reading Project. They identified a subset of 37 MZ and 37 same-sex DZ twin pairs in which one of the pair had been diagnosed with ADHD by a structured diagnostic interview. Using a basic regression model, they found 79% concordance for MZ twins and 32% for DZ twins. In addition, they attempted to determine the extent to which the variance in ADHD symptoms was due to individual differences in IQ or reading performance. However, controlling for these two factors did not significantly alter their results. Thus, the authors concluded that ADHD is highly heritable independently of its comorbidity with reading problems.

In another study of reading-disabled twin pairs from the Colorado Reading Project, Gilger, Pennington, and DeFries (1992) identified 81 MZ and 52 same-sex DZ twin pairs. This group included the sample studied by Gillis and colleagues (1992). They found that 81% of the MZ twin pairs were concordant for ADHD in contrast to 29% of the DZ twin pairs. The concordance rate for both reading disability (RD) and ADHD was 44% for MZ twins and 30% for DZ twins, while that for RD alone was 84% for MZ twins and 66% for DZ twins. The authors concluded that independent genetic factors may play a role in both ADHD and RD.

Other investigators have focused on the heritability of various symptoms of ADHD. MZ twin pairs have been found to be more similar to each other than DZ pairs in psychomotor activity (Hechtman, 1996; Rutter, Korn, & Birch, 1963) and in attentional problems (Edelbrock, Rende, Plomin, & Thompson, 1995; Stevenson, 1992). Thus, the data on concordance rates for individual symptoms of ADHD also support the importance of family-genetic factors in the development of ADHD.

Adoption studies have also suggested a possible genetic basis for ADHD. Morrison and Stewart (1973) showed that biological relatives of ADHD children were more likely to have ADHD than were adoptive relatives of ADHD children. Alberts-Corush, Firestone, and Goodman (1986) studied 176 biological and adoptive parents of ADHD and normal control children; biological parents of ADHD children performed more poorly on several standardized attentional measures than did biological parents of controls or adoptive parents of ADHD or control children. These data further support the role of genetics in the development of ADHD.

Studies of Comorbid Samples

Studies of comorbid populations may also help clarify the etiology of ADHD. Genetic studies of ADHD are complicated by the presence of genetic heterogeneity. One indicator of this heterogeneity is the high comorbidity between ADHD and other psychiatric disorders (Cantwell, 1996; see also Chapter 2, this volume). In the 1970s, families of ADHD children were observed to have high rates of other disorders. As noted earlier, Morrison and Stewart (1971) and Cantwell (1972) found higher rates of alcoholism, hysteria, and sociopathy in biological parents of ADHD children. Biederman and colleagues (1992), in a study of 140 children with ADHD, 120 normal controls, and 822 first-degree relatives, reported that ADHD probands were more likely than controls to have comorbid CD, major depressive disorder (MDD), or anxiety disorders (ANX), but almost half (49%) had no comorbidity. Relatives of the ADHD probands were more likely than relatives of normal controls to have ADHD, depressive disorders, substance dependence, ANX, and antisocial disorders.

Grouping ADHD probands according to the presence of comorbid disorders may help identify more homogenous subgroups and better characterize the association between ADHD and those disorders. Biederman and colleagues (1992) tested three major hypotheses regarding the familial transmission of ADHD and various comorbid disorder or disorders (CM):

1. If ADHD and the CM are independently transmitted, higher rates of ADHD should be found in the relatives of both ADHD probands and ADHD+CM probands than in normal controls. However, only the families of the ADHD+CM group should have higher rates of the CM; in these families, different individuals should account for the risks for ADHD and the CM (i.e., the two disorders should not cosegregate). This transmission pattern fit the data for ADHD and ANX.

2. If ADHD and the CM share the same familial etiologic factors, high rates of both ADHD and the CM should be found in the relatives of ADHD probands and ADHD+CM probands compared with relatives of normal controls. As in the first hypothesis, the two disorders should not cosegregate. This transmission pattern was observed for ADHD and MDD.

3. If ADHD+CM is a distinct subtype, the pattern should be similar to that in hypothesis 1: There should be higher rates of ADHD in relatives of both ADHD probands and ADHD+CM probands compared to normal controls, with high rates

of CM only in relatives of the ADHD+CM group. However, the frequency of comorbidity in the relatives should be greater than that expected by chance alone; that is, the two disorders should tend to occur in the same family members, indicating that the two disorders are transmitted together rather than independently. In other words, ADHD and CM should cosegregate. This transmission pattern was observed for ADHD and CD (Biederman et al., 1992).

Lahey and colleagues (1988) also examined families of children with ADHD only (n = 18), CD only (n = 14), ADHD+CD (n = 23), and clinic controls (n = 30). The children ranged in age from 6 to 13 years, and were predominantly white and male. One custodial, biological parent was interviewed in each family, although data were gathered regarding both biological parents. Information included symptoms and questions about parental antisocial behavior (i.e., fighting, arrests, and incarceration). Parents of ADHD children (regardless of whether the child had comorbid CD) did not show elevated rates of any psychiatric diagnosis. Compared to parents of control children, ADHD children's mothers and fathers showed higher rates of antisocial behaviors; however, this pattern was due to high rates of fighting and arrests among the parents of children with ADHD+CD. Among the families of ADHD-only children, there were no reports of maternal antisocial behaviors, and fathers' rates were below that of clinic controls. The CD children who showed the greatest amount of physically aggressive and otherwise illegal behaviors were the CD+ADHD group. The fathers of CD+ADHD children were significantly more likely than fathers of CD-only, ADHD-only, and control children to have frequent physical fights, arrests, and imprisonment.

At least two groups of investigators have examined the association between ADHD and learning disabilities (LD). Gilger and colleagues (1992) hypothesized that if the cross-concordance rates for ADHD and RD were significantly greater in MZ twins than in DZ twins, the comorbidity between the two disorders could be due to a common genetic etiology. The within-pair cross-concordances between ADHD and RD were larger (44%) for MZ than for DZ twins (30%), but not significantly so ($p < 0.10$). Thus, their data suggested that RD and ADHD may be genetically independent.

More recently, Faraone, Biederman, Lehman, Keenan, and colleagues (1993) assessed LD in 140 ADHD children, 120 normal controls, and their 822 first-degree relatives. They found that relatives of ADHD probands and relatives of ADHD+LD probands had higher risks for ADHD than did relatives of control children. The risk for LD was higher in relatives of ADHD+LD probands than in families of ADHD-only children. Among relatives of ADHD+LD children, ADHD and LD did not cosegregate. Thus, the data of these investigators supported the independent transmission of ADHD and LD, a finding consistent with those of Gilger and colleagues (1992). Further, Faraone, Biederman, Lehman, Keenan, and colleagues reported that spouses of ADHD individuals had greater rates of LD than did spouses of non-ADHD individuals, and they suggested that the two disorders may co-occur as a result of nonrandom mating.

The relationship between tic disorders and ADHD has been controversial. Knell and Comings (1993) proposed that ADHD and Tourette's syndrome (TS) may be produced by the same set of genes. In support of this hypothesis, they reported significantly higher rates of ADHD, with or without tics, in the first-degree relatives of TS probands than in relatives of controls. Pauls, Leckman, and Cohen (1993) also examined this potential relationship. Like Knell and Comings, they postulated that if ADHD and TS were variant expressions of the same genes, ADHD should occur more frequently in relatives of TS probands than in relatives of controls. In addition, the rates of ADHD should be the same in relatives of TS probands and in relatives of TS+ADHD probands. In contrast to the findings of Knell and Comings, Pauls and colleagues found no significant differences between ADHD rates in families of TS probands and rates in families of controls. ADHD occurred more frequently in first-degree relatives of TS+ADHD probands (15.9%) than in relatives of TS-only probands (3.2 %) or in those of controls (4.4%). Thus, their data were not consistent with the hypothesis that ADHD and TS are expressions of the same genes.

Pauls and colleagues (1993) also suggested that the sequence of onset of ADHD and TS may distinguish important subgroups among TS+ADHD probands. Relatives of probands in whom ADHD preceded TS were twice as likely (25%) to have ADHD alone as were relatives of probands with ADHD concurrent or following TS (12.2%). They suggested that early-onset ADHD may be more likely to be independent of TS whereas later-onset ADHD may occur secondary to the expression of TS. The significance of this finding is limited by the retrospective nature of their data about age at onset; future investigations should use a prospective design. More research is needed to clarify the nature of the relationship between these disorders.

Studies of Susceptibility Genes

Efforts are under way to search for common susceptibility genes in ADHD. A number of investigators have begun to examine candidate gene associations in ADHD (Smalley, 1997). Cook and colleagues (1995) reported a significant association between an allelic variant at the dopamine transporter gene (DAT1) and ADHD. In a recent abstract, Waldman and colleagues (1996) described a replication study supporting this association. In particular, they suggested that the DAT1 480bp allele may be associated with the combined type of ADHD. Palmer and colleagues (1997) failed to replicate the association of the DAT1 with any ADHD subtype. LaHoste and colleagues (1996) reported an association between ADHD and the dopamine D4 receptor gene (DRD4), which has been linked to novelty seeking and risk-taking behavior. Bailey and colleagues (1997) also investigated the link between one of the alleles of the DRD4 in 77 families of children and adolescents with ADHD. They found that this allele was significantly associated with ADHD in families where the ADHD child had no affected first-degree relatives (the sporadic type), but not in families where the proband had at least one affected first-degree relative (the familial type).

The association of several specific genetic syndromes with ADHD has suggested other directions for the search for candidate genes. Generalized resistance to thyroid hormone (GRTH), a rare, autosomal dominant disorder, has been studied in 18 families by Hauser and colleagues (1993). Using blinded structured interviews, the authors found that 61% (30 of 49) of the GRTH patients had ADHD compared to 13% (7 of 55) of unaffected family members. Mutations were identified in 13 of the 18 families. Further study of GRTH, which may be the first molecular model of ADHD, may provide clues to the pathophysiology of ADHD. Fragile X syndrome has also been linked to ADHD. However, few studies have controlled for IQ. Einfeld, Hall, and Levy (1991) compared 45 mentally retarded fragile X subjects with controls matched for age, sex, and IQ. They reported no differences between groups on ratings of hyperactivity, inattention, impulsivity, or aggression. Therefore, the association between fragile X and ADHD symptoms may be due to the mental retardation that is common in this group. (See Chapter 8, this volume, for additional discussion of susceptibility gene studies.)

FAMILY-ENVIRONMENT RISK FACTORS

Global Risks and Outcomes

The familial nature of ADHD has been well documented; however, not all children with a familial vulnerability to ADHD develop the disorder. Many disorders run in families because of environmental factors rather than (or in addition to) genetic ones. Perhaps because ADHD has not generally been considered to be psychogenic, the impact of pathogenic environments on the development of ADHD is less well studied than are the genetic risk factors previously discussed.

Rutter, Cox, Tupling, Berger, and Yule (1975) and Rutter and Quinton (1977) in their classic work on the Isle of Wight and the inner borough of London described six family-environment risk factors which were significantly associated with child psychopathology: (1) severe marital discord, (2) low SES, (3) large family size, (4) criminality in fathers, (5) mental illness in mothers, and (6) foster placement. They found that the sum of these factors rather than any single one correlated with dysfunction.

Velez, Johnson, and Cohen (1989) performed a 2-year prospective longitudinal study of risk factors for psychopathology in a community sample of individuals ages 9–18 and then assessed the group for both externalizing and internalizing disorders 2 years later. Those found at time 1 to have low SES, single-parent families, parental sociopathy, many stressful life events, and school failure were more likely to have developed externalizing disorders, but not internalizing disorders, after 2 years.

Several investigators have studied protective factors against general psychopathology in children. In a 32-year longitudinal study, Werner (1989) followed a group of infants in Kauai at high risk due to perinatal stress, low SES, family discord or divorce, and parental mental disorder or alcoholism. As adults, one third had had more positive life experiences than the rest and were considered resilient. This group was described in grade school as getting along well with peers, having good reasoning and reading skills, and having many interests and hobbies. The resilient individuals came from smaller families, had fewer separations from their primary caretaker, and had extrafamilial emotional support. All of these factors seemed to protect these high-risk individuals from negative life outcomes.

Rae-Grant, Thomas, Offord, and Boyle (1989) identified family and parental problems as risk factors for ADHD, CD, neurosis, and somatization disorders. They found that those who got along with others, did well academically, and participated in at least two activities had lower risk for any disorder. In another study of risk and protective factors for disruptive behavior disorders (DBD), Grizenko and

Pawliuk (1994) used a matched control design to study 50 children with DBD and 50 controls. Significant factors associated with illness included hyperactivity as an infant, learning disability, school failure, perinatal complications, and a history of maternal depression. Social variables associated with development of DBD included frequent moving or changing schools, having immigrant parents, and family violence. Protective factors that distinguished DBD and control children were the presence of a positive relationship with grandparents and having at least two hobbies. Psychological protective factors included the ability to adapt to change, to cope with stress, and to express feelings easily.

Thus, the data show that an individual's general competence and personality characteristics, positive relationships, and participation in outside activities seem to be protective against general psychopathology both in community samples and in high-risk children.

Family-Environment Risks for ADHD

Much less research has been done on family-environment risk factors specific to ADHD and associated symptoms. In the Dunedin longitudinal study, McGee, Williams, and Silva (1985) found that ADHD was associated with family factors such as maternal psychological health, marital problems, and poor family relationships. Biederman, Milberger, Faraone, Kiely, Guite, Mick, Ablon, Warburton, and Reed (1995) examined ADHD children for the presence of Rutter's six indicators of adversity (Rutter & Quinton, 1977). They reported that the risk for ADHD and related psychopathology correlated with the number of adversity factors present. In addition, Biederman, Milberger, Faraone, Kiely, Guite, Mick, Ablon, Warburton, Reed, and Davis (1995) also used dimensional measures of adversity to further characterize environmental risk factors for ADHD. Specifically, they used measures of family conflict and parental psychopathology to determine whether these factors were associated with ADHD. Families of ADHD children had higher levels of parental conflict, less fam-

ily cohesion, and increased exposure to parental psychopathology compared to control families. These differences could not be accounted for by SES. Higher levels of adversity in the home predicted lower adaptive functioning. Moreover, chronic family conflict affected children more significantly than did exposure to parental psychopathology. One limitation of their cross-sectional design is that associations do not indicate causal or even temporal relationships. In fact, if the children already have ADHD, it may be questioned whether these factors are indeed risk factors, or simply concurrent markers of psychopathology.

Interestingly, Biederman, Milberger, Faraone, Kiely, Guite, Mick, Ablon, Warburton, Reed, and Davis (1995) found that exposure to maternal psychopathology correlated more strongly with ADHD than did exposure to paternal psychopathology. This finding is consistent with that of Goodman and Stevenson (1989), who found ADHD to be associated with maternal malaise, coldness to the child, and criticism of the child. However, the impact of maternal illness and behavior may appear more important in both investigations simply because mothers were more likely to be major informants than were fathers (see also Chapter 6, this volume). Moreover, because mothers may be more likely to work in the home than fathers, they may be much more affected by having an ADHD child.

In the investigation by Biederman, Milberger, Faraone, Kiely, Guite, Mick, Ablon, Warburton, Reed, and Davis (1995), the harmful impact of these adversity factors was demonstrated independently of the ADHD diagnosis, supporting the idea that adversity can affect functioning of children with or without a psychiatric diagnosis. However, family-environment adversity factors did not seem to increase the risk of comorbid disorders in ADHD children. This is surprising given the findings that such factors may have a significant role in the development of CD and criminality (Kolvin, Miller, Fleeting, & Kolvin, 1988; see also Chapter 19, this volume). The absence of increased comorbidity in ADHD children with greater adversity factors supports the notion that ADHD-associated CD may be less influenced by family-environment risk factors than is CD without ADHD.

How strong is the association between adverse family-environment factors and ADHD? In their twin study, Goodman and Stevenson (1989) found modest correlations between ADHD and seven measures of adverse family factors, including marital discord, parental malaise, coldness to the child, and criticism of the child. However, when these factors were considered simultaneously in a multiple-regression analysis, less than 10% of the variance in ADHD could be explained. Goodman and Stevenson contrasted this with the much stronger link they found between ADHD and genetic factors, and concluded that the contribution of family-environment variables may be relatively minor.

What is the direction of the link between ADHD or hyperactivity and family adversity? Goodman and Stevenson (1989) proposed several hypotheses which could explain the association: (1) family adversity could be a cause of ADHD; (2) family adversity and ADHD could be linked by common antecedent genetic variables, since families share genes; (3) the two could also be linked by common environmental variables such as low SES or environmental toxins; or (4) ADHD may lead to adverse family factors such as parental criticism and coldness and family conflict. This last hypothesis is supported by the work of Schachar, Taylor, Wieselberg, Thorley, and Rutter (1987), who found that stimulant treatment of ADHD children resulted in increased maternal warmth and contact and decreased maternal criticism (see Chapter 10, this volume). More research is needed to clarify and test these hypotheses.

PRENATAL AND PERINATAL RISK FACTORS

Obstetric and Birth Complications

Other variables that have been considered in the development of ADHD are complications during pregnancy, delivery, and early infancy. Such factors have been associated with various forms of psychopathology in children. For instance, high rates of prenatal adversity have been significantly associated with TS (Leckman et al., 1990) and increased perinatal complications have been found in children with LD (Colletti, 1979) and incarcerated delinquent children (Lewis & Shanok, 1979).

A number of investigators have studied the impact of these variables on the development of ADHD and related symptoms. The data reveal conflicting findings. One frequently cited early study by Pasamanick, Rogers, and Lilienfeld (1956) reported retrospective data from birth and hospital records of more than 1000 children with "behavior disturbance" and matched controls. The disordered children had significantly higher rates of exposure to maternal pregnancy complications (particularly toxemia) than did controls. They were also more likely to have been born preterm than controls, even when those with maternal complications were excluded. When Pasamanick and colleagues compared a subset who were "confused, disorganized, and hyperactive" with controls, they found even greater differences. Conners (1975) also reported that mothers of ADHD children had high rates of toxemia and history of prior abortions.

Hartsough and Lambert (1985) studied prenatal variables in a large sample of ADHD children and matched controls. They were able to discriminate the ADHD group based on eight factors: (1) poor maternal health during pregnancy, toxemia, or eclampsia; (2) low maternal age at the child's birth; (3) first pregnancy; (4) fetal postmaturity; (5) long labor; (6) fetal distress during labor or delivery; (7) congenital problems; and (8) health problems in the child during infancy. Pre- and perinatal factors that did not significantly distinguish between groups included prior miscarriages, prematurity, low birth weight, and Rh incompatibility.

Minde, Webb, and Sykes (1968) found that mothers of ADHD children were more likely to have had extremely short or prolonged labor, and forceps delivery than were mothers of control children. However, they found no significant differences between groups in all other pre- and perinatal variables examined including toxemia, maternal age, prior abortions, prenatal illnesses, labor duration, delivery complications, birth weight, fetal distress, or APGAR scores.

Sprich-Buckminster, Biederman, Milberger, Faraone, and Lehman (1993) examined the role of pre- and perinatal complications in ADHD and further studied the influence of comorbidity and familiality. They compared 73 ADHD boys ages 6–17 with 26 psychiatric controls and 26 healthy control children. The examiners found that 52% of the ADHD probands, 65% of the psychiatric controls and 35% of the normal controls ($p > 0.05$) had a history of *any* pregnancy, delivery, or infancy complication (PDIC). Thus, the risk of any PDIC was high for both ADHD children (odds ratio = 2.1) and psychiatric controls (odds ratio = 3.6, $p < .05$) in comparison to normal controls, consistent with the hypothesis that PDIC may be nonspecific risk factors for general psychopathology.

Further, ADHD boys were four times more likely than normal controls to have had a delivery complication, six times more likely to have had an infancy complication and two times as likely to have had any PDIC. When the investigators subdivided ADHD children by comorbidity status with ANX, CD, or MDD, they found that the association between ADHD and PDIC was strongest for those with comorbidity; conversely, non-comorbid ADHD boys had PDIC rates more similar to controls. When they stratified ADHD probands by family history for ADHD, they found that the link between ADHD and PDIC was strongest for those with nonfamilial ADHD. The familial ADHD children had PDIC rates more similar to normal controls. They concluded that PDIC are risk factors for ADHD with comorbidity and for nonfamilial ADHD. The strong link between PDIC and comorbid ADHD may relate to the role of PDIC as risk factors for general psychopathology as well as for ADHD. If the comorbid disorders were predominantly CD, then the PDIC may have added additional disinhibiting behavior traits to those individuals. The authors suggested further that PDIC may affect the number of disorders present.

Sprich-Buckminster and colleagues (1993) also studied the interaction between family history and comorbidity. They noted higher rates of PDIC in comorbid ADHD children only if they lacked a family history of ADHD. Among children with nonfamilial ADHD, those with a history of any PDIC were 22 times more likely to have comorbidity than those with no PDIC. They suggested that PDIC may contribute to the development of phenotypically similar but nongenetic forms of ADHD in some children.

Low birth weight (LBW) (≤2500 g) has been identified as a risk factor for developmental deficits in children. Studies of school-age very-low-birth-weight (VLBW) (≤1500 g) and extremely-low-birth-weight (ELBW) (≤1000 g) children without severe neurologic impairment have shown significant academic and behavior problems (McCormick, Brooks-Gunn, Workman-Daniels, Turner, & Peckham, 1992; Teplin, Burchinal, Johnson-Martin, Humphry, & Kraybill, 1991), including inattention and hyperactivity (Hack *et al.*, 1992). Szatmari, Saigal, Rosenbaum, Campbell, and King (1990) reported increased rates of ADHD in 5-year-old ELBW children. A number of investigations have suggested that higher risk for behavioral disturbance is also present in the larger group of LBW children (McCormick *et al.*, 1992; The Scottish Low Birthweight Study Group, 1992), but there is little information on specific psychiatric disorders in this population.

Breslau and colleagues (1996) studied a large sample of LBW 6-year-old children without severe neurologic impairment in two populations (urban and suburban) and assessed them for psychiatric disorders using a structured parent interview. Compared to their matched normal-birth-weight (NBW) controls, the LBW children had higher rates of ADHD. This association was not accounted for by perinatal risk factors such as single motherhood, maternal history of substance abuse or dependence, and smoking during pregnancy. They noted no association between LBW and ANX or ODD. Because SES and ethnic status are associated with biological risk factors for LBW (maternal age, parity, birth interval, infections, tobacco and alcohol consumption, and poor nutrition;

Kramer, 1987) and because SES itself is a risk factor for child psychopathology, the authors tried to limit the potentially confounding effects of SES and ethnicity by comparing LBW children to NBW controls in two populations—urban and middle-class suburban. They found that LBW was more strongly linked to ADHD in the socially disadvantaged urban population than in the suburban group, and suggested that social environment may modify the effect of LBW on the development of ADHD, and thus function as a protective factor.

Other research has failed to link pre- and perinatal factors with ADHD. For instance, Werner, Bierman, and French (1971), in their epidemiological study of children in Kauai, found that the severity of "emotional problems" at age 10 was unrelated to the severity of perinatal stress. McGee, Williams, and Silva (1984) also conducted an epidemiological study comparing a subset with problems such as aggressiveness and hyperactivity with the remainder of their community sample. They reported no between-group differences in mode of birth, birth weight, head circumference, or prenatal maternal health problems. However, neither of these studies examined children diagnosed with ADHD, only children with broadly defined categories of dysfunction such as "emotional problems" and "behavioral disturbance."

In another epidemiological investigation, this one of 8-year-old children, Schmidt and colleagues (1987) compared a subgroup with minimal brain dysfunction (MBD) with the remainder of their sample. They reported that the two groups did not differ significantly on risk scores based on pre- and perinatal complications.

Some investigators have used twin and sibling studies to examine genetic and perinatal contributions to the development of ADHD. Goodman and Stevenson (1989) in their large study of 13-year-old twins found no significant association between perinatal adversity specific to twins and hyperactivity. They reported that second-born twins experience relatively more perinatal problems than their firstborn co-twins, as do lighter twins compared to their heavier co-twins. In their sample, hyperactivity

and inattention measures were similar regardless of birth order or relative birth weight. However, their findings may not generalize to singletons, since the perinatal adversity experienced by twins may be unique to twins.

Levy, Hay, McLaughlin, Wood, and Waldman (1996) emphasized the usefulness of comparing psychological development and behavior of twins and singletons in testing the generalizability of data from twin samples to the general population. They studied a nonselected sample of 1938 families with children ages 4–12 years and looked at maternal ratings of symptoms of ADHD, ODD, CD, and Separation Anxiety (SA) using a questionnaire. The questionnaire was validated by a structured parent interview, and also contained measures of speech and reading problems. Their final sample consisted of 1919 male twins, 1915 female twins, 597 male siblings, and 594 female siblings. Twins had significantly more ADHD symptoms and higher scores on measures of speech and reading problems than did singletons, but no differences were found for CD, ODD, or SA symptoms.

Twins may have more ADHD symptoms than singletons for reasons other than genetics. Many perinatal complications are more common or more severe in twins than in singletons. In the Levy and colleagues (1996) study, twins had significantly lower gestational age and birth weight than their singleton siblings. Levy and colleagues found no differences in ADHD symptom number, speech problems, gestational age, or birth weight between MZ male pairs, DZ male pairs, and DZ male twins from opposite-sex pairs. They also noted no such differences among the corresponding female twin groups.

In summary, multiple investigators have linked pre- and perinatal factors to the development of many forms of psychopathology. On balance, more evidence supports the role of pre- and perinatal factors than opposes such a role. There is some evidence that such factors may place individuals at risk for ADHD with comorbidity and for nonfamilial ADHD. Pre- and perinatal complications may lead to the ADHD phenotype by a different mechanism than occurs with the genetic form of ADHD. The role of specific PDIC is even less clear. Some data supports a specific link between LBW and ADHD, and the protective role of social environment on development of ADHD. Additional data on the role of PDIC must be collected to further clarify this pathway and to help shape intervention strategies.

Prenatal Exposure to Teratogens

Alcohol

Streissguth, Barr, Sampson, and Bookstein (1994) conducted a prospective, longitudinal, population-based study that followed a community birth cohort of 500 children through their first 14 years of life to evaluate the long-term effects of prenatal alcohol exposure. Because the study began in the early 1970s when alcohol was not commonly known to have prenatal health effects, the authors thought that the mothers would be less likely to minimize their alcohol consumption than would a comparable sample today. Women were recruited in their fifth month of pregnancy to ensure that they were receiving good prenatal care. The investigators quantified the severity of alcohol use in multiple dimensions (ounces of absolute alcohol per day, volume and pattern of use, and three different measures of binge drinking) both before pregnancy recognition and during pregnancy. Children were blindly examined as neonates, at 8 months, 18 months, and at 4, 7, and 14 years of age. Teacher evaluations were obtained at ages 8 and 11. At age 14, 82% of the original cohort was retained. The investigators used laboratory and teacher behavior ratings, computerized vigilance tasks, measures of IQ and academic achievement, and other neurobehavioral measures.

Streissguth and colleagues (1994) noted alcohol-related deficits in vigilance test performance at ages 4, 7, and 14 (both omission and commission errors), indicating difficulties with sustained attention and response inhibition. Behavior ratings (in the laboratory at age 7 and by teachers at ages 8 and 11) showed increased

impulsivity, trouble focusing and maintaining attention, and slower speed of processing information. At age 14, there were continued alcohol-related difficulties with attention and response inhibition. Learning problems, especially in attention and in speed of information processing, were noted across the 14-year period; lower performance in arithmetic scores were observed at 7 and 14 years of age. Using multiple-regression techniques the authors controlled for a large number of potential confounds such as maternal nutrition, other prenatal drug and medication use, family education and sociodemographic characteristics, mother–child interaction, major life stress, and maternal nicotine use. For most outcomes, binge drinking had more serious consequences than steady drinking and drinking early in pregnancy had more serious consequences than the same pattern of drinking in mid-pregnancy. There was no evidence for a threshold level of prenatal drinking.

Boyd, Ernhart, Greene, Sokol, and Martier (1991) failed to replicate Streissguth and colleagues' (1994) finding of significantly impaired attention on a vigilance task in their prospective study of preschool-age children with prenatal alcohol exposure. They controlled for sociodemographic variables, life stress, other prenatal drug use, and maternal IQ. The contradictory findings in this study and that of Streissguth and colleagues (1994) may be due to a number of factors. Boyd and colleagues' sample was drawn from a more disadvantaged population and had a greater proportion of African American children (34.7% vs. 6.6%). Although both controlled for maternal education, Boyd and colleagues also controlled for maternal IQ. Streissguth and colleagues conducted their computerized vigilance task in the laboratory, whereas Boyd and colleagues conducted theirs in the children's homes, where it may have been more difficult to control for distracting stimuli. The most significant links to ADHD symptoms found by Streissguth and colleagues were binge drinking and drinking early in pregnancy. Boyd and colleagues measured amount of drinking with an index of alcohol consumption per day averaged across the pregnancy period; this index may not have accurately reflected the severity of drinking in binge drinkers and may have masked significant effects of drinking at certain periods in pregnancy. In contrast, Streissguth and colleagues accounted for steady and binge patterns of drinking in their index of drinking severity, and distinguished between exposure to alcohol in early and late pregnancy.

Brown and colleagues (1991) also longitudinally studied the effects of prenatal alcohol exposure at school age in a smaller sample selected from a predominantly low-income, African American population. Sixty-eight mother–child pairs were divided roughly equally into three groups: (1) women who never drank during pregnancy, (2) women who reported using alcohol throughout pregnancy, and (3) those who drank an equivalent amount of absolute alcohol per week in early pregnancy but who stopped drinking after educational intervention in their second trimester. Drinking cessation was confirmed by family and medical staff. Children were then studied at mean age 5 years and 10 months with a parent and teacher checklist, computerized vigilance tasks, a measure of impulsivity, and an assessment of free-play activity level and maternal–child interaction via videotaped observation in the laboratory (the reliability of coding was kept at ≥0.80). They found that teachers reported more externalizing behaviors and internalizing behaviors (especially depression) in the children of the "continued to drink" group. However, when current alcohol use was covaried, these effects were significant only for the externalizing behaviors. Children in the "continued to drink" group performed less well than the others in ratings of school performance, learning, hard work, and appropriate behavior even when current drinking was covaried. Children of mothers who "continued to drink" also showed difficulties with sustained attention; however, these results were no longer significant when current maternal alcohol was covaried. *No* differences between groups were seen on observational measures.

In the Brown and colleagues (1991) study, on computerized vigilance tasks, the children of "continued to drink" mothers made more errors of omission, suggesting attentional deficits. However, this effect disappeared when Brown and colleagues controlled for current maternal drinking. They found no differences between groups on impulsivity measures. Thus, consistent with findings of Streissguth and colleagues (1994), they found prenatal alcohol effects on externalizing behaviors (disruptive behaviors) as measured by teacher ratings. However, consistent with Boyd and colleagues (1991), they did not find effects on attention.

The results of the Brown and colleagues (1991) study highlight the importance of controlling for current maternal alcohol use; many of the findings from prior studies may have been confounded by this postnatal environmental factor. On the other hand, the sample size of the study by Brown and colleagues may not have been large enough to reach statistical significance on the same measures. Also, Brown and colleagues did not note the mean amount of prenatal alcohol intake in their drinking groups. Since there is some evidence of a dose–response relationship, if their sample drank significantly less absolute alcohol per unit time (or had fewer or less severe episodes of binge drinking) than did the sample of Streissguth and colleagues (1994), this may also explain their negative findings. Thus, there does appear to be a significant relationship between prenatal alcohol use and ADHD-related psychopathology, but the data must be interpreted with some caution because of the difficulty in controlling for environmental variables such as ongoing maternal drinking.

Heroin

Heroin exposure during pregnancy has also been suggested as a risk factor for ADHD-related psychopathology. The most consistent finding for prenatal exposure to heroin (and other illicit drugs) is low birth weight, which may, in turn, be a risk factor for ADHD.

Studies on prenatal heroin exposure have been confounded by maternal polydrug use and on-going (postnatal) maternal drug use. The effects of prenatal heroin use were examined by Ornoy, Michailevskaya, Lukashov, Bar-Hamburger, and Harel (1996) in 83 children born to heroin-dependent mothers (44 of these children were adopted after birth), and compared with 76 children born to heroin-dependent fathers and three control groups: 50 children with environmental deprivation and neglect, 50 normal children from a moderate to high SES background (no deprivation), and 80 healthy normal children from local schools and nurseries. The children born to heroin-dependent mothers had high rates of hyperactivity and inattention. However, 42% of the children born to heroin-dependent fathers also had hyperactivity and inattention. Hyperactivity was found in only 20% of the prenatally heroin-exposed children who had been adopted in contrast to 74% of those who were not adopted and living with biological parents. This study has some methodologic problems including a wide age range in the subjects, the lack of standardized measures of behavior and attention, and questionable blindedness of the examiners, but points out a potentially very significant role for the social and home environment in mediating the outcome for children at biological risk. It also suggests the need for replication of the findings using blinded observational data and standardized measures of attention and behavior.

Nicotine

Prenatal nicotine exposure has also been examined as a possible risk factor for ADHD. Nichols and Chen (1981) collected data on a large community sample of children and found increased rates of hyperactivity and impulsivity in the 7-year-old children of smokers. The number of cigarettes smoked per day was the strongest predictor and accounted for 10% of the variance. Nichols and Chen found that maternal smoking had some effect on hyperactivity and impulsivity, but that it was relatively weak

(as were the effects of other pre- and perinatal factors). In other investigations, prenatal exposure to cigarettes has been associated with poorer performance on response-inhibition tasks and with increased errors of comission on vigilance tasks (Fried, Watkinson, & Gray, 1992; Kristjansson, Fried, & Watkinson, 1989).

Cocaine

In recent years, cocaine use in North America has climbed and concern has increased about the effects of prenatal cocaine use on children's development (Richardson, Conroy, & Day, 1996). Studies of prenatal cocaine effects on later behavioral and cognitive outcomes have been limited in number. Azuma and Chasnoff (1993) and Griffith, Azuma, and Chasnoff (1994) followed for 3 years children of cocaine-, alcohol-, and marijuana-using mothers, and nonusing mothers. Drug-exposed groups had significantly lower verbal reasoning scores on intelligence testing and more aggressive behaviors than nonexposed groups. Cocaine exposure predicted significantly more externalizing problems after controlling for other substance use. However, study subjects were poorly retained and the authors did not control for aspects of the current caregiving environment, including caregiver substance use and foster placement.

Richardson and colleagues (1996) conducted a 6-year prospective follow-up study of 28 prenatally cocaine-exposed infants with infants of non–cocaine-using females. Mothers of the first group were light to moderate users. Compared to controls, the cocaine-exposed children made significantly more omission errors on a vigilance task, suggesting differences on attention between the two groups. This finding was significant even when the authors controlled for the child's age, IQ, grade in school, and for mother's race, self-esteem, and first trimester noncocaine substance use. The authors found no effects of cocaine exposure on academic achievement, teacher rated behavior, intellectual ability, or growth. The cocaine-using mothers were generally Caucasian, were light to moderate users of powder cocaine who mainly used in early pregnancy; women who received no prenatal care were excluded. Thus, the findings may not be generalizable to off-spring of heavier users, users of crack cocaine, or non-Caucasian women.

In summary, the data on potential links between prenatal substance exposure and ADHD are limited and have been confounded by polydrug exposure and by ongoing maternal substance use. There is some evidence that pre-natal alcohol exposure may predispose children to ADHD-related psychopathology, especially in early pregnancy and with binge drinking; however, the data should be interpreted cau-tiously, given that many studies have not con-trolled for ongoing maternal drinking. The data on other substance exposure is even more limited. Prenatal heroin exposure is associated with low birth weight, which may, in turn, be a risk factor for ADHD. Children of heroin-dependent mothers have high rates of ADHD symptoms; however, the role of the social and home environment in mediating the outcome for these at-risk children may be very signifi-cant. Cigarette smoking during pregnancy has been associated with hyperactivity and im-pulsivity, and prenatal cocaine use may be associated with both inattentiveness and exter-nalizing behaviors. More prospective studies using both dimensional variables (inattention, hyperactivity) and categorical variables (ADHD by structured interview) are needed to confirm the findings just described.

TEMPERAMENT AND DEVELOPMENTAL RISK FACTORS

A number of investigators have examined the role of infant temperament, or behavioral style, in the development of ADHD. Because differences in temperament can be identified very early in life, it is generally considered to have a constitutional basis. Differences in tem-perament are often based on characteristics such as activity level, emotional responsiveness, and adaptability. "Easy" children are character-ized by low-intensity reactions to stimuli and adaptability to change whereas "difficult" chil-dren often demonstrate high-intensity reactions and difficulty adapting to change. An impor-tant role has been established for temperament in behavior problems in ODD and CD (see Chapter 18, this volume).

In the New York Longitudinal Study, a difficult temperament was found to be a predic-tor of later behavior problems (recently sum-marized in Chess & Thomas, 1996). Cameron (1977, 1978) reanalyzed these data and reported that temperament measures in the first year of life predicted only mild behavior problems. However, parental intolerance, inconsistency, and conflict were associated with negative tem-perament changes; when combined with initial temperament, these changes predicted moderate to severe behavior problems in girls. Rothbart and Bates (1998) reviewed the literature linking certain temperament characteristics to later in-ternalizing or externalizing behaviors. Early in-hibition predicted internalizing problems; early "unmanageability" predicted externalizing problems; early negative affect predicted both types of behaviors.

Other investigators have studied the role of temperament in ADHD symptomatology. Sanson, Smart, Prior, and Oberklaid (1992) conducted a prospective longitudinal study of early characteristics of ADHD children from in-fancy to 8 years of age. They identified four groups of children: those who were ADHD, those who were aggressive, those who were both ADHD and aggressive, and a normal control group. The two aggressive groups had more dif-ficult temperaments and behaviors and more significant life stress from infancy on (compared to the purely ADHD and control groups.) This was most evident in the ADHD-aggressive group. By contrast, the ADHD-only group did not develop problems that distinguished them from controls until or after age 3–4 years. The authors proposed a transactional model of devel-opment in which aggression with or without ADHD may result when a difficult early tem-perament interacts with high life stress. They suggested that these temperament factors may help to identify infants and children at high risk for poor adaptation later in life and for whom early intervention may be possible (see Chapter 18, this volume, for further discussion of this study).

Other developmental variables have also been linked to the development of inattentiveness and hyperactivity in children. Carlson, Jacobvitz, and Sroufe (1995) examined such factors in an 11-year, prospective longitudinal study of 191 children of low-SES mothers. They used measures of infant temperament and development, maternal personality, quality of early maternal caregiving (caregiver intrusiveness and sensitivity), and context (maternal relationship states and emotional support), as well as observational ratings of distractibility and hyperactivity. Distractibility at $3\frac{1}{2}$ years predicted hyperactivity in early elementary years (ages 6–8, $p < .01$) and hyperactivity remained stable throughout the elementary years ($p < .001$). Maternal personality characteristics and quality of caregiving independently ($p < .01$) and in combination ($p < .02$) significantly predicted distractibility at age $3^{1}/_{2}$; the most important predictor was the quality of caregiving. In the early elementary years (ages 6–8), early caregiving characteristics and contextual variables independently predicted hyperactivity ($p < .02$), and this relationship remained even after controlling for early distractibility. Hyperactivity at ages 6–8 was the best predictor of hyperactivity at age 11. Caregiving and contextual variables also predicted later hyperactivity ($p < .04$); this held true even after controlling for earlier hyperactivity. These factors seemed to contribute to the stability of hyperactivity throughout this period.

Such data are consistent with the idea that multiple pathways are likely to lead to the development of ADHD. In some children, overstimulating and intrusive parenting or parental isolation and lack of social support may be the most important risk factors. For others, genetic or other biological factors may be primary. For still others, broader environmental factors may be most influential. Moreover, in some, a trans-

actional model with combined influences of more than one of the variables just mentioned may best describe the development of ADHD.

CHILDHOOD NUTRITION AND DIET

Sucrose

In the 1970s, Feingold (1975) claimed that many ADHD children could be relieved of their symptoms with a diet eliminating food additives such as artificial colors and flavors. This generated much public interest and became the impetus for research studying the role of food additives in ADHD. Conners (1980) reviewed a number of uncontrolled positive studies and later negative studies that were controlled and concluded that food additives are likely to be relevant risk factors in a very small number of cases.

Sucrose has also received some public attention as a possible contributor to disruptive behavior. Prinz, Roberts, and Hantman (1980) reported an association between sucrose intake and aggressive, restless behavior during free play in 28 ADHD children. Their findings were not replicated in a double-blind randomized controlled study by Behar, Rapoport, Adams, Berg, and Cornblath (1984). Behar and colleagues recruited children with a reported history of ADHD-Hyperactive type reactions to sucrose in order to maximize the likelihood of positive findings. They were given sucrose, glucose, or saccharin-flavored placebo. No increases in activity or differences in behavioral ratings or cognitive measures three hours after ingestion of sucrose or glucose were found.

Lead

Unlike food additives and sugar, lead has clearly been shown to be neurotoxic at high doses. The effect of chronic low-dose lead exposure has been under debate since Needleman and colleagues (1979) reported on ADHD symptoms and dentine lead levels from deciduous teeth of 2335 first and second graders in the Boston area. Classroom ratings of deviant behavior increased significantly with lead levels; the strongest correlation was with distractibility. Thomson and colleagues (1989) reported similar findings in a sample of 501 Edinburgh (Scotland) children ages 6–9 years. They found a significant relationship between blood lead levels and ADHD and aggressive behavior ratings even after controlling for possible confounds such as SES, sex, age, and numerous child and parent variables. Moreover, they noted a dose–response relationship between blood lead levels and behavior ratings with no evidence for a threshold.

More recently, Tuthill (1996) studied ADHD symptoms cross-sectionally in 277 first graders and attempted to relate them to hair lead levels. He reported a highly significantly dose–response relationship between lead levels and increased ADHD symptoms on a teacher rating scale, even after controlling for gender, ethnicity, age, and SES. The association was even stronger in children who had a prior diagnosis of ADHD. They also reported no safe threshold level for lead.

In contrast, other investigators (Dietrich et al., 1987, Dietrich, Succop, Berger, Hammond, & Bornschein, 1991) reported few correlations in their prospective study of 258 children. They reported that higher infant lead levels were associated with poorer performance on an intellectual assessment battery, but only for those from the poorest families. Fergusson, Fergusson, Horwood, and Kinzett (1988), in a longitudinal prospective study reported a significant relationship between lead levels and inattention and restlessness in children but noted that it accounted for less than 1% of the variance after controlling for confounds.

Overall, the data suggest that chronic low-level lead exposure is a risk factor for ADHD symptoms but also that it is likely one of many factors that interact with SES to produce ADHD-related psychopathology. However, factors that are frequently associated with low SES, such as low parental education levels, family adversity, and prenatal alcohol exposure,

may be so harmful that they mask the effects of lead (Castellanos & Rapoport, 1992).

CONCLUSIONS

Family studies provide convincing evidence for a significant genetic contribution to the genesis of ADHD. In twin studies, genetic factors have been found to account for a substantial proportion of differences in ADHD symptoms (at least 50% of the explainable variance). The remaining variance may be due to family adversity, pre- and perinatal events, temperament, developmental factors, and toxin exposure. However, all these factors are likely to interact in complex ways to result in the ADHD phenotype.

Figure 1 is an example of a working model for these influences. As previously noted, protective factors can act at many points by blocking pathways to dysfunction, modifying effects of risk factors, or preventing the occurrence of risk factors. Some family-environment risk factors (such as parent characteristics) could be linked to ADHD by common antecedent genetic variables, since family members share genes; they could also be linked by common environmental variables, such as poverty. ADHD may also lead to adverse developmental events such as parental criticism, coldness, and family conflict. This concept is supported by the finding that stimulant treatment of ADHD children leads to increased maternal warmth and decreased maternal coldness (Schachar et al., 1987). Future models should reflect the remarkably complex interactions between risk and protective factors. These models should also reflect the fact that the timing of these interactions in an individual's development matters; even genetic influences may act differently at varying points in development.

It is important to remember that these influences are mediated by underlying neurophysiological mechanisms. However, what exactly is inherited or what is damaged (by prenatal substance exposure, lead ingestion, or

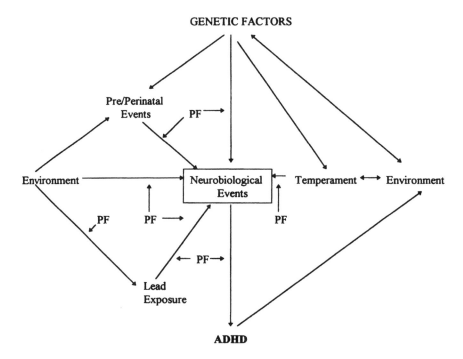

FIGURE 1.   Working model for risk and protective factors (PF).

family adversity) is not well understood. There is increasing evidence that impaired executive function and inhibitory processes underlie many ADHD behaviors (Quay, 1997). The neurochemical and neurophysiologic mechanisms involved in these functional systems are also poorly understood, but multiple anatomic regions of the brain and several neurotransmitter systems are likely to be involved (Hechtman, 1994; see also Chapter 8, this volume).

The present data have many limitations. Many investigations have been confounded by heterogeneity of samples and inadequate controls for environmental and parental characteristics. Researchers should focus on adequate sampling methods to maximize generalizability and on multiple measurement techniques, as well as on prospective and longitudinal designs. As with most research on ADHD, work in the area of risk and resilience has been concentrated on boys. More work is needed on girls, and gender differences in risk and protective factors must be studied. In addition, populations need to be assessed using both dimensional variables (hyperactivity, inattention) and categorical variables (ADHD diagnosis); both have an important role.

Risk factors for ADHD must be studied in conjunction with protective influences, resilience, and competence. Research into protective factors has been limited, as have studies of interventions aimed at fostering resilience. Interventions may be directed toward identified high-risk groups or may be universally enacted to promote competence in large populations. Interventions that target only one factor may have limited effects, since multiple processes are likely to be involved in series or in parallel. For this reason, future interventions may need to target multiple risk and protective factors simultaneously. Since risk factors frequently co-occur and poor outcomes also co-occur, future researchers must move away from investigations of single factors or isolated outcomes (Masten, in press).

The study of risk and protective factors for ADHD and other disorders is essential to understanding the developmental pathways to dysfunction. This review suggests that much can be gained by analyzing these influences using integrated, multidimensional models. Such research can provide a basis for intervention strategies designed to reduce risk, foster resilience, and prevent or ameliorate psychopathology.

REFERENCES

Alberts-Corush, J., Firestone, P., & Goodman, J. T. (1986). Attention and impulsivity characteristics of the biological and adoptive parents of hyperactive and normal control children. *American Journal of Orthopsychiatry, 56,* 413–423.

Azuma, S. D., & Chasnoff, I. J. (1993). Outcome of children prenatally exposed to cocaine and other drugs: A path analysis of three year data. *Pediatrics, 92,* 396–402.

Bailey, J. N., Palmer, C. G. S., Ramsey, C., Cantwell, D., Kim, K., Woodward, J. A., McGough, J., Asarnow, J. A., Asarnow, R. F., Nelson, S., & Smalley, S. L. (1997, October). *DRD4 Gene and susceptibility to ADHD: Differences in familial and sporadic cases.* Paper presented at the International Congress on Psychiatric Genetics, Santa Fe, NM.

Behar, D., Rapoport, J. L., Adams, A. J., Berg, C. J., & Cornblath, M. (1984). Sugar challenge testing with children considered behaviorally "sugar reactive." *Nutrition and Behavior, 1,* 277–288.

Biederman, J., Faraone, S. V., Keenan K., Knee, D., & Tsuang, M. T. (1990). Family-genetic and psychosocial risk actors in DSM-III attention deficit disorder. *Journal of the American Academy of Child and Adolescent Psychiatry, 29,* 526–533.

Biederman, J., Faraone, S. V., Keenan, K., Benjamin, J., Krifcher, B., Moore, C., Sprich-Buckminster, S., Ugaglia, K., Jellinek, M. S., Steingard, R., Spencer, T., Norman, D., Kolodny, R., Kraus, I., Perrin, J., Keller, M. B., & Tsuang, M. T. (1992). Further evidence for family-genetic risk factors in attention deficit hyperactivity disorder: Patterns of comorbidity in probands and relatives in psychiatrically and pediatrically referred samples. *Archives of General Psychiatry, 49,* 728–738.

Biederman, J., Milberger, S., Faraone, S. V., Kiely, K., Guite, J., Mick, E., Ablon, S., Warburton, R., & Reed, E. (1995). Family–environment risk factors for attention deficit hyperactivity disorder: A test of Rutter's indicators of adversity. *Archives of General Psychiatry, 152,* 464–470.

Biederman, J., Milberger, S., Faraone, S. V., Kiely, K., Guite, J., Mick, E., Ablon, S., Warburton, R., Reed, E., & Davis, S. G. (1995). Impact of adversity on functioning and comorbidity in children with attention deficit hyperactivity disorder. *Journal of the American Academy of Child and Adolescent Psychiatry, 34,* 1495–1503.

Boyd, T. A., Ernhart, C. B., Greene, T. H., Sokol, R. J., & Martier, S. (1991). Prenatal alcohol exposure and sus-

tained attention in the preschool years. *Neurotoxicology and Teratology, 13,* 49–55.

Breslau, N., Brown, G. G., DelDotto, J. E., Kumar, S., Ezhuthachan, S., Andreski, P., & Hufnagle, K. G. (1996). Psychiatric sequelae of low birth weight at 6 years of age. *Journal of Abnormal Child Psychology, 24,* 385–400.

Brown, R. T., Coles, C. D., Smith, I. E., Platzman, K. A., Silverstein, J., Erickson, S., & Falek, A. (1991). Effects of prenatal alcohol exposure at school age: II. Attention and behavior. *Neurotoxicology and Teratology, 13,* 369–376.

Cameron, J. R. (1977). Parental treatment, children's temperament, and the risk of childhood behavioral problems: 1. Relationships between parental characteristics and changes in children's temperament over time. *American Journal of Orthopsychiatry, 47,* 568–576.

Cameron, J. R. (1978). Parental treatment, children's temperament, and the risk of childhood behavioral problems: 2. Initial temperament, parental attitudes and the incidence and form of behavioral problems. *American Journal of Orthopsychiatry, 48,* 140–147.

Cantwell, D. P. (1972) Psychiatric illness in the families of hyperactive children. *Archives of General Psychiatry, 27,* 414–417.

Cantwell, D. P. (1996). Attention deficit disorder: A review of the past ten years. *Journal of the Academy of Child and Adolescent Psychiatry, 35,* 978–987.

Carlson, E. A., Jacobvitz, D., & Sroufe, L. A. (1995). A developmental investigation of inattentiveness and hyperactivity. *Child Development, 66,* 37–54.

Castellanos, F. X., & Rapoport, J. L. (1992). Etiology of attention deficit hyperactivity disorder. *Child and Adolescent Psychiatric Clinics of North America, 1,* 373–384.

Chess, S., & Thomas, A. (1996). Temperament. In M. Lewis (Ed.), *Child and adolescent psychiatry: A comprehensive textbook* (2nd ed., pp. 170–181). Baltimore: Williams & Wilkins.

Coie, J. D., Watt, N. F., West, S. G., Hawkins, J. D., Asarnow, J. R., Markman, H. J., Ramey, S. L., Shure, M. B., & Long, B. (1993). The science of prevention: A conceptual framework and some directions for a national research program. *American Psychologist, 48,* 1013–1022.

Colletti, L. F. (1979). Relationship between pregnancy and birth complications and the later development of learning abilities. *Journal of Learning Disabilities, 12,* 659–663.

Conners, C. K. (1975). Controlled trial of methylphenidate in preschool children with minimal brain dysfunction. *International Journal of Mental Health, 4,* 61–74.

Conners, C. K. (1980). *Food additives and hyperactive children.* New York: Plenum.

Cook, E. H., Stein, M. A., Krasowski, M. D., Cox, N. J., Olkon, D. M., Kieffer, J. E., & Leventhal, B. L. (1995). Association of attention deficit disorder and the dopamine transporter gene. *American Journal of Human Genetics, 56,* 993–998.

Dietrich, K. N., Krafft, K. M., Bornschein, R. L., Hammond, P. B., Berger, O., Succop, P. A., Bier, M. (1987). Low level fetal lead exposure effect on neurobehavioral development in early infancy. *Pediatrics, 80,* 721–730.

Dietrich, K. N., Succop, P. A., Berger, O., Hammond, P. B., & Bornschein, R. L. (1991). Lead exposure and the cognitive development of urban preschool children: The Cincinnati Lead Study cohort at age 4 years. *Neurotoxicology and Teratology, 13,* 203–211.

Edelbrock, C., Rende, R., Plomin, R., & Thompson, L. A. (1995). A twin study of competence and problem behavior in childhood and early adolescence. *Journal of Child Psychology and Psychiatry, 36,* 775–785.

Einfeld, S., Hall, W., & Levy, F. (1991). Hyperactivity and the Fragile X Syndrome. *Journal of Abnormal Child Psychology, 19,* 253–262.

Faraone, S. V., Biederman, J., Lehman, B. K., Keenan, K., Norman, D., Seidman, L. J., Kolodny, R., Kraus, I., Perrin, J., & Chen, W. J. (1993). Evidence for the independent familial transmission of attention deficit hyperactivity disorder and learning disabilities: Results from a family genetic study. *American Journal of Psychiatry, 150,* 891–895.

Faraone, S. V., Biederman, J., Lehman, B. K., Spencer, T., Norman, D., Seidman, L. J., Krause, I., Perrin, J., Chen, W. J., & Tsuang, M. T. (1993). Intellectual performance and school failure in children with attention deficit hyperactivity disorder and in their siblings. *Journal of Abnormal Psychology, 102,* 616–623.

Faraone, S. V., Biederman, J., & Milberger, S. (1994) An exploratory study of ADHD among second-degree relatives of ADHD children. *Biological Psychiatry, 35,* 398–402.

Feingold, B. F. (1975). Hyperkinesis and learning disabilities linked to artificial food flavors and colors. *American Journal of Nursing, 75,* 797–803.

Fergusson, D. M., Fergusson, J. E., Horwood, L. J., & Kinzett, N. G. (1988). A longitudinal study of dentine lead levels, intelligence, school performance, and behavior. *Journal of Child Psychology and Psychiatry, 29,* 811–824.

Fried, P. A., Watkinson, B., & Gray, R. (1992). A follow-up study of attentional behavior in 6-year old children exposed prenatally to marihuana, cigarettes, and alcohol. *Neurotoxicology and Teratology, 14,* 299–311.

Gilger, J. W., Pennington, B. F., & DeFries, J. C. (1992). A twin study of the etiology of comorbidity: Attention-deficit hyperactivity disorder and dyslexia. *Journal of the American Academy of Child and Adolescent Psychiatry, 31,* 343–348.

Gillis, J. J., Gilger, J. W., Pennington, B. F., & DeFries, J. C., (1992). Attention deficit disorder in reading-disabled twins: Evidence for a genetic etiology. *Journal of Abnormal Child Psychology, 20,* 303–315.

Goodman, R., & Stevenson, J. (1989). A twin study of hyperactivity: II. The aetiological role of genes, family relationships and perinatal adversity. *Journal of Child Psychology and Psychiatry, 30,* 691–709.

Griffith, D. R., Azuma, S. D., & Chasnoff, I. J. (1994). Three-year outcome of children exposed prenatally to drugs. *Journal of the American Academy of Child and Adolescent Psychiatry, 33,* 20–27.

Grizenko, N., & Pawliuk, N. (1994). Risk and protective factors for disruptive behavior disorders in children. *American Journal of Orthopsychiatry, 64,* 534–544.

Hack, M., Breslau, N., Aram, D., Weissman, B., Klein, N., & Borawski-Clark, E. (1992). The effect of very low birth weight and social risk on neurocognitive abilities at school age. *Journal of Developmental and Behavioral Pediatrics, 13,* 412–420.

Hartsough, C. S., & Lambert, N. M. (1985). Medical factors in hyperactive and normal children: Prenatal, developmental, and health history findings. *American Journal of Orthopsychiatry, 55,* 190–201.

Hauser, P., Zametkin, A. J., Martinez, P., Vitiello, B., Matochik, J. A., Mixson, A. J., & Weintraub, B. D. (1993). Attention deficit hyperactivity disorder in people with generalized resistance to thyroid hormone. *New England Journal of Medicine, 328,* 997–1001.

Hechtman, L. (1994). Genetic and neurobiological aaspects of attention deficit hyperactivity disorder: A review. *Journal of Psychiatry and Neuroscience, 19,* 193–201.

Hechtman, L. (1996) Families of children with attention deficit hyperactivity disorder: A review. *Canadian Journal of Psychiatry, 41,* 350–360.

Knell, E. R., & Comings, D. E. (1993). Tourette's syndrome and attention deficit hyperactivity disorder: Evidence for a genetic relationship. *Journal of Clinical Psychiatry, 54,* 331–337.

Kolvin, J., Miller, F., Fleeting, M., & Kolvin, P. (1988). Risk/protective factors for offending with particular reference to deprivation. In M. Rutter (Ed.), *Studies of psychosocial risk: The power of longitudinal data* (pp. 77–95). Cambridge, England: Cambridge University Press.

Kramer, M. S. (1987). Determinants of low birthweight: Methodological assessment and meta-analysis. *Bulletin of the World Health Organization, 65,* 663–737.

Kristjansson, E. A., Fried, P. A., & Watkinson, B. (1989). Maternal smoking during pregnancy affects children's vigilance performance. *Drug and Alcohol Dependence, 24,* 11–19.

Lahey, B. B., Piacentini, J. C., McBurnett, K., Stone, P., Hartdagen, S., & Hynd, G. (1988). Psychopathology in the parents of children with conduct disorder and hyperactivity. *Journal of the American Academy of Child and Adolescent Psychiatry, 27,* 163–170.

LaHoste, G. J., Swanson, J. M., Wigal, S. B., Glabe, C., Wigal, T., King, N., & Kennedy, J. L. (1996). Dopamine D4 receptor gene polymorphism is associated with attention deficit hyperactivity disorder. *Molecular Psychiatry, 1,* 121–124.

Leckman, J. F., Dolnansky, E. S., Hardin, M. T., Clubb, M., Walkup, J. T., Stevenson, J., & Pauls, D. L. (1990). Perinatal factors in the expression of Tourette's Syndrome: An exploratory study. *Journal of the American Academy of Child and Adolescent Psychiatry, 29,* 220–226.

Levy, F., Hay, D., McLaughlin, M., Wood, C., & Waldman, I. (1996). Twin–sibling differences in parental reports of ADHD, speech, reading and behavior problems. *Journal of Child Psychology and Psychiatry, 37,* 569–578.

Lewis, D. O., & Shanok, S. S. (1979). A comparison of the medical histories of incarcerated delinquent children and a matched sample of non-delinquent children. *Child Psychiatry and Human Development, 9,* 210–214.

Masten, A. S. (1994). Resilience in individual development: Successful adaptation despite risk and adversity. In M. Wang & E. Gordon (Eds.), *Risk and resilience in inner city America: Challenges and prospects* (pp. 3–25). Hillsdale, NJ: Erlbaum.

Masten, A. S. (in press). Resilience comes of age: Reflections on the past and outlook for the next generation of research. In M. D. Glantz, J. Johnson, & L. Huffman (Eds.), *Resilience and development: Positive life adaptations.* New York: Plenum.

Masten, A. S., & Wright, M. O. (1998). Cumulative risk and protection models of child maltreatment. *Journal of Aggression, Maltreatment, and Trauma, 2,* 7–30.

McCormick, M. C., Brooks-Gunn, J., Workman-Daniels, K., Turner, J., & Peckham, G. (1992). The health and developmental status of very low-birth-weight children at school age. *Journal of the American Medical Association, 267,* 2204–2208.

McGee, R., Williams, S., & Silva, P. A. (1984). Background characteristics of aggressive, hyperactive, and aggressive-hyperactive boys. *Journal of the American Academy of Child and Adolescent Psychiatry, 23,* 280–284.

McGee, R., Williams, S., & Silva, P. A. (1985). Factor structure and correlates of ratings of inattention, hyperactivity, and antisocial behavior in a large sample of 9 year old children from the general population. *Journal of Consulting and Clinical Psychology, 53,* 480–490.

Minde, K., Webb, G., & Sykes, D. (1968). Studies on the hyperactive child: VI. Prenatal and paranatal factors associated with hyperactivity. *Developmental Medicine and Child Neurology, 10,* 355–363.

Morrison J. R., & Stewart M. A. (1971). A family study of the hyperactive child syndrome. *Biological Psychiatry, 3,* 189–195.

Morrison, J. R., & Stewart, M. A. (1973). The psychiatric status of the legal families of adopted hyperactive children. *Archives of General Psychiatry, 28,* 888–891.

Needleman, H. L., Gunnoe, C., Leviton, A., Reed, R., Peresie, H., Maher, C., & Barnett, P. (1979). Deficits in psychologic and classroom performance of children with elevated dentine levels. *New England Journal of Medicine, 300,* 689–695.

Nichols, P. L., & Chen, T. C. (1981). *Minimal brain dysfunction: A prospective study.* Hillsdale, NJ: Erlbaum.

Ornoy, A., Michailevskaya, V., Lukashov, I., Bar-Hamburger, R., & Harel, S. (1996). The developmental outcome of children born to heroin dependent mothers, raised at home or adopted. *Child Abuse and Neglect, 20,* 385–396.

Palmer, C. G. S., Bailey, J. N., Ramsey, C., Cantwell, D., Del'Homme, M., McGough, J., Woodward, J. A., Asarnow, R., Asarnow, J., Smalley, S. L., & Nelson, S. (1997, October). *Possible evidence of DAT1 gene by sex interaction in susceptibility to ADHD.* Paper presented at the International Congress on Psychiatric Genetics, Santa Fe, NM.

Pasamanick, B., Rogers, M. E., & Lilienfeld, A. M. (1956). Pregnancy experience and the development of behavior disorders in children. *American Journal of Psychiatry, 112,* 613–618.

Pauls, D. L., Leckman, J. F., & Cohen, D. J. (1993). Familial relationship between Gilles de La Tourette's syndrome, attention deficit disorder, learning disabilities, speech disorders, and stuttering. *Journal of the American Academy of Child and Adolescent Psychiatry, 32,* 1044–1050.

Prinz, R. J., Roberts, W. A., & Hantman, E. (1980) Dietary correlates of hyperactive behavior in children. *Journal of Consulting and Clinical Psychology, 48,* 760–769.

Quay, H. C. (1997). Inhibition and attention deficit hyperactivity disorder. *Journal of Abnormal Child Psychology, 25,* 7–13.

Rae-Grant, N., Thomas, B. H., Offord, D. R., & Boyle, M. H. (1989). Risk, protective factors, and the prevalence of behavioral and emotional disorders in children and adolescents. *Journal of the American Academy of Child and Adolescent Psychiatry, 28,* 262–268.

Richardson, G. A., Conroy, M. L., & Day, N. L. (1996). Prenatal cocaine exposure: Effects on the development of school age children. *Neurotoxicology and Teratology, 18,* 627–634.

Rothbart, M. K., & Bates, J. E. (1998). Temperament. In W. Damon (Series Ed.) & N. Eisenberg (Vol. Ed.), *Handbook of Child Psychology: Volume 3. Social, emotional and personality development* (5th ed., pp. 105–176). New York: Wiley.

Rutter, M. (1985). Resilience in the face of adversity: Protective factors and resistance to psychiatric disorder. *British Journal of Psychiatry, 147,* 598–611.

Rutter, M., & Quinton, D. (1977). Psychiatric disorder: Ecological factors and concepts of causation. In H. McGurk (Ed.), *Ecological factors in human development* (pp. 173–187). Amsterdam, The Netherlands: North Holland.

Rutter, M., Korn, S., & Birch, H. G. (1963). Genetic and environmental factors in the development of "primary reaction patterns. " *British Journal of Social and Clinical Psychology, 2,* 162–173.

Rutter, M., Cox, A., Tupling, C., Berger, M., & Yule, W. (1975). Attainment and adjustment in two geographical areas: The prevalence of psychiatric disorders. *British Journal of Psychiatry, 126,* 493–509.

Rutter, M., Yule, B., Quinton, D., Rowlands, O., Yule, W., & Berger, M. (1975). Attainment and adjustment in two geographical areas: Some factors accounting for area differences. *British Journal of Psychiatry, 126,* 520–533.

Safer, D. J. (1973). A familial factor in minimal brain dysfunction. *Behavior Genetics, 3, 175–186.*

Sanson, A., Smart, D., Prior, M., & Oberklaid, F. (1992). Precursors of hyperactivity and aggression. *Journal of the American Academy of Child and Adolescent Psychiatry, 32,* 1207–1216.

Schachar, R., Taylor, E., Wieselberg, M., Thorley, G., & Rutter, M. (1987). Changes in family function and relationships in children who respond to methylphenidate. *Journal of the American Academy of Child and Adolescent Psychiatry, 26,* 728–732.

Schmidt, M. H., Esser, G., Allehoff, W., Geisel, B., Laucht, M., & Woerner, W. (1987). Evaluating the significance of minimal brain dysfunction—Results of an epidemiological study. *Journal of Child Psychology and Psychiatry, 28,* 803–821.

The Scottish Low Birth Weight Study Group. (1992). The Scottish Low Birth Weight Study: II. Language attainment, cognitive status, and behavioural problems. *Archives of Disease in Childhood, 67,* 682–686.

Smalley, S. L. (1997). Genetic influences in childhood-onset psychiatric disorders: Autism and attention deficit disorder. *American Journal of Human Genetics, 60,* 1276–1282.

Sprich-Buckminster, S., Biederman, J., Milberger, S., Faraone, S. V., & Lehman, B. K. (1993). Are perinatal complications relevant to the manifestation of ADD? Issues of comorbidity and familiality. *Journal of the American Academy of Child and Adolescent Psychiatry, 32,* 1032–1037.

Stevenson, J. (1992). Evidence for a genetic etiology in hyperactivity in children. *Behavior Genetics, 22,* 337–43.

Stewart, M. A., Pitts, F. N., Craig, A. G., & Dieruf, W. (1966). The hyperactive child syndrome. *American Journal of Orthopsychiatry, 36,* 861–867.

Stewart, M. A., DeBlois, C. S., & Cummings, C. (1980). Psychiatric disorder in the parents of hyperactive boys and those with conduct disorder. *Journal of Child Psychology and Psychiatry, 21,* 283–292.

Streissguth, A. P., Barr, H. M., Sampson, P. D., & Bookstein, F. L. (1994). Prenatal alcohol and offspring development: The first fourteen years. *Drug and Alcohol Dependence, 36,* 89–99.

Szatmari, P., Saigal, S., Rosenbaum, P., Campbell, D., & King, S. (1990). Psychiatric disorders at five years among children with birthweights <1000 grams: A regional perspective. *Developmental Medicine and Child Neurology, 32,* 954–962.

Teplin, S. W., Burchinal, M., Johnson-Martin, N., Humphry, R. A., & Kraybill, E. N. (1991). Neurodevelopmental, health, and growth status at age 6 years of children with birth weights less than 1001 grams. *Journal of Pediatrics, 118,* 768–777.

Thomson, G. O. B., Raab, G. M., Hepburn, W. S., Hunter, R., Fulton, M., & Laxen, D. P. H. (1989). Blood lead levels and children's behavior—Results from the Edinburgh Lead Study. *Journal of Child Psychology and Psychiatry, 30,* 515–528.

Tuthill, R. W. (1996). Hair lead levels related to children's classroom attention deficit behavior. *Archives of Environmental Health, 51,* 214–220.

Velez, C. N., Johnson, J., & Cohen, P. (1989). A longitudinal analysis of selected risk factors for childhood psychopathology. *Journal of the American Academy of Child and Adolescent Psychiatry, 28,* 861–864.

Waldman, I. D., Rowe, D. C., Abramowitz, A., Kozel, S., Mohr, J., Sherman, S. L., Cleveland, H. H., Sanders, M. L., & Stever, C. (1996). Association of the dopamine transporter gene (DAT1) and attention deficit hyperactivity disorder in children. *American Journal of Human Genetics, 59* (Suppl. 10), A25.

Welner, Z., Welner, A., Stewart, M., Palkes, H., & Wish, E. (1977) A controlled study of siblings of hyperactive children. *Journal of Nervous and Mental Disease, 165,* 110–117.

Werner, E. E. (1989). High risk children in young adulthood: A longitudinal study from birth to 32 years. *American Journal of Orthopsychiatry, 59,* 72–81.

Werner, E. E., Bierman, J. M., & French, F. E. (1971). *The children of Kauai: A longitudinal study from the prenatal period to age ten.* Honolulu: University of Hawaii Press.

10

Pharmacological Treatment of Attention-Deficit/Hyperactivity Disorder

RUSSELL SCHACHAR and ABEL ICKOWICZ

INTRODUCTION

A vast body of research and clinical experience about the pharmacological treatment of Attention-Deficit/Hyperactivity Disorder (ADHD) has been gathered over several decades. In this chapter's review of this literature, we particularly emphasize the role and effects of psychostimulants, the most commonly prescribed medications for children with ADHD and the most extensively studied. We examine the current role of medication in the treatment of ADHD, summarize the contemporary concepts of the neurochemical rationale for the effects of the various drugs used to treat ADHD, and comment on the benefits and limitations of each class of medication. Although we emphasize the clinical implications of existing knowledge about drug effects, we do not provide a guide to clinical practice for the treatment of children with ADHD.

THE PREVALENCE OF MEDICATION USE AMONG CHILDREN WITH ADHD

The number of prescriptions for children with ADHD has more than doubled over the past two decades, rising from 2 million in 1990 to 5 million in 1994 in the United States (Swanson, Lerner, & Williams, 1995). Currently, as many as 1.5 million children in North America receive medication for ADHD (Safer, Zito, & Fine, 1996). Most of these prescriptions are for stimulants, in particular methylphenidate (MPH: Ritalin; Safer & Krager, 1988; Safer & Zito, 1996; Swanson, Lerner & Williams, 1995), but dextroamphetamine (DEX) is also widely prescribed. Although the prevalence of stimulant use in Canada may be lower than it is in the United States (Ruel & Hickey, 1992; Szatmari, Offord, & Boyle, 1989a), Canada has also experienced a rapid increase in the amount of MPH consumed. Consumption of MPH increased fivefold between 1982 and 1996 and threefold between 1993 and 1996 (J. M. Ruel, personal communication, November 1997). Stimulants are prescribed far less often in Europe and Australia, but their use is increasing.

RUSSELL SCHACHAR and ABEL ICKOWICZ • Department of Psychiatry, The Hospital for Sick Children, Toronto, Ontario, Canada M5G 1X8

Handbook of Disruptive Behavior Disorders, edited by Quay and Hogan. Kluwer Academic/Plenum Publishers, New York, 1999.

This steady rise in rate of use of medication is attributable to a number of factors. ADHD is being diagnosed in more girls, adolescents, and adults than before because research and clinical experience has demonstrated that ADHD is not a transient disorder that is limited to elementary-school-aged boys (Klein & Mannuzza, 1991). There is a growing tendency to prescribe medication three times per day 7 days per week, rather than twice per day 5 days per week, to manage the social and behavioral problems of persons with ADHD that are evident in the evening and on weekends (Greenhill et al., 1996). Fewer physicians recommend drug holidays, because recent research evidence questions the idea that stimulant medication retards growth (Spencer, Biederman, Harding, et al., 1996). There may also be a trend toward the administration of higher doses of stimulant medication (Borcherding, Keysor, Cooper, & Rapoport, 1989). The increasing prevalence of the use of medication may also be linked to physicians', educators', and parents' greater familiarity with and acceptance of the medication and the absence of convincing evidence that nonpharmacological interventions are as effective as those involving medication (Richters et al., 1995; see also Chapter 11, this volume). Moreover, community physicians seem to rely heavily on medication for the treatment of ADHD: As many as 88% of children having a diagnosis of ADHD are prescribed medication (Kwasman, Tinsley, & Lepper, 1995; Wolraich et al., 1990).

Changes in the diagnostic criteria for ADHD may also contribute to an increase in the use of medication. First, the *Diagnostic and Statistical Manual of Mental Disorders* (4th edition) (DSM-IV; American Psychiatric Association, 1994) now permits a subcategory of ADHD defined predominantly by the presence of inattentiveness. This subtype may allow diagnosis of a large number of children whose primary problems arise from learning rather than behavioral problems (Wolraich, Hannah, Pinnock, & Baumgaertel, 1996). Second, the DSM-IV specifies that the diagnosis of ADHD pertains only to children with evidence of pervasive impairment. Yet the criteria for determining pervasive impairment have not been specified in DSM-IV. Consequently, children whose difficulties are primarily academic may have a diagnosis of ADHD and be medicated largely on the basis of behavioral problems that are evident primarily or exclusively in the school setting.

Furthermore, stimulant response is nonspecific: The activity of both normal children and those with ADHD is reduced and their attentiveness increased with MPH treatment (Rapoport et al., 1980). Consequently, as more children are given medication, more seem to respond and to warrant continued treatment.

Not only is medication used more often, but it also appears to be used in an inconsistent and potentially inappropriate manner for some children. For example, the rate of use of medication varies widely across otherwise similar communities, even though professionals assume that the prevalence of ADHD does not vary. In some communities, the rates of use of medication are very high; in others, the rates (6% of school children) approximate the prevalence of ADHD in the population (Safer & Krager, 1988; see Chapter 2, this volume); and in others, the rate is lower than the prevalence of the disorder (Rappley, Gardiner, Jetton, & Houang, 1995; Safer et al., 1996; Sherman & Hertzig, 1991; Szatmari, Offord, & Boyle, 1989b). Variable rates of use of medication could reflect differences in access to resources as much as over- or underprescription; these rates could indicate that for some children the potential role of medication in their care is not being adequately assessed (Szatmari et al., 1989b).

THE PHARMACOLOGICAL BASIS FOR MEDICATION EFFECTS

Although the effect of stimulants on children's behavior was discovered by serendipity rather than by clarification of the mechanisms of ADHD, our current understanding of ADHD provides a tentative rationale for the beneficial effects of stimulant medication. The core aberration in ADHD appears to be a deficit in the executive control processes of the cognitive system (Douglas, Barr, Amin, O'Neill, & Britton, 1988; Pennington & Ozonoff, 1996; Schachar & Logan, 1990) that arises from abnormalities in the neurochemical and neurophysiological substrates of information processing and behavioral self-regulation.

There is evidence of abnormality in children with ADHD in each of the catecholamine systems that have been implicated in the regulation of attention and behavior. Moreover, medications that have an impact on the manifestations of ADHD are known to affect these catecholamine systems (Pliszka, McCracken, & Maas, 1996); however, the relationship among neurotransmitter function, attention, and behavior is complex.

Developments in cognitive neuroscience and neuroimaging have begun to elucidate the neural networks involved in attentional functions. Attention may be viewed as a set of networks that carry out different functions, including orientation to sensory stimuli, exercise of executive control, and maintenance of an alert state (Posner & Petersen, 1990). The attentional network is like an interactive aggregate in which a posterior system is responsible for the orientation toward new stimuli and an anterior executive system coordinates the frontal-lobe functions necessary for the analysis, selection, and initiation of responses.

Normally, the act of preparing for a target quiets the sensory system. When the level of background activity is less, targets can be more effectively recognized and amplified. Norepinephrine appears to reduce background noise and enhance target-induced activity at the cellular level. Attentional deficits may result, in part, from a problem with this preparatory mechanism (Posner & Raichle, 1994). A disregulated central norepinephrine system in persons with ADHD may not efficiently prime the posterior attention system to external stimuli (Pliszka *et al.*, 1996).

In contrast, the anterior system, which is responsible for executive functions (inhibitory control and working memory), is to a great extent dopaminergic. Evidence indicates that dopamine plays a major role in regulating the excitability of the cortical circuitry on which the working memory function of the prefrontal cortex depends (Goldman-Rakic, 1996). Inadequate dopaminergic activity at prefrontal synapses may lead to a dysfunction in inhibitory control and working memory—putative core deficits in persons with ADHD (Barkley, 1997). Dopamine is not restricted to anterior (frontal lobe) functions, but is involved also in the mesolimbic circuits mediating sensitivity to reward (Quay, 1997) and in cerebellar activity (Volkow *et al.*, 1997). The cerebellum has been classically associated with motor coordination, and increasing evidence suggests that it also plays an important role in higher cognitive functions, including memory, learning, and attention (Leiner, Leiner, & Dow, 1989).

Molecular genetics studies are beginning to elucidate the contribution of the genes to the expression of the symptoms associated with ADHD, including variations in the gene that encodes the D4 dopamine receptor (LaHoste *et al.*, 1996) and the anomalies of the dopamine transporter gene (Cook *et al.*, 1995; Gill, Daly, Heron, Hawi, & Fitzgerald, 1997). These findings suggest a genetic substrate associated with dopaminergic dysfunction (see Chapter 8, this volume).

Also, the role of central and peripheral epinephrine may be critical in the response to stimulant medication. Both central epinephrine and peripheral epinephrine systems are involved in a person's response to information through their effects on the locus ceruleus. The locus ceruleus is an essential part of the preparatory mechanisms for attention described previously. Central epinephrine inhibits the locus ceruleus directly, and the peripheral effects of epinephrine (increased heart rate and blood pressure) may reset the locus ceruleus to a lower level of activity (Pliszka *et al.*, 1996; Shenker, 1992). The role of epinephrine in the stimulants' mechanism of action is supported by the fact that both MPH and DEX increase epinephrine metabolites in urine (Elia *et al.*, 1990).

Results of pharmacological probes in children with ADHD using different medications suggest that the drug effects are related to both noradrenergic and dopaminergic activity. As discussed later in the chapter, stimulants and monoamine oxidase (MAO) inhibitors are among the most effective agents. Drugs that target specific cathecolamine systems have smaller effects. For example, children using imipramine and desipramine show relatively less efficacy on cognitive tasks than those using stimulants, which may be explained, in part, by the fact that these tricyclic antidepressants are much less potent in their ability to inhibit the uptake of dopamine than of norepinephrine (Shenker, 1992). Similarly, the apparent lack of effect of clonidine on measures of inhibitory control and working memory in children with ADHD could be explained by clonidine's selective adrenergic activity and lesser dopaminergic activity (Ickowicz, Masellis, & Tannock, 1996). Drugs that selectively target the dopaminergic system are also less effective. A summary of the relative effectiveness of the drugs used in the treatment of children with ADHD is provided in Table 1.

STIMULANTS

Pharmacology

Stimulants are sympathomimetic amines that closely resemble neurotransmitters. The stimulants MPH and DEX both indirectly activate central catecholamine receptors by increasing the concentrations of the endogenous agonist in the synaptic cleft (Zametkin & Rapoport, 1987). The mechanism of the action of DEX includes direct neuronal release of dopamine and norepinephrine, as well as the blockade of catecholamine reuptake. It also has a weak MAO-inhibitory effect. Weak antagonism of the α_2-adrenergic receptors may also contribute to the central effects of the amphetamine (Shenker, 1992). Generally, the D-isomer is several times more active than the L-isomer. The molecule is rapidly absorbed from the intestine and readily penetrates the brain. The

TABLE 1.   The Relationship between the Mechanism of Action and the Effectiveness of Pharmacological Agents Used in the Treatment of ADHD

Clinical efficacy	Drug	Proposed mechanism of action
Very effective	Dextroamphetamine Methylphenidate Pemoline	Indirect agonist at multiple DA and NE receptors
	Clorgyline	MAO-A inhibitor
	Tranylcypromine	MAO-A&B inhibitor
Moderately effective	Desipramine Imipramine Clomipramine Carbamazepine	NE-uptake inhibitors, weak DA-uptake inhibitors
	Clonidine Guanfacine	α2-adrenoreceptor agonists
	Haloperidol Chlorpromazine Thioridazine	DA and α-adrenoreceptor antagonists
Minimally or not effective	Levodopa	DA agonist
	Deprenyl	MAO-B inhibitor
	Piribedil	DA agonist
	Mianserin	α-adrenoreceptor antagonist and NE-uptake inhibitor

MAO = monoamine oxidase, NE = norepinephrine, DA = dopamine.
Note. Adapted from Shenker (1992).

onset of clinical effects is rapid; peak plasma levels after oral administration are achieved in 1 to 3 hr. The plasma half-life is 6.8 hr (Brown, Hunt, Ebert, Bunney, & Kopin, 1979). Urinary acidification reduces the half-life.

Structurally, MPH is related to DEX, although MPH is considered a milder stimulant. The mechanism of MPH's action is similar to that of DEX, but it has been shown to act on a different pool of vesicular dopamine. MPH is also rapidly absorbed and easily crosses the blood–brain barrier. Effects occur in 30 min, with a peak plasma level in 1 to 2 hr, falling to a half-peak level in less than 3 hr (Shaywitz, Hunt, & Jatlow, 1982). MPH absorption is unaffected by food (Chan et al., 1983). The primary clinical implications of the pharmacological profile of MPH and DEX are that their effects are short-lived and, therefore, the medication must be taken repeatedly.

Despite their different half-lives, these stimulants reach their peak therapeutic effect during the absorption phase of the kinetic curve. The absorption phase parallels the acute release of neurotransmitters into the synapse. This phenomenon may explain the transient mood elevation or euphoria observed in some of the children treated with stimulants, as well as the development of rebound.

Clinical Effects of Stimulants

Behavioral Effects

The most immediate and obvious, and arguably the most beneficial effect of stimulant therapy is the rapid improvement in the behavioral manifestations of ADHD, such as restlessness, inattentiveness, and impulsiveness. These effects have been known for decades and have been replicated in numerous randomized controlled trials (see Spencer, Biederman, Wilens, et al., 1996, for review). Reduced activity and improved attentiveness are evident in structured situations (e.g., while playing baseball) (Pelham, McBurnett, et al., 1990; Porrino et al., 1983). Activity during free play or unstructured situations may actually increase, although the intensity of the activity decreases

(Henker, Astor-Dubin, & Varni, 1986). In general, this behavioral effect increases with a higher dose of MPH, in the range of 5 to 20 mg (Rapport, Denney, DuPaul, & Gardner, 1994). A beneficial impact on behavior is observed in approximately 70% of treated children (see Spencer, Biederman, Wilens, et al., 1996, for review), but only 25% to 50% of children show normalization of teacher-rated behavior scores (DuPaul & Rapport, 1993; Rapport et al., 1994). In general, all stimulants have equivalent effectiveness (Greenhill, 1992), yet some children may respond better to one than to another (Elia, Borcherding, Rapoport, & Keysor, 1991; Greenhill et al., 1996).

If both MPH and DEX at a range of doses are tried, the rate of behavioral nonresponse may be no more than 5% (Arnold, Christopher, Huestis, & Smeltzer, 1978; Elia et al., 1991). Greater severity of ADHD symptoms, younger age, and absence of symptoms of anxiety predict a more favorable clinical response (Buitelaar, Van der Gaag, Swaab-Barneveld, & Kuiper, 1995; DuPaul, Barkley, & McMurray, 1994; Pliszka, 1989; Taylor et al., 1987). An abnormal neurological examination and electroencephalogram are not reliable predictors of a favorable response (Halperin, Gittelman, Katz, & Struve, 1986; Zametkin & Rapoport, 1987), but disinhibition may predict a favorable response (Quay, 1997).

The behavioral effects of stimulants are limited to a 1- to-4-hr period of pharmacological activity; there is no evidence of any carryover effect to periods in which the medication is not pharmacologically active. For example, the typical regimen of twice-daily dosing does not result in any significant behavioral effects during the after-school period (Schachar, Tannock, Cunnigham, & Corkum, 1997). Moreover, there is no evidence that even prolonged therapy leads to the internalization of self-control; the beneficial effects of stimulant therapy dissipate rapidly upon discontinuation of treatment (Brown, Borden, Wynne, Schleser, & Clingerman, 1986).

Tolerance to the effect of MPH may develop in some children over months or years of continuous therapy (e.g., Charles, Schain, &

Guthrie, 1979; Kupietz, Winsberg, Richardson, Maitinsky, & Mendell, 1988; Sleator, Von Neumann, & Sprague, 1974) and an increased dose may be required in about one third of children with ADHD (Satterfield, Satterfield, & Cantwell, 1981; Sleator et al., 1974). However, few children seem to lose their initial favorable response completely, even after extended periods of therapy (Safer & Allen, 1989).

Cognitive Effects

There has been considerable debate about the possible adverse impact of stimulants on cognition, such as a decrease in the flexibility of problem solving, an increase in perseveration of inappropriate responses, an overfocus on limited aspects of available information, and an inability to think divergently and creatively. The likelihood of these effects is thought to increase with increasing task complexity and dosage of the stimulant (Brown & Sleator, 1979; Brown, Slimmer, & Wynne, 1984; Sprague & Sleator, 1977; Tannock, Schachar, Carr, Chajczyk, & Logan, 1989). In theory, even subtle adverse cognitive effects could have important ramifications when averaged over many years on medication, creating a well-behaved child at the expense of more important cognitive functions.

Rather than causing an adverse effect on the performance of cognitive tasks, MPH, according to laboratory research, generally has a beneficial effect on many of the cognitive processes that are deficient in children with ADHD. MPH decreases reaction time, decreases response variability, improves accuracy of performance, facilitates detection and correction of errors, improves the ability to focus on the most relevant aspects of information, and decreases impulsive responding (Krusch et al., 1996; Losier, McGrath, & Klein, 1996). Moreover, MPH reduces the decrement in performance after a failure, decreases the tendency to quit working on very difficult tasks, increases the effort expended to obtain a reward, and increases the tolerance of frustration (Douglas et al., 1988; Haenlein & Caul, 1987; Milich, Licht, Murphy, & Pelham, 1989; Milich, Carl-

son, Pelham, & Licht, 1991; Wilkison, Kirsher, McMahon, & Sloane, 1995). These apparent improvements are not only evident on boring, simple sustained-attention tasks, but also on a range of demanding, divergent thinking tasks. Indeed, MPH improves higher-order executive functions more clearly than it does more basic processes such as encoding and memory search (de Sonneville, Njiokiktjien, & Bos, 1994; Douglas et al., 1988; Douglas, Barr, Desilets, & Sherman, 1995; Rapport & Kelly, 1991; Solanto & Wender, 1989; Tannock, Schachar, Carr, Chajczyk, & Logan, 1989; Vyse & Rapport, 1989). There is scant evidence of state-dependent learning, namely, that information learned while a child is receiving medication is recalled less easily when the child is off medication (Becker-Mattes, Mattes, Abikoff, & Brandt, 1985).

However, clinicians typically titrate the dosage of MPH according to behavioral rather than cognitive responses because cognitive responses are much more complicated to assess. Theoretically, this practice could result in doses of MPH that optimize behavior, but reduce cognitive function. However, there is minimal evidence to support this concern within the range of doses typical of clinical and research practice (i.e., 0.3 to 1.0 mg/kg). The effects of higher doses have not been subject to the same rigorous evaluation. In general, performance on cognitive tasks improves in a linear fashion with doses of MPH up to 1.0 mg/kg (typically considered a large dose; see Douglas et al., 1995, for review), although there is some evidence that higher doses have little incremental effect on behavior beyond the effect of moderate doses (Brown & Sleator, 1979; Brown et al., 1984; Rapport et al., 1994; Sprague & Sleator, 1977; Tannock, Schachar, Carr, Chajczyk, & Logan, 1989; Tannock, Schachar, Carr, & Logan, 1989). Moreover, there is little evidence that a definable subgroup of children who exhibit adverse drug effects across multiple cognitive measures exists (Douglas et al., 1995; Solanto & Wender, 1989). The one exception may be the subgroup of children with ADHD and comorbid anxiety discussed later in this chapter: They may not show the same magnitude of improvement in cognition that is observed in nonanxious children with ADHD.

Academic Effects

Children with ADHD experience serious and impairing academic difficulties. They fail more grades, achieve lower marks, are more likely to drop out of school, and often have a diagnosis of a learning disability (Klein & Mannuzza, 1991). Academic underachievement figures prominently in the referral and diagnostic processes (Copeland, Wolraich, Lindgren, Milich, & Woolson, 1987). In general, MPH treatment results in marked improvement in classroom behavior, attention to academic tasks, persistence, and effort (Rapport et al., 1994). Across all groups of treated children, MPH improves academic productivity, as judged by the percentage of problems completed and completed correctly. Performance on measures of mathematical computation, word discovery, verbal retrieval, letter search, and reading improve (Balthazor, Wagner, & Pelham 1991; Pelham, Swanson, Furman, & Schwindt, 1995; Rapport et al., 1994; Richardson, Kupietz, Winsberg, Maitinsky, & Mendell, 1988; Tannock, Schachar, Carr, & Logan, 1989). Stimulant therapy may even have a beneficial impact on school grades (Famularo & Fenton, 1987; cf. Wolraich, Drummond, Salomon, O'Brien, & Sivage, 1978).

However, there are important individual differences in responsiveness to stimulants. A far greater proportion of medicated children exhibit clinically significant improvement in classroom behavior (94%) than in attention to task (76%) or in academic efficiency (53%; Rapport et al., 1994). Increasing the dose of medication may result in further improvement in behavior and attention in all but 5% of children, but has no incremental impact on academic efficiency in a substantial number of children. This dissociation of learning and behavioral effects that appears in some cases may explain why no long-term benefit of the use of MPH has been demonstrated for academic performance (see Schachar & Tannock, 1993, for review). For some children who fail to respond to one stimulant, switching to a second may result in additional behavioral improvement (Elia et al., 1991). The same is unlikely to be true for academic performance because behavioral response does not predict academic response with a high degree of precision (Rapport et al., 1994).

Social Effects

ADHD has a significant impact on children's relationships with peers, family, and adults. Very often, children with a diagnosis of ADHD are disruptive, interfering, intrusive, abrupt, impatient, and both verbally and physically aggressive. They are more socially busy, intrusive, critical, and overbearing, and less attuned to the social agenda of their peers. They are inattentive to subtle social cues and procedures for entering a peer group, and they have a tendency to attribute hostile motives to others (Buhrmester, Whalen, Henker, MacDonald, & Hinshaw, 1992; Murphy, Pelham, & Lang, 1992; see also Chapters 6 and 7, this volume). As a result of these characteristics, children with ADHD experience high levels of rejection by their peers and teachers, and their parents respond to them in a controlling and negative fashion (e.g., Barkley, Karlsson, Strzelecki, & Murphy, 1984). These undesirable social interactions play a significant role in the impairment that children with ADHD experience. Also, these interactions are stable (Parker & Asher, 1987) and may be a major determinant of poor outcomes in adolescence (Barkley, Fischer, Edelbrock, & Smallish, 1990; Taylor, Chadwick, Heptinstall, & Danckaerts, 1996; see also Chapter 12, this volume).

Treatment with stimulants results in a substantial and immediate improvement in the quality of the children's social interactions with their peers, parents, and teachers. Treatment reduces the frequency of negative verbalizations, such as teasing and swearing, and of conduct problems, such as physical aggression, lying, stealing, and destruction of property. Medicated children are less dominating and annoying and initiate fewer negative social interactions with their peers. They are more cooperative with their peers (they follow rules more frequently), as well as with parents and teachers (Hinshaw, Henker, Whalen, Erhardt, & Dunnington, 1989). They are less disruptive in the classroom (e.g., they call out less frequently). Their social standing in the eyes of their peers improves (e.g., they are more often rated as fun to be with, as cooperative, or as someone's best friend; Cunningham, Siegel, & Offord, 1991; Hinshaw & McHale 1991; Hinshaw, Buhrmester, & Heller, 1989; Hinshaw, Henker, et al., 1989; Pelham & Bender, 1982; Pelham et al., 1991; Whalen, Henker, Buhrmester, et al., 1989). Parents and teachers respond to this altered social behavior with a reciprocal decrease in their own controlling, critical, and punitive behavior toward these medicated children with ADHD (Cunningham et al., 1991). Parents and siblings are more positive and less critical of them, and family members spend more time together (Barkley & Cunningham, 1979; Schachar, Taylor, Wieselberg, Thorley, & Rutter, 1987).

However, marked individual variation in response is evident. One quarter of children with ADHD who are aggressive before treatment do not show an increase in prosocial behavior (Hinshaw, Henker, et al., 1989; Whalen, Henker, Buhrmester, et al., 1989). Moreover, improvement in the quality of social interactions seems to be a consequence of the reduced severity of the core behavioral deficits of ADHD; children with minimal behavioral response to medication show little change in social interaction (Schachar et al., 1987).

More important, several aspects of social behavior are relatively unresponsive to MPH. Medication has a variable effect on socially appropriate behavior (Buhrmester et al., 1992; Granger, Whalen, & Henker, 1993; Murphy et al., 1992). Medicated children with ADHD may not cease their aggressive response when provoked (Pelham et al., 1991). Medication has minimal effects on processing of social information by these children, including their typical attribution of hostile intentions to their peers. Simultaneously, there may be an increase in socially inhibited behavior, social withdrawal, and dysphoria. These behaviors

may decrease the extent to which the children are liked by their peers or adults because the behaviors may be perceived as socially unresponsive (Buhrmester et al., 1992; Granger et al., 1993; Whalen & Henker, 1991; Whalen, Henker, & Granger, 1989; Whalen, Henker, & Granger, 1990). Perhaps as a consequence of these unresolved social difficulties, peers are much less responsive to the alterations in behavior arising from medication than are adults (Cunningham et al., 1991; Granger et al., 1993; Whalen et al., 1990).

Doses as low as 0.3 mg/kg may be sufficient to reduce many types of aggressive behavior in a particular child, although, generally, higher doses result in greater improvement (Murphy et al., 1992; cf. Cunningham et al., 1991). Doses of approximately 0.6 mg/kg may be necessary to decrease intentional aggression or aggressive responses to provocation (Barkley, McMurray, Edelbrock, & Robbins, 1989; Casat, Pearson, Van Davelaar, & Cherek, 1995; Hinshaw, Henker, & Whalen, 1984b; Murphy et al., 1992), to achieve a reduction in maternal directiveness and negative interactions with mothers (Barkley, Karlsson, Pollard, & Murphy, 1985), and to alter peer responses to a child with ADHD (Cunningham et al., 1991; Hinshaw et al., 1984b). There are very few studies of the effects of twice-daily doses higher than 0.6 mg/kg in the social domain (Hinshaw & McHale, 1991).

There is no carryover of the effect of daytime treatment on the child's social behavior in the evening (Schachar et al., 1997). As a result, parent–child interactions may not improve, and hostile and dysfunctional interactions may persist and have an adverse impact on outcome of ADHD. To some extent, this limitation can be minimized through the use of a third dose that covers the after-school and early evening period (this is discussed later in this chapter).

The social effects of MPH seem to be similar for younger and older ADHD children (Hinshaw, Buhrmester, & Heller, 1989). Comparable social effects have been noted for both aggressive and nonaggressive children with ADHD (Barkley et al., 1989; Klorman et al., 1989; Klorman, Brumaghim, Fitzpatrick, Borgstedt,

& Strauss, 1994), although, as expected, greater improvement in aggressive behavior is observed among those who are more aggressive before treatment (also Barkley *et al.*, 1989).

Psychological and Mood Effects

Most children with ADHD feel increased vigor and decreased fatigue when they are medicated; in a substantial proportion of children, their mood improves (e.g., Ahmann *et al.*, 1993; Barkley, McMurray, Edelbrock, & Robbins, 1990; Klorman *et al.*, 1994). However, some children do experience increased irritability and depressed mood on medication (see side effects later in this chapter). Euphoria, particularly immediately after taking MPH, has been described occasionally (Corrigall & Ford, 1996).

The majority of children understand why they are taking medication and feel that it is helpful (Whalen & Henker, 1991). Yet many adolescents complain that they want to try managing their difficulties without pills, which suggests that some experience medication as an undesirable form of external control.

Stimulant medication does not seem to engender an external locus of control in children with ADHD, namely, an enduring belief that their success is attributable to external factors instead of their own personal effort. Rather, as the children's behavior improves, so does their self-esteem (Abikoff & Gittelman, 1984) and the likelihood that they will attribute their success to personal effort. Moreover, medicated children do not give up after an experience with a problem that they cannot solve (Milich *et al.*, 1989, 1991; Pelham *et al.*, 1992). This pattern suggests that medicated children evaluate their performance more accurately.

We do not know the effects of medication on children's attributions about aspects of their performance other than that on academic tasks, the effects of prolonged treatment on these psychological variables, or the effect of medication when it is taken in combination with other treatments. In contrast with the favorable attributional effects of medication on the child with ADHD in experimental situations, teachers and peers appear to attribute the success of a medicated child to the effect of the medication and the success of an unmedicated child to high effort (Amirkhan, 1982).

There is no evidence that MPH treatment generates dependence on MPH or that MPH treatment reduces the risk of the substance use and drug dependence that characterize persons with ADHD (Hechtman, 1985). Occasionally, clinicians observe older students who demand a great deal of themselves and feel that they would be unable to succeed academically without MPH. Typically, these students are happy to stop taking the medication over the summer and during school holidays, a finding that suggests that they are psychologically, not physiologically, dependent on the medication.

Age and Development Effects

MPH has its clearest impact on elementary-school-aged children. Among these children, those who are younger respond as well (Buitelaar *et al.*, 1995) or somewhat better (Taylor *et al.*, 1987) than those who are older. The academic, social, cognitive, and long-term effects of stimulants have been studied far less often in preschoolers, adolescents, and adults with ADHD than in elementary-school-aged children. In general, preschoolers are less responsive to stimulants than school-aged children and may be more likely to have side effects such as irritability, sadness, and insomnia (Mayes, Crites, Bixler, Humphrey, & Mattison, 1994).

Adolescents have the same robust response to stimulants as elementary-school-aged children, but many parents describe their adolescents as not substantially better or as somewhat worse (e.g., Klorman, Coons, & Borgstedt, 1987). Rather than abuse of or habituation to stimulants, noncompliance seems to be a bigger problem in the treatment of adolescents (Biederman, Wilens *et al.*, 1995). They complain about the cyclical effect of the medication and their dislike of taking pills, particularly at school. Long-acting preparations may be advantageous for this reason.

Few studies of the effects of stimulants in adults have been conducted. Existing studies

(Spencer, Biederman, Wilens, *et al.*, 1996) show somewhat less effect in adults than in children. Adults have more irritability, sedation (i.e., zombie-like feeling), anxiety, and insomnia (e.g., Wender, Reimherr, Wood, & Ward, 1985). The benefits of stimulants are evident in reduced core behavioral symptoms, as well as in improved occupational performance and marital relationships (Wender *et al.*, 1985). The duration of the action may be shorter in adults, who may require either higher doses or long-acting preparations.

Children with neurodevelopmental delay associated with ADHD respond as favorably to MPH as those without such delay (Mayes *et al.*, 1994).

Side Effects

Physiological Side Effects

The most common side effects of stimulants are physiological complaints such as loss of appetite, insomnia, headache, and stomachache. These symptoms occur in approximately half of treated children with ADHD, significantly more often than in those treated with a placebo (Ahmann *et al.*, 1993; Barkley, McMurray, *et al.*, 1990; Schachar *et al.*, 1997). Appetite suppression results in a rapid reduction in weight gain and, in some cases, in actual weight loss. For example, Klorman and colleagues (1994) reported that children treated with MPH at a low dose lost 0.5 kg in 21 days, whereas children on the placebo gained 0.5 kg over the same period. Appetite suppression may be managed with the consumption of high-calorie snacks, the addition of late-evening meals, a decrease in the dose of the medication before meals, or a change in the timing of the late-day dose so that it follows a meal.

Stomachache may be treated with a change in the timing or type of medication: Medication may be taken after meals (Swanson, Sandman, Deutsch, & Baren, 1983) with an antacid or be switched to a sustained-release preparation that is absorbed more slowly. Not every case of appetite suppression is associated with stomachache, however: Appetite suppres-

sion may be a result of the direct drug effects on appetite regulation (Schachar *et al.*, 1997).

The weight loss associated with taking stimulants does not dissipate, but persists over at least 4 months of treatment (Schachar *et al.*, 1997). However, no reliable effect on height or weight over prolonged periods of treatment has been demonstrated (Spencer, Biederman, Harding, *et al.*, 1996; Zeiner, 1995). Spencer, Biederman, Harding, and colleagues (1996) argue that any difference in the eventual stature of children with ADHD who have been medicated is evidence of the developmental delay associated with ADHD and is not a function of the dose or duration of the drug treatment. They argue that growth will normalize spontaneously with or without medication.

Nevertheless, the possibility of growth suppression will require reevaluation because of the growing trend to prescribe stimulants three times daily 7 days per week without drug holidays. Caution should be exercised when stimulant medication is prescribed, especially at higher doses for prolonged periods, and for children of very short stature. Drug holidays may be useful because several studies (Klein, Landa, Mattes, & Klein, 1988; Safer & Allen, 1973; Safer, Allen, & Barr, 1975) have found that rebound growth occurs during these holidays. However, drug holidays must be arranged at times when academic or social function will not be adversely affected.

Some disruption of sleep (e.g., delayed sleep onset) is evident with twice-daily dosing (Greenhill, Puig-Antich, Goetz, Hanlon, & Davies, 1983; Kent, Blader, Koplewicz, Abikoff, & Foley, 1995; cf. Busby & Pivik, 1985; Nahas & Krynicki, 1977) and even with a single morning dose of MPH (Tirosh, Sadeh, Munvez, & Lavie, 1993). The issue of drug-induced sleep disturbance is increasingly important, given the current trend to the use of three daily doses of MPH to achieve behavioral control in the evening (Greenhill *et al.*, 1996). A thrice-daily dosing schedule seems to effectively reduce ADHD symptoms in the evening and, for the majority of children, does not result in an increase in side effects or delayed sleep onset (Kent *et al.*, 1995). However, even twice-daily dosing may be associated with a decrease in total sleep duration and an increase in tiredness upon awakening in some children (Haig, Schroeder, & Schroeder, 1974; Kent *et al.*, 1995; Stein *et al.*, 1996). Clinicians would be wise to monitor the effect of a late-day dose of MPH on sleep since all current studies of thrice-daily dosing have been short-term.

For most children with ADHD, dose-related minimal increases in heart rate and blood pressure are the only cardiovascular effects observed (Kelly, Rapport, & DuPaul, 1988). Children with ADHD and comorbid anxiety (Urman, Ickowicz, Fulford, & Tannock, 1995; Zeiner, 1995) and black male adolescents (Brown & Sexson, 1989) may have a greater increase in blood pressure after taking MPH.

Overall, the prevalence of sleep and appetite disturbances among children with ADHD is similar for MPH and DEX.

Tics, Dystonic Movements, and Obsessive-Compulsive Behavioral Side Effects

Motor tics (e.g., blinking), vocal tics, dystonic movements (e.g., tongue thrusting), and obsessive–compulsive behaviors (e.g., picking at the fingernails, preoccupation with particular activities) are common consequences of stimulant therapy (found in approximately 20% of cases; Barkley, McMurray *et al.*, 1990; Ickowicz, Tannock, Fulford, Purvis, & Schachar, 1993). They are not usually severe and typically subside with a decrease in the dosage or the discontinuation of the medication; they rarely result in the discontinuation of treatment (only in approximately 2%; Borcherding, Keysor, Rapoport, Elia, & Amass, 1990; Denckla, Bemporad, & MacKay, 1976; Lipkin, Goldstein, & Adesman, 1994). These side effects are observed more frequently in systematic clinical trials (i.e., in 76% of cases; Borcherding *et al.*, 1990) than in typical clinical practice (i.e., in 8%; Lipkin *et al.*, 1994), an observation that suggests they are difficult to detect without training.

Tourette's syndrome, a pattern of severe and persistent vocal and motor tics that occurs as a consequence of the stimulant treatment and persists after the discontinuation of the medication has rarely been reported (e.g., Bachman, 1981; Lowe, Cohen, Detlor, Kremenitzer, & Shaywitz, 1982). Tics and abnormal movements are not dose-dependent; they occur at low as well as high doses (Borcherding *et al.*, 1990). Consequently, careful and direct examination of the child for tics and abnormal movements before and after the initiation of stimulants is essential, as is the education of parents and teachers about the nature of tics.

Tics may occur early in the treatment or after several months of treatment with stimulants. If tics or obsessive–compulsive behavior is noted during treatment, the child should be monitored for several days before the dose is reduced or the treatment discontinued to determine whether these behaviors will dissipate spontaneously. If the tics do not dissipate spontaneously, a different stimulant should be tried before the treatment is discontinued. Stimulants should be used with extra caution in children with a personal or family history of tics or Tourette's syndrome because of the increased likelihood of exacerbating tics.

In general, DEX and MPH are equally likely to cause abnormal movements (Borcherding *et al.*, 1990). However, DEX may be more likely to cause overly meticulous behavior, and MPH, dysphoria, nervous habits, and mannerisms (Elia *et al.*, 1991).

Rebound

It is common for parents to complain that their medicated children with ADHD experience a period of rebound, typically at the end of the day. In some instances, parents may complain about their child's behavior reverting to its original, unmedicated levels as the medication wears off (Schachar *et al.*, 1997). In other cases, parents report that their child's behavior is worse after a day of medication than it is after a day without medication. When Johnston, Pelham, Hoza, and Sturges (1988) investigated behavioral rebound directly, they concluded that there was little evidence of behavioral rebound across a group of medicated children. However, as many as one third of children in their study showed some behavioral rebound.

An increase in side effects at the end of the day may also prompt parents to complain about rebound. Even with twice-daily administration of the drug, side effects seem to be more frequent or severe at the end of the day than during the day (Barkley, McMurray, *et al.*, 1990; Schachar *et al.*, 1997), although the frequency of side effects seems greater when MPH is taken thrice daily rather than twice daily (Ahmann *et al.*, 1993).

Psychological and Mood Side Effects

An increase in sadness and anxiety occurs in a significant proportion of medicated children with ADHD at low (0.3 mg/kg; Whalen, Henker, & Granger, 1989) and moderate (0.6 mg/kg; Buhrmester *et al.*, 1992) doses. This effect is not evident when medicated children are observed at play, so careful assessment is necessary to detect the signs of dysphoria (Hinshaw, Buhrmester, & Heller, 1989). In contrast, many children experience decreased irritability, crying, anger, and unhappiness (Ahmann *et al.*, 1993; Klorman *et al.*, 1994) and may report feeling significantly better about themselves (Pelham *et al.*, 1992). Euphoria is not observed often (Barkley, McMurray, *et al.*, 1990; Corrigall & Ford, 1996) but does occur rarely in some children within 30 min of taking medication.

Onset and Persistence of Side Effects

Rather than dissipating with continued treatment, as has been suggested in the literature (Cantwell, 1996; Golinko, 1984), initial physiological side effects tend to persist for at least 4 months (Schachar *et al.*, 1997). Other side effects may have a delayed onset. For example, affective symptoms with MPH are not evident immediately after starting treatment but are first evident after 4 months of treatment (Schachar *et al.*, 1997), and abnormal movements with pemoline are first evident after 1 month of treatment (Sallee, Stiller, Perel, & Everett, 1989).

Of the few long-term trials of stimulants that have been conducted, a minority of investigators (Brown *et al.*, 1986; Gittelman-Klein, Klein, Katz, Saraf, & Pollack, 1976; Rie, Rie, Stewart, & Ambuel, 1976a, 1976b; Schain & Reynard, 1975) have commented on side effects. These existing long-term studies document an increase in physical side effects, somberness, and, in one study (Rie *et al.*, 1976a), social withdrawal. Even prolonged treatment with stimulants does not seem to increase the risk of drug use or abuse (Weiss, Hechtman, Milroy, & Perlman, 1985).

Dose-Related Side Effects

Side effects occur even at low doses of MPH and are more frequent as the dose increases (Ahmann *et al.*, 1993). Although the goal of a recent treatment study (Schachar *et al.*, 1997) was to reach a twice-daily dose of 0.7 mg/kg of MPH, the dosage of MPH was adjusted according to the incidence of side effects. As a result, the target dose could not be reached or had to be reduced in a significant proportion of children; the final average dose of MPH was approximately 0.5 mg/kg twice daily. Safer and Allen (1989) suggested that titration to a dose in milligrams per kilogram could result in doses that are too high for heavier children. However, in the study of Schachar and colleagues (1997), the target dose could not be reached for children of any weight. The standard practice of titrating the dose according to body mass may not be supportable: Wide variation in the absorption, metabolism, and excretion, and high inter- and intraindividual variation among children is independent of weight (Rapport & Denney, 1997).

Long-Term Effects of Stimulants

The long-term effects of stimulants are less well investigated than the short-term, possibly because of the greater difficulty conducting randomized clinical trials of extended treatments. Schachar and Tannock (1993) identified 18 studies of stimulants that involved active treatment of 3 months or longer. Only 11 of these studies were controlled in any systematic fashion. Many methodological limitations are evident in this body of research, including lack of randomization, diagnostic heterogeneity, high and unspecified attrition from the studies, lack of compliance with treatment, failure to ensure optimal stimulant treatment, lack of control over adjunctive nonpharmacological therapy, and a narrow range of outcome measures.

Across the 11 well-controlled trials that Schachar and Tannock (1993) identified, the finding that prolonged treatment with stimulants improves core behavioral symptoms was generally consistent, although few subjects progressed sufficiently to be considered normalized (e.g., Conrad, Dworkin, Shai, & Tobiessen, 1971). Benefits were noted with both low-dose (Brown, Wynne, & Medenis, 1985) and high-dose (Gittelman-Klein et al., 1976) therapy, although a significant impact on aggression was found only at a twice-daily dose of 0.7 mg/kg (not at 0.3 mg/kg or 0.5 mg/kg; Kupietz et al., 1988). Studies in which the dose was titrated according to the patient's response to the medication yielded more consistent benefits than studies that used fixed doses (Schachar & Tannock, 1993). Benefits dissipate rapidly, even after prolonged therapy (e.g., Brown et al., 1986), and there may be a deterioration in behavior over 6 months of therapy, even in continuously medicated children (Kupietz et al., 1988). There appears to be no carryover of daytime treatment (i.e., twice-daily dosing) into the evening, even after extended treatment (Schachar et al., 1997).

The existing extended-treatment studies identified by Schachar and Tannock (1993) provide little evidence of a beneficial effect of stimulants on academic attainment, conduct disturbance, peer relationships, or self-esteem, and no evidence that medication reduces the overall impairment associated with ADHD. Available extended MPH treatment studies find no evidence for an increased external locus of control (Horn et al., 1991) or a differential response among the subtypes of ADHD. Very few studies have contrasted the effectiveness of various medications. In one such study (Quinn & Rapoport, 1975), stimulants were of greater benefit than the tricyclic antidepressant imipramine.

The apparent paradox between the immediate short-term benefit and the general absence of long-term benefit may be attributable to limitations in the design of the existing research (Schachar & Tannock, 1993), poor adherence to treatment (Brown, Borden, Wynne, Spunt, & Clingerman, 1987), or ineffectively managed treatment (Sherman & Hertzig, 1991). It may be that the suppression of core behavioral symptoms such as restlessness, inattentiveness, and impulsiveness is not all that is necessary to mitigate long-term impairment in persons with ADHD. Continued troubled parent–child relationships, peer problems, or academic underachievement may be more salient predictors of outcome (Barkley & Cunningham, 1978; Whalen, Henker, & Granger, 1989).

Long-Acting Stimulants

Long-acting stimulants (Ritalin SR, Dexedrine spansules, and pemoline) provide coverage over the course of the day without a midday dose and with less fluctuation in effect than short-acting stimulants. Supervision of the midday dose is obviated and the possibility of social stigmatization at school is reduced. The effects of these long-acting preparations may be sufficiently persistent to cover behavior at the end of the day. The effect of Dexedrine spansules lasts 9 hr (Pelham, Greenslade, et al., 1990). However, Ritalin SR, which is designed to have the same impact as 10 mg of regular MPH taken twice daily, has a variable and slow onset of effect (3 hr) that may last only 5 hr (Pelham et al., 1987; Pelham, Greenslade, et al., 1990). Moreover, individual responsiveness to long-acting forms of DEX and MPH is highly variable (Pelham et al., 1987; Pelham, Greenslade, et al., 1990).

Pemoline effects increase with time after ingestion over a period of 4 to 5 hr; its effects persist for 7 hr after ingestion. Pemoline at a dose of 56.25 mg ($1\frac{1}{2}$ tablets) has effects similar to those reported for short-acting MPH (10 mg, twice daily), Dextroamphetamine spansule (10 mg, given in the morning), or Ritalin SR (20 mg given in the morning) (Pelham, Greenslade, et al., 1990). At this dose, pemoline may have cognitive, academic, and behavioral effects in 1 or 2 hr, not several weeks, as previously believed (Pelham, Greenslade, et al., 1990; Pelham et al., 1995; Sallee, Stiller, & Perel, 1992). The effects increase when the dose is increased to 112.5 mg, with minimal side effects. However, the late onset of choreoathetoid movements may be a concern (Sallee et al., 1992). Pemoline has been recommended because it has a lower potential for abuse than MPH (Riggs, Thompson, Mikulich, Whitmore, & Crowley, 1996), but there is no systematic evidence that pemoline is effective for children who fail to respond to MPH.

Considerable doubt has been raised about the role of pemoline since the recent advisory concerning its association with life-threatening hepatic failure (McCurry & Cronquist, 1997; Shevell & Schreiber, 1997; Sterling, Kane, & Grace, 1996). The risk of hepatic failure is serious but low. The earliest onset of hepatic abnormalities occurs 6 months after the initiation of therapy and may occur without prodromal symptoms preceding the onset of jaundice (Berkovitch, Pope, Phillips, & Koren, 1995). The earliest manifestations may be nausea, vomiting, anorexia, fatigue, or jaundice. Assessments of liver function before the initiation of treatment, after the establishment of treatment, and at regular intervals, possibly every 6 months, are recommended, but have not been shown to predict acute liver failure (Shevell & Schreiber, 1997). Pemoline should be discontinued immediately if clinically significant hepatic dysfunction is observed.

NONSTIMULANT MEDICATIONS

Approximately 30% of children with ADHD have an inadequate behavioral response to or impairing side effects with stimulants (e.g., Spencer, Biederman, Wilens, et al., 1996; Wilens & Biederman, 1992). For many of these children, a change to a nonstimulant medication may be useful.

Consultation with a colleague experienced in child psychopharmacology may be advisable

before the initiation of these nonstimulant treatments because none of these medications has been investigated as extensively as the stimulants. The effects of nonstimulants on the full scope of ADHD behavioral, learning, and cognitive symptoms and on long-term outcome have not been explored in detail.

The effectiveness of many of these medications is described in the following sections, but clinicians are advised to investigate the details of pretreatment assessment, contraindications, initial and maintenance dosage, drug interactions, and monitoring before prescribing these medications for their patients with ADHD. For some medications, specific investigations (as described in the following paragraphs) will be necessary.

Antidepressants

Tricyclic Antidepressants

Imipramine, desipramine, clomipramine, and nortriptyline are the most commonly used and extensively investigated of tricyclic antidepressants for the treatment of ADHD. Tricyclic antidepressants increase plasma norepinephrine by blocking the reuptake of norepinephrine and have virtually no effect on the dopamine system. The primary impact of tricyclic antidepressants is on the behavioral manifestations of ADHD; tricyclic antidepressants have less benefit for cognitive and academic functions (Gualtieri, Keenan, & Chandler, 1991). Tricyclic antidepressants have the potential advantage of a long half-life, a reduced need for a midday dose, no potential for abuse, and the possibility of monitoring compliance through the assessment of levels of the drug in the blood. They also have potential usefulness in the presence of comorbid conditions because of their established efficacy in the treatment of obsessive–compulsive symptoms (Leonard et al., 1989), tic disorders (Singer et al., 1995), and anxiety (Klein, Koplewicz, & Kanner, 1992). Tricyclic antidepressants are, however, less effective for the treatment of ADHD than stimulants (Biederman, Baldessarini, Wright, Knee, & Harmatz, 1989).

Tricyclic antidepressants may cause side effects such as dry mouth, dizziness, nausea, constipation, palpitations, drowsiness, perspiration, and tremor. More important, tricyclic antidepressants may cause increased systolic and diastolic blood pressure; increased heart rate (14 to 20 beats per min, evidence of sinus tachycardia); and prolongation of electrocardiogram-conduction variables, indicating an intraventricular conduction delay of the right bundle–branch block type. Clomipramine has a greater impact on cardiac conduction than desipramine (Leonard et al., 1995). Since these effects are not typically associated with clinical consequences (Wilens et al., 1996), few subjects must discontinue treatment because of tachycardia (Leonard et al., 1995).

However, serious questions have been raised about the clinical role of tricyclic antidepressants because of seven sudden deaths of apparently healthy children taking this medication who had no established history of cardiovascular problems (Riddle, Geller, & Ryan, 1993; Swanson, Jones, Krasselt, Denmark, & Ratti, 1997; Varley & McClellan, 1997; Werry, Biederman, Thisted, Greenhill, & Ryan, 1995). Such sudden deaths are rare, may not exceed the incidence of sudden death in the general pediatric population (Biederman, Thisted, Greenhill, & Ryan, 1995), and seem impossible to predict, even with careful monitoring. The mechanism of these cardiac effects is unknown, but may arise from conduction abnormalities caused in predisposed persons by changes in the parasympathetic and sympathetic input to the heart (Riddle et al., 1993). No relationship between the dosage of tricyclic antidepressants and cardiac effects has been noted (Leonard et al., 1995). Adverse cardiac effects may be exaggerated by the combination of the stimulant medication with other medications such as thioridazine or terfenadine (Seldane, Marion Merrell Dow, Kansas City, MO), which, by themselves, have been shown to prolong cardiac conduction. These effects may be more marked in children with comorbid anxiety who may have an increased sensitivity to augmented noradrenergic function (Urman et al., 1995).

Consequently, treatment with tricyclic antidepressants should be undertaken cautiously and with careful monitoring (see Wilens et al., 1996, for guidelines). Recommendations for the safe use of tricyclic antidepressants include a baseline electrocardiogram, family history for premature cardiac disease, and, possibly, cardiological consultation. Cardiogram and tricyclic antidepressant plasma levels should be repeated several days after the patient reaches a daily dose of 2.5 mg/kg per day and repeated again after subsequent increases. Evidence of lightheadedness or headaches indicates a need to check vital signs (Wilens et al., 1996). Several persons who did not have tachycardia during acute treatment did have it after more prolonged therapy, indicating the need for continuous monitoring of cardiac effects. Tricyclic antidepressants should not be discontinued abruptly.

Specific Serotonin Reuptake Inhibitors

Specific serotonin reuptake inhibitors (SSRI) are commonly used in the treatment of depression, anxiety, and obsessive–compulsive symptoms. Information about the effects of SSRI in children with ADHD is limited to case reports and open trials. In general, these studies suggest that fluoxetine may be useful for the behavioral and affective symptoms associated with ADHD, but is less effective in improving attention (Barrickman, Noyes, Kuperman, Schumacher, & Verda, 1991; Gammon & Brown, 1993). Gammon and Brown reported that fluoxetine and MPH in combination may be a safe and effective alternative in children with ADHD and comorbid anxiety or depressive symptoms who do not respond to monotherapy. Similarly, Findling (1996) reported good results with the combined use of psychostimulants with sertraline or fluoxetine in the management of comorbid depression and ADHD. Although the safety and side-effect profile of SSRI is more benign than that of tricyclic antidepressants, SSRI are not free of adverse effects, including sleep disturbance, restlessness, social disinhibition, and subjective sensation of excitation, that may be difficult to differentiate from core ADHD symptoms (Riddle *et al.*, 1990–1991). These side effects may be avoided by the initiation of treatment with lower doses or ameliorated with dose reduction when they develop.

Monoamine Oxidase Inhibitors

MAO inhibitors are primarily used to treat adults with depressive disorders that are unresponsive to other antidepressants. Type A MAO is involved in the metabolism of norepinephrine and serotonin; type B MAO metabolizes dopamine and phenylethylamine. Both clorgyline, a selective MAO-A inhibitor, and tranylcipromine, a combined MAO-A+B inhibitor, were as effective as DEX in a double-blind crossover study of 14 boys with ADHD (Zametkin, Rapoport, Murphy, Linnoila, & Ismond, 1985). In contrast, deprenyl, a selective MAO-B inhibitor had little effect (Zametkin & Rapoport, 1987), suggesting that the pharmacological action of MAO inhibitors on ADHD symptoms is mediated by noradrenergic mechanisms. The side effects and drug interactions of the MAO inhibitors, coupled with the dietary constraints associated with the therapeutic use of these drugs, however, result in serious limitations of the use of this type of medication for the management of children with ADHD.

Bupropion

Bupropion is an antidepressant with a pharmacological profile similar to that of stimulants. Presumably, it acts by decreasing whole-body norepinephrine turnover. Conners and colleagues (1996) reported significant improvement in core ADHD symptoms with bupropion without any concomitant deterioration in cognitive performance and without serious side effects. A direct comparison (Barrickman *et al.*, 1995) found that bupropion was less effective than MPH in improving attention, but otherwise had rather comparable effects. In that study, the majority of subjects

continued on MPH rather than bupropion after the trial because, unlike bupropion, MPH can be taken on weekdays only and because many subjects had previous positive responses to MPH. The initial dosage of bupropion was 1.5 mg/kg per day, increasing to a maximum of 5 to 6 mg/kg over several weeks in divided doses.

α2-Adrenergic Agonists

Clonidine

Clonidine acts predominantly as an α2-adrenergic agonist through direct activation of the presynaptic receptor, suppressing the release of norepinephrine and reducing the firing of the locus ceruleus. Peak plasma levels occur between 3 and 5 hr after ingestion; the plasma half-life is between 8 and 12 hr in adolescents and is much shorter in preadolescent children (ranging from 4 to 6 hr; Leckman *et al.*, 1985).

Clonidine was first used by child psychiatrists two decades ago as a treatment of Tourette's syndrome (Cohen, Detlor, Young, & Shaywitz, 1980; Leckman *et al.*, 1991). More recently, clonidine has been shown to reduce the symptoms of ADHD (Hunt, Minderaa, & Cohen, 1985, 1986). Available evidence suggests that clonidine results in a positive behavioral response and increased tolerance to frustration, with lesser effects on cognition (Hunt, 1987). However, in healthy adults, a small but significant decrease in attention capacity, together with a decline in the speed of processing, follows clonidine administration (Clark, Geffen, & Geffen, 1987). Likewise, clonidine impairs attentional and working memory functions in healthy young adults (Coull, Middleton, Robbins, & Sahakian, 1995a, 1995b) and may also result in discrete impairment of executive control in children with ADHD and comorbid anxiety (Ickowicz *et al.*, 1996).

Clonidine is probably most clearly indicated when the target symptoms are related to hyperarousal and poor tolerance of frustration. It clearly plays an important role in the management of tic disorders and Tourette's syndrome. Clonidine has been used effectively in the treatment of sleep disorders in persons with ADHD (Rubinstein, Silver, & Licamele, 1994; Swanson, Flockhart, Udrea, & Cantwell, 1995; Wilens, Biederman, & Spencer, 1994) and of sleep disturbances arising from treatment with stimulants (Prince, Wilens, Biederman, Spencer, & Wozniak, 1996).

Clonidine is generally well tolerated, but may cause sedation, fatigue, and hypotension, especially at the outset of treatment. These side effects are not usually a problem (Leckman *et al.*, 1991) and can be minimized by careful titration of the dose. Clonidine should be avoided for children and adolescents with past or present depressive symptoms or a family history of mood disorders (Hunt, Capper, & O'Connell, 1990). Several cases of electrocardiographic abnormalities have been reported with concurrent use of clonidine and other psychotropic medication (Chandran, 1994).

Clonidine treatment starts with doses of 25 to 50 µg per day, with increases of 25 to 50 µg every third day to a maximum daily dose of 3 to 6 µg/kg. Clonidine should not be withdrawn suddenly because of the attendant risk of hypertension.

Guanfacine

Guanfacine is a long-acting α2-adrenergic agonist that preferentially binds postsynaptic receptors that are concentrated in the prefrontal cortical regions (Arnsten, 1997; Arnsten, Steere, & Hunt, 1996). Guanfacine causes less sedation and hypotension than clonidine (Chappell *et al.*, 1995). Guanfacine has proven effective and safe in a small number of subjects with ADHD (Hunt, Arnsten, & Asbell, 1995) and may be effective for children with ADHD and comorbid tic disorder (Chappell *et al.*, 1995). As with clonidine, preliminary evidence suggests that guanfacine is less effective for cognition than is typically observed with stimulants (Crook, Wilner, & Rothwell, 1992). The initial dose of guanfacine is 0.5 mg per day, increased every 3 or 4 days up to about 1.5 mg per day given in morning, after-school, and bedtime doses.

Mood Stabilizers (Antimanics)

Lithium Carbonate

Lithium carbonate is a mood stabilizer commonly used to treat mania in adults. It is of questionable or no value for the treatment of the behavioral or cognitive manifestations of ADHD, but may effect modest reduction in the symptoms of aggression and conduct disorder in children and adolescents (see Alessi, Naylor, Ghaziuddin, & Zubieta, 1994, for review; Campbell *et al.*, 1995; DeLong & Aldershof, 1987). Lithium has been used experimentally to augment the stimulant treatment of ADHD associated with manialike symptoms (Carlson, Rapport, Kelly, & Pataki, 1992). In 60% of children, side effects occur, the most common of which are central nervous system (tremor, drowsiness, ataxia, confusion), gastrointestinal (abdominal discomfort, nausea, vomiting, diarrhea), genitourinary (polydipsia or polyuria, secondary enuresis), and ocular effects (blurred vision) (Hagino *et al.*, 1995). These side effects tend to occur during the first week of treatment and are associated with higher lithium levels. Hagino and colleagues (1995) did not report any increase in the frequency of side effects or increase in lithium levels in children taking concurrent medication such as stimulants, imipramine, or antibiotics.

The starting dose for lithium is 300 or 600 mg/day with increases to 1200 mg/day, adjusted to achieve serum levels between 0.6 and 1.2 mEq/L (see Weller, Weller, & Fristad, 1986, for a guide to lithium dosage). Lithium levels should be obtained 24 hr after the first test dose, 12 hr after each change of dose at 8:00 A.M., and 5 days after the maintenance dose is achieved.

Carbamazepine

Carbamazepine is an anticonvulsant that is structurally related to tricyclic antidepressants. A recent meta-analytic review (Silva, Munoz, & Alpert, 1996) of the literature on carbamazepine suggested that close to 70% of patients experience at least marked improvement in their ADHD symptoms with carbamazepine. This finding should be interpreted with caution because only 3 of the 10 reviewed studies used a placebo-control design, few subjects were involved in these studies (total N = 53), and the operational definitions of ADHD varied. Little effect on aggressive symptoms has been observed with the use of carbamazepine for children with a primary diagnosis of Conduct Disorder (Cueva et al., 1996). Carbamazepine may play a role in the management of comorbid ADHD and mood disorders.

Carbamazepine has a long half-life and attainment of steady-state levels may require 3 to 6 weeks (Silva et al., 1996). The oral dose is in the range of 200 to 600 mg/day (20 mg/kg per day) and stabilization takes up to 2 months. The most common side effects are sedation, ataxia, tremor, headache, diplopia, incoordination, slurred speech, and dizziness, which are all mild and transient. Since carbamazepine can cause hematological changes and liver abnormalities, monitoring of these systems is indicated.

Antipsychotics

The majority of studies evaluating the effectiveness of antipsychotics in children with hyperactive behaviors were done two and three decades ago. Double-blind studies found that some of these drugs were effective treatments for children many of whom would meet present criteria for ADHD. Chlorpromazine was superior to a placebo in a double-blind, 8-week trial of 39 hyperactive children (Werry, Weiss, Douglas, & Martin, 1966). Chlorpromazine resulted in marked improvement in hyperactive behavior, yet intellectual functioning and symptoms of distractibility, aggressiveness, and excitability did not seem to be particularly responsive. Frequent side effects were sedation and photosensitivity. Thioridazine was superior to a placebo in children with ADHD, but not as effective as MPH alone or a combination of thioridazine plus MPH (Gittelman-Klein et al., 1976). Haloperidol's efficacy was also evaluated in children with symptoms of inattention and

hyperactivity. Werry and Aman (1975) conducted a double-blind crossover study comparing the effects of MPH (0.3 mg/kg), two doses of haloperidol (0.025 and 0.05 mg/kg), and a placebo on attention, memory, and activity in 24 children. MPH, and to a lesser extent low-dose haloperidol, improved the cognitive functions of vigilance and short-term memory, whereas high-dose haloperidol may have caused a deterioration in performance.

Given the serious risks associated with both acute and long-term use (e.g., tardive dyskinesia), the indication for antipsychotics for the management of ADHD is restricted to extreme cases in which severe symptoms and impairment persist, even after exhaustive investigation of treatment alternatives known to be both safer and more effective.

COMBINATIONS AND AUGMENTATION

Combinations of medications are used because of a lack of response to a single medication or because of the presence of comorbid psychiatric disorders in children with ADHD, particularly in the most seriously disturbed (Wilens, Spencer, Biederman, Wozniak, & Connor, 1995; see also Chapter 2, this volume). Interactions among drugs are a concern with combinations of medications because one drug may alter the absorption, distribution, metabolism, or excretion of another. Combinations of medications may increase the proportion of unbound pharmacologically active drug and, therefore, the frequency of side effects. These drug interactions are likely to be complex and are generally unknown.

For example, MPH decreases the metabolic clearance of imipramine, resulting in increased circulating concentrations of imipramine and increased risk of side effects. Children treated with combined MPH and desipramine are more likely than those treated with MPH alone to experience nausea, dry mouth, tremor, headaches, anorexia, feelings of tiredness, and higher ventricular heart rate (Pataki, Carlson, Kelly, Rapport, & Biancaniello, 1993). There have been no cases of behavioral or cognitive deterioration with combined MPH and desipramine therapy, and none of the reported side effects seem to preclude continuation of treatment (Pataki et al., 1993). MPH can increase blood levels of anticonvulsants and SSRI, which may cause agitation; a combination of MPH and MAO antidepressants can cause a serious elevation in blood pressure; and a combination of MPH and theophylline can cause agitation and dizziness. SSRI may raise the blood levels of tricyclic antidepressants and carbamazepine. Antihistamines such as terfenadine (Seldane) have cardiovascular effects and may have a synergistic effect when combined with other medications.

Careful monitoring of blood levels and side effects is necessary with combined drug treatment (see Greenhill, 1992). The combination of MPH and clonidine is frequently used for the sleep problems associated with ADHD or those that result from stimulant therapy (Wilens et al., 1994). There have been 23 serious reactions reported with this combination: 4 fatal and 19 nonfatal (Swanson, Flockhart, et al., 1995). There is a clear need for research into the efficacy and safety of various combinations of medications for ADHD.

PHARMACOLOGICAL CONSIDERATIONS FOR ADHD SUBTYPES

It is quite common for children with ADHD to have one or more comorbid disorders (Biederman, Newcorn, & Sprich, 1991). The effect of stimulants on these comorbid cases is clinically and theoretically important.

ADHD and Conduct Disorder

Comorbid Conduct Disorder or marked Oppositional Defiant Disorder, which is present in about 25% of patients with ADHD in clinic samples, can be treated with MPH. MPH has comparable effects on aggressive and nonaggressive ADHD (Barkley et al., 1989; Klorman et al., 1994) although, as might be expected, greater improvement in aggression is observed among those who are more aggressive before treatment (also Barkley et al., 1989).

ADHD and Anxiety

Anxiety Disorder is evident in 25% of persons with ADHD (Anderson, Williams, McGee, & Silva, 1987; Bird, Gould, & Staghezza, 1993). Compared with their nonanxious ADHD peers, these comorbid patients have a differential response to MPH, especially at higher doses, that is characterized by a less robust behavioral response and possibly a greater incidence of side effects (DuPaul et al., 1994; Pliszka, 1992; Tannock, Ickowicz, & Schachar, 1995; Taylor et al., 1987). However, two thirds of children with comorbid ADHD and anxiety respond favorably to stimulants (Ickowicz & Tannock, 1997); stimulants likely constitute the first line of pharmacologic treatment for these persons. Although a combination of SSRI and stimulants may be helpful (Gammon & Brown, 1993), clonidine does not seem to be particularly effective for the ADHD–anxiety comorbid group (Ickowicz et al., 1996).

ADHD and Tic Disorders

As many as 10% to 20% of unmedicated children with ADHD exhibit tics (Barkley, McMurray et al., 1990), and about 25% of children with Tourette's syndrome have ADHD (Dykens et al., 1990). Many children with Tourette's syndrome experience substantial impairment from their ADHD symptoms (Comings & Comings, 1987a, 1987b). Behavior and the quality of social interaction tend to improve with MPH treatment, but normalization of behavior is uncommon (Nolan & Gadow, 1997). Stimulant treatment may increase the severity of preexisting tics in a substantial proportion of patients (see Chappell, Scahill, & Leckman, 1997, for review) but in many others the tics, particularly vocal tics, actually improve (Gadow, Nolan, Sprafkin, & Sverd, 1995; Gadow, Sverd, Sprafkin, Nolan, & Ezor, 1995). In some cases, tics that have developed during stimulant treatment may diminish with continued treatment (Castellanos *et al.,* 1997).

Neuroleptics seem to be of little value for the treatment of ADHD symptoms in children with Tourette's syndrome (Shapiro, Shapiro, & Fulop, 1987; Shapiro *et al.,* 1989) but tricyclic antidepressants seem effective (Riddle, Hardin, Cho, Woolston, & Leckman, 1988; Singer *et al.,* 1995; Spencer, Biederman, Kerman, Steingard, & Wilens, 1993). Clonidine may be helpful for the treatment of a tic disorder that is comorbid with ADHD, although the impact on the ADHD symptoms is greater than that on the tics (Leckman *et al.,* 1991; Singer *et al.,* 1995, Steingard, Biederman, Spencer, Wilens, & Gonzalez, 1993). Bupropion targets ADHD symptoms, but may exacerbate the tics (Spencer, Biederman, Steingard, & Wilens, 1993). An open trial (Steingard, Goldberg, Lee, & De-Maso, 1994) indicated that clonazepam may be a useful adjunctive pharmacological agent for augmenting the MPH treatment of children in whom tics persist. The combination was well tolerated; early mild sedation dissipated with time. Observed behavioral disinhibition needed to be monitored. The mean dose of clonazepam was in the range of 0.25 to 2 mg/day, given at bedtime or in divided doses twice daily.

ADHD and Bipolar Disorder

The controversial diagnosis of comorbid mania in children with ADHD is not easily established because of the extent to which the diagnostic features of the disorders overlap (E. B. Weller, Weller, & Fristad, 1995; R. A. Weller, Weller, Tucker, & Fristad, 1986; Wozniak, Biederman, Kiely, *et al.,* 1995). The most obvious and troublesome mood manifestations among ADHD subjects are very severe persistent irritability, affective storms, and prolonged, aggressive, and violent outbursts rather than the euphoria that is more typical of mania among adults. There may be a positive family history for mania (Wozniak, Biederman, Mundy, Mennin, & Faraone, 1995). Currently, stimulants are thought to be the first line of treatment for these children because of their beneficial effect on irritability and mood, as well as on the

symptoms of ADHD and aggressiveness; because of the ease of assessment of their effect; and because of their low risk for serious side effects. Careful monitoring for exacerbation of mood symptoms is essential. In other cases, irritability may be exacerbated as a consequence of stimulant therapy, indicating a need for dose reduction or discontinuation of the medication.

The role of tricyclic antidepressants in the treatment of children with ADHD and a bipolar or major depressive disorder has not been established. The combination of desipramine and MPH may result in a clinically meaningful improvement in behavior (in self-control, attention, hyperactivity, and aggression) beyond that observed with either drug alone. However, the combination of drugs does not have an additional effect on mood symptoms (Carlson, Rapport, Kelly, & Pataki, 1995; Pataki *et al.,* 1993; Rapport, Carlson, Kelly, & Pataki, 1993). The effectiveness of this combination may be greater with a longer period of desipramine treatment. The clearest advantage of desipramine was evident in the late afternoon and early evening when the MPH effect had dissipated. Monitoring mood symptoms is necessary if tricyclic antidepressants are used because they may precipitate mania or a rapid-cycling mood disturbance. It may be preferable to give these children mood stabilizers (e.g., lithium, valproic acid, carbamazepine) before a tricyclic antidepressant if a bipolar mood disorder is strongly suspected.

CLINICAL IMPLICATIONS

Limitations of Medication and the Logic of Multimodal Therapy

The preceding review highlights the many benefits of medication, particularly stimulants, in the treatment of ADHD. However, it also reveals many of the potential limitations of medication. A substantial number of children with ADHD have an unfavorable response to stimulants (Spencer, Biederman, Wilens, *et al.,* 1996). Although few children fail to have a positive behavioral response if a range of doses and both MPH and DEX are tried (Arnold, 1996; Elia *et al.*, 1991), many respond only at a dose that engenders unacceptable side effects (Ahmann *et al.*, 1993; Barkley, McMurray, *et al.*, 1990; Elia *et al.*, 1991). These side effects result in the discontinuation of medication in a substantial proportion of cases (10%; Schachar *et al.*, 1997). Even for those who have a favorable behavioral response, medication does not normalize all aspects of the disorder. For example, stimulants may improve but do not necessarily normalize peer relationships (Hinshaw, Henker, & Whalen, 1984a; Whalen, Henker, Buhrmester, *et al.*, 1989), classroom behavior (Abikoff & Gittelman, 1984; Elia *et al.*, 1991; Rapport *et al.*, 1994), academic achievement (Barkley & Cunningham, 1978; Rapport *et al.*, 1994; Wolraich *et al.*, 1978), or the sense of personal competence (Pelham *et al.*, 1992) for all children. Some children with ADHD may be less likely to benefit than others; for example, children with ADHD and concurrent anxiety respond less well and with more side effects than nonanxious children with ADHD (Ickowicz & Tannock, 1997; Pliszka, 1989; Tannock *et al.*, 1995).

Furthermore, the medication is effective only when it is pharmacologically active: It has no carryover to the later part of the day or to weekends when homework must be done and family and peer interactions are common (Schachar *et al.*, 1997). Expanding the period of active medication by prescribing a third dose of MPH, which has been little researched, may be associated with an increase in the prevalence and severity of side effects (Kent *et al.*, 1995; Stein *et al.*, 1996; Tirosh *et al.*, 1993). Moreover, various aspects of child behavior and adjustment may be affected differently by a particular dose of medication (Sprague & Sleator, 1977). Doses that optimize child behavior may not necessarily optimize academic performance in every child (Rapport *et al.*, 1994).

The effects of medication dissipate rapidly on discontinuation of treatment (Brown *et al.*, 1986), suggesting that little enduring benefit for the child's self-regulatory capacity is derived from the period when symptoms are suppressed by the medication.

This is a serious deficiency of MPH, given that ADHD may be a lifelong condition (Klein & Mannuzza, 1991; Mannuzza *et al.*, 1991); that compliance with medication may be a problem (Brown *et al.*, 1987; Firestone & Witt, 1982; Kauffman, Smith-Wright, Reese, Simpson, & Jones, 1981); and that many persons discontinue medication and treatment of any kind after several months or years (Barkley, McMurray, *et al.*, 1990; Firestone, 1982). Little evidence exists for the extended benefit of medication (Hechtman, Weiss, & Perlman, 1984; see Schachar & Tannock, 1993, for review). Various methodological limitations in existing follow-up studies could account for the apparent lack of long-term benefits of MPH (Schachar & Tannock, 1993). Poor compliance (Brown *et al.*, 1987; Firestone, 1982), premature termination (Firestone, 1982), habituation to the effects of medication (Kupietz *et al.*, 1988; Winsberg, Matinsky, Kupietz, & Richardson, 1987), treatment of cases with uncertain diagnoses (Copeland *et al.*, 1987), and inconsistent medical management (Sherman & Hertzig, 1991) could also account for the reduced efficacy in some cases. The long-term outcome of ADHD also may not be altered by drug treatment because the acute effects of MPH (e.g., on core symptoms) are not those (e.g., impaired parent–child, adult, and peer relationships; learning disability) that are crucial determinants of the long-term outcome (Parker & Asher, 1987).

Another less obvious limitation of medication may be that, for many families, educators, and children, medication is not an acceptable intervention for ethical, medical, or other reasons. Those who find drug treatment acceptable may refer themselves to clinics that are known for their use of medication, creating an impression that medication is a highly acceptable form of treatment. Those who do not find drugs acceptable may seek assistance where family or behavioral therapies are primarily used. Once children started on medication, Firestone, Crowe, Goodman, and McGrath (1986) noted that it was common for families to discontinue the medication, in most instances, without consulting their physician. The major reason for nonadherence to treatment with medication was that the families were not comfortable with the idea of medicating their children or that their children were reluctant to take their medication. The authors also noted that several children were pressured to discontinue their medication by their teachers, despite its apparent benefit. Younger children, females, those with lower scores on intelligence tests, and those children with younger parents who themselves had lower scores on intelligence tests were more likely to discontinue medication. Those who discontinued medication did not seem any less likely to have benefited from MPH.

Finally, medication makes little sense as a primary intervention at an early stage in the development of ADHD or for children with a less severe disturbance.

Each of these limitations supports the logic of combining pharmacological and nonpharmacological interventions for ADHD children and their families. Combinations of medication and psychosocial therapy (e.g., behavioral parent training, classroom behavior modification, and cognitive self-control training) could enhance treatment effects, result in greater coverage of symptoms over the course of the day, have an impact on a broader range of impairments, permit the use of lower doses of medication (Horn et al., 1991), facilitate the persistence of therapeutic effects after the discontinuation of medication (Ialongo et al., 1993), or enhance the adherence to treatment.

However, clinicians must vigilantly monitor for possible negative interactions between drug and nondrug treatments. For example, immediate behavioral improvement accruing from medication may undermine parents' efforts to alter their parenting practices and family environment. Drug-induced changes may imply that their child's problems are completely biological and that parenting, scholastic, or social factors play no role in either the cause or treatment of the disturbance. This process could lead to a diminished commitment to nonpharmacological interventions. Alternatively, parents may feel that they are being hasty if they institute drug treatment when there are psychosocial interventions that they have not tried. Medication could undermine efforts to alter parenting practices by increasing the children's irritability, dysphoria, insomnia, or the frequency of other side effects that may have an adverse impact on the children's behavior (Schachar et al., 1997). The cognitive effects of MPH, such as overfocusing, may impair the children's ability to learn new self-regulatory strategies. Much more research must be done on the effectiveness of various combinations of pharmacological and nonpharmacological therapies.

Practical Guidelines

Typically, treatment for ADHD is initiated with a stimulant. Regular-acting stimulants permit the adjustment and timing of individual doses throughout the day. The failure of one stimulant to produce the desired clinical effect or the development of unmanageable side effects is a reasonable justification for switching to another. Long-acting preparations play an important role in management when compliance is an issue, when stigmatization at school is a concern, or when the child complains about the waxing and waning effects of short-acting preparations.

The initiation of treatment involves the slow increase of the dose to some target dose, often in the range of 0.7 mg/kg given twice daily at the start. However, the dose based on a milligram-per-kilogram calculation may result in doses that are too high for older or heavier children. Conversely, fixed doses (e.g., a target of 10 or 15 mg twice daily) could result in doses that are too high for younger or lighter children. Some hybrid approach is optimal, such as targeting a dose of 0.7 mg/kg, but stopping at a maximum single dose of 20 mg. There is a growing trend toward the use of a third dose of MPH toward the end of the day but little research has been done on the effects of this treatment regimen. For the present, careful monitoring of the effect of the third dose on sleep, appetite, and side effects is necessary.

The presence of physical complaints such as headaches and insomnia, which might incorrectly be construed as side effects once treatment starts, must be assessed before the start of medication. Side effects must be monitored continuously because many have a late onset (Schachar et al., 1997). Some side effects such as overfocusing, perseveration, and dystonia are subtle and unreliably reported by teachers and parents. Direct observation is important. A useful strategy for monitoring the effects of the medication is to have the child attend the follow-up visit at a time of the peak medication effect, such as 1 to 2 hr after an oral dose of medication. Systematic observation for tics, stereotypical movements, perseveration, overfocusing, and other side effects can be conducted during the course of these routine office visits, in addition to eliciting the reports of parents and teachers. Regular contact with the child's teacher is useful and can be organized by having the parents take a behavior-rating and side-effects scale to the teacher before each follow-up visit. If medication is given twice daily 5 days per week, the parents may not actually see their child when the effects of the medication are at their peak.

Poor compliance can be an important reason for ineffective treatment and can be difficult to assess without a thorough discussion with the child and family. Physicians must guard against families who try to obtain repeats of medication by telephone without attending follow-up appointments. Drug holidays must be planned for times when they are likely to succeed. The need for medication should be reassessed on an annual basis.

The Role of the Systematic Trial of Medication

Various authorities (e.g., Greenhill et al., 1996) have recommended that a double-blind, placebo-controlled trial be an essential part of the process by which medication is initiated in clinical practice. A systematic trial is justified primarily on the grounds that there is a differential dose–response relationship for various aspects of the outcome of treatment and that performance across different doses is clearly individualistic and task specific (Rapport et al., 1994). Consequently, the optimum dose that is established through a systematic trial involving a range of formal behavioral, cognitive, and academic measures may differ from the dose that is established through informal titration in response to reports of behavioral improvement. In addition, side effects such as dystonic movements are more readily discerned during systematic trials with close observation by trained staff (Borcherding et al., 1990; Ickowicz & Tannock, 1997) than in typical office visits (Lipkin et al., 1994). Since many parents are reassured by the rigor of a systematic trial (Fine & Johnston, 1993), this factor alone could be ample justification for the effort involved in instituting a systematic trial.

For most children with ADHD, however, there is little evidence of a differential dose–response relationship across various aspects of the outcome of treatment with stimulants. Most children show a linear dose response for a range of outcomes; there is little evidence of deterioration in response to increasing doses of stimulants (Douglas et al., 1995; Rapport et al., 1994). Furthermore, there is evidence that the optimum dose established in the context of a systematic open trial that uses an increasing dosage approximates the optimum doses established through acute, double-blind trials with systematic measurement of attention and behavior. In double-blind, placebo-controlled, laboratory-based trials, most children showed optimal behavioral, academic, and cognitive responses on approximately 0.4 mg/kg of MPH per dose (Ickowicz & Tannock, 1997). Open titration over several months in a separate sample found that doses of 0.5 mg/kg twice daily provided the optimal trade-off between benefits and side effects (Schachar et al., 1997).

Systematic, randomized placebo-controlled trials play an important role in investigational protocols; in clinical practice these trials are indicated in cases in which the efficacy of the medication (effects versus side effects) and optimal dose is questioned.

CONCLUSIONS

Medication in the treatment of ADHD is neither a poison nor a panacea. For the majority of children, the behavioral improvement associated with stimulant therapy, in particular, is not purchased at the expense of important cognitive or social skills. Medication can provide an opportunity to implement other essential aspects of therapy. Yet the overall benefits even of stimulants, which are the most effective medications, may be limited in important ways. The behavior, academic performance, and social competencies of a substantial number of children are not normalized by medication, and medication may not confer the necessary and desired long-term improvement in social functioning, family interaction, or academic attainment. Side effects of stimulants are frequent but they are not usually serious. However, they may lead to premature discontinuation of treatment.

The majority of children with ADHD derive substantial benefit from the medications currently in use. However, there are many limitations of these treatments. For most children, a combination of pharmacological and non-pharmacological interventions is essential.

REFERENCES

Abikoff, H., & Gittelman, R. (1984). Does behavior therapy normalize the classroom behavior of hyperactive children? *Archives of General Psychiatry, 41,* 449–454.

Ahmann, P. A., Waltonen, S. J., Olson, K. A., Theye, F. W., Van Erem, A. J., & LaPlant, R. J. (1993). Placebo-controlled evaluation of Ritalin side effects. *Pediatrics, 91,* 1101–1106.

Alessi, N., Naylor, M. W., Ghaziuddin, M., & Zubieta, J. K. (1994). Update on lithium carbonate therapy in children and adolescents. *Journal of the American Academy of Child and Adolescent Psychiatry, 33,* 291–304.

American Psychiatric Association. (1994). *Diagnostic and statistical manual of mental disorders* (4th ed.). Washington, DC: Author.

Amirkhan, J. (1982). Expectations and attributions for hyperactive and medicated hyperactive students. *Journal of Abnormal Child Psychology, 10,* 265–276.

Anderson, J. C., Williams, S., McGee, R., & Silva, P. A. (1987). DSM-III disorders in preadolescent children: Prevalence in a large sample from the general population. *Archives of General Psychiatry, 44,* 69–76.

Arnold, L. E. (1996). Responders and nonresponders. *Journal of the American Academy of Child and Adolescent Psychiatry, 35,* 1569–1570.

Arnold, L. E., Christopher, J., Huestis, R., & Smeltzer, D. J. (1978). Methylphenidate vs. dextroamphetamine vs. caffeine in minimal brain dysfunction: Controlled comparison by placebo washout design with Bayes' analysis. *Archives of General Psychiatry, 35,* 463–473.

Arnsten, A. F. (1997). Catecholamine regulation in the prefrontal cortex. *Journal of Psychopharmacology, 11,* 151–162.

Arnsten, A. F., Steere, J. C., & Hunt, R.D. (1996). The contribution of alpha 2-noradrenergic mechanisms to prefrontal cortical cognitive function: Potential significance for attention-deficit hyperactivity disorder. *Archives of General Psychiatry, 53,* 448–455.

Bachman, D. S. (1981). Pemoline-induced Tourette's disorder: A case report. *American Journal of Psychiatry, 138,* 1116–1117.

Balthazor, M. J., Wagner, R. K., & Pelham, W. E. (1991). The specificity of the effects of stimulant medication on classroom learning-related measures of cognitive processing for attention deficit disorder children. *Journal of Abnormal Child Psychology, 19,* 35–52.

Barkley, R. A. (1997). Behavioral inhibition, sustained attention, and executive functions: Constructing a unifying theory of ADHD. *Psychological Bulletin, 121,* 65–94.

Barkley, R. A., & Cunningham, C. E. (1978). Do stimulant drugs improve the academic performance of hyperkinetic children? A review of outcome studies. *Clinical Pediatrics, 17,* 85–92.

Barkley, R. A., & Cunningham, C. E. (1979). The effects of methylphenidate on the mother–child interactions of hyperactive children. *Archives of General Psychiatry, 36,* 201–208.

Barkley, R. A., Karlsson, J., Strzelecki, E., & Murphy, J. V. (1984). Effects of age and Ritalin dosage on the mother–child interactions of hyperactive children. *Journal of Consulting and Clinical Psychology, 52,* 750–758.

Barkley, R. A., Karlsson, J., Pollard, S., & Murphy, J. V. (1985). Developmental changes in the mother–child interactions of hyperactive boys: Effects of two dose levels of Ritalin. *Journal of Child Psychology & Psychiatry, 26,* 705–715.

Barkley, R. A., McMurray, M. B., Edelbrock, C. S., & Robbins, K. (1989). The response of aggressive and nonaggressive ADHD children to two doses of methylphenidate. *Journal of the American Academy of Child and Adolescent Psychiatry, 28,* 873–881.

Barkley, R. A., Fischer, M., Edelbrock, C. S., & Smallish, L. (1990). The adolescent outcome of hyperactive children diagnosed by research criteria: I. An 8-year prospective follow-up study. *Journal of the American Academy of Child and Adolescent Psychiatry, 29,* 546–557.

Barkley, R. A., McMurray, M. B., Edelbrock, C. S., & Robbins, K. (1990). Side effects of methylphenidate in children with attention deficit hyperactivity disorder: A systemic, placebo-controlled evaluation. *Pediatrics, 86,* 184–192.

Barrickman, L., Noyes, R., Kuperman, S., Schumacher, E., & Verda, M. (1991). Treatment of ADHD with fluoxetine: A preliminary trial. *Journal of the American Academy of Child and Adolescent Psychiatry, 30,* 762–767.

Barrickman, L. L., Perry, P. J., Allen, A. J., Kuperman, S., Arndt, S. V., Herrmann, K. J., & Schumacher, E. (1995). Bupropion versus methylphenidate in the treatment of attention-deficit hyperactivity disorder. *Journal of the American Academy of Child and Adolescent Psychiatry, 34,* 649–657.

Becker-Mattes, A., Mattes, J. A., Abikoff, H., & Brandt, L. (1985). State-dependent learning in hyperactive children receiving methylphenidate. *American Journal of Psychiatry, 142,* 455–459.

Berkovitch, M., Pope, E., Phillips, J., & Koren, G. (1995). Pemoline-associated fulminant liver failure: Testing the evidence for causation. *Clinical Pharmacology & Therapeutics, 57,* 696–698.

Biederman, J., Baldessarini, R. J., Wright, V., Knee, D., & Harmatz, J. S. (1989). A double-blind placebo controlled study of desipramine in the treatment of ADD: I. Efficacy. *Journal of the American Academy of Child and Adolescent Psychiatry, 28,* 777–784.

Biederman, J., Newcorn, J., & Sprich, S. (1991). Comorbidity of attention deficit hyperactivity disorder with conduct, depressive, anxiety, and other disorders. *American Journal of Psychiatry, 148,* 564–577.

Biederman, J., Thisted, R. A., Greenhill, L. L., & Ryan, N. D. (1995). Estimation of the association between desipramine and the risk for sudden death in 5- to 14-year-old children. *Journal of Clinical Psychiatry, 56,* 87–93.

Biederman, J., Wilens, T., Mick, E., Milberger, S., Spencer, T. J., & Faraone, S. V. (1995). Psychoactive substance use disorders in adults with attention deficit hyperactivity disorder (ADHD): Effects of ADHD and psychiatric comorbidity. *American Journal of Psychiatry, 152,* 1652–1658.

Bird, H. R., Gould, M. S., & Staghezza, B. M. (1993). Patterns of diagnostic comorbidity in a community sample of children aged 9 through 16 years. *Journal of the American Academy of Child and Adolescent Psychiatry, 32,* 361–368.

Borcherding, B. G., Keysor, C. S., Cooper, T. B., & Rapoport, J. L. (1989). Differential effects of methylphenidate and dextroamphetamine on the motor activity level of hyperactive children. *Neuropsychopharmacology, 2,* 255–263.

Borcherding, B. G., Keysor, C. S., Rapoport, J. L., Elia, J., & Amass, J. (1990). Motor/vocal tics and compulsive behaviors on stimulant drugs: Is there a common vulnerability? *Psychiatry Research, 33,* 83–94.

Brown, G. L., Hunt, R. D., Ebert, M. H., Bunney, W. E., & Kopin, I. J. (1979). Plasma levels of D-amphetamine in hyperactive children. *Psychopharmacology, 62,* 133–140.

Brown, R. T., & Sexson, S. B. (1989). Effects of methylphenidate on cardiovascular responses in attention deficit hyperactivity disordered adolescents. *Journal of Adolescent Health Care, 10,* 179–183.

Brown, R. T., & Sleator, E. K. (1979). Methylphenidate in hyperkinetic children: Differences in dose effects on impulsive behavior. *Pediatrics, 64,* 408–411.

Brown, R. T., Slimmer, L. W., & Wynne, M. E. (1984). How much stimulant medication is appropriate for hyperactive school children?. *Journal of School Health, 54,* 128–130.

Brown, R. T., Wynne, M. E., & Medenis, R. (1985). Methylphenidate and cognitive therapy: A comparison of treatment approaches with hyperactive boys. *Journal of Abnormal Child Psychology, 13,* 69–87.

Brown, R. T., Borden, K. A., Wynne, M. E., Schleser, R., & Clingerman, S. R. (1986). Methylphenidate and cognitive therapy with ADD children: A methodological reconsideration. *Journal of Abnormal Child Psychology, 14,* 481–497.

Brown, R. T., Borden, K. A., Wynne, M. E., Spunt, A. L., & Clingerman, S. R. (1987). Compliance with pharmacological and cognitive treatments for attention deficit disorder. *Journal of the American Academy of Child and Adolescent Psychiatry, 26,* 521–526.

Buhrmester, D., Whalen, C. K., Henker, B., MacDonald, V., & Hinshaw, S. P. (1992). Prosocial behavior in hyperactive boys: Effects of stimulant medication and comparison with normal boys. *Journal of Abnormal Child Psychology, 20,* 103–121.

Buitelaar, J. K., Van der Gaag, R. J., Swaab-Barneveld, H., & Kuiper, M. (1995). Prediction of clinical response to methylphenidate in children with attention-deficit hyperactivity disorder. *Journal of the American Academy of Child and Adolescent Psychiatry, 34,* 1025–1032.

Busby, K., & Pivik, R. T. (1985). Auditory arousal thresholds during sleep in hyperkinetic children. *Sleep, 8,* 332–341.

Campbell, M., Adams, P. B., Small, A. M., Kafantaris, V., Silva, R. R., Shell, J., Perry, R., & Overall, J. E. (1995). Lithium in hospitalized aggressive children with conduct disorder: A double-blind and placebo-controlled study. *Journal of the American Academy of Child and Adolescent Psychiatry, 34,* 445–453.

Cantwell, D. P. (1996). Attention deficit disorder: A review of the past 10 years. *Journal of the American Academy of Child and Adolescent Psychiatry, 35,* 978–987.

Carlson, G. A., Rapport, M. D., Kelly, K. L., & Pataki, C. S. (1992). The effects of methylphenidate and lithium on attention and activity level. *Journal of the American Academy of Child and Adolescent Psychiatry, 31,* 262–270.

Carlson, G., Rapport, M. D., Kelly, K. L., & Pataki, C. S. (1995). Methylphenidate and desipramine in hospitalized children with comorbid behavior and mood disorders: Separate and combined effects on behavior and mood. *Journal of Child and Adolescent Psychopharmacology, 5,* 191–204.

Casat, C. D., Pearson, D. A., Van Davelaar, M. J., & Cherek, D. R. (1995). Methylphenidate effects on a laboratory aggression measure in children with ADHD. *Psychopharmacology Bulletin, 31,* 353–356.

Castellanos, F. X., Giedd, J. N., Elia, J., Marsh, W. L., Ritchie, G. F., Hamburger, S. D., & Rapoport, J. L. (1997). Controlled stimulant treatment of ADHD and comorbid Tourette's syndrome: Effects of stimulant and dose. *Journal of the American Academy of Child and Adolescent Psychiatry, 36,* 589–596.

Chan, Y. P., Swanson, J. M., Soldin, S. S., Thiessen, J. J., Macleod, S. M., & Logan, W. (1983). Methylphenidate hydrochloride given with or before breakfast: II. Effects on plasma concentration of methylphenidate and ritalinic acid. *Pediatrics, 72,* 56–59.

Chandran, K. S. (1994). ECG and clonidine. *Journal of the American Academy of Child and Adolescent Psychiatry, 33,* 1351–1352.

Chappell, P. B., Riddle, M. A., Scahill, L., Lynch, K. A., Schultz, R., Arnsten, A., Leckman, J. F., & Cohen, D. J. (1995). Guanfacine treatment of comorbid attention-deficit hyperactivity disorder and Tourette's syndrome: Preliminary clinical experience. *Journal of the American Academy of Child and Adolescent Psychiatry, 34,* 1140–1146.

Chappell, P. B., Scahill, L. D., & Leckman, J. F. (1997). Future therapies of Tourette syndrome. *Neurologic Clinics, 15,* 429–450.

Charles, L., Schain, R. J., & Guthrie, D. (1979). Long-term use and discontinuation of methylphenidate with hyperactive children. *Developmental Medicine and Child Neurology, 21,* 758–764.

Clark, C. R., Geffen, G. M., & Geffen, L. B. (1987). Catecholamines and attention: II. Pharmacological studies in normal humans. *Neuroscience and Biobehavioral Reviews, 11,* 353–364.

Cohen, D. J., Detlor, J., Young, J. G., & Shaywitz, B. A. (1980). Clonidine ameliorates Gilles de la Tourette syndrome. *Archives of General Psychiatry, 37,* 1350–1354.

Comings, D. E., & Comings, B. G. (1987a). A controlled study of Tourette syndrome: I. Attention-deficit disorder, learning disorders, and school problems. *American Journal of Human Genetics, 41,* 701–741.

Comings, D. E., & Comings, B. G. (1987b). Tourette's syndrome and attention deficit disorder with hyperactivity. *Archives of General Psychiatry, 44,* 1023–1026.

Conners, C. K., Casat, C. D., Gualtieri, C. T., Weller, E., Reader, M., Reiss, A., Weller, R. A., Khayrallah, M., & Ascher, J. (1996). Bupropion hydrochloride in attention deficit disorder with hyperactivity. *Journal of the American Academy of Child and Adolescent Psychiatry, 35,* 1314–1321.

Conrad, W. G., Dworkin, E. S., Shai, A., & Tobiessen, J. E. (1971). Effects of amphetamine therapy and prescriptive tutoring on the behavior and achievement of lower class hyperactive children. *Journal of Learning Disabilities, 4,* 509–517.

Cook, E. H., Jr., Stein, M. A., Krasowski, M. D., Cox, N. J., Olkon, D. M., Kieffer, J. E., & Leventhal, B. L. (1995). Association of attention-deficit disorder and the dopamine transporter gene. *American Journal of Human Genetics, 56,* 993–998.

Copeland, L., Wolraich, M., Lindgren, S., Milich, R., & Woolson, R. (1987). Pediatricians' reported practices in the assessment and treatment of attention deficit disorders. *Journal of Developmental and Behavioral Pediatrics, 8,* 191–197.

Corrigall, R., & Ford, T. (1996). Methylphenidate euphoria. *Journal of the American Academy of Child and Adolescent Psychiatry, 35,* 1421.

Coull, J. T., Middleton, H. C., Robbins, T. S., & Sahakian, B. J. (1995a). Clonidine and diazepam have differential effects on tests of attention and learning. *Psychopharmacology, 122,* 322–332.

Coull, J. T., Middleton, H. C., Robbins, T. S., & Sahakian, B. J. (1995b). Contrasting effects of clonidine and diazepam on tests of working memory and planning. *Psychopharmacology, 122,* 311–321.

Crook, T., Wilner, E., & Rothwell, A. (1992). Noradrenergic intervention in Alzheimer's Disease. *Psychopharmacology Bulletin, 28,* 67–70.

Cueva, J. E., Overall, J. E., Small, A. M., Armenteros, J. L., Perry, R., & Campbell, J. (1996). Carbamazepine in aggressive children with conduct disorder: A double-blind and placebo-controlled study. *Journal of the American Academy of Child and Adolescent Psychiatry, 35,* 480–490

Cunningham, C. E., Siegel, L. S., & Offord, D. R. (1991). A dose-response analysis of the effects of methylphenidate on the peer interactions and simulated classroom performance of ADD children with and without conduct problems. *Journal of Child Psychology & Psychiatry, 32,* 439–452.

de Sonneville, L. M., Njiokiktjien, C., & Bos, H. (1994). Methylphenidate and information processing: Part 1. Differentiation between responders and nonresponders; Part 2. Efficacy in responders. *Journal of Clinical and Experimental Neuropsychology, 16,* 877–897.

DeLong, G. R., & Aldershof, A. L. (1987). Long-term experience with lithium treatment in childhood: Correlation with clinical diagnosis. *Journal of the American Academy of Child and Adolescent Psychiatry, 26,* 389–394.

Denckla, M. B., Bemporad, J. R., & MacKay, M. C. (1976). Tics following methylphenidate administration: A report of 20 cases. *Journal of the American Medical Association, 235,* 1349–1351.

Douglas, V. I., Barr, R. G., Amin, K., O'Neill, M. E., & Britton, B. G. (1988). Dosage effects and individual responsivity to methylphenidate in attention deficit disorder. *Journal of Child Psychology & Psychiatry, 29,* 453–475.

Douglas, V. I., Barr, R. G., Desilets, J., & Sherman, E. (1995). Do high doses of stimulants impair flexible thinking in attention-deficit hyperactivity disorder? *Journal of the American Academy of Child and Adolescent Psychiatry, 34,* 877–885.

DuPaul, G. J., & Rapport, M. D. (1993). Does methylphenidate normalize the classroom performance of children with attention deficit disorder? *Journal of the American Academy of Child and Adolescent Psychiatry, 32,* 190–198.

DuPaul, G. J., Barkley, R. A., & McMurray, M. B. (1994). Response of children with ADHD to methylphenidate: Interaction with internalizing symptoms. *Journal of the American Academy of Child and Adolescent Psychiatry, 33,* 894–903.

Dykens, E., Leckman, J., Riddle, M., Hardin, M., Schwartz, S., & Cohen, D. (1990). Intellectual, academic, and adaptive functioning of Tourette syndrome children with and without attention deficit disorder. *Journal of Abnormal Child Psychology, 18,* 607–615.

Elia, J., Borcherding, B. G., Potter, W. Z., Mefford, I. N., Rapoport, J. L., & Keysor, C. S. (1990). Stimulant drug treatment of hyperactivity: Biochemical correlates. *Clinical Pharmacology & Therapeutics, 48,* 57–66.

Elia, J., Borcherding, B. G., Rapoport, J. L., & Keysor, C. S. (1991). Methylphenidate and dextroamphetamine treatments of hyperactivity: Are there true nonresponders? *Psychiatry Research, 36,* 141–155.

Famularo, R., & Fenton, T. (1987). The effect of methylphenidate on school grades in children with attention deficit disorder without hyperactivity: A preliminary report. *Journal of Clinical Psychiatry, 48,* 112–114.

Findling, R. L. (1996). Open-label treatment of comorbid depression and attentional disorders with co-administration of serotonin reuptake inhibitors and psychostimulants in children, adolescents and adults: A case series. *Journal of Child and Adolescent Psychopharmacology, 6,* 165–175.

Fine, S., & Johnston, C. (1993). Drug and placebo side effects in methylphenidate–placebo trial for attention deficit hyperactivity disorder. *Child Psychiatry and Human Development, 24,* 25–30.

Firestone, P. (1982). Factors associated with children's adherence to stimulant medication. *American Journal of Orthopsychiatry, 52,* 447–457.

Firestone, P., & Witt, J. E. (1982). Characteristics of families completing and prematurely discontinuing a behavioral parent-training program. *Journal of Pediatric Psychology, 7,* 209–222.

Firestone, P., Crowe, D., Goodman, J. T., & McGrath, P. (1986). Vicissitudes of follow-up studies: Differential effects of parent training and stimulant medication with hyperactives. *American Journal of Orthopsychiatry, 56,* 184–194.

Gadow, K. D., Nolan, E., Sprafkin, J., & Sverd, J. (1995). School observations of children with attention-deficit hyperactivity disorder and comorbid tic disorder: Effects of methylphenidate treatment. *Journal of Developmental and Behavioral Pediatrics, 16,* 167–176.

Gadow, K. D., Sverd, J., Sprafkin, J., Nolan, E. E., & Ezor, S. N. (1995). Efficacy of methylphenidate for attention-deficit hyperactivity disorder in children with tic disorder. *Archives of General Psychiatry, 52,* 444–455.

Gammon, G. D., & Brown, T. E. (1993). Fluoxetine and methylphenidate in combination for treatment of attention deficit disorder and comorbid depressive disorder. *Journal of Child and Adolescent Psychopharmacology, 3,* 1–10.

Gill, M., Daly, G., Heron, S., Hawi, Z., & Fitzgerald, M. (1997). Confirmation of association between attention deficit hyperactivity disorder and a dopamine transporter polymorphism. *Molecular Psychiatry, 2,* 311–313.

Gittelman-Klein, R., Klein, D. F., Katz, S., Saraf, K., & Pollack, E. (1976). Comparative effects of methylphenidate and thioridazine in hyperkinetic children. *Archives of General Psychiatry, 33,* 1217–1231.

Goldman-Rakic, P. S. (1996). Regional and cellular fractionation of working memory. *Proceedings of the National Academy of the Sciences of the United States of America, 93,* 13473–13480.

Golinko, B. E. (1984). Side effects of dextroamphetamine and methylphenidate in hyperactive children—A brief review. *Progress in Neuro-Psychopharmacology and Biological Psychiatry, 8,* 1–8.

Granger, D. A., Whalen, C. K., & Henker, B. (1993). Malleability of social impressions of hyperactive children. *Journal of Abnormal Child Psychology, 21,* 631–647.

Greenhill, L., Puig-Antich, J., Goetz, R., Hanlon, C., & Davies, M. (1983). Sleep architecture and REM sleep measures in prepubertal children with attention deficit disorder with hyperactivity. *Sleep, 6,* 91–101.

Greenhill, L. L. (1992). Pharmacologic treatment of attention deficit hyperactivity disorder. *Psychiatric Clinics of North America, 15,* 1–27.

Greenhill, L. L., Abikoff, H. B., Arnold, L. E., Cantwell, D. P., Conners, C. K., Elliott, G., Hechtman, L., Hinshaw, S. P., Hoza, B., Jensen, P. S., March, J. S., Newcorn, J., Pelham, W. E., Severe, J. B., Swanson, J. M., Vitiello, B., & Wells, K. (1996). Medication treatment strategies in the MTA Study: Relevance to clinicians and researchers. *Journal of the American Academy of Child and Adolescent Psychiatry, 35,* 1304–1313.

Gualtieri, C. T., Keenan, P. A., & Chandler, M. (1991). Clinical and neuropsychological effects of desipramine in children with attention deficit hyperactivity disorder. *Journal of Clinical Psychopharmacology, 11,* 155–159.

Haenlein, M., & Caul, W. F. (1987). Attention deficit disorder with hyperactivity: A specific hypothesis of reward dysfunction. *Journal of the American Academy of Child and Adolescent Psychiatry, 26,* 356–362.

Hagino, O. R., Weller, E. B., Weller, R. A., Washing, D., Fristad, M. A., & Kontras, S. B. (1995). Untoward effects of lithium treatment in children aged four through six years. *Journal of the American Academy of Child and Adolescent Psychiatry, 34,* 1584–1590.

Haig, J. R., Schroeder, C. S., & Schroeder, S. R. (1974). Effects of methylphenidate on hyperactive children's sleep. *Psychopharmacologia, 37,* 185–188.

Halperin, J. M., Gittelman, R., Katz, S., & Struve, F. A. (1986). Relationship between stimulant effect, electroencephalogram, and clinical neurological findings in hyperactive children. *Journal of the American Academy of Child Psychiatry, 25*, 820–825.

Hechtman, L. (1985). Adolescent outcome of hyperactive children treated with stimulants in childhood: A review. *Psychopharmacology Bulletin, 21*, 178–191.

Hechtman, L., Weiss, G., & Perlman, T. (1984). Young adult outcome of hyperactive children who received long-term stimulant treatment. *Journal of the American Academy of Child Psychiatry, 23*, 261–269.

Henker, B., Astor-Dubin, L., & Varni, W. J. (1986). Psychostimulant medication and percieved intensity in hyperactive children . *Journal of Abnormal Child Psychology, 14*, 105–114.

Hinshaw, S. P., & McHale, J. P. (1991). Stimulant medication and the social interactions of hyperactive children. In D. G. Gilbert and J. J. Connolly (Eds.), *Personality, social skills, and psychopathology: An individual differences approach* (pp. 229–253). New York: Plenum.

Hinshaw, S. P., Henker, B., & Whalen, C. K. (1984a). Cognitive-behavioral and pharmacologic interventions for hyperactive boys: Comparative and combined effects. *Journal of Consulting and Clinical Psychology, 52*, 739–49.

Hinshaw, S. P., Henker, B., & Whalen, C. K. (1984b). Self-control in hyperactive boys in anger-inducing situations: Effects of cognitive-behavioral training and of methylphenidate. *Journal of Abnormal Child Psychology, 12*, 55–77.

Hinshaw, S. P., Buhrmester, D., & Heller, T. (1989). Anger control in response to verbal provocation: Effects of stimulant medication for boys with ADHD. *Journal of Abnormal Child Psychology, 17*, 393–407.

Hinshaw, S. P., Henker, B., Whalen, C. K., Erhardt, D., & Dunnington, R. E., Jr. (1989). Aggressive, prosocial, and nonsocial behavior in hyperactive boys: Dose effects of methylphenidate in naturalistic settings. *Journal of Consulting and Clinical Psychology, 57*, 636–643.

Horn, W. F., Ialongo, N. S., Pascoe, J. M., Greenberg, G., Packard, T., Lopez, M., Wagner, A., & Puttler, L. (1991). Additive effects of psychostimulants, parent training, and self-control therapy with ADHD children. *Journal of the American Academy of Child and Adolescent Psychiatry, 30*, 233–240.

Hunt, R. D. (1987). Treatment effects of oral and transdermal clonidine in relation to methylphenidate: An open pilot study in ADD-H. *Psychopharmacology Bulletin, 23*, 111–114.

Hunt, R. D., Minderaa, R. B., & Cohen, D. J. (1985). Clonidine benefits children with attention deficit disorder and hyperactivity: Report of a double-blind placebo-crossover therapeutic trial. *Journal of the American Academy of Child and Adolescent Psychiatry, 24*, 617–629.

Hunt, R. D., Minderaa, R. B., & Cohen, D. J. (1986). The therapeutic effect of clonidine in attention deficit with hyperactivity: A comparison with placebo and methylphenidate. *Psychopharmacology Bulletin, 22*, 229–236.

Hunt, R. D., Capper, L., & O'Connell, P. (1990). Clonidine in child and adolescent psychiatry. *Journal of Child and Adolescent Psychopharmacology, 1*, 87–101.

Hunt, R. D., Arnsten, A. F. T., & Asbell, M. D. (1995). An open trial of guanfacine in the treatment of attention deficit–hyperactivity disorder. *Journal of the American Academy of Child and Adolescent Psychiatry, 34*, 50–54.

Ialongo, N. S., Horn, W. F., Pascoe, J. M., Greenberg, G., Packard, T., Lopez, M., Wagner, A., & Puttler, L. (1993). The effects of a multimodal intervention with attention-deficit hyperactivity disorder children: A 9-month follow-up. *Journal of the American Academy of Child and Adolescent Psychiatry, 32*, 182–189.

Ickowicz, A., & Tannock, R. (1997). *Predictors of clinical response to methylphenidate in children with ADHD.* Poster presented at the 44th annual meeting of the American Academy of Child and Adolescent Psychiatry, Toronto, Ontario, Canada.

Ickowicz, A., Tannock, R., Fulford, P., Purvis, K., & Schachar, R. (1993). Transient tics and compulsive behaviors following methylphenidate: Evidence from a placebo controlled double blind clinical trial. *Journal of the American Academy of Child and Adolescent Psychiatry, 32*, 884.

Ickowicz, A., Masellis, M., & Tannock, R. (1996). *Clonidine in comorbid ADHD and anxiety: Behavioral and Cognitive effects.* Poster presented at the 43rd annual meeting of the American Academy of Child and Adolescent Psychiatry, Philadelphia.

Johnston, C., Pelham, W. E., Hoza, J., & Sturges, J. (1988). Psychostimulant rebound in attention deficit disordered boys. *Journal of the American Academy of Child and Adolescent Psychiatry, 27*, 806–810.

Kaufman, R. E., Smith-Wright, D., Reese, C. A., Simpson, R., & Jones, F. (1981). Medication compliance in hyperactive children. *Pediatric Pharmacology, 1*, 231–237.

Kelly, K. L., Rapport, M. D., & DuPaul, G. J. (1988). Attention deficit disorder and methylphenidate: A multi-step analysis of dose–response effects on children's cardiovascular functioning. *International Clinical Psychopharmacology, 3*, 167–181.

Kent, J. D., Blader, J. C., Koplewicz, H. S., Abikoff, H., & Foley, C. A. (1995). Effects of late-afternoon methylphenidate administration on behavior and sleep in attention-deficit hyperactivity disorder. *Pediatrics, 96*, 320–325.

Klein, R. G., & Mannuzza, S. (1991). Long-term outcome of hyperactive children: A review. *Journal of the American Academy of Child and Adolescent Psychiatry, 30*, 383–387.

Klein, R. G., Landa, B., Mattes, J. A., & Klein, D. F. (1988). Methylphenidate and growth in hyperactive children: A controlled withdrawal study. *Archives of General Psychiatry, 45*, 1127–1130.

Klein, R. G., Koplewicz, H. S., & Kanner, A. (1992). Imipramine treatment of children with separation anxiety disorder. *Journal of the American Academy of Child and Adolescent Psychiatry, 31*, 21–28.

Klorman, R., Coons, H. W., & Borgstedt, A. D. (1987). Effects of methylphenidate on adolescents with a childhood history of attention deficit disorder: I. Clinical findings. *Journal of the American Academy of Child and Adolescent Psychiatry, 26,* 363–367.

Klorman, R., Brumaghim, J. T., Salzman, L. F., Strauss, J., Borgstedt, A. D., McBride, M. C., & Loeb, S. (1989). Comparative effects of methylphenidate on attention-deficit hyperactivity disorder with and without aggressive/noncompliant features. *Psychopharmacology Bulletin, 25,* 109–113.

Klorman, R., Brumaghim, J. T., Fitzpatrick, P. A., Borgstedt, A. D., & Strauss, J. (1994). Clinical and cognitive effects of methylphenidate on children with attention deficit disorder as a function of aggression/oppositionality and age. *Journal of Abnormal Psychology, 103,* 206–221.

Krusch, D. A., Klorman, R., Brumaghim, J. T., Fitzpatrick, P. A., Borgstedt, A. D., & Strauss, J. (1996). Methylphenidate slows reactions of children with attention deficit disorder during and after an error. *Journal of Abnormal Child Psychology, 24,* 633–650.

Kupietz, S. S., Winsberg, B. G., Richardson, E., Maitinsky, S., & Mendell, N. (1988). Effects of methylphenidate dosage in hyperactive reading-disabled children: I. Behavior and cognitive performance effects. *Journal of the American Academy of Child and Adolescent Psychiatry, 27,* 70–77.

Kwasman, A., Tinsley, B. J., & Lepper, H. S. (1995). Pediatricians' knowledge and attitudes concerning diagnosis and treatment of attention deficit and hyperactivity disorders: A national survey approach. *Archives of Pediatrics & Adolescent Medicine, 149,* 1211–1216.

LaHoste, G. J., Swanson, J. M., Wigal, S. B., Glabe, C., Wigal, T., King, N., & Kennedy, J. L. (1996). Dopamine D4 receptor gene polymorphism is associated with attention deficit hyperactivity disorder. *Molecular Psychiatry, 1,* 121–124.

Leckman, J. F., Detlor, J., Harcherik, D. F., Ort, S., Shaywitz, B. A., & Cohen, D. J. (1985). Short and long-term treatment of Tourette's syndrome with clonidine: A clinical perspective. *Neurology, 35,* 345–351.

Leckman, J. F., Hardin, M. T., Riddle, M. A., Stevenson, J., Ort, S. I., & Cohen, D. J. (1991). Clonidine treatment of Gilles de la Tourette's syndrome. *Archives of General Psychiatry, 48,* 324–328.

Leiner, H. C., Leiner, A. L., & Dow, R. S. (1989). Reappraising the cerebellum: Does the hindbrain contribute to the forebrain? *Behavioral Neuroscience, 103,* 998–1008.

Leonard, H. L., Swedo, S. E., Rapoport, J. L., Koby, E. V., Lenane, M. C., Cheslow, D. L., & Hamburger, S. D. (1989). Treatment of obsessive-compulsive disorder with clomipramine and desipramine in children and adolescents: A double-blind crossover comparison. *Archives of General Psychiatry, 46,* 1088–1092.

Leonard, H. L., Meyer, M. C., Swedo, S. E., Richter, D., Hamburger, S. D., Allen, A. J., Rapoport, J. L., &

Tucker, E. (1995). Electrocardiographic changes during desipramine and clomipramine treatment in children and adolescents. *Journal of the American Academy of Child and Adolescent Psychiatry, 34,* 1460–1468.

Lipkin, P. H., Goldstein, I. J., & Adesman, A. R. (1994). Tics and dyskinesias associated with stimulant treatment in attention-deficit hyperactivity disorder. *Archives of Pediatrics & Adolescent Medicine, 148,* 859–861.

Losier, B. J., McGrath, P. J., & Klein, R. M. (1996). Error patterns on the continuous performance test in non-medicated and medicated samples of children with and without ADHD: A meta-analytic review. *Journal of Child Psychology & Psychiatry, 37,* 971–987.

Lowe, T. L., Cohen, D. J., Detlor, J., Kremenitzer, M. W., & Shaywitz, B. A. (1982). Stimulant medications precipitate Tourette's syndrome. *Journal of the American Medical Association, 247,* 1168–1169.

Mannuzza, S., Klein, R. G., Bonagura, N., Malloy, P., Giampino, T. L., & Addalli, K. A. (1991). Hyperactive boys almost grown up: V. Replication of psychiatric status. *Archives of General Psychiatry, 48,* 77–83.

Mayes, S. D., Crites, D. L., Bixler, E. O., Humphrey, F. J., 2nd, & Mattison, R. E. (1994). Methylphenidate and ADHD: Influence of age, IQ and neurodevelopmental status. *Developmental Medicine and Child Neurology, 36,* 1099–1107.

McCurry, L., & Cronquist, S. (1997). Pemoline and hepatotoxicity. *American Journal of Psychiatry, 154,* 713–714.

Milich, R., Licht, B. G., Murphy, D. A., & Pelham, W. E. (1989). Attention-deficit hyperactivity disordered boys' evaluations of and attributions for task performance on medication versus placebo. *Journal of Abnormal Psychology, 98,* 280–284.

Milich, R., Carlson, C. L., Pelham, W. E., Jr, & Licht, B. G. (1991). Effects of methylphenidate on the persistence of ADHD boys following failure experiences. *Journal of Abnormal Child Psychology, 19,* 519–536.

Murphy, D. A., Pelham, W. E., & Lang, A. R. (1992). Aggression in boys with attention deficit–hyperactivity disorder: Methylphenidate effects on naturalistically observed aggression, response to provocation, and social information processing. *Journal of Abnormal Child Psychology, 20,* 451–466.

Nahas, A. D., & Krynicki, V. (1977). Effect of methylphenidate on sleep stages and ultradian rhythms in hyperactive children. *Journal of Nervous and Mental Disease, 164,* 66–69.

Nolan, E. E., & Gadow, K. D. (1997). Children with ADHD and tic disorder and their classmates: Behavioral normalization with methylphenidate. *Journal of the American Academy of Child and Adolescent Psychiatry, 36,* 597–604.

Parker, J. G., & Asher, S. R. (1987). Peer relations and later personal adjustment: Are low-accepted children at risk? *Psychological Bulletin, 102,* 357–389.

Pataki, C. S., Carlson, G. A., Kelly, K. L., Rapport, M. D., & Biancaniello, T. M. (1993). Side effects of methylphenidate and desipramine alone and in combination in children. *Journal of the American Academy of Child and Adolescent Psychiatry, 32,* 1065–1072.

Pelham, W. E., & Bender M.E. (1982). Peer relationships in hyperactive children: Description and treatment. In K. Gadow & I. Bialer (Eds.), *Advances in learning and behavioral disabilities* (Vol. 1, pp. 365–436). Greenwich, CT: JAI.

Pelham, W. E., Jr, Sturges, J., Hoza, J., Schmidt, C., Bijlsma, J. J., Milich, R., & Moorer, S. (1987). Sustained release and standard methylphenidate effects on cognitive and social behavior in children with attention deficit disorder. *Pediatrics, 80,* 491–501.

Pelham, W. E., Jr, Greenslade, K. E., Vodde-Hamilton, M., Murphy, D. A., Greenstein, J. J., Gnagy, E. M., Guthrie, K. J., Hoover, M. D., & Dahl, R. E. (1990). Relative efficacy of long-acting stimulants on children with attention deficit–hyperactivity disorder: A comparison of standard methylphenidate, sustained-release methylphenidate, sustained-release dextroamphetamine, and pemoline. *Pediatrics, 86,* 226–237.

Pelham, W. E., Jr, McBurnett, K., Harper, G. W., Milich, R., Murphy, D. A., Clinton, J., & Thiele, C. (1990). Methylphenidate and baseball playing in ADHD children: Who's on first? *Journal of Consulting and Clinical Psychology, 58,* 130–133.

Pelham, W. E., Milich, R., Cummings, E. M., Murphy, D. A., Schaughency, E. A., & Greiner, A. R. (1991). Effects of background anger, provocation, and methylphenidate on emotional arousal and aggressive responding in attention-deficit hyperactivity disordered boys with and without concurrent aggressiveness. *Journal of Abnormal Child Psychology, 19,* 407–426.

Pelham, W. E., Murphy, D. A., Vannatta, K., Milich, R., Licht, B. G., Gnagy, E. M., Greenslade, K. E., Greiner, A. R., & Vodde-Hamilton, M. (1992). Methylphenidate and attributions in boys with attention-deficit hyperactivity disorder. *Journal of Consulting and Clinical Psychology, 60,* 282–292.

Pelham, W. E., Jr, Swanson, J. M., Furman, M. B., & Schwindt, H. (1995). Pemoline effects on children with ADHD: A time–response by dose–response analysis on classroom measures. *Journal of the American Academy of Child and Adolescent Psychiatry, 34,* 1504–1513.

Pennington, B. F., & Ozonoff, S. (1996). Executive functions and developmental psychopathology. *Journal of Child Psychology and Psychiatry, 37,* 51–87.

Pliszka, S. R. (1989). Effect of anxiety on cognition, behavior, and stimulant response in ADHD. *Journal of the American Academy of Child and Adolescent Psychiatry, 28,* 882–887.

Pliszka, S. R. (1992). Comorbidity of attention-deficit hyperactivity disorder and overanxious disorder. *Journal of the American Academy of Child and Adolescent Psychiatry, 31,* 197–203.

Pliszka, S. R., McCracken, J. T., & Maas, J. W. (1996). Catecholamines in attention-deficit hyperactivity disorder: Current perspectives. *Journal of the American Academy of Child and Adolescent Psychiatry, 35,* 264–272.

Porrino, L. J., Rapoport, J. L., Behar, D., Sceery, W., Ismond, D. R., & Bunney, W. E., Jr. (1983). A naturalistic assessment of the motor activity of hyperactive boys: I. Comparison with normal controls. *Archives of General Psychiatry, 40,* 681–687.

Posner, M. I., & Petersen, S. E. (1990). The attention system of the human brain. *Annual Review of Neuroscience, 13,* 25–42.

Posner, M. I., & Raichle, M. E. (1994). *Images of mind.* New York: Scientific American Library.

Prince, J. B., Wilens, T. E., Biederman, J., Spencer, T. J., & Wozniak, J. R. (1996). Clonidine for sleep disturbances associated with attention-deficit hyperactivity disorder: A systematic chart review of 62 cases. *Journal of the American Academy of Child and Adolescent Psychiatry, 35,* 599–605.

Quay, H. C. (1997). Inhibition and attention deficit hyperactivity disorder. *Journal of Abnormal Child Psychology, 25,* 7–13.

Quinn, P. O., & Rapoport, J. L. (1975). One-year follow-up of hyperactive boys treated with imipramine or methylphenidate. *American Journal of Psychiatry, 132,* 241–245.

Rapoport, J. L., Buchsbaum, M. S., Weingartner, H., Zahn, T. P., Ludlow, C., & Mikkelsen, E. J. (1980). Dextroamphetamine: Its cognitive and behavioral effects in normal and hyperactive boys and normal men. *Archives of General Psychiatry, 37,* 933–943.

Rappley, M. D., Gardiner, J. C., Jetton, J. R., & Houang, R. T. (1995). The use of methylphenidate in Michigan. *Archives of Pediatrics & Adolescent Medicine, 149,* 675–679.

Rapport, M. D., & Denney, C. (1997). Titrating methylphenidate in children with attention-deficit/ hyperactivity disorder: Is body mass predictive of clinical response? *Journal of the American Academy of Child and Adolescent Psychiatry, 36,* 523–530.

Rapport, M. D., & Kelly, K. L. (1991). Psychostimulant effects on learning and cognitive function: Findings and implications for children with attention deficit hyperactivity disorder. *Clinical Psychology Review, 11,* 61–92.

Rapport, M. D., Carlson, G. A., Kelly, K. L., & Pataki, C. (1993). Methylphenidate and desipramine in hospitalized children: I. Separate and combined effects on cognitive function. *Journal of the American Academy of Child and Adolescent Psychiatry, 32,* 333–342.

Rapport, M. D., Denney, C., DuPaul, G. J., & Gardner, M. J. (1994). Attention deficit disorder and methylphenidate: Normalization rates, clinical effectiveness, and response prediction in 76 children. *Journal of the American Academy of Child and Adolescent Psychiatry, 33,* 882–893.

Richardson, E., Kupietz, S. S., Winsberg, B. G., Maitinsky, S., & Mendell, N. (1988). Effects of methylphenidate dosage in hyperactive reading-disabled children: II. Reading achievement. *Journal of the American Academy of Child and Adolescent Psychiatry, 27,* 78–87.

Richters, J. E., Arnold, L. E., Jensen, P. S., Abikoff, H., Conners, C. K., Greenhill, L. L., Hechtman, L., Hinshaw, S. P., Pelham, W. E., & Swanson, J. M. (1995). NIMH collaborative multisite multimodal treatment study of children with ADHD: I. Background and rationale. *Journal of the American Academy of Child and Adolescent Psychiatry, 34,* 987–1000.

Riddle, M. A., Hardin, M. T., Cho, S. C., Woolston, J. L., & Leckman, J. F. (1988). Desipramine treatment of boys with attention-deficit hyperactivity disorder and tics: Preliminary clinical experience. *Journal of the American Academy of Child and Adolescent Psychiatry, 27,* 811–814.

Riddle, M. A., King, R. A., Hardin, M. T., Scahil, L., Ort, S. I., Chappell, P., Rasmusson, A., & Leckman, J. F. (1990–1991). Behavioral side effects of fluoxetine in children and adolescents. *Journal of Child and Adolescent Psychopharmacology, 1,* 193–198.

Riddle, M. A., Geller, B., & Ryan, N. (1993). Another sudden death in a child treated with desipramine. *Journal of the American Academy of Child and Adolescent Psychiatry, 32,* 792–797.

Rie, H. E., Rie, E. D., Stewart, S., & Ambuel, J. P. (1976a). Effects of methylphenidate on underachieving children. *Journal of Consulting and Clinical Psychology, 44,* 250–260.

Rie, H. E., Rie, E. D., Stewart, S., & Ambuel, J. P. (1976b). Effects of Ritalin on underachieving children: A replication. *American Journal of Orthopsychiatry, 46,* 313–322.

Riggs, P. D., Thompson, L. L., Mikulich, S. K., Whitmore, E. A., & Crowley, T. J. (1996). An open trial of pemoline in drug-dependent delinquents with attention-deficit hyperactivity disorder. *Journal of the American Academy of Child and Adolescent Psychiatry, 35,* 1018–1024.

Rubinstein, S., Silver, L. B., & Licamele, W. L. (1994). Clonidine for stimulant-related sleep problems. *Journal of the American Academy of Child and Adolescent Psychiatry, 33,* 281–282.

Ruel, J. M., & Hickey, C. P. (1992). Are too many children being treated with methylphenidate? *Canadian Journal of Psychiatry, 37,* 570–572.

Safer, D. J., & Allen, R. P. (1973). Factors influencing the suppressant effects of two stimulant drugs on the growth of hyperactive children. *Pediatrics, 51,* 660–667.

Safer, D. J., & Allen, R. P. (1989). Absence of tolerance to the behavioral effects of methylphenidate in hyperactive and inattentive children. *Journal of Pediatrics, 115,* 1003–1008.

Safer, D. J., & Krager, J. M. (1988). A survey of medication treatment for hyperactive/inattentive students. *Journal of the American Medical Association, 260,* 2256–2258.

Safer, D., & Zito, J. M. (1996). *Increased methylphenidate usage for attention deficit disorder in the 1990's.* Paper presented at the 43rd annual meeting of the American Academy of Child and Adolescent Psychiatry, Philadelphia.

Safer, D. J., Allen, R. P., & Barr, E. (1975). Growth rebound after termination of stimulant drugs. *Journal of Pediatrics, 86,* 113–116.

Safer, D. J., Zito, J. M., & Fine, E. M. (1996). Increased methylphenidate usage for attention deficit disorder in the 1990s. *Pediatrics, 98,* 1084–1088.

Sallee, F. R., Stiller, R. L., Perel, J. M., & Everett, G. (1989). Pemoline-induced abnormal involuntary movements. *Journal of Clinical Psychopharmacology, 9,* 125–129.

Sallee, F. R., Stiller, R. L., & Perel, J. M. (1992). Pharmacodynamics of pemoline in attention deficit disorder with hyperactivity. *Journal of the American Academy of Child and Adolescent Psychiatry, 31,* 244–251.

Satterfield, J. H., Satterfield, B. T., & Cantwell, D. P. (1981). Three-year multimodality treatment study of 100 hyperactive boys. *Journal of Pediatrics, 98,* 650–655.

Schachar, R., & Logan, G. D. (1990). Implulsivity and inhibitory control in normal development and childhood psychopathology. *Developmental Psychology, 26,* 710–720.

Schachar, R., & Tannock, R. (1993). Childhood hyperactivity and psychostimulants: A review of extended treatment studies. *Journal of Child and Adolescent Psychopharmacology, 3,* 81–97.

Schachar, R., Taylor, E., Wieselberg, M., Thorley, G., & Rutter, M. (1987). Changes in family function and relationships in children who respond to methylphenidate. *Journal of the American Academy of Child and Adolescent Psychiatry, 26,* 728–732.

Schachar, R., Tannock, R., Cunningham, C., & Corkum, P. (1997). Behavioral, situational, and temporal effects of treatment of ADHD with methylphenidate. *Journal of the American Academy of Child and Adolescent Psychiatry, 36,* 1–10.

Schain, R. J., & Reynard, C. L. (1975). Observations on effects of a central stimulant drug (methylphenidate) in children with hyperactive behavior. *Pediatrics, 55,* 709–716.

Shapiro, A. K., Shapiro, E., & Fulop, G. (1987). Pimozide treatment of tic and Tourette disorders. *Pediatrics, 79,* 1032–1039.

Shapiro, E., Shapiro, A. K., Fulop, G., Hubbard, M., Mandeli, J., Nordlie, J., & Phillips, R. A. (1989). Controlled study of haloperidol, pimozide and placebo for the treatment of Gilles de la Tourette's syndrome. *Archives of General Psychiatry, 46,* 722–730.

Shaywitz, S. E., Hunt, R. D., & Jatlow, P. (1982). Psychopharmacology of attention deficit disorder: Pharmacokinetic, neuroendocrine and behavioral measures following acute and chronic treatment with methylphenidate. *Pediatrics, 69,* 688–694.

Shenker, A. (1992). The mechanism of action of drugs used to treat Attention-Deficit Hyperactivity Disorder: Focus on catecholamine receptor pharmacology. *Advances in Pediatrics, 39,* 337–382.

Sherman, M., & Hertzig, M. E. (1991). Prescribing Practices of Ritalin: The Suffolk County, New York Study. In L. L. Greenhill & B. B. Osman (Eds), *Ritalin: Theory and patient management* (pp. 187–193). New York: Liebert.

Shevell, M., & Schreiber, R. (1997). Pemoline-associated hepatic failure: A critical analysis of the literature. *Pediatric Neurology, 16,* 14–16.

Silva, R. R., Munoz, D. M., & Alpert, M. (1996). Carbamazepine use in children and adolescents with features of attention-deficit hyperactivity disorder: A meta-analysis. *Journal of the American Academy Child and Adolescent Psychiatry, 35*, 352–358.

Singer, H. S., Brown, J., Quaskey, S., Rosenberg, L. A., Mellits, E. D., & Denckla, M. B. (1995). The treatment of attention-deficit hyperactivity disorder in Tourette's syndrome: A double-blind placebo-controlled study with clonidine and desipramine. *Pediatrics, 95*, 74–81.

Sleator, E. K., Von Neumann, A., & Sprague, R. L. (1974). Hyperactive children: A continuous long-term placebo-controlled follow-up. *Journal of the American Medical Association, 229*, 316–317.

Solanto, M. V., & Wender, E. H. (1989). Does methylphenidate constrict cognitive functioning? *Journal of the American Academy of Child and Adolescent Psychiatry, 28*, 897–902.

Spencer, T., Biederman, J., Kerman, K., Steingard, R., & Wilens, T. (1993). Desipramine treatment of children with attention-deficit hyperactivity disorder and tic disorder or Tourette's syndrome. *Journal of the American Academy of Child and Adolescent Psychiatry, 32*, 354–360.

Spencer, T., Biederman, J., Steingard, R., & Wilens, T. (1993). Bupropion exacerbates tics in children with attention-deficit hyperactivity disorder and Tourette's syndrome. *Journal of the American Academy of Child and Adolescent Psychiatry, 32*, 211–214.

Spencer, T. J., Biederman, J., Harding, M., O'Donnell, D., Faraone, S. V., & Wilens, T. E. (1996). Growth deficits in ADHD children revisited: Evidence for disorder-associated growth delays? *Journal of the American Academy of Child and Adolescent Psychiatry, 35*, 1460–1469.

Spencer, T., Biederman, J., Wilens, T., Harding, M., O'Donnell, D., & Griffin, S. (1996). Pharmacotherapy of attention-deficit hyperactivity disorder across the life cycle. *Journal of the American Academy of Child and Adolescent Psychiatry, 35*, 409–432.

Sprague, R. L., & Sleator, E. K. (1977). Methylphenidate in hyperkinetic children: Differences in dose effects on learning and social behavior. *Science, 198*, 1274–1276.

Stein, M. A., Blondis, T. A., Schnitzler, E. R., O'Brien, T., Fishkin, J., Blackwell, B., Szumowski, E., & Roizen, N. J. (1996). Methylphenidate dosing: Twice daily versus three times daily. *Pediatrics, 98*, 748–756.

Steingard, R., Biederman, J., Spencer, T., Wilens, T., & Gonzalez, A. (1993). Comparison of clonidine response in the treatment of attention-deficit hyperactivity disorder with and without comorbid tic disorders. *Journal of the American Academy of Child and Adolescent Psychiatry, 32*, 350–353.

Steingard, R. J., Goldberg, M., Lee, D., & DeMaso, D. R. (1994). Adjunctive clonazepam treatment of tic symptoms in children with comorbid tic disorders and ADHD. *Journal of the American Academy of Child and Adolescent Psychiatry, 33*, 394–399.

Sterling, M. J., Kane, M., & Grace, N. D. (1996). Pemoline-induced autoimmune hepatitis. *American Journal of Gastroenterology, 91*, 2233–2234.

Swanson, J. M., Sandman, C. A., Deutsch, C., & Baren, M. (1983). Methylphenidate hydrochloride given with or before breakfast: I. Behavioral, cognitive, and electrophysiologic effects. *Pediatrics, 72*, 49–55.

Swanson, J. M., Flockhart, D., Udrea, D., & Cantwell, D. (1995). Clonidine in the treatment ADHD: Questions about safety and efficacy. *Journal of Child and Adolescent Psychopharmacology, 5*, 301–304.

Swanson, J. M., Lerner, M., & Williams, L. (1995). More frequent diagnosis of attention deficit-hyperactivity disorder. *New England Journal of Medicine, 333*, 944.

Swanson, J. R., Jones, G. R., Krasselt, W., Denmark, L. N., & Ratti, F. (1997). Death of two subjects due to imipramine and desipramine metabolite accumulation during chronic therapy: A review of the literature and possible mechanisms. *Journal of Forensic Sciences, 42*, 335–339.

Szatmari, P., Offord, D. R., & Boyle, M. H. (1989a). Correlates, associated impairments and patterns of service utilization of children with attention deficit disorder: Findings from the Ontario Child Health Study. *Journal of Child Psychology & Psychiatry, 30*, 205–217.

Szatmari, P., Offord, D. R., & Boyle, M. H. (1989b). Ontario Child Health Study: Prevalence of attention deficit disorder with hyperactivity. *Journal of Child Psychology & Psychiatry, 30*, 219–230.

Tannock, R., Schachar, R. J., Carr, R. P., Chajczyk, D., & Logan, G. D. (1989). Effects of methylphenidate on inhibitory control in hyperactive children. *Journal of Abnormal Child Psychology, 17*, 473–491.

Tannock, R., Schachar, R. J., Carr, R. P., & Logan, G. D. (1989). Dose–response effects of methylphenidate on academic performance and overt behavior in hyperactive children. *Pediatrics, 84*, 648–457.

Tannock, R., Ickowicz, A., & Schachar, R. (1995). Differential effects of methylphenidate on working memory in ADHD children with and without comorbid anxiety. *Journal of the American Academy of Child and Adolescent Psychiatry, 34*, 886–896.

Taylor, E., Schachar, R., Thorley, G., Wieselberg, H. M., Everitt, B., & Rutter, M. (1987). Which boys respond to stimulant medication? A controlled trial of methylphenidate in boys with disruptive behaviour. *Psychological Medicine, 17*, 121–143.

Taylor, E., Chadwick, O., Heptinstall, E., & Danckaerts, M. (1996). Hyperactivity and conduct problems as risk factors for adolescent development. *Journal of the American Academy of Child and Adolescent Psychiatry, 35*, 1213–1226.

Tirosh, E., Sadeh, A., Munvez, R., & Lavie, P. (1993). Effects of methylphenidate on sleep in children with attention-deficient hyperactivity disorder: An activity monitor study. *American Journal of Diseases of Children, 147*, 1313–1315.

Urman, R., Ickowicz, A., Fulford, P., & Tannock, R. (1995). An exaggerated cardiovascular response to methylphenidate in ADHD children with anxiety. *Journal of Child and Adolescent Psychopharmacology, 5,* 29–37.

Varley, C. K., & McClellan, J. (1997). Case study: Two additional sudden deaths with tricyclic antidepressants. *Journal of the American Academy of Child and Adolescent Psychiatry, 36,* 390–394.

Volkow, N. D., Wang, G. J., Fowler, J. S. , Logan, J., Burton, A., Hitzeman, R., Lieberman, J., & Pappas, N. (1997). Effects of methylphenidate on regional brain glucose metabolism in human: Relationship to dopamine D2 receptors. *American Journal of Psychiatry, 154,* 50–55.

Vyse, S. A., & Rapport, M. D. (1989). The effects of methylphenidate on learning in children with ADDH: The stimulus equivalence paradigm. *Journal of Consulting and Clinical Psychology, 57,* 425–435.

Weiss, G., Hechtman, L., Milroy, T., & Perlman, T. (1985). Psychiatric status of hyperactives as adults: A controlled prospective 15-year follow-up of 63 hyperactive children. *Journal of the American Academy of Child Psychiatry, 24,* 211–220.

Weller, E. B., Weller, R. A., & Fristad, M. A. (1986). Lithium dosage guide for prepubertal children: A preliminary report. *Journal of the American Academy of Child Psychiatry, 25,* 92–95.

Weller, E. B., Weller, R. A., & Fristad, M. A. (1995). Bipolar disorder in children: Misdiagnosis, underdiagnosis, and future directions. *Journal of the American Academy of Child and Adolescent Psychiatry, 34,* 709–714.

Weller, R. A., Weller, E. B., Tucker, S. G., & Fristad, M. A. (1986). Mania in prepubertal children: Has it been underdiagnosed? *Journal of Affective Disorders, 11,* 151–154.

Wender, P. H., Reimherr, F. W., Wood, D., & Ward, M. (1985). A controlled study of methylphenidate in the treatment of attention deficit disorder, residual type, in adults. *American Journal of Psychiatry, 142,* 547–552.

Werry, J. S., & Aman, M. G. (1975). Methylphenidate and haloperidol in children: Effects on attention, memory and activity. *Archives of General Psychiatry, 32,* 790–795.

Werry, J. S., Weiss, G., Douglas, V., & Martin, J. (1966). Studies on the hyperactive child: III. The effect of chlorpromazine upon behavior and learning ability. *Journal of the American Academy of Child Psychiatry, 5,* 292–312.

Werry, J. S., Biederman, J., Thisted, R., Greenhill, L., & Ryan, N. (1995). Resolved: Cardiac arrhythmias make desipramine an unacceptable choice in children. *Journal of the American Academy of Child and Adolescent Psychiatry, 34,* 1239–1245 (Discussion 1245–1248).

Whalen, C. K., & Henker, B. (1991). Therapies for hyperactive children: Comparisons, combinations, and compromises. *Journal of Consulting and Clinical Psychology, 59,* 126–137.

Whalen, C. K., Henker, B., Buhrmester, D., Hinshaw, S. P., Huber, A., & Laski, K. (1989). Does stimulant medication improve the peer status of hyperactive children? *Journal of Consulting and Clinical Psychology, 57,* 545–549.

Whalen, C. K., Henker, B., & Granger, D. A. (1989). Ratings of medication effects in hyperactive children: Viable or vulnerable? *Behavioral Assessment, 11,* 179–199.

Whalen, C. K., Henker, B., & Granger, D. A. (1990). Social judgment processes in hyperactive boys: Effects of methylphenidate and comparisons with normal peers. *Journal of Abnormal Child Psychology, 18,* 297–316.

Wilens, T. E., & Biederman, J. (1992). The stimulants. *Psychiatric Clinics of North America, 15,* 191–222.

Wilens, T. E., Biederman, J., & Spencer, T. (1994). Clonidine for sleep disturbances associated with attention-deficit hyperactivity disorder. *Journal of the American Academy of Child and Adolescent Psychiatry, 33,* 424–426.

Wilens, T. E., Spencer, T., Biederman, J., Wozniak, J., & Connor, D. (1995). Combined pharmacotherapy: An emerging trend in pediatric psychopharmacology. *Journal of the American Academy of Child and Adolescent Psychiatry, 34,* 110–112.

Wilens, T. E., Biederman, J., Baldessarini, R. J., Geller, B., Schleifer, D., Spencer, T. J., Birmaher, B., & Goldblatt, A. (1996). Cardiovascular effects of therapeutic doses of tricyclic antidepressants in children and adolescents. *Journal of the American Academy of Child and Adolescent Psychiatry, 35,* 1491–1501.

Wilkison, P. C., Kircher, J. C., McMahon, W. M., & Sloane, H. N. (1995). Effects of methylphenidate on reward strength in boys with attention-deficit hyperactivity disorder. *Journal of the American Academy of Child and Adolescent Psychiatry, 34,* 897–901.

Winsberg, B., Matinsky, S., Kupietz, S., & Richardson, E. (1987). Is there dose-dependent tolerance associated with chronic methylphenidate therapy in hyperactive children: Oral dose and plasma considerations. *Psychopharmacology Bulletin, 23,* 107–110.

Wolraich, M., Drummond, T., Salomon, M. K., O'Brien, M. L., & Sivage, C. (1978). Effects of methylphenidate alone and in combination with behavior modification procedures on the behavior and academic performance of hyperactive children. *Journal of Abnormal Child Psychology, 6,* 149–161.

Wolraich, M. L., Lindgren, S., Stromquist, A., Milich, R., Davis, C., & Watson, D. (1990). Stimulant medication use by primary care physicians in the treatment of attention deficit hyperactivity disorder. *Pediatrics, 86,* 95–101.

Wolraich, M. L., Hannah, J. N., Pinnock, T. Y., & Baumgaertel, A. (1996). Comparison of diagnostic criteria for attention-deficit hyperactivity disorder in a country-wide sample. *Journal of the American Academy of Child and Adolescent Psychiatry, 35,* 319–324.

Wozniak, J., Biederman, J., Kiely, K., Ablon, J. S., Faraone, S. V., Mundy, E., & Mennin, D. (1995). Mania-like symptoms suggestive of childhood-onset bipolar disorder in clinically referred children. *Journal of the American Academy of Child and Adolescent Psychiatry, 34,* 867–876.

Wozniak, J., Biederman, J., Mundy, E., Mennin, D., & Faraone, S. V. (1995). A pilot family study of childhood-onset mania. *Journal of the American Academy of Child and Adolescent Psychiatry, 34,* 1577–1583.

Zametkin, A. J., & Rapoport, J. L. (1987). Neurobiology of attention deficit disorder with hyperactivity: Where have we come in 50 years. *Journal of the American Academy of Child and Adolescent Psychiatry, 26,* 676–686.

Zametkin, A. J., Rapoport, J. L., Murphy, D. L., Linnoila, M., & Ismond, D. (1985). Treatment of hyperactive children with monoamine oxidase inhibitors: I. Clinical efficacy. *Archives of General Psychiatry, 42,* 962–966.

Zeiner, P. (1995). Body growth and cardiovascular function after extended treatment (1.75 years) with methylphenidate in boys with attention-deficit hyperactivity disorder. *Journal of Child and Adolescent Psychopharmacology, 5,* 129–138.

11

Behavioral Intervention in Attention-Deficit/Hyperactivity Disorder

WILLIAM E. PELHAM, JR., and DANIEL A. WASCHBUSCH

INTRODUCTION

Attention-Deficit/Hyperactivity Disorder (ADHD) is a chronic disorder of childhood characterized by abnormally high levels of inattention, impulsivity, and overactivity (American Psychiatric Association, 1994). ADHD children have serious impairment in many domains of functioning, including school, family, and peer domains, that not only highlight the seriousness of ADHD as a childhood problem but also predict the development of even more serious problems and a poor outcome in adolescence and adulthood (see Chapter 12, this volume). Thus, effective treatment for childhood ADHD is a major public health agenda.

A wide variety of treatments have been tried and are widely used for ADHD, including traditional one-to-one therapy, restrictive or supplemental diets, allergy treatments, chiropractics, biofeedback, perceptual-motor training, treatment for inner ear problems, and pet therapy. However, none of these interventions

are effective in treating ADHD. Only three treatments have been validated as effective short-term treatments for ADHD: (1) behavior modification; (2) drugs, mainly central nervous system stimulants (see Chapter 10, this volume); and (3) the combination of (1) and (2). We discuss two of these validated treatments, behavioral and combined interventions. Behavioral interventions have been used for children specifically diagnosed as having ADHD for more than 20 years (O'Leary, Pelham, Rosenbaum, & Price, 1976), and they have been used for 30 years to treat disruptive children, some of whom, although not diagnosed as ADHD, very likely had the disorder (O'Leary & Becker, 1967). Further, many early studies of treatment for conduct disordered (CD) children (e.g., Patterson, 1974) included a high percentage of children who were also diagnosed as ADHD (or the diagnostic equivalent of that time). Thus, there is an extensive literature on behavioral treatments for ADHD.

We examine behavioral treatments by separating them into five categories (Pelham & Murphy, 1986): (1) clinical behavior therapy, (2) direct contingency management, (3) cognitive-behavioral interventions, (4) intensive, packaged behavioral treatments, and (5) combined behavioral and pharmacological treatments. These categories are discussed separately

WILLIAM E. PELHAM, JR. • Department of Psychology, State University of New York at Buffalo, Buffalo, New York 14260-4110.   DANIEL A. WASCHBUSCH • Department of Psychology, Dalhousie University, Halifax, Nova Scotia, Canada B3H 4J1.

Handbook of Disruptive Behavior Disorders, edited by Quay and Hogan. Kluwer Academic/Plenum Publishers, New York, 1999.

because they differ in the nature and efficacy of their interventions. The chapter concludes with a brief discussion of future directions for research on the behavioral treatment of ADHD.

PHARMACOLOGICAL INTERVENTION

Any discussion of psychosocial treatments for ADHD must begin with a brief review of pharmacological treatments, which are ubiquitously employed and therefore provide the contrast or background for behavioral treatment of ADHD. Pharmacological interventions for ADHD are reviewed in Chapter 10 (this volume), and the efficacy for stimulants is therefore not discussed here. However, we touch on the limitations of pharmacotherapy, as those limitations are central to the question of the utility of psychosocial treatments with ADHD.

First, it is important to note that despite their clear beneficial effects on classroom performance (e.g., on task behavior and academic productivity), evidence that stimulants cause long-term changes in academic achievement does not exist (Swanson, McBurnett, Christian, & Wigal, 1995). Similarly, although stimulants clearly improve disruptive social behavior and peer interactions in acute studies (Hinshaw, 1991), there is no evidence that stimulants effect changes in long-term interpersonal relationships.

Further, even in studies where large beneficial drug effects on academic and social domains are found, only approximately 70% to 80% of ADHD children respond positively to the stimulant regimen, but the remaining quarter show either an adverse response or no response (Swanson *et al.,* 1995). Of those children who do respond, only a minority show sufficient improvement for their behavior to fall entirely within the normal range; the rest are improved but their behavior is not normalized, often remaining a standard deviation above the norm (Pelham & Murphy, 1986). One variable on which the degree of a child's response to a stimulant drug depends is the ad-

ministered dose. There is considerable controversy regarding what dose of stimulant is best for ADHD children. Generally, the larger the dose, the larger the drug effect, and the dose–response relationship is usually linear up to .6 mg/kg or slightly higher (Pelham, Swanson, Furman, & Schwindt, 1995; Rapport & Kelly, 1991). However, there are large individual differences in the size and topography of the drug response among the three fourths of ADHD children who respond to stimulants (Pelham & Milich, 1991). Response to stimulants varies both across and within children and depends on dose, dependent measure, and the child's target symptoms. On many dependent measures, the group data for drug response do not accurately reflect dose effects for the individuals who make up the group, and no measures reliably predict drug response in individuals.

Despite the evidence documenting their beneficial short-term effects, several additional limitations of drug treatment are noted. For example, although stimulants positively affect ADHD children's behavior during structured parent–child interactions in analog settings (e.g., Barkley, 1988; Barkley, Karlsson, Strzelecki, & Murphy, 1984; Barkley, Karlsson, Pollard, & Murphy, 1985), families of ADHD children are often dysfunctional in multiple domains, including maternal stress and depression, paternal alcohol abuse, and inappropriate parental discipline (see Fischer, 1990; Mash & Johnston, 1990, for reviews) and there is little reason to believe that providing a stimulant to the ADHD child will resolve such family problems. Even if medication had a beneficial effect on family functioning, there are difficulties in prescribing medication in the home setting. In order to avoid growth suppressant effects that may accompany high dosages administered daily without drug "holidays," psychostimulants are now most often administered during school hours, and their effects do not last through the evening hours. Parents are thus often left to their own means to control their children's behavior during nonschool hours.

The major limitation of stimulant therapy is that studies that have followed children treated with psychostimulant medication for periods up to 5 years have failed to provide any evidence that the drugs improve ADHD children's long-term prognosis (Charles & Schain, 1981; Satterfield, Hoppe, & Schell, 1982; Weiss & Hechtman, 1993; see also Chapter 12, this volume). Although their methodological inadequacies require that these studies be interpreted cautiously, beneficial treatment effects do not appear to be maintained when psychostimulant medication, as typically administered, is used as a long-term treatment for the average ADHD child.

The explanation for this failure is not clear. Perhaps the drugs are not prescribed on a regular basis. A recent survey of all prescriptions in one county for a year (Sherman & Hertzig, 1991) revealed that the majority of ADHD children for whom physicians prescribed stimulants received only one or two prescriptions. Given that ADHD is a chronic condition often requiring ongoing pharmacological treatment, these data suggest that most physicians or parents or both in this survey were terminating medication prematurely. Alternatively, although there is no documentation for this speculation, it is our clinical impression that when a child is a positive responder to medication, both parents and teachers are inclined to rely on medication as the sole form of treatment. That is, when medication works, the psychosocial and psychoeducational treatments to which the medication is supposed to be an adjunct are less likely to be employed. Perhaps it is the failure to employ concurrent psychosocial interventions that limits long-term stimulant efficacy. Shortcomings such as these have given rise to the investigation of psychosocial treatment for ADHD—primarily behavioral interventions—for the home and school.

CLINICAL BEHAVIOR THERAPY

Applications of traditional, outpatient-based, clinical behavior therapy have typically involved training parents to implement contingency-management programs with their children and often consulting with the children's teachers with the same goal (e.g., Anastopoulos, Shelton, DuPaul, & Guevremont, 1993; O'Leary & Pelham, 1978; Pelham et al., 1988). In typical behavioral treatment programs, parents are given assigned readings and in a series of 8 to 20 weekly group sessions are taught standard behavioral techniques such as time-out, point systems, and contingent attention (Barkley, 1995; Cunningham, Bremner, & Secord-Gilbert, 1994; Forehand & Long, 1996; Forgatch & Patterson, 1989). Similarly, therapists work with teachers to develop (1) classroom management strategies that can be implemented by the teacher with the target children and (2) daily report cards that provide feedback to parents on the children's school performance, for which parents provide a consequence at home (DuPaul & Stoner, 1994; Kelly & McCain, 1995).

For example, to establish a daily report card, which should be considered an essential component of school-based treatment of ADHD, a consultant (e.g., psychologist, physician, school counselor) meets with the teachers and other school staff involved with the child to assess the domains of functioning in which the child is impaired at school. It is important to specifically assess functioning in all relevant domains and settings as treatment response may vary widely across these variables (Waschbusch, Kipp, & Pelham, 1998). The purpose of the assessment is to identify general goals (e.g., improving academic performance), and these goals are then defined in terms of specific behaviors that can be changed to accomplish the identified goal (e.g., having necessary classwork materials, completing assigned tasks accurately, completing and returning homework). Three to five such specific target behaviors are typically included on a child's daily report card (DRC). The consultant and teacher must then decide what criteria a child must meet for each target behavior to earn a positive evaluation. Baseline rates of behavior (e.g., how much of a child's work he or she typically is completing), the amount a child must improve (e.g., a child who never completes assignments has a long way to go), and shaping (e.g., rewarding small increments of improvement starting with baseline level) are considered in selecting initial goals and adjusting them during treatment. Form 1 illustrates a typical DRC for an ADHD child.

After meeting with the school staff and setting up appropriate goals, the consultant or therapist meets with the parents to help them establish rewards at home for the child's daily performance at school. Keeping in mind that rewards need to be selected so that the child will work hard to meet the goals, parents could use privileges that had previously been noncontingent (e.g., television, video games, weekend activities). It works well to have a menu of rewards and to have them broken into several levels or units, so the child can earn partial reward for improvement short of the goal. We also recommend that parents employ concurrent weekly rewards and longer-term reinforcers so the child has some long-term motivation (e.g., saving points for a new bicycle) along with the daily reward. This may also help teach the child the importance of delayed

gratification, which some evidence suggests is a deficit that is specific to externalizing disorders of childhood (Krueger, Caspi, Moffitt, White, & Stouthamer-Loeber, 1996).

Treating professionals need to remember that implementation of behavioral interventions can be complicated; ongoing monitoring and modification are the rule. Consultant-established classroom interventions in which teachers have one or two consultation sessions and are then left to their own devices have been shown to be ineffective (Fuchs & Fuchs, 1989). Therefore, the therapist needs to be available initially for at least weekly consultations with the parents and teachers, either by phone or in person. Once the intervention is in place and running smoothly, contact gradually may become less frequent or may be turned over to the parent in order to begin generalizing the treatment past the clinician-consultant's participation.

The efficacy of clinical behavior therapy approaches has been evaluated in a number of studies. Typically, these outcome studies lasted 8 to 20 weeks and many can be traced

FORM 1.   Sample Daily Report Card (DRC)

Child's Name: _____ Date: _____									
	Special		LA		Math		Reading		SS/Science	
Follows class rules with no more than 3 rule violations per period.	Y	N	Y	N	Y	N	Y	N	Y	N
Completes assignments within the designated time.	Y	N	Y	N	Y	N	Y	N	Y	N
Completes assignments at 80% accuracy.	Y	N	Y	N	Y	N	Y	N	Y	N
Complies with teacher requests (no more than 3 instances of noncompliance per period).	Y	N	Y	N	Y	N	Y	N	Y	N
No more than 3 instances of teasing per period.	Y	N	Y	N	Y	N	Y	N	Y	N
OTHER										
Follows lunch rules.	Y	N								
Follows recess rules.	Y	N								
Total Number of Yeses:	_____									
Teacher's Initials										
Comments: _____										

to the O'Learys' laboratory at the State University of New York at Stony Brook (e.g., O'Leary & Pelham, 1978; Pelham, Schnedler, Bologna, & Contreras, 1980; Pelham *et al.,* 1988). The format of therapy in these studies generally consisted of weekly sessions with parents in the clinic and weekly visits to teachers, during which basic behavior management skills were taught by therapists. Impact in these studies was typically measured from pre- to posttreatment with ratings and direct observations. In general, the clinical behavior therapy examined in these studies consistently revealed considerable improvement on the measures examined, and this was true in both classroom and home settings. Similarly, a number of studies have found that standard behaviorally based parent training decreases ADHD children's overall rate of behavior problems (e.g., Anastopolous *et al.,* 1993; Barkley, Guevremont, Anastopoulos, & Fletcher, 1992; Firestone, Kelly, Goodman, & Davey, 1981; Horn, Ialongo, Greenberg, Packard, & Smith-Winberry, 1990; Pisterman *et al.,* 1992). These results are generally similar to those reported in early studies of behavioral treatments of CD children (e.g., Kent & O'Leary, 1976; Patterson, 1974), many of whom also had comorbid ADHD.

Thus, clinical behavior therapy of the sort that is likely to be implemented by therapists in community mental health, primary care, and private practice settings (e.g., 8 to 12 weekly sessions) results in clinically important improvement on multiple measures in home and school settings for most children with ADHD who receive treatment. However, the improvements obtained with clinical behavioral interventions typically are not as strong as those obtained with medication. For example, Gittelman and colleagues (1980) showed that clinical behavior therapy alone, while effective, was inferior to methylphenidate (MPH) alone on direct observations of disruptive behavior in the classroom for ADHD children treated over 8 weeks. More intensive behavioral treatments or combined treatments (see later sections) are often required to maximize the impact of behavioral treatments on ADHD children.

CONTINGENCY MANAGEMENT

In contrast to clinical behavior therapy, contingency management approaches are characterized by relatively more intensive interventions. Although the treatment components may be the same as or similar to those implemented in clinical behavior therapy, contingency management approaches are implemented directly in the setting of interest and typically by a paraprofessional or consulting professional rather than a parent or teacher. Instead of being conducted in outpatient settings, contingency management programs usually take place in specialized treatment facilities or in demonstration classroom settings where greater control can be gained over treatment implementation. The techniques employed in contingency management programs range from relatively more potent components such as point-token economy reward systems, time-out, and response-cost to relatively less potent components such as manipulations of teacher attention and removal of privileges.

Efficacy studies of contingency management have been conducted using a variety of methodologies, including both case studies and group studies. For example, in a classic study by Rapport and colleagues (Rapport, Murphy, & Bailey, 1980), a response-cost program was implemented with two children in regular classroom settings. They employed a flip-card system in which the child and teacher had cards with numbers in descending order from 20 to 0. The child was told he could earn up to 20 min of free time but if the child was not working, then the teacher flipped a card down, and the child lost 1 min of free time. The child monitored the teacher's number on the flip card and matched it on his flip card. This response-cost system showed clearly beneficial effects on both classroom work and classroom behavior. In fact, the effects of response-cost treatment were greater than or equal to those obtained with substantial doses of stimulant medication (MPH). Group studies (Carlson, Pelham, Milich, & Dixon, 1992; Pelham *et al.,* 1993), as well as other case studies (Abramowitz, Eckstrand, O'Leary, & Dulcan, 1992; Atkins, Pelham, & White, 1989; DuPaul, Guevremont, & Barkley, 1992; Hoza, Pelham, Sams, & Carlson, 1992; Kelly & McCain, 1995; Rapport, Murphy, & Bailey, 1982; Schell *et al.,* 1986) have shown similar results.

A major question of interest in the contingency management studies has been whether negative procedures such as punishment are necessary components of contingency management programs. Behavioral clinicians who have worked with CD children have long argued that the effective use of punishment is the key to parent management of CD children (Patterson, 1982). The same conclusion appears to apply to ADHD children. O'Leary and colleagues (Abramowitz, O'Leary, & Rosen, 1987; Abramowitz, O'Leary, & Futtersak, 1988; Acker, & O'Leary, 1987; Pfiffner, & O'Leary, 1987; Pfiffner, O'Leary, Rosen, & Sanderson, 1985; Pfiffner, Rosen, & O'Leary, 1985; Rosen, O'Leary, Joyce, Conway, & Pfiffner, 1984) have found that prudent negative consequences (verbal reprimands backed up with time-out and loss of privileges) are an effective and necessary component of classroom behavioral interventions, whereas positive consequences are not. Interestingly, this appears to be particularly true for the maintenance of treatment effects after behavioral interventions are withdrawn.

As might be expected given that contingency management approaches are often implemented in controlled settings by trained individuals, treatment effects are typically larger than those obtained in clinical behavior therapy studies. The major question regarding contingency management studies has long been how to facilitate maintenance of treatment effects when the initial treatment structures are withdrawn (see discussion of limitations later in this chapter).

COGNITIVE-BEHAVIORAL TREATMENT

Many different types of cognitive-behavioral treatments have been applied to children with ADHD, including verbal self-instructions, problem-solving strategies, cognitive

modeling, self-monitoring, self-evaluation, and self-reinforcement (Abikoff, 1987, 1991). The underlying theme of these types of treatments is the promotion of self-controlled behavior through the enhancement of problem-solving strategies (Hinshaw, & Erhardt, 1991). Beginning with a seminal article by Meichenbaum and Goodman (1971), a great deal of attention has been directed toward the development of cognitive behavioral therapy for treatment of ADHD. Typical intervention involves a series of sessions, usually once or twice weekly, in which a therapist or paraprofessional works with an individual child and attempts to teach the child cognitive techniques that the child can use to control his or her inattention and impulsive behavior problems in other settings. For example, for social problem solving, the child is taught to "stop, look, and listen" in order to identify the problem, brainstorm about possible solutions, evaluate possible solutions, and enact the best solution in a nonimpulsive manner. These techniques are taught didactically and rehearsed through role-play and supervised practice. The child is encouraged to use the skills in home and school settings. Cognitive therapy was designed in part to provide internal mediators that would facilitate generalization and maintenance of effects of behavioral treatment. Because the absence of such internal mediators appears to characterize ADHD, cognitive-behavioral treatments appeared a natural match for the disorder. However, controlled studies have not supported this contention.

There have been many investigations examining the effectiveness of cognitive-behavioral treatments for ADHD. For example, Abikoff and colleagues (Abikoff *et al.,* 1988) administered 16 weeks of intensive cognitive training to children with ADHD and found essentially no positive effects in comparison with attention control and no-training groups, and this was true across multiple measures of academic, cognitive, and behavioral functioning. The results of this study, and many other studies like it (e.g., Bloomquist, August, Cohen, Doyle, & Everhart, 1997; Brown, Borden, Wynne, Spunt, & Clingerman, 1987) are remarkably consistent in showing that cognitive-behavioral treatment of ADHD generally does not provide clinically important changes in the behavior and academic performance of children with ADHD. Despite the high face validity of cognitive treatments for ADHD and despite the fact that there is some demonstrated efficacy of cognitive treatments for other childhood disorders (Dujovne, Barnard, & Rapoff, 1995; Kendall, & Gosch, 1994; Lochman, 1992), there is no demonstrated efficacy for cognitive treatment of ADHD.

There may be three exceptions to this conclusion; cognitive training may have some clinical efficacy in the treatment of ADHD, especially when combined with intensive, multicomponent treatment packages. First, social skills training that is adjunctive to operant behavioral or clinical behavioral interventions may be beneficial (Pelham & Hoza, 1996; Pelham *et al.*, 1988; Pfiffner & McBurnett, 1997). Second, teaching anger control in the context of intensive behavioral interventions may also be useful (Hinshaw, & Erhardt, 1991). Third, problem-solving training might help aggressive children with ADHD if it is combined with parent training (Kazdin, 1996; Lochman, & Lenhart, 1993). Finally, although the hypothesis has not been tested, it might reasonably be argued that cognitive interventions could have enhanced adjunctive value in *maintenance and generalization* in the context of a lengthy and very intensive behavioral and pharmacological treatment program. Although cognitive behavioral interventions were originally developed to facilitate maintenance of operant interventions, not as treatments sufficient unto themselves, no studies have addressed that issue.

INTENSIVE TREATMENTS

Given these shortcomings of behavioral, medication, and combined treatments, it is not surprising that there is beginning to be a consensus among professionals that regular outpatient treatment may not be adequate for many if not most ADHD children, and that intensive treatment programs are necessary. The Chil-

dren's Summer Treatment Program (STP) that we shall discuss is one such intensive treatment program and another is the University of California at Irvine Child Development Center School (Swanson, 1992). The STP was developed over the past two decades by the first author (WEP), and STPs have been successfully implemented in a number of academic and community settings, including locations in Atlanta, Tallahassee, Nashville, New York City, Ottawa, Denver, Houston, Pittsburgh, and Buffalo. In addition, the STP was a central component of psychosocial treatment in the National Institute of Mental Health's Multisite Treatment Study of ADHD (MTA; Richters *et al.*, 1995), and was implemented in the seven North America sites of that study.

The STP is based on the premise that combining an intensive summer day treatment program with a school year, outpatient follow-up program will provide a maximally effective intervention for ADHD (Pelham *et al.*, 1996). The STP runs for 9 hr on weekdays for 8 weeks. In the context of a summer-camp or summer-school–like program with a broad treatment focus, children are placed in groups with 12 children of similar age and five clinical staff persons. These groups stay together throughout the day, so that children receive intensive experience in functioning as a group and in making friends. Each group spends 2 hr daily in classrooms in which appropriately individualized paper-and-pencil and computer-assisted instruction is also provided. The remainder of each day consists of recreation-based group activities during which treatment strategies are implemented. Detailed descriptions of the program components and procedures are operationalized in the Children's Summer Treatment Program Manual (Pelham, Greiner, & Gnagy, 1997).

The backbone of the behavioral intervention in the STP is a point system with both reward and cost components that is implemented in every setting throughout the day. Points are exchanged for privileges (e.g., weekly field trips), social honors, and home-based rewards. Children are disciplined for certain behaviors, with discipline taking the form of loss of privileges or time out from ongoing activities.

Treatment also includes daily training in social skills and engaging in cooperative group tasks designed to foster friendship reciprocity. In addition children are taught anger management and group problem-solving skills, and are given intensive coaching and supervised practice in sports and game skills. The sports skills training is integrated with the other treatment components to provide a comprehensive intervention for peer relationship difficulties. Children receive a DRC on which their progress in individualized target behaviors is tracked and rewarded by parents at home. Finally, if the standard interventions do not produce the desired behavior change for a child, a functional analysis of the problematic behavior is conducted and an individualized program is developed.

Information gathered daily on children's behavior and response to treatment from the point systems, academic assignments, counselor, teacher, and parent ratings and direct observational measures is entered into a database and is available to staff members to monitor children's response to treatment and also serve as dependent measures in studies of treatment efficacy (e.g., Pelham, Bender, Caddell, Booth, & Moorer, 1985; Pelham *et al.,* 1993). Staff members receive daily supervision during which children's response is evaluated and treatment strategies are monitored, if necessary. Extensive procedures for assessing and ensuring treatment adherence and fidelity are built into the STP structure (Pelham, Greiner, & Gnagy, 1997).

One of the key features of the STP is that it was expressly developed to focus on treatments for difficulties in peer relationships. Although clinical behavior therapy and medication have many salutary effects, peer rejection is not an area in which they have been shown to have a major impact on ADHD children. This is important because it has become clear that deficits in peer relationships are arguably the most severe area of impairment for ADHD children (Milich, & Landau, 1982; Pelham, & Bender, 1982; see also Chapter 7, this volume). ADHD children are annoying and aggressive toward peers, and this results in their being actively rejected and having few if any friends. Given that peer relations are widely believed to be the key mediator of adult adjustment (Hartup, 1983; Parker, & Asher, 1987), any comprehensive intervention for ADHD must have as a central component an effective intervention for peer deficits. To date, the primary technique that has been tried in treating peer relations is social skills training (SST). SST usually involves a combination of social learning–based techniques such as modeling, coaching, role-playing, and practice given in individual or small-group settings over a number of sessions (e.g., Oden, & Asher, 1977; see also Chapter 20, this volume). These methods, however, have not achieved a great deal of success when applied to socially rejected children (see, e.g., Coie, & Krehbiel, 1984). ADHD children are no exception. In particular, little evidence exists that these methods, or any other office-based treatment method used alone or in combination (e.g., with medication, cognitive training), can normalize the peer relations of ADHD children.

In contrast to office-based social skills sessions or groups, the STP integrates treatment for peer difficulties into the daily activities of children with their peers (e.g., soccer, basketball), thus affording greater opportunity to observe and directly modify a child's dysfunctional peer interactions in a context close to the natural contexts in which children interact with peers.

No randomized trial has been conducted with the STP or any other intensive treatment package for ADHD. However, Pelham and Hoza (1996) reported pre- to post measures of functioning for a sample of 258 ADHD boys of normal intelligence between the ages of 5 and 12 who attended STPs conducted at the University of Pittsburgh from 1987 through 1992. The sample was ethnically and socioeconomically diverse, and 58% were comorbid for aggressive disorders. Treatment responsiveness to the STP was measured in numerous ways, including parent, teacher, and staff ratings of improvement; standardized parent ratings of disruptive behavior; direct observations of social and academic behaviors; self-esteem; parental satisfaction; and measures of social validity.

Very large effects of treatment were obtained on all of these measures. For example, 96% of the parents rated the children as improved and 93% said that they would recommend the program to other parents. Comparisons of the effect sizes of pre- to posttreatment gains with other studies in the literature revealed that changes in self-concept and disruptive behavior yielded effect sizes that were twice the size of those reported in studies employing clinical behavior therapy. Notably, these positive treatment effects were equivalent for ADHD children with and without comorbid aggression, for ADHD children from single-parent and two-parent households, and for ADHD children from low- versus middle- or upper-income families. These three characteristics predict poor response to treatment in the extant literature (see the following discussion), suggesting that the STP effects are sufficiently potent to overcome variables that interfere with treatment in other contexts. It should be noted that a major difference between this intensive packaged summer program and most other treatment programs is that the STP dropout rate is extremely low— 3% over the years in which these data were gathered, compared to rates up to 50% that characterize other treatment approaches such as clinical behavioral parent training (Miller, & Prinz, 1990). Since attendance at therapy is a prerequisite to changing, the STP would appear to offer a unique advantage to other forms of behavioral intervention.

In summary, while these data are uncontrolled, they certainly suggest that intensive treatment packages such as the STP are a powerful treatment for ADHD. The low dropout rate, excellent parent satisfaction ratings, and children's overall improvement are all superior to those generally reported for psychosocial treatment programs for ADHD boys. At the same time, the STP alone is clearly an insufficient treatment for ADHD. It must be combined with parent training, which is a component of the STP, and school-based follow-up. As we discuss briefly later, that package—STP, parent training, and school-based intervention—constitutes the psychosocial treatment package for the MTA Study.

SHORTCOMINGS OF BEHAVIORAL INTERVENTIONS

The shortcomings of behavioral interventions with ADHD children are similar to those of psychostimulant medication (Pelham, & Murphy, 1986). First, although the studies we reviewed showed that standard clinical behavior therapy and direct contingency management are effective in improving parent and teacher ratings on standardized rating scales and observations of ADHD, they do not normalize children. In fact, as is the case with studies of stimulant medication, posttreatment levels are usually one SD above normative means (e.g., Pelham et al., 1988). Also, as with psychostimulant medication, the short-term effects of behavioral interventions are limited to the period when the programs are actually in effect; that is, no studies have yet shown maintenance of treatment gains beyond a few months after therapy is terminated.

Furthermore, a substantial minority of children (comparable to the proportion cited for stimulant medication) fail to show improvement (e.g., Pelham et al., 1988). In many cases such failure may be attributable to the unwillingness or inability of parents and teachers to implement the behavioral programs as directed. A major problem is that many teachers, who are not obligated to cooperate with outside consultants, will not implement a complicated behavioral intervention (Witt, 1986) and do not continue them after initiation without ongoing consultation (Fuchs & Fuchs, 1989). In addition, many parents, up to half of those beginning treatment discontinue parent training against therapeutic advice (Firestone et al., 1981). Even when parents and teachers apparently comply with treatment, therapist contact in standard clinical behavior therapy is typically limited to once per week and manipulation checks of whether parents and teachers actually follow through with treatment are almost never conducted. For example, single mothers with relatively lower levels of education, income, and contact with other adults have great difficulty implementing and maintaining treatment, with meager treatment outcomes (Wahler, 1980).

Just as some of the limitations of medication can be removed by increasing the dosage, the effects of behavior therapy can be maximized by increasing the power and comprehensiveness of the intervention. The standard clinical behavior therapy approach involving weekly contact with parents and teachers is less potent than are highly structured, closely monitored contingency management programs. Because it is quite time-consuming and difficult to conduct such systems unassisted, however, regular classroom teachers are typically much less willing to implement complex contingency management programs, particularly those that involve negative consequences. In summary, the efficacy of behavior therapy depends on the motivation and capabilities of the significant adults in the child's life and on the skills of the interveners in overcoming such obstacles. If key adults are unwilling or unable to implement the interventions, and if the objections or obstacles to intervention cannot be overcome, then behavior therapy will not be effective.

A final possible limitation of behavior therapy with ADHD children—again similar to a limitation of stimulant effects—is the lack of evidence for long-term effects. No studies have been conducted that examine long-term effects of behavioral interventions with ADHD children. Demonstration of the maintenance of treatment effects over time is one of the major concerns of those employing behavioral interventions with children, and research regarding how to maintain effects in the long run has not been conducted. All of these limitations have led to the growing practice of combining behavioral treatments with pharmacological interventions for ADHD.

COMBINED PHARMACOLOGICAL AND BEHAVIORAL INTERVENTIONS

Theoretically, the effects of combined treatments, such as combined pharmacological and behavioral treatments, can differ from the effects of the component treatments in several different ways: potentiation, inhibition, reciprocation, or addition. Alternatively, the two interventions can have complementary effects, each affecting different symptoms such that the combined intervention affects a greater range of symptomatology than does either treatment alone (Pelham, & Murphy, 1986). Thus, there is strong theoretical rationale to combine behavioral and pharmacological treatments for treatment of mental health problems.

More specifically, there are a number of advantages of combining behavioral and pharmacological treatments of ADHD. First, the behavioral component of treatment can usually be reduced in scope and complexity if combined with low dosages of medication (Atkins et al., 1989). Second, because less complex treatments are also less expensive, the cost-effectiveness of treatment is improved with a combined intervention. For example, a powerful, maximally effective contingency management intervention in a referred child's classroom might require daily therapist trips to the school compared to the single weekly trip characteristic of standard clinical behavior therapy. At $100 per visit, the more powerful behavioral intervention would cost $500 per week. In contrast, the addition of a low dose of psychostimulant medication to a typical clinical behavioral intervention might also maximize improvement but would cost less than $5 per week. Such concerns are major influences on whether parents seek out and follow through with treatment.

Third, these treatments often have complementary effects. For example, parent training is a standard component of a behavioral intervention for ADHD, thus ensuring that a treatment is available for the times of the day that are typically not addressed by medication for a child on a twice-a-day (b.i.d.) schedule. Similarly, psychostimulant medication can reduce problematic behaviors that are very difficult to treat with practical behavioral programs, such as low-rate, peer-directed aggression and stealing that occurs in the absence of adult authority (Hinshaw, Henker, Whalen, Erhardt, & Dunnington, 1989; Hinshaw, Heller, & McHale, 1992). Further, medication effects on prosocial and antisocial behaviors appear to be facilitated when behavioral contingencies supporting social behavior are in effect (Pelham, & Hoza, 1987). In several ways, then, a combined intervention is more comprehensive in coverage than either treatment alone.

Finally, there are several reasons to speculate that long-term maintenance of treatment effects might be improved with a combined intervention. First, it is clear that ADHD children suffer from a lack of cognitive and behavioral skills that are necessary for academic and social adjustment. To the extent that these skills must be acquired for successful long-term outcome, medication alone, which does not teach a child alternative behaviors for coping with problematic situations, would not be a sufficient treatment. The addition of a behavioral intervention that focuses in part on teaching such skills should improve the long-term outcome that would be achieved with medication alone. Similarly, to facilitate maintenance of behavioral treatment effects, the child's parents or teachers should be able to continue the intervention for a protracted time and maintain it by using naturally occurring contingencies following therapy termination. Because the addition of a low dose of psychostimulant medication makes relatively greater effects possible with less restrictive and more natural behavioral programs, a combined intervention may be more likely to be maintained by parents and teachers following termination of therapeutic contact.

In 1986, we reviewed the 19 studies that existed at that time in which a combination of behavioral and stimulant treatments had been used with ADHD children and we drew several conclusions (Pelham, & Murphy, 1986). First, 13 of the 19 independent studies (68%) showed superiority for a combined treatment on at least one classroom-based task or motor or social measure. For those studies in which a behavioral or pharmacological effect was found, only very rarely was either of these treatments alone superior to their combination. If order of condition means, rather than statistical significance, was used to interpret results, the combination treatment was superior to component treatments in almost every study reviewed. For the average ADHD child treated in these stud-

ies, a combined intervention resulted in greater improvement than did either treatment alone.

Consider, for example, the study reported by Gittelman and colleagues (1980). In an 8-week investigation, they compared (1) a clinical behavioral intervention (mainly teacher rather than parent training), (2) stimulant medication, and (3) both treatments combined. On a variety of measures the combined treatment group came closer to normalization of functioning than did either treatment alone, with stimulant treatment alone next in efficacy and behavioral treatment a distant third, despite the significant within-subject gains for this clinical behavior therapy intervention alone (see Figure 1). As Figure 1 shows, global evaluations of improvement made by mothers, teachers, and psychiatrists were always best for the combined behavioral and pharmacological treatment.

A number of studies conducted since 1986 have reached similar conclusions, and we review several of them. Several single-subject studies have shown that low (e.g., .3 mg/kg) doses of MPH and behavioral treatments have additive effects (e.g., Atkins et al., 1989; Pelham et al., 1980; Schell et al., 1986), yielding a larger treatment effect than either medication or behavioral intervention alone.

One study conducted in our laboratory (Pelham et al., 1988) was designed to determine whether these enhancing effects of a low dose of MPH would be obtained if combined with a clinical behavioral intervention over a longer period of time than the brief probes of the previous studies. This study, then, involved a 5-month behavioral intervention that included parent training, a school intervention, and Saturday social skills training groups. One group of subjects also received .3 mg/kg MPH b.i.d., while the other group received placebo. The low dose of medication had a clearly beneficial additive effect, even though its additional effect did not last after the medication was withdrawn. Interestingly, the level of final functioning that these children showed was similar to that obtained in the Gittelman and colleagues (1980) study's medication group but with half the dose of medication.

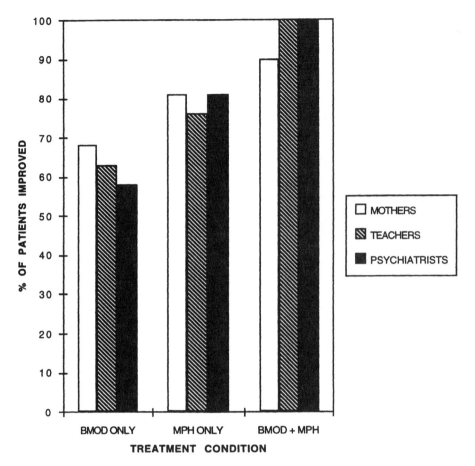

FIGURE 1.   Percentage of patients improved as rated by mothers, teachers, and psychiatrists as a function of treatment (data from Gittelman *et al.*, 1980).

Despite the fact that clinically important levels of improvement were obtained in this study, the final levels of functioning were far from acceptable. For example, 75% of the children were still one *SD* above their class means on negative peer nominations at posttreatment. Only 2 of the 20 treated children were within normal levels on all measures—parent and teacher ratings, peer nominations, and classroom observations—at treatment close. Thus, even a combination of low-dose stimulant therapy and clinical behavior therapy with social skills training groups over 5 months did not normalize treated children, particularly in the domain of peer relationships. This highlights the need for even more intensive behavioral treatments such as the STP discussed earlier.

Two other recent studies examined the combined effects of behavioral interventions and medication in STP classroom settings. Carlson and colleagues (1992) conducted a 2-week, within-subject evaluation of the concurrent effects of a behavioral intervention and .3 and .6 mg/kg MPH with 26 ADHD boys for 2 weeks in the STP classroom. Compared to a no–behavior modification ("regular classroom") condition, the full behavioral intervention included a reward and cost point system, a daily report card, and time-out. Behavioral conditions were alternated on a weekly basis, and medication was varied daily within the behavioral manipulation. Dependent measures included observations of on-task, disruptive, and rule-following behavior in the classroom, as well as numerous measures of academic productivity and accuracy. As in the studies of Pelham and colleagues (1988) and Gittelman and colleagues (1980), both the behavioral intervention and MPH had salutary effects on on-task, disruptive, and rule-following behavior. The effects of the behavioral intervention and .3 mg/kg were equivalent and additive on these measures of behavior, such that the combination of the two resulted in behavioral improvement equal to the .6 mg/kg dose of MPH (see Figure 2 for a graphical example of the effect). *In other words, the effective dose of MPH could be cut in half when the behavioral program was in effect in the classroom,* and there was no incremental value of the higher dose given the behavioral intervention. Interestingly, complementary effects were also observed in this study. The drug effect was significant for all six measures of academic productivity and accuracy but the behavioral intervention had no effect on any of these measures. Although behavior modifica-

tion was effective in changing social behavior, the pharmacological intervention was a necessary adjunct to produce academic changes in these ADHD boys.

Pelham and colleagues (1993) expanded on the Carlson and colleagues (1992) study by including a sufficient number of days per condition to make possible an assessment of individual differences in response to the behavioral intervention, MPH, and their combination. The design was the same as that employed by Carlson and colleagues but the study lasted 6 weeks, affording a relatively stable estimate of each individual's response to (1) behavioral treatment, (2) MPH, and (3) the combined treatment. In addition to standard dependent measures, we computed individual effect sizes (each child's treatment mean minus his no-treatment mean, divided by his SD over no-treatment days) that were weighted according to children's baseline symptom severity, and we also measured normalization of response.

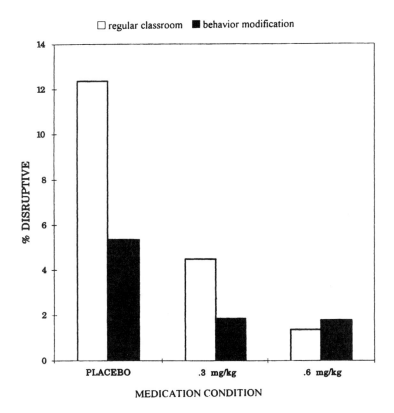

FIGURE 2.   Average percentage of disruptive behavior as a function of treatment (data from Carlson *et al.*, 1992).

Results for the group analyses were similar to our own and previous studies. That is, both treatments were effective but MPH was superior to behavioral treatment on most measures, particularly when individual effect sizes and normalization of functioning were examined (see Figure 3). Although there was no significant additive effect of the behavioral and drug treatments at the group level, the individual difference results regarding the incremental value of combined treatment revealed that 41% of the boys showed incremental improvement with combined treatment over their MPH-alone response, while 78% showed incremental improvement with combined treatment over their behavior-modification-alone response. Thus, despite the fact that MPH had twice the impact of behavior modification at the group level of analysis, and despite the fact that the combined treatment was not significantly superior to the single treatments, a sub-

stantial proportion of individuals clearly benefited from combined treatments.

One additional study conducted in the STP classroom (Hoza *et al.*, 1992) examined whether the potency of the behavioral treatment in the classroom could be enhanced by increasing the dose of behavioral treatment. Two children whose behavior was not controllable using our standard classroom intervention were treated with contingencies that were more powerful and showed an improved response to psychosocial treatment. Thus, this study showed that, just as the effect of medication can be increased by increasing the dose, so can the effect of a psychosocial treatment.

As indicated in these three studies, there are individual differences in response to behavioral and combined treatments that are as salient as the individual differences in response to psychostimulant medication. Notably, the standard deviations of the effect sizes shown in Figure 3

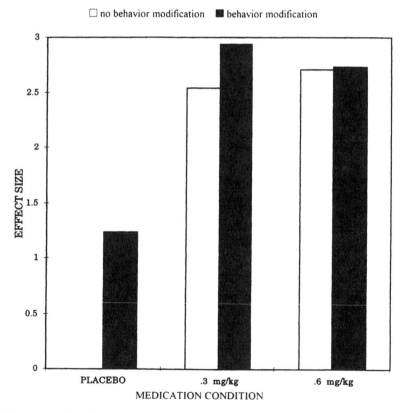

FIGURE 3. Average effect size for normalization ratings as a function of treatment (data from Pelham *et al.*, 1993).

ranged from 2 to 4. As Pelham and colleagues (1993) showed, some children derive benefit from a combined treatment regimen; others do not. This raises an important question: How does a clinician select among different doses and combinations of medication and behavioral treatments to ensure the best possible treatment for an individual child? The answer is through systematic assessment, using ecologically valid, individualized measures of behavioral functioning. As we have argued, treatment for ADHD should begin with the behavioral interventions listed in Table 1, including a DRC from the teacher to the parents (see example in Figure 1), which is a standard component of treatment for ADHD. For some children a DRC will be sufficient to normalize classroom behavior; for others (the majority), additional interventions will be necessary. However, if further behavioral interventions prove insufficient or cannot be conducted, then medication may be considered as an adjunctive treatment. One highly sensitive and ecologically valid method of assessing whether medication yields additional benefits beyond behavioral interventions is to use the child's DRC as an index of medication response. The teacher has already identified on the DRC the most salient target behaviors for that child, so those are the most relevant targets for medication response. By examining the child's DRC performance as a function of different doses of medication, the child's need for medication and the most appropriate dose can easily be determined.

Consider a child being treated in our clinic for whom the therapist determined that the behavioral treatments were not sufficiently effective. A clinical medication assessment was then conducted. Figure 4 shows a plot of the percentage of daily yeses achieved by the child (i.e., "proportion positive") on two of his DRC goals (i.e., "completes assignments accurately" and "follows instructions from the teacher") as a function of different medication conditions (placebo, .3 mg/kg, .6 mg/kg MPH), which were varied daily (see Pelham, 1993, for a complete description of this school-based medication assessment procedure). Conclusions about the incremental benefit of medication for this child were made by comparing the three medication

conditions that are represented by the three different lines in each of the two graphs. Three results are immediately clear. First, there is a low proportion positive on placebo days, suggesting that behavioral treatment alone was insufficient.

TABLE 1. Components of Effective, Comprehensive Treatment for ADHD

Parent training
    Behavioral approach
    Focus on behavior and family relationships
    Parent implemented
    Group-based, weekly sessions with therapist initially, then contact faded
    Provided over 2 or 3 years
    Program for maintenance and relapse prevention (e.g., develop plans for dealing with concurrent cyclic parental problems, such as maternal depression and parental substance abuse)

School intervention
    Behavioral approach
    Focus on classroom behavior, academic performance, and peer relationships
    Teacher implemented
    Consultant work with teacher—initial weekly sessions, then contact faded
    Provided over 2 or 3 years
    Program for maintenance and relapse prevention (e.g., train all school staff, including administrators; eventually train parent to implement and monitor)

Child intervention
    Behavioral and developmental approach
    Focus on teaching academic, recreational, and social/behavioral compentencies, decreasing aggression, developing close friendships, and buiilding self-efficacy
    Paraprofessional implemented
    Intensive treatments such as summer treatment programs (9 hours daily for 8 weeks), with school-year, after-school, and Saturday (6 hours) sessions
    Provided over 2 or 3 years
    Program for generalization and relapse prevention (e.g., integrate with school and parent treatments)

Concurrent psychostimulant medication
    Need determined following initiation of behavioral treatments
    Individualized, randomized, school-based medication trial conducted to determine need and minimal dose to complement the behavioral intervention
    Need for t.i.d. or long-acting medication also determined during initial assessment based on child's impairment across settings
    Repeated annual trials to adjust dosages and justify continued need

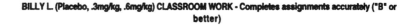

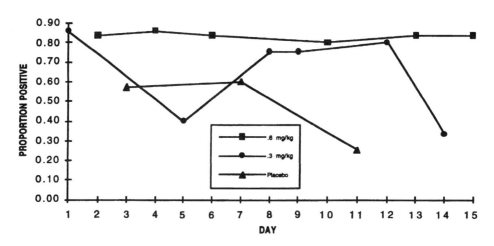

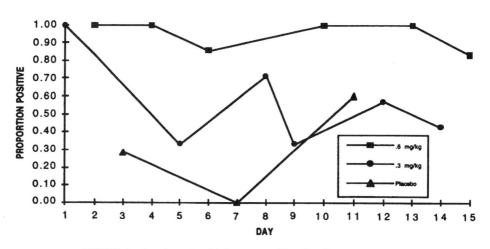

FIGURE 4.   Sample results of daily report card-based medication assessment.

Second, there was some, but not sufficient, improvement with the .3 mg/kg dose. Third, there was a consistently higher proportion positive on .6 mg/kg days, clearly demonstrating that this child benefited from the addition of that dose of medication to his treatment regimen. That this child needed the higher of two doses of MPH illustrates the individual differences in response to combined treatment, as most children are maximally responsive to the lower dose (Pelham, & Milich, 1991).

This case example is a good illustration of how a component of the behavioral treatment, the DRC, can be used to determine the child's concurrent medication dose, providing another way in which a combined approach to treatment can be uniquely effective. Indeed, children's individualized DRC targets as indicators of drug response yield clearer evidence of drug effects for ADHD children in regular classroom settings than do teacher ratings, the most commonly used way of measuring stimulant responsivity in ADHD children (Pelham, Hoza, *et al.,* 1997).

In summary, extant studies provide strong evidence for the efficacy of combining psychostimulant medication and behavioral therapy in treating children with ADHD. At the same time, several qualifications are in order. One of them is that, compared to the large numbers of subjects who have been studied over considerably longer time periods with pharmacological interventions, the combined intervention is relatively unstudied. Only 167 children were treated in the 19 studies reviewed by Pelham and Murphy (1986), and the median duration of treatment was less than 3 weeks. Only approximately 100 additional ADHD children have been treated with combined treatments in published studies in the decade since our original review, and most of the studies have been single-subject, crossover designs. Much more evidence is required before adequate knowledge is obtained regarding the effects of combined treatments and the procedures that will ensure maximal responsiveness, but it is our firm belief that the combined approach shows more promise than any other form of intervention with ADHD children.

In all studies, the incremental beneficial effects of the combined treatments does not last after either component is withdrawn. In the only study of its type, Pelham and colleagues (1988) discontinued the medication component of combined treatment and found that only the effects of the behavioral treatment remained. Although such a result could be viewed as a glass half empty, the fact that the behavioral treatment effects remained following medication is quite important. Gittelman, Abikoff, and colleagues (Abikoff, & Hechtman, 1996; Gittelman *et al.,* 1980) argued that combined treatments have no advantage over medication alone, but all of their studies have measured endpoint outcome *only while subjects were receiving medication.* If medication is discontinued—and this appears quite likely for most ADHD children at some time (Sherman, & Hertzig, 1991)—then a combination regimen of behavioral and low-dose pharmacological treatments will yield better functioning than a medication-only regimen. Studies that evaluate combined treatment effects without consideration of this obvious methodological issue (Abikoff, & Hechtman, 1996; Gittelman *et al.,* 1980) are missing the point of the potential of combined treatment. Surprisingly, all existing studies of combined treatment regimens have focused on acute effects rather than maintenance. Whether a systematic medication withdrawal and maintenance program could maintain the obviously beneficial effects of the combined treatment over the long term has yet to be investigated. No controlled, long-term outcome studies of combined interventions have yet been conducted.

SUMMARY

In this chapter, we have described and reviewed evidence for the efficacy of different types of behavioral treatment for ADHD, including clinical behavior therapy, contingency management, cognitive-behavioral treatment, combined pharmacological and behavioral treatment, and intensive treatments. We have also presented the strengths and weakness of the treatments. Our review has been an informal one, but more formal reviews have also drawn the conclusion that behavioral interventions are effective for ADHD. For example, Weisz, Weiss, Han, Granger, and Morton (1995) conducted a meta-analysis of the effects of child treatment in which they concluded that behavioral treatments (typically conducted in controlled settings) were effective for children with externalizing disorders and that clinic-based, typically nonbehavioral treatments were not.

Recently, a task force of Division 12 of the American Psychological Association has been addressing the validity of currently used treatment for mental health disorders (Task Force on Promotion and Dissemination for Psychological Procedures, 1995). The task force has focused on adult disorders. Using the criteria from this task force, a recent Task Force of the Section on Child Clinical Psychology of Division 12 reported on a systematic evaluation of the treatment literature for all *childhood* disorders (Lonigan, Elbert, & Johnson, 1998). With respect to ADHD, behavioral parent training and classroom interventions met criteria for the "empirically supported treatment" category of this task force (Pelham, Wheeler, & Chronis, 1998).

These various reviews have not analyzed the *components* of effective behavioral treatments for ADHD, but, based on our review and others, we believe a comprehensive treatment for ADHD is a multicomponent intervention that includes the facets listed in Table 1, namely, parent training, school intervention, child-based treatment, and concurrent medication. Key points about these components are noted in Table 1.

FUTURE DIRECTIONS

We conclude this chapter with a discussion of key questions that remain to be answered and problems that remain to be solved. We also discuss current initiatives and trends in the field that influence psychosocial treatments for ADHD. First, there is one ongoing clinical trial that will provide important information relevant to this chapter. It is noteworthy that the multicomponent approach to treatment that we summarize in Table 1 is precisely what the Multisite Study for ADHD (MTA) utilized (Richters *et al.*, 1995). That study employed an intensive psychosocial treatment package consisting of the components listed in Table 1 and crossed that treatment with stimulant medication to yield four groups in a large, controlled clinical trial lasting 14 months with a 10-month follow-up period: (1) psychosocial treatment alone, (2) pharmacological treatment alone, (3) combined psychosocial and pharmacological treatment, and (4) community comparison (control) treatment. With 144 ADHD children per cell, it will provide information on psychosocial and combined treatments for nearly as many children as have been studied in all previous studies. It is the largest clinical trial ever conducted by the National Institute of Mental Health, and it comprises the largest, most intensive, and longest treatment study of a childhood disorder that has ever been conducted. Within the limitations of its design, it will thus answer important questions about psychosocial and combined treatments for ADHD. Results should be forthcoming in the new millennium.

One question regarding behavioral treatment of ADHD concerns whether children's response to treatment may be predicted a priori. Few studies to date have addressed this question. The one or two studies that have addressed predictors of treatment response show that, consistent with earlier research (Wahler, 1980), behavioral treatment is more effective for children with mothers who have higher levels of social support (Firestone, & Witt, 1982; Horn, Ialongo, Popovich, & Peradotto, 1987). Interestingly, other reports suggest that parent training in turn reduces the amount of stress experienced by parents (Anastopoulos *et al.*, 1993; Pisterman *et al.*, 1992). Recent laboratory studies have documented that ADHD children cause extreme levels of subjective and physiologically measured distress in their parents, particularly their mothers, and that mothers with dysfunctional coping styles may respond to this distress with elevated alcohol consumption (Lang, Pelham, Atkeson, & Murphy, 1998; Molina, Pelham, & Lang, 1997; Pelham, Lang, *et al.*, 1997, 1998). Thus, dysfunctional parent characteristics may predict their child's response to treatment, require intervention as a part of treatment, and predict response to behavioral parent training. Studies of the mediational and moderational effects of various parent characteristics on treatment outcome for ADHD children are needed. However, given the lack of research on the predictors of treatment response for children with ADHD, these conclusions must be considered preliminary.

A second question that remains to be answered is whether the different types of behavioral treatments have differing efficacy for different types of children. One of the most important individual difference variables to be examined is age. Given that younger and older ADHD children have been shown to differ on at least some studies of cognitive and social functioning (Barkley *et al.*, 1984; Hoza, & Pelham, 1995), it may be that younger and older ADHD children differ in response to behavioral treatments. For example, perhaps older (i.e., young adolescents) ADHD children are more responsive to adjunct treatments (e.g., problem solving, self-monitoring) than are younger ADHD children. Similar arguments could be made for differential treatment response for ADHD children with comorbid aggressive or defiance (e.g., ODD or CD), and for ADHD children with comorbid learning disorders. We are aware of only two studies that have examined the response of children comorbid for aggression to behavioral treatments, and both showed that comorbid aggressive ADHD boys responded as well as nonaggressive boys to behavioral treatments (Pelham & Hoza, 1996; Pelham *et al.*, 1993). The absence of well-validated, empirically sound predictors of treatment response makes comprehensive, objective, and systematic evaluation of treatment responses all the more necessary and important.

A third question that remains to be addressed concerning behavioral treatment of ADHD is cost-effectiveness relative to other types of treatments. Behavioral treatments are much less cost-effective than administering stimulant medication, given that medications are administered only once or twice per day at a cost measured in cents, whereas behavioral treatments need to be constantly administered by professionals, teachers, and parents at considerably greater cost in effort and money. Long-term positive or negative impacts of the types and combinations of treatments also must be considered when assessing cost–benefit ratios. For example, intensive treatments such as that provided in the STP may have relatively high initial costs (e.g., the STP costs $2500 per child in 1997 dollars) that are offset by long-term savings. As we noted previously, however, adding a low dose of medication to an ongoing behavioral treatment may avoid the need for a more intensive and more expensive behavioral treatment. Unfortunately, we know of no data that differentiates these competing hypotheses.

It is becoming increasingly important to answer cost–benefit questions in the current era of managed care and health care reform, especially given our increasingly familiar experience that many insurance companies are refusing to pay for treatment of ADHD (or, at the least, severely constraining treatments).

A fourth area for future research is examination of differences in treatment response as a function of domain and settings. That is, children's response to behavioral and pharmacological treatment may vary as a function of the measure that is being examined and the setting in which it is being examined (Waschbusch *et al.*, 1998). For example, as noted earlier, Carlson and colleagues (1992) found that the combination of behavior modification and a low dose of stimulants was as effective as a high dose of stimulants in treating ADHD boys' disruptive behavior, but that only medication was effective in treating their academic work. Similar or analogous results have been obtained in other studies (Firestone *et al.*, 1981; Horn *et al.*, 1990, 1991; Pisterman *et al.*, 1992). Such results emphasize the potential benefit of the complementary effects of combined treatments. While these types of differences in individual treatment response are becoming increasingly well documented, the reasons for these differences remain unexplored. Only one study has examined whether responses to stimulant medication and response to behavioral treatments are related, an important question for both theoretical and practical perspectives. That study found that responses to the behavioral and pharmacological treatments were highly correlated, suggesting that similar brain mechanisms may control responses to these different treatment modalities (Pelham *et al.*, 1993).

A virtually unstudied aspect of behavioral and combined treatment concerns dosage effects and which components of treatment are necessary. Although it is widely viewed that school intervention is a necessary component of treatment for ADHD, perhaps the combination of medication and parent training will be sufficient for some ADHD children (Horn *et al.*, 1990). Perhaps only prudent negative consequences (versus positive programs) are sufficient for most ADHD children, as the O'Leary studies cited earlier would suggest, and the time and expense of parent training, teacher training, or both could be reduced by eliminating the sessions teaching positive control techniques. Could some components of intensive treatment packages, such as the STP, be eliminated or the length of treatment be reduced, thereby reducing the complexity and cost of treatment? Do higher (versus lower) doses of medication interfere with concurrent psychosocial treatment implementation, as we suggested earlier? There are no studies addressing such questions regarding treatment parameters, and they are needed.

A related question concerns the sequencing of treatment components. For example, should behavioral and pharmacological treatments be begun simultaneously in a combined treatment regimen or, as we have argued, should medication lag the behavioral treatment? How would different sequencing arrangements affect maintenance of treatment effects?

An important but unstudied aspect of behavioral treatments for ADHD is their exportability to clinic settings—the issue of efficacy versus effectiveness (Hoagwood, Hibbs, Brent, & Jensen, 1995; Weisz, Donenberg, Han, & Weisz, 1995). With very few exceptions (e.g., Pelham, & Hoza, 1996), most studies of behavioral and combined treatments for ADHD have been conducted in controlled university settings using highly homogeneous samples rather than in settings that are part of the mental health system and with samples that are more representative of those seen in "real-world" settings. As Weisz, Weiss, and colleagues (Weisz, Weiss, et al., 1995) noted, that fact likely overestimates the effectiveness of behavioral treatments for ADHD as they are likely to be conducted in the mental health system. Research on the exportability of behavioral treatment needs to be conducted and excellent suggestions are available (Weisz, Donenberg, et al., 1995).

One area in which behavioral treatments for ADHD are far superior to other forms of treatment for childhood disorders is the relatively long history of reliance on treatment man-

uals. Most forms of behavioral parent training, for example, have long been well manualized, as have teacher interventions and intensive treatment programs. The use of manualized treatments has many advantages that should serve behavioral treatments well as they are exported into community settings (Wilson, 1996).

Finally, and perhaps most important, the long-term effects of different types of behavioral and combinations of behavioral and pharmacological therapy need to be studied. The short-term efficacy of most types of behavior therapy is well documented. However, few studies have yet examined whether these short-term improvements have any substantial impact, either alone or in combination with medication, on the long-term outcome of children with ADHD. Given the chronicity and poor outcome of ADHD, the answer to this question is critical. As we have discussed, it may differ depending on the intensity of the behavioral treatment, the consistency with which it was administered, its duration, and whether appropriate pharmacological treatments were adjunctively applied.

REFERENCES

Abikoff, H. (1987). An evaluation of cognitive behavior therapy for hyperactive children. In B. B. Lahey, & A. E. Kazdin (Eds.), *Advances in clinical child psychology* (pp. 171–216). New York: Plenum.

Abikoff, H. (1991). Cognitive training in ADHD children: Less to it than meets the eye. *Journal of Learning Disabilities, 24,* 205–209.

Abikoff, H., & Hechtman, L. (1996). Multimodal therapy and stimulants in the treatment of children with attention deficit hyperactivity disorder. In E. D. Hibbs, & P. S. Jensen (Eds.), *Psychosocial treatments for child and adolescent disorders: Empirically based strategies for clinical practice* (pp. 341–369). Washington, DC: American Psychological Association.

Abikoff, H., Ganeles, D., Reiter, G., Blum, C., Foley, C., & Klein, R. G. (1988). Cognitive training in academically deficient ADDH boys receiving stimulant medication. *Journal of Abnormal Child Psychology, 16,* 411–432.

Abramowitz, A. J., O'Leary, S. G., & Rosen, L. A. (1987). Reducing off-task behavior in the classroom: A comparison of encouragement and reprimands. *Journal of Abnormal Child Psychology, 15,* 153–163.

Abramowitz, A. J., O'Leary, S. G., & Futtersak, M. W. (1988). The relative impact of long and short reprimands on children's off-task behavior in the classroom. *Behavior Therapy, 19,* 243–247.

Abramowitz, A. J., Eckstrand, D., O'Leary, S. G., & Dulcan, M. K. (1992). ADHD children's responses to stimulant medication and two intensities of a behavioral intervention. *Behavior Modification, 16,* 193–203.

Acker, M. M., & O'Leary, S. G. (1987). Effects of reprimands and praise on appropriate social behavior in the classroom. *Journal of Abnormal Child Psychology, 5,* 549–557.

American Psychiatric Association. (1994). *Diagnostic and statistical manual of mental disorders* (4th ed.). Washington, DC: Author.

Anastopoulos, A. D., Shelton, T. L., DuPaul, G. J., & Guevremont, D. C. (1993). Parent training for attention-deficit hyperactivity disorder: Its impact on parent functioning. *Journal of Abnormal Child Psychology, 21,* 581–596.

Atkins, M. S., Pelham, W. E., & White, K. J. (1989). Hyperactivity and attention deficit disorders. In M. Hersen (Ed.), *Psychological aspects of developmental and physical disabilities: A casebook* (pp. 137–156). Newbury Park, CA: Sage.

Barkley, R. A. (1988). The effects of methylphenidate on the interactions of preschool ADHD children with their mothers. *Journal of the American Academy of Child and Adolescent Psychiatry, 27,* 336–341.

Barkley, R. A. (1995). *Taking charge of ADHD: The complete, authoritative guide for parents.* New York: Guilford.

Barkley, R. A., Karlsson, J., Strzelecki, E., & Murphy, J. V. (1984). Effects of age and ritalin dosage on the mother–child interactions of hyperactive children. *Journal of Consulting and Clinical Psychology, 52,* 739–749.

Barkley, R. A., Karlsson, J., Pollard, S., & Murphy, J. (1985). Developmental changes in the mother–child interactions of hyperactive boys: Effects of two doses of Ritalin. *Journal of Child Psychology and Psychiatry, 26,* 705–715.

Barkley, R. A., Guevremont, D. C., Anastopoulos, A. D., & Fletcher, K. E. (1992). A comparison of three family therapy programs for treating family conflicts in adolescents with attention-deficit hyperactivity disorder. *Journal of Consulting and Clinical Psychology, 60,* 450–462.

Bloomquist, M. L., August, G. J., Cohen, C., Doyle, A., & Everhart, K. (1997). Social problem solving in hyperactive-aggressive children: How and what they think in conditions of automatic and controlled processing. *Journal of Clinical Child Psychology, 26,* 172–180.

Brown, R. T., Borden, K. A., Wynne, M. E., Spunt, A. L., & Clingerman, S. R. (1987). Compliance with pharmacological and cognitive treatment for attention deficit disorder. *Journal of the American Academy of Child and Adolescent Psychiatry, 26,* 521–526.

Carlson, C. L., Pelham, W. E., Milich, R., & Dixon, J. (1992). Single and combined effects of methylphenidate and behavior therapy on the classroom perfor-

mance of children with ADHD. *Journal of Abnormal Child Psychology, 20,* 213–232.

Charles, L., & Schain, R. (1981). A four-year follow-up study of the effects of methylphenidate on the behavior and academic achievement of hyperactive children. *Journal of Abnormal Child Psychology, 9,* 495–505.

Coie, J. D., & Krehbiel, G. (1984). Effects of academic tutoring on the social status of low-achieving, socially rejected children. *Child Development, 55,* 1465–1478.

Cunningham, C. E., Bremner, R., & Secord-Gilbert, M. (1994). *The community parent education (COPE) program: A school based family systems oriented course for parents of children with disruptive behavior disorders.* Unpublished manuscript, McMaster University and Chedoke-McMaster Hospitals, Hamilton, Ontario, Canada.

Dujovne, V. F., Barnard, M. U., & Rapoff, M. A. (1995). Pharmacological and cognitive-behavioral approaches in the treatment of childhood depression: A review and critique. *Clinical Psychology Review, 15,* 589–611.

DuPaul, G. J., & Stoner, G. D. (1994). *ADHD in the schools: Assessment and intervention strategies.* New York: Guilford.

DuPaul, G. J., Guevremont, D. C., & Barkley, R. A. (1992). Behavioral treatment of attention-deficit hyperactivity disorder in the classroom: The use of the attention training system. *Behavior Modification, 16,* 204–225.

Firestone, P., & Witt, J. E. (1982). Characteristics of families completing and prematurely discontinuing a behavioral parent-training program. *Journal of Pediatric Psychology, 7,* 209–222.

Firestone, P., Kelly, M. J., Goodman, J. T., & Davey, J. (1981). Differential effects of parent training and stimulant medication with hyperactives. *Journal of the American Academy of Child Psychiatry, 20,* 135–147.

Fischer, M. (1990). Parenting stress and the child with attention deficit hyperactivity disorder. *Journal of Clinical Child Psychology, 19,* 337–346.

Forehand, R., & Long, N. (1996). *Parenting the strong-willed child.* Chicago: Contemporary Books.

Forgatch, M., & Patterson, G. R. (1989). *Parents and adolescents living together: Part 2. Family problem solving.* Eugene, OR: Castalia.

Fuchs, D., & Fuchs, L. S. (1989). Exploring effective and efficient prereferral interventions: A component analysis of behavioral consultation. *School Psychology Review, 18,* 260–283.

Gittelman, R., Abikoff, H., Pollack, E., Klein, D. F., Katz, S., & Mattes, J. (1980). A controlled trial of behavior modification and methylphenidate in hyperactive children. In C. K. Whalen, & B. Henker (Eds.), *Hyperactive children: The social ecology of identification and treatment* (pp. 221–243). New York: Academic Press.

Hartup, W. (1983). Peer relations. In P. H. Mussen (Ed.), *Handbook of child psychology: Socialization, personality, and social development* (Vol. 4, pp. 103–196). New York: Wiley.

Hinshaw, S. P. (1991). Stimulant medication and the treatment of aggression in children with attentional deficits. *Journal of Clinical Child Psychology, 20,* 301–312.

Hinshaw, S. P., & Erhardt, D. (1991). Attention-deficit hyperactivity disorder. In P. Kendall (Ed.), *Child and adolescent therapy: Cognitive-behavioral procedures* (pp. 98–128). New York: Guilford.

Hinshaw, S. P., Henker, B., Whalen, C. K., Erhardt, D., & Dunnington, R. E. (1989). Aggressive, prosocial, and nonsocial behavior in hyperactive boys: Dose effects of methylphenidate in naturalistic settings. *Journal of Consulting and Clinical Psychology, 57,* 636–643.

Hinshaw, S. P., Heller, T., & McHale, J. P. (1992). Covert antisocial behavior in boys with attention deficit hyperactivity disorder: External validation and effects of methylphenidate. *Journal of Consulting and Clinical Psychology, 60,* 274–281.

Hoagwood, K., Hibbs, E., Brent, D., & Jensen, P. (1995). Introduction to the special section: Efficacy and effectiveness in studies of child and adolescent psychotherapy. *Journal of Consulting and Clinical Psychology, 63,* 683–687.

Horn, W. F., Ialongo, N., Popovich, S., & Peradotto, D. (1987). Behavioral parent training and cognitive-behavioral self-control therapy with ADD-H children: Comparative and combined effects. *Journal of Clinical Child Psychology, 16,* 57–68.

Horn, W. F., Ialongo, N., Greenberg, G., Packard, T., & Smith-Winberry, C. (1990). Additive effects of behavioral parent training and self-control therapy with ADHD children. *Journal of Clinical Child Psychology, 19,* 98–110.

Horn, W. F., Ialongo, N., Pascoe, J. M., Greenberg, G., Packard, T., Lopez, M., Wagner, A., & Puttler, L. (1991). Additive effects of psychostimulants. parent training, and self-control therapy with ADHD children: A 9-month follow-up. *Journal of the American Academy of Child and Adolescent Psychiatry, 32,* 182–189.

Hoza, B., & Pelham, W. E. (1995). Social-cognitive predictors of treatment response in children with ADHD. *Journal of Social and Clinical Psychology, 14,* 23–35.

Hoza, B., Pelham, W. E., Sams, S. E., & Carlson, C. (1992). An examination of the dosage effects of both behavior therapy and methylphenidate on the classroom performance of two ADHD children. *Behavior Modification, 16,* 164–192.

Kazdin, A. E. (1996). Problem solving and parent management in treating aggressive and antisocial behavior. In E. D. Hibbs, & P. S. Jensen (Eds.), *Psychosocial treatments for child and adolescent disorders: Empirically based strategies for clinical practice* (pp. 377–408). Washington, DC: American Psychological Association.

Kelly, M. L., & McCain, A. P. (1995). Promoting academic performance in inattentive children: The relative efficacy of school–home notes with and without response cost. *Behavior Modification, 19,* 357–375.

Kendall, P. C., & Gosch, E. A. (1994). Cognitive-behavioral interventions. In T. H. Ollendick, N. J. King, & W. Yule (Eds.), *International handbook of phobic and anxiety disorders in children and adolescents* (pp. 415–438). New York: Plenum.

Kent, R. N., & O'Leary, K. D. (1976). A controlled evaluation of behavior modification with conduct problem children. *Journal of Consulting and Clinical Psychology, 44,* 586–596.

Krueger, R. F., Caspi, A., Moffitt, T. E., White, J., & Stouthamer-Loeber, M. (1996). Delay of gratification, psychopathology, and personality: Is low self-control specific to externalizing problems? *Journal of Personality, 64,* 107–129.

Lang, A. R., Pelham, W. E., Atkeson, B. M., & Murphy, D. A. (1998). Effects of alcohol intoxication on parenting in interactions with child confederates exhibiting normal or deviant behaviors. *Journal of Abnormal Child Psychology, 1,* 103–114.

Lochman, J. E. (1992). Cognitive-behavioral intervention with aggressive boys: Three-year follow up and preventive effects. *Journal of Consulting and Clinical Psychology, 60,* 426–432.

Lochman, J. E., & Lenhart, L. A. (1993). Anger coping intervention for aggressive children: Conceptual models and outcome effects. *Clinical Psychology Review, 13,* 785–805.

Lonigan, G., Elbert, J. C., & Johnson, S. B. (1998). Empirically supported psychosocial interventions for children: An overview. *Journal of Clinical Child Psychology, 27,* 138–145.

Mash, E. J., & Johnston, C. (1990). Determinants of parenting stress: Illustrations from families of hyperactive children and families of physically abused children. *Journal of Clinical Child Psychology, 19,* 313–328.

Meichenbaum, D., & Goodman, J. (1971). Training impulsive children to talk to themselves: A means of developing self-control. *Journal of Abnormal Psychology, 77,* 115–126.

Milich, R., & Landau, S. (1982). Socialization and peer relations in the hyperactive child. In K. Gadow, & I. Bialer (Eds.), *Advances in learning and behavioral disabilities* (Vol. 1, pp. 283–339). Greenwich, CT: JAI.

Miller, G. E., & Prinz, R. J. (1990). Enhancement of social learning family interventions for childhood conduct disorder. *Psychological Bulletin, 108,* 291–307.

Molina, B., Pelham, W. E., & Lang, A. (1997). Alcohol expectancies and drinking characteristics in parents of children with attention deficit hyperactivity disorder. *Alcoholism: Clinical and Experimental Research, 21,* 557–566.

Oden, S., & Asher, S. R. (1977). Coaching children in social skills for friendship making. *Child Development, 48,* 495–506.

O'Leary, K. D., & Becker, W. C. (1967). Behavior modification of an adjustment class: A token reinforcement program. *Exceptional Children, 33,* 637–642.

O'Leary, K. D., Pelham, W. E., Rosenbaum, A., & Price, G. (1976). Behavioral treatment of hyperkinetic children: An experimental evaluation of its usefulness. *Clinical Pediatrics, 15,* 510–515.

O'Leary, S. G., & Pelham, W. E. (1978). Behavior therapy and withdrawal of stimulant medication with hyperactive children. *Pediatrics, 61,* 211–217.

Parker, J. G., & Asher, S. R. (1987). Peer relations and later personal adjustment: Are low-accepted children at risk? *Psychological Bulletin, 102,* 357–389.

Patterson, G. R. (1974). Intervention for boys with conduct problems: Multiple settings, treatment, and criteria. *Journal of Consulting and Clinical Psychology, 42,* 471–481.

Patterson, G. R. (1982). *Coercive family process.* Eugene, OR: Castalia.

Pelham, W. E. (1993). Pharmacotherapy for children with attention-deficit hyperactivity disorder. *School Psychology Review, 22,* 199–227.

Pelham, W. E., & Bender, M. E. (1982). Peer relationships in hyperactive children: Description and treatment. In K. Gadow, & I. Bialer (Eds.), *Advances in learning and behavior disabilities* (Vol. 1, pp. 365–436). Greenwich, CT: JAI.

Pelham, W. E., & Hoza, J. (1987). Behavioral assessment of psychostimulant effects in ADD children in a Summer Day Treatment Program. In R. Prinz (Ed.), *Advances in behavioral assessment of children and families* (Vol. 3, pp. 3–33). Greenwich, CT: JAI.

Pelham, W. E., & Hoza, B. (1996). Intensive treatment: A summer treatment program for children with ADHD. In E. Hibbs, & P. Jensen (Eds.), *Psychosocial treatments for child and adolescent disorders: Empirically based strategies for clinical practice* (pp. 311–340). New York: American Psychological Association Press.

Pelham, W. E., & Milich, R. (1991). Individual differences in response to Ritalin in classwork and social behavior. In L. L. Greenhill, & B. B. Osman (Eds.), *Ritalin: Theory and patient management* (pp. 203–221). New York: Liebert.

Pelham, W. E., & Murphy, H. A. (1986). Attention deficit and conduct disorder. In M. Hersen (Ed.), *Pharmacological and behavioral treatment: An integrative approach* (pp. 108–148). New York: Wiley.

Pelham, W. E., Schnedler, R. W., Bologna, N., & Contreras, A. (1980). Behavioral and stimulant treatment of hyperactive children: A therapy study with methylphenidate probes in a within-study design. *Journal of Applied Behavioral Analysis, 13,* 221–236.

Pelham, W. E., Bender, M. E., Caddell, J., Booth, S., & Moorer, S. (1985). The dose–response effects of methylphenidate on classroom academic and social behavior in children with attention-deficit disorder. *Archives of General Psychiatry, 42,* 948–952.

Pelham, W. E., Schnedler, R. W., Bender, M. E., Miller, J., Nilsson, D., Budrow, M., Ronnei, M., Paluchowski, C., & Marks, D. (1988). The combination of behavior therapy and methylphenidate in the treatment of hyperactivity: A therapy outcome study. In L. M. Bloomingdale (Ed.), *Attention deficit disorders* (Vol. 3, pp. 29–48). London: Pergamon.

Pelham, W. E., Carlson, C., Sams, S. E., Vallano, G., Dixon, M. J., & Hoza, B. (1993). Separate and combined effects of methylphenidate and behavior modification on boys with ADHD in the classroom. *Journal of Consulting and Clinical Psychology, 61,* 506–515.

Pelham, W. E., Swanson, J. M., Furman, M. B., & Schwindt, H. (1995). Pemoline effects on children with ADHD: A time–response by dose–response analysis on classroom measures. *Journal of the American Academy of Child and Adolescent Psychiatry, 34,* 1504–1513.

Pelham, W. E., Greiner, A. R., Gnagy, E. M., Hoza, B., Martin, L., Sams, S. E., & Wilson, T. (1996). A summer treatment program for children with ADHD. In M. Roberts, & A. LaGreca (Eds.), *Model programs for service delivery for child and family mental health* (pp. 193–212). Hillsdale, NJ: Erlbaum.

Pelham, W. E., Greiner, A. R., & Gnagy, E. M. (1997). *Children's summer treatment program manual.* Buffalo, NY: Comprehensive Treatment for Attention Deficit Disorder, Inc.

Pelham, W. E., Hoza, B., Pillow, D. R., Gnagy, E. M., Kipp, H. L., Greiner, A. R., Trane, S. T., Greenhouse, J., Wolfson, L., & Fitzpatrick, E. (1997, July). *Effects of MPH and expectancy on children with ADHD: Behavior, academic performance, and attributions in a summer treatment program and regular classroom setting.* Poster presented at the annual meeting of the International Society for Research in Child and Adolescent Psychopathology, Paris.

Pelham, W. E., Lang, A. R., Atkeson, B., Murphy, D. A., Gnagy, E. M., Greiner, A. R., Vodde-Hamilton, M., & Greenslade, K. E. (1997). Effects of deviant child behavior on parental distress and alcohol consumption in laboratory interactions. *Journal of Abnormal Child Psychology, 25,* 413–424.

Pelham, W. E., Wheeler, T., & Chronis, A. (1998). Empirically supported psychosocial treatments for ADHD. *Journal of Clinical Child Psychology, 27,* 189–204.

Pelham, W. E., Lang, A. R., Atkeson, B., Murphy, D. A., Gnagy, E. M., Greiner, A. R., Vodde-Hamilton, M., & Greenslade, K. E. (1998). Effects of deviant child behavior on parental alcohol consumption: Stress-induced drinking in parents of ADHD children. *American Journal on Addictions, 7,* 103–114.

Pfiffner, L. J., & McBurnett, K. (1997). Social skills training with parent generalization: Treatment effects for children with ADD/ADHD. *Journal of Consulting and Clinical Psychology, 65,* 749–757.

Pfiffner, L. J., & O'Leary, S. G. (1987). The efficacy of all-positive management as a function of the prior use of negative consequences. *Journal of Applied Behavior Analysis, 20,* 265–271.

Pfiffner, L. J., O'Leary, S. G., Rosen, L. A., & Sanderson, W. C., Jr. (1985). A comparison of the effects of continuous and intermittent response cost and reprimands in the classroom. *Journal of Clinical Child Psychology, 14,* 348–352.

Pfiffner, L. J., Rosen, L. A., & O'Leary, S. G. (1985). The efficacy of an all-positive approach to classroom management. *Journal of Applied Behavior Analysis, 18,* 257–261.

Pisterman, S., Firestone, P., McGrath, P., Goodman, J. T., Webster, I., Mallory, R., & Goffin, B. (1992). The role of parent training in treatment of preschoolers with ADD-H. *American Journal of Orthopsychiatry, 62,* 397–408.

Rapport, M. D., & Kelly, K. L. (1991). Psychostimulant effects on learning and cognitive functions: Findings and implications for children with attention deficit hyperactivity disorder. *Clinical Psychology Review, 11,* 61–92.

Rapport, M. D., Murphy, H. A., & Bailey, J. S. (1980). The effects of a response cost treatment tactic on hyperactive children. *Journal of School Psychology, 18,* 98–111.

Rapport, M. D., Murphy, H. A., & Bailey, J. S. (1982). Ritalin vs. response cost in the control of hyperactive children: A within-subjects comparison. *Journal of Applied Behavior Analysis, 15,* 205–216.

Richters, J. E., Arnold, L. E., Jensen, P. S., Abikoff, H., Conners, C. K., Greenhill, L. L., Hechtman, L., Hinshaw, S. P., Pelham, W. E., & Swanson, J. M. (1995). The National Institute of Mental Health collaborative multisite multimodal treatment study of children with Attention-Deficit/Hyperactivity Disorder (MTA): I. Background and rationale. *Journal of the American Academy of Child, and Adolescent Psychiatry, 34,* 987–1000.

Rosen, L. A., O'Leary, S. G., Joyce, S. A., Conway, G., & Pfiffner, L. J. (1984). The importance of prudent negative consequences for maintaining the appropriate behavior of hyperactive students. *Journal of Abnormal Child Psychology, 12,* 581–604.

Satterfield, J. H., Hoppe, C. M., & Schell, A. M. (1982). A prospective study of delinquency in 110 adolescent boys with attention deficit disorder and 88 normal adolescents. *American Journal of Psychiatry, 139,* 795–798.

Schell, R. M., Pelham, W. E., Bender, M. E., Andree, J., Law, T., & Robbins, F. (1986). The concurrent assessment of behavioral and psychostimulant interventions: A controlled case study. *Behavioral Assessment, 8,* 373–384.

Sherman, M., & Hertzig, M. E. (1991). Prescribing practices of Ritalin: The Suffolk County, New York study.

In L. L. Greenhill & B. B. Osman (Eds.), *Ritalin: Theory and patient management* (pp. 187–193). New York: Liebert.

Swanson, J. M. (1992). *School-based assessments and interventions for ADD students.* Irvine, CA: K. C. Publishing.

Swanson, J. M., McBurnett, K., Christian, D. L., & Wigal, T. (1995). Stimulant medication and treatment of children with ADHD. In T. H. Ollendick, & R. J. Prinz (Eds.), *Advances in clinical child psychology* (Vol. 17, pp. 265–322). New York: Plenum.

Task Force on Promotion and Dissemination of Psychological Procedures. (1995). Training in and dissemination of empirically validated psychological treatments: Report and recommendations. *The Clinical Psychologist, 48,* 3–24.

Wahler, R. G. (1980). The insular mother: Her problems in parent–child treatment. *Journal of Applied Behavior Analysis, 13,* 207–219.

Waschbusch, D. A., Kipp, H. L., & Pelham, W. E. (1998). Generalization of behavioral and pharmacological treatment of attention-deficit/hyperactivity disorder (ADHD): Discussion and examples. *Behavior Research and Therapy, 36,* 675–694.

Weiss, G., & Hechtman, L. (1993). *Hyperactive children grown up* (2nd ed.). New York: Guilford.

Weisz, J. R., Donenberg, G. R., Han, S. S., & Weisz, B. (1995). Bridging the gap between laboratory and clinic in child and adolescent psychotherapy. *Journal of Consulting and Clinical Psychology, 63,* 688–701.

Weisz, J. R., Weiss, B., Han, S. S., Granger, D. A., & Morton, T. (1995). Effects of psychotherapy with children and adolescents revisited: A meta-analysis of treatment outcome studies. *Psychological Bulletin, 117,* 450–468.

Wilson, G. T. (1996). Manual-based treatments: The clinical application of research findings. *Behaviour Research and Therapy, 34,* 295–314.

Witt, J. C. (1986). Teachers' resistance to the use of school-based interventions. *Journal of School Psychology, 24,* 37–44.

12

Adolescent and Adult Outcomes in Attention-Deficit/Hyperactivity Disorder

SALVATORE MANNUZZA and RACHEL G. KLEIN

INTRODUCTION

Follow-up studies of childhood disorders are valuable for multiple reasons. Knowledge of which symptoms are likely to persist and what secondary complications are likely to develop is important to families of affected children, as well as to the design of long-term interventions. Knowledge of the course and outcome of a disorder also contributes to the assessment of diagnostic validity. Furthermore, longitudinal studies can be used to identify early predictors of later functioning. The fate of children with Attention-Deficit/ Hyperactivity Disorder (ADHD)* is especially important because the disorder is one of the most prevalent (see Chapter 2, this volume), and is associated with impairment in multiple functional domains in childhood (Arnold & Jensen, 1995; Barkley, 1996).

This chapter reports on the adolescent and adult outcomes of children with ADHD. Our focus primarily is on controlled, prospective follow-up studies that have been published during the past 15 years. The reader is referred to previous reviews for coverage of earlier prospective and retrospective studies, and for detailed discussions of methodological issues in longitudinal research (Brown & Borden, 1986; Hechtman, 1996; Klein & Mannuzza, 1989, 1991; Thorley, 1984; Weiss, 1996; Weiss & Hechtman, 1993. In addition, only brief mention is made of studies with short follow-up intervals (e.g., 1–4 years) and those with relatively young follow-up ages (e.g., 11–14 years) because these studies do not provide data relevant to outcome much beyond the peak of the age-risk period for diagnosis. For example, mean age at follow-up in the study by Barkley, Fischer, Edelbrock, & Smallish (1990) was 14.9 years,

*The DSM-IV (American Psychiatric Association, 1994) and DSM-III-R (American Psychiatric Association, 1987) term Attention-Deficit/Hyperactivity Disorder (ADHD) is used throughout this chapter for consistency. However, because this chapter focuses on follow-up studies, most of which began prior to 1987, children necessarily met criteria for diagnoses in earlier systems of nomenclature, that is, DSM-III Attention Deficit Disorder with Hyperactivity (American Psychiatric Association, 1980) and DSM-II Hyperkinetic Reaction of Childhood (American Psychiatric Association, 1968). There is little doubt that children with any of these diagnoses overlap substantially in their clinical profiles. However, the criteria for these diagnoses are not identical and, therefore, could conceivably identify slightly different clinical groups.

SALVATORE MANNUZZA and RACHEL G. KLEIN • Department of Clinical Psychology, Columbia University, and New York State Psychiatric Institute, New York, New York 10032.

Handbook of Disruptive Behavior Disorders, edited by Quay and Hogan. Kluwer Academic/Plenum Publishers, New York, 1999.

and follow-up duration in the study by Bieder-man and colleagues (1996) was only 4 years.

DSM-IV (American Psychiatric Associa-tion, 1994) distinguishes three types of ADHD, predominantly inattentive, predominantly hy-peractive-impulsive, and combined. As a func-tion of the classification system extant when projects were initiated, the studies reviewed in this chapter include children who, today, would be diagnosed as having either the predomi-nantly hyperactive-impulsive or the combined type. To date, there has been no long-term prospective follow-up study of ADHD children who are predominantly inattentive.

Terms such as "adolescence," "young adult-hood," and "adulthood" have been used in the literature with varying standards that have led to some confusion regarding the persistence of childhood symptoms "into adulthood." In this chapter, we operationalize such terms (generally referring to mean age at follow-up) as follows: early adolescence = early to mid teens (13–15 years); late adolescence = late teens (16–19 years); adulthood = age 20 and beyond. The ra-tionale for these divisions is twofold. First, the extent of certain deficits changes over time. For example, the prevalence of ADHD symptoms in late adolescence is substantially different from that in adulthood. Therefore, classifying late adolescent and adult follow-up studies together would distort findings. Second, and perhaps more important, separating studies into these three epochs makes good developmental and clinical sense. As mentioned previously, short-term follow-up studies into early adolescence combine concurrent difficulties and immediate consequences of the disorder with outcome. For most individuals, late adolescence marks a major transition, for example, completing high school, starting college, leaving home, and beginning a career. By adulthood, for the most part, priori-ties and objectives have been set.

A universal finding among epidemiologi-cal and clinical studies of ADHD children is that boys are greatly overrepresented (McGee & Feehan, 1991; Szatmari, 1992). Consequently, most studies have either restricted their sam-ples to boys (Biederman et al., 1996; Gittel-man, Mannuzza, Shenker, & Bonagura, 1985;

Mannuzza et al., 1991) or have reported results that largely reflect the outcome of ADHD males (Weiss & Hechtman, 1993). Similarly, ethnic composition has been exclusively, or nearly exclusively white (Barkley et al., 1990; Biederman et al., 1996; Gittelman et al., 1985; Loney, Kramer, & Milich, 1981; Mannuzza et al., 1991; Satterfield, Hoppe, & Schell, 1982; Weiss & Hechtman, 1993). Therefore, the re-sults presented in this chapter are based on studies of predominantly white ADHD boys.

Most follow-up studies of ADHD chil-dren did not assess the role of comorbid Con-duct Disorder (CD) in the initial childhood cohort. Although the disorder was well estab-lished and had been the subject of multiple studies, it was not until 1980, with the advent of DSM-III (American Psychiatric Association, 1980), that criteria for CD were first intro-duced. It has been estimated that 30%–50% of children with ADHD have comorbid CDs (Biederman, Newcorn, & Sprich, 1991). Conse-quently, outcome in certain studies may have been affected. For example, Satterfield, Satter-field, and Schell (1987) estimate that their childhood sample had a 75% rate of CD. Be-cause multiple studies have shown that symp-toms of CD in childhood (i.e., antisocial, aggressive behavior) predict similar problems at follow-up (August, Stewart, & Holmes, 1983; Fischer, Barkley, Fletcher, & Smallish, 1993; Loney et al., 1981; Weiss, Minde, Werry, Douglas, & Nemeth, 1971) and that early CD predicts adult Antisocial Personality Disorder (APD) (Robins, 1974), antisocial behaviors found in the long-term outcome of ADHD children may be a function of the earlier CD cases. However, standards for diagnosing CD have changed over the past 15 years. The DSM-III, DSM-III-R, and DSM-IV all require a per-vasive pattern of rule-breaking behavior to diagnose CD, but in DSM-III, a single behav-ior sufficed to meet criteria and this could con-sist of lying exclusively. Criteria became more rigorous in DSM-III-R and DSM-IV. For exam-ple, both of these systems require three behav-iors, and DSM-IV added an impairment criterion. The New York Study (described later) systematically screened ADHD children to be free of antisocial behavior (without the opportunity of applying specific criteria for CD, since these did not exist) because, at that time, the investigators believed that ADHD and CD were distinct, unrelated conditions. It is possible that follow-up studies of ADHD children included a substantial proportion of children with CD as defined in DSM-III. It is highly unlikely, however, that the syndrome as defined in DSM-IV was prevalent to any meaningful extent in all of these studies.

In contrast, the same cannot be averred for oppositional behaviors. These are very common among children referred for ADHD, and the prevalence of Oppositional Defiant Disorder (ODD) is likely to have been elevated in the initial cohorts of children who have been followed. However, these behaviors may represent an index of severity and chronicity of the ADHD syndrome, rather than the occurrence of an independent maladaptive pathological process. In that sense, the co-occurrence of ODD and ADHD may not reflect the usual concept of comorbidity. Nevertheless, these issues must be kept in mind when interpreting the results of outcome studies of ADHD.

EARLY ADOLESCENT OUTCOME (AGES 13–15)

Prospective, controlled follow-up studies of ADHD children into early adolescence have shown that, at average ages 13–15, relative deficits are apparent in several areas. In school, these youngsters fail more courses, obtain lower grades, and more often repeat grades than controls (Ackerman, Dykman, & Peters, 1977; Biederman et al., 1996; Fischer, Barkley, Edelbrock, & Smallish, 1990; Weiss et al., 1971). The formerly ADHD adolescents also perform worse on cognitive tests than controls (Biederman et al., 1996; Cohen, Weiss, & Minde, 1972; Hoy, Weiss, Minde, & Cohen, 1978). In addition, low self-esteem and poor social functioning are common (Ackerman et al., 1977; Hoy et al., 1978; Weiss et al., 1971). For example, in one study, 30% of former ADHD children were described by their mothers as having

no steady friends at the average age of 13 (Weiss et al., 1971).

Early studies showed that a substantial, significant proportion of probands exhibit antisocial behaviors and continue to show symptoms of the childhood syndrome, that is, distractibility, impulsivity, and hyperactivity (Ackerman et al., 1977; Minde, Weiss, & Mendelson, 1972; Weiss et al., 1971). Moreover, using DSM-III-R criteria (American Psychiatric Association, 1987), two recent studies reported the following rates of disorder in probands and controls, respectively, at mean follow-up ages 14–15 years: CD, 28%–43% versus 2%–6%; ADHD, 65%–71% versus 3% (Barkley et al., 1990; Biederman et al., 1996). Notably, Barkley and colleagues (1990) reported that the majority of their cases showed aggressive or oppositional symptoms in childhood; Biederman and colleagues (1996) reported that 22% of their probands had CD and 65% had ODD in childhood.

In summary, short-term follow-up studies of children with ADHD fairly consistently have shown that these children experience significant academic, cognitive, and behavioral difficulties in their early to mid teens. Two thirds to three quarters continue to exhibit the full ADHD syndrome, and pervasive conduct problems are common.

LATE ADOLESCENT OUTCOME (AGES 16–19)

Two controlled, prospective follow-up studies of ADHD children, one in Montreal and the other in New York, have generated most of the systematic, comprehensive data on the late adolescent and adult outcomes of these children.

Overview of Major Studies

The Montreal Study

Weiss and Hechtman (1993) conducted 5-, 10-, and 15-year follow-up studies of a sample of ADHD children. The initial cohort consisted of 104 nonpsychotic, cross-situationally hyperactive children of average intelligence who were between 6 and 12 years of age. All were clinically diagnosed at the Department of Psychiatry of Montreal Children's Hospital in the early to mid 1960s and entered in a series of drug treatment studies.

At 5-year follow-up (mean age = 13–15 years), approximately 88% of the initial childhood cohort were evaluated. At 10-year follow-up (mean age = 19 years), about 73% were evaluated. And at 15-year follow-up (mean age = 25 years), 49% to 61% were assessed, depending on the outcome measure. Evaluations were conducted by clinicians.

A control group was recruited via advertising in the same schools that the ADHD cases attended. Subjects were accepted as controls if both parents and teachers agreed that they did not exhibit behavioral problems at home or in school, and if they had never failed a grade. Thirty-five controls were recruited at 5-year follow-up. An additional 10 controls (same criteria) were recruited at 10-year follow-up by asking existing controls for names of acquaintances at work or school.

Positive features of the Montreal Study included a prospective, controlled design, a respectable sample size, and assessments at multiple time points by clinicians (childhood, early adolescence, late adolescence, and adulthood).

The New York Study

We conducted 9- and 16-year follow-up studies of ADHD children (Gittelman *et al.*, 1985; Mannuzza, Klein, Bessler, Malloy, & LaPadula, 1993). The initial cohort consisted of 115 nonpsychotic, cross-situationally hyperactive children of average intelligence who were between 6 and 12 years of age. All were clinically diagnosed as having hyperkinetic reaction of childhood (American Psychiatric Association, 1968) at a child psychiatric research clinic in the 1970s. These children participated in a treatment study primarily restricted to pharmacotherapy (Gittelman-Klein, Klein, Katz, Saraf, & Pollack, 1976).

Children were not accepted if a primary reason for referral involved aggressive or antisocial behaviors. Therefore, we suspect that the initial childhood cohort was relatively pure with respect to CD but not oppositional behaviors.

At 9-year follow-up (mean age = 18 years), 98% were evaluated. At 16-year follow-up (mean age = 25 years), 90% were assessed.

A control group was recruited during the adolescent follow-up. These individuals were identified via chart reviews from nonpsychiatric departments in the same medical center where probands were seen. Subjects were accepted as controls if no behavior problems were noted prior to age 13 in their charts and if parents indicated that elementary school teachers never complained about their child's behavior. One hundred controls were recruited. All adolescent and adult follow-up assessments were made by trained clinicians who were blind to the subject's group membership (proband or control).

Like the Montreal Study, the New York Study included several positive features, for example, prospective, controlled, respectable sample size, and assessments at multiple time points by clinicians (childhood, late adolescence, and adulthood). In addition, assessments were conducted without knowledge of childhood diagnosis. The New York Study also included an independent replication sample of 111 additional ADHD children who were seen at the same clinic and recruited using the same inclusion and exclusion criteria as the first cohort (Gittelman *et al.*, 1980). This second cohort was also followed up in late adolescence (Mannuzza *et al.*, 1991) and adulthood (Mannuzza, Klein, Bessler, Malloy, & Hynes, 1997; Mannuzza, Klein, Bessler, Malloy, & LaPadula, 1998;). At 11-year follow-up (mean age = 18 years), 89% of the childhood sample were evaluated; at 17-year follow-up (mean age = 24 years), 83% were assessed. A control group of 78 subjects was also recruited during the adolescent follow-up of the replication cohort. As with the first cohort, all follow-up assessments were made by clinicians blind to group membership.

Outcome in Late Adolescence

Academic Performance

As noted, several investigators have reported academic difficulties among ADHD children in early adolescence. In their 10-year follow-up, Weiss and colleagues (Weiss, Hechtman, Perlman, Hopkins, & Wener, 1979) found that at mean age 19 ADHD probands continued to fare relatively poorly in the academic arena. Compared to controls, probands completed less formal schooling, achieved lower grades, failed more courses, and were more often expelled. Similarly, the New York Study found that at mean age 18, compared to controls, ADHD probands obtained worse scores on standardized achievement tests (Piacentini, Mannuzza, & Klein, 1987) and more often repeated a grade, failed courses, and were expelled (Klein & Mannuzza, 1989).

Cognitive Functioning

The Montreal Study reported that deficits on cognitive tasks observed in early adolescence (Cohen et al., 1972; Hoy et al., 1978) continued through late adolescence. At average age 19, ADHD probands scored significantly worse on tests of vigilance and visual motor integration, including the Matching Familiar Figures Test (MFFT), the Embedded Figures Test, and the Stroop Color Test (Hopkins, Perlman, Hechtman, & Weiss, 1979).

The New York Study failed to obtain findings consistent with pervasive cognitive deficit as obtained in the Montreal Study. At mean age 18, subjects were tested on measures presumed to reflect attentional processes (MFFT, Cancellation Task, Trail Making Test). Of the 9 scores obtained, a group difference was found on only one (Trail Making, Part B, Latency), in disfavor of probands (Piacentini et al., 1987). Unfortunately, our battery and that of the Montreal Study shared only one task (the MFFT). However, it should be noted that at a subsequent follow-up (mean age = 22 years) the Montreal Study did not obtain significant group differ-

ences on two of three tasks (MFFT and Stroop Test) (Hechtman, Weiss, & Perlman, 1984b). The pattern of results suggests that cognitive deficits may normalize over time.

Self-Esteem and Social Functioning

Low self-esteem and poor social functioning among ADHD subjects have been consistent findings in early adolescence (Ackerman et al., 1977; Hoy et al., 1978; Weiss et al., 1971). These deficits continued to be observed in late adolescence. At average age 18–19 years, compared to controls, former ADHDs had fewer friends, scored more poorly on social skills and self-esteem tests, and were rated by clinicians as having poorer psychosocial adjustment (Hechtman, Weiss, & Perlman, 1980; Slomkowski, Klein, & Mannuzza, 1995; Weiss, Hechtman, & Perlman, 1978; Weiss et al., 1979).

We note later that ADHD children are at significantly increased risk for having a mental disorder in late adolescence. Therefore, it is not surprising that they also have displayed poor self-esteem and impaired social functioning. In our late adolescent follow-up (mean age = 18 years) we found that when comparisons were limited to individuals who did not have a current diagnosis, probands and controls were strikingly similar on a host of measures. Although "not ill" probands continued to show significant difficulties in academic functioning, they did not differ from "not ill" controls in numerous other areas, for example, temperament, occupational adjustment, alcohol and non-alcohol substance use and abuse, and several antisocial activities (Mannuzza, Klein, Bonagura, Konig, & Shenker, 1988). In an effort to determine whether poor self-esteem and functional impairment (including academic, behavioral, and social adjustment) characterized former ADHD probands independent of late adolescent mental status, we compared subjects without any ongoing mental disorder. Small yet significant group differences in disfavor of probands remained on self-rated measures of self-esteem and clinician-rated measures of overall adjustment (Slomkowski et al., 1995). The findings suggest that psychiatric diagnosis at follow-up accounts for much of the probands' functional disadvantage, but that poor self-esteem may be a particular feature of the longitudinal course of ADHD.

Arrest History

Arrest history is clearly not independent of psychiatric status (reviewed later). Individuals with CD or APD are at increased risk for having an arrest history. However, since arrest history is, in a sense, an objective index of the severity of antisocial behavior and, more important, provides some indication of cost to society, it is treated separately.

Satterfield and colleagues (1982) were the first to report the arrest histories of ADHD youths in a controlled, prospective study. Official arrest records were obtained for all subjects who resided in Los Angeles County, California, during the 8-year follow-up interval. At follow-up, the 110 ADHD boys and 88 normal controls had a mean age of 17 years. Arrest rates for probands and controls were 36%–58% versus 2%–11%, depending on social class, and for multiple arrests, 25%–45% versus 0%–6%. Furthermore, 25% of probands versus 1% of controls were institutionalized for delinquent behavior. All contrasts were significant in disfavor of probands. These investigators estimate that 75% of their initial sample had CD in addition to ADHD as children (Satterfield *et al.,* 1987). However, the criteria employed in arriving at this estimate are unclear.

The Montreal Study reported very different findings. At follow-up (mean age = 19 years), ADHD probands tended to report more court referrals than controls during the 5 years, but not during the 1 year preceding the follow-up interview. Also, there was no excess among probands in the number and seriousness of reported offenses (Hechtman, Weiss, & Perlman, 1984a).

Weiss and Hechtman (1993) suggested that perhaps sociocultural differences between Los Angeles and Montreal accounted for the discrepant findings. However, it seems improbable that such differences completely account for relative, between-group differences in criminality.

Satterfield and colleagues (1982) suggested that differences were attributed to attrition (28% in the Montreal Study and 0% in their study) and methodology (interviews in the Montreal Study and official arrest records in their study).

In the New York Study, we obtained the official arrest records of all subjects who resided in New York State during the follow-up interval (Mannuzza, Klein, Konig, & Giampino, 1989). Results showed that significantly more probands than controls had been arrested (39% vs. 20%), convicted (28% vs. 11%), and incarcerated (9% vs. 1%). In addition, significantly more probands than controls had multiple arrests (26% vs. 8%), multiple convictions (20% vs. 2%), and had been charged with an aggressive offense (i.e., robbery, assault, vandalism, or weapon use, 18% vs. 7%), a felony (25% vs. 7%), and multiple felonies (12% vs. 3%). Furthermore, the presence of an antisocial disorder (i.e., CD or APD) in late adolescence almost completely accounted for the increased risk of criminality in ADHD probands. Stated differently, when subjects without an antisocial disorder were compared, ADHD proband and control groups did not differ in rates of criminality (28% vs. 16%). Therefore, antisocial disorder was a powerful mediating factor regarding arrest history. We also compared arrest histories based on judicial records with arrests reported by subjects in our late adolescent follow-up; 83% of arrested subjects reported having been arrested. Those who denied being arrested had been charged with minor offenses (e.g., trespassing, criminal mischief, petit larceny). Therefore, subject interviews provided a reasonably valid index of criminality. These results suggest that methodological differences in assessing criminality are unlikely to yield strikingly different rates.

Mental Status

Antisocial and Substance Use Disorders. Thus far, the New York Study has been the only investigation to report rates of clinical diagnoses in late adolescence (mean = 18 years). Since this study predated DSM-III-R and DSM-IV, only DSM-III diagnoses were available.

Overall, approximately half of the probands versus one fifth of controls had an ongoing mental disorder at follow-up (48% vs. 20%, $p < .001$). Three disorders significantly discriminated probands from controls: Attention Deficit Disorder (ADD) (40% vs. 3%), antisocial disorders (27% vs. 8%), and nonalcohol substance use disorder (16% vs. 3%). These three disorders aggregated significantly in the same individuals. Ongoing mood and anxiety disorders were rare in both groups of these male subjects (Gittelman et al., 1985).

The independent cohort of the New York Study provided a powerful replication of these findings (Mannuzza et al., 1991). As in the previous study, significantly more probands than controls were diagnosed as having ADD (43% vs. 4%), antisocial disorders (32% vs. 8%), and nonalcohol substance use disorder (10% vs. 1%) at mean age 18 years. Also, ongoing anxiety and mood disorders were rare.

ADHD Symptoms and Syndromes. In the Montreal Study, Weiss and colleagues (1979) reported that, at average age 19 years, significantly more probands than controls reported feeling restless and were observed to be restless during the interview. In addition, impulsivity was suggested by several findings. For example, compared to controls, ADHD probands had more car accidents, changed residences more frequently, had a higher rate of impulsive personality traits (Weiss et al., 1979), and were significantly more impulsive on cognitive tests (Hopkins et al., 1979). No data were reported on inattention, concentration difficulties, distractibility, and so on.

In the New York Study, hyperactivity-restlessness, impulsivity, and inattention were all significantly more common in probands than controls at mean age 18 years regardless of whether rates were based on parent or self-reports (Gittelman & Mannuzza, 1985). Prevalence rates for probands derived from self-reports ranged from 16% to 21%, depending on the symptom; derived from parent reports, 32%–41%; and for controls, 0%–4%. It is important to emphasize that assessment of ADHD symptoms was made by clinicians who were blind to group status. Also, symptoms were not considered present unless they resulted in clinically significant distress or impairment. For example, if a subject reported "occasional distractibility" that was "not a big deal" and never resulted in any problems, inattention was not rated. However, if a subject indicated that concentration difficulties affected his schoolwork, the symptom was considered present.

We also derived prevalence rates for syndromal clusters of the three core symptoms based on parent *and* self reports (i.e., counting symptoms as present if *either* informant endorsed them as resulting in clinically significant distress or impairment). At late adolescent follow-up (mean age = 18 years), 31% of probands versus 3% of controls had the full syndrome, that is, all three core symptoms. In addition, 40% of probands versus 3% of controls had at least two of the three symptoms (Gittelman et al., 1985). These findings are very similar to those obtained in our replication sample, that is, 43% versus 4% with at least two of three symptoms (Mannuzza et al., 1991).

These results and those of follow-up studies into early adolescence, clearly put to rest the belief that ADHD is a childhood condition that disappears by adolescence (Laufer & Denhoff, 1957). However, about half of ADHD cases showed no evidence of any mental disorder at follow-up, including the full or partial ADHD syndrome.

ADULT OUTCOME

Only two prospective, controlled studies have followed ADHD children into adulthood, the Montreal Study and the New York Study. These have focused primarily on the following variables: educational achievement, work history, symptoms of the childhood syndrome, and psychiatric status.

Educational Attainment

It is not surprising that significant deficits in educational achievement have been a consistent finding. In the Montreal and New

York Studies (both cohorts), probands completed significantly 2–3 years less formal schooling than controls, on average (Mannuzza *et al.,* 1993, 1997; Weiss, Hechtman, Milroy, & Perlman, 1985). Results across studies showed that one quarter to one third of probands (vs. 1%–9% of controls) dropped out of high school. Only 3% of probands (vs. 15%–16% of controls) were enrolled in or had completed a graduate degree at average age 24–25 years and only about 15% of probands (vs. half of the controls) had completed a bachelor's degree or higher. It is usually in the school environment that the symptoms of ADHD exact their highest toll, a phenomenon that might explain the relatively early school termination.

Occupational History

Occupational Rank

Occupational rank is an important index of compromised adaptation in chronic disorders. The Montreal and New York Studies both found that probands had significantly lower occupational rankings (Hollingshead & Redlich, 1958) than controls at average age 25 years (Mannuzza *et al.,* 1993; Weiss & Hechtman, 1993). In the independent cohort of the New York Study, this comparison was only at the level of a trend in disfavor of probands (Mannuzza *et al.,* 1997).

The most common profession among probands in the New York Studies (both cohorts) was skilled workers, for example, carpenters, electricians, plumbers, painters, machinists, and mechanics (Mannuzza *et al.,* 1993, 1997). The Montreal Study did not report specific professions.

Performance on the Job

As part of their 15-year follow-up (mean age = 25 years), Weiss and Hechtman (1993) mailed a 7-item questionnaire to the employers of study subjects. Employers rated probands significantly worse than controls on work adequacy, working independently, completing tasks, and getting along well with supervisors. There were no proband–control differences on getting along with coworkers or punctuality. However, there was a trend for employers not to want to rehire probands compared to controls.

Also in the Montreal Study, subjects were interviewed to obtain additional information on work history during the past 3 years. Based on these data, probands reported being "laid off," but not fired, significantly more often than controls (Weiss & Hechtman, 1993). As the authors indicated, the distinction between being fired and laid off might be simply a semantic difference resulting from employer preference. Also, subjects might use these terms interchangeably.

Gainful Employment

In the Montreal and New York Studies (both cohorts), rate of employment was not different for probands and controls (Mannuzza *et al.,* 1993, 1997; Weiss & Hechtman, 1993). A full 90% of probands from both New York cohorts were either gainfully employed or full-time students at adult follow-up.

The Montreal Study found no difference between probands and controls regarding annual income (Weiss & Hechtman, 1993). (The New York Study did not systematically collect these data.) This finding is intriguing in view of the significant difference in occupational rank.

Self-Esteem and Social Skills

Problems in self-esteem and social functioning continue into adulthood. The Montreal Study administered the same self-esteem and social skills tests to subjects at 10- and 15-year follow-ups. As in late adolescence, probands scored significantly worse than controls in adulthood (Weiss & Hechtman, 1993).

Unfortunately, the New York Study did not obtain data on these variables. It is not known whether these deficits were associated with mental status at adult follow-up in the Montreal Study. Because low self-esteem and poor social adjustment were independent of psychiatric status in late adolescence (Slomkowski *et al.,* 1995), it is possible that these problems do not result entirely from current mental disorders in adulthood.

Mental Status

Antisocial and Substance Use Disorders

A preponderance of probands with APD in adulthood has been a consistent finding. The Montreal Study reported that, at mean age 25 years, APD was the only DSM-III (American Psychiatric Association, 1980) diagnosis that was significantly more prevalent in probands than controls (23% vs. 2%) (Weiss et al., 1985).

The New York Study (both cohorts) found that one third of probands versus less than one fifth of controls had an ongoing DSM-III-R (American Psychiatric Association, 1987) diagnosis at adult follow-up. In both samples, APD was significantly more prevalent in probands than controls (12%–18% vs 2%–3%) (Mannuzza et al., 1993, 1998). Several factors strongly suggest that this finding could not have resulted from a preponderance of DSM-IV CD in the ADHD childhood cohorts. First, for both New York Study samples, children were excluded if the principal reason for referral involved aggressive or other antisocial acts. Second, in the replication sample (Mannuzza et al., 1998), child psychiatrists systematically recorded DSM-II (American Psychiatric Association, 1968) diagnoses on the NIMH Children's Diagnostic Classification form (National Institute of Mental Health [NIMH], 1973). Of the 104 boys in the initial sample, only one was diagnosed as DSM-II unsocialized aggressive reaction, and none as DSM-II group delinquent reaction, the diagnoses that approximate CD. Furthermore, other clinical data document the absence of antisocial symptoms in this cohort (Klein & Abikoff, 1997). Therefore, childhood CD was virtually absent in this sample.

Loney, Whaley-Klahn, Kosier, and Conboy (1983) evaluated 22 former ADHD individuals and their non-ADHD brothers between 21 and 23 years of age. They found that 45% of probands versus 18% of siblings had APD ($p < .05$).

Findings regarding drug abuse in adulthood have been less consistent. The New York Study reported that nonalcohol substance use disorder was significantly more prevalent in probands than controls (16% vs. 4%) (Mannuzza et al., 1993). This finding was replicated on the independent cohort (12% vs. 4%) (Mannuzza et al., 1998). However, neither Weiss and colleagues (1985) nor Loney and colleagues (1983) found an excess of substance abuse among probands. This is surprising since both studies report an increased risk for antisocial disorder among probands, a disorder which regularly is highly associated with substance abuse syndromes.

ADHD Symptoms and Syndromes

The Montreal Study assessed ADHD symptoms at adult follow-up in three ways. First, subjects were asked whether restlessness, distractibility, or impulsivity was mildly, moderately, or severely disabling, if at all. About 36% of probands versus only one of 41 controls reported that at least one symptom was moderately or severely disabling. Second, subjects were asked whether they "felt restless." About 64% of probands versus 29% of controls responded affirmatively. Third, two psychiatrists rated amount of movement during the interview. About 44% of probands versus 10% of controls were rated as restless. All of these contrasts were significant. The authors concluded that "about half" of former ADHD probands were still experiencing some aspects of the childhood syndrome at the mean age of 25 (Weiss et al., 1985).

In the New York Study, full DSM-III-R (American Psychiatric Association, 1987) ADHD criteria were met for 8% of probands and 1% of controls at adult follow-up. An additional 3% of probands reported that one or more ADHD symptoms resulted in clinically significant distress or impairment. Therefore, in total, 11% of probands versus 1% of controls ($p < .05$) had ongoing ADHD symptoms or syndromes at mean age 25 years (Mannuzza et al., 1993). In the replication sample of the New York cohort (Mannuzza et al., 1998), ADHD was even more rare. Only 4% of probands (vs. no controls) had the full syndrome at mean age 24 years, and no subject from either group reported clinically impair-ing symptoms in the absence of DSM-III-R ADHD.

Several factors clarify discrepant findings of the Montreal and New York Studies. It is tempting to conjecture that the loss of nearly 40% of the sample to follow-up (Weiss et al., 1985) contributed to a higher rate of ADHD symptoms because, according to these investigators, those who refused participation appeared to represent "a healthier group" (p. 217). However, even if ADHD symptoms were absent in all uninterviewed subjects, the rate of ADHD in the Montreal Study would remain high, that is, 21% (22/104).

The nature of the evaluations may have contributed to different study outcomes. Whereas our assessments were conducted blind to group status, those in the Montreal Study were not. Therefore, it is possible that unintentional procedural differences found their way into the evaluations (e.g., asking probands more questions than controls). Our ascertainment procedures also differed. We first asked subjects about symptoms in childhood. For ADHD symptoms that were at least moderately distressing or impairing in childhood, their presence in adolescence and adulthood was explored. Therefore, if symptoms were retrospectively reported as only mildly disturbing, or no problem at all, their status in adolescence and adulthood was not assessed. Weiss and colleagues (1985) asked about current (i.e., adult) functioning regardless of previous functioning. Thus, we might have missed cases in whom childhood symptoms were denied due to poor recall. Or Weiss and colleagues might have counted symptoms that were not continuously present since childhood. For example, if an individual had childhood ADHD that had remitted by age 16, but at age 25 reported poor attention secondary to current marital conflict, should this be considered a continuing symptom of the syndrome?

Results of the Montreal and New York Studies suggest that there is no "true" or universal rate of adult ADHD in individuals who were clinically diagnosed as having ADHD in childhood. Instead, persistence of the childhood syndrome is likely to be dependent on a multitude of interacting factors.

ADULT ADHD

Special mention should be made of "adult ADHD," which has attracted considerable media attention during the past 5 years (Hales & Hales, 1996; Talan, 1995; Vega, 1995; Wallis, 1994). Support groups such as Children and Adults with Attention Deficit Disorder have been formed, popular books have been published on the subject (Hallowell & Ratey, 1994; Nadeau, 1996; Solden, 1995), and one individual, who was previously diagnosed with adult ADHD, founded the Adult Attention Deficit Foundation, a clearinghouse for information on the condition. Scales have been marketed to evaluate adult ADHD (e.g., McCarney, 1996) and certain centers specialize in its systematic assessment and treatment, for example, the University of Utah Medical School, Salt Lake City, and the University of Massachusetts Medical Center, Worcester (Kane, Mikalac, Benjamin, & Barkley, 1990).

Some believe that adult ADHD is a valid syndrome (Biederman et al., 1994; Spencer, Biederman, Wilens, & Faraone, 1994), whereas others are more skeptical (Shaffer, 1994). A critical review of literature pertaining to the validity of adult ADHD is beyond the scope of this chapter. However, we discuss some of the issues that are relevant to adult outcome of children with ADHD.

What is adult ADHD? Before answering this question, we should address another: What is adulthood? The New York Study has been cited as showing that up to 40% of children with ADHD continue to demonstrate signs of the syndrome in "adulthood." This statement is somewhat misleading since it refers to results of our late adolescent follow-up studies (Gittelman et al., 1985; Mannuzza et al., 1991). The distinction between adolescence and adulthood is not trivial. First, most individuals' lives are in a state of flux in their late teens. Many leave their parental home, some begin college, others start their first "real" job, and so on. Most of these major transitions are behind them by their mid-20s. Second, as we reviewed earlier, there are differences in outcome between late adolescence and adulthood. Third, follow-up studies with *mean* ages of 18 or 19 include younger subjects as well (e.g., 16- and 17-year-olds). Does it make sense to combine outcome at age 16 with outcome at 30 (the upper range of the adult New York cohorts)? Extrapolating from the late adolescent and adult findings, some have estimated that the prevalence of adult ADHD is as high as 2% in the general population (Spencer *et al.*, 1996). This rate can be questioned on the basis of one's definition of adulthood.

Interest in adult ADHD grew out of Paul Wender's pioneering work in the 1970s on treating adults with ADD symptoms (Kane *et al.*, 1990). These adults were purported to suffer from a continuation of the childhood syndrome. Their favorable response to psychostimulants further reinforced this belief, as did their endorsement of childhood symptoms. However, some have expressed reservations as to whether these adult studies reflect ADHD children grown up (Hechtman, 1996; Shaffer, 1994). The adult treatment studies are based on retrospective diagnoses of childhood ADHD. In addition, many were based exclusively on the subject's recollections and parental reports were not obtained. Also, several disorders share symptoms with ADHD (e.g., major depression, generalized anxiety disorder, hypomania, and certain personality disorders), complicating an adult differential diagnosis of ADHD. Furthermore, contrary to findings in children, males and females appear to be equally represented in adult treatment studies (Biederman *et al.*, 1994).

There is little doubt that childhood ADHD persists into adulthood in a proportion of children with the syndrome and that adult ADHD exists. However, at this time, it is unclear what percentage of childhood cases is likely to continue to exhibit ADHD symptoms into adulthood. Ongoing, prospective, controlled studies of ADHD children (Barkley *et al.*, 1990; Biederman *et al.*, 1996), rather than retrospectively diagnosed adults presenting with ADHD symptoms are best suited to address this question. As has been noted, it would be informative to determine whether adults complaining of ADHD symptoms but *denying* childhood ADHD histories respond to stimulants (Klein & Wender, 1995). However, to date, no systematic, placebo-controlled study has addressed this issue.

DIFFERENTIAL OUTCOME OF BOYS AND GIRLS

We reported the only controlled, prospective follow-up study of a clinical sample of ADHD girls (Mannuzza & Gittelman, 1984). All 12 females from the first cohort were evaluated at mean age 17 years. These were compared to 24 ADHD males and 24 male controls matched for age and social class. In this small study, no significant differences were found between ADHD females and males on any of the follow-up measures, including academic, behavioral, and social adjustment in junior high and high school, and rates of specific and overall mental disorders. When compared to normal male controls, female probands were rated significantly lower on academic, behavioral, and social functioning. These results in adolescence did not change when the 7 girls from the second cohort were added to the initial sample (total $N = 19$) (Klein, 1990). However, at adult follow-up, female probands appeared to have a more favorable outcome than their male counterparts, at least regarding antisocial personality and substance abuse.

These findings must be viewed cautiously since the female sample was necessarily small. The relative lack of knowledge about ADHD girls is likely to change in the near future; a concerted research effort is being made to clarify sex differences (Arnold, 1996).

CHILDHOOD PREDICTORS OF OUTCOME

A consistent finding is that, despite its well-established therapeutic gains in childhood, stimulant treatment does not alter the adolescent or adult outcome of ADHD (see reviews by Hechtman, 1985; Jacobvitz, Sroufe, Stewart, & Leffert, 1990).

We previously reviewed three studies that examined the relationship between a large number of childhood and outcome variables (Mannuzza & Klein, 1992). To date, these are the only prediction studies of clinic samples of ADHD children in which outcome measures were obtained in late adolescence or adulthood and in which multiple predictor variables were examined.

Loney and colleagues (1983) evaluated ADHD boys at ages 21 to 23 years. The 14 (childhood) predictor variables spanned four domains: treatment (age at referral), individual (e.g., academic problems), ecological (e.g., urban or rural residence), and familial (e.g., parental psychopathology). The 39 (adult) outcome variables primarily focused on antisocial behaviors and substance use and abuse. Outcome measures were significantly associated with IQ (negative association), childhood aggression (positive), urban residence (positive), and parent mental disorder (positive). Regarding two major outcome variables, APD and alcoholism, it is disconcerting that the proportion of variance accounted for by the childhood predictors was less than 10%.

Hechtman, Weiss, Perlman, and Amsel (1984) examined childhood predictors of outcome in their late adolescent follow-up (mean age = 19 years). As in the study by Loney and colleagues (1983), childhood variables spanned several domains, and outcome variables primarily reflected factors relevant to APD and substance abuse (e.g., police contacts, car accidents, alcohol use, grades failed). Lower IQ, parental mental disorder, and lower SES were significantly associated with multiple adult variables. Unfortunately, certain analyses represented as little as 50% of the childhood cohort due to attrition and missing data. Also, significant differences are difficult to interpret because nearly 300 correlations were calculated.

We also examined childhood predictors of outcome in our late adolescent follow-up at mean age 18 years (Mannuzza, Klein, Konig, & Giampino, 1990). As in the Loney and col-

leagues (1983) and Hechtman, Weiss, Perlman, and Amsel (1984) studies, childhood variables represented multiple domains: clinical (e.g., parent, teacher, and clinician ratings), cognitive (aptitude and achievement tests), and familial-environmental (parental mental disorder, social class, and family stability). These measures were entered into discriminant function analyses, with late adolescent mental status distinguishing the outcome groups. Results were discouraging. Despite multiple discriminant analyses, all childhood variables, in combination, did not significantly predict membership in the late adolescent diagnostic groups. Also, we did not replicate the findings of Loney and colleagues and Hechtman and colleagues that IQ and parental mental disorder were important predictors of outcome. Finally, when data were reanalyzed controlling for biased associations, there were dramatic reductions in the percentage of subjects correctly classified. This finding stresses the importance of using appropriate statistical controls in studies of this type.

In our review of prediction studies (Mannuzza & Klein, 1992), we concluded that follow-up studies of ADHD children have yet to identify convincing predictors of late adolescent and adult outcome, and the present state of knowledge has not changed since then. Perhaps the reason that sturdy childhood predictors have been so elusive is that, as suggested by Loney and colleagues (1983) and Hechtman, Weiss, Perlman, and Amsel (1984), it is unlikely that single childhood measures will carry much weight by themselves. Instead, multiple interactive factors are likely to account for eventual fate, and these might be more difficult to tease out.

A recent examination of the data from the Montreal Study (Herrero, Hechtman, & Weiss, 1994) illustrates this point. Several longitudinal studies of ADHD children into early adolescence have suggested that antisocial, aggressive behaviors in childhood predict similar problems at follow-up (August et al., 1983; Fischer et al., 1993; Loney et al., 1981; Weiss et al., 1971). Herrero and colleagues conducted an extensive chart review of the childhood (baseline), and the 5-, 10-, and 15-year follow-up data from the Montreal Study to assess the history of antisocial disorders and factors associated with their development. They found that the absence of childhood behavior problems (e.g., fighting, lying, stealing) predicted the absence of antisocial disorders in adulthood. However, the presence of childhood behavior problems did not predict an adult antisocial outcome. Also, the data suggested that familial mental health was a protective factor in children with behavior problems at initial intake. Aggressive ADHD children with mentally ill family members tended to exhibit antisocial behaviors or an antisocial personality disorder at 15-year follow-up, whereas even more aggressive ADHD children with "well" relatives tended not to be associated with an adult antisocial outcome. This study underscores the potential complexity of interactive factors.

SUMMARY AND CONCLUSIONS

The late adolescent fate of ADHD children is plagued with difficulties. Extrapolating from groups studied so far (consisting mainly of white males), about two fifths of these children will continue to experience symptoms of the childhood syndrome to a clinically significant degree in their late teens. One quarter to one third will exhibit an antisocial disorder, and two thirds of these individuals will become known to the criminal justice system. Drug abuse is also a problem among a significant minority of these youths.

Although half will not have a diagnosable mental disorder in late adolescence, they will not escape certain other problems. The school environment will continue to present difficulties, as it has since childhood. In addition, low self-esteem and poor peer relationships will continue. However, those with no mental disorder will be indistinguishable from their non-ADHD counterparts regarding alcohol and other substance use and abuse, occupational functioning, temperament, and a host of antisocial activities and behaviors.

Childhood ADHD will continue to affect important functional domains in adulthood.

Compared to their non-ADHD counterparts, these individuals will complete less formal schooling, hold lower-ranking positions, and will more often be considered inferior by their employers. In addition, they will continue to be at an increased risk for having APD and, perhaps, a substance use disorder. They will also continue to suffer from poor self-esteem and deficits in social skills. Up to half of these individuals will not entirely outgrow all aspects of their childhood syndrome by their mid-20s.

On the other hand, the overwhelming majority of these individuals will be gainfully employed as adults. Furthermore, compared to their adolescent fate, substantially fewer will experience emotional and behavioral problems as adults. Indeed, a full two thirds of these children will show no evidence of any mental disorder in adulthood. Finally, childhood ADHD will not regularly preclude the chances of obtaining a higher-level education or profession; some will attend law school and medical school, while others will become accountants and stockbrokers.

Studies attempting to identify childhood predictors of later fate have been disconcerting. It appears that outcome is not likely to be associated with any single variable. Instead, multiple interactive factors are probably operative. Given the importance of this area, the search for sturdy, convincing predictors of later outcome will continue.

REFERENCES

Ackerman, P. T., Dykman, R. A., & Peters, J. E. (1977). Teenage status of hyperactive and non-hyperactive learning disabled boys. *American Journal of Orthopsychiatry, 47,* 577–596.

American Psychiatric Association. (1968). *Diagnostic and statistical manual of mental disorders* (2nd ed.). Washington, DC: Author.

American Psychiatric Association. (1980). *Diagnostic and statistical manual of mental disorders* (3rd ed.). Washington, DC: Author.

American Psychiatric Association. (1987). *Diagnostic and statistical manual of mental disorders* (3rd ed., rev.). Washington, DC: Author.

American Psychiatric Association. (1994). *Diagnostic and statistical manual of mental disorders* (4th ed.). Washington, DC: Author.

Arnold, L. E. (1996). Sex differences in ADHD: Conference summary. *Journal of Abnormal Child Psychology, 24,* 555–569.

Arnold, L. E., & Jensen, P. S. (1995). Attention-deficit disorders. In H. I. Kaplan & B. J. Sadock (Eds.), *Comprehensive textbook of psychiatry* (6th ed., Vol. 2, pp. 2295–2310). Baltimore: Williams & Wilkins.

August, G. J., Stewart, M. A., & Holmes, C. S. (1983). A four-year follow-up of hyperactive boys with and without conduct disorder. *British Journal of Psychiatry, 143,* 192–198.

Barkley, R. A. (1996). Attention-deficit/hyperactivity disorder. In E. J. Mash & R. A. Barkley (Eds.), *Child psychopathology* (pp. 63–112). New York: Guilford.

Barkley, R. A., Fischer, M., Edelbrock, C. S., & Smallish, L. (1990). The adolescent outcome of hyperactive children diagnosed by research criteria. *Journal of the American Academy of Child and Adolescent Psychiatry, 29,* 546–557.

Biederman, J., Newcorn, J., & Sprich, S. (1991). Comorbidity of attention deficit hyperactivity disorder with conduct, depressive, anxiety, and other disorders. *American Journal of Psychiatry, 148,* 564–577.

Biederman, J., Faraone, S. V., Spencer, T., Wilens, T., Mick, E., & Lapey, K. A. (1994). Gender differences in a sample of adults with attention deficit hyperactivity disorder. *Psychiatry Research, 53,* 13–29.

Biederman, J., Faraone, S., Milberger, S., Guite, J., Mick, E., Chen, L., Mennin, D., Marrs, A., Ouellette, C., Moore, P., Spencer, T., Norman, D., Wilens, T., Kraus, I., & Perrin, J. (1996). A prospective 4-year follow-up study of attention-deficit hyperactivity and related disorders. *Archives of General Psychiatry, 53,* 437–446.

Brown, R. T., & Borden, K. A. (1986). Hyperactivity at adolescence: Some misconceptions and new directions. *Journal of Clinical Child Psychology, 15,* 194–209.

Cohen, N. J., Weiss, G., & Minde, K. (1972). Cognitive styles in adolescents previously diagnosed as hyperactive. *Journal of Child Psychology and Psychiatry, 13,* 203–209.

Fischer, M., Barkley, R. A., Edelbrock, C. S., & Smallish, L. (1990). The adolescent outcome of hyperactive children diagnosed by research criteria. *Journal of Consulting and Clinical Psychology, 58,* 580–588.

Fischer, M., Barkley, R. A., Fletcher, K. E., & Smallish, L. (1993). The adolescent outcome of hyperactive children. *Journal of the American Academy of Child and Adolescent Psychiatry, 32,* 324–332.

Gittelman, R., & Mannuzza, S. (1985). Diagnosing ADD-H in adolescents. *Psychopharmacology Bulletin, 21,* 237–242.

Gittelman, R., Abikoff, H., Pollack, E., Klein, D. F., Katz, S., & Mattes, J. (1980). A controlled trial of behavior modification and methylphenidate in hyperactive children. In C. Whalen & B. Henker (Eds.), *Hyperactive children: The social ecology of identification and treatment* (pp. 221–243). Orlando, FL: Academic Press.

Gittelman, R., Mannuzza, S., Shenker, R., & Bonagura, N. (1985). Hyperactive boys almost grown up: I. Psychiatric status. *Archives of General Psychiatry, 42,* 937–947.

Gittelman-Klein, R., Klein, D. F., Katz, S., Saraf, K., & Pollack, E. (1976). Comparative effects of methylphenidate and thioridazine in hyperkinetic children. *Archives of General Psychiatry, 33,* 1217–1231.

Hales, D., & Hales, R. E. (1996, January 7). Finally, I know what's wrong. *Newsday, Parade Magazine,* pp. 8, 11.

Hallowell, E., & Ratey, J. J. (1994). *Driven to distraction: Recognizing and coping with attention deficit disorder from childhood through adulthood.* New York: Simon and Schuster.

Hechtman, L. (1985). Adolescent outcome of hyperactive children treated with stimulants in childhood: A review. *Psychopharmacology Bulletin, 21,* 178–191.

Hechtman, L. (1996). Attention-deficit hyperactivity disorder. In L. Hechtman (Ed.), *Do they grow out of it? Long-term outcomes of childhood disorders* (pp. 17–38). Washington, DC: American Psychiatric Press.

Hechtman, L., Weiss, G., & Perlman, T. (1980). Hyperactives as young adults: Self-esteem and social skills. *Canadian Journal of Psychiatry, 25,* 478–483.

Hechtman, L., Weiss, G., & Perlman, T. (1984a). Hyperactives as young adults: Past and current substance abuse and antisocial behavior. *American Journal of Orthopsychiatry, 54,* 415–425.

Hechtman, L., Weiss, G., & Perlman, T. (1984b). Young adult outcome of hyperactive children who received long-term stimulant treatment. *Journal of the American Academy of Child Psychiatry, 23,* 261–269.

Hechtman, L., Weiss, G., Perlman, T., & Amsel, R. (1984). Hyperactives as young adults: Initial predictors of adult outcome. *Journal of the American Academy of Child Psychiatry, 23,* 250–260.

Herrero, M. E., Hechtman, L., & Weiss, G. (1994). Antisocial disorders in hyperactive subjects from childhood to adulthood: Predictive factors and characteristics of subgroups. *American Journal of Orthopsychiatry, 64,* 510–521.

Hollingshead, A. B., & Redlich, F. C. (1958). *Social class and mental illness: A community study.* New York: Wiley.

Hopkins, J., Perlman, T., Hechtman, L., & Weiss, G. (1979). Cognitive style in adults originally diagnosed as hyperactives. *Journal of Child Psychology and Psychiatry, 20,* 209–216.

Hoy, E., Weiss, G., Minde, K., & Cohen, N. (1978). The hyperactive child at adolescence. *Journal of Abnormal Child Psychology, 6,* 311–324.

Jacobvitz, D., Sroufe, L. A., Stewart, M., & Leffert, N. (1990). Treatment of attentional and hyperactivity problems in children with sympathomimetic drugs. *Journal of the American Academy of Child and Adolescent Psychiatry, 29,* 677–688.

Kane, R., Mikalac, C., Benjamin, S., & Barkley, R. A. (1990). Assessment and treatment of adults with ADHD. In R. A. Barkley (Ed.), *Attention-deficit hyperactivity disorder* (pp. 613–654). New York: Guilford.

Klein, R. G. (1990). *Relationship between childhood hyperactivity and adult affective, antisocial and substance use disor-*

ders. Paper presented at the third annual research conference of the New York State Office of Mental Health, Albany, NY.

Klein, R. G., & Abikoff, H. (1997). *Behavior therapy and methylphenidate in the treatment of children with ADHD.* Manuscript submitted for publication.

Klein, R. G., & Mannuzza, S. (1989). The long-term outcome of the attention-deficit disorder/hyperkinetic syndrome. In T. Sagvolden & T. Archer (Eds.), *Attention deficit disorder: Clinical and basic research* (pp. 71–91). Hillsdale, NJ: Erlbaum.

Klein, R. G., & Mannuzza, S. (1991). Long-term outcome of hyperactive children: A review. *Journal of the American Academy of Child and Adolescent Psychiatry, 30,* 383–387.

Klein, R. G., & Wender, P. (1995). The role of methylphenidate in psychiatry. *Archives of General Psychiatry, 52,* 429–433.

Laufer, M. W., & Denhoff, E. D. (1957). Hyperkinetic behavior syndrome in children. *Journal of Pediatrics, 50,* 467–473.

Loney, J., Kramer, J., & Milich, R. (1981). The hyperkinetic child grows up. In K. Gadow & J. Loney (Eds.), *Psychosocial aspects of drug treatment for hyperactivity* (pp. 381–415). Boulder, CO: Westview.

Loney, J., Whaley-Klahn, M. A., Kosier, T., & Conboy, J. (1983). Hyperactive boys and their brothers at 21. In K. T. Van Dusen & S. A. Mednick (Eds.), *Prospective studies of crime and delinquency* (pp. 181–206). Boston: Kluwer-Nijhoff.

Mannuzza, S., & Gittelman, R. (1984). The adolescent outcome of hyperactive girls. *Psychiatry Research, 13,* 19–29.

Mannuzza, S., & Klein, R. G. (1992). Predictors of outcome of children with attention deficit hyperactivity disorder. *Child and Adolescent Psychiatric Clinics of North America, 1,* 567–578.

Mannuzza, S., Klein, R. G., Bonagura, N., Konig, P. H., & Shenker, R. (1988). Hyperactive boys almost grown up: II. Status of subjects without a mental disorder. *Archives of General Psychiatry, 45,* 13–18.

Mannuzza, S., Klein, R. G., Konig, P. H., & Giampino, T. L. (1989). Hyperactive boys almost grown up: IV. Criminality and its relationship to psychiatric status. *Archives of General Psychiatry, 46,* 1073–1079.

Mannuzza, S., Klein, R. G., Konig, P. H., & Giampino, T. L. (1990). Childhood predictors of psychiatric status in the young adulthood of hyperactive boys. In L. N. Robins & M. Rutter (Eds.), *Straight and devious pathways from childhood to adulthood* (pp. 279–299). New York: Cambridge University Press.

Mannuzza, S., Klein, R. G., Bonagura, N., Malloy, P., Giampino, T. L., & Addalli, K. A. (1991). Hyperactive boys almost grown up: V. Replication of psychiatric status. *Archives of General Psychiatry, 48,* 77–83.

Mannuzza, S., Klein, R. G., Bessler, A., Malloy, P., & La-Padula, M. (1993). Adult outcome of hyperactive boys: Educational achievement, occupational rank, and psychiatric status. *Archives of General Psychiatry, 50,* 565–576.

Mannuzza, S., Klein, R. G., Bessler, A., Malloy, P., & Hynes, M. E. (1997). Educational and occupational outcome of hyperactive boys grown up. *Journal of the American Academy of Child and Adolescent Psychiatry, 36,* 1222–1227.

Mannuzza, S., Klein, R. G., Bessler, A., Malloy, P., & La-Padula, M. (1998). Adult psychiatric status of hyperactive boys grown up. *American Journal of Psychiatry, 155,* 493–498.

McCarney, S. B. (1996). *Adult attention deficit disorders evaluation scale.* Columbia, MO: Hawthorne Educational Services.

McGee, R., & Feehan, M. (1991). Are girls with problems of attention underrecognized? *Journal of Psychopathology and Behavioral Assessment, 13,* 187–198.

Minde, K., Weiss, G., & Mendelson, N. (1972). A 5-year follow-up study of 91 hyperactive school children. *Journal of the American Academy of Child Psychiatry, 11,* 595–619.

Nadeau, K. G. (1996). *Adventures in fast forward: Life, love, work for the ADHD adult.* New York: Brunner/Mazel.

National Institute of Mental Health Psychopharmacology Research Branch. (1973). *ECDEU assessment battery.* Rockville, MD: U.S. Department of Health, Education and Welfare.

Piacentini, J., Mannuzza, S., & Klein, R. (1987). *Cognitive functioning of young adult males previously diagnosed as hyperactive.* Paper presented at the annual meeting of the American Psychological Association, New York.

Robins, L. N. (1974). *Deviant children grown up.* Huntington, NY: Krieger.

Satterfield, J. H., Hoppe, C. M., & Schell, A. M. (1982). A prospective study of delinquency in 110 adolescent boys with attention-deficit disorder and 88 normal adolescent boys. *American Journal of Psychiatry, 139,* 795–798.

Satterfield, J. H., Satterfield, B. T., & Schell, A. M. (1987). Therapeutic interventions to prevent delinquency in hyperactive boys. *Journal of the American Academy of Child and Adolescent Psychiatry, 26,* 56–64.

Shaffer, D. (1994). Attention deficit hyperactivity disorder in adults. *American Journal of Psychiatry, 151,* 633–638.

Slomkowski, C., Klein, R. G., & Mannuzza, S. (1995). Is self-esteem an important outcome in hyperactive children? *Journal of Abnormal Child Psychology, 23,* 303–315.

Solden, S. (1995). *Women with attention deficit disorder.* New York: Underwood.

Spencer, T., Biederman, J., Wilens, T., & Faraone, S. V. (1994). Is attention-deficit hyperactivity disorder in adults a valid disorder? *Harvard Review of Psychiatry, 1,* 326–335.

Spencer, T., Biederman, J., Wilens, T., Harding, M., O'Donnell, D., & Griffin, S. (1996). Pharmacotherapy of attention-deficit hyperactivity disorder across the life cycle. *Journal of the American Academy of Child and Adolescent Psychiatry, 35,* 409–432.

Szatmari, P. (1992). The epidemiology of attention-deficit hyperactivity disorders. *Child and Adolescent Psychiatric Clinics of North America, 1*, 361–371.

Talan, J. (1995, June 21). Attention disorder not "just for kids." *Newsday*, p. A17.

Thorley, G. (1984). Review of follow-up and follow-back studies of childhood hyperactivity. *Psychological Bulletin, 96*, 116–132.

Vega, W. (1995, February 24–26). Pay attention to this article. *Rockland Journal News. USA Weekend*, p.12.

Wallis, C. (1994, July 18). An epidemic of attention deficit disorder. *Time*, pp. 43–50.

Weiss, G. (1996). Research issues in longitudinal studies. In L. Hechtman (Ed.), *Do they grow out of it? Long-term outcomes of childhood disorders* (pp. 1–16). Washington, DC: American Psychiatric Press.

Weiss, G., & Hechtman, L. T. (1993). *Hyperactive children grown up* (2nd ed.). New York: Guilford.

Weiss, G., Minde, K., Werry, J. S., Douglas, V., & Nemeth, E. (1971). Studies on the hyperactive child: VIII. Five-year follow-up. *Archives of General Psychiatry, 24*, 409–414.

Weiss, G., Hechtman, L., & Perlman, T. (1978). Hyperactives as young adults: School, employer, and self-rating scales obtained during ten-year follow-up evaluation. *American Journal of Orthopsychiatry, 48*, 438–445.

Weiss, G., Hechtman, L., Perlman, T., Hopkins, J., & Wener, A. (1979). Hyperactives as young adults: A controlled prospective ten-year follow-up of 75 children. *Archives of General Psychiatry, 36*, 675–681.

Weiss, G., Hechtman, L., Milroy, T., & Perlman, T. (1985). Psychiatric status of hyperactives as adults. *Journal of the American Academy of Child and Adolescent Psychiatry, 24*, 211–220.

13

Theories of Attention-Deficit/Hyperactivity Disorder

RUSSELL A. BARKLEY

INTRODUCTION

Attempts to explain the nature of the central problems involved in Attention-Deficit/Hyperactivity Disorder (ADHD) date back to the turn of the 19th century (Still, 1902). Such attempts go beyond mere descriptions of the deficits and excesses of behavior and cognition demonstrated by those diagnosed as ADHD and constitute efforts to explain or understand why those deficits and excesses exist as they do. The descriptions these conceptualizations attempt to explain are often reported as being the "symptoms" of the disorder, implying that some larger, underlying difficulty, construct, or set of constructs exist that comprise the "core" of ADHD and that account for the appearance of these overt symptoms. Over this past century, a number of notable attempts have been made at such explanations or conceptualizations of ADHD. They do not, however, rise to the level of a formal theory as scientific theories are defined but remain at the level of hypothetical conceptualizations or viewpoints. Much more is required of them before they could be granted the status of a psychological theory of ADHD, as I demonstrate here.

The purpose of this chapter is to discuss the most prominent conceptualizations that may have risen to the level of a theory of ADHD. Such developments in theory construction are an encouraging sign in the science of ADHD for they indicate a maturational progress from one of description and simple hypotheses to one of true theoretical construction (Taylor, 1996). This milestone is the culmination of almost 90 years of mostly descriptive research found in thousands of scientific papers, book chapters, and professional textbooks.

The Limitations of This Chapter

It is not my intent to review the history of ADHD, though some early historical viewpoints are mentioned along the way. More detailed reviews of the history of ADHD and its precursors (e.g., hyperactivity, minimal brain dysfunction) can be found elsewhere (Barkley, 1998; Kessler, 1980; Ross & Ross, 1976; Schachar, 1986; Walters & Barrett, 1993; Werry, 1992). Nor do I review every attempt that has been made to explain the nature of ADHD, particularly as these may have been offered in the popular media. Instead, for many reasons including those of space limitations, I have selected for discussion what I consider to be the most serious scientific attempts at accounting for the psychological nature of the disorder.

RUSSELL A. BARKLEY • Department of Psychiatry, University of Massachusetts Medical Center, Worcester, Massachusetts 01655.

Handbook of Disruptive Behavior Disorders, edited by Quay and Hogan. Kluwer Academic/Plenum Publishers, New York, 1999.

I do not discuss the possible biological etiologies of ADHD for several reasons. First, they are discussed in more detail in Chapters 8 and 9 (this volume). And second, they do not constitute theories at the psychological level of analysis. Instead, they are efforts at reduction to a more basic level of causal explanation, and they currently constitute *hypotheses* about potential biological causes of ADHD, derived from empirical observations of biological structure and function. Nevertheless, there needs to be some biological underpinnings to any theory of ADHD in view of both the repeated associations of neurological and genetic factors with this disorder and the substantial percentage of ADHD children who respond well to stimulant medications. A few efforts to explain the causes of ADHD, however, have moved in the other direction by attempting to explain the nature of the disorder at the next level, that being a sociological or social psychological one (e.g., parent–child interactions, see Chapter 6, this volume). These, however, are not actually psychological theories of ADHD but again are hypotheses about the biological or social psychological origins that give rise to the psychological difficulties or symptoms manifest by those with the disorder. Therefore, I restrict my review to conceptualizations of the disorder and theory-building at the individual psychological level of analysis. To appreciate the distinctions made here between description, conceptualization, and theory, it will help to define the nature of a theory so that we can see whether previous and current conceptualizations of the disorder rise to that august status in science.

Defining a Scientific Theory

The term "theory" is often invoked incorrectly in the literature on ADHD. In many instances, the authors usually mean that they have a particular hypothesis, explanation, or construct by which to conceptualize ADHD. These are typically a single order of inference removed, or one level up, from the actual empirical observations on which they might be based. For example, the current clinical consensus view that ADHD is primarily a deficit in attention (American Psychiatric Association, 1987, 1994) or a combination of deficits in attention and hyperactive-impulsive behavior is not a scientific theory. It is primarily a statement of the constructs that seem to be involved in the disorder along with lists describing the behaviors (symptoms) thought to comprise these constructs. Such an approach at best qualifies as a statement of the principal psychological constructs involved in the disorder, but it is not a theory. It may rise to the level of a hypothesis when it is used to predict that problems of inattention will be found to occur in groups of children diagnosed as ADHD on specific measures. But this is unimpressive as we know that both the construct of inattention as it is used in ADHD and this prediction are founded on past instances of observing children display these behaviors. The reasoning here is circular and not worthy of the status of a theory, much less a hypothesis.

Likewise, to claim that ADHD represents a deficit in response inhibition (Schachar, Tannock, & Logan, 1993) or self-regulation (Douglas, 1988) is not to specify a theory of ADHD but to specify the construct believed to be at the heart of the disorder. Such statements may qualify as psychological explanations. In some cases, they may even be hypotheses provided that their constructs are operationally defined to a sufficient degree to put them to empirical test and that the hypothesis or prediction is not of the circular form noted previously. Even these hypotheses remain at a rather primitive level of explanation because they are simply one order of inference removed from the empirical data that instantiates them. Theories involve levels or orders of inference beyond this first level. Consequently these statements about inhibition or self-regulation being central to ADHD are not scientific theories, and may not even be hypotheses unless they can be extended beyond the class of observations upon which they were initially based (Turner, 1967).

A scientific theory appears to have at least three distinctive features, according to Turner (1967). A theory (1) "embodies propositions, principles, and syntactical structure such that its corpus is sufficient for deriving experimental hypotheses in the form of empirical laws" (p. 226). The experiment that is suggested by the theory becomes a means of instantiating that law. Such laws are empirical generalizations made from observations or classes of observations (Carnap, 1966). They come to form our expectations about events, being statements of what we should find to be correct about those events when the expectation is put to the test in an experiment (Turner, 1967). In a sense, such laws are statements of the regularities observed in events in nature. A theory (2) also "involves presumptive hypotheses (i.e., theoretical constructs), which are not completely interpretable in terms of the observation language" (p. 226). The hypotheses may not be completely empirically verifiable, remaining to some degree in the realm of inference. For instance, I may create a construct termed "antisocial" or "delinquent" that is based on the intercorrelation of parent ratings of aggression, teacher ratings of aggression, self-reported aggression, police record of delinquent acts, and even number of traffic citations while driving. No single measure constitutes the delinquent construct in the model as it is a latent construct embedded in the shared variance of these diverse measures. Such constructs are the means by which theoretical inferences are often proposed. And (3) "a theory pulls together some set of laws" (p. 226). It performs a synthetic function such that its set of assumptions permits the inference of these laws. Theories, in short, seek to provide explanations for the regularities observed in nature, often stated as empirical laws or empirical generalizations, by construing these as manifestations of entities, constructs, or processes that lie behind or beneath these observed regularities. Those theoretical entities, constructs, or processes are themselves governed by certain theoretical principles or theoretical laws (Hempel, 1966). Such theoretical laws differ from empirical ones in that they are not directly derived from observations. The entities, constructs, processes, and their governing principles must be specified with as much clarity and precision as possible, otherwise the theory is unable to serve its scientific purpose (Hempel, 1966). In short, a good theory places its bets. It specifies a set of conditional relations among its elements with sufficient precision to make them testable.

It is safe to say that few conceptualizations regarding the nature of ADHD and its central constructs over the past century could be granted the honorific title of a theory by this definition. Nevertheless, some have aspired to do so and they shall be examined here. A few of these theories are in many respects compatible, rather than competing or conflicting. Of these, one has been developed by the author over the past 5 years. It is the most recent, comprehensive. and far-reaching of the theories to be reviewed here; consequently, it receives more attention in the following sections than some of the other, less comprehensive ones.

My goal is not to review all of the evidence that may be available in the literature on ADHD as it may weigh in for or against each theory. That task is a far more comprehensive one than space limitations will permit. Even so, along the way some empirical findings are mentioned if they provide important supportive or contradictory evidence to some of the predictions made by a theory. My intent, instead, is to evaluate each of these conceptualizations relative to acceptable scientific standards for what comprises a theory. Also, for space reasons, I do not review the efforts of Sergeant and van der Meere to use information-processing theory as a means of delineating the stage of processing at which the deficit in ADHD may arise, or the energetic factors that may also be involved, as these are reviewed in Chapter 4 (this volume).

PSYCHOLOGICAL THEORIES OF ADHD

There have been numerous attempts over the past century to try to conceptualize the psychological nature of ADHD. The first of these occurred in the scientific papers by George Still (1902) who is credited with also being the first to describe clinic-referred children having this disorder.

Still's Theory of Defective Moral Control

Still's (1902) papers are an impressive effort of logical reasoning for its time or any other. The three speeches that comprise his papers were based on only the observations of this astute clinician. No statistics were employed, just thoughtful analysis, careful reasoning, and numerous instantiations of his points with his clinical cases. He reported on a group of 43 children in his clinical practice whom he defined as having a deficit in "volitional inhibition" (p. 1008) or a "defect in moral control" (p. 1009) over their own behavior. Twenty-three of these children suffered from mental retardation and 20 were not so intellectually impaired. Thus, while Still recognized that the disorder could arise as a result of intellectual delays or mental illness, he focused much of his three lectures on the notion that defective volitional inhibition and moral regulation could arise independently of intellectual delay.

To Still (1902), the moral control of behavior meant "the control of action in conformity with the idea of the good of all" (p. 1008). Today, this might be interpreted to mean the regulation of behavior by rules or principles of conduct (see Berkowitz, 1982; Hayes, Gifford, & Ruckstuhl, 1996; Peterson, 1982). In Still's opinion, moral control arises out of a cognitive or conscious comparison of the individual's volitional activity with that of the good of all, a comparison that he termed moral consciousness. Such a comparison inherently involves the capacity to hold forms of information about oneself and one's actions in mind along with that of the context so as to make such a comparison. Still did not specifically identify these inherent aspects of the comparative process but it is clearly implied in the manner in which he uses the term "conscious" in describing this process. He stipulated that this process of comparison of proposed action to a rule concerning the greater good involved the critical element of the conscious or cognitive relation of the individual to their environment, or self-awareness. Intellect played a part in moral consciousness but the notion of volition was just as or more important. The latter is where Still believed the impairment arose in many of those with defective moral control who suffered no intellectual delay. Volition was viewed as being primarily inhibitory in nature, in that a stimulus to act must be overpowered by the stimulus of the idea of the greater good of all.

Both volitional inhibition and the moral regulation of behavior founded upon it were believed to develop gradually in children, such that younger children would find it more difficult to resist acting on impulse than would older children. Thus, judging a child defective in volitional inhibition and moral control of behavior meant making a comparison to same-age normal children and taking into account the degree of appeal of the stimulus. Even at the same age, inhibition and moral control varied across children, owing in part to environmental factors, but also, Still proposed, to differences in these innate capacities.

Still (1902) noted that this condition persisted into adulthood in some cases but he believed it to be ideally studied during childhood. Aggressive, passionate, lawless, vindictive, spiteful or cruel, destructive, inattentive, impulsive, and overactive were descriptions he applied to these children, many of whom today would be diagnosed not only as ADHD but also as having Oppositional Defiant Disorder (ODD) and some even Conduct Disorder (CD). The immediate gratification of the self was proposed as being the "keynote" quality of these attributes. And among all of them, it was passion (or heightened emotionality) that was the most commonly observed attribute and the most noteworthy. Still noted further that an insensitivity to punishment characterized many of these cases for they would be punished, evenly physically so, yet engage in the same infraction within a matter of hours. And he was particularly impressed by the serious problems with sustained attention that these cases often manifested, agreeing with William James (1890/1992) that such attention may be another important element in the moral control of behavior. Still concluded that a defect in moral control, therefore, could arise as a function of three distinct impairments: "(1) defect of cognitive relation to the environment; (2) defect of moral consciousness; and (3) defect in inhibitory volition" (p. 1011). He placed these in a hierarchical relation to each other in that order, arguing that impairments in lower levels would affect those levels above it and ultimately the moral control of behavior.

This description can be considered a theory of sorts. It goes well beyond a single order of inference up from the observations that gave rise to these concepts or constructs of volitional inhibition and moral control. It stipulates the processes (cognitive comparisons) that are involved in these constructs and even some moderating variables (intelligence, environment, innate capacities) that may be involved in the moral regulation of behavior. And these constructs and processes were proposed and defined with some clarity or precision. Indeed, many of the elements that comprise the current list of symptoms for ADHD (and ODD) were noted by Still (1902), these being poor sustained attention, impulsiveness, and hyperactivity (see Chapter 1, this volume). A hierarchical and even conditional set of relations among the constructs also was set forth making them testable. And he carefully and logically distinguished this impairment in moral control from that which might occur simply as a function of general cognitive delay; his lectures, in fact, are a most thoughtful demonstration of differential diagnosis. Finally, Still discussed those constructs and processes that are involved in the normal development of the moral control of behavior before describing how these may be impaired in the group of children that were the focus of his work.

It would be almost 70 years before another serious attempt was made at constructing a theory of ADHD. By the time scientific attention returned on a more consistent basis to the problems of these children following two world wars, Still's (1902) syndrome of defective moral control had become the brain-injured child syndrome (Strauss & Lehtinen, 1947), then minimal brain damage, and eventually minimal brain dysfunction (see Rie & Rie, 1980). When this term proved overly inclusive to the point of losing any clinical specificity or utility it may have had (Rie & Rie, 1980), the

term hyperactive child syndrome had come to replace it (Chess, 1960). And even that syndrome would soon evolve into the clinical syndrome known as hyperkinetic reaction of childhood (American Psychiatric Association, 1968). For the most part, all of these psychological conceptualizations remained at the level of description of symptoms believed to comprise the syndrome. One notable exception was the early work of Paul Wender.

Wender's Conceptualization of Minimal Brain Dysfunction

Wender (1971) described the essential psychological characteristics of children with minimal brain dysfunction (MBD) as comprising six clusters of symptoms: (1) motor behavior, (2) attentional-perceptual cognitive function, (3) learning difficulties, (4) impulse control, (5) interpersonal relations, and (6) emotion. Many of the characteristics first reported by Still (1902) would be echoed by Wender in his six domains of functioning, described in the following paragraphs.

1. Within the realm of motor behavior, the essential features were hyperactivity and poor motor coordination. Excessive speech, colic, and sleeping difficulties were related to the hyperactivity. Foreshadowing the later DSM-III designation of a group of children with attentional problems who would not be hyperactive (ADD without Hyperactivity; American Psychiatric Association, 1980), Wender suggested that some of these children were hypoactive and listless while still demonstrating an attentional disturbance. He argued that they should be included because of their manifestation of many of the other difficulties thought to characterize the syndrome.

2. Short attention span and poor concentration were described as the most striking deficit in the attentional and perceptual-cognitive domain. Distractibility, daydreaming, and poor organization of ideas and precepts were also included with these attentional disturbances.

3. Learning difficulties were the third domain of dysfunction, with most of these children observed to be doing poorly in their

academic performance. A large percentage were described as having specific difficulties with learning to read, with handwriting, and with reading comprehension and arithmetic. We now recognize that specific learning disabilities are separate disorders from that of ADHD but may be comorbid with it in a large minority of cases (Barkley, 1998).

4. Impulse-control problems, or a decreased ability to inhibit behavior, were identified as a fourth characteristic of most MBD children. Within this general category, Wender (1971) included low frustration tolerance, an inability to delay gratification, antisocial behavior, and lack of planning, forethought, or judgment, as well as poor sphincter control leading to enuresis and encopresis. Disorderliness, or lack of organization, and recklessness, particularly with regard to bodily safety were also listed in this domain of dysfunction.

5. In the area of interpersonal relations, Wender (1971) singled out the unresponsiveness of these children to social demands as the most serious. Extroversion, excessive independence, obstinence, stubbornness, negativism, disobedience, noncompliance, sassiness, and imperviousness were some of the characteristics that instantiated the problem with interpersonal relations.

6. Last, in the domain of emotional difficulties, Wender (1971) included increased lability of mood, altered reactivity, increased anger, aggressiveness, temper outbursts, and dysphoria. The dysphoria of these children involved the more specific difficulties of anhedonia, depression, low self-esteem, and anxiety. A diminished sensitivity to pain and punishment were also felt to typify this area of dysfunction in children with MBD. All of these symptoms bear a striking resemblance to the case descriptions Still (1902) had provided earlier.

Wender (1971) theorized that these six domains of dysfunction could be best accounted for by three primary deficits: (1) a decreased experience of pleasure and pain, (2) a generally high and poorly modulated level of activation, and (3) extroversion. A consequence of (1) is that MBD children would prove less sensitive to both rewards and punishments,

making them less susceptible to social influence. The generally high and poorly modulated level of activation were thought to be aspects of poor inhibition. Hyperactivity, of course, was the consummate demonstration of this high level of activation. The problems with poor sustained attention and distractibility were conjectured to be secondary aspects of high activation. Emotional overreactivity, low frustration tolerance, quickness to anger, and temper outbursts resulted from the poor modulation of activation. These three primary deficits, then, created a cascading of effects into the larger social ecology of the child, resulting in numerous interpersonal problems and academic performance difficulties.

This, then, constitutes an attempt at theory construction for the syndrome of MBD. Wender (1971) considered that these three primary deficits accounted for the myriad of other problems MBD children might demonstrate as part of this syndrome. He specified some conditional relations that ought to be evident in his model (primary vs. secondary deficits) and even went so far as to speculate at the biological level of analysis what deficiencies might give rise to these three primary deficits (brain damage or genetic predisposition that affect monoamine metabolism). However, Wender did not stipulate precisely how the secondary symptoms arise from the primary ones.

Like Still (1902), Wender (1971) gave a prominent role to the construct of poor inhibition. It is believed to explain both the activation difficulties and the attentional problems that stem from them, as well as the excessive emotionality, low frustration tolerance, and hot temperedness of these children. It is therefore unclear why deficient inhibition was not made a primary symptom in this theory in place of high activation and poor modulation of activation.

Unlike Still's (1902) attempt at a theory, however, Wender (1971) did not say much about normal developmental processes with respect to the three primary areas of deficit and so did not clarify more precisely what may be going awry in them to give rise to these characteristics of MBD. The exception is his discussion of a diminished sensitivity in those with ADHD to the reasonably well-understood processes of reinforcement and punishment. A higher than normal threshold for pleasure and pain, as already noted, was thought to create these insensitivities to behavioral consequences.

Wender's (1971) theory is also unclear about a number of issues. For instance, how do the three primary deficits account for the difficulties with motor coordination that occurred alongside hyperactivity in his category of motor control problems? It is doubtful that a high level of activation that is said to cause the hyperactivity also causes these motor deficits. Nor is it clear just how the academic achievement deficits in reading, math, and handwriting can arise from the three primary deficits in the model. It is also unclear why the construct of extroversion needs to be proposed at all if what is meant by its use is reduced social inhibition. This might just as parsimoniously be explained by the deficit in behavioral inhibition already posited in the model. And the meaning of the term *activation* in the model is not clearly specified. Does it refer to excessive behavior, in which case hyperactivity would have sufficed? Or does it refer to level of central nervous system arousal, which ample subsequent evidence has not found to be the case (Hastings & Barkley, 1978; Rosenthal & Allen, 1978)? To his credit, Wender recognized the abstract nature of the term activation as he employed it in this theory but retained it as he felt it could be used to incorporate both the hyperactive and hypoactive child. It is never made clear just how this could be the case, however.

It is also evident that Wender was combining the symptoms of ODD (and even CD) in with those of ADHD to form a single disorder. Still (1902) did very much the same thing. This is understandable given that clinic-referred cases served as the starting point for both theories and many clinic-referred cases are comorbid for both disorders (ADHD/ODD/CD). Sufficient evidence now exists, however, to show that these are not the same disorder (August & Stewart, 1983; Hinshaw, 1987; Stewart, deBlois, & Cummings, 1980; see also Chapter 1, this volume).

Douglas's Model of Cognitive Deficits

In 1972, in her presidential address to the Canadian Psychological Association, Virginia Douglas (1972) reviewed a multitude of findings from her own research and that of her students on the nature of the cognitive deficits in hyperactive children (see also Chapter 5, this volume). Unlike previous theoretical papers, in which the authors either summarized their clinical cases or the research of others, Douglas had actually conducted experimental studies of hyperactive children using psychological tests of a variety of cognitive abilities. During the previous two decades of research, the field had shifted toward an emphasis on hyperactivity as the central feature of the disorder, although authors of these earlier studies often commented on the inattentive and impulsive symptoms of their subjects. Douglas demonstrated in her studies that there were more cognitive deficits associated with the disorder than the symptom of hyperactivity was able to explain. Problems of poor sustained attention, distractibility, and poor impulse control appeared to be equally important deficits in these children, leading Douglas to describe their problem as one of an inability to "stop, look, and listen." Like Still (1902) and Wender (1971), Douglas observed difficulties with motor coordination in addition to the difficulties with hyperactivity, inattention, and impulsiveness. She also found evidence, in agreement with Still again, that moral development appeared to be delayed in these children. She further instantiated this claim by reporting the results of another research team that found actual observations of cheating behavior in the classroom to correlate with measures of inattention and impulsiveness. Although Douglas's paper reiterated a number of the deficits that earlier theorists associated with ADHD, it is of historical importance because of the substantial empirical research she marshaled in support of these conclusions. Her work and that of her students subsequently served as a major impetus to the renaming of the disorder in DSM-III as Attention Deficit Disorder (ADD; American Psychiatric Association, 1980), in which problems with attention were now accorded more emphasis than the difficulties with hyperactive and impulsive behavior. Indeed, children could now be diagnosed as having this disorder even in the absence of the latter symptoms, much as Wender had argued should be the case.

Douglas's (1972) review paper had not proposed a model, much less a theory, of ADHD as yet. But as her research and that of her colleagues progressed, along with that of other investigators, Douglas began to identify a pattern of deficits she felt accounted for a great proportion of the cognitive impairments associated with the disorder (Douglas, 1983, Douglas & Peters, 1979). This pattern included four major deficits: (1) poor investment and maintenance of effort, (2) deficient modulation of arousal to meet situational demands, (3) a strong inclination to seek immediate reinforcement, and (4) the originally proposed difficulties with impulse control (Douglas, 1983).

Douglas eventually progressed to the conclusion that these four deficiencies in ADHD arose from a more central impairment in self-regulation (Douglas, 1988). This deficiency resulted in difficulties with planning, organization, executive functions, metacognition, adapting cognitive sets (flexibility), self-monitoring, and self-correction. Although no place in this revised model of ADHD was made for them, deficits in motor control and perceptual-motor performance continued to be identified by Douglas as being associated with this disorder.

Whereas Wender (1971) had hypothesized an insensitivity to both reinforcement and punishment as one feature of the disorder, Douglas hypothesized an unusually strong inclination to seek immediate, salient rewards combined with unusually low levels of intrinsic motivation. Although an early review of the literature on the response of ADHD children to reinforcement seemed to support Wender's opinion (Haenlein & Caul, 1987), later research clarified this problem further. That research eventually suggested that the unusually low level of effort and intrinsic motivation tends to account for the performance of ADHD children under varying reward and punishment schedules (August, 1987; Barber, Milich, & Welsh,

1996; Borcherding et al., 1988; Douglas & Benezra, 1990; van der Meere, Hughes, Borger, & Sallee, 1995; Milich, 1994; Wilkison, Kircher, McMahon, & Sloane, 1995). Indeed, the subjects in the Wilkison and colleagues (1995) study made thousands of responses under relatively unreinforcing conditions. The research to date would be more consistent with Douglas's other hypothesis that difficulties with effort allocation and intrinsic motivation characterize the performance of ADHD children on many cognitive tasks; the more tasks demand such effortful attention and self-generated motivation, the more ADHD children would be deficient on the task relative to normal children.

Although Douglas's initial and revised model of ADHD were very helpful to the field in distilling the myriad cognitive deficits into a pattern, and this pattern might be considered to be a rudimentary scientific theory, the model has some difficulties as a theory. Granted, Douglas made several predictions about the task performance of ADHD children that could be considered hypothetical in nature (i.e., the degree of effort required by a task would determine the degree of deficits shown by ADHD children; those with ADHD have an unusually strong inclination to immediate rewards). These were testable predictions, the latter of which would eventually be shown by Douglas's own research to be incorrect (Douglas, Barr, Desilets, & Sherman, 1995).

But this pattern of deficits seems to fall short as a theory for several reasons. For one thing, many of the constructs in this model are poorly defined, if at all. Terms such as *self-regulation, executive functions, metacognition,* and *arousal* are not clarified or operationalized. In fairness to Douglas, however, these terms are just as poorly defined in the literature of neuropsychology and developmental psychology (Barkley, 1996). Nor is it specified to any appreciable degree how the processes at work among these constructs give rise to the symptoms. This model also does not articulate the normal developmental processes involved in each of these areas of deficits and how they may go awry in those with the disorder. And what is it that they have in common that might provide a clue to the deeper and more central nature of the impairment that comprises ADHD? To say that this central problem is one of self-regulation is helpful only if the nature of self-regulation itself and the manner in which these deficits are related to it are more clearly articulated. Regrettably, they are not.

The Quay/Gray Theory of Behavioral Inhibition

At approximately the same time that Douglas was moving on to conceptualize ADHD as a disorder of self-regulation, Herbert Quay adopted Jeffrey Gray's neuropsychological model of anxiety (Gray, 1982, 1987, 1994) to explain the origin of the poor inhibition evident in ADHD (Quay, 1988a, 1988b, 1997). Gray identified a behavioral inhibition system and a behavioral activation system as being critical to understanding instrumental learning and certain emotions. He also stipulated mechanisms for basic nonspecific arousal and for the appraisal of incoming information that must be critical elements of any attempt to model the emotional functions of the brain.

According to this theory, signals of reward serve to increase activity in the behavioral activation system (BAS), thus giving rise to approach behavior and the maintenance of such behavior. Active avoidance and escape from aversive consequences (negative reinforcement) likewise serve to activate this system. Signals of impending punishment (particularly conditioned punishment) as well as frustrative nonreward serve to increase activity in the behavioral inhibition system (BIS). Another system is the fight–flight system, which reacts to unconditioned punitive stimuli.

Quay's use of this model for ADHD stated that the impulsiveness characterizing the disorder arises from diminished activity in the brain's behavioral inhibition system (BIS). This model predicts that those with ADHD should prove less sensitive to such signals, particularly in passive avoidance paradigms (Quay, 1988b). The theory also specifies predictions that can be used to test and even falsify the model as it ap-

plies to ADHD, as some have recently tried to do with only partial success (Milich, Hartung, Martin, & Haigler, 1994). For example, Quay (1988a, 1988b) predicted that there should be greater resistance to extinction following periods of continuous reinforcement in those with ADHD but less resistance when training conditions involved partial reward. They should also demonstrate a decreased ability to inhibit behavior in passive avoidance paradigms when avoidance of the punishment is achieved through the inhibition of responding. There should also be diminished inhibition to signals of pain and novelty as well as to conditioned signals of punishment. Finally, Quay predicted that there should be increased rates of responding by those with ADHD under fixed-interval or fixed-ratio schedules of consequences.

This is a simple theory to understand. The components of the system are reasonably well specified by Gray's model (1982, 1987, 1994) and the manner in which poor inhibition arises in ADHD is made explicit by Quay (1997) sufficient to make predictions that can serve as hypotheses for experiments to test the theory. A problem for this view of ADHD, however, arises in that Gray's theory posits that anxiety disorders arise from an overactivity of the BIS. If that is true, then Quay's use of Gray's theory to explain ADHD would imply that children with ADHD cannot demonstrate an anxiety disorder. Logically, it is difficult to see how one could have both an over- and an underactive BIS in the same person. Research, however, has shown that children with ADHD can have anxiety disorders or higher than normal levels of internalizing symptoms (Biederman, Faraone, & Lapey, 1992; Tannock, in press). Yet they still manifest greater impulsiveness than normal, although such impulsiveness tends to be less than that evident in ADHD children without high levels of internalizing symptoms (Tannock, in press). Such findings seem to contradict Quay's assertion about ADHD or they indicate that children having both anxiety disorders and ADHD do not really have true ADHD but a pseudo-ADHD that arises somehow from their anxiety disorder. I am unaware of anyone who has advanced such a notion nor am I confident that it could withstand critical scrutiny in view of the evidence that such comorbid children do have deficits in inhibition.

Alternatively, it is possible that this coexistence of ADHD with anxiety implies that the forms of anxiety in this comorbid group may arise from a different brain system than the BIS. Perhaps it is the fight or flight system. This system automatically evaluates the potentially threatening nature of stimuli. It imparts to them an affective bias early in their midbrain unconscious processing before such stimuli undergo further higher level and more conscious information processing, perhaps at the cortical level. Such an appraisal–affective bias (i.e., threat–anxiety) placed on information before it influences the BAS and BIS early in unconscious information processing would increase activity in the BIS that is downstream from this early event appraisal system. Thus, ADHD children who are deficient in behavioral inhibition, if possessed of an appraisal–affect system that imparts such a threat–anxiety bias to events early in their processing, could display findings identical to those seen in the extant, albeit limited, literature on those having both ADHD and high anxiety levels. They would still be less inhibited than normal but more inhibited than ADHD children without high levels of anxiety. This is because the early appraisal of threat–anxiety can still increase activity in the BIS although that system is underfunctioning in these children relative to normal. Moreover, such an explanation would clearly permit the two disorders to coexist without being theoretical contradictions to each other, as seems to be the case in the current Quay/Gray model of ADHD.

The Barkley/Bronowski Theory of Executive Functions

Recently (Barkley, 1994, 1997b, 1997c), I have combined Bronowski's theory of the unique properties of human language that arise from the prefrontal cortex (Bronowski, 1977) with the views of Fuster (1985, 1989, 1995, 1997) and Goldman-Rakic (1995) on the functions of that prefrontal cortex. This hybrid model provides a unifying theory of behavioral inhibition, executive functions, and self-regulation. It also can be used as a model of ADHD.

Increasing evidence suggests that ADHD may arise from deficiencies in the development, structure, and function of the prefrontal cortex and its networks with other brain regions, especially with the striatum (Casey et al., 1997; Castellanos et al., 1994; Castellanos et al., 1996; Lou, Henriksen, & Bruhn, 1984; Lou, Henriksen, Bruhn, Borner, & Nielsen, 1989; Zametkin et al., 1990; see also Chapter 8, this volume). A model of prefrontal executive functions should therefore offer some promise as a model for understanding ADHD as well.

Like Quay (1988b, 1997), I believe that a deficit in behavioral inhibition is central to ADHD. The hybrid model, however, goes further than Quay's theory in positing that behavioral inhibition makes a fundamental contribution to the effective performance of four executive functions: nonverbal working memory, verbal working memory (internalized speech), the self-regulation of affect/motivation/arousal, and reconstitution. Each of these represents a form of behavior that was originally public and outer-directed in form but comes to be covert, internalized, or "privatized" across development. This progressive developmental internalization of behavior permits the developing human to engage in private, eventually unobservable forms of self-directed behavior that are used to simulate possible response options to events, to modify the individual's initial prepotent responses, and to generally bring behavior under the control of such internally represented information. That information includes a sense of time, past, and the hypothetical or anticipated future. In essence, across child development the control of behavior is being transferred from that of the immediate context and temporal present to that of internally represented behavior, time, and the anticipated future (Barkley, 1997b, 1997c).

The four executive functions depend on the inhibition of the prepotent response (that which would gain immediate reinforcement) to an event so as to allow for a delay in responding. During such delays, the executive functions (self-directed covert behaviors) occur and must be protected from disruption by ongoing external and internal events (interference control) (Fuster, 1989, 1997). They function to wrest behavior from its more primitive state of being controlled and determined by the immediate environment (the temporal present) and bring such behavior under the control and guidance of internally represented information. That information provides a sense of time, timing, and timeliness to behavior, directs behavior away from the moment and toward future hypothetical events or goals, and serves to sustain behavior toward those events and goals. Such goal-directed persistence occurs even in the absence of immediate rewards for doing so and may also occur despite the presence of immediately aversive consequences or self-imposed deprivation. This is because the individual is capable of covertly motivating themselves to sustain goal-directed activities. These are the functions that provide for the human will and volition (Bastian, 1892; James, 1890/1992; Still, 1902)—behavior that is characterized as intentional, purposive, future-oriented, self-disciplined, and reasoned.

Given this relationship of inhibition to executive functioning, the hybrid theory predicts that the deficiency in behavioral inhibition that characterizes ADHD diminishes the effective deployment of these four executive abilities that subserve self-control and goal-directed behavior. This inhibitory deficit disrupts the control of goal-directed motor behavior through its detrimental effects on these executive functions and the internally represented information they generate. As a consequence, the behavior of those with ADHD is controlled by the immediate context and its consequences more than is seen in others. The behavior of others, in contrast, tends to be controlled by internally represented information, such as hindsight, forethought, time, plans, rules, and self-motivating information. These capacities ultimately provide for the direction of behavior toward anticipated future events and the maximization of future net outcomes.

The predictions of the model for those with ADHD and the available evidence sup-porting many of them have been discussed at length elsewhere (Barkley, 1997b). That evidence is compelling for many of these predicted deficits and it is at least suggestive for most of the others. Although I use the terms *deficit* or *deficiency* here interchangeably, I intend to connote a relative delay in the development of the abilities under discussion.

Each executive function noted previously and its subfunctions have been rephrased in Figure 1 into their negative or impaired states. This is done to make clear the deficiencies expected to arise in each function that are secondary to the principal delay in behavioral inhibition.

Nonverbal Working Memory

Figure 1 illustrates how a delay in development of behavioral inhibition, as is found in ADHD, should lead to secondary deficiencies in nonverbal working memory and its subfunctions. In contrast to others, those with ADHD cannot hold in mind as well information that would govern their responses to ongoing events. They are also unable to protect the activities of working memory and its informational contents from being disrupted by competing sources of interference or behavioral control. As normal children become able to act on and manipulate the contents of working memory, those with ADHD are found to be less able to do so for much the same reasons. This likely explains their deficits in speed and accuracy of mental computation (see Barkley, 1997b, 1997c).

This relative deficiency in the power to mentally represent information, manipulate it, and use it to guide behavior also should interfere with the ADHD child's capacity to imitate novel, complex behaviors demonstrated by others. That is because the template required for imitating those behaviors resides in the capacity for representational memory and that memory is being disrupted by ADHD. Some research findings using motor imitation tasks are consistent with such a prediction (Breen, 1989; Mariani & Barkley, 1997).

Two important subprocesses involved in working memory should be less proficient in

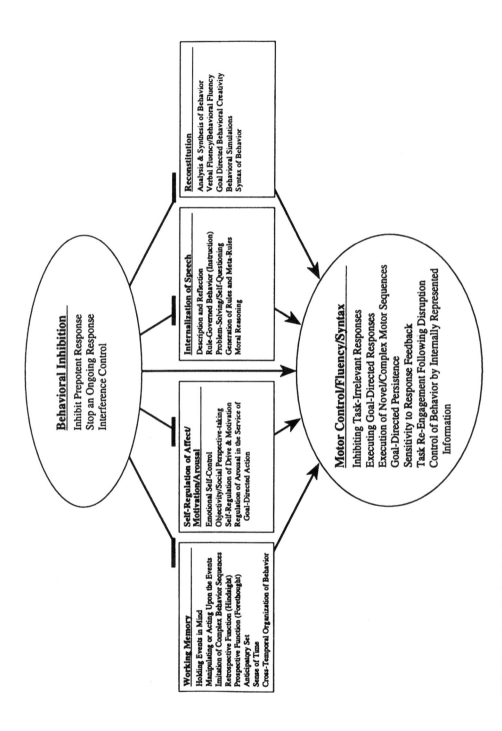

FIGURE 1. A model of the impairments in executive functions predicted to be associated with the deficits in behavioral inhibition that characterize ADHD. From R. A. Barkley (1997). *ADHD and the nature of self-control*. New York: Guilford. Copyright by Guilford Publications. Reprinted with permission.

those with ADHD than in normal peers. These processes are the retrospective (re-sensing) and prospective (preparatory motor) functions (Fuster, 1989, 1995, 1997) that give rise to a sense of the past and, from it, a sense of the future (Bronowski, 1977). Such carrying forward of information on past behavior so as to guide future behavior creates a sensitivity to errors, a sensitivity found to be diminished in those with ADHD (Sergeant & van der Meere, 1988). Moreover, hindsight, forethought, and the working memory on which they are based create self-awareness (Kopp, 1982, 1989). If this is so, then those with ADHD should show a diminished capacity for hindsight, forethought, and self-awareness relative to normal individuals.

Inherent in conceptualizations of working memory is the capacity to represent events in their proper temporal order (Fuster, 1995; Godbout & Doyon, 1995). The model of ADHD in Figure 1 suggests that those with ADHD should show difficulties not only with retaining information in working memory, but also with sequencing it in its proper temporal order. Like patients with frontal lobe injuries (Godbout & Doyon, 1995; Milner, 1995), those with ADHD should demonstrate difficulties with sequencing information recalled from memory, as well as with incoming new information that must be retained in a proper temporal sequence; this seems to be the case (Tannock, 1996). As a result, planning and the sequencing of goal-directed actions to which it leads, should be haphazard, erratic, temporally disorganized, and far less effective in those with ADHD than in normal peers, as indeed, research finds it to be (Pennington, Grossier, & Welsh, 1993).

These retrospective and prospective functions of working memory give rise to the execution of anticipatory or preparatory behaviors founded on them. Such behavior should be less evident in those with ADHD. Consequently, they are less prepared to meet the arrival of future events that others would have anticipated and for which they have prepared (Douglas, 1983). And the timing of those preparatory behaviors they do initiate also may be deficient.

Working memory does nothing if it does not impart time, timing, and timeliness to behavior and its cross-temporal organization (Fuster, 1989, 1995).

As Figure 1 further suggests, those with ADHD should show a developmental delay in the psychological sense of time because that sense of time is founded, at least in part, on the retention of sequences of events in working memory (Michon, 1985). Those with ADHD should be found to make judgments of temporal intervals that are more variable in their accuracy such that they are more typical of those of a younger stage of normal development, as my own research suggests (Barkley, Koplowicz, Anderson, & McMurray, 1997). When asked to wait, those with ADHD should perceive the interval as lasting longer than it does or than is perceived by same-age individuals. When asked to do something within a time period, those with ADHD should act as if they have more time available to do the work than they actually do, thus being seen to procrastinate and be wasteful of their time. And when asked to be at a certain place at a certain time, they are less likely than other individuals to be punctual for the appointment.

If sense of past, future, and time in general is deficient in those with ADHD, then they should display less control of behavior by time and more deficient organization of behavior relative to time. And given that working memory provides the means by which behavior is organized across time so as to bridge delays and create cross-temporal behavioral structures (Fuster, 1989, 1997), the performance of those with ADHD under cross-temporal contingencies will be less effective. They cannot bridge the delays in the contingencies using internally represented information as well as others. The longer the delays in time that separate the components of a behavioral contingency (events, responses, and their consequences), the less successful those with ADHD will be in effectively managing those tasks. This means that ADHD is associated with a form of *temporal myopia* or *blindness to time* concerning the direction of behavior toward conjectured future events.

There also should be less ability to successfully persist in goal-directed behavior in those with ADHD given that such goal-directed persistence is predicated on and guided by information that is internally represented in working memory. And even when goal-directed behavior is undertaken by those with ADHD, it should be subject to greater interference by sources of disruption in both the external and internal environments, resulting in less success at attaining goals. *The problem, then, for those with ADHD is not one of knowing what to do, but one of DOING what they know WHEN it would be most adaptive to do so.*

Internalization of Speech (Verbal Working Memory)

Figure 1 predicts a delay in the internalization of speech or verbal working memory in those with ADHD. Three studies have, indeed, noted such a delay (see Barkley, 1997b; Berk & Potts, 1991). This creates widespread difficulties for them in the use of self-speech for self-regulation. Preschool children with ADHD should not be employing self-speech as much as other-speech at the point where normal children are making this transition from speech to others to speech to self. Even when ADHD preschool children make this transition, it will be delayed not only in its onset but also in its ability to regulate behavior and assist with problem solving. Self-speech is especially critical to the management of task failures, leading not so much to improvement at the moment as to improvement in the future performance of similar tasks, as it has been shown to do in young normal children (Berk, 1992). At that stage in which self-speech progresses to becoming quieter, those with ADHD will remain delayed, manifesting more public self-speech characteristic of younger normal children. Ultimately, those with ADHD should be found to be delayed in the eventual internalization of speech to its covert (unobservable) stage where it comes to form verbal thought. This suggests that even the verbal thinking of those with ADHD is more public and disorganized and less likely to result in the verbal regulation of behavior than in others.

Given this deficiency in the progression to internalized speech, those with ADHD would be predicted to rely less on description and reflection to themselves through covert speech before responding to events. And because self-speech is becoming increasingly wedded to motor control as children mature (Diaz & Berk, 1992), children with ADHD should find their own self-speech as well as the directions given to them by others less effective in controlling their motor behavior (rule-governed behavior) (Berk & Potts, 1991). Rule-governed behavior provides a means of sustaining behavior across large gaps in time among the units of a behavioral contingency (event–response–outcome) (Hayes, 1989); those with ADHD should be less capable of such cross-temporal bridging as a result of their poor rule-governed behavior. ADHD should also interfere with the capacity of the individual to formulate and execute their own rules. Rules are unable to provide the template for constructing lengthy sequences of behavioral chains for those with ADHD as they do for others, such that behavior cannot be as easily guided toward the attainment of a future goal by internalized language. This leads to the prediction that those with ADHD are less likely to formulate strategies (problem solving) and, even if strategies are formulated, less able to apply them effectively in their own task performance (Conte & Regehr, 1991; Greve, Williams, & Dickens, 1996).

Another deficit that should exist in those with ADHD can be discerned from this delay in the privatization of speech. The interaction of nonverbal working memory with that of verbal working memory or private speech contributes to the capacity for reading comprehension. What is silently read to the self via internalized speech must also be held in mind so as to extract its semantic and inferential content. The deficits predicted to exist in both of these executive functions due to ADHD ought to create a diminution in the powers of reading comprehension in those with the disorder and, indeed, they seem to do so (see Barkley, 1997b; Brock & Knapp, 1996).

The control of behavior by the sense of past and future, as well as by the more general rules or meta-rules formulated from them or acquired via socialization, most likely makes some contribution to the development of conscience and moral reasoning. If this is so, then this model predicts that those with ADHD will be delayed in the stages of moral development, as has also been shown to be the case (see Barkley, 1997b, 1997c).

Self-Regulation of Affect, Motivation, and Arousal

An integral aspect of private, self-directed sensing and speech is the associations such mentally represented forms of information will have with affective, motivational, appetitive, and even arousal states (Damasio, 1994, 1995). This provides the drive in the absence of external rewards that fuels the individual's persistence in cross-temporal behaviors and thereby bridges the delay to the future reinforcer. ADHD should therefore create a condition in which those with the disorder are unable to covertly emote and motivate themselves. Thus, they should also be less capable of bridging delays in contingencies and especially delays to reinforcers (Campbell & Ewing, 1990; Rapport, Tucker, DuPaul, Merlo, & Stoner, 1986). This makes them more dependent on external forms of immediate reinforcement in order to persist at tasks and activities.

The diminished power to inhibit prepotent responses to events in those with ADHD brings with it a diminished power to delay their emotional reactions that are associated with those prepotent responses. Less time is granted the person with ADHD for a period for internally generated and self-directed actions (e.g., imagery, private speech) that would modulate their eventual emotional expression to an event. As a consequence, children with ADHD are less able to create more positive emotional and motivational states in themselves when angered, frustrated, disappointed, saddened, anxious, or bored because they are less able to covertly manipulate the variables of which such negative states and their positive alternatives are a function. The developmental progression in the internalization of emotion is likely to be delayed in those with ADHD, leaving them to manifest their emotions impulsively and publicly far longer in their development than normal children, most surely to their social detriment.

Reconstitution

Reconstitution involves the analysis and synthesis of internally represented information and the behavioral structures associated with that information. By taking apart such information, one automatically takes apart the behaviors associated with it (analysis). These dismembered units of information and behavior can then be recombined (synthesis) to create entirely new behavioral sequences and their hierarchies in response to problems or to attain future goals. This grants to humans a tremendous generative capacity for behavioral creativity in pursuit of goals. I have elsewhere (Barkley, 1997b) likened this process to a form of internalized play. The model in Figure 1 stipulates that those with ADHD should be less able to take apart the units of previously acquired behavioral sequences in their repertoire and so they are less able to recombine such units to create novel behavior out of previously learned responses. This problem should be evident not only in their speech (verbal fluency) when it must be goal-directed (Grodzinsky & Diamond, 1992; Tannock, Purvis, & Schachar, 1992) but also in nonverbal forms of fine and gross motor behavior, such as design fluency, when these abilities are needed to solve a problem or achieve a goal. The disorder therefore can be expected to exact a toll on goal-directed behavioral flexibility and creativity, the power to assemble multiple potential responses for the resolution of a problem or the attainment of a future goal.

The combining of units of behavior must be based on a syntax or set of rules governing the temporal sequencing of such units and especially their contingent "if–then" relations. This would suggest that those with ADHD should have more difficulties with that syntax, making their behavior more disorganized in their attempts to assemble complex, hierarchically arranged, goal-directed behavioral structures aimed toward the future.

Motor Control, Fluency, and Syntax

Across human development, internal, covert forms of self-directed behavior and the information they generate increasingly control the motor programming and execution systems. By doing so behavior is brought under the control of time and the likely future. This shift to internally represented information concerning past, future, plans, and time gives behavior not only an increasingly deliberate, reasoned, and dispassionate nature but also a more purposive, intentional, and future-oriented one. All of this would be expected to be disrupted by the inhibitory deficits associated with ADHD.

Distinguishing Two Forms of Sustained Attention

This model of ADHD argues for a critical distinction between two forms of sustained attention (persistence); that distinction is between persistence that is *contingency-shaped* and that which is *self-regulated and goal-directed* (Barkley, 1997b, 1997c). The former is largely a function of immediate contextual factors, such as the schedule of reinforcement associated with the task, the novelty of the task, and the close temporal contiguity of the elements of the contingency. The second type of sustained attention is controlled by covert, self-directed actions that permit much longer, more complex, and more novel chains of responses to be created and executed toward achieving later goals. These goal-directed behavioral structures do not require immediate reward for execution because the motivation driving them is self-created. It is this self-regulatory type of sustained attention that is developmentally delayed in ADHD children, not the type that is contingency-shaped.

Conclusion

There undoubtedly is much about this theory that requires both clarification and verification. Although many of the constructs and their processes and relationships are specified and the model is clearly linked to the literature in both developmental psychology and neuropsychology, some of those processes and relationships need to be better specified. Yet here is a theory that places its bets. Out of such a theory come a number of new and testable hypotheses about the nature of ADHD that have not previously been predicted to be associated with this disorder by any prior theory of it.

The theory of ADHD espoused here is the only one that asserts that the very process by which forms of external behavior become internalized and give rise to comparable forms of thought is delayed in those with the disorder. Therefore, understanding the very nature of the process of the developmental internalization of behavior and that of directing behavior toward the future is absolutely critical to achieving a more complete understanding of the nature of ADHD and its cognitive and social impairments. The implications for clinical practice from such a shift of perspective on this disorder are substantial (see Barkley, 1997b). Yet such a paradigm shift is not as radical as it may seem at first, for it was anticipated nearly a century ago in Still's (1902) original theory in which he postulated that inhibition and the guidance of behavior by internal information were at the heart of this disorder.

REFERENCES

American Psychiatric Association. (1968). *Diagnostic and statistical manual of mental disorders* (2nd ed.). Washington, DC: Author.

American Psychiatric Association. (1980). *Diagnostic and statistical manual of mental disorders* (3rd ed.). Washington, DC: Author.

American Psychiatric Association. (1987). *Diagnostic and statistical manual of mental disorders* (3rd ed., rev.). Washington, DC: Author.

American Psychiatric Association. (1994). *Diagnostic and statistical manual of mental disorders* (4th ed.). Washington, DC: Author.

August, G. J. (1987). Production deficiencies in free recall: A comparison of hyperactive, learning-disabled, and normal children. *Journal of Abnormal Child Psychology, 15,* 429–440.

August, G. J., & Stewart, M. A. (1983). Family subtypes of childhood hyperactivity. *Journal of Nervous and Mental Disease, 171,* 362–368.

Barber, M. A., Milich, R., & Welsh, R. (1996). Effects of reinforcement schedule and task difficulty on the performance of attention deficit hyperactivity disordered and control boys. *Journal of Clinical Child Psychology, 25,* 66–76.

Barkley, R. A. (1994). Impaired delayed responding: A unified theory of attention deficit hyperactivity disorder. In D. K. Routh (Ed.), *Disruptive Behavior Disorders: Essays in honor of Herbert Quay* (pp. 11–57). New York: Plenum.

Barkley, R. A. (1996). Linkages between attention and executive functions. In G. R. Lyon & N. A. Krasnegor (Eds.), *Attention, memory, and executive function* (pp. 307–326). Baltimore: Brookes.

Barkley, R. A. (1997a). *ADHD and the nature of self-control.* New York: Guilford.

Barkley, R. A. (1997b). *ADHD, self-control, and time: A unifying theory of executive functions and its clinical implications.* New York: Guilford.

Barkley, R. A. (1997c). Behavioral inhibition, sustained attention, and executive functions: Constructing a unifying theory of ADHD. *Psychological Bulletin, 121,* 65–94.

Barkley, R. A. (1998). *Attention deficit hyperactivity disorder: A handbook for diagnosis and treatment* (2nd ed.). New York: Guilford.

Barkley, R. A., Koplowicz, S., Anderson, T., & McMurray, M. B. (1997). Sense of time in children with ADHD: Two preliminary studies. *Journal of the International Neuropsychological Society, 3,* 359–369.

Bastian, H. C. (1892). On the neural processes underlying attention and volition. *Brain, 15,* 1–34.

Berk, L. E. (1992). Children's private speech: An overview of theory and the status of research. In R. M. Diaz & L. E. Berk (Eds.), *Private speech: From social interaction to self-regulation* (pp. 17–54). Mahwah, NJ: Erlbaum.

Berk, L. E., & Potts, M. K. (1991). Development and functional significance of private speech among attention-deficit hyperactivity disorder and normal boys. *Journal of Abnormal Child Psychology, 19,* 357–377.

Berkowitz, M. W. (1982). Self-control development and relation to prosocial behavior: A response to Peterson. *Merrill-Palmer Quarterly, 28,* 223–236.

Biederman, J., Faraone, S. V., & Lapey, K. (1992). Comorbidity of diagnosis in attention-deficit hyperactivity disorder. In. G. Weiss (Ed.), *Child and adolescent psychiatry clinics of North America: Attention deficit disorder* (pp. 335–360). Philadelphia: Saunders.

Borcherding, B., Thompson, K., Krusei, M., Bartko, J., Rapoport, J. L., & Weingartner, H. (1988). Automatic and effortful processing in attention deficit/hyperactivity disorder. *Journal of Abnormal Child Psychology, 16,* 333–345.

Breen, M. J. (1989). ADHD girls and boys: An analysis of attentional, emotional, cognitive, and family variables. *Journal of Child Psychology and Psychiatry, 30,* 711–716.

Brock, S. W., & Knapp, P. K. (1996). Reading comprehension abilities of children with attention-deficit/hyper-activity disorder. *Journal of Attention Disorders, 1,* 173–186.

Bronowski, J. (1977). Human and animal languages. *A sense of the future* (pp. 104–131). Cambridge, MA: MIT Press.

Campbell, S. B., & Ewing, L. J. (1990). Follow-up of hard-to-manage preschoolers: Adjustment at age nine years and predictors of continuing symptoms. *Journal of Child Psychology and Psychiatry, 31,* 891–910.

Carnap, R. (1966). *The philosophy of science.* New York: Basic Books.

Casey, B. J., Castellanos, F. X., Giedd, J. N., Marsh, W. L., Hamburger, S. D., Schubert, A. B., Vauss, Y. C., Vaituzis, A. C., Dickstein, D. P., Sarfatti, S. E., & Rapoport, J. L. (1997). Implication of right frontostriatal circuitry in response inhibition and attention-deficit/hyperactivity disorder. *Journal of the American Academy of Child and Adolescent Psychiatry, 36,* 374–383.

Castellanos, F. X., Giedd, J. N., Eckburg, P., Marsh, W. L., Vaituzis, C., Kaysen, D., Hamburger, S. D., & Rapoport, J. L. (1994). Quantitative morphology of the caudate nucleus in attention deficit hyperactivity disorder. *American Journal of Psychiatry, 151,* 1791–1796.

Castellanos, F. X., Giedd, J. N., Marsh, W. L., Hamburger, S. D., Vaituzis, A. C., Dickstein, D. P., Sarfatti, S. E., Vauss, Y. C., Snell, J. W., Lange, N., Kaysen, D., Krain, A. L., Ritchie, G. F., Rajapakse, J. C., & Rapoport, J. L. (1996). Quantitative brain magnetic resonance imaging in attention-deficit hyperactivity disorder. *Archives of General Psychiatry, 53,* 607–616.

Chess, S. (1960). Diagnosis and treatment of the hyperactive child. *New York State Journal of Medicine, 60,* 2379–2385.

Conte, R., & Regehr, S. M. (1991). Learning and transfer of inductive reasoning rules in overactive children. *Cognitive Therapy and Research, 15,* 129–139.

Damasio, A. R. (1994). *Descartes' error: Emotion, reason, and the human brain.* New York: Putnam.

Damasio, A. R. (1995). On some functions of the human prefrontal cortex. In J. Grafma, K. J. Holyoak, & F. Boller (Eds.), *Structure and functions of the human prefrontal cortex: Vol. 769. Annals of the New York Academy of Sciences* (pp. 241–251). New York: New York Academy of Sciences.

Diaz, R. M., & Berk, L. E. (1992). *Private speech: From social interaction to self-regulation.* Mahwah, NJ: Erlbaum.

Douglas, V. I. (1972). Stop, look, and listen: The problem of sustained attention and impulse control in hyperactive and normal children. *Canadian Journal of Behavioural Science, 4,* 259–282.

Douglas, V. I. (1983). Attention and cognitive problems. In M. Rutter (Ed.), *Developmental neuropsychiatry* (pp. 280–329). New York: Guilford.

Douglas, V. I. (1988). Cognitive deficits in children with attention deficit disorder with hyperactivity. In. L. M. Bloomingdale & J. A. Sergeant (Eds.), *Attention deficit disorder: Criteria, cognition, intervention* (pp. 65–82). London: Pergamon.

Douglas, V. I., & Benezra, E. (1990). Supraspan verbal memory in attention deficit disorder with hyperactivity, normal, and reading disabled boys. *Journal of Abnormal Child Psychology, 18,* 617–638.

Douglas, V. I., & Peters, K. G. (1979). Toward a clearer definition of the attentional deficit of hyperactive children. In G. A. Hale & M. Lewis (Eds.), *Attention and cognitive development* (pp. 173–248). New York: Plenum.

Douglas, V. I., Barr, R. G., Desilets, J., & Sherman, E. (1995). Do high doses of stimulants impair flexible thinking in attention-deficit hyperactivity disorder? *Journal of the American Academy of Child and Adolescent Psychiatry, 34,* 877–885.

Fuster, J. M. (1985). *The prefrontal cortex.* New York: Raven.

Fuster, J. M. (1989). *The prefrontal cortex* (2nd ed.). New York: Raven.

Fuster, J. M. (1995). Memory and planning: Two temporal perspectives of frontal lobe function. In H. H. Jasper, S. Riggio, & P. S. Goldman-Rakic (Eds.), *Epilepsy and the functional anatomy of the frontal lobe* (pp. 9–18). New York: Raven.

Fuster, J. M. (1997). *The prefrontal cortex* (3rd ed.). New York: Raven.

Godbout, L., & Doyon, J. (1995). Mental representation of knowledge following frontal-lobe or post-rolandic lesions. *Neuropsychologia, 33,* 1671–1696.

Goldman-Rakic, P. S. (1995). Architecture of the prefrontal cortex and the central executive. In J. Grafman, K. J. Holyoak, & F. Boller (Eds.), *Structure and functions of the human prefrontal cortex: Vol. 769. Annals of the New York Academy of Sciences* (pp. 71–83). New York: New York Academy of Sciences.

Gray, J. A. (1982). *The neuropsychology of anxiety.* New York: Oxford University Press.

Gray, J. A. (1987). *The psychology of fear and stress* (2nd ed.). Cambridge, England: Cambridge University Press.

Gray, J. A. (1994). Three fundamental emotional systems. In P. Ekman & R. J. Davidson (Eds.), *The nature of emotion: Fundamental questions* (pp. 243–247). New York: Oxford University Press.

Greve, K. W., Williams, M. C., & Dickens, T. J., Jr. (1996, February). *Concept formation in attention disordered children.* Poster presented at the meeting of the International Neuropsychological Society, Chicago.

Grodzinsky, G. M., & Diamond, R. (1992). Frontal lobe functioning in boys with attention-deficit hyperactivity disorder. *Developmental Neuropsychology, 8,* 427–445.

Haenlein, M., & Caul, W. F. (1987). Attention deficit disorder with hyperactivity: A specific hypothesis of reward dysfunction. *Journal of the American Academy of Child and Adolescent Psychiatry, 26,* 356–362.

Hastings, J. E., & Barkley, R. A. (1978). A review of psychophysiological research with hyperkinetic children. *Journal of Abnormal Child Psychology, 6,* 413–447.

Hayes, S. (1989). *Rule-governed behavior.* New York: Plenum.

Hayes, S. C., Gifford, E. V., & Ruckstuhl, J. (1996). Relational frame theory and executive function: A behavioral analysis. In G. R. Lyon & N. A. Krasnegor (Eds.), *Attention, memory, and executive function* (pp. 279–306). Baltimore: Brookes.

Hempel, C. G. (1966). *Philosophy of natural science.* Englewood Cliffs, NJ: Prentice-Hall.

Hinshaw, S. P. (1987). On the distinction between attentional deficits/hyperactivity and conduct problems/aggression in child psychopathology. *Psychological Bulletin, 101,* 443–447.

James, W. (1890/1992). *Principles of psychology.* Chicago: Encyclopedia Britannica.

Kessler, J. W. (1980). History of minimal brain dysfunction. In H. Rie & L. Rie (Eds.), *Handbook of minimal brain dysfunctions: A critical view* (pp. 18–52). New York: Wiley.

Kopp, C. B. (1982). Antecedents of self-regulation: A developmental perspective. *Developmental Psychology, 18,* 199–214.

Kopp, C. B. (1989). Regulation of distress and negative emotions: A developmental view. *Developmental Psychology, 25,* 343–354.

Lou, H. C., Henriksen, L., & Bruhn, P. (1984). Focal cerebral hypoperfusion in children with dysphasia and/or Attention Deficit Disorder. *Archives of Neurology, 41,* 825–829.

Lou, H. C., Henriksen, L., Bruhn, P., Borner, H., & Nielsen, J. B. (1989). Striatal dysfunction in attention deficit and hyperkinetic disorder. *Archives of Neurology, 46,* 48–52.

Mariani, M. A., & Barkley, R. A. (1997). Neuropsychological and academic functioning in preschool boys with attention deficit hyperactivity disorder. *Developmental Neuropsychology, 13,* 111–129.

Meere, J. van der, Hughes, K. A., Borger, N., & Sallee, F. R. (1995). The effect of reward on sustained attention in ADHD children with and without CD. In J. A. Sergeant (Ed.), *Eunethydis: European approaches to hyperkinetic disorder* (pp. 241–253). Zurich, Switzerland: Fotorator.

Michon, J. A. (1985). Introduction. In J. Michon & T. Jackson (Eds.), *Time, mind, & behavior.* Berlin, Germany: Springer-Verlag.

Milich, R. (1994). The response of children with ADHD to failure: If at first you don't succeed, do you try, try again? *School Psychology Review, 23,* 11–28.

Milich, R., Hartung, C. M., Martin, C. A., & Haigler, E. D. (1994). Behavioral disinhibition and underlying processes in adolescents with disruptive behavior disorders. In D. K. Routh (Ed.), *Disruptive behavior disorders in childhood* (pp. 109–138). New York: Plenum.

Milner, B. (1995). Aspects of human frontal lobe function. In H. H. Jasper, S. Riggio, & P. S. Goldman-Rakic (Eds.), *Epilepsy and the functional anatomy of the frontal lobe* (pp. 67–81). New York: Raven.

Pennington, B. F., Grossier, D., & Welsh, M. C. (1993). Contrasting cognitive deficits in attention deficit disorder versus reading disability. *Developmental Psychology, 29,* 511–523.

Peterson, L. (1982). Altruism and the development of internal control: An integrative model. *Merrill-Palmer Quarterly, 28,* 197–222.

Quay, H. C. (1988a). Attention deficit disorder and the behavioral inhibition system: The relevance of the neuropsychological theory of Jeffrey A. Gray. In L. M. Bloomingdale & J. Sergeant (Eds.), *Attention deficit disorder: Criteria, cognition, intervention* (pp. 117–126). New York: Pergamon.

Quay, H. C. (1988b). The behavioral reward and inhibition systems in childhood behavior disorder. In L. M. Bloomingdale (Ed.), *Attention Deficit Disorder: III. New research in treatment, psychopharmacology, and attention* (pp. 176–186). New York: Pergamon.

Quay, H. C. (1997). Inhibition and attention deficit hyperactivity disorder. *Journal of Abnormal Child Psychology, 25,* 7–13.

Rapport, M. D., Tucker, S. B., DuPaul, G. J., Merlo, M., & Stoner, G. (1986). Hyperactivity and frustration: The influence of control over and size of rewards in delaying gratification. *Journal of Abnormal Child Psychology, 14,* 181–204.

Rie, H., & Rie, L. (Eds.). (1980). *Handbook of minimal brain dysfunctions: A critical view.* New York: Wiley.

Rosenthal, R. H., & Allen, T. W. (1978). An examination of attention, arousal, and learning dysfunctions of hyperkinetic children. *Psychological Bulletin, 85,* 689–715.

Ross, D. M., & Ross, S. A. (1976). *Hyperactivity: Research, theory and action.* New York: Wiley.

Schachar, R. J. (1986). Hyperkinetic syndrome: Historical development of the concept. In E. Taylor (Ed.), *The overactive child* (pp. 19–40). Philadelphia: Lippincott.

Schachar, R. J., Tannock, R., & Logan, G. (1993). Inhibitory control, impulsiveness, and attention deficit hyperactivity disorder. *Clinical Psychology Review, 13,* 721–739.

Sergeant, J. A., & Meere, J. van der. (1988). What happens when the hyperactive child commits an error? *Psychiatry Research, 24,* 157–164.

Stewart, M. A., deBlois, S., & Cummings, C. (1980). Psychiatric disorder in the parents of hyperactive boys and those with conduct disorder. *Journal of Child Psychology and Psychiatry, 21,* 283–292.

Still, G. F. (1902). Some abnormal psychical conditions in children. *Lancet, 1,* 1008–1012, 1077–1082, 1163–1168.

Strauss, A. A., & Lehtinen, L. E. (1947). *Psychopathology and education of the brain-injured child.* New York: Grune & Stratton.

Tannock, R. (1996, January). *Discourse deficits in ADHD: Executive dysfunction as an underlying mechanism?* Paper presented at the annual meeting of the International Society for Research in Child and Adolescent Psychopathology, Santa Monica, CA.

Tannock, R. (in press). Attention deficit disorders with anxiety disorders. In T. E. Brown (Ed.), *Subtypes of attention deficit disorders in children, adolescents, and adults.* Washington, DC: American Psychiatric Press.

Tannock, R., Purvis, K. L., & Schachar, R. J. (1992). Narrative abilities in children with attention deficit hyperactivity disorder and normal peers. *Journal of Abnormal Child Psychology, 21,* 103–117.

Taylor, E. (1996, January). *Discussion of current theories of ADHD.* Paper presented at the annual meeting of the International Society for Research in Child and Adolescent Psychopathology, Los Angeles.

Turner, M. B. (1967). *Philosophy and the science of behavior.* New York: Appleton-Century-Crofts.

Walters, A. S., & Barrett, R. P. (1993). The history of hyperactivity. In J. Matson (Ed.), *Handbook of hyperactivity* (pp. 1–10). Needham Heights, MA: Allyn & Bacon.

Wender, P. H. (1971). *Minimal brain dysfunction in children.* New York: Wiley.

Werry, J. S. (1992). History, terminology, and manifestations at different ages. In G. Weiss (Ed.), *Child and adolescent psychiatry clinics of North America: Attention deficit disorder* (pp. 297–310). Philadelphia: Saunders.

Wilkison, P. C., Kircher, J. C., McMahon, W. M., & Sloane, H. N. (1995). Effects of methylphenidate on reward strength in boys with attention-deficit hyperactivity disorder. *Journal of the American Academy of Child and Adolescent Psychiatry, 34,* 877–885.

Zametkin, A. J., Nordahl, T. E., Gross, M., King, A. C., Semple, W. E., Rumsey, J., Hamburger, S., & Cohen, R. M. (1990). Cerebral glucose metabolism in adults with hyperactivity of childhood onset. *New England Journal of Medicine, 323,* 1361–1366.

III

Oppositional Defiant Disorder and Conduct Disorder

14

Cognitive Functioning in Children with Oppositional Defiant Disorder and Conduct Disorder

ANNE E. HOGAN

INTRODUCTION

This chapter reviews evidence regarding the cognitive functioning of children with Conduct Disorder (CD) and Oppositional Defiant Disorder (ODD). General topics include overall intellectual functioning as assessed by IQ tests, as well as executive function abilities, social-cognitive development, and information processing.

The label *CD* is used throughout the chapter to refer to subjects' Disruptive Behavior Disorder (DBD) status; however, a substantial number of studies reviewed did not use psychiatric diagnoses. Studies are included in which youth were diagnosed as CD or ODD; categorized as aggressive, antisocial, delinquent; or identified as having heterogeneous externalizing behavior problems. Problems were variously reported by parents, teachers, peers, the subjects themselves, or some combination. While some studies gave thorough information regarding subjects' comorbid attentional or internalizing problems, the majority did not.

ANNE E. HOGAN • Department of Psychology, University of Miami, Coral Gables, Florida 33124-0721.

Handbook of Disruptive Behavior Disorders, edited by Quay and Hogan. Kluwer Academic/Plenum Publishers, New York, 1999.

CD AND IQ

Perhaps the most frequently examined question regarding cognitive functioning in youth with CD has been whether they demonstrate low IQs. The exact form of the question has varied. Correlational-regression designs have been used to assess the strength and significance of the expected negative correlation between CD and IQ, and ANOVA-type designs have been used to test whether CD subjects have lower IQs than contrast groups. The type of IQ score used has varied, including use of Full Scale (FSIQ), Verbal (VIQ), Performance (PIQ) scores, or combinations, and various short forms. Different types of CD groups have also been used: occasionally purely CD subjects but more typically heterogeneous CD or delinquent (DELQ) subjects. Commonly, then, results reflect the performance of subjects likely comorbid for Attention-Deficit/Hyperactivity Disorder (ADHD) and other disorders. Contrast groups have also varied, with "normal" controls in many epidemiological or school-based studies, and clinic group comparisons in clinic-referral or inpatient studies.

Because many variables are correlated with IQ and CD, additional measures have often been included (e.g., SES, global measures of environmental adversity; parental variables such as IQ or education). Because ADHD is often found in ODD/CD subjects (see Chapter 2, this volume), relevant symptoms may have been assessed; some studies have distinguished subjects as being "pure" CD versus CD+ ADHD. Results regarding the CD–IQ relation have then been interpreted after statistically controlling for the influence of demographic, familial, and ADHD variable or variables.

Not surprisingly, variability in how researchers have asked the CD–IQ question has led to a mixed picture. In general, the link between lower IQ and CD has been observed most often when (1) comorbid ADHD symptoms were not measured, (2) the subjects were adolescents, or under both conditions. Another issue has been whether the IQ deficit for children with CD is specific to VIQ. Finally, correlational evidence has been examined to explore possible causal links between intellectual functioning and CD. The following section reviews these findings in more detail.

Control for Comorbid ADHD Symptoms

Overall, of 27 studies reviewed, 16 studies did not assess or did not control for ADHD in their CD subjects. Of these, 12 (indicated with an asterisk) reported a significant relationship between CD and lower IQ (Beitchman, Patterson, Gelfand, & Minty, 1982; *Chandler & Moran, 1990; *Fergusson, Lynskey, & Horwood, 1996; *Frick, O'Brien, Wootton, & McBurnett, 1994; *Goodman, Simonoff, & Stevenson, 1995; Hodges & Plow, 1990; *Kandel et al., 1988; Lochman, Wayland, & White, 1993; *Lochman, Bierman, & McMahon, 1997; *Nagin, Farrington, & Moffitt, 1995; *Noam, Paget, Valiant, Borst, & Bartok, 1994; *Pianta & Caldwell, 1990; *Schonfeld, Shaffer, O'Connor, & Portnoy, 1988; Sonuga-Barke, Lamparelli, Stevenson, Thompson, & Henry, 1994; *White, Moffitt, & Silva, 1989; *White et al., 1994).

Varied samples were examined; seven of the studies used exclusively male subjects. Lower IQs were found in (1) DELQ and adult offender groups (Chandler & Moran, 1990; Kandel et al., 1988; Nagin et al., 1995; White et al., 1989), (2) clinic-based groups of CD boys (Frick et al., 1994; Noam et al., 1994), and (3) longitudinal studies of high-risk CD youth (Schonfeld et al., 1988; White et al., 1994). In epidemiological and school samples, CD was negatively associated with IQ (Fergusson et al., 1996; Goodman et al., 1995). Two studies reported that declines in CD behavior in early elementary school were linked to higher IQ (Lochman et al., 1997; Pianta & Caldwell, 1990).

Three studies did not assess ADHD symptoms in the CD group and reported no evidence for a relationship between low IQ and CD. All included girls and two used clinic-based comparison groups (Beitchman et al., 1982; Hodges & Plow, 1990). Beitchman and colleagues reported mixed findings; their CD group did not differ from neurotic or mixed-problem groups. Without normal controls, the CD group was compared to a population mean IQ of 100 and found to be significantly lower. Given the modest demographic information provided, the appropriateness of that comparison was questionable. One third of these reports used a preschool sample (Sonuga-Barke et al., 1994).

Ten studies that reported CD–IQ analyses attempted to control for comorbid ADHD symptoms using correlational techniques or by constructing groups of pure CD subjects to contrast with other groups (Anderson, Williams, McGee, & Silva, 1989; Fergusson, Horwood, & Lynskey, 1993; Frick et al., 1991; Goodman, 1995; Lahey et al., 1995; Loeber, Green, Keenan, & Lahey, 1995; Lynam, Moffitt, & Stouthamer-Loeber, 1993; Moffitt, 1990; Schachar & Tannock, 1995; Taylor, Chadwick, Heptinstall, & Danckaerts, 1996). Paternite, Loney, and Roberts (1995) used a similar strategy to examine IQ performance in a pure ODD group. Of these 11 studies, 3 found IQ–CD links after controlling for ADHD problems (Fergusson et al., 1993; Goodman, 1995; Lynam et al., 1993). Two studies had mixed results (Lahey et al., 1995; Loeber et al., 1995); the remaining 6 found no evidence of IQ deficits in pure CD youth.

Providing perhaps the strongest evidence for a pure CD–IQ link, Fergusson and colleagues (1993) used a structural modeling approach to examine predictive links among CD, ADHD, juvenile offending, and scholastic attainment. Modeling analyses controlled for the substantial correlation between CD and ADHD (estimated correlation $r = .79$), and included a measure of IQ. CD and IQ showed significant, unique relationships; lower IQ at age 8 was associated with greater CD at ages 6, 8, and 10 (estimated correlations ranged from $-.33$ to $-.40$).

While not measuring ADHD symptoms per se, Lynam and colleagues (1993) included a composite measure of impulsivity. Impulsivity was significantly related to both VIQ and DELQ; however, it did not account for the observed relationship between VIQ and DELQ. Goodman (1995) found CD was negatively related to IQ ($r = -.21$); the correlation remained significant even when controlling for an "immaturity" variable (ratings of restlessness and high activity).

Two reports of the developmental course of CD onset and persistence found differences in the CD–IQ link over time. In predicting the *onset* of CD, Loeber and colleagues (1995) found that boys who subsequently became CD differed in IQ from boys who did not; in contrast, these groups did not differ on ADHD symptoms. The subsequent-CD boys had lower FSIQ, VIQ, and PIQ; however, in regression analyses, IQ did not add to the prediction of CD-onset when SES, parental substance abuse, and ODD were in the equation. Lahey and colleagues (1995) compared boys who did or did not meet criteria for CD diagnosis and found no significant difference in *concurrent* VIQ when SES was controlled. However, Lahey and colleagues also found an interaction between VIQ and parental psychopathology in predicting *persistence* of CD. CD symptoms declined over time only when boys had both higher VIQs and parents without Antisocial Personality Disorder (APD); the presence of either low VIQ, parental APD, or both was associated with continued CD. Thus, after controlling for demographic and family variables, lower VIQs

were not uniquely linked to CD prior to onset or at time of diagnosis; however, lower VIQ appeared to play a role in continuing CD after the boy had been diagnosed.

The last five reports in this set of studies included pure CD groups as well as CD+ADHD or mixed disorder groups. Anderson and colleagues (1989) found pure CD children (diagnosis at age 11) did not differ significantly from normal controls on IQ at ages 5, 7, 9, or 11, while the ADHD and mixed-disorder groups scored more poorly. Moffitt (1990) reported that DELQ males (by self-report at ages 13 and 15) without ADHD did not significantly differ from nondisordered controls on IQ at age 5 or VIQ at ages 7, 9, 11, and 13. Only the DELQ+ADHD showed IQ deficits: lower than controls at all ages, and lower than pure DELQ at ages 11 and 13. Taylor and colleagues (1996) also reported IQ deficits at ages 8 and 16–18 only for children with *both* CD and ADHD problems; children with CD only did not differ from controls at either age. Schachar and Tannock (1995) found no significant IQ differences among CD-only, ADHD-only, CD+ADHD, and clinic-referred controls. Frick and colleagues (1991) also reported nonsignificant differences among CD, ADHD, and clinic controls. The CD children's mean IQs in these latter two studies were 107 and 99, respectively; thus, the failure to find lower IQs in CD groups was not due to general low IQs among all clinic groups. Similarly, Paternite and colleagues (1995) found that boys with pure ODD did not differ in IQ from non-DBD controls; the ODD group had a mean FSIQ of 102.

In summary, nearly 60% of the CD–IQ studies reviewed here reported significant associations. Among those significant findings, 80% of the studies did not include assessment of ADHD symptoms; these studies may often have included subjects comorbid for symptoms of ADHD. Among studies controlling for comorbid ADHD, 73% did not find CD uniquely linked to lower IQ. The reports of significant CD–IQ patterns with accompanying controls for ADHD symptoms had large samples and were correlational in design (these studies are discussed further in the section on causal links). When pure CD subject *groups* have been studied, they have not shown mean IQ deficits; in contrast, CD+ADHD children have often shown mean IQ deficits.

Subject Age

The link between low IQ and CD has been found more frequently in studies with older subjects. This general pattern is consistent with Hinshaw's (1992) extensive review; he concluded that poorer cognitive functioning had been more closely linked to attentional problems in childhood and to antisocial problems in adolescence.

For the *preschool* stage, two studies have reported no significant concurrent link between low IQ and disruptive behavior. Sonuga-Barke and colleagues (1994) found no relationship between CD and IQ for boys, and a rather surprising *positive* link between CD and IQ for girls. Similarly, Campbell, Pierce, March, Ewing, and Szumowski (1994) found no significant IQ deficit in their sample of hard-to-manage boys, whose symptoms included both attentional and oppositional behavior problems.

The findings for *middle childhood* ages have been mixed. As noted previously, Anderson and colleagues (1989) and Moffitt (1990) reported no deficits for pure CD or pure DELQ groups across ages 5 to 11. Some comparisons of clinic groups have yielded no significant deficit for CD (e.g., as already noted, Beitchman *et al.,* 1982; Frick *et al.,* 1991; Hodges & Plow, 1990; Lahey *et al.,* 1995; Paternite et al, 1995; Schachar & Tannock, 1995).

In contrast to these results, Frick and colleagues (1994) reported that the CD group (without accompanying psychopathy) had a lower mean IQ than clinic-referred controls. Nagin and colleagues (1995) reported IQ data from a longitudinal study of different offender groups from ages 8 to 32. Groups were nonoffenders, adolescent-limited offenders, and chronic (i.e., life-course persistent) offenders. At age 10, chronic offenders had shown lower PIQs and VIQs than nonoffenders; adolescent-limited offenders had lower PIQs, but not VIQs, relative to nonoffenders. And as noted,

Fergusson and colleagues (1993) found significant, negative correlations between IQ at age 8 and CD at ages 6, 8, and 10 (with control for ADHD and demographic variables).

During *adolescence,* the pattern shifts. Goodman and colleagues (1995) found significant negative correlations between IQ and CD in a sample of 13-year-old-twins. Noam and colleagues (1994) reported that inpatient subjects ages 11–17 with CD had lower IQs than inpatients with affective disorders. Chandler and Moran (1990) found lower IQs in adjudicated DELQ subjects ages 14–17 relative to controls. In Nagin and colleagues' (1995) comparison of nonoffenders, adolescent-limited offenders, and chronic offenders, at age 14, both offender groups had significantly lower PIQs and VIQs than the nonoffenders. In predicting CD at ages 15–16, Fergusson and colleagues (1996) found IQ at age 8 contributed uniquely even when measures of CD at age 8 and ages 14–15 were in the equation (however, measures of ADHD were not). As already noted, Lynam and colleagues (1993) reported an association between DELQ at ages 12–13 with lower VIQ that could not be accounted for by race, SES, or impulsivity. With the data used by Lynam and colleagues, White and colleagues (1994) reported that IQ at ages 12–13 was related to prior delinquency (i.e., age 10) as well; the correlation ($r = -.30$) remained significant with SES controlled. In a recent review, Loeber and Hay (1997) concluded that although aggressive children typically become delinquent regardless of their IQ, low IQ is nevertheless a risk factor for later delinquency. In contrast, Lochman and colleagues (1993) found no IQ differences between teacher-rated aggressive and nonaggressive high school students.

Three studies with a wide age range are of special interest here. Schonfeld and colleagues' (1988) longitudinal study of IQ and CD (diagnosed in adolescence) reported no initial IQ difference at age 4; however, at ages 7 and 17, the CD boys had significantly lower IQs than non-CD controls. Goodman (1995) found CD associated with lower IQ in a sample of 5- to 16-year-olds. Although the IQ–CD correlations were of similar magnitude for both genders, the correlation was significant for teenagers but fell short of significance for the younger subjects (rs −.31 vs. −.13). Behaviors found to most strongly account for the IQ–CD link included "truancy/staying out late" and "stealing" (more characteristic of adolescent-onset CD; see Chapter 1, this volume).

White and colleagues (1989) reported on an epidemiological data set that included IQ at age 5, a CD problem measure at age 5 that was collapsed into a binary "risk" variable (i.e., the highest scoring 33% of the sample was considered high-risk; remaining subjects were considered low-risk), and a self-report measure of DELQ at ages 13 and 15; subjects were then classified as DELQ or non-DELQ. Results indicated that DELQ status was related to IQ, but risk status was not. Thus, within the same sample, there was no link between antisocial behavior problems and IQ *concurrently* in childhood; however, retrospectively, the DELQ adolescents had shown lower IQs at age 5.

Overall these results suggest that the IQ–CD link is most evident in older or DELQ subjects but it should be noted that many of the studies described with adolescent samples did not assess ADHD symptomatology. The developmental pattern, however, may not be entirely artifactual. Adolescents with a history of CD may also have a history of poor school adjustment and attendance. For some, the *accumulating* intellectual deficit relative to age mates may be detectable only after years of schooling (or lack thereof) (see Chapter 16, this volume; Ceci, 1991).

Is VIQ the Particular Problem?

Rather than a global intellectual deficit, VIQ and language ability have been suggested as key deficits among children with DBD, with concerns for low VIQ, a large discrepancy of VIQ < PIQ, or both (cf. Hinshaw, 1992; Moffitt, 1993). Hodges and Plow (1990) reported that the CD group in their inpatient sample had IQ subscale scores comparable to comparison groups (i.e., were not significantly lower, even on the Verbal subscales); however, the CD group was the only group to show a significant VIQ <

PIQ discrepancy (VIQ mean = 92.6, PIQ mean = 101.8). That is, the CD subjects did not have verbal deficits relative to *other* subjects, only relative to their own nonverbal abilities.

In contrast to Hodges and Plow (1990), two studies have reported CD–IQ links specific to VIQ. In Beitchman and colleagues' (1982) comparison of IQ scores to an estimated population mean of 100, they found the CD group had significantly lower VIQ, but not PIQ. As noted, Schonfeld and colleagues (1988) found significant VIQ deficits at ages 7 and 17 for CD subjects relative to non-CD controls in their urban sample of black male youth. The results for PIQ were of marginal significance ($p < .10$) at both ages, in the direction of poorer scores for CD youth. Lynam and colleagues (1993) found DELQ was more strongly linked to VIQ than to PIQ among white subjects.

Difficulties in PIQ for CD children sometimes have been reported as well. Frick and colleagues (1994) examined a sample using separate measures of ODD/CD symptoms and psychopathy and found a negative relationship between ODD/CD and PIQ (but not VIQ). As noted earlier, Nagin and colleagues (1995) results indicated that chronic offenders showed consistent VIQ *and* PIQ deficits, whereas the adolescent-limited offenders showed a PIQ deficit *earlier* than a VIQ deficit.

Two similar studies examined IQ as a protective factor among individuals at risk for antisocial behavior (Kandel *et al.*, 1988; White *et al.*, 1989). Although not analyzed for VIQ–PIQ differences, the CD groups' VIQ and PIQ deficits were comparable. In Kandel and colleagues' study, among the high risk groups, relative to noncriminals, criminals' VIQ and PIQ deficits were 12.6 and 12.4 points, respectively. (VIQ and PIQ means for low-risk groups were within 1 point). White and colleagues provided means separately for males and females. Across risk groups, relative to non-DELQ boys, DELQ boys had 6- to 7-point VIQ deficits and 5- to 7-point PIQ deficits; relative to non-DELQ girls, DELQ girls had 5- to 7-point VIQ deficits and 4- to 10-point PIQ deficits.

Thus, results from several studies have failed to support the notion that the intellectual deficit of CD youth is exclusively or primarily in the area of VIQ. Rather, when deficits have been observed, PIQ scores have often been lower as well.

Questions of Causality

Of the studies already reviewed, many also included questions regarding possible *causal* links between low IQ and CD. Although these types of data sets cannot answer questions of causality *directly,* correlational techniques have been used to examine the relative plausibility of different causal paths: (1) low IQ as a cause of CD, (2) CD as a cause of low IQ, and (3) a third variable as a cause of both CD and low IQ.

Results of two reports have supported the notion of low IQ contributing to CD. Schonfeld and colleagues (1988) interpreted their findings as indicating support for the hypothesis that low IQ contributes to CD, and failing to support the hypothesis that early aggression contributes to low IQ. In path analysis, IQ made a significant, independent contribution to predicting CD at age 17, whereas early aggression was not significantly related to later IQ once the link between early aggression and IQ at age 7 was controlled. As possible third variables, parental psychopathology and environmental disadvantage failed to account for the link between IQ and CD. In this urban sample of black male youth, environmental disadvantage was unrelated to CD, and aggression at age 7 only modestly predicted later CD. Hinshaw (1992) noted that shared method and rater variance may have affected the IQ–aggression correlations (as the IQ tester also rated aggression within the test context). Correlations may also have been affected by sample characteristics, which in turn would affect path analyses or attempts at causal modeling.

Goodman and colleagues (1995) studied a large sample of 13-year-old twins to contrast explicitly the plausibility of IQ as cause versus consequence of CD hypotheses. Additional potential predictors included twin IQ, parent IQ, and SES to address possible "third variable" causes. Correlations between IQ and CD were

−.21 and −.28 for parent and teacher ratings, respectively. With all predictors included, parent-rated CD was significantly predicted by child's IQ and SES; teacher-rated CD was predicted solely by child's IQ. Results were interpreted as most supportive of the "IQ as cause" hypothesis, as potential alternate causes failed to account for the link between IQ and CD.

Very different results were reported by Fergusson and colleagues (1993) and Loeber and colleagues (1995). Fergusson and colleagues found a relationship between low IQ and CD in childhood; however, in predicting adolescent offending, IQ did *not* add to the prediction from prior CD. In other words, the low IQ–CD link was already present by age 8, and then early antisocial problems alone predicted later antisocial problems. Loeber and colleagues reported that VIQ failed to contribute significantly in predicting CD onset. Instead, the combination of low SES, an earlier diagnosis of ODD, and parental substance abuse predicted a subsequent CD diagnosis, with low SES the strongest predictor in the equation.

Based on her findings, Moffitt (1990) concluded that lower VIQ could not be considered a contributing cause to pure delinquency in boys, that is, delinquency in the absence of comorbid attention problems. The pure DELQ group had never shown lower VIQs in prior assessments. On the other hand, the group that was DELQ+ADHD had shown consistently lower VIQ, as well as many other early developmental and environmental disadvantages. Regression analyses results indicated that, for the comorbid boys, low VIQ was a significant independent predictor. Thus, in this study, lower VIQ did not appear to be a contributing cause to pure delinquency, but was a factor in antisocial outcomes for boys with both CD *and* attention problems.

In evaluating competing causal hypotheses, there appears to be little support in any of these findings for viewing CD as a cause of low IQ. The data are mixed regarding low IQ as a cause for CD; this highlights in part how study design differences may influence results. Low IQ appeared causally linked to CD when ADHD was not assessed (as in Schonfeld *et al.,*

1988), and in a nonlongitudinal study (Goodman et al., 1995), which could not evaluate the developmental timing of CD onset with IQ patterns. The three longitudinal studies that included ADHD measures did not find low IQ to have a causal path to CD from childhood through adolescence, given that ADHD was statistically controlled (Fergusson et al., 1993; Loeber et al., 1995; Moffitt, 1990).

If CD and IQ are already correlated in childhood, as data such as Fergusson and colleagues (1993) indicated, the question arises of when and how that relationship emerges. A recent longitudinal study is relevant to the question, and the findings suggest a complex pattern. Lyons-Ruth, Easterbrooks, and Cibelli (1997) reported on a small sample ($N = 50$) for whom they had measures of mental development and mother–infant attachment at age 18 months, mothers' mental health, and ratings of externalizing (EXT) behaviors at age 7 years. Toddler mental development was significantly, negatively correlated to EXT at age 7 (–.31 and –.33 for mother and teacher ratings, respectively). In multivariate analyses to predict EXT, mental development did not contribute uniquely. However, there was a significant interaction between mental development and attachment quality; the combination of poorer mental development and disorganized-insecure attachment yielded the most EXT elevations.

CD AND EXECUTIVE FUNCTIONS AND SELF-REGULATION

Although much empirical attention has been given to the IQ test performance of CD youth, findings of IQ deficits provide little insight into the precise nature of their cognitive limitations. Some researchers have turned to the study of executive function (EF) tasks from a neuropsychological perspective for a clearer picture of what the CD-associated cognitive problems are. (See reviews by Moffitt, 1993, and Pennington & Ozonoff, 1996, for more comprehensive coverage of conceptual issues and research findings; for EF patterns in ADHD, see Chapters 5 and 13, this volume.)

In brief, EF tasks tap the individual's regulation of goal-directed behavior, including the planning of and persisting in task-relevant activities and the inhibiting of task-irrelevant thoughts and actions. EF abilities are more reflective of *how* one solves a problem, rather than one's acquired knowledge. Thus, one might hypothesize that part of what underlies the antisocial and disinhibited behavior of CD youth is poor or immature executive functioning, rather than a lack of general ability or knowledge per se.

Moffitt (1993) suggested that CD youth have difficulties in verbal abilities, which limit their capacity to use language as a means for self-control, as well as difficulties in EF. Recently, this suggestion received empirical support: Nigg, Quamma, Greenberg, and Kusche (1997) found EF performance uniquely contributed a modest but significant amount to subsequent aggression ratings, even when prior aggression was entered earlier in the regression equation.

Pennington and Ozonoff (1996) came to somewhat different conclusions regarding EF skills in CD youth. Although they agreed with Moffitt (1993) on the presence of verbal difficulties in CD subjects, they disagreed regarding EF abilities. They found many studies had reported EF deficits for ADHD youth; however, findings of EF problems for CD youth occurred only when subjects were selected without ruling out comorbid ADHD. Thus, Pennington and Ozonoff concluded that there has been no evidence for EF deficits in pure CD subjects. Schachar and Tannock's (1995) results (not reviewed by Pennington and Ozonoff, 1996) paralleled that summary, with EF deficits for ADHD and ADHD+CD groups; the pure CD group and controls did not differ, and showed better EF performance than the groups with ADHD. The Nigg and colleagues (1997) study described earlier did not adjust for ADHD symptoms; it sheds no further light on whether the EF difficulties in CD youth are present only for those who have accompanying ADHD problems.

More generally, executive functions include skills in self-monitoring and self-control (including delay of gratification and resistance to temptation); failure in these processes may result in antisocial and aggressive behaviors. Recent reviews have outlined conceptual frameworks, with supporting evidence, that highlight potential problem areas in learning, self-monitoring, and self-regulation for CD children (Lynam, 1996; Newman & Wallace, 1993; Quay, 1993). An extended review cannot be provided here but common features and parallel findings are noted.

Newman and Wallace (1993), Quay (1993), and Lynam (1996) consider the presence of reinforcement or rewards to be especially salient for CD children, and to interfere with their self-regulation. Heightened arousal and attention to rewards may negatively affect the child, in part by reducing attention to other environmental cues. For example, CD subjects have shown perseverative responding for reward in the face of changing contingencies and increasing punishment (e.g., Daugherty & Quay, 1991; Newman, Patterson, & Kosson, 1987; Shapiro, Quay, Hogan, & Schwartz, 1988); that is, they continued to seek reinforcement even when it was less and less available (by experimental manipulation). O'Brien and Frick (1996) found that nonanxious CD 6- to 13-year-olds (who may have had ADHD as well) showed more perseverative responding than groups of pure ADHD children, CD+Anxious children, and normal controls.

This pattern has not always been replicated: Milich, Hartung, Martin, and Haigler (1994) failed to find a significant correlation between CD symptoms and perseverative responding in a sample of 90 adolescents. CD symptoms were rated by both the subjects and their mothers; the sample consisted of 60 psychiatry outpatient clinic–referred youth and 30 adolescents from an alternative school for youth with disruptive behavior problems.

There are some differences in the hypothesized underpinnings of sensitivity to reward, and the nature of its interference with learning, among the conceptualizations of Quay (1993), Newman and Wallace (1993), and Lynam (1996). All, however, describe the pattern as (1) having psychobiological roots, (2) contributing to the stability of antisocial and disinhibited behavior across childhood to adulthood, and (3) occurring in subgroups of the population considered to be CD. Quay has concentrated on accounting for the subgroup of CD considered to be "undersocialized" (and thus overlapping most with childhood-onset CD); Lynam has described this pattern as occurring in the comorbid CD+ADHD subgroup; Newman and Wallace have focused on accounting for psychopathic subgroups of offenders and delinquents. No doubt these subgroups have considerable overlap.

Three studies with younger subjects have reported relations between resistance to temptation and heterogeneous behavior problems (BP). Cole, Usher, and Cargo (1993) found poorer resistance to temptation in preschool children rated as high in BP by their mothers and teachers; moderate and low BP groups did not differ in how long they resisted touching the "forbidden" candy jar. Campbell and colleagues (1994) also found their preschool BP group showed poorer resistance to temptation, as well as more aggression in play. Winsler and colleagues (1997) found teacher ratings of normal preschoolers' BP were significantly related to resistance to temptation at both the beginning and end of the school year. No relation, however, was found between BP and delay of gratification at either time.

It should be noted that skills in resisting temptation and delaying gratification typically develop across the preschool years and into middle childhood in normal children. Thus, studies with younger children may sometimes fail to find group differences or correlations with CD symptoms because of wide variability among young, typically developing subjects who are in the process of acquiring these self-regulation skills. Differences may be more obvious in samples with older children, when normal or non-CD clinic controls have mastered these basic self-monitoring and self-regulation skills. As examples, among third to sixth graders, Crick (1997) found that peer-rated aggressive children reported having more difficulty with self-restraint relative to comparison children. Krueger, Caspi, Moffitt, White, and

Stouthamer-Loeber (1996) found difficulties in delay of gratification among 12- to 13-year-old CD boys. Relative to boys with internalizing problems or nondisordered controls, CD boys were less likely to choose a longer delay interval for greater monetary reward.

CD AND SOCIAL COGNITION

Another broad area of inquiry regarding cognition in children with CD has been whether the pervasive social adjustment problems seen in CD youth can be accounted for by what or how they think about themselves and others. Two theoretical perspectives have guided most of this research, and the methods used have reflected these different views: cognitive-developmental approaches and information-processing approaches.

Cognitive-Developmental Perspectives

The cognitive-developmental perspective emphasizes age-related changes in children's thinking. In brief, in addition to quantitative changes in how much children know, there are several ways in which the *quality* of children's thinking shifts from preschool through adolescence. Important changes include (1) increasing ability to form abstract concepts and beliefs; (2) increasing ability to consider multiple perspectives simultaneously (i.e., others' views as well as one's own); (3) increasing ability to consider psychological and interpersonal attributes when thinking about self and others; and (4) increasing ability to engage in hypothetical, future-oriented reasoning, including consideration of multiple actions and related consequences.

Several areas of social-cognitive development have been examined to determine whether CD youth show difficulties or developmental immaturity, including emotion concept knowledge, beliefs about antisocial behavior, empathy and perspective-taking skills, and moral reasoning. A number of studies have found poorer functioning in children with DBD; these findings are briefly reviewed.

Emotion Concept Knowledge

Two early studies reported that errors in emotion labeling were asssociated with DELQ and aggression (McCown, Johnson, & Austin, 1986; Nasby, Hayden, & DePaulo, 1980). More recently, Lochman and Dodge (1994) found that aggressive (Ag) and violent (VIOL) adolescent groups differed from nonaggressive (NA) controls on use of the label "Happy" to stimulus vignettes; the NA group used the Happy label significantly *less* often than the other two groups, who did not differ. No differences were found in use of Fear, Anger or Sad. In a study of first and second graders, Cook, Greenberg, and Kusche (1994) identified children as high, medium, or low in parent-rated disruptive behaviors. With VIQ controlled, the groups did not differ on recognizing emotion cues, but the high-problem group was significantly less able to talk appropriately about the basic emotions of Happy and Sad. Cole and colleagues (1993) failed to find emotion labeling differences between preschoolers with heterogeneous behavior problems (by a combination of parent and teacher ratings) and controls. In interpreting the nonsignificant difference, the authors noted that there were many errors in *both* groups, suggesting that a labeling deficit may not emerge until later in development (i.e., when typically developing children have mastered the emotion concepts, but DBD children have not).

Beliefs about Antisocial Behavior

Some studies have reported that young children expect undetected, antisocial acts (e.g., theft, cheating, harm to other) will result in positive feelings for the actor (e.g., Arsenio & Kramer, 1992; Dunn, Brown, & Maguire, 1995). This has been interpreted as the child's focusing on positive, concrete outcomes for the actor, coupled with difficulty in simultaneously taking the perspective of both the actor and the victim. Generally, from roughly ages 4 to 8, children begin to acknowledge negative feelings for both the actor and the victim; that is, by middle childhood, children typically expect engaging in an antisocial act would lead to some negative feeling for the *actor.*

Several studies have reported links between positive beliefs about antisocial behavior and CD in middle childhood and adolescence. Miller (1997) found a modest, positive correlation between boys' beliefs about the acceptability of aggression (e.g., "It's OK to hit if . . .") and teacher-rated aggression in a sample of second to fourth graders; no link was found for girls. In a sample of third to sixth graders, Boldizar, Perry, and Perry (1989) asked peer-nominated aggressive (Ag) children and nonaggressive controls about possible outcomes of aggression. Relative to controls, Ag children attached greater value to controlling the victim and lower values to possible social rejection or the victim's suffering. Thus, while the groups did not differ on the importance of getting a tangible reward, Ag children were less concerned with the negative social consequences of aggression.

Two recent studies with delinquents examined the relationship between antisocial behavior and cognitive distortions that rationalize aggression. Barriga and Gibbs (1996) found that greater endorsement of cognitive distortions (e.g., "If someone is careless enough to lose a wallet, they deserve to have it stolen") correlated significantly with self-reports of aggression and delinquency (rs of .54 and .46, respectively). Liau, Barriga, and Gibbs (1997) found more specific links between distortions and behavior. Path analyses revealed that distortion regarding the acceptability of overt aggression was uniquely related to self-reports of overt aggressive behavior and distortion regarding covert aggression was uniquely related to covert acts.

Zhang, Loeber, & Stouthamer-Loeber (1997) examined links between attitudes toward delinquent acts (stealing, violence toward others) and self-reports of those acts in a large longitudinal study of boys ages 6–17. Overall, attitudes toward the delinquent acts become more tolerant across the age span. As in Liau and colleagues (1997), there was higher correspondence between tolerant attitudes and behaviors within domains than across; that is, favorable attitudes toward theft were more strongly associated with higher self-reports of theft than of aggression and favorable attitudes toward physical aggression were more strongly associated with higher rates of self-reported aggression than of theft.

Empathy and Perspective-Taking

In an earlier review, Hogan and Quay (1984) reported that CD subjects had frequently demonstrated difficulties in empathy and perspective-taking skills. Lee and Prentice (1988) reported mixed findings in examining empathy and perspective-taking: DELQ subjects showed poorer perspective-taking than controls (with VIQ controlled); there were no differences on the empathy measures. Chandler and Moran (1990) also failed to find differences in an empathy measure between incarcerated DELQ and controls (with IQ controlled). However, the link between poor perspective-taking and CD problems was more recently replicated by Lenhart and Rabiner (1995), who found that teacher-rated aggression was significantly related to perspective-taking in a high school sample.

In accounting for previous mixed findings on empathy measures, Cohen and Strayer (1996) suggested that DELQ groups may be so heterogeneous that empathy deficits might not always be observed, but that pure CD groups should show empathy deficits. In contrasting CD adolescents in a residential setting to community controls, the CD group performed more poorly on both the affective and cognitive components of the empathy tasks. In response to videotaped stimuli, the CD group showed poorer emotion recognition, reported fewer emotion matches, and, when they *did* report an emotion match, provided less cognitively complex reasoning and attributions when asked to explain the emotional response. Although IQ was not statistically controlled, Cohen and Strayer noted the CD subjects had IQs that were average or above (i.e., 89 or higher).

Moral Reasoning

Hogan and Quay's (1984) review found some initial support for the expected pattern of less mature moral reasoning among DELQ groups. Since then, that pattern has been replicated. Chandler and Moran (1990) found incarcerated delinquents showed less mature levels of moral reasoning with IQ controlled. Nelson, Smith, and Dodd (1990) reported a meta-analysis on 15 studies of moral reasoning in delinquents, and concluded that delinquents as a group show less mature moral reasoning. Among the 15 studies, 13 used IQ matches, 13 used SES matches, and 13 matched on both IQ and SES; thus, the results did not appear to be solely attributable to general cognitive or demographic factors.

Overall, a variety of evidence has demonstrated social cognitive difficulties for CD youth. Deficits in knowledge and immature thinking have been shown in their understanding of emotions and interpersonal consequences of aggressive acts, as well as their reasoning about other's feelings and perspectives and moral dilemmas. The general developmental pattern in these results suggests that these areas of social reasoning may be difficult for most children during the preschool period; however, with the transition through middle childhood to adolescence, CD youth show increasing problems relative to non-CD youth.

Social Information-Processing Perspectives

The work of Dodge and his colleagues has provided a considerable corpus of evidence regarding social information–processing difficulties in children with CD. For an extensive review of the earlier studies, the reader is referred to Dodge's (1986) description of the original model (which summarized early evidence), and Crick and Dodge's (1994) more recent review and revision of the model.

The initial model identified five major steps in the processing sequence: Encoding, Representation, Response Search, Response Decision, and Enactment. Given a social cue or stimulus, the child must perceive and attend to the cue (Encoding), interpret and give meaning to the cue (Representation), mentally generate possible actions for response (Response Search), evaluate the possible actions regarding their relative effectiveness and consequences and select one (Response Decision), and perform the response (Enactment).

Crick and Dodge's (1994) revision of the model provided a much more complex view of the child as a social-information processor. All steps from the prior model were retained; although there was some elaboration of Representation (step 2), now relabeled Interpretation of Cues, the summary in the preceding paragraph regarding the major cognitive activity at each step is still valid. However, one step was added, and the inclusion of the child's background knowledge was made much more central to the model. The additional step occurs between Interpretation (step 2) and Response (Search) Access and Construction (now step 4). Clarification of Goals has been added as Step 3. After Encoding and Interpreting the available cues, the child sets a goal for the interaction; the goal is an organizing guide for Response Search. This adds considerable complexity because emotional arousal and self-regulatory processes enter the model directly via the Goal step.

Highlighting of the child's background social knowledge and experience was indicated by bidirectional effects between processing and background knowledge at each step. Thus, the child's social memories, "scripts" and skills may directly enhance or impede effective processing at each step. Social script knowledge refers to "event packages," that is, knowledge of an entire sequence of highly familiar actions or interactions. Learning the sequence initially may require conscious thinking and action; with frequent practice, the behavior sequence can become automatic (i.e., "scripted"). Although such scripts could support positive, adaptive social exchanges, Crick and Dodge (1994) emphasize the negative potential for preemptive processing, or maladaptive script patterns that aggressive children may develop and use (leading to further social difficulties). The following section reviews recent research organized by processing step.

Step 1: Encoding

Assessment of this step measures the child's attention to and immediate memory for social cues. An early study by Milich and

Dodge (1984) contrasted four clinic groups plus a normal control group (NC). The clinic groups were Hyperactive+Aggressive (H+Ag), Aggressive only (Ag), Hyperactive only (H), and non-Hyperactive+non-Aggressive clinic controls (CC). Poorer performance was predicted for the H+Ag group relative to all other groups; no predictions were made for the Ag group. Subjects heard a large set of storylike stimuli (19 in all); story cue types were hostile, neutral, or benevolent. H+Ag boys recalled fewer *neutral* cues relative to all other groups; they did not differ in recall of hostile or benevolent cues. Statistical control for the H+Ag group's lower IQs did not account for their poorer performance. The Ag group was not contrasted to the CC or NC groups; the means showed modest differences.

Two recent studies also reported encoding deficits for groups with more severe problems. In Lochman and Dodge (1994), two groups were from school samples: boys identified by teachers as Aggressive (Ag) or Non-Aggressive (NA); the third group consisted of boys from a state program serving youth who had shown violent or assaultive behavior (VIOL). The VIOL boys showed encoding deficits; they recalled fewer cues than the Ag or NA groups, who did not differ. Again, although the VIOL group had a lower mean IQ, that general deficit did not account for their poorer encoding skills.

Dodge, Lochman, Harnish, Bates, and Pettit (1997) studied whether information-processing difficulties vary as a function of subtypes of aggression. For the elementary school sample, teacher ratings were used to assess Proactive (e.g., instrumental, bullying) and Reactive (e.g., angry, defensive) forms of aggression. For the juvenile offenders, case file information was rated for reactive and proactive behaviors. Elementary school subjects were sorted based on whether their aggression was predominantly Reactive (RA), predominantly Proactive (PA), or both (R+P); the juvenile offenders as either predominantly Reactive (RA) or predominantly Proactive (PA). Encoding problems were predicted only for the RA subjects. In the school sample, only the R+P group showed encoding deficits; the RA and PA subgroups did not differ. In contrast, among the juvenile offenders, as predicted, the RA subgroup showed poorer recall than the PA subgroup.

Summary. Encoding problems have emerged most often in more severely aggressive and comorbid youth (i.e., violently or pervasively aggressive, aggressive+hyperactive). These subjects may also have shown lower IQs but that did not appear to account for their processing difficulties at this step.

Step 2: Interpretation

Assessment of this step measures how the child interprets the social cues just encoded. Most often, children judge whether the cues indicate hostile, benign, or neutral intentions on the part of the actor in the stimuli vignettes.

Milich and Dodge (1984) reported only modest differences in Interpretation among their H+Ag, H, Ag, CC, and NC groups. Relative to the NC group, the H+Ag group showed the hostile attribution bias only when the question was asked in an open-ended format. None of the clinic groups differed from each other.

A stronger pattern of results was reported by Guerra and Slaby (1989) and Dodge, Price, Bacharowski, and Newman (1990). In an elementary school setting, Guerra and Slaby found that teacher-rated aggressive boys were more likely than nonaggressive controls to perceive hostility in social vignettes. Dodge and colleagues studied a sample of incarcerated adolescents and found significant correlations (rs from .20 to .25) between hostile attribution bias and several indices of CD (including rating scale measures of aggression and number of violent crimes). These relations remained significant after controlling for IQ, SES, and race. Of note was the pattern of correlations suggesting that the link between attribution bias and CD was specific to undersocialized CD and violent crime, rather than to Socialized Aggression and nonviolent crime. Dodge and colleagues interpreted this as indicating that hostile attribution biases may be linked specifically to their construct of Reactive Aggression rather than Proactive Aggression. This pattern may also suggest that hostile attribution bias is associated more strongly with childhood-onset CD than with adolescent-onset CD.

Quiggle, Garber, Panak, and Dodge (1992) also found evidence using a school sample categorized as Aggressive, Depressed, both, or controls. Main effects were found for both Aggression and Depression; problems with either were linked to showing a hostile attribution bias. Waldman (1996) reported on school-age boys categorized as Aggressive, Isolated, both, or controls based on peer ratings and nominations. Children were shown both hostile and nonhostile cues. The Aggressive groups showed a bias in attributing hostility to non-hostile cues even when attention and impulsivity problems were statistically controlled.

These links between aggression and attribution bias, however, have not always been successfully replicated. Crick and Dodge (1996) used school-based groups categorized as Reactively Aggressive (RA), Proactively Aggressive (PA), Both (R+P), or non-Aggressive (NA) by teacher ratings. In grades three and four, there were no group differences in Interpretation measures. At grades five and six, the RA group showed greater hostile interpretation than the NA group. However, the RA group did not differ from the PA group as predicted. Dodge and colleagues (1997) found no evidence for a hostile interpretive bias in the two samples examined: no differences were found among the school children categorized as RA, PA, R+P, or NA; nor between violent juvenile offenders characterized as predominantly RA or PA. Miller-Johnson and Maumary-Gremard (1997) found no link between aggression and attribution bias among first and second graders.

Additional variables that may affect whether the hostile attribution bias is shown include gender of the subject, target of the attribution, and the subject's emotional arousal. Boys have been more likely to show a pattern of hostile attribution than girls (e.g., Feldman & Dodge, 1987; Jakubowyc, 1997). The bias may be more likely when the attribution is about a peer rather than the subject's mother (Bickett, Milich, & Brown, 1996) or a nonhostile authority figure (Lochman & Dodge, 1994). Negative emotional arousal may also contribute to the hostile attribution bias (Craven & Lochman, 1997; Dodge & Somberg, 1987).*

Summary. As with Encoding, Interpretation difficulties appeared most frequently in more severely aggressive youth, multiproblem youth, or both. In the pattern of mixed findings, no single type of aggression clearly emerged as linked to hostile attribution biases, nor was this bias found to be unique to conduct problems. This bias pattern may be more characteristic of boys than girls and seen more often when peers are the target of the attribution or when children are negatively aroused.

Step 3: Clarification of Goals

Three recent studies have explicitly measured the goal-setting step and found that differences in goal type were linked to aspects of children's aggression. Lochman and colleagues (1993) studied adolescent males who had previously served as controls in a larger intervention study for aggressive youth. Subjects were presented with hypothetical ambiguous provocations, and asked what their social goals would be in that context. Goals of revenge and dominance were positively correlated to self-reports of crimes against persons and marijuana use. In addition, group comparisons indicated that aggressive males placed higher value on dominance and revenge goals.

Crick and Dodge (1996) reported that Proactively Aggressive (PA) children reported different goals. Compared to nonproactively aggressive children (including both nonaggressive and purely reactive aggressive groups), the PA reported more instrumental goals in a conflict situation. Erdley and Asher (1996) identified a large group of children who showed a hostile attribution bias, and then categorized them based on whether their response would be aggressive. They then looked for differences in

*Of related interest, Keltner, Moffitt, and Stouthamer-Loeber (1995) reported that boys rated as high in externalizing problems by teachers demonstrated more facial expressions of anger during a standardized testing situation than nonproblem youth, suggesting the possibility that CD youth may more often be negatively aroused and "primed" for hostile biases.

goals between children who endorsed aggressive responses and children who said their response to hostile provocation would be to withdraw or try to solve the problem. Aggressive responders endorsed negative goals (e.g., "get back" or "make the other feel bad") more strongly than the other subjects. The nonaggressive responders, even in the face of a perceived hostile provocation, strongly endorsed more prosocial goals (e.g., "getting along with the other").

Step 4: Response Access

Assessment at this step measures the child's suggestions for possible actions in response to the social "challenge" provided in the stimuli vignettes.

Rabiner, Lenhart, and Lochman (1990) examined whether aggressive children's poorer response access might be due to quick, automatic processing (e.g., through negative scripts from prior experience). They hypothesized that slowing down the response pattern might enable children to engage in more reflective and deliberate generation of response alternatives. Aggressive children were more likely to suggest enlisting others' help (considered a less mature response) and less likely to suggest assertive responses. As poorer performance was seen in a *delay* condition, the authors concluded that simply encouraging aggressive children to think more about what to do in social situations is unlikely to lead to more optimal problem solving.

Rudolph and Heller (1997) explored whether 10 preschoolers with teacher-rated externalizing problems (EXT) would benefit from more directive prompts when asked for solutions to hypothetical social problems. As expected, without a direct prompt for a prosocial solution, relative to controls, the EXT preschoolers gave fewer prosocial solutions. While the prompts (for the "nicest" action possible) led to more prosocial responses for both groups, the EXT children continued to give significantly fewer prosocial responses.

As in previous steps, more severe problem groups may have more difficulty at this step.

Milich and Dodge (1984) found their H+Ag group generated significantly more aggressive responses than normal control boys; however, there were no differences among the various clinic groups. Lochman and Dodge (1994) reported the VIOL groups were less effective at response access than the Ag and NA groups; the latter two did not differ significantly. In looking at subtypes, Dodge and colleagues (1997) also found that both P+R and RA groups suggested more aggressive responses than controls (and the PA group did not differ from controls).

Not all studies have found Response Access problems linked to aggressive status. Quiggle and colleagues (1992) found no group differences at this step. In a study of girls' information processing, Weiser and Foster (1997) found no aggression-related deficits in response access.

Results of two studies revealed context effects. Bickett and colleagues (1996) reported CD boys accessed more aggressive responses when vignettes were about peers or teachers; however, they rarely mentioned aggressive responses when vignettes were about their mothers, and did not differ from controls in this latter context. Perhaps the most interesting context effect was observed by Waldman (1996). When boys perceived the vignette actor's intent as hostile, aggressive and nonaggressive groups were similar in the aggressiveness of their suggested responses. However, when perceiving *non*hostile intent, aggressive boys suggested more aggressive responses; that is, they suggested aggression *regardless* of the social cues they perceived.

Summary. As with the earlier steps, problems at this step have been demonstrated more clearly for subjects who were more severely aggressive had comorbid attentional difficulties, or both, and may be more likely to occur in boys. Context effects reported by Bickett and colleagues (1996) and Waldman (1996) suggested a pattern of "scripts" in aggressive boys: a possibly more optimal script for interactions with their mothers (few aggressive responses regardless of her intentions) and a less optimal script with peers (more aggressive responses even in the face of neutral intentions).

Step 5: Response Decision

The individual's cognitive processes at this step include generating expectations about the outcomes of responses accessed in the previous step and evaluating how effective one might be at enacting those responses. Optimal processing would included choosing a response that leads to accomplishing the goal (set at Step 3) and that one could successfully perform.

Guerra and Slaby's (1989) aggressive boys generated fewer consequences for aggressive responses compared to controls. They summarized the pattern of aggressive boys' thinking as one of failure to anticipate negative consequences for aggression and less sensitivity to consequences for the social partner.

Positive expectations for aggression have typically been found in samples that included females. Among studies already noted, Weiser and Foster (1997) found in their all-girl sample that aggressive girls differed *most* in their positive evaluation of aggressive interaction strategies; Jakubowyc (1997) reported that girls', but not boys', aggressive response selection was concurrently related to self-reports of delinquency and aggression. With respect to aggression subtypes, Crick and Dodge (1996) and Dodge and colleagues (1997) found that PA groups of school-aged children expected more positive outcomes than non-PA groups.

Surprisingly, two reports of male-only samples found a weaker pattern of results with respect to positive outcome expectations for aggression. In their adolescent sample of violent offenders, Dodge and colleagues (1997) failed to find the expected difference of more positive expectations for aggression in the PA group. Lochman and Dodge (1994) failed to find significant differences in expectations among their VIOL, Ag, and NA subjects.

In addition to assessing outcome expectations, several of these studies also asked the subjects how confident they would be in performing these aggressive responses (to assess self-efficacy). Quiggle and colleagues (1992) and Erdley and Asher (1996) both reported aggressive children feeling confident about performing aggressive actions. Dodge and col-

leagues (1997) found that both PA and RA children had greater feelings of self-efficacy regarding aggression relative to nonaggressive controls.

Feelings of self-efficacy have sometimes differentiated among types of aggressive subjects. PA subjects reported greater self-efficacy regarding aggression when compared to non-PA school-age children by Crick and Dodge (1996). Dodge and colleagues (1997) failed to replicate this pattern in their school-age sample, but did find it when comparing groups of PA versus RA male adolescent offenders.

Summary. Unlike findings for other Social Information Processing (SIP) steps, links between response decision patterns and aggression have not emerged primarily for the most severely aggressive subjects. Although positive expectations and feelings of self-efficacy regarding aggression have been found in several studies, it is not yet clear if this pattern is unique to a particular type of aggression. Gender differences at this step may be worth further investigation.

CONCLUSION

Overall, what has this literature suggested about the cognitive functioning of children with CD? It appears that for childhood-onset CD there are two cognitive patterns. The majority of early-onset cases also have attentional problems. These children typically show cognitive difficulties from early an early age: They have lower IQs, have academic trouble at school onset and continuing onward (see Chapter 16, this volume), have problems developing age-appropriate social knowledge, and often show biased and maladaptive social information processing. In addition, they usually show executive function deficits and trouble in self-regulation. These cognitive limitations are also correlated with a wide range of other risk factors, including genetic, developmental, familial, and ecological variables associated with poor long-term adjustment. Thus, the cognitive difficulties of the CD+ADHD child are often part of a larger problematic picture.

The cognitive data also suggest a second, much smaller group of early-onset CD subjects. These children do not show the pervasive cognitive difficulties of the CD+ADHD children. Rather, their IQs are often comparable to normal controls, at least into early adolescence. They may also be less prone to encoding errors and hostile biases in social information processing. Nevertheless, they may be less likely to develop the social and emotional knowledge and skills required for adequate social adjustment in middle childhood, placing greater value on outcomes of aggressive acts, and minimizing aggression's negative social consequences. Heightened sensitivity to rewards and difficulty in delaying gratification may contribute to disinhibited and interpersonally maladaptive behavior patterns. Through childhood into adolescence, pure CD children's disruptive behavior may interfere in a cumulative fashion with social and academic adjustment, so that by adolescence IQ and achievement difficulties may begin to emerge.

The currently available data are difficult to interpret regarding "unique" patterns for adolescent-onset CD because most samples of adolescents would have included both child-onset and adolescent-onset cases. Overall, however, the most consistent findings of links between cognitive and social-cognitive difficulties and antisocial behavior (CD symptoms, delinquency markers) have been in this age range.

Methodologically, the frequent failure to assess ADHD symptoms has made teasing apart the CD–ADHD confound in cognitive performance data very difficult. Although many of the more recent IQ studies have included measures of ADHD, the majority of social-cognitive studies have not. Clearly, future studies must more carefully address this design issue.

Most of the literature here also provides little help in clarifying potential causal patterns between CD and cognition. There is ample evidence of various types of cognitive and social-cognitive difficulties throughout childhood and adolescence for youth with CD but CD measures and cognitive markers typically share 5%–15% of the variance regardless of the type of cognitive marker. To assess how cognitive factors contribute to developing or desisting from CD, we may need designs that enable researchers to study possible *interactions* between cognitive factors and other variables. For example, studies reviewed here found that family factors interacted with cognitive variables both to increase EXT symptoms, as when poorer toddler mental development combined with nonoptimal attachment relationships with their mothers (Lyons-Ruth *et al.*, 1997), and to decrease CD symptoms, as when boys' higher VIQs combined with better parental mental health (Lahey *et al.*, 1995). These findings hint that a fuller understanding of developmental patterns of both increases and decreases in CD will require a fuller picture of the child's family context and family relations as well as the child's cognitive and social cognitive profiles.

Regardless of the *causal* patterns, however, it is clear that children with CD frequently have cognitive and social-cognitive difficulties that no doubt contribute to ongoing social adjustment problems. These areas may be useful targets for intervention even if these deficits did not cause the disorder (see also Chapter 25, this volume), and they are worthy of much further study.

REFERENCES

Anderson, J., Williams, S., McGee, R., & Silva, P. A. (1989). Cognitive and social correlates of DSM-III disorders in preadolescent children. *Journal of the American Academy of Child and Adolescent Psychiatry, 28,* 842–846.

Arsenio, W., & Kramer, R. (1992). Victimizers and their victims: Children's conceptions of the mixed emotional consequences of moral transgressions. *Child Development, 63,* 915–927.

Barriga, A. Q., & Gibbs, J. C. (1996). Measuring cognitive distortion in antisocial youth: Development and preliminary validation of the "How I Think" Questionnaire. *Aggressive Behavior, 22,* 333–343.

Beitchman, J. H., Patterson, P., Gelfand, B., & Minty, G. (1982). IQ and child psychiatric disorder. *Canadian Journal of Psychiatry, 27,* 23–28.

Bickett, L. R., Milich, R., & Brown, R. T. (1996). Attributional styles of aggressive boys and their mothers. *Journal of Abnormal Child Psychology, 24,* 457–472.

Boldizar, J. P., Perry, D. G., & Perry, L. C. (1989). Outcome values and aggression. *Child Development, 60,* 571–579.

Campbell, S. B., Pierce, E. W., March, C. L., Ewing, L. J., & Szumowski, E. K. (1994). Hard to manage preschool boys: Symptomatic behavior across contexts and time. *Child Development, 65*, 836–851.

Ceci, S. J. (1991). How much does schooling influence general intelligence and its cognitive components? A reassessment of the evidence. *Developmental Psychology, 27*, 703–722.

Chandler, M., & Moran, T. (1990). Psychopathy and moral development: A comparative study of delinquent and nondelinquent youth. *Development and Psychopathology, 2*, 227–246.

Cohen, D., & Strayer, J. (1996). Empathy in conduct disordered and comparison youth. *Developmental Psychology, 32*, 988–998.

Cole, P. M., Usher, B. A., & Cargo, A. P. (1993). Cognitive risk and its association with risk for disruptive behavior disorders in preschoolers. *Journal of Clinical Child Psychology, 22*, 154–164.

Cook, E. T., Greenberg, M. T., & Kusche, C. (1994). The relations between emotional understanding, intellectual functioning and disruptive behavior problems in elementary school-aged children. *Journal of Abnormal Child Psychology, 22*, 205–220.

Craven, S. V., & Lochman, J. E. (1997, April). *A study of boys' physiological, emotional, and attributional processes in response to peer provocation at 3 levels of aggression.* Poster presented at the meeting of the Society for Research in Child Development, Washington, DC.

Crick, N. R. (1997). Engagement in gender normative versus nonnormative forms of aggression: Links to social-psychological adjustment. *Developmental Psychology, 33*, 610–617.

Crick, N. R., & Dodge, K. A. (1994). A review and reformulation of social information-processing mechanisms in children's social adjustment. *Psychological Bulletin, 115*, 74–101.

Crick, N. R., & Dodge, K. A. (1996). Social information processing mechanisms in reactive and proactive aggression. *Child Development, 67*, 993–1002.

Daugherty, T. K., & Quay, H. C. (1991). Response perseveration and delayed responding in childhood behavior disorders. *Journal of Child Psychology and Psychiatry, 32*, 453–461.

Dodge, K. A. (1986). A social information processing model of social competence in children. In M. Perlmutter (Ed.), *The Minnesota symposium on child psychology* (Vol. 18, pp. 77–125). Hillsdale, NJ: Erlbaum.

Dodge, K. A., & Somberg, D. R. (1987). Hostile attribution biases among aggressive boys are exacerbated under conditions of threat to the self. *Child Development, 58*, 213–224.

Dodge, K. A., Price, J. M., Bacharowski, J., & Newman, J. P. (1990). Hostile attribution biases in severely aggressive adolescents. *Journal of Abnormal Psychology, 99*, 385–392.

Dodge, K. A., Lochman, J. E., Harnish, J. D., Bates, J. E., & Pettit, G. S. (1997). Reactive and proactive aggres-

sion in school children and psychiatrically impaired chronically assaultive youth. *Journal of Abnormal Psychology, 106*, 37–51.

Dunn, J., Brown, J. R., & Maguire, M. (1995). The development of children's moral sensibility: Individual differences and emotion understanding. *Developmental Psychology, 31*, 645–659.

Erdley, C. A., & Asher, S. R. (1996). Children's social goals and self-efficacy perceptions as influences on their responses to ambiguous provocations. *Child Development, 67*, 1329–1344.

Feldman, E., & Dodge, K. A. (1987). Social information processing and sociometric status: Sex, age, and situational effects. *Journal of Abnormal Child Psychology, 15*, 211–227.

Fergusson, D. M., Horwood, L. J., & Lynskey, M. T. (1993). The effects of conduct disorder and attention deficit in middle childhood on offending and scholastic ability at age 13. *Journal of Child Psychology and Psychiatry, 34*, 899–916.

Fergusson, D. M., Lynskey, M. T., & Horwood, L. J. (1996). Origins of comorbidity between conduct and affective disorders. *Journal of the American Academy of Child and Adolescent Psychiatry, 35*, 451–460.

Frick, P. J., Kamphaus, R. W., Lahey, B. B., Loeber, R., Christ, M. A. G., Hart, E. L., & Tannebaum, L. E. (1991). Academic underachievement and the disruptive behavior disorders. *Journal of Consulting and Clinical Psychology, 59*, 289–294.

Frick, P. J., O'Brien, B. S., Wootton, J. M., & McBurnett, K. (1994). Psychopathy and conduct problems in children. *Journal of Abnormal Psychology, 103*, 700–707.

Goodman, R. (1995). The relationship between normal variation in IQ and common childhood psychopathology: A clinical study. *European Child and Adolescent Psychiatry, 4*, 187–196.

Goodman, R., Simonoff, E., & Stevenson, J. (1995). The impact of child IQ, parent IQ, and sibling IQ on child behavioral deviance scores. *Journal of Child Psychology and Psychiatry, 36*, 409–425.

Guerra, N. G., & Slaby, R. G. (1989). Evaluative factors in social problem-solving by aggressive boys. *Journal of Abnormal Child Psychology, 17*, 277–289.

Hinshaw, S. P. (1992). Externalizing behavior problems and academic underachievement in childhood and adolescence: Causal relationships and underlying mechanisms. *Psychological Bulletin, 111*, 127–155.

Hodges, K., & Plow, J. (1990). Intellectual ability and achievement in psychiatrically hospitalized children with conduct, anxiety and affective disorders. *Journal of Consulting and Clinical Psychology, 58*, 589–595.

Hogan, A. E., & Quay, H. C. (1984). Cognition in child and adolescent behavior disorders. In B. B. Lahey & A. E. Kazdin (Eds.), *Advances in clinical child psychology* (Vol. 7, pp. 1–34). New York: Plenum.

Jakubowyc, N. J. (1997, April). *Social-cognitive processes as predictors of social adjustment in urban, inner-city boys and girls.* Poster presented at the meeting of the Society for Research in Child Development, Washington, DC.

Kandel, E., Mednick, S. A., Kirkegaard-Sorenson, L., Hutchings, B., Knop, J., Rosenberg, R., & Schulsinger, F. (1988). IQ as a protective factor for subjects at high risk for antisocial behavior. *Journal of Consulting and Clinical Psychology, 56,* 224–226.

Keltner, D., Moffitt, T. E., & Stouthamer-Loeber, M. (1995). Facial expression of emotion and psychopathology in adolescent boys. *Journal of Abnormal Psychology, 104,* 644–652.

Krueger, R. F., Caspi, A., Moffitt, T. E., White, J., & Stouthamer-Loeber, M. (1996). Delay of gratification, psychopathology, and personality: Is low self-control specific to externalizing problems? *Journal of Personality, 64,* 107–129.

Lahey, B. B., Loeber, R., Hart, E. L., Frick, P. J., Applegate, B., Zhang, Q., Green, S. M., & Russo, M. F. (1995). Four year longitudinal study of conduct disorder in boys: Patterns and predictors of persistence. *Journal of Abnormal Psychology, 104,* 83–93.

Lee, M., & Prentice, N. M. (1988). Interrelations of empathy, cognition, and moral reasoning with dimensions of juvenile delinquency. *Journal of Abnormal Child Psychology, 16,* 127–139.

Lenhart, L. A., & Rabiner, D. L. (1995). An integrative approach to the study of social competence in adolescence. *Development and Psychopathology, 7,* 543–561.

Liau, A. K., Barriga, A. Q., & Gibbs, J. C. (1997, April). *Relations between self-serving cognitive distortions and overt vs. covert antisocial behavior in adolescents.* Poster presented at the meeting of the Society for Research in Child Development, Washington, DC.

Lochman, J. E., & Dodge, K. A. (1994). Social-cognitive processes of severely violent, moderately aggressive, and nonaggressive boys. *Journal of Consulting and Clinical Psychology, 62,* 366–374.

Lochman, J. E., Wayland, K. K., & White, K. J. (1993). Social goals: Relationship to adolescent adjustment and to social problem-solving. *Journal of Abnormal Child Psychology, 21,* 135–151.

Lochman, J. E., Bierman, K. L., & McMahon, R. J. (1997, April). Predictors of outcome: Parent characteristics, child characteristics, and intervention dosage. In *Prevention of antisocial behavior: Initial findings from the Fast Track Project.* Symposium conducted at the meeting of the Society for Research in Child Development, Washington, DC.

Loeber, R., & Hay, D. (1997). Key issues in the development of aggression and violence from childhood to early adolescence. *Annual Review of Psychology, 48,* 317–410.

Loeber, R., Green, S. Keenan, K., & Lahey, B. B. (1995). Which boys will fare worse? Early predictors of the onset of conduct disorder in a six year longitudinal study. *Journal of the American Academy of Child and Adolescent Psychiatry, 34,* 499–509.

Lynam, D. (1996). Early identification of chronic offenders: Who is the fledgling psychopath? *Psychological Bulletin, 120,* 209–234.

Lynam, D., Moffitt, T. E., & Stouthamer-Loeber, M. (1993). Explaining the relation between IQ and delinquency: Class, race, test motivation, school failure or self-control? *Journal of Abnormal Psychology, 102,* 187–196.

Lyons-Ruth, K., Easterbrooks, M. A., & Cibelli, C. D. (1997). Infant attachment strategies, infant mental lag, and maternal depressive symptoms: Predictors of internalizing and externalizing problems at age 7. *Developmental Psychology, 33,* 681–692.

McCown, W., Johnson, J., & Austin, S. (1986). Inability of delinquents to recognize facial affects. *Journal of Social Behavior and Personality, 1,* 489–496.

Milich, R., & Dodge, K. A. (1984). Social information processing in child psychiatric populations. *Journal of Abnormal Child Psychology, 12,* 471–490.

Milich, R., Hartung, C. M., Martin, C. A., & Haigler, E. D. (1994). Behavioral disinhibition and underlying processes in adolescents with disruptive behavior disorders. In D. K. Routh (Ed.), *Disruptive behavior disorders in childhood* (pp. 109–138). New York: Plenum.

Miller, L. (1997, April). *Girls' and boys' aggressive and prosocial behavior: The role of normative beliefs about aggression.* Paper presented at the meeting of the Society for Research in Child Development, Washington, DC.

Miller-Johnson, S., & Maumary-Gremard, A. (1997). *Peer rejection and aggression and early starter models of conduct disorder.* Poster presented at the meeting of the Society for Research in Child Development, Washington, DC.

Moffitt, T. E. (1990). Juvenile delinquency and attention deficit disorder: Developmental trajectories from age 3 to age 15. *Child Development, 61,* 893–910.

Moffitt, T. E. (1993). The neuropsychology of conduct disorder. *Development and Psychopathology, 5,* 135–152.

Nagin, D. S., Farrington, D. P., & Moffitt, T. E. (1995). Life-course trajectories of different types of offenders. *Criminology, 33,* 111–139.

Nasby, W., Hayden, B., & DePaolo, B. M. (1980). Attributional bias among aggressive boys to interpret unambiguous social stimuli as displays of hostility. *Journal of Abnormal Psychology, 89,* 459–468.

Nelson, J. R., Smith, D. J., & Dodd, J. (1990). The moral reasoning of juvenile delinquents: A meta-analysis. *Journal of Abnormal Child Psychology, 18,* 231–239.

Newman, J. P., & Wallace, J. F. (1993). Diverse pathways to deficient self-regulation: Implications for disinhibitory psychopathology in children. *Clinical Psychology Review, 13,* 699–720.

Newman, J. P., Patterson, C. M., & Kosson, D. S. (1987). Response perseveration in psychopaths. *Journal of Abnormal Psychology, 96,* 145–148.

Nigg, J. T., Quamma, J. P., Greenberg, M. T., & Kusche, C. A. (1997, April). *A two year longitudinal study of neuropsychological performance in relation to competence and symptoms in elementary school children.* Poster presented at the meeting of the Society for Research in Child Development, Washington, DC.

Noam, G. G., Paget, K., Valiant, G., Borst, S., & Bartok, J. (1994). Conduct and affective disorders in developmental perspective: A systematic study of adolescent psychopathology. *Development and Psychopathology, 6,* 519–532.

O'Brien, B. S., & Frick, P. J. (1996). Reward dominance: Associations with anxiety, conduct problems, and psychopathy in children. *Journal of Abnormal Child Psychology, 24,* 223–240.

Paternite, C. E., Loney, J., & Roberts, M. A. (1995). External validation of oppositional disorder and attention deficit disorder with hyperactivity. *Journal of Abnormal Child Psychology, 23,* 453–471.

Pennington, B. F., & Ozonoff, S. (1996). Executive functions and developmental psychopathology. *Journal of Child Psychology and Psychiatry, 37,* 51–87.

Pianta, R. D., & Caldwell, C. B. (1990). Stability of externalizing symptoms from kindergarten to first grade and factors related to instability. *Development and Psychopathology, 2,* 247–258.

Quay, H. C. (1993). The psychobiology of undersocialized aggressive conduct disorder: A theoretical perspective. *Development and Psychopathology, 5,* 165–180.

Quiggle, N. L., Garber, J., Panak, W. F., & Dodge, K. A. (1992). Social information processing in aggressive and depressed children. *Child Development, 63,* 1305–1320.

Rabiner, D. L., Lenhart, L., & Lochman, J. E. (1990). Automatic versus reflective social problem-solving in relation to children's sociometric status. *Developmental Psychology, 26,* 1010–1016.

Rudolph, K. D., & Heller, T. L. (1997). Interpersonal problem solving, externalizing behavior, and social competence in preschoolers: A knowledge–performance discrepancy? *Journal of Applied Developmental Psychology, 18,* 107–118.

Schachar, R., & Tannock, R. (1995). Test of four hypotheses for the co-morbidity of attention-deficit hyperactivity and conduct disorder. *Journal of the American Academy of Child and Adolescent Psychiatry, 34,* 639–648.

Schonfeld, I. S., Shaffer, D., O'Connor, P., & Portnoy, S. (1988). Conduct disorder and cognitive functioning: Testing three causal hypotheses. *Child Development, 59,* 993–1007.

Shapiro, S. K., Quay, H. C., Hogan, A. E., & Schwartz, K. P. (1988). Response perseveration and delayed responding in undersocialized aggressive conduct disorder. *Journal of Abnormal Psychology, 97,* 371–373.

Sonuga-Barke, E. J. S., Lamparelli, M., Stevenson, J., Thompson, M., & Henry, A. (1994). Behavior problems and preschool intellectual attainment: The associations of hyperactivity and conduct problems. *Journal of Child Psychology and Psychiatry, 35,* 949–960.

Taylor, E., Chadwick, O., Heptinstall, E., & Danckaerts, M. (1996). Hyperactivity and conduct problems as risk factors for adolescent development. *Journal of the American Academy of Child and Adolescent Psychiatry, 35,* 1213–1226.

Waldman, I. D. (1996). Aggressive boys' hostile perceptual and response biases: The role of attention and impulsivity, *Child Development, 67,* 1015–1033.

Weiser, P. H., & Foster, S. L. (1997, April). *Withdrawal and rejection as predictors of girls' information processing in peer entry and failure situations.* Poster presented at the meeting of the Society for Research in Child Development, Washington, DC.

White, J. L., Moffitt, T. E., & Silva, P. A. (1989). A prospective study replication of the protective effects of IQ in subjects at high risk for juvenile delinquency. *Journal of Consulting and Clinical Psychology, 57,* 719–724.

White, J. L., Moffitt, T. E., Caspi, A., Bartusch, D. J., Needles, D. J., & Stouthamer-Loeber, M. (1994). Measuring impulsivity and examining its relationship to delinquency. *Journal of Abnormal Psychology, 103,* 192–205.

Winsler, A., De Leon, J. R., Carlton, M. P., Barry, M. J., Jenkins, T. M., & Carter, K. L. (1997, April). *Components of self regulation in the preschool years: Stability, validity and relationship to classroom behavior.* Poster presented at the meeting of the Society for Research in Child Development, Washington, DC.

Zhang, Q., Loeber, R., & Stouthamer-Loeber, M. (1997). Developmental trends of delinquent attitudes and behaviors: Replications and synthesis across domains, time, and samples. *Journal of Quantitative Criminology, 13,* 181–216.

15

The Child with Oppositional Defiant Disorder and Conduct Disorder in the Family

CARYN L. CARLSON, LEANNE TAMM, and ANNE E. HOGAN

INTRODUCTION

In this chapter, we begin with a review of literature examining the child with Conduct Disorder (CD) or Oppositional Defiant Disorder (ODD) in the family setting, focusing on research using groups defined by DSM criteria. Next, we provide an integrative summary of findings in various domains, including marital discord and status, family functioning, parenting characteristics, parent–child interactions, and parental characteristics and psychopathology. We then identify methodological issues that may affect interpretation of results. We conclude with a discussion of theoretical models, including coercion theory (e.g., Patterson, 1976, 1982), attachment theory (e.g., Greenberg, Speltz, & DeKlyen, 1993), and a model of genotype–environment interaction (e.g., Scarr, 1989, 1992; Scarr & McCartney, 1983). We propose that the latter model offers a promising framework within which to conceptualize family influences on causal pathways and correlates of CD and ODD.

CARYN L. CARLSON and LEANNE TAMM • Department of Psychology, University of Texas at Austin, Austin, Texas 78712-1189.   ANNE E. HOGAN • Department of Psychology, University of Miami, Coral Gables, Florida 33124-0721.

Handbook of Disruptive Behavior Disorders, edited by Quay and Hogan. Kluwer Academic/Plenum Publishers, New York, 1999.

Many studies have used terms including "conduct problem," "behavior problem," "aggressive," "noncompliant," "at risk," and "delinquent," to describe children with a variety of disruptive behavior disorders (DBD); consequently, many presumed correlates of "conduct problems" identified in these studies may not be specific to CD or ODD but rather to CD or ODD comorbid with Attention-Deficit/ Hyperactivity Disorder (ADHD). Therefore, this review attempted to limit its focus to those studies using the terms ODD and CD. Although we initially attempted to confine the review to studies using DSM criteria to define groups, we also included studies using specified cutoff scores on standardized rating scales (see Chapter 3, this volume). Few studies explicitly excluded children with ADHD; however, we did not include studies that identified children as *primarily* ADHD if ODD/CD groups were not also examined.

REVIEW OF LITERATURE

Many of the relevant studies included dependent or outcome variables or both from a variety of domains, making it difficult to organize the review by topic. Instead, studies are grouped by method, that is, whether the study employed report measures, observational measures, or both. Although some studies included both boys and girls and both mothers and fathers, the majority of samples consisted of male subjects and their mothers. When studies included girls or fathers or both, a special note is made. Also, unless otherwise noted, inclusion in the CD/ ODD groups was based on DSM-III (American Psychiatric Association, 1980) or DSM-III-R (American Psychiatric Association, 1987) diagnoses. Information relevant for CD subtyping was rarely provided.

Report-Based Studies

Fendrich, Warner, and Weissman (1990) examined the effect of family discord on psychopathology in children of depressed and nondepressed parents. Participants were 91 families with a total of 220 offspring (48% male, and ranging in age from 6 to 23 years). Among the offspring, 20% were diagnosed with CD, 64% were diagnosed with depression or anxiety disorders, and 30% had no psychiatric diagnosis. Of the 220 children examined, 153 were from 65 families with one or both parents exhibiting depression and 67 from 26 families with neither parent exhibiting depression. Parents provided information on divorce, parent–child discord, marital adjustment (Short Marital Adjustment Test [SMAT]; Locke & Wallace, 1959), family cohesion (Family Adaptability and Cohesion Evaluation Scale [FACES]; Olson, Sprenkle, & Russell, 1979), and "affectionless control" (i.e., parenting characterized by low caring plus high control rated on the Parental Bonding Instrument ([PBI]; Parker, Tupling, & Brown, 1979). High rates of parent–child discord, parental depression, and divorce were associated with a diagnosis of CD. Low family cohesion was associated with childhood diagnoses of both depression and CD. Parent–child discord and parental divorce were more important as risk factors for CD than for anxiety or depression.

Haddad, Barocas, and Hollenbeck (1991) examined the relationships among situational characteristics, maternal cognitive variables, family environment dimensions, and CD by comparing CD (n = 23), Anxiety Disorder (n = 20), and clinic control boys (n = 25) on demographic and family functioning measures. Boys ranged in age from 9 to 13 years. Controls were found to have higher SES and a higher percentage of intact families than the clinical groups. The groups did not differ on maternal cognitive variables, levels of organization and control (assessed by the Family Environment Scale [FES]; Moos & Moos, 1976), or family emphasis on moral concerns or personal growth. With SES, family status, stress level, and satisfaction with marital and family roles controlled, mothers and sons in the CD group reported lower family cohesion and more conflict than the control and Anxiety Disorder groups. The CD group had a lower active-recreational orientation than the controls but did not differ from the Anxiety Disorder group. The authors concluded that quality of family relations is the best predictor of boys' antisocial behavior, and that family discord, rather than family disruption (e.g., divorce or separation) itself, increases the risk for the development of CD.

Lahey, Hartdagen, and colleagues (1988) examined the relationships among divorce, parental Antisocial Personality Disorder (APD), and CD. They hypothesized that the findings that have linked the development of CD to marital discord or divorce have been confounded with parental psychopathology and, in particular, APD. A clinic sample was used, with 28 CD boys and 34 boys with other diagnoses; age range was 6–13. A multivariate analysis revealed that divorce was not directly associated with CD beyond the variance accounted for by parental (primarily paternal) APD. The authors concluded that there is no direct relationship between CD and divorce but rather that APD is strongly related to both. Two limitations of the study were the small number of married parents with APD (n = 2), and that paternal diagnoses were most often based on maternal report.

The following five studies examined differences in family variables among DBD subgroups; subjects had single diagnoses of CD, ODD, ADHD, or were comorbid for CD+ADHD or ODD+ADHD. Schachar and Wachsmuth (1991) examined family dysfunction and psychosocial adversity in the families of ADHD

(n = 18), ODD/CD (n = 15), ADHD+CD (n = 25), Emotional Disorder (ED; n = 20), Learning Disabled (LD; n = 22), and nondiagnosed control boys (n = 20). Children were 7–11 years of age; both parents provided ratings of family functioning using the Family Assessment Measure (FAM; Skinner, Steinhauer, & Santa-Barbara, 1983). Relative to other groups, the ADHD+CD and ODD/CD groups reported greater weaknesses on numerous dimensions of family functioning by both parents' reports. Specifically, these findings suggest lack of agreement regarding role expectations, insufficient or masked communications, rigid or destructive efforts at control often characterized by overt or covert power struggles, and an absence of shared values and norms in the families of children with ODD/CD (with or without accompanying ADHD). The greatest psychosocial adversity was associated with the ED and ODD/CD groups. In particular, these groups had fewer intact families than ADHD and ADHD+CD subjects; ED and ODD/CD groups had parental divorce rates double that of the ADHD+CD and ADHD groups. Family violence reported by the children was higher for all diagnostic groups than controls, but this was partially accounted for by the comparatively high rate of marital violence in the ODD/CD and ADHD+CD groups. The authors concluded that pathological family interactions are more characteristic of CD children than ADHD children.

In investigating the distinction between ODD and ADHD, Paternite, Loney, and Roberts (1995) measured a large set of behavioral, cognitive, and family variables. Subjects included ODD (n = 9), ADHD (n = 20), ODD+ADHD (n = 40), and control (n = 28) boys from 6 to 12 years of age. With respect to the family variables, the authors hypothesized that the boys with ODD would differ from non-ODD boys on family measures (SES and family functioning). Although there were no pure ODD effects on any family measure, the ODD+ADHD group reported greater family conflict than the ODD and control groups, and less family cohesion than the ADHD and control groups.

Lahey, Piacentini, and colleagues (1988) compared parental psychopathology and anti-social behaviors in a clinic sample of 6- to 14-year-old children with CD (n = 14), with ADHD (n = 18), with CD+ADHD (n = 23), and non-CD/non-ADHD clinic controls (n = 30). Custodial biological parents were interviewed; for 95% of subjects, mothers provided information on both parents. Mothers of children with CD (regardless of the child's ADHD status) reported more depression and APD; they were also more likely to report engaging in physical fighting and having served a prison sentence. Similarly, children with CD fathers showed greater APD, fighting, and incarceration, as well as greater substance abuse. Although data on most of the fathers was by maternal report, nevertheless the findings supported the association of higher rates of psychopathology and antisocial behavior among both mothers and fathers of CD children than among parents of clinic-referred children without CD.

Frick and colleagues (1992) examined parental psychopathology (in both mothers and fathers) and maternal parenting styles in the families of ODD and CD boys. Children ranged in age from 7 to 12; there were 70 ODD boys, 68 CD boys, and 39 control boys. Parental adjustment was assessed utilizing structured DSM-III-R (American Psychiatric Association, 1987) clinical interviews including the modules for Major Depressive Episode, APD, alcohol abuse, and drug abuse. To assess parenting styles, mothers provided information about (1) supervision, (2) consistency in discipline, (3) time spent together, and (4) frequency of discussions. Neither ODD nor CD was associated with a parental affective disorder. However, the CD group had a significantly higher proportion of APD parents than did ODD children; both groups differed significantly from controls. The parents in the CD group had a significantly higher rate of substance abuse than controls, but did not differ significantly from the parents in the ODD group (which fell intermediate to the CD and control groups). Further, it was revealed that these associations were accounted for by *paternal* diagnoses; no maternal diagnosis was associated with ODD or CD. When compared on maternal parenting variables, the ODD and CD groups did not differ on time spent together or frequency of discussions. However, the CD group's mothers reported significantly less supervision and persistence with discipline than controls. The ODD group did not differ significantly from either group, but again fell in the intermediate range between the two. Multivariate analyses to predict diagnostic status revealed that there was a main effect only for paternal APD; maternal parenting and interaction terms were not significant. The authors concluded that paternal APD appears to be a significant risk factor for a child to develop CD, independent of maternal parenting behavior.

Schachar and Wachsmuth (1990) compared CD (*n* = 22), ODD (*n* = 21), and control (*n* = 20) groups of 7- to 11-year-old boys on a number of variables, including child and demographic characteristics, family dysfunction (FAM), psychosocial adversity, and parental psychopathology. Mothers in the ODD group reported more problematic marital relationships than mothers in the CD and control groups. Mothers in both the ODD and CD groups reported more dysfunction in their relationship with their sons than did mothers of controls. Fathers in the ODD and CD groups rated their families as more dysfunctional than did fathers of controls. On measures of psychosocial adversity, the groups differed on separation from father (CD > ODD), and family violence (CD = ODD > control). Analyses of a mean composite score of family adversity revealed that the ODD group fell between CD and control groups but did not differ significantly from either. Compared to controls, ODD and CD groups had higher rates of paternal psychopathology (most commonly substance abuse, alcoholism, and APD), but the three groups did not differ on maternal psychopathology. Overall, the ODD group had higher rates of paternal psychopathology, LD, social difficulties, and family dysfunction than controls, and were indistinguishable from CD children.

Johnson and O'Leary (1987) examined demographic characteristics, marital satisfaction, parental aggression, and parenting style in families of CD and control girls recruited through a newspaper advertisement. In this study, girls were identified as CD using the Conduct Problem subscale of the Revised Behavior Problem Checklist (RBPC; Quay & Pe-

terson, 1983, 1996), with 25 in the CD group and 17 controls. The girls ranged in age from 9 to 11. Data were gathered from daughters, mothers, and fathers. The groups did not differ on demographic variables except mothers' ages: CD girls' mothers were younger. Children's perceptions of their parents' marriage was also assessed. Parents and girls in both groups had similar perceptions of the parental marriage. Parents of CD girls rated themselves as more hostile and aggressive. Specifically, mothers of CD girls were more openly hostile toward their spouses than the mothers of controls, and fathers of CD girls were more aggressive than fathers of controls. The mothers' behavior patterns tended to be more closely associated with children's behavior patterns than were fathers' (i.e., children's CD scores were significantly correlated with mothers' self-report of negative behavior and aggression).

Rey and Plapp (1990) examined parenting styles as reported by CD, ODD, and control 12- to 16-year-olds. The CD group had 62 subjects (54% male); the ODD group had 42 subjects (54% male); the control group had 62 subjects (63% male). Adolescents rated their parents using the PBI (Parker *et al.,* 1979). ODD and CD groups differed from controls on maternal care (ODD < control) and paternal overprotection (ODD > control); the CD group also differed from controls on maternal overprotection (CD > control) and paternal care (CD < control). There were no differences between the CD and ODD group ratings of parental care and protection.

Holcomb and Kashani (1991) examined the personality style, expressed concerns, and behavioral correlates of adolescents attending public school. A subsample (representing 7% of all adolescents attending school in Columbia, Missouri; overall, 50% male) was divided into CD (*n* = 13) and non-CD (*n* = 137) groups by structured interview. Both groups completed the Millon Adolescent Personality Inventory (MAPI; Millon, Green, & Meagher, 1984). The CD group rated their family life as less satisfactory, as less nurturing, and as having greater conflict than the non-CD group.

In an effort to extend Patterson's family coercion model (Patterson, 1976, 1982), Baden and Howe (1992) hypothesized that parental attributions about the etiology of child behavior problems and parental expectancies regarding the effectiveness of their parenting techniques contribute to coercive exchanges. Subjects were 40 mothers of clinic-referred CD adolescents and 40 mothers of matched nonreferred control adolescents (ages 11–18; 82% male). CD status was determined using the Eyberg Child Behavior Inventory (ECBI; Eyberg & Ross, 1978) conduct problem scale. The sample was predominantly Caucasian, of lower SES, and less well educated than national norms; the two groups did not differ on demographic characteristics except that controls tended to have more years of schooling and a higher income. Analyses comparing clinic and control group mothers revealed that mothers of CD children viewed their child's misbehavior as intentional, and ascribed the causes of misbehavior as global, stable, and beyond their control. The two groups of mothers did not differ in their beliefs regarding the effectiveness of parenting techniques, but mothers of CD adolescents were less likely to believe the techniques would be effective when applied to their own children. The authors described their results as consistent with Patterson's model, in which parents engaging in coercive interactions tend to blame their children for their misbehavior. Blame is likely to become part of a cognitive-affective set that contributes to further initiation of coercive cycles. The authors attempted to extend Patterson's model by suggesting that a stance of helplessness in the parent is an additional component of the coercive interaction.

Bickett, Milich, and Brown (1996) examined whether aggressive boys and their mothers shared a propensity to infer hostility in ambiguous interpersonal situations. Participants included 25 mothers of 7- to 12-year-old boys diagnosed with DBD (i.e., 5 CD, 1 CD+ ADHD, 2 ODD, 10 ADHD+ODD, and 7 ADHD children) who had a score greater than 70 on the Aggressive factor of the CBCL (Achenbach, 1978) and 25 mothers of control children, recruited from an outpatient pediatric clinic, who were not exhibiting behavioral or psychiatric problems. The groups were matched on race, SES, age, and verbal ability.

Mothers were asked to complete attribution scales involving both negative and ambiguous outcomes after the following two sets of conditions: (1) hypothetical situations involving maternal interactions with a peer, her partner, and her son; and (2) hypothetical situations involving her son's interactions with a classmate and teacher. Children were presented with five hypothetical situations in which the child was described as the recipient of a negative outcome at the hands of his mother, teacher, or classmate. Children were also asked two open-ended questions (why it had occurred and what they would do) after each situation; responses were coded for hostile versus benign attributions and aggressive versus nonaggressive responses. Mothers of aggressive boys were more likely to make hostile attributions about their child's behavior than control mothers; however, the groups did not differ on aggressiveness of response. Further, mothers of aggressive boys tended to make more hostile attributions in both hostile and ambiguous situations, compared with control mothers who tended not to rate ambiguous situations as hostile. Similarly, aggressive boys made more hostile attributions than controls and indicated a significantly higher propensity to respond aggressively. The authors tentatively suggested that the hostile attributional bias, rather than aggressive responses, may be modeled and reinforced by mothers of aggressive children.

Observation-Based Studies

Anderson, Lytton, and Romney (1986) observed mothers' reactions to children (ages 6–11) during three laboratory tasks. Subjects included 32 mother–child dyads (16 clinic-referred CD boys, 16 Boy Scout controls), with subjects matched on demographic characteristics. In three 15-min sessions (5 min each of free play, cleanup, and computations), mothers were videotaped interacting with their own child, with another child from same group, and with a child from the other group. Interactions were coded every 10 s for positive, negative, and neutral responses; mother requests and child compliance were also tallied. Mothers in both groups made more negative responses and more requests to CD children than to controls. Further, an interaction revealed that CD mothers were more negative with their own CD child than with other CD children. CD children complied less than controls across conditions (e.g., with mothers of another CD child, their own mother, and control mothers). The authors concluded that interactions are "driven mainly by the child and not the mother" (p. 607), and that neither maternal behavior alone nor the combination of child–mother behavioral styles determines the expression of CD.

Brunk and Henggeler (1984) experimentally examined a model of parent–child bidirectionality that proposes that members of dyadic systems maintain an equilibrium by behaving in a certain fashion. Specifically, the model suggests that when the rate of a behavior by one member falls below a certain threshold, the other member will act to elicit that behavior (lower limit control). Alternatively, when one member's behavior goes above a certain threshold, the other member will act to reduce this behavior (upper limit control). Two 10-year-old boys with similar appearances and above average IQs were trained and paid as confederates. One was trained to behave as a child with an Anxiety Disorder and one was trained to behave as a child with CD. Examples of anxious behaviors included avoiding looking at, smiling at, or talking to the adult, quiet and passively noncompliant behavior, downcast eyes, poor posture, and a downturned mouth. CD behaviors included being aggressively noncompliant, avoiding looking at the adult, refusing every command, doing things his own way, glaring, acting cocky, and noncooperative behavior. Subjects included 32 middle-class mothers who were videotaped playing checkers with the confederate, and instructed to use their own control strategies. After the session, the adults were interviewed and debriefed. Both mothers and confederates were scored for verbal responsiveness and response to directives, boys' changes in activity level were coded, and adults' upper and lower limit controls were coded. Interestingly, the results supported the model of bidirectionality. Overall, adults exhibited more stimulating controls (helping and rewards) with the "anxious" child

and more restrictive controls (ignoring, commands, and discipline) with the "CD" child. An analysis of sequential measures revealed that when both confederates emitted the same behavior, the mothers responded differentially (e.g., the "CD" child's compliance elicited discipline but not reward; the "anxious" child's compliance elicited reward and not discipline). The authors suggested that the adults formed a cognitive set early in the session and then maintained the behavioral style to retain control over the child.

Snyder, Schrepferman and St. Peter (1997) conducted a test of two theoretical models of socialization, negative reinforcement and affect dysregulation, and their respective contributions to the development of childhood antisocial behavior. A sample of 57 boys referred for treatment of conduct problems and their families were observed interacting in their home for at least six fifteen minute sessions on four different occasions. Parent–child and sibling interactions were coded using the Family Process Code. These codes were subsequently collapsed into content (aversive and non-aversive) and affect (positive and negative) summary categories. Results indicated that the boys's initiation and reciprocation of aggressive behavior was directly and linearly related with the probability that parents negatively reinforced aggressive behavior during conflict. A similar pattern was found for affect dysregulation, such that boys were most likely to reciprocate aggressive behavior when in a negative affect state, and this was more probable given their parents's negative affect state. These findings held true for sibling interactions also. Tests of the two theoretical models indicated that both contributed significantly to the development of antisocial behavior, as assessed by three follow-up measures (placement outside of home, arrest records, and school discipline incidents) assessed two years after study completion. The authors concluded that both models likely interact in a synergistic fashion in their contribution to the development of conduct problems, such that negative affective states increase the probability of conflict, which potentially sets up a negative reinforcement contingency and increases the likelihood that parents and children will resort to aggressive measures to deal with the conflict.

The next three studies reviewed were conducted by Dadds, Sanders, and colleagues, and based on a common sample of approximately 70 children. The first study described reported on only observational data. The remaining two are described in the following section, as they reported findings from both report and observational measures.

Dadds, Sanders, Morrison, and Rebgetz (1992) examined family interaction patterns in the homes of 73 7- to 14-year-olds (88% males). Diagnostic groups were CD (n = 27), depressed (n = 18), comorbid CD+depressed (n = 12), and control children (n = 16). The authors hypothesized that parents in the clinical groups would exhibit more aversive behaviors than control parents but that, consistent with Patterson's model of reciprocality, only the CD (with or without depression) children would respond in kind. Parents and children were coded for aversive behavior; children were also coded for deviant behavior. Parents of CD children directed more aversive behavior (questions, instructions, and social attention deemed aversive because of content or tone of voice) to their children than control parents, but did not differ significantly from parents of comorbid CD+depressed and depressed children. The CD children and their siblings exhibited more deviant behavior (demanding, noncompliant, oppositional) than the children in the other three groups. Surprisingly, the CD+depressed children did not differ from the depressed or control groups in deviant behavior. Mothers in all three clinical groups engaged in less smiling than control mothers. The authors concluded that the aversive behavior displayed by the CD child is reciprocated by parents and siblings, and the CD family system is marked by negativity and coercion, consistent with Patterson's model. Further, they noted that parental aversiveness is a better predictor of clinical outcome than lack of positive behaviors. The authors suggested that the pure CD group may be more likely to display oppositional behavior in a scrutinized setting, with co-occurring depression limiting the expression of aggression.

Studies Combining Report and Observation

Sanders, Dadds, Johnston, and Cash (1992) examined marital satisfaction, self-reported depression, and mother–child interactions in families with CD, depressed, comorbid CD+ depressed, and nonclinic control children (same group sizes as in Dadds et al., 1992). Groups were matched as closely as possible on demographic variables; however, the control group mothers had a higher SES. Mother–child dyads were videotaped for 10 min: 5 min discussing an issue designated as problematic for the child and 5 min discussing an issue designated as problematic for the parent. The interactions were coded for positive solution, aversive content, and affective codes (based on nonverbal behaviors). At the end of each interaction, the mother and child completed a Likert scale rating the other's affect during the interaction. CD mothers expressed a lower level of marital satisfaction than all other groups; however, their mean scores fell in the nondistressed range. During the problem-solving interactions, both CD children and their mothers had higher levels of aversive content and angry affect and fewer positive problem solutions. In addition, CD children demonstrated higher rates of depressed affect. CD mothers rated their children as showing more angry and less happy affect than comparison mothers. The authors highlighted the centrality of interpersonal problem-solving deficits in CD and suggested that CD children reciprocate the level of angry affect and aversive verbal behavior displayed by their parents.

Sanders and Dadds (1992) examined reports from both mothers and fathers and the mother–child dyadic interaction data just described. Contrast groups were the ODD/CD group (n = 25) and normal controls (n = 17). ODD/CD mothers rated themselves as more depressed and less satisfied with their marriage than control mothers. ODD/CD fathers also reported lower levels of marital satisfaction than controls, but did not differ from controls on self-rated depression. Compared to controls, ODD/CD children and their mothers showed less optimal cognitions about the family (i.e., fewer positive and more negative cognitions). The ODD/CD parents also tended to rate their child more negatively during problem-focused discussions. The authors suggested that the parents' negative self-cognitions may interfere with accurate information processing during problem solving and may result in an inability to generate constructive solutions. They further suggested that the mother may "escalate reciprocally in the face of child hostility" (p. 377).

Field and colleagues (1987) compared CD, depressed, and normal control boys' play interactions with their mothers in order to examine differences in temperament and behavior; maternal characteristics were also compared. Subjects were 56 mother–child dyads: 38 recruited from a developmental follow-up clinic (18 CD, 20 depressed) and 18 normal controls. Boys were 4–8 years of age and matched on demographic characteristics. Mothers provided demographic information and completed questionnaires on parenting characteristics, their own depression, temperament, locus of control, and child behavior. In addition, mother-and-child play interactions were videotaped in four situations: mother–child free play, child–mother teaching task, child solitary free play, and child solitary puzzle completion. The interactions were coded for social and disciplinary behaviors modeled, aggressive behavior, and physical affection. Children wore an activity bracelet monitor to establish the global activity levels in each interaction. Mothers of CD children rated themselves as more depressed, as having an external locus of control, as being more disapproving, and as being less nurturant in child-rearing practices. CD children and their mothers were rated as less interactive in the sessions. In addition, CD mothers rated their children as having more active temperaments and, in fact, CD children demonstrated more motoric activity and off-task behavior during the sessions.

Slee (1996) examined maternal perceptions of the family climate in 19 mothers of CD children (79% boys) and 19 control mothers. All mothers completed the FES (Moos & Moos, 1976). In addition, a subsample of 9 mother–child dyads from each group were observed interacting in the home. Compared to controls, mothers of CD children rated their families as less cohesive, less expressive of feelings, expressing more open conflict, less encouraging of independence, less involved in active recreational pursuits, less organized, and more control oriented. CD mothers viewed their families as lacking in structure and clarity regarding familial roles and rules. Mothers also rated the family in which they were raised; CD mothers rated their families of origin as less cohesive and less encouraging of independence than control mothers. No significant differences were observed between groups on discrete behavior categories (i.e., comment, instruct, question, and silence). On ratings of control and warmth, CD mothers were significantly more controlling than control mothers, but did not differ on ratings of warmth. The authors suggested that the maternal perceptions of the family climate may be influenced by the presence of a CD child in the family for an extended period of time. Further, they suggested that the current results were consistent with systems theory, which posits the influence of intergenerational influence in families.

Vuchinich, Wood, and Vuchinich (1994) examined family problem-solving styles of CD, at risk for CD, and control groups. They hypothesized that the strength of the parent–child and mother–father coalitions, as well as parental warmth, were associated with family problem solving. Subjects were from 188 families with children ranging in age from 8 to 13. CD status was determined by elevated scores (> 70th percentile) on the Aggression, Delinquency, or Externalizing subscales of the RCBCL (Achenbach, 1991). The at-risk group included a subset of children and their families with the children attending schools with the highest rates of juvenile delinquency (above the 66th percentile) as determined by examining police records. The CD group consisted of 30 children and their families, the at-risk group consisted of 68 children and their families, and there were 90 controls. Overall, the CD group demonstrated less effective problem-solving skills than the at-risk and control groups; the at-risk group also demonstrated less effective problem solving than controls. Further, the CD group was found to have lower SES, lower marital satisfaction, and less parental warmth than the at-risk and control groups. Multiple regression results, with all psychosocial and experimental variables entered simultaneously, revealed that (1) parental warmth was positively associated with family problem solving in all three groups, (2) stronger parental coalitions were "significantly linked to fewer beneficial problem-solving processes" (p. 418) in the CD and at-risk groups, and (3) the parent–child coalitions had no significant effects in any of the three groups. The authors concluded that the findings are consistent with a scapegoating pattern in which the parents side with each other in blaming the child for problems in the family. However, they noted that further longitudinal studies are needed to isolate the specific mechanism through which parental coalitions are linked to family problem solving.

SUMMARY OF FINDINGS

Marital Status and Discord

Of the five studies reviewed that examined marital status, three found CD to be associated with higher divorce rates (Fendrich et al., 1990; Lahey, Hartdagen, et al., 1988; Schachar & Wachsmuth, 1991). Sanders and Dadds (1992) and Schachar and Wachsmuth (1990) did not find rates of divorce to be higher in CD families. In the only study to also contrast CD and ODD groups, Schachar and Wachsmuth (1990) found no difference in divorce rates. It should be noted that relatively low divorce rates were reported for all groups in the three studies conducted outside the United States. Given the mixed results, no definitive conclusions about divorce in CD/ODD families can be drawn.

Of the seven studies examining marital discord or satisfaction, five reported more marital distress in parents of CD children (Fendrich et al., 1990; Sanders & Dadds, 1992; Sanders et al., 1992; Schachar & Wachsmuth, 1991; Vuchinich et al., 1994). Schachar and Wachsmuth (1990) reported mixed results, and although Johnson and O'Leary (1987) found no differences in global marital satisfaction between CD

and controls, CD mothers reported more hostility toward their spouses. When mothers and fathers were examined separately, Sanders and Dadds (1992) found lower rates of satisfaction in both parents of CD children, whereas Johnson and O'Leary (1987) reported that pattern for mothers only. In Fendrich and colleagues (1990) poorer marital adjustment was not specific to the CD group, and was also found in the other non-DBD clinical groups. Although the mothers of children in Sanders and colleagues' (1992) study reported poorer marital adjustment than mothers of depressed or control children, their scores were in the nondistressed range. Finally, both studies that examined marital violence found higher rates in parents of ODD/CD children (Schachar & Wachsmuth, 1990, 1991). Overall, these findings support a relationship between marital distress and CD/ODD that is consistent with Campbell's (1995) review of research on global, externalizing behavior problems in preschool children, which indicated greater marital dissatisfaction in these families.

Ratings of Family Functioning

Seven studies examined family functioning variables. Schachar and Wachsmuth (1990, 1991) reported no differences between CD/ODD versus control families on maternal ratings of general family functioning; these two studies had some divergent findings as well. Schachar and Wachsmuth (1990) found poorer paternal-rated family functioning in CD/ODD families relative to controls, but no differences in parent ratings of parent–child relationships. In contrast, Schachar and Wachsmuth (1991) found no differences in paternal ratings of family functioning; however, parents of ODD/CD children rated their relationship with their child as more dysfunctional. Haddad and colleagues (1991) and Slee (1996) both found higher conflict and less cohesion in CD families relative to controls. While Slee also found CD families to be less expressive, less encouraging of independence, and more control-oriented, Haddad and colleagues' results did not show this pattern. Paternite and colleagues (1995) found that ODD+ADHD but not ODD-only families showed higher conflict and less cohesion than controls. Fendrich and colleagues (1990) found that families of CD children reported less cohesion and more mother–child fighting. Finally, Holcomb and Kashani (1991) found that CD adolescents reported more family conflict and rated their family life as less nurturant and satisfactory.

Overall, a clear pattern of poorer family functioning is associated with CD/ODD, with most consistent findings emerging in the dimensions of low cohesion and high conflict. Again, this suggestion is consistent with that of Campbell (1995), who concluded that disruptive preschoolers come from more dysfunctional families.

Parenting Characteristics

A variety of methodologies and measures have been used to evaluate the parenting characteristics of CD children's parents. Mothers of CD children have been found to report a more external locus of control both for themselves (Field *et al.*, 1987) and with respect to their children's misbehavior (Baden & Howe, 1992). Relative to controls, mothers of CD children have also reported themselves to be less nurturant (Field *et al.*, 1987) , to provide less supervision and consistent discipline (Frick *et al.*, 1992), and to believe their parenting efforts will be less effective (Baden & Howe, 1992). Not surprisingly, parents of CD girls expected their daughters to engage in more CD behavior (Johnson & O'Leary, 1987).

Results have been inconsistent regarding the parental pattern of "affectionless control." Fendrich and colleagues (1990) found no evidence for this pattern in CD parents. Rey & Plapp (1990) found that both CD children and parents endorsed this pattern of low caring and high control as characteristic of their family; ODD children, but not their parents, also reported this pattern.

Some parenting variables have not differentiated between ODD/CD and control groups. For example, maternal reports of time spent and discussions with children were comparable across groups (Frick *et al.*, 1992), as were beliefs regarding parenting techniques (Baden & Howe, 1992).

Overall, inconsistent findings characterize the studies on parenting variables. Although parents of CD/ODD children spend time and discuss issues with their children, they may be less consistent in their parenting styles, may show negative expectations, and tend to be less nurturant. Various forms of negative parenting styles (which include uninvolved, rejecting, or harsh parenting) have been linked to behavior problems in preschoolers as well (Campbell, 1995).

Behavioral Interactions

Among the studies reviewed, nine reports on six samples included behavioral observations. Across these, there has been ample evidence of more negative and fewer positive behaviors from both CD children and the adults with whom they interact; these patterns have been seen in both problem solving and play interactions.

In interaction with their parents, CD children have shown more negative cognitions and negative affect (Sanders & Dadds, 1992; Snyder, Schrepferman, & St. Peter, 1997), greater activity and less positive affect (Field *et al.*, 1987; Snyder, Schrepferman, & St. Peter, 1997), and more deviant behavior (Dadds *et al.*, 1992). Children with CD also complied less with female adults (Anderson *et al.*, 1986).

In interaction with their CD children, parents have also shown more negative cognitions (Sanders & Dadds, 1992), greater negativity (Anderson *et al.*, 1986), more aversive behavior (Dadds *et al.*, 1992; Snyder, Schrepferman, & St. Peter, 1997), a more controlling style (Slee, 1996), and lower rates of interaction in play (Field *et al.*, 1987). Overall, relative to controls, CD families have demonstrated less effective problem solving (Vuchinich *et al.*, 1994).

The three studies that attempted to separate child and parent effects in these negative exchanges concluded that parent behavior was strongly affected by child behavior (Anderson *et al.*, 1986; Brunk & Henggeler, 1984; Snyder, Schrepferman, & St. Peter, 1997); similarly, one study showed that child behavior was strongly affected by parent behavior (Snyder, Schrepferman, & St. Peter, 1997). Overall, CD children were found to evoke greater negative behaviors from their own mothers and from comparison mothers.

In summary, CD families demonstrated deficiencies in problem-solving skills, with interactions generally characterized by more disapproval and negative affect, less positive expressiveness, and more efforts at parental control; both children and parents have fewer positive cognitions about their interactions. This negative and controlling interaction pattern has also been shown to characterize the mother–child interactions of preschool children with behavior problems (Campbell, 1995).

Parental Characteristics and Psychopathology

Nine studies assessed parental psychopathology or related characteristics in families of CD children. Among four studies that examined depression, three found evidence of greater depression in mothers of CD children than comparison mothers (Field *et al.*, 1987; Lahey, Piacentini, *et al.*, 1988; Sanders & Dadds, 1992), whereas Frick and colleagues (1992) failed to find greater depression in parents of children with CD or ODD relative to controls. Campbell's (1995) review also found greater depression among parents of preschoolers with behavior problems.

Several studies included measures relevant to maternal aggression and antisocial behaviors. Compared to controls, mothers of CD children have demonstrated hostile attribution biases (Bickett *et al.*, 1996); evidence for aggressive behavior has been mixed. No differences in self-reports regarding aggression were found by Bickett and colleagues (1996) and Johnson and O'Leary (1987), whereas Lahey, Piacentini, and colleagues (1988) found a greater number of self-reports of physical fighting among CD mothers. Findings have also been mixed for diagnoses of APD among mothers of CD children; Lahey, Piacentini, and colleagues (1988) found more APD diagnoses among CD mothers, but Frick and colleagues (1992) and Schachar and Wachsmuth (1990) did not.

In contrast, fathers of CD children have consistently been found to demonstrate greater aggressive and antisocial behavior. Higher rates

of APD and substance abuse diagnoses have been reported by Frick and colleagues (1992); Lahey, Hartdagen, and colleagues (1988); Lahey, Piacentini, and colleagues (1988); and Schachar and Wachsmuth (1990). Lahey, Piacentini, and colleagues (1988) also found CD fathers to report more fighting. Johnson and O'Leary (1987) found fathers of CD girls reported themselves to be more aggressive than fathers of control girls.

Thus, among families of CD children, fathers have frequently shown higher rates of a wide range of aggressive and antisocial behavior patterns. The evidence for maternal psychopathology is mixed, however, with both depression and antisocial patterns sometimes emerging.

METHODOLOGICAL ISSUES

Gender

Of the studies reviewed, ten included boys only, and nine had girls and boys (in percentages ranging from 12% to 52%) but did not analyze findings separately by gender. Thus, only Johnson and O'Leary (1987) provided data specifically about family factors in CD/ODD girls; this study used lenient inclusion criteria. This study did not find the parents of CD girls to report more marital dissatisfaction, although CD mothers reported more hostility toward their spouses. Further, fathers of CD girls reported a more aggressive behavior style. Although these findings suggest that, for girls, paternal aggression and maternal hostility toward spouse are linked to CD/ODD behavior and that general marital satisfaction and parenting attitudes are not, these conclusions are clearly preliminary due to the scarcity of data.

CD–ODD Distinction

The studies reviewed varied widely on their inclusion criteria and on whether CD and ODD were separated. Of the studies reviewed, one included only ODD subjects, ten included CD subjects only, six included a mixed CD/

ODD sample, and three separately examined ODD and CD. The mixed pattern of results makes definitive conclusions difficult; overall, however, ODD groups show evidence of impaired family functioning relative to controls. In some domains, the ODD groups' levels of impairment equaled that of CD groups (paternal-rated family dysfunction in Schachar & Wachsmuth, 1990; child-rated "affectionless control" in Rey & Plapp, 1990). In other domains, the ODD group fell intermediate to that of CD and control families (parenting variables of maternal supervision and inconsistent discipline in Frick *et al.*, 1992; parent ratings of "affectionless control" in Rey & Plapp, 1990). Although paternal psychopathology was linked to ODD in both studies that examined it, one study found ODD and CD to show equivalent rates on a general psychopathology measure (Schachar & Wachsmuth, 1990); the other found that both ODD and CD fathers had more substance abuse than controls, but that only the CD fathers had more APD (Frick *et al.*, 1992).

Comorbidity with ADHD

Given the high comorbidity among DBD, obtaining pure samples of DBD children is important for delineating the relationship between specific disorders and their correlates. The vast majority of studies reviewed did not specifically exclude ADHD children from their groups: Only three studies examined pure ODD or CD groups, with one comparing pure ODD to comorbid ODD/ ADHD (Paternite *et al.*, 1995), one comparing pure ODD and pure CD groups (Rey & Plapp, 1990), and one comparing ODD/CD, ADHD, and comorbid ODD/ CD/ADHD (Schachar & Wachsmuth, 1991). Of the two studies that examined comorbid groups, one compared ODD to ODD/ ADHD and found the comorbid group to have higher family dysfunction (Paternite *et al.*, 1995); the other compared a mixed CD/ODD group to a mixed CD/ODD/ ADHD group and found similar rates of family dysfunction in the groups (Schachar & Wachsmuth, 1991). Since most studies in this review probably included ADHD children in their samples, it is difficult to draw conclusions about the extent to which specific family findings are correlates of ODD/ CD or ADHD. It does appear that not all effects can be attributed to the presence of ADHD since the study that used only pure ODD and CD groups found evidence of dysfunctional parenting relative to controls (Rey & Plapp, 1990). However, it may be that CD alone is sufficient to induce family dysfunction regardless of the presence of ADHD (Schachar & Wachsmuth, 1991), whereas ODD alone does not result in dysfunction unless accompanied by ADHD (Paternite *et al.*, 1995). This conclusion is clearly tentative given the little existing data and the small sample size (9 pure ODD children) in the Paternite and colleagues study (see also Chapter 6, this volume).

THEORETICAL MODELS

This final section presents three theoretical perspectives that continue to help organize research with CD children and families. The first, coercion theory, highlights a behavioral level of analysis to understand negative and antisocial behaviors and their development. The second, attachment theory, highlights the quality of family relationships as a level of analysis to understand the development of DBD. Finally, the third, theory of genotype–environment effects, highlights the use of multiple levels of analysis to include explicitly genetic as well as environmental contributions to DBD. We propose that this third theory can account for the findings linking parental psychopathology, parenting characteristics, and family environment to CD/ODD and that it can suggest causal mechanisms underlying covariance among these factors.

Coercion Theory

Coercive family process theory (Patterson, 1976, 1982) has long been the prevailing conceptual model linking parenting styles to aggression in children. Although individual differences are acknowledged, family interaction is emphasized as the primary cause of children's aggressive behavior. Forming its theoretical basis in operant conditioning, coercion theory focuses on the reciprocal influences between child and parent behavior, with the child viewed as both "the victim and architect" (Patterson, 1976) of the maladaptive interactional patterns that arise as a result of coercive processes. Negative reinforcement is posited to be a particularly important factor contributing to such coercive processes, with children and parents shaped to behave in ways that result in the termination of unpleasant behavior in the other. Thus, children's tantrums are likely to increase when they result in parent's attempts to stop them by offering a treat, both because the child has been positively reinforced by the treat, and because the parent has been negatively reinforced by the cessation of the tantrum. This kind of reciprocal interaction, termed a "coercion trap" or reinforcement trap, is viewed as contributing to an escalating pattern of maladaptive interactions in families of CD children.

In explaining how this pattern arises in some families and not others, Patterson (1982) cited data suggesting that, in families with a problem child versus control families, parents are more likely to start and continue aversive episodes, and the child is more frequently negatively reinforced. A number of studies in this review presented data consistent with Patterson's model (Baden & Howe, 1992; Dadds *et al.*, 1992; Rey & Plapp, 1990; Sanders & Dadds, 1992; Sanders *et al.*, 1992; Snyder, Schrepferman, & St. Peter, 1997). However, this model does not specify the mechanisms that account for the fact that such patterns of coercive interactions arise in some families but not others.

Attachment Theory

Based in part on the seminal work of John Bowlby, Greenberg and colleagues have applied attachment theory to conceptualizing the early development of DBD (e.g., Greenberg *et al.,* 1993). From an attachment theory perspective, children form concepts of both self and others that guide expectations for how the self and others help regulate negative feelings. A general lack of warmth or inconsistency in

responding on the part of the caregiver is thought to lead the child to an insecure attachment; the child expects continuity of negative feelings in close relationships and does not receive supportive models for handling negative emotions. These expectations can be modified with experience; nevertheless, they provide a "working model" that leads to continuity in the child's behavior. If negative, this model may lead to coercive behavioral cycles and difficulty in mastering age-appropriate self-control. In parallel fashion, the caregiver develops expectations regarding the child, which, if positive, can support patient responding even in the face of young children's challenging behaviors. Alternatively, a more negative model might lead to insensitive or adverse emotional responding to the child.

Recent work by Greenberg, Speltz, and colleagues yielded findings regarding attachment quality for both children and mothers. Children with DBD were more likely to show insecure attachments toward their mothers than were community controls in two independent samples (84% vs. 28% in Speltz, Greenberg, & DeKlyen, 1990; 80% vs. 28% in Greenberg, Speltz, DeKlyen, & Endriga, 1991). In the latter sample, DeKlyen (1996) examined mothers' attachment classification through interviews about relationships in their families of origin; like their children, mothers of DBD subjects were more likely to be classified as nonsecure.

Greenberg and colleagues considered insecure attachment to be a risk factor for DBD, but not a necessary or sufficient cause (Greenberg *et al.,* 1993; Greenberg, DeKlyen, Speltz, & Endriga, 1997). In conjunction with additional risk factors that interfere with family functioning or normal development, however, insecure attachments may be associated with DBD. For example, Lyons-Ruth, Easterbrooks, and Cibelli (1997) reported greater externalizing problems at age 7 for children who had *both* insecure attachments and low developmental quotients as toddlers. Thus, although the attachment perspective may be a useful addition to larger, explanatory models of DBD, it is unlikely to account fully for the range of findings presented in this chapter.

A Theory of Genotype–Environment Correlations

In a series of papers, Scarr (e.g., 1989, 1992; Scarr & McCartney, 1983) discussed the role of genotype–environment correlations in development. The theory of genotype–environment effects (Plomin, DeFries, & Loehlin, 1977) suggests that genotypes drive experiences, such that individuals create their own environments that are uniquely correlated with their genetically based individual differences. This theory, which has been applied to intelligence (e.g., Scarr, 1992) and to the continuity of antisocial behavior (Caspi & Moffitt, 1995), provides what we believe to be a viable framework for synthesizing the existing literature on family influences on the ODD/CD child.

Three specific types of genotype–environment correlations are passive, evocative, and active (Scarr, 1992). Passive effects are related to biological parents' providing both the genes and the home environment to children, resulting in a correlation between the two. Evocative effects refer to the responses received from others that are related to certain child characteristics; for example, a fussy infant may elicit more controlling responses from a parent than a calm one. Finally, active effects occur when people's choices about what environments to experience are related to their genetically determined characteristics, such as when a naturally gifted athlete chooses to spend long hours engaged in sports activities. All three of these effects can help account for the relationships among parental, family, and child characteristics of ODD/CD children, although passive and evocative effects may be particularly relevant. This model is not inconsistent with Patterson's coercion theory or attachment theory. However, the genotype–environment effects model considers a broader range of influences (e.g., passive, active), and integrates the data supporting the role of genetic-biological factors in the etiology of ODD/CD (see Chapters 17, 18, & 19, this volume). Further supporting this notion, Plomin & Bergeman (1991) reviewed a number of behavior-genetic studies documenting a genetic influence on a number of measures similar to those used by studies in the current review, including parent–child videotaped interactions and ratings of family environment. Although these measures were typically conceptualized by authors as socialization or environmental variables, the Plomin & Bergeman paper suggests that genetic factors may have contributed to findings.

The model of genotype–environment effects ascribes causative roles to both environmental and genetic factors, but suggests that genetic variations drive environmental ones. In the current review, externalizing behavior (e.g., APD, aggression, substance abuse) was consistently found to characterize the fathers of CD/ODD children, suggesting the presence of genetic factors (see also Chapters 18 & 19, this volume). The poorer parenting style found to characterize CD parents could represent a passive effect, such that, associated with their pathology, APD fathers provide to their children inconsistent and less nurturing parenting. Similarly, the hostile attributional style demonstrated by mothers of aggressive children may directly influence the development of this style by their children (Bickett et al., 1996).

Alternatively, CD/ODD children may evoke poorer parenting from parents; such evocative effects could also help explain the generally poorer family functioning and negative pattern of behavioral interaction seen in the families of CD/ODD children. The potential evocative effects of child behavior on the parents of CD children is particularly compelling in explaining maternal behavior (since maternal pathology, which has been less consistently linked to CD/ODD, is less suggestive of passive effects). This conclusion is consistent with the results of studies showing that CD confederate boys evoked more negative responses from normal mothers. Further supportive evidence comes from Wootton, Frick, Shelton, and Silverthorn (1997), who found that ineffective maternal parenting was unrelated to severity of conduct problems for children who displayed callous and unemotional traits (perhaps suggestive of a more pure genetic-biological etiology); however, for children without these traits, ineffective parenting was associated with higher rates of conduct problems.

CONCLUSIONS AND DIRECTIONS FOR FUTURE RESEARCH

Despite some discrepancies across studies, this review found consistent evidence suggesting that paternal antisocial behavior, marital discord, poor parenting strategies, and impaired patterns of interaction characterize the families of CD/ODD children. Many of the same factors have been found in research examining behavior problems in preschool children (Campbell, 1995). These patterns are consistent with a model of genotype–environment effects, whereby genetic-biological factors drive environmental variability; specifically, CD/ODD children are affected by the passive environments provided by parents, and evoke dysfunctional reactions from their families. Of particular need in future research examining family functioning in CD/ODD children are studies that examine girls, consider comorbidity, explore the role of maternal psychopathology, and utilize multivariate designs to allow further refinement of our understanding of etiological factors.

REFERENCES

Achenbach, T. M. (1978). The child behavior profile: I. Boys aged 6–11. *Journal of Consulting and Clinical Psychology, 46,* 478–488.

Achenbach, T. M. (1991). *Manual for the Child Behavior Checklist/4–18 and 1991* Profile. Burlington: University of Vermont, Department of Psychiatry.

American Psychiatric Association. (1980). *Diagnostic and statistical manual of mental disorders* (3rd ed.). Washington, DC: Author.

American Psychiatric Association. (1987). *Diagnostic and statistical manual of mental disorders* (3rd ed., rev.). Washington, DC: Author.

American Psychiatric Association. (1994). *Diagnostic and statistical manual of mental disorders* (4th ed.). Washington, DC: Author.

Anderson, K. E., Lytton, H., & Romney, D. M. (1986). Mothers' interactions with normal and conduct disordered boys: Who affects whom? *Developmental Psychology, 22,* 604–609.

Baden, A. D., & Howe, G. W. (1992). Mothers' attributions and expectancies regarding their conduct-disordered children. *Journal of Abnormal Child Psychology, 20,* 467–485.

Bickett, L. R., Milich, R., & Brown, R. T. (1996). Attributional styles of aggressive boys and their mothers. *Journal of Abnormal Child Psychology, 24,* 457–472.

Brunk, M. A., & Henggeler, S. W. (1984). Child influences on adult controls: An experimental investigation. *Developmental Psychology, 20,* 1074–1081.

Campbell, S. B. (1995). Behavior problems of preschool children: A review of recent research. *Journal of Child Psychology and Psychiatry, 36,* 113–149.

Caspi, A., & Moffitt, T. E. (1995). The continuity of maladaptive behavior: From description to understanding in the study of antisocial behavior. In D. Cicchetti & D. J. Cohen (Eds.), *Developmental psychopathology* (Vol. 2, pp. 472–511). New York: Wiley.

Dadds, M. R., Sanders, M. R., Morrison, M., & Rebgetz, M. (1992). Childhood depression and conduct disorder: II. An analysis of family interaction patterns in the home. *Journal of Abnormal Psychology, 101,* 505–513.

DeKlyen, M. (1996). Disruptive behavior disorder and intergenerational attachment patterns: A comparison of clinic-referred and normally functioning preschoolers and their mothers. *Journal of Consulting and Clinical Psychology, 64,* 357–365.

Eyberg, S. M., & Ross, A. W. (1978). Assessment of child behavior problems: The validation of a new inventory. *Journal of Clinical Child Psychology, 7,* 113–116.

Fendrich, M., Warner, V., & Weissman, M. M. (1990). Family risk factors, parental depression, and psychopathology in offspring. *Developmental Psychology, 26,* 40–50.

Field, T. M., Sandberg, D., Goldstein, S., Garcia, R., Vega-Lahr, N., Porter, K., & Dowling, M. (1987). Play interactions and interviews of depressed and conduct disorder children and their mothers. *Child Psychiatry and Human Development, 17,* 213–234.

Frick, P. J., Lahey, B. B., Loeber, R., Stouthamer-Loeber, M., Christ, M. A. G., & Hanson, K. (1992). Familial risk factors to oppositional defiant disorder and conduct disorder: Parental psychopathology and maternal parenting. *Journal of Consulting and Clinical Psychology, 60,* 49–55.

Greenberg, M. T., Speltz, M. L., DeKlyen, M., & Endriga, M. C. (1991). Attachment security in preschoolers with and without externalizing behavior problems: A replication. *Development and Psychopathology, 3,* 413–430.

Greenberg, M. T., Speltz, M. L., & DeKlyen, M. (1993). The role of attachment in the early development of disruptive behavior problems. *Development and Psychopathology, 5,* 191–213.

Greenberg, M. T., DeKlyen, M., Speltz, M. L., & Endriga, M. (1997). The role of attachment processes in externalizing psychopathology in young children. In L. Atkinson & E. Zucker (Eds.), *Attachment and psychopathology* (pp. 196–222). New York: Guilford.

Haddad, J. D., Barocas, R., & Hollenbeck, A. R. (1991). Family organization and parent attitudes of children with conduct disorder. *Journal of Clinical Child Psychology, 20,* 152–161.

Holcomb, W. R., & Kashani, J. H. (1991). Personality characteristics of a community sample of adolescents with conduct disorders. *Adolescence, 26,* 579–586.

Johnson, P. L., & O'Leary, K. D. (1987). Parental behavior patterns and conduct disorders in girls. *Journal of Abnormal Child Psychology, 15,* 573–581.

Lahey, B. B., Hartdagen, S. E., Frick, P. J., McBurnett, K., Connor, R., & Hynd, G. (1988). Conduct disorder: Parsing the confounded relation to parental divorce and antisocial personality. *Journal of Abnormal Psychology, 97,* 334–337.

Lahey, B. B., Piacentini, J. C., McBurnett, K., Stone, P., Hartdagen, S., & Hynd, G. (1988). Psychopathology in the parents of children with conduct disorder and hyperactivity. *Journal of the American Academy of Child and Adolescent Psychiatry, 27,* 163–170.

Locke, H. J., & Wallace, K. M. (1959). Short marital adjustment and prediction tests: Their reliability and validity. *Marriage and Family Living, 21,* 251–255.

Lyons-Ruth, K., Easterbrooks, M. A., & Cibelli, C. D. (1997). Infant attachment strategies, infant mental lag, and maternal depressive symptoms: Predictors of internalizing and externalizing problems at age 7. *Developmental Psychology, 33,* 681–692.

Millon, T., Green, C. J., & Meagher, R. B. (1984). *Millon Adolescent Personality Inventory manual.* Minneapolis, MN: Interpretive Scoring Systems.

Moos, R. H., & Moos, B. S. (1976). *Family Environment Scale manual.* Palo Alto, CA: Consulting Psychologists Press.

Olson, D. H., Sprenkle, D. H., & Russell, C. S. (1979). Circumplex model of marital and family systems: 1. Cohesion and adaptability dimensions, family types, and clinical applications. *Family Process, 18,* 3–28.

Parker, G., Tupling, H., & Brown, L. B. (1979). A parental bonding instrument. *British Journal of Medical Psychology, 52,* 1–10.

Paternite, C. E., Loney, J., & Roberts, M. (1995). External validation of oppositional disorder and attention deficit disorder with hyperactivity. *Journal of Abnormal Child Psychology, 23,* 453–471.

Patterson, G. R. (1976). The aggressive child: Victim and architect of a coercive system. In L. A. Hammerlynck, L. C. Handy, & E. J. Mash (Eds.), *Behavior modification and families: Theory and research* (Vol. 1, pp. 267–316). New York: Brunner/Mazel.

Patterson, G. R. (1982). *A social learning approach: Vol. 3. Coercive family process.* Eugene, OR: Castalia.

Plomin, R., & Bergeman, C. S. (1991). The nature of nurture: Genetic influences on "environmental" measures. *Behavioral and Brain Sciences, 14,* 373–427.

Plomin, R., DeFries, J. C., & Loehlin, J. C. (1977). Genotype–environment interaction and correlation in the analysis of human behavior. *Psychological Bulletin, 84,* 309–322.

Quay, H. C., & Peterson, D. R. (1983, 1996). *Manual for the Revised Behavior Problem Checklist.* Odessa, FL: PAR.

Rey, J. M., & Plapp, J. M. (1990). Quality of perceived parenting in oppositional and conduct disordered adolescents. *Journal of the American Academy of Child and Adolescent Psychiatry, 29,* 382–385.

Sanders, M. R., & Dadds, M. R. (1992). Children's and parents' cognitions about family interaction: An evaluation of video-mediated recall and thought listing procedures in the assessment of conduct-disordered children. *Journal of Clinical Child Psychology, 21,* 371–379.

Sanders, M. R., Dadds, M. R., Johnston, B. M., & Cash, R. (1992). Childhood depression and conduct disorder: I. Behavioral, affective, and cognitive aspects of family problem-solving interactions. *Journal of Abnormal Psychology, 101,* 495–504.

Scarr, S. (1989). How genotypes and environments combine: Development and individual differences. In G. Downey, A. Caspi, & N. Bolger (Eds.), *Interacting systems in human development* (pp. 217–244). New York: Cambridge University Press.

Scarr, S. (1992). Developmental theories for the 1990s: Development and individual differences. *Child Development, 63,* 1–19.

Scarr, S., & McCartney, K. (1983). How people make their own environments: A theory of genotype–environment effects. *Child Development, 54,* 424–435.

Schachar, R. J., & Wachsmuth, R. (1990). Oppositional disorder in children: A validation study comparing conduct disorder, oppositional disorder, and normal control children. *Journal of Child Psychology and Psychiatry, 31,* 1089–1102.

Schachar, R. J., & Wachsmuth, R. (1991). Family dysfunction and psychosocial adversity: Comparison of attention deficit disorder, conduct disorder, normal, and clinical controls. *Canadian Journal of Behavioral Science, 23,* 332–348.

Skinner, H. A., Steinhauer, P. D., & Santa-Barbara, J. (1983), The family assessment measure. *Canadian Journal of Community Mental Health, 2,* 91–105.

Slee, P. T. (1996). Family climate and behavior in families with conduct disordered children. *Child Psychiatry and Human Development, 26,* 255–266.

Snyder, J., Schrepferman, L., and St. Peter, C. (1997). Origins of antisocial behavior: Negative reinforcement and affect dysregulation of behavior as socialization mechanisms in family interaction. *Behavior Modification, 21,* 187–215.

Speltz, M. L., Greenberg, M. T., & DeKlyen, M. (1990). Attachment in preschoolers with disruptive behavior: A comparison of clinic-referred and nonproblem children. *Development and Psychopathology, 2,* 31–46.

Vuchinich, S., Wood, B., & Vuchinich, R. (1994). Coalitions and family problem-solving with preadolescents in referred, at-risk, and comparison families. *Family Process, 33,* 409–424.

Wootton, J. M., Frick, P. J., Shelton, K. K., & Silverthorn, P. (1997). Ineffective parenting and childhood conduct problems: The moderating role of callous-unemotional traits. *Journal of Consulting and Clinical Psychology, 65,* 301–308.

16

Children and Adolescents with Oppositional Defiant Disorder and Conduct Disorder in the Community

Experiences at School and with Peers

JANE E. LEDINGHAM

INTRODUCTION

This chapter examines the life of Oppositional Defiant (ODD) and Conduct Disordered (CD) children and adolescents as they emerge into the world beyond their families of origin. It documents how they function in school and in the larger community, how they relate to peers, and finally how they deal with intimate relationships and with children of their own. In addition to focusing on the behavior of these individuals, the reactions of significant others in the social context are explored, because these reactions often markedly alter the trajectory of the ODD/CD children's development.

Because very little research in these areas has focused on samples who have been formally diagnosed as either ODD or CD, the literature dealing with a number of groups similar on many dimensions will be explored. Thus, terms such as "aggressive," "aggressive-disruptive," "delinquent," "antisocial," and "externalizing

JANE E. LEDINGHAM • School of Psychology, University of Ottawa, Ottawa, Ontario, Canada K1N 6N5.

Handbook of Disruptive Behavior Disorders, edited by Quay and Hogan. Kluwer Academic/Plenum Publishers, New York, 1999.

problems" are used here in a roughly interchangeable fashion for ODD and CD. Although studies that use subject selection criteria that are not tied to formal diagnoses tend to use community-based rather than clinical samples and thus generally choose individuals with less severe problems, many of the participants in these studies may in fact meet criteria for ODD/CD diagnoses and others may show precursor forms of these disorders. Subjects may also meet criteria for other disorders, particularly Attention-Deficit/Hyperactivity Disorder (ADHD). Studies in which CD/ODD subjects are comorbid for other disorders are discussed later in this chapter. However, the means by which investigators identified these children with Disruptive Behavior Disorders (DBD) is routinely indicated and, whenever the nature of the target sample selection procedures has potentially important implications for the generalizability of the findings, this is noted.

Traditionally, researchers in this area of research have focused almost exclusively on ODD/CD males. However, there is a growing body of literature that addresses the course of women's life histories and the consequences of ODD/CD diagnoses for females as well. These studies highlight the significance of gender for the course of ODD and CD disorders and emphasize the different courses that the sexes pursue as a result of continuing behavior problems (see also Chapter 28, this volume).

ACADEMIC PERFORMANCE AND SCHOOL EXPERIENCES

School provides the first main arena for the child outside of the family and the first public venue in which children can demonstrate their skills in both cognitive and interpersonal domains. We examine the success of CD children at school in terms of their school attainment and the way in which other features of the school environment shape their experiences.

Academic Achievement

There is substantial agreement among studies that a correlation exists between CD and academic achievement (ACH). Across a variety of indices of CD and ACH, different samples, and varying ages, the magnitude of the correlations is consistent but modest, in the order of −.10 to −.30, and thus accounts for only a very small proportion of the variance (Feshbach & Price, 1984; Olweus, 1983; Williams & McGee, 1994). Whether this relationship is mediated by IQ is not clear. Goodman and colleagues (Goodman, 1995; Goodman, Simonoff, & Stevenson, 1995) reported that reading scores did not add to the prediction of conduct problems once IQ was entered into the equation. However, Frick and colleagues (1991) found that IQ did *not* account for the significant negative correlation between CD/ODD symptoms and math ACH. Lynam, Moffitt, and Stouthamer-Loeber (1993) found different results as a function of race. For the white sample, with verbal IQ taken into account, the link between ACH and delinquency was nonsignificant. However, for blacks, ACH mediated the relationship between verbal IQ and delinquency.

Despite evidence that some sort of association exists between CD and ACH, there is no consistent evidence demonstrating that CD children have lower ACH scores than other children in any *specific* domain. Anderson, Williams, McGee, and Silva (1989) found that pure CD subjects diagnosed at age 11 did not differ significantly from controls on reading scores at ages 7, 9, or 11 or on spelling scores at 9 or 11. Hodges and Plow (1990) reported that their CD group did not differ from inpatient controls on measures of ACH in reading, math, written language, or general knowledge. Shachar and Tannock's (1995) CD group was significantly lower in math but not in reading skills relative to clinic controls.

When one moves from considering ACH in specific scholastic domains to overall grade point average at school, there is evidence for a link with CD. In a large Finnish birth cohort, delinquents were overrepresented among those with poor grades regardless of their family's social class (SES), level of social mobility, or intactness (Jarvelin, Laara, Rantakallio, Moilanen, & Isohanni, 1994). Ouston (1984), in a study of inner city children, also found that delinquency rates were higher among those who had lower grades, as well as among those who had changed schools between 14 and 16 years of age, had poorer attendance records, and had left school early at age 16. Delinquency rates for both sexes in this study were also higher among those who had lower reading scores. However, poor reading ability only increased the subsequent risk of delinquency among those who had been rated *low* on antisocial behavior by teachers at the age of 10; reading ability did *not* differentiate later delinquents and nondelinquents among those who had been rated *high* on antisocial behavior at age 10. In this sample, apparent differences between delinquents and nondelinquents on IQ and grades were substantially reduced or eliminated once group differences on variables such as SES and early behavior in school were taken into account.

Results from a number of studies suggest that the apparent association between CD and ACH is in fact attributable to coexisting problems of attention. Frick and colleagues (1991) found no evidence for underachievement (i.e., ACH lower than that expected for IQ) in a pure CD group, although CD children with comorbid ADHD demonstrated significant underachievement. Moffitt (1990) reported that subjects later identified as pure delinquents had not previously differed from controls on reading ACH at any age. In contrast, delinquents with concomitant attentional problems had shown poorer reading ability than controls at ages 7, 11, and 13. Maughan, Pickles, Hagell, Rutter, and Yule (1996) compared CD behaviors in children identified as either poor readers or controls. At age 10, once attentional problems had been accounted for, reading groups did not differ on ratings of CD.

The duration of CD problems may also have implications for their relation to ACH. In a large longitudinal study in which CD problems were identified at a very young age, Kingston and Prior (1995) identified four groups of children: those who had been consistently aggressive since the age of 2, those who had been aggressive from ages 2 to 4 but whose aggression had declined during the preschool years, those who had not been aggressive from ages 2 to 4 but whose aggression had increased with school entry, and those who had never shown high levels of aggression. In grade 2, the group which had been consistently aggressive from age 2 had significantly lower reading levels, with the average score falling a full standard deviation below the mean for the nonaggressive group.

Pianta and Caldwell (1990) also examined ACH and CD problems in young children. They found that poorer academic performance and CD behavior were correlated even in kindergarten. In grade 1, children who had scored higher on ACH in kindergarten showed lower than expected rates of externalizing problems, suggesting that more academically able children had improved behaviorally over time. Children with externalizing problems in kindergarten who had improved behaviorally by grade 1 had also been rated as having more affectionate interactions with their mothers in kindergarten.

Thus, both higher ACH and good relationships with parents may serve as protective factors in the development of CD.

Is There a Specific Causal Pattern that Accounts for the CD–ACH Relationship?

Associations between CD and ACH could be due to three possible mechanisms. First, CD could lead to poor ACH through the disruption of relationships with teachers and other students and absences from school. Second, poor ACH could lead to CD: Proponents of strain theory, for example, argue that not doing well academically at school leads to CD as a result of frustration and alienation (Agnew, 1985). Finally, a third variable could be responsible for the apparent connection between CD and ACH: Those espousing the social control hypothesis argue that weak bonds tying the child to individuals and to the goals of conventional society lead both to CD and to lack of involvement in and commitment to the school experience and thus lower ACH (Fagan & Pabon, 1990).

Krohn, Thornberry, Collins-Hall, and Lizotte (1995) prospectively studied a sample heavily weighted for males and individuals from areas with high rates of arrest, testing them first in grade 8 or 9 and subsequently at 6-month intervals until they reached grade 10 or 11. They found that dropping out of school was predicted by a low GPA, low commitment to school, low expectations for attending college, and prior drug use, but was unrelated to family structure, attachment to parents, parental supervision, and prior serious delinquency. Delinquency was predicted only by prior delinquency and being male, but not by family or school variables. In short, the study provided no support for strain theory, since poor grades did not predict CD or school dropout; it also provided no support for a direct causal link from CD to dropping out of school. There was some support for social control theory, in that ties to schooling but not to parents predicted subsequent dropout rates.

Fergusson and Horwood (1995) used structural equation modeling to evaluate the link between poor ACH and delinquency. Using data from a large birth cohort, they measured CD, ADHD, and IQ at 8 years of age, scholastic ability at 13, and delinquency at 15. They concluded that when the effects of earlier behavior and IQ are taken into account scholastic ability and delinquency are essentially independent. The same model was supported for both males and females. At age 8, CD, ADHD, and IQ were all significantly correlated, and there were significant paths from both ADHD and IQ at age 8 to ACH at age 13 and from CD at age 8 to delinquency at age 15. However, consistent with the results of Krohn and colleagues (1995), ACH at 13 and delinquency at 15 were uncorrelated once the remaining relationships among variables were taken into account. Fergusson and Horwood speculated that the apparent association between ACH and CD in fact may be attributable to common antecedent variables that affect them both.

In a study that included a measure of one potentially common causal antecedent (parental academic ACH), DeBaryshe, Patterson, and Capaldi (1993) also examined the links between antisocial behavior and ACH in a sample of boys. Ineffective parental discipline and antisocial behavior of boys were measured when the boys were in grade 6, academic engagement was measured in grade 7, and academic ACH was measured in grade 8. The model that best fit the data included significant paths between parental ACH and both ineffective discipline and child antisocial behavior in grade 6, as well as a reciprocal relationship between ineffective discipline and child antisocial behavior. There were also significant paths between ineffective discipline measured in grade 6 and the child's subsequent academic engagement and between academic engagement and later ACH. In general, these results agree substantially with those of Krohn and colleagues (1995) and Fergusson and Horwood (1995) by indicating that poor academic performance and antisocial behavior represent essentially distinct outcomes. Thus, these studies provide no evidence that a causal link exists either from CD to ACH or from ACH to CD. In contrast, there is fairly convincing support for the idea that a third variable influences both CD and ACH.

Sex Differences in the CD–ACH Association

A number of studies suggest that CD and ACH may be related in different ways for boys and girls. Williams and McGee (1994) used causal modeling techniques to evaluate competing hypotheses that reading failure causes CD, CD causes reading failure, or environmental disadvantage acts as a third variable to affect both reading ability and CD. Literacy and CD behaviors were measured at ages 7 and 9, and literacy and delinquency were measured at age 15. A composite measure of family disadvantage was collected at all ages. The specific model of the CD–literacy relationship that was supported by the data differed as a function of how the variables were defined. When both reading ability and CD were treated as continuous variables, there was no evidence that reading problems contributed to the development of CD at ages 9 or 15. However, there was support for the hypothesis that CD affects reading ability. A significant negative path was found between CD at age 9 and literacy at age 15, indicating that childhood CD problems predicted poorer reading skills in adolescence. These patterns remained unchanged when reading scores were adjusted for IQ, and the same pattern held for both boys and girls. In contrast, when reading disability and CD were treated as categorical variables in order to contrast true cases of reading disability and CD with all other subjects, early reading disability was found to predict later CD, but only for boys. Across these analyses, then, there was no consistent support for either the hypothesis that CD leads to poor reading or the hypothesis that poor reading leads to CD. In addition, there was no clear evidence as to whether CD and reading ability are related in the same way for both sexes. Nevertheless, in both continuous and categorical variable analyses, family disadvantage was found to predict both CD and reading ability for both boys and girls.

Maughan and colleagues (1996) studied a sample of poor readers and controls from childhood into adulthood. They also reported gender differences in the CD–reading relationship. However, their findings differed from those of Williams and McGee (1994). In Maughan and colleagues' sample, both poor reading at age 10 and social disadvantage contributed to CD outcomes at age 14 for females (adult antisocial outcomes for women were too infrequent to analyze). For males, a more complex pattern emerged. Poor reading at age 10 was not associated with concurrent CD, and reading ability did not affect antisocial outcomes directly in either adolescence or adulthood. Rather, the effect of reading was indirect and mediated through school attendance. That is, poor male readers attended school less often, and lower attendance was linked to greater juvenile, but not adult, offending. In this study, males' adult antisocial outcomes were predicted directly only by childhood and adolescent CD.

Tremblay and colleagues (1992) used structural equation modeling to assess the links between CD and ACH separately for each sex. Aggressive-DBD was measured at age 7, ACH was measured at ages 7 and 10, and delinquent behavior was assessed at age 14. For boys, although aggressive-DBD and ACH were associated at age 7, early ACH predicted later ACH but not delinquency and early aggressive-DBD predicted later delinquency but not later ACH. For girls, aggressive-DBD and ACH were also related at age 7. However, both aggressive-DBD and ACH at age 7 predicted ACH at age 10, although neither predicted delinquency at age 14. This suggests that the progression of antisocial behavior is less stable for girls.

Clearly, there is very little consistency among the findings of studies that have examined sex differences in causal models. However, overall, the results of these studies support the notion that the relationship between these variables is quite possibly different for boys and girls.

The School Context

Beyond involvement in academic tasks, children's experiences at school are shaped by routine transactional exchanges with school personnel and influenced by characteristics of the school such as the composition of the student body.

Teachers play an important role in the identification of ODD/CD children. Although teachers report fewer problem behaviors than do parents, their ratings are more strongly predictive of subsequent outcomes (Hart, Lahey, Loeber, & Hanson, 1994; Verhulst, Koot, & Van der Ende, 1994). Very early in elementary school, teachers begin to respond differently to disruptive boys. They spatially segregate them, assigning them more often to seats in the front or rear of the classroom, and these extreme seat positions persist over time (Charlebois, Berneche, LeBlanc, Gagnon, & Larivee, 1995). Having an extreme seat position is also associated with more teacher talk but less teacher attention, and with greater teacher aversiveness. Such spatial isolation of antisocial children by teachers may contribute to their marginalization and serve to decrease further their commitment to education.

A compelling demonstration that the school context exerts an important influence on the development of DBD comes from a study by Caspi and his colleagues (Caspi, Lynam, Moffitt, & Silva, 1993). This study was carried out in New Zealand, where girls had a choice of entering either an all-girl or a coeducational school at the age of 13. The sample of girls came from a longitudinal study of a birth cohort on which multiple waves of evaluation had been carried out. Approximately half of the sample chose to attend an all-girl school and half a mixed-sex school. While there were some differences between groups choosing the two alternatives, with same-sex school girls having higher IQs and coming from families of higher SES and different family climates, these differences tended to be small in magnitude. Nevertheless, the two groups did not differ on their levels of behavior problems at the age of 9. However, they did differ in rates of self-reported delinquency at ages 13 and 15 as a function of their menarcheal status: Girls who were early maturers scored higher on delinquency when they were attending mixed-sex schools than when they were attending same-sex schools.

Girls who were average in their menarcheal age also tended to report more delinquency in mixed-sex schools than in same-sex schools at age 15; late-onset menarcheal groups did not differ in rates of delinquency at either age as a function of the type of school they attended. Delinquent behavior was also more stable from age 13 to age 15 in the coeducational than in the all-girl school. In summary, the risk of delinquency was higher in girls when they were attending schools with both sexes, particularly when they experienced early menarche. These investigators have argued that coeducational schools facilitate delinquent behavior in early-maturing girls in several ways: They may put less emphasis on control and discipline and provide exposure to boys, who model higher rates of delinquency than do girls and exert more pressure for norm violations.

NEIGHBORHOOD INFLUENCES

In addition to family and school influences, the larger community seems to exert an influence on DBD (see also Chapter 19, this volume). Kupersmidt, Griesler, DeRosier, Patterson, and Davis (1995) examined children's aggression scores as a function of both family type (black or white, single parent or intact family, high or low income) and neighborhood type (middle or low SES). Besides main effects for family type, aggression scores were affected by a significant family type by neighborhood type interaction: Children in African American, lower income, single-parent families scored higher on aggression if they lived in low SES neighborhoods than if they lived in middle SES neighborhoods. Thus, neighborhood influences may protect the child and reduce the risk of aggression.

The ratio of adult males to females in a community and rates of employment for both sexes were also shown to be related to rates of delinquency: Figueira-McDonough (1993) found that, in an urban center with generally high poverty rates, areas with lower ratios of males to females had higher rates of employment for males and lower rates of delinquency. How-

ever, areas with higher rates of employment for *both* males and females had higher rates of delinquency, possibly because there were lower rates of supervision with adults at work during the day. These results indicate that characteristics of the larger community go beyond family and school influences to shape rates of antisocial behavior.

RELATIONSHIPS WITH PEERS

From early childhood, interactions with other children form an increasingly important part of the child's social world and how a child is regarded by his or her peer group is an important predictor of later adjustment (Parker & Asher, 1987). In addition to general peer acceptance, however, the formation of close, predominantly same-sex friendships with peers is an important developmental task for elementary-school-aged children.

Aggression–Rejection Links

Aggression is one of the strongest correlates of peer rejection. About 50% of children who are classified as rejected by their peers score high on aggression (Cillessen, IJzendoorn, van Lieshout, & Hartup, 1992; French, 1988). Strauss, Lahey, Frick, Frame, and Hynd (1988) found that 50% of children diagnosed with CD were identified as rejected by their classmates, as compared to 6% of children diagnosed with anxiety disorders. Furthermore, aggressive-rejected children are more likely to retain their rejected status over time than are other rejected children (Cillessen *et al.,* 1992).

However, not all aggressive children are rejected. Bierman, Smoot, and Anmiller (1993) estimated that at least one third of aggressive children do not receive extreme scores on rejection from their peers. Aggressive boys who *were* rejected were not more physically aggressive or less prosocial than aggressive boys who were not rejected, but they were more argumentative, disruptive, and inattentive. Aggressive children who also score high on withdrawal are more disliked by peers than are those who score high only on aggression (Ledingham, 1981; Milich & Landau, 1984).

Somewhat surprisingly, aggressive children do not rate themselves as less popular than other children (Cairns, Cairns, Neckerman, Gest, & Gariepy, 1988). Zakriski and Coie (1996) compared aggressive-rejected and non-aggressive-rejected children's guesses about how many classmates would say they liked them the most and how many would say they liked them the least; actually these two groups had received equal numbers of "like most" and "like least" nominations from peers. Aggressive-rejected children attributed many fewer "like least" nominations to themselves than did nonaggressive-rejected children and, in fact, did not differ in their estimates from average children. However, when estimating how many "like most" and "like least" votes were given to other children, they proved to be *more* accurate than either average or nonaggressive-rejected children, indicating that they are not just poorer judges of peer acceptance and rejection overall.

It was possible that aggressive-rejected children's poorer accuracy in judging their own popularity was not due to a self-protective rating bias but was a result of the fact that peers were less willing to give them unmistakable cues of their dislike for fear of retaliation. In this latter case, differences in aggressive-rejected children's ratings might be due solely to differences in the clarity of the message given to them by peers. Zakriski and Coie (1996) subsequently had subjects characterize unequivocally negative or ambiguous feedback delivered both to another individual and to themselves. Aggressive-rejected children rated the feedback directed toward another as more negative than did nonaggressive-rejected or average children but rated feedback given to themselves no differently than did the other groups. Thus, they showed a larger self-favoring discrepancy between perceptions of feedback given to themselves and to others. Whether the feedback was unequivocally negative did not influence judgments of the aggressive-rejected group relative to other peer status groups. In short, there did appear to be a defen-

sive bias operating in this group which was most evident in how the aggressive-rejected child interpreted reactions directed toward others. Epkins (1994) has described the existence of a similar bias which she labeled projection: Children who score high on aggression also rate other peers higher on aggression than do children who score average or low. This finding suggests that aggressive children see others as more aggressive than do nonaggressive children (see also Chapter 14, this volume).

Because aggression and peer rejection overlap substantially, it is possible that many aspects of poor adjustment that are attributed to aggression are actually a consequence of peer rejection. Although this issue remains open to debate, Kupersmidt and Coie (1990) have reported data that are relevant to the question. They followed a group of fifth-grade children over a 7-year period. Suspension, truancy, grade retention, early school withdrawal, and police contacts were used as outcome measures. Deviance on both aggression and peer rejection in grade 5 predicted both later contacts with the police and experiencing *at least* one negative outcome from the poor school record and police contact measures. However, deviance on the aggression measure but not on the peer rejection measure predicted being kept back in a grade, truancy, and dropping out of school in subsequent years. In contrast to the Kupersmidt and Coie findings, Coie, Terry, Zakriski, and Lochman (1995) found that measures of social preference were unrelated to subsequent delinquency when measured either early, in grade 3, or late, in grade 8. These studies, taken together, suggest that aggression may be a more powerful predictor of subsequent problems than is peer rejection.

Does behaving aggressively decrease liking by peers or does being disliked by peers result in more aggressive behavior? There is very little research dealing specifically with this question. Vuchinich, Bank, and Patterson (1992) found no evidence longitudinally in support of either hypothesis, although aggressive behavior did predict peer relations contemporaneously in this sample of boys. At least one study suggests that different relationships exist between aggression and peer likability for boys and girls. Coie and colleagues (1995) reported that, for boys in grade 8, higher levels of aggression predicted greater association with deviant peers, which in turn predicted, rather surprisingly, *higher* liking by peers. In contrast, for girls, being disliked by peers in grade 3 predicted more delinquency before grade 8, which subsequently predicted both higher levels of aggression and lower liking by peers in grade 8. Thus, aggression for boys appears to have a positive but indirect influence on peer likability, while for girls peer acceptance is negatively related to aggression. This finding is consistent with the generally greater centrality of aggression to the male role.

Friendship and Peer Groups

It has been argued that global peer group acceptance may be less important for adjustment when the child has a best friend (Price & Ladd, 1986). Aggressive children appear to be similar to other children in terms of the number of nominations they receive from classmates as a best friend (Cairns *et al.*, 1988) and the number of times they and a classmate reciprocally identify each other as a best friend (Cairns *et al.*, 1988; Feltham, Doyle, Schwartzman, Serbin, & Ledingham, 1985). However, the nature and quality of their friendships are different from those of comparison groups. Children and their friends tend to be similar on dimensions such as sex, race, family income, academic achievement, withdrawal, and aggression, and aggressive children thus are more likely to have friends who are also aggressive (Dishion, Andrews, & Crosby, 1995; Kupersmidt, DeRosier, & Patterson, 1995), although this may be more true of boys' than of girls' friendships, especially at younger ages (Cairns *et al.*, 1988). Moreover, similarities on problem behaviors tend to precede the actual beginnings of friendship, although friends become increasingly similar over time (Kandel, 1978).

Antisocial children are also more likely to have friends that come not from the school context but from the neighborhood (Dishion *et al.*, 1995), and nonschool friendships are associated

with higher self-reported loneliness, lower relationship satisfaction, and higher levels of aggression among aggressive boys (Dishion *et al.*, 1995; East & Rook, 1992). In interactions with their friends, antisocial boys are not different on rates of prosocial behaviors from nonantisocial boys, but they make more commands and are judged by observers to be more noxious and less socially skilled (Dishion *et al.*, 1995). CD children, especially boys, display less empathy for others than do nondisordered children (Cohen & Strayer, 1996). These differences may help to explain why antisocial boys' friendships tend to be of shorter duration (Dishion *et al.*, 1995).

Given the fact that aggressive children's friendships seem to be of lower quality in many ways than those of nonaggressive children, it is not surprising that having a friend has not been shown to improve the outcome of aggressive children. Kupersmidt, Burchinal, and Patterson (1995) reported that rejection predicted aggression better when children had a best friend than when they did not. Furthermore, other things being equal, students who had a best friend were more likely to become delinquent than those who did not have a best friend. These authors concluded that a positive relationship with a friend did not reduce the risk of antisocial outcomes. Tremblay, Masse, Vitaro, and Dobkin (1995) also found that neither the friend's likability nor the friend's aggressiveness predicted delinquent behavior in a target child 1 year later. These data suggest that having a best friend, regardless of what that friend is like, does not protect the individual from later problems with the law.

In addition to not serving as a protective factor, however, several researchers have hypothesized that relationships with other antisocial individuals may actually increase the risk of poor outcomes. Deviant peer association theory (Sutherland & Cressey, 1970) argues that choosing to associate with peers who are engaged in illegal activities leads the individual into increasingly more deviant behavior as a result of the social influence process. In fact, for young offenders, affiliations with deviant peers predict serious crime independently of family variables (Hoge, Andrews, & Leschied, 1994). For boys, whose social groups generally include more peers than do those of girls (Waldrop & Halverson, 1975), at least prior to adolescence, the importance of the larger peer group may be as great as or greater than the importance of a best friend. To test this hypothesis, many researchers have evaluated the significance for later deviant behavior of having friends who are deviant. Keenan, Loeber, Zhang, Stouthamer-Loeber, and Van Kammen (1995), for example, collected data every 6 months on six occasions for boys in grades 4 and 7. Boys who reported that they were involved with deviant peers were also more likely to report beginning to engage in many kinds of delinquent acts over the next 6 months. Huizenga (1995) also found that the proportion of friends who were deviant predicted transitions from nondelinquent status to delinquent status for both boys and girls.

Fergusson and Horwood (1996) assessed conduct problems at age 8 and deviant peer associations and offending at ages 14 and 16. They found that conduct problems at age 8 predicted both deviant peer associations and offending at age 14. Both at 14 and at 16 deviant peer associations predicted offending contemporaneously more strongly than offending predicted deviant peer associations. However, earlier deviant peer affiliations did not predict later offending directly and earlier offending did not predict later deviant peer associations directly. Coie and colleagues (1995) also reported results indicating that deviant peer relations have very little influence on subsequent delinquency for boys or girls and that aggression predicts later associations with deviant peers. These findings suggest that, although consorting with antisocial peers may have some effect on later offending, early conduct problems contribute largely both to offending and to affiliations with deviant peers.

The fact that prior problem behavior predicts consorting with peers who have similar problems suggests that it is not generally the case that innocent children are being led astray by bad friends as deviant peer association theory predicts. Rather, such results are more in line with a theory arguing that similarity is an important factor governing the formation of interpersonal bonds and alliances. Such a theory is consistent with the view that individuals select particular niches in the environment that are conducive to their specific behavioral profiles (Fergusson, Lynskey, & Horwood, 1996; Scarr & McCartney, 1983). There seems to be a developmental trend for niche picking to be more characteristic of adolescents than of younger children; similarity between friends and among members of a group is greater in grade 8 than in grade 6 (Cairns et al., 1988; Coie et al., 1995). Perhaps as a result of this, Coie and colleagues (1995) have speculated that deviant peer associations may be more important for understanding adolescent-onset time-limited offending (see Chapter 1, this volume).

Despite the fact that there is little evidence to support the *global* importance of deviant associations, this factor has been demonstrated to be extremely important for girls experiencing early pubertal development. Caspi and colleagues (1993) indicated that familiarity with delinquent peers was strongly related to norm violations both for girls who had a history of externalizing problems and for those who did not.

TRANSITION TO ADULT ROLES

The onset of puberty presents a unique series of challenges to the adolescent and begins the process of developing adult patterns of behavior. During this period bodily changes make adjustments in both self-image and social roles necessary, and patterns of relationships with the opposite sex alter dramatically.

Timing of Puberty

That puberty is a function of biological factors is a well-accepted fact, but it also appears that the timing of puberty may be a function of social factors as well, at least for girls. Moffitt, Caspi, Belsky, and Silva (1992) explored the importance of family structure and atmosphere for the onset of menarche in girls.

Father absence was determined from maternal reports when the index child, drawn from a large birth cohort, was born and at 3, 5, 7, 9, and 11 years of age. Family conflict was measured when the child was 7. Both father absence and family conflict predicted an earlier onset of menarche significantly but modestly. Moffitt and colleagues (1992) pointed out that the observed relationship might be due not to social factors but to the operation of genetic factors. Since early-maturing girls are more likely to date, become sexually active, and have children earlier and since early marriages are more likely to dissolve, it is possible that the mother's early onset of menarche was the true cause of the daughter's early menarche rather than the correlated factors of father absence and family conflict.

Japel, Tremblay, Vitaro, and Boulerice (1997) also related timing of menarche to family structure and father absence. However, in contrast to the findings of Moffitt and colleagues (1992), they found that girls from divorced families had *lower* pubertal status at age 11 than children from intact families when mother's SES and age at the birth of her first child and the child's age at parental separation were controlled for. Girls whose mothers had not remarried continued to have lower pubertal status than children from intact families at age 13. Thus, while there is evidence that menarcheal onset is related to family structure, the exact *nature* of that relationship is not yet clear.

Romantic and Sexual Relationships

Numerous studies have examined the importance of same-sex peer relationships for DBD but there is very little research on the importance of relationships with the opposite sex, and almost all of it focuses only on sexual involvement. Neeman, Hubbard, and Masten (1995) studied the importance of interest and involvement in romantic relationships for adjustment from childhood to adolescence. Subjects were tested first at ages 8 to 12 and again at ages 14 to 19. A composite score for romantic involvement was based on both children's and parents' reports of the child's interest in the

opposite sex and whether he or she had a girlfriend or boyfriend. Measures of social and academic competence, rule breaking (which included contraventions of the law), and job competence were also collected. Path analyses indicated that early interest or involvement in romantic relationships had negative implications for later development: Involvement in romantic relationships in childhood predicted rule breaking and was negatively associated with academic competence in adolescence. In contrast, later involvement with the opposite sex was associated with better adjustment at an earlier age: Greater social competence in childhood predicted involvement in romantic relationships that began only in adolescence.

Choice of partners in intimate relationships is a function of diagnostic status. Quinton, Pickles, Maughan, and Rutter (1993) found that a diagnosis of CD in childhood predicted being involved with a partner in early adulthood who was antisocial or a substance abuser, and that this effect was especially marked for women, who in general had a much higher risk of having a deviant partner, probably because of the higher prevalence of CD in men than in women. Whether an individual had a partner who was supportive and nondeviant substantially determined whether CD was stable from childhood into adulthood: Those who as adults lacked such a partner generally continued to be diagnosed with CD, whereas almost all of those *with* such a partner no longer carried such a diagnosis in adulthood. Risk for being involved with a deviant partner was greater among boys who had deviant peer associations and among girls who were less planful in their behavior, came from less harmonious families, and had had a teenage pregnancy.

The age at which adolescents first engage in sexual intercourse is predictive of later delinquency. In a prospective longitudinal study that followed boys and girls in grades 10 and 11 over a 2-year period, Tubman, Windle, and Windle (1996) found that later delinquency and problems with alcohol were associated with earlier onset of and continuing reports of sexual intercourse; the time that sexual intercourse first occurred was associated with a subsequent acceleration in reports of delinquency. However, Moffitt (1993) pointed out that there is a group of delinquents whose problems with the law begin in adolescence, but whose deviance does not persist into adult life (see also Chapter 24, this volume). This suggests that the delinquency reported by Tubman and colleagues may have been time limited. This interpretation is made less likely by the fact that retrospectively reported externalizing problems in childhood were higher for those who reported having sexual intercourse consistently across the 2-year period than for those who remained sexually inactive. While grade point averages were higher for adolescents reporting later sexual involvement, academic performance and the onset of sexual activity appeared to be relatively independent.

Bingham and Crockett (1996) examined the link between timing of first sexual intercourse and adjustment in a sample of boys and girls followed from initial testing in grades 7 to 9 through grade 12. Groups with early-, middle-, or late-onset sexual involvement differed on rates of minor deviance and drunkenness, with the early-intercourse group showing the most problem behaviors and greater drug use. However, after the results were adjusted for prior levels of behavioral adjustment, timing of intercourse did not predict poorer adjustment. These results are thus in agreement with those of Tubman and colleagues (1996) in suggesting that early sexual involvement is a consequence of earlier behavior problems.

Capaldi, Crosby, and Stoolmiller (1996) followed a group of boys from grade 6 to grade 12. Age at first sexual intercourse was predicted by family SES, the number of changes in parental figures in the family, parental antisocial behavior, and levels of parental monitoring, as well as by characteristics of the boy himself (deviant peer associations, antisocial behavior, substance use, physical maturity, and academic skill). These results provide more evidence for the association of early antisocial behavior with early sexual involvement. As in the case of the Moffitt and colleagues (1992) study, it is unclear whether these results indicate the importance of family instability or whether, in

fact, parental antisocial behavior was the critical factor. It may be that antisocial fathers pass on to their sons a genetic component for both antisocial behavior and early physical maturity, and that early physical maturity also leads to earlier and less stable marriages.

Several additional studies have focused on the importance of behavior problems for sexual involvement and pregnancy in girls. Bardone, Moffitt, Caspi, Dickson, and Silva (1996) compared groups of girls who had been diagnosed with CD, depression, or no psychiatric problems at the age of 15 in terms of their functioning at the age of 21. CD at the age of 15 predicted adult Antisocial Personality Disorder, substance dependence, illegal behavior, dependence on multiple welfare sources, early departure from the family of origin, multiple cohabitation partners, and the experience of physical violence by partners at the age of 21. Depression at the age of 15 predicted depression at the age of 21. Both CD and depression diagnoses at the age of 15 predicted anxiety disorder, multiple drug use, early school leaving, low school attainment, cohabitation, pregnancy, and early childbearing by the age of 21. It thus appears that both externalizing and internalizing problems in adolescence may be associated for girls with a number of poor outcomes, including early pregnancy. However, in a follow-up study of girls seen in childhood for depression or other disorders, Kovacs, Krol, and Voti (1994) reported that only early-onset CD and not depression predicted pregnancy at an earlier age.

Stiffman, Earls, Robins, Jung, and Kulbok (1987) interviewed girls aged 13 to 18 from low-SES areas who were attending a health care clinic but were not currently pregnant. Girls who were sexually active scored higher on lifetime diagnoses of CD and had higher rates of substance abuse than sexually inactive girls. Girls who had been pregnant were much more likely to have dropped out of school and to have come from less stable homes than both girls who were sexually active but had never been pregnant and sexually inactive girls.

Serbin, Peters, McAffer, and Schwartzman (1991) obtained information on gynecological treatment received in adolescence and early adulthood by girls originally identified in grades 1, 4, or 7 as aggressive (A), withdrawn (W), aggressive-withdrawn (AW), or nondeviant (ND). This study relied on government records of medical treatment provided in Quebec, where medicare paid for the costs of treatment for all individuals. The information on treatment was provided from government archives by groups, with no data identified as belonging to a given individual subject. Because individual consents were thus not required, the results from this study probably include information on more deviant individuals who might have refused permission for the researchers to examine their files or proved to be untraceable had their collaboration been solicited on an individual basis.

Serbin and colleagues (1991) compared each behaviorally deviant group of girls separately to the ND contrast group at a given grade level (no comparisons were made between different deviant groups). They found that both A and AW girls who had been identified initially in grade 1 were more than twice as likely as ND contrasts to have been provided with methods of birth control between the ages of 11 and 17. A girls first identified in grade 4 were more likely to have been treated for sexually transmitted diseases between the ages of 14 and 20 than ND girls of the same age and AW girls in this age group were more likely to have become pregnant and given birth than ND girls. A girls originally seen in grade 7 were significantly more likely than ND contrasts to have been pregnant between the ages of 17 and 23. In this sample it was not merely the existence of a pattern of deviant behavior that predicted gynecological events: W girls did not differ from ND girls on measures of types of gynecological treatment at any age.

Parenting

A history of aggressive behavior during childhood has also been shown to affect the adequacy of parenting in women who became parents during adolescence or early adulthood. Serbin and colleagues (1991) reported that mothers' childhood aggression and withdrawal scores predicted their emotional and verbal responsiveness to their young children; children's levels of developmental delay were predicted by maternal aggression scores in childhood as well as by mother's age at first pregnancy, the quality of the home environment, and age of the child.

In a subsequent and expanded follow-up of the same sample, Serbin, Peters, and Schwartzman (1996) examined emergency ward visits for the children of young adult mothers identified in childhood as A, W, AW, or ND. Again, because of constraints due to sample size, records for children of A, W, and AW mothers were compared only to those for children of ND mothers. Mothers originally classified as A or AW took their children up to age 4 to the emergency ward more times per year than did ND mothers; rates for mothers originally classified as W did not differ from those of the contrast group. That this difference was not the result of parents taking children to the emergency ward instead of making appointments in doctors' offices is indicated by the fact that there were no group differences in rates of nonemergency medical consultations. Sons of A mothers were more likely to have injury-related diagnoses than sons of ND mothers; daughters of AW mothers tended to be more likely than the daughters of ND mothers to have injury-related diagnoses. The children of AW mothers were also significantly more likely than the children of ND mothers to be seen on two or more occasions for infections and other acute illnesses. These results suggest that preventive monitoring of children's health and well-being by A and AW mothers may be poorer, although, at least for the children of A mothers, characteristics of the child such as impulsiveness and risk taking may also have influenced accident rates.

Lewis and colleagues (1991) followed up a sample of 21 delinquent girls who had been incarcerated in a juvenile correctional facility. Originally the average age in the sample was 15, and follow-up information was collected from 7 to 12 years later. Although there was no control group included for comparison in this study, these authors reported very high rates of dysfunctional mothering in the sample. There was evidence of child abuse or neglect in the histories of 12 of the 15 women who had had children, and 8 of these mothers had given up custody of at least one child. These findings, along with those of Serbin and colleagues (1996), indicate the high risk of abuse and neglect for the offspring of DBD women.

THE IMPORTANCE OF COEXISTING PROBLEMS FOR THE COURSE OF ODD AND CD

A large proportion of children or adolescents diagnosed with ODD or CD have additional problems. In a sample of 11-year-olds, Anderson, Williams, McGee, and Silva (1987) found that 49% of children with diagnoses of ODD or CD had also been assigned another diagnosis. The most common were ADHD and anxiety disorders. When the same birth cohort was rediagnosed at the age of 15, 26% of those diagnosed with ODD or CD were found to be comorbid for at least one other disorder, with the most frequently identified comorbid disorders being depression or dysthymia and anxiety disorders (McGee et al., 1990). Thus, earlier-onset CD is more strongly associated with coexisting problems, and the nature of the comorbid conditions changes with age. Comorbidity with both ADHD and internalizing symptomatology has been shown to have important consequences for the course of CD.

It is more often the case that children with CD are comorbid for ADHD than that children with ADHD are comorbid for CD (Abikoff & Klein, 1992). Although both disorders are associated with underachievement at school, several authors have concluded that it is the comorbidity with ADHD that is largely responsible for poor academic performance in CD children (Frick et al., 1991; Hinshaw, 1992). Children diagnosed with both CD and ADHD also demonstrate greater symptom severity, an increased risk for later antisocial disorders, greater parental psychopathology and family adversity, higher rates of peer rejection, and greater deficits in social information processing

than children diagnosed with CD alone (Abikoff & Klein, 1992; see also Chapter 24, this volume).

A large number of studies have demonstrated that coexisting internalizing problems are important for the prognosis of individuals diagnosed with CD, but there is still some question about whether comorbid internalizing problems are associated with better or poorer outcomes. Children diagnosed with CD but no anxiety disorder are more likely than CD children *with* comorbid anxiety disorder to receive more concurrently measured "fights more" and "meanest" nominations from peers and to have had more school suspensions and contacts with the police (Walker et al., 1991). However, a pattern of simultaneous externalizing and internalizing problems has been found in a number of studies to be more predictive of *subsequent* antisocial behavior than externalizing problems alone. Boys and girls described as both aggressive and anxious were more likely to remain aggressive over time than children who were only aggressive (Ialongo, Edelsohn, Werthamer-Larsson, Crockett, & Kellam, 1996). McCord (1987) reported that boys characterized by teachers as both shy and aggressive in early elementary school were more likely than aggressive-only or shy-only boys to have criminal records as juveniles and as adults, and were also the most likely to have records for criminal behavior and alcoholism. Kellam and his colleagues (Ensminger, Kellam, & Rubin, 1983; Kellam, Brown, Rubin, & Ensminger, 1983) conducted analyses that indicate that a combination of aggression and shyness in grade 1 predicts higher levels of self-reported delinquency, physical assault, and substance use in adolescence than high scores on either of these dimensions alone. Douglas (1966) and Farrington, Gallagher, Morley, St Ledger, and West (1988) similarly reported higher rates of crime later in life for children characterized as both nervous, shy, or withdrawn *and* aggressive than for children characterized by only one of these patterns.

Part of the answer to the question of how additional problems of an internalizing nature affect the course of CD may be found in how the internalizing problems are identified. Kerr, Tremblay, Pagani, and Vitaro (1997) differentiated between behavioral inhibition, characterized by shyness and fearfulness, and social withdrawal, or the preference for solitary activity and a failure to be rewarded by social interaction and the approval of others. They found that boys identified as high on aggressive-disruptive behavior between the ages of 10 and 12 were more likely to report more delinquent acts between the ages of 13 and 15 and more depression at age 15 if they had also been rated as high on social withdrawal between the ages of 10 and 12. However, being rated as high on behavioral inhibition resulted in *lower* rates of later delinquency for *all* boys, regardless of whether they had originally scored high on aggressive-disruptive behavior. Thus, behavioral inhibition appears to act as a protective factor against later antisocial behavior, whereas social withdrawal in conjunction with aggressive-disruptive behavior appears to serve as a risk factor for subsequent delinquency and depression.

In addition to the greater risk of continuing externalizing problems among children who are both aggressive and socially withdrawn, there appear to be more negative consequences in the realms of peer relations and school achievement. Aggressive-withdrawn children are rated as less likable by their peers (Ledingham, 1981), have fewer reciprocal friends (Feltham et al., 1985), and have higher subsequent rates of school failure and special class placement than do aggressive children (Ledingham & Schwartzman, 1984). However, comorbid anxiety, as opposed to social withdrawal, does *not* appear to increase the risk of poorer peer relations: Walker and colleagues (1991) reported no difference in nominations by peers of who was liked most or liked least in boys diagnosed with CD as a function of whether they had a comorbid anxiety disorder.

Being aggressive appears to increase the risk of both concurrent (Cole & Carpentieri, 1990) and later depression (Panak & Garber, 1992) but at least part of this effect seems to be mediated by poor relations with peers (Panak & Garber, 1992; Patterson & Stoolmiller, 1991). These findings suggest that CD

in conjunction with peer rejection results in higher levels of subsequent depression than CD alone. Both CD and depression are further associated with higher levels of substance use (Henry et al., 1993).

In summary, it is clear that coexisting problems of ADHD, internalizing disorders, and peer rejection contribute in an important way to the outcome of CD children. Moreover, the co-occurrence of such problems is not a low-frequency event. Thus, assessing individuals on these additional dimensions should improve our understanding of the course of CD and also give us more insight into the causal mechanisms operating. Gjone and Stevenson (1997), using data from identical and fraternal twins, reported results suggesting that genetic factors are more important for explaining pure internalizing or externalizing problems and shared environmental factors are more important for concurrent internalizing and externalizing problems.

CONCLUSIONS

CD children do poorly in a number of social arenas outside the family. They receive poorer grades at school, are more often placed in special classes or fail a grade, and drop out of school early. Much of their early academic trouble appears to be due to coexisting problems of ADHD. However, their aversive interaction patterns with both peers and teachers probably also decrease their commitment to continuing in school. Aggressive children are generally more disliked than other children but aggressive behavior may result in greater peer rejection for girls than for boys. Aggressive children are as likely as other children to have friends and be part of a social group but the friendships appear to be less satisfying and over time their social networks are increasingly likely to include others with similar levels of antisocial behavior.

The onset of puberty is associated with the beginning of distinctly different trajectories for antisocial boys and girls. Aggressive girls are more likely than aggressive boys to enter into a relationship with a deviant partner; being involved with a deviant partner is highly associated with the likelihood that antisocial behavior will remain stable into adulthood. For boys, whether their *same-sex* affiliations are deviant seems to be a more important determinant of continuing deviance than is the nature of their intimate opposite-sex relationships. Although a history of conduct problems predicts earlier sexual involvement for both boys and girls, the consequences of sexual behavior are more serious for girls as they become pregnant, drop out of school, and begin to parent, often with no support from a partner. Clearly the social worlds and levels of responsibility of antisocial boys and girls can be quite different as they enter adulthood.

Researchers such as Neeman and colleagues (1995) and Quinton and colleagues (1993) have begun to explore the significance of romantic relationships for CD, but much remains to be learned about variations in the quality and course of such relationships and in levels of commitment made to them. This information may prove to be important for a greater understanding of how outcomes diverge for different individuals.

Several investigators have demonstrated that various different *types* of aggression have different consequences, although the ultimate significance of these types remains largely unspecified. Price and Dodge (1989), for example, demonstrated that reactive, or hostile, aggression in young children was associated with peer rejection, whereas proactive, or instrumental, aggression was associated with more positive peer perceptions.

Crick and Grotpeter (1995) have recently highlighted the importance of relational aggression, which includes acts such as exclusion from play, threatened withdrawal of friendship, and hostile rumor spreading, and is said to be more characteristic of girls. They have documented how relational aggression relates to contemporaneous adjustment, but there is to date no information on what the long-term consequences of this type of aggression are relative to the consequences of physical aggression. Since girls spend much of their time in dyadic interactions, it is possible that relational aggression serves the adaptive purpose of prevent-

ing intrusions into intimate interactions with a best friend and in the long run is *not* linked to poorer outcomes. However, there is a need for research demonstrating that individuals can be reliably differentiated in terms of the specific manner in which they express their aggression, and that such differences are stable over time. Such work should prove an important addition to our understanding of how antisocial behavior develops, particularly in girls.

REFERENCES

Abikoff, H., & Klein, R. G. (1992). Attention-deficit hyperactivity and conduct disorder: Comorbidity and implications for treatment. *Journal of Consulting and Clinical Psychology, 60,* 881–892.

Agnew, R. (1985). A revised strain theory of delinquency. *Social Forces, 64,* 151–167.

Anderson, J., Williams, S., McGee, R., & Silva, P. A. (1987). DSM-III disorders in pre-adolescent children: Prevalence in a large sample from the general population. *Archives of General Psychiatry, 44,* 69–76.

Anderson, J., Williams, S., McGee, R., & Silva, P. A. (1989). Cognitive and social correlates of DSM-III disorders in preadolescent children. *Journal of the American Academy of Child and Adolescent Psychiatry, 28,* 842–846.

Bardone, A. M., Moffitt, T. E., Caspi, A., Dickson, N., & Silva, P. A. (1996). Adult mental health and social outcomes of adolescent girls with depression and conduct disorder. *Development and Psychopathology, 8,* 811–825.

Bierman, K. L., Smoot, D. L., & Anmiller, K. (1993). Characteristics of aggressive-rejected, aggressive (nonrejected), and rejected (nonaggressive) boys. *Child Development, 64,* 139–151.

Bingham, C. R., & Crockett, L. J. (1996). Longitudinal adjustment patterns of boys and girls experiencing early, middle, and late sexual intercourse. *Developmental Psychology, 32,* 647–658.

Cairns, R. B., Cairns, B. D., Neckerman, H. J., Gest, S., & Gariepy, J.-L. (1988). Peer networks and aggressive behavior: Social support or social rejection? *Developmental Psychology, 24,* 320–330.

Capaldi, D. M., Crosby, L., & Stoolmiller, M. (1996). Predicting the timing of first sexual intercourse for at-risk adolescent males. *Child Development, 67,* 344–359.

Caspi, A., Lynam, D., Moffitt, T. E., & Silva, P. A. (1993). Unravelling girls' delinquency: Biological, dispositional, and contextual contributions to adolescent misbehavior. *Developmental Psychology, 29,* 19–30.

Charlebois, P., Berneche, F., LeBlanc, M., Gagnon, C., & Larivee, S. (1995). Classroom seating and juvenile delinquency. In J. McCord (Ed.), *Coercion and punish-*

ment in long-term perspectives (pp. 198–212). New York: Cambridge University Press.

Cillessen, A. N. H., IJzendoorn, H. W., van Lieshout, C. F. M., & Hartup, W. W. (1992). Heterogeneity among peer-rejected boys: Subtypes and stabilities. Child Development, 63, 893–905.

Cohen, D., & Strayer, J. (1996). Empathy in conduct-disordered and comparison youth. Developmental Psychology, 32, 988–998.

Coie, J. D., Terry, R., Zakriski, A., & Lochman, J. (1995). Early adolescent social influences on delinquent behavior. In J. McCord (Ed.), Coercion and punishment in long-term perspectives (pp.229–244). New York: Cambridge University Press.

Cole, D. A., & Carpentieri, S. (1990). Social status and the comorbidity of child depression and conduct disorder. Journal of Consulting and Clinical Psychology, 58, 748–757.

Crick, N. R., & Grotpeter, J. K. (1995). Relational aggression, gender, and social-psychological adjustment. Child Development, 66, 710–722.

DeBaryshe, B. D., Patterson, G. R., & Capaldi, D. M. (1993). A performance model for academic achievement in early adolescent boys. Developmental Psychology, 29, 795–804.

Dishion, T. J., Andrews, D. W., & Crosby, L. (1995). Antisocial boys and their friends in early adolescence: Relationship characteristics, quality, and interactional process. Child Development, 66, 139–151.

Douglas, J. W. B. (1966). The school progress of nervous and troublesome children. British Journal of Psychiatry, 112, 1115–1116.

East, P. L., & Rook, K. G. (1992). Compensatory patterns of support among children's peer relationships: A test using school friends, nonschool friend, and siblings. Developmental Psychology, 28, 163–172.

Ensminger, M. E., Kellam, S. G., & Rubin, B. R. (1983). School and family origins of delinquency: Comparisons by sex. In K. T. Van Dusen & S. A. Mednick (Eds.), Prospective studies of crime and delinquency (pp. 73–97). Boston: Kluwer-Nijhoff.

Epkins, C. C. (1994). Peer ratings of depression, anxiety, and aggression in inpatient and elementary school children: Rating biases and influence of rater's self-reported depression, anxiety, and aggression. Journal of Abnormal Child Psychology, 22, 611–628.

Fagan, J., & Pabon, E. (1990). Contributions of delinquency and substance use to school dropout among inner city youths. Youth and Society, 21, 306–354.

Farrington, D. P., Gallagher, B., Morley, L., St Ledger, R. J., & West, D. J. (1988). Are there any successful men from criminogenic backgrounds? Psychiatry, 51, 116–130.

Feltham, R. F., Doyle, A. B., Schwartzman, A. E., Serbin, L. A., & Ledingham, J. E. (1985). Friendships in normal and socially deviant children. Journal of Early Adolescence, 5, 371–382.

Fergusson, D. M., & Horwood, L. J. (1995). Early disruptive behavior, IQ, and later school achievement and

delinquent behavior. Journal of Abnormal Child Psychology, 23, 183–199.

Fergusson, D. M., & Horwood, L. J. (1996). The role of adolescent peer affiliations in the continuity between childhood behavioral adjustment and juvenile offending. Journal of Abnormal Child Psychology, 24, 205–222.

Fergusson, D. M., Lynskey, M. T., & Horwood, L. J. (1996). Factors associated with continuity and changes in disruptive behavior patterns between childhood and adolescence. Journal of Abnormal Child Psychology, 24, 533–553.

Feshbach, S., & Price, J. (1984). Cognitive competence and aggressive behavior: A developmental study. Aggressive Behavior, 10, 185–200.

Figueira-McDonough, J. (1993). Residence, dropping out, and delinquency rates. Deviant Behavior, 14, 109–132.

French, D. C. (1988). Heterogeneity of peer-rejected boys: Aggressive and nonaggressive subtypes. Child Development, 59, 976–985.

Frick, P. J., Kamphaus, R. W., Lahey, B. B., Loeber, R., Christ, M. A. G., Hart, E. L., & Tannenbaum, L. E. (1991). Academic underachievement and the disruptive behavior disorders. Journal of Consulting and Clinical Psychology, 59, 289–294.

Gjone, H., & Stevenson, J. (1997). The association between internalizing and externalizing behavior in childhood and early adolescence: Genetic or environmental common influences? Journal of Abnormal Child Psychology, 25, 277–286.

Goodman, R. (1995). The relationship between normal variation in IQ and common childhood psychopathology: A clinical study. European Child and Adolescent Psychiatry, 4, 187–196.

Goodman, R., Simonoff, E., & Stevenson, J. (1995). The impact of child IQ, parent IQ, and sibling IQ on child behavioral deviance scores. Journal of Child Psychology and Psychiatry, 36, 409–425.

Hart, E. L., Lahey, B. B., Loeber, R., & Hanson, K. S. (1994). Criterion validity of informants in the diagnosis of disruptive behavior disorders in children: A preliminary study. Journal of Consulting and Clinical Psychology, 62, 410–414.

Henry, B., Feehan, M., McGee, R., Stanton, W., Moffitt, T. E., & Silva, P. (1993). The importance of conduct problems and depressive symptoms in predicting adolescent substance use. Journal of Abnormal Child Psychology, 21, 469–480.

Hinshaw, S. P. (1992). Academic underachievement, attention deficits, and aggression: Comorbidity and implications for intervention. Journal of Consulting and Clinical Psychology, 60, 893–903.

Hodges, K., & Plow, J. (1990). Intellectual ability and achievement in psychiatrically hospitalized children with conduct, anxiety, and affective disorders. Journal of Consulting and Clinical Psychology, 58, 589–595.

Hoge, R. D., Andrews, D. A., & Leschied, A. W. (1994). Tests of three hypotheses regarding the predictors of delinquency. Journal of Abnormal Child Psychology, 22, 547–559.

Huizenga, D. (1995). Developmental sequences in delinquency: Dynamic typologies. In L.J Crockett & A. C. Crouter (Eds.), *Pathways through adolescence* (pp. 15–34). Mahwah, NJ: Erlbaum.

Ialongo, N., Edelsohn, G., Werthamer-Larsson, L.,Crockett, L., & Kellam, S. (1996). The course of aggression in first-grade children with and without comorbid anxious symptoms. *Journal of Abnormal Child Psychology, 24,* 445–456.

Japel, C., Tremblay, R. E., Vitaro, F., & Boulerice, B. (1977). Effects of early family transitions on girls' psychosocial adaptation and pubertal development between 9 and 13 years of age. Unpublished Manuscript.

Jarvelin, M.-R., Laara, E., Rantakallio, P., Moilanen, I., & Isohanni, M. (1994). Juvenile delinquency, education, and mental disability. *Exceptional Children, 61,* 230–241.

Kandel, D. B. (1978). Similarity in real-life adolescence friendship pairs. *Journal of Personality and Social Psychology, 36,* 306–312.

Keenan, K., Loeber, R., Zhang, Q., Stouthamer-Loeber, M., & Van Kammen, W. B. (1995). The influence of deviant peers on the development of boys' disruptive and delinquent behavior: A temporal analysis. *Development and Psychopathology, 7,* 715–726.

Kellam, S. G., Brown, C. H., Rubin, B. R., & Ensminger, M. E. (1983). Paths leading to teenage psychiatric symptoms and substance use: Developmental epidemiological studies in Woodlawn. In S. B. Guze, F. J. Earls, & J. E. Barrett (Eds.), *Childhood psychopathology and development* (pp. 17–51). New York: Raven.

Kerr, M., Tremblay, R. E., Pagani, L., & Vitaro, F. (1997). Boys' behavioral inhibition and the risk of later delinquency. *Archives of General Psychiatry, 54,* 809–816.

Kingston, L., & Prior, M. (1995). The development of patterns of stable, transient, and school-age onset aggressive behavior in young children. *Journal of the Academy of Child and Adolescent Psychiatry, 34,* 348–358.

Kovacs, M., Krol, R. S. M., & Voti, L. (1994). Early onset psychopathology and the risk for teenage pregnancy among clinically referred girls. *Journal of the American Academy of Child and Adolescent Psychiatry, 33,* 106–113.

Krohn, M. D., Thornberry, T. P., Collins-Hall, L., & Lizotte, A. J. (1995). School dropout, delinquent behavior, and drug use: An examination of the causes and consequences of dropping out of school. In H. B. Kaplan (Ed.), *Drugs, crime, and other deviant adaptations: Longitudinal studies* (pp. 163–183). New York: Plenum.

Kupersmidt, J. B., & Coie, J. D. (1990). Preadolescent peer status, aggression, and school adjustment as predictors of externalizing problems in adolescence. *Child Development, 61,* 1350–1362.

Kupersmidt, J. B., Burchinal, M., & Patterson, C. J. (1995). Developmental patterns of childhood peer relations as predictors of externalizing behavior problems. *Development and Psychopathology, 7,* 825–843.

Kupersmidt, J. B., DeRosier, M. E., & Patterson, C. P. (1995). Similarity as the basis for children's friendships: The roles of sociometric status, aggressive and withdrawn behavior, academic achievement, and demographic characteristics. *Journal of Social and Personal Relationships, 12,* 439–452.

Kupersmidt, J. B., Griesler, P. C., De Rosier, M. E., Patterson, C. J., & Davis, P. W. (1995). Childhood aggression and peer relations in the context of family and neighborhood factors. *Child Development, 66,* 360–375.

Ledingham, J. E. (1981). Developmental patterns of aggressive and withdrawn behavior in childhood: A possible method for identifying preschizophrenics. *Journal of Abnormal Child Psychology, 9,* 1–22.

Ledingham, J. E., & Schwartzman, A. E. (1984). A 3-year follow-up of aggressive and withdrawn behavior in childhood: Preliminary findings. *Journal of Abnormal Child Psychology, 12,* 157–168.

Lewis, D. O., Yeager, C. A., Cobham-Portorreal, C. S., Klein, N., Showalter, C., & Anthony, A. (1991). A follow-up of female delinquents: Maternal contributions to the perpetuation of deviance. *Journal of the American Academy of Child and Adolescent Psychiatry, 30,* 197–201.

Lynam, D., Moffitt, T. E., & Stouthamer-Loeber, M. (1993). Explaining the relation between IQ and delinquency: Class, race, test motivation, school failure, or self-control? *Journal of Abnormal Psychology, 102,* 187–196.

Maughan, B., Pickles, A., Hagell, A., Rutter, M., & Yule, W. (1996). Reading problems and antisocial behavior: Developmental trends in comorbidity. *Journal of Child Psychology and Psychiatry, 37,* 405–418.

McCord, J. (1987, April). *Aggression and shyness as predictors of problems: A longterm view.* Paper presented at the biennial meeting of the Society for Research in Child Development as part of the symposium "Aggression and Withdrawal: Prospective Studies of Childhood Deviance," Baltimore.

McGee, A. R., Feehan, M., Williams, S., Partridge, F., Silva, P. A., & Kelly, J. (1990). DSM-III disorders in a large sample of adolescents. *Journal of the American Academy of Child and Adolescent Psychiatry, 29,* 611–619.

Milich, R., & Landau, S. (1984). A comparison of the social status and social behavior of aggressive and aggressive/withdrawn boys. *Journal of Abnormal Child Psychology, 12,* 277–288.

Moffitt, T. E. (1990). Juvenile delinquency and attention deficit disorder: Developmental trajectories from age 3 to age 15. *Child Development, 61,* 893–910.

Moffitt, T. E. (1993). Adolescence-limited and life-course-persistent antisocial behaviour: A developmental taxonomy. *Psychological Review, 100,* 674–701.

Moffitt, T. E., Caspi, A., Belsky, J., & Silva, P. A. (1992). Childhood experience and the onset of menarche: A test of a sociobiological model. *Child Development, 63,* 47–58.

Neeman, J., Hubbard, J., & Masten, A. S. (1995). The changing importance of romantic relationship involvement to competence from late childhood to late adolescence. *Development and Psychopathology, 7,* 727–750.

Olweus, D. (1983). Low school achievement and aggressive behavior in adolescent boys. In D. Magnusson & V. L. Allen (Eds.), *Human development: An interactional perspective* (pp. 353–365). San Diego, CA: Academic Press.

Ouston, J. (1984). Delinquency, family background, and educational attainment. *British Journal of Criminology, 24,* 2–26.

Panak, W. F., & Garber, J. (1992). Role of aggression, rejection, and attributions in the prediction of depression in children. *Development and Psychopathology, 4,* 145–165.

Parker, J. G., & Asher, S. R. (1987). Peer relations and later personal adjustment: Are low-accepted children at risk? *Psychological Bulletin, 102,* 357–389.

Patterson, G. R., & Stoolmiller, M. (1991). Replications of a dual failure model for boys' depressed mood. *Journal of Consulting and Clinical Psychology, 59,* 491–498.

Pianta, R. D., & Caldwell, C. B. (1990). Stability of externalizing symptoms from kindergarten to first grade and factors related to instability. *Development and Psychopathology, 2,* 247–258.

Price, J. M., & Dodge, K. A. (1989). Reactive and proactive aggression in childhood: Relations to peer status and social context dimensions. *Journal of Abnormal Child Psychology, 17,* 455–471.

Price, J. M., & Ladd, G. W. (1986). Assessment of children's friendships: Implications for social competence and social adjustment. *Advances in Behavioral Assessment of Children and Families, 2,* 121–149.

Quinton, D., Pickles, A., Maughan, B., & Rutter, M. (1993). Partners, peers, and pathways: Assortative pairing and continuities in conduct disorder. *Development and Psychopathology, 5,* 763–783.

Scarr, S., & McCartney, K. (1983). How people make their own environments: A theory of genotype environmental effects. *Child Development, 54,* 424–435.

Schachar, R., & Tannock, R. (1995). Test of four hypotheses for the comorbidity of attention deficit hyperactivity and conduct disorder. *Journal of the American Academy of Child and Adolescent Psychiatry, 34,* 639–648.

Serbin, L., Peters, P. L., McAffer, V. J., & Schwartzman, A. E. (1991). Childhood aggression and withdrawal as predictors of adolescent pregnancy, early parenthood, and environmental risk for the next generation. *Canadian Journal of Behavioral Science, 23,* 318–331.

Serbin, L. A., Peters, P. L., & Schwartzman, A. E. (1996). Longitudinal study of early childhood injuries and acute illnesses in the offspring of adolescent mothers who were aggressive, withdrawn, or aggressive-withdrawn in childhood. *Journal of Abnormal Psychology, 105,* 500–507.

Stiffman, A. R., Earls, F., Robins, L. N., Jung, K. G., & Kulbok, P. (1987). Adolescent sexual activity and pregnancy: Socioenvironmental problems, physical health, and mental health. *Journal of Youth and Adolescence, 16,* 497–509.

Strauss, C. C., Lahey, B. B., Frick, P., Frame, C. L., & Hynd, G. W. (1988). Peer social status of children with anxiety disorders. *Journal of Consulting and Clinical Psychology, 56,* 137–141.

Sutherland, E. H., & Cressey, D. R. (1970). *Principles of criminology* (6th ed.). New York: Lippincott.

Tremblay, R. E., Masse, B., Perron, D., Leblanc, M., Schwartzman, A. E., & Ledingham, J. E. (1992). Early disruptive behavior, poor school achievement, delinquent behavior, and delinquent personality: Longitudinal analyses. *Journal of Consulting and Clinical Psychology, 60,* 64–72.

Tremblay, R. E. Masse, L. C., Vitaro, F., & Dobkin, P. L. (1995). The impact of friends' deviant behavior on early onset of delinquency: Longitudinal data from 6 to 13 years of age. *Development and Psychopathology, 7,* 649–667.

Tubman, J. G., Windle, M., & Windle, R. C. (1996). The onset and cross-temporal patterning of sexual intercourse in middle adolescence: Prospective relations with behavioral and emotional problems. *Child Development, 67,* 327–343.

Verhulst, F. C., Koot, H. M., & Van der Ende, J. (1994). Differential predictive value of parents' and teachers' reports of children's problem behaviors: A longitudinal study. *Journal of Abnormal Child Psychology, 22,* 531–546.

Vuchinich, S., Bank, L., & Patterson, G. R. (1992). Parenting, peers, and the stability of antisocial behavior in preadolescent boys. *Developmental Psychology, 28,* 510–521.

Waldrop, M. F., & Halverson, C. F. (1975). Intensive and extensive peer behavior: Longitudinal and cross-sectional analyses. *Child Development, 46,* 19–25.

Walker, J. L., Lahey, B. B., Russo, M. F., Frick, P. J., Christ, M. A., McBurnett, K., Loeber, R., Stouthamer-Loeber, M., & Green, S. M. (1991). Anxiety, inhibition, and conduct disorder in children: I. Relations to social impairment. *Journal of the American Academy of Child and Adolescent Psychiatry, 30,* 187–191.

Williams, S., & McGee, R. (1994). Reading attainment and juvenile delinquency. *Journal of Child Psychology and Psychiatry, 35,* 441–459.

Zakriski, A. L., & Coie, J. D. (1996). A comparison of aggressive-rejected and nonaggressive-rejected children's interpretations of self-directed and other-directed rejection. *Child Development, 67,* 1048–1070.

17

The Psychobiology of Oppositional Defiant Disorder and Conduct Disorder

STEVEN R. PLISZKA

INTRODUCTION

As discussed in Chapter 1 (this volume), DSM-IV (American Psychiatric Association, 1994) subtypes Conduct Disorder (CD) by age of onset, but biological research has most often relied on the undersocialized aggressive subtype as described in earlier DSMs. It has been assumed that this subtype is most likely to be related to psychobiological factors, especially those that might provide a basis for both disinhibition and reward seeking (Quay, 1993). In current thinking, biological factors are more likely to be linked to a pattern of antisocial behavior that involves (1) early onset, (2) pervasive antisocial behavior over time and different settings, (3) impulsive aggression toward people and property, (4) severe and early onset of alcohol and substance abuse, and (5) a positive family history of antisocial behavior and alcohol or substance abuse (DiLalla & Gottesman, 1989; Dolan, 1994; Linnoila & Virkkunen, 1992; Virkkunen & Linnoila, 1993). It is highly likely that this constellation of behav-

iors comprises what most investigators classified as "undersocialized-aggressive" (with or without benefit of formal DSM diagnoses) in earlier studies.

Since the early-onset CD may suggest a greater role for biological factors, it is important to make note of the comorbidity of Attention-Deficit/Hyperactivity Disorder (ADHD) in early-onset CD. No study has yet been able to identify a population of early-onset (before age 10) CD children who did not also meet criteria for ADHD (Halperin, Newcorn, Schwartz, et al., 1997; Kruesi et al., 1990; Reeves, Werry, Elkind, & Zametkin, 1987). The psychobiology of ADHD was reviewed in Chapter 8 (this volume). However, increasing evidence suggests that ADHD and ADHD with comorbid CD are distinct subtypes, perhaps even at the genetic level (Biederman et al., 1992). Medical and perinatal history does not distinguish ADHD from ADHD/CD children (August & Stewart, 1983; McGee, Williams, & Silva, 1984a, 1984b; Moffitt, 1990; Reeves et al., 1987), but studies have consistently shown that ADHD children with CD have a much stronger family history of antisocial behavior in their first-degree relatives compared with children with ADHD alone (Biederman, Munir, & Knee, 1987; Biederman et al., 1992; Faraone, Biederman, Keenan, & Tsuang, 1991; Lahey

STEVEN R. PLISZKA • Department of Psychiatry, The University of Texas Health Science Center at San Antonio, San Antonio, Texas 78284-7792.

Handbook of Disruptive Behavior Disorders, edited by Quay and Hogan. Kluwer Academic/Plenum Publishers, New York, 1999.

et al., 1988). Indeed, for children who have ADHD alone, the rate of antisocial behavior in relatives does not exceed that of control children. Biederman and colleagues (1992) examined the rate of psychiatric diagnosis among the relatives of a large sample of ADHD and ADHD/CD children. The risk for ADHD was the same in both groups of relatives, but the ADHD/CD children had an elevated number of relatives with CD (26%) compared to the ADHD-only group (13%). Furthermore, relatives with CD also tended to have ADHD; that is, the two disorders cosegregated, indicating that ADHD/CD is a distinct familial subtype. This confirms an earlier study (August & Stewart, 1983) that also found that ADHD/CD children were more likely to have siblings who suffered from both ADHD and CD, while the siblings of children with ADHD alone had only hyperactivity. Although ADHD by itself conveys some risk for adult antisocial behavior, it is when the ADHD child has a comorbid CD that the risk of adult antisocial personality and criminal conviction rises sharply (Mannuzza, Klein, Konig, & Giampino, 1989; Mannuzza et al., 1991).

GENETICS OF ANTISOCIAL BEHAVIOR IN YOUTH AND ADULTS

There are different genetic effects on juvenile CD* and adult antisocial behavior. Also, genetic studies of antisocial behavior must take into account separate genetic effects on alcoholism and substance abuse, of which crime can be a secondary factor. Genetic factors can be assessed through twin and adoptee studies. In the near future, molecular genetic studies may help identify specific genes involved in antisocial behavior (Virkkunen, Goldman, & Linnoila, 1996). In terms of adult criminality, monozygotic (MZ) twins have shown a higher concordance rate for antisocial behavior and criminal conviction than dizygotic (DZ) twins. Thirty-five percent of MZ twins were concordant for criminality compared to 13% of DZ twins (Christiansen, 1977). Gottesman and Goldsmith (1994) pooled twin studies of adult criminality carried out worldwide since 1931: male MZ twins showed a 52% concordance rate compared to 23% for DZ twins. Nearly 16,000 twin pairs were studied as part of the National Academy of Sciences–National Research Council World War II Veteran Twin Registry (Centerwall & Robinette, 1989). The MZ concordance rate for dishonorable discharge (highly correlated with antisocial behavior) was 15%, in contrast to 1.6% for DZ twins.

Adoptee studies are also consistent in showing a genetic effect on adult criminality. Adoptees from a biological parent with a criminal conviction show an elevated rate of criminality relative to adoptees whose biological parents do not have antisocial behavior, even when separated from their biological parents at birth (Cadoret & Cain, 1980; Crowe, 1978; Hutchings & Mednick, 1974; Schulsinger, 1972).

In terms of juvenile delinquency, the genetic picture is less clear, with much more evidence that environment plays a major role. For many years, twin studies have tended to show similar rates of juvenile delinquency in MZ and DZ twins (McGuffin & Gottesman, 1985). Other studies have shown modest heritability for juvenile delinquency (Grove et al., 1990; Rowe, 1983; Rowe & Osgood, 1984). Recently, Lyons and colleagues (1995) performed structured interviews for CD and adult Antisocial Personality Disorder (APD) in more than 3000 twins. The authors relied on the subjects' recall of their youthful antisocial behavior. The heritability of CD behavior was quite small (.07) but genetics explained over 40% of the variance of adult antisocial traits. This study involved men who enlisted for military service and thus may have excluded individuals who were severely conduct disordered and not eligible for military service. More than 2600 Australian adult twins were interviewed by telephone about their childhood CD behaviors

*In this chapter I use Conduct Disorder (CD) as a general term to subsume what investigators may have referred to as juvenile antisocial behavior. It should be borne in mind, however, that many legally defined juvenile delinquents do not meet either clinical or psychometric criteria for CD or any other disorder (see Quay, 1987)

(Slutske *et al.*, 1997). In contrast to Lyons and colleagues, significant effects of genetics of CD were found: 53% of male MZ twins were concordant for CD, as opposed to 37% of the DZ twins. Heritability of CD was calculated at .71. The authors argued that their broader sample, compared to the Lyons and colleagues sample, accounted for the different findings. It is also possible that in Australia, with a more ethnically homogeneous population and fewer extremes of social problems (ghettos, drugs, urban decay), there is less environmental push toward CD behavior. Therefore, those who develop CD are more likely to have a genetic diathesis toward it.

Cadoret, Yates, Troughton, Woodworth, and Stewart (1995b) used an adoption paradigm to study genetic effects on juvenile antisocial behavior. Clear gene by environment interactions were found for childhood aggressivity, childhood diagnosis of CD, and adolescent aggressivity. In the absence of an antisocial biological parent, the adoptee had no risk for these three conditions even when reared in a dysfunctional environment. For children of biological parents with antisocial behavior, the risk of childhood or adolescent CD increased as a function of the adversity of the adoptive home environment (marital stress, alcohol and drug problems, legal problems, divorce, mental illness in adoptive parent). Thus, there is a genetic effect on childhood disruptive behavior, though it is considerably smaller than that for adult antisocial behavior. There is also a gene by environment interaction for CD behavior not seen for adult criminality.

A crucial issue for the study of genetics of antisocial behavior is the overlap with substance and alcohol abuse, which have their own genetic factors (Cloninger, 1989). At one point, it was suggested that the entire genetic effect on adult crime was accounted for by alcoholism (Bohman, 1978). Alcohol abuse would clearly make crime more likely. Follow-up studies showed that there were increased criminal convictions in the adopted sons of biological nonalcoholic criminal fathers who were not alcoholic relative to controls (Rutter & Giller, 1983).

Cloninger (1989) has distinguished two types of alcoholism. In Type I (the less severe type), age of onset of drinking is later, more women are affected, there is an absence of antisocial behavior, and there is substantial guilt over drinking. Type II alcoholism is almost exclusively male, is associated with fighting and antisocial behavior, and has an early age of onset. The genetic patterns of these two types are quite different. Adopted-away children of biological parents with Type I alcoholism do not show an increased risk of alcohol abuse unless they are raised by an alcoholic adoptive parent. That is, Type I alcoholism shows a clear gene by environment interaction. In contrast, about 18% of adopted-away children of Type II alcoholics develop severe alcohol abuse regardless of the alcohol abuse history of the adoptive parent. Interestingly, if a child who does not have a Type II alcoholic biological parent is raised by a Type II adoptive parent, his risk of alcoholism does not exceed that of a control group (Cloninger, 1989). This indicates that there is no effect of the environment on Type II alcoholism.

Cadoret, Yates, Troughton, Woodworth, and Stewart (1995a) studied 95 male adoptees, 46 of whom had biological parents with either APD or alcohol and substance abuse. A log linear analysis showed two pathways to substance abuse. One was direct: Alcohol and substance abuse in the biological parent was related to these problems in the adoptee, independent of aggression or CD behavior. The second began with APD in the biological parent and led to the early onset of aggression and CD in the adoptee. These symptoms in turn led to APD in the adoptee, finally ending in alcohol and substance abuse. These two patterns are highly consistent with Cloninger's (1989) dichotomy of Type I and Type II alcoholism. It is likely that genetic factors are most important for continuous antisocials, who are more likely to show both early onset of antisocial behavior and Type II alcoholism. Genetic studies of early CD and adult antisocial behavior are likely to show strong genetic effects, as there is continuity in these conditions. In contrast, a study of adolescent delinquents would include a large number of socialized aggressives in whom genetic effects are negligible.

THE SEROTONERGIC SYSTEM IN IMPULSE CONTROL AND AGGRESSION

Serotonin (5-HT) is one of the most widely distributed systems in the brain. The cell bodies of the 5-HT system reside in nine major groups in the brainstem (B1–B9), though most originate in the raphe nuclei (Nieuwenhuys, 1985). The axons of these neurons project to both rostral and caudal targets, reaching nearly every area of the brain. The 5-HT neurons pass through the median forebrain bundle and then diverge to inervate the entire cortex, the dorsal and neostriatum, the amygdala, hippocampus, and the septal nuclei. A caudal projection inervates the spinal cord, with specific input to the interiomediolateral cell column (IML), which controls sympathetic outflow. 5-HT neurons project to the hypothalamus, where they modulate the activity of the various hypothalamic releasing factors. This in turn influences pituitary output of hormones such as prolactin and adenocorticotropin hormone (ACTH). Drugs such as fenfluramine affect the secretion of these hormones, thus testing the "responsiveness" of the 5-HT system.

Particularly important for the study of behavior, the 5-HT neurons of the raphe project to the dopaminergic neurons of the ventral tegmental area (VTA) and the substantia nigra (Kapur & Remington, 1996; Nieuwenhuys, 1985). The dopamine (DA) VTA neurons project to the prefrontal cortex and the nucleus accumbens, which are critical in mediating the organism's response to reward (discussed later in the chapter). 5-HT neurons synapse directly on the neurons of the substantia nigra and inhibit their firing (Kelland, Freeman, & Chiodo, 1990). The 5-HT neurons also synapse on the terminal axons of the DA neurons in the substantia nigra and decrease the release of DA there (Waldmier & Delini-Stula, 1979). Similarly, neurons which project to the nucleus accumbens synapse on

the terminal axons of the DA neurons that project there, releasing 5-HT onto "heteroreceptors," also inhibiting DA release from those neurons (Hetey, Kudrin, Shemanow, Rayevsky, & Oelssner, 1985).

This would suggest an overall inhibitory action of 5-HT on DA, although it may not be that straightforward. In both human and nonhuman primates, there is, in fact, a strong positive correlation (>.70) of 5-hydroxyindoleacetic acid (5-HIAA), the principal metabolite of 5-HT and homovanillic acid (HVA), the principal metabolite of DA in cerebrospinal fluid (CSF) (Agren, Mefford, Rudorfer, Linnoila, & Potter, 1986; Kraemer & Clarke, 1996; Kraemer, Ebert, Schmidt, & McKinney, 1989). Statistical modeling is consistent with a strong facilitory effect of 5-HT on DA (Agren *et al.,* 1986). To help resolve this issue, Agren and colleagues examined the correlations of 5-HIAA and HVA and found it to be positive in all brain regions except the caudate and nucleus accumbens, where it was negative. To date no studies have emerged that explain the contradiction in findings regarding the relationship of DA and 5-HT in the behaving organism. Figure 1 shows a method of visualizing these complex relationships for the purpose of this chapter.

Spoont (1992) reviewed the animal literature on the role of 5-HT in behavior and noted that the effects of 5-HT agonists and antagonists on behavior are most consistent when studied in the context of DA transmission. It is well established that amphetamine enhances locomotor activity in rodents; concomitant administration of 5-HT consistently abolishes this effect of DA (Gerson & Baldessarini, 1980). Exploratory behavior is increased by lesions of the 5-HT systems; administering a DA agonist to these animals further enhances such behavior, with a greater likelihood of the animal degenerating into stereotyped hyperlocomotion (Gately, Poon, Segal, & Geyer, 1985). Spoont also reviewed data showing that the 5-HT activity disrupts the reward-enhancing effects of DA in the nucleus accumbens and decreases startle responses. Spoont hypothesized that the principal role of the 5-HT sys-

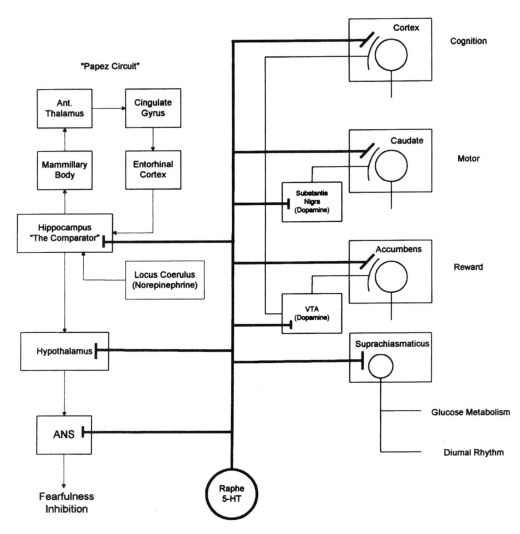

FIGURE 1. The hippocampal circuit is hypothesized by Gray (1982) to be instrumental in comparing current stimuli to representations in long-term memory. If the stimulus is novel or has been associated with punishment in the past, the output from the hippocampus may activate the ANS, resulting in anxiety and inhibition. The norepinephrine and 5-HT input to the hippocampus may enhance this inibitory response. 5-HT input to the cortex, caudate, accumbens, and suprachiasmaticus may influence inhibitory control via influence on dopamine input. See text for details.

tem is to constrain signals, both internal to the organism (DA-facilitated reward) and external (startle to noises). Thus, 5-HT does not play a role in any single behavior, but constrains the organism's response to stimuli. This is consistent with Soubrie's (1986) earlier hypothesis that the 5-HT system plays an overall role in inhibitory control. A wide body of data has now emerged in both humans and nonhuman primates that implicates the 5-HT system in disinhibition and aggression.

Studies in Adult Nonhuman Primates

In rhesus monkeys, 5-HIAA levels are under substantial genetic control (>50% of the variance) and are highly consistent within individuals over time (Clarke *et al.,* 1995; Higley, Suomi, & Linnoila, 1992; Higley *et al.,* 1993; Higley, King, *et al.,* 1996; Kraemer *et al.,* 1989). Nonetheless, environmental factors can affect the development of the 5-HT system, as we see in the next section. In adult rhesus monkeys, CSF 5-HIAA is highly associated with measures of aggression and social competence. CSF 5-HIAA is negatively correlated with rates of prolonged, inappropriate aggression in both males and females (Higley, King, et al., 1996; Raleigh & McGuire, 1994; Yodyingyuad, De La Riva, Abbott, Herbert, & Keverne, 1985). Fenfluramine, when administered acutely, acts as a potent 5-HT agonist. It blocks the reuptake of 5-HT and induces the neuron to actively release 5-HT. (It is thus a more potent 5-HT agonist than the "specific serotonin reuptake inhibitors," which only block reuptake.) With chronic administration, fenfluramine gradually depletes neurons of 5-HT. In Old World species of monkeys, fenfluramine lowered 5-HIAA and increased aggression (Raleigh et al., 1986). In rhesus monkeys living in the wild, CSF 5-HIAA was positively correlated with prosocial behaviors such as grooming and physical proximity to other monkeys (Mehlman et al., 1995). In contrast, low CSF 5-HIAA was associated with increased intensity of aggression, more physical wounds and greater risk taking. Low CSF 5-HIAA monkeys were more likely to take long leaps from trees at dangerous heights (Mehlman et al., 1994).

Higley, Mehlman, and colleagues (1996) collected CSF 5-HIAA from monkeys and followed them in the wild over a 3-year period; 46% of the monkeys in the low 5-HIAA group were dead at follow-up, most likely because of increased aggression. When monkeys with a high number of wounds were identified and compared with control monkeys with no or few wounds, the wounded monkeys showed lower CSF 5-HIAA (Higley, Mehlman, et al., 1992). Finally, monkeys who showed a low prolactin response to fenfluramine made more threatening gestures when shown slides of other monkeys than animals with a high prolactin response (Kyes, Botchin, Kaplan, Manuck, & Mann, 1995).

Genetics are not the only factors influencing CSF 5-HIAA in monkeys. CSF 5-HIAA rose in monkeys who were introduced to a new social group, as well as when a new monkey was placed in an established group (Higley, King, et al., 1996). Interestingly, diet has recently been shown to influence both CSF 5-HIAA and aggression in nonhuman primates. Studies of the relationship of cholesterol and aggression were stimulated by the finding that human subjects on cholesterol-lowering diets showed increased mortality from violence and suicide (Muldoon, Manuck, & Matthews, 1990). Kaplan and colleagues (1994) randomized cynomolgus monkeys to a high- or low-cholesterol diet for an 8-month period. The monkeys on a high-cholesterol diet had plasma cholesterol levels nearly three times higher than those on the low-cholesterol diet. The low-cholesterol group had significantly lower CSF 5-HIAA and higher ratings of aggression than the high-cholesterol group. This finding was replicated by Fontenot, Kaplan, Shively, Manuck, and Mann (1996) in a different species of monkey.

The results are contrary to the stereotype of impulsive, aggressive children consuming too much fat or sugar, and may have relevance for institutional dietary policies. Equally important is the effect of season; in adult humans CSF 5-HIAA is 40% lower in the late winter and early spring than in the summer and fall (Brewerton, Berrettini, Nurnberger, & Linnoila, 1987), although this seasonal pattern is not seen in children (Swedo et al., 1989).

5-HT Developmental Studies in Nonhuman Primates

Kraemer and colleagues (1989) first studied the effects of social rearing on the development of biogenic amine systems in rhesus monkeys. Twelve infant male rhesus monkeys were reared by their mothers until the age of 10–14 months. This group was subdivided into those who continued to live with their mothers but were peer deprived and those who continued to live with their mothers and have contact with peers. Another group of 6 infant monkeys were deprived of both mother and peer contact. These monkeys were finally introduced to peers at age 15–21 months. The mother-reared and peer-deprived monkeys were also introduced to peers at age 21–22 months. Serial measurements of CSF 5-HIAA, norepinephrine (NE), and HVA were made throughout the monkeys' development.

5-HIAA declined steadily from birth to age 24 months for all the infant monkeys regardless of social rearing group. CSF HVA did not discriminate the groups nor did it change with age. 5-HIAA did not change when the juvenile monkeys were introduced to a new social group, contrary to the increases seen in adult monkeys (Higley, King, et al., 1996). The effects of social rearing were most pronounced on the correlations of 5-HT indices with the measures of the DA and NE systems. By 22 months, monkeys reared with mothers showed strong, positive correlations of 5-HIAA with HVA (.96) but no such correlation was noted in the other two groups of monkeys. These correlations suggest that social deprivation may disrupt the "entraining" of the DA and 5-HT systems.

In a second study (Kraemer & Clarke, 1996), 48 infant rhesus monkeys were divided into mother-reared or peer-reared groups and CSF amine metabolites were assessed as in Kraemer and colleagues (1989). No differences were found in CSF 5-HIAA between the two groups, and there was no overall difference in aggressive behavior. 5-HIAA was positively correlated with NE and HVA in the mother-reared group, but only with HVA in the peer-reared group. Negative correlations between aggression and 5-HIAA were found in the mother-reared group (consistent with adult studies), but no such correlation emerged in the peer-reared group.

In contrast to the studies just described, Higley, Suomi, and Linnoila (1991) found that peer rearing increased CSF 5-HIAA relative to mother-reared monkeys in males but not females, though a disproportionate number of the monkeys in this study came from one father, possibly biasing the results. In the next study (Higley, Suomi, et al., 1992), peer-reared males had increased CSF 5-HIAA levels relative to peer-reared females but peer-reared females had lower CSF 5-HIAA concentrations compared to female mother-reared monkeys. This difference was apparent only at age 1 year; there were no effects of either rearing status or

sex on 5-HIAA in 2-year-old monkeys. Further studies (Higley, Suomi, & Linnoila, 1996a, 1996b) randomized 29 infant rhesus monkeys to mother-reared or peer-reared conditions. They were given free access to alcohol. At ages 6 and 50 months, they underwent a series of four 4-day separations followed by reunion to their home cages. CSF biogenic amines were measured at baseline and during the first and fourth separation. Before separation, peer-reared monkeys had lower CSF 5-HIAA than mother-reared monkeys; they also consumed more alcohol. During the first separation (regardless of the age of the monkey), all the monkeys had an increase in CSF 5-HIAA, but showed a decline in this metabolite when exposed to the fourth separation. There was no interaction with rearing status. CSF 5-HIAA correlated negatively with aggression in both mother-reared and peer-reared groups. The data suggested an interaction between low CSF 5-HIAA and peer rearing such that these monkeys were particularly aggressive and socially inept. It can be seen that the development of the 5-HT system is complex. The factors affecting it include genetics, sex, early rearing experiences, diet, and age. The results of the infant monkey 5-HT studies are more complex and less consistent than the studies of 5-HT in adult monkeys. A similar pattern is emerging in human studies.

5-HT Studies in Adult Humans

Studies of 5-HIAA in adult personality disorders show a striking consistency with those in nonhuman primates. A high negative correlation (−.78) between CSF 5-HIAA and ratings of aggression and suicide attempts was found in men discharged from the military for inappropriate behavior (Brown, Goodwin, Ballenger, Goyer, & Major, 1979; Brown et al., 1982). Lower 5-HIAA was found in impulsive personality disorders relative to paranoid or passive aggressive personality disorders (Linnoila et al., 1983). Men who impulsively murdered a sex partner or their own children had lower CSF 5-HIAA than other violent criminals (Lidberg, Tuck, Asberg, Scalia-Tomba, &

Bertilsson, 1985) and CSF 5-HIAA correlated negatively with ratings of hostility in normal volunteers (Roy, Adinoff, & Linnoila, 1986). Criminals with high rates of recidivism and a history of suicide attempts had lower CSF 5-HIAA than less chronic offenders (Linnoila, Delong, & Virkkunen, 1989). Impulsive offenders with early-onset alcoholism and arsonists also showed low levels of CSF 5-HIAA (Virkkunen & Linnoila, 1993; Virkkunen, Nuutila, Goodwin, & Linnoila, 1987; Virkkunen et al., 1994). In the latter study (Virkkunen et al., 1994), four groups were compared: 23 men with APD, 20 men with Intermittent Explosive Disorder (IED) (both of these groups were highly impulsive), 15 nonimpulsive offenders, and 21 control subjects. CSF HVA and 3-methoxy, 4-hydroxyphenylglycol (MHPG, a metabolite of NE) did not distinguish the groups. CSF 5-HIAA was significantly lower in the APD than in the control group and the nonimpulsive offenders were significantly higher in CSF 5-HIAA than the controls. The offenders with IED also had a very low glucose nadir during a glucose tolerance test compared to the other groups. Both impulsive groups showed higher mean activity levels as measured by actometer counts, as well as a loss of the normal diurnal rhythm of activity. Testosterone was elevated in the APD group relative to healthy volunteers.

Based on such studies, a model of 5-HT dysfunction in impulsive, alcoholic individuals has been proposed (Linnoila & Virkkunen, 1992; Virkkunen & Linnoila, 1993). As shown in Figure 1, it is hypothesized that there is decreased 5-HT input into the nucleus suprachiasmaticus, a principal hypothalamic nucleus responsible for the maintenance of circadian rhythms that also plays a role in glucose metabolism. These authors suggested that deficient 5-HT input to the suprachiasmaticus resulted in disturbed sleep, increased activity, and a tendency for glucose to fall to an abnormally low level. The dysphoria resulting from this disturbed state would then lower the threshold for impulsive, aggressive behavior. It might also result in an increased craving for alcohol to relieve the dysphoria.

Does low CSF 5-HIAA necessarily indicate decreased release of 5-HT in the brain? We cannot be certain without measuring 5-HT itself in the CSF, which is technically not possible. CSF 5-HIAA correlates positively with the amount of prolactin released in response to fenfluramine (Mann, McBride, Brown, et al., 1992). More prolactin would mean more 5-HT had been released and that more was metabolized to 5-HIAA. Thus, it would be reasonable to interpret a low prolactin response as suggestive of low 5-HT release. On the other hand, a family has been identified in which males suffer from an X-linked disorder consisting of borderline mental retardation and impulsive aggression. They have a selective deficiency of monoamine oxidase A (MAOA), which catalyzes the breakdown of 5-HT into 5-HIAA. These patients show excess rates of urinary amines, including 5-HIAA (Brunner, Nelen, Breakfield, Ropers, & van Oost, 1993; Brunner, Nelen, van Zandvoort, et al., 1993). (CSF has not yet been obtained on members of this family.)

Recently a rodent model of MAOA deficiency has been developed; these mice show highly abnormal levels of aggression (Cases et al., 1995). Their brains show strikingly high levels of 5-HT and abnormally low levels of 5-HIAA. 5-HIAA is low not because there is a deficient release of 5-HT, but because 5-HT cannot be broken down. This will most likely prolong the action of 5-HT at the postsynaptic receptor. Prolonged action of 5-HT at the postsynaptic receptor would lead to downregulation, and this might account for the blunted prolactin response. Not all aggressive patients have a deficiency of MAOA, but these findings should remind us that low 5-HIAA does not automatically mean low 5-HT activity.

5-HT Neuroendocrine Probe Studies in Adults

Fenfluramine is an indirect central 5-HT agonist. It enhances release of 5-HT from neurons, blocks the reuptake of 5-HT, and stimulates postsynaptic 5-HT receptors. These actions in the hypothalamus ultimately cause the pituitary to release a large bolus of prolactin which can be measured in the plasma. There are a wide variety of serotonin receptors distributed throughout the brain, but it is not known which receptors are specifically involved in the prolactin response. These 5-HT receptor subtypes are summarized in Table 1 (Mansour, Chalmers, Fox, Meador-Woodruff & Watson, 1996).

Coccaro and colleagues (1989) used this methodology in patients with personality disorders. Male patients with impulsive personality disorders and history of suicide attempts showed a blunted prolactin response relative to controls and nonimpulsive depressed patients. A negative correlation was found between the peak prolactin level in plasma and ratings of aggression and hostility on several standardized ratings scales. A group of violent offenders with antisocial personality also showed blunted prolactin responses to fenfluramine (O'Keane et al., 1992).

Fishbein, Lozovsky, and Jaffe (1989) performed the fenfluramine stimulation test in a population of mixed substance abusers and found elevated prolactin response in "impulsive, aggressive" subjects. Later, Handelsman, Holloway, Shiekh, Sturiano, and Bernstein (1993) examined the relationship between the prolactin response to fenfluramine and ratings of hostility in alcohol and cocaine abusers. They found that alcohol abusers showed negative correlations of the prolactin response with ratings of hostility; the cocaine abusers showed positive correlations of the prolactin response with such ratings. Thus, history of alcohol or substance abuse is a crucial factor in the outcome of these studies. It is not known whether cocaine changes the nature of the 5-HT response to agonists or whether substance-abusing persons with personality disorders have a different defect in the 5-HT system from those who abuse alcohol.

Other 5-HT agonists have been used in the prolactin stimulation test. MCPP, a postsynaptic 5-HT agonist, was administered to patients with APD and controls; investigators also found an inverse relationship between peak prolactin and assaultive behavior (Moss, Yao, & Panzak, 1990). The APD groups as a whole had blunted responses, even though they had a history of substance abuse. Coccaro, Gabriel, and Siever (1990) and Coccaro, Kavoussi, and Hauger (1995) used the 5-HT1A receptor agonists buspirone and ipsapirone and found blunted prolactin and thermal responses, respectively. Fenfluramine enhances release of 5-HT, therefore a blunted prolactin response to it can be interpreted as decreased release of 5-HT in the impulsive patients. Decreased release should lead to postsynaptic hypersensitivity. The 5-HT1A agonists work directly on the postsynaptic receptor; the blunted response to

TABLE 1.   Neuroanatomical Distribution of Serotonin Receptor Messenger RNA

Receptor subtype	Anatomic distribution
5-HT_{1A}	Limbic brain areas, hippocampus, septum, amygdala, and raphe nuclei. Found pre- and postsynaptically
5-HT_{1B}	Raphe neurons and hippocampus, striatum and neocortex. Found pre- and postsynaptically
5-HT_{1C}	Choroid plexus, subiculum, hypothalamus, and dorsal raphe
5-HT_{1D}	Hippocampus, striatum, and amygdala
5-HT_{1E}	Human neocortex
5-HT_{1F}	Neocortex, hippocampus, dorsal raphe
5-HT_{2}	Neocortex, claustrum, pontine nuclei, and hippocampus. Primarily postsynaptic
5-HT_{3}	Neocortex, hippocampus, amygdala, and dorsal raphe. A ligand gated ion channel, can depolarize neurons
5-HT_{4}	Hippocampus and midbrain
5-HT_{5}	Neocortex, hippocampus, and cerebellum. Primarily postsynaptic.
5-HT_{6}	Hippocampus. Primarily postsynaptic.
5-HT_{7}	Hippocampus, amygdala, and raphe nuclei. Found pre- and postsynaptically.

Note. Adapted from Mansour et al., 1996.

them suggests 5-HT1A receptor subsensitivity, which would be consistent with a chronic excessive release of 5-HT. Further studies are needed to resolve these issues.

Molecular Genetic Studies of the 5-HT system

Genomic DNA can be isolated from white blood cells and through modern techniques the genes for neurotransmitter receptors and the enzymes that control their production and metabolism can be identified. Researchers can look for mutant genes in disturbed populations. As noted earlier in this chapter, a family has been identified who show an X chromosome–linked behavior disorder and mild mental retardation (Brunner, Nelen, Breakfield, et al., 1993; Brunner, Nelen, van Zandvoort, et al., 1993). A point mutation was identified in the MAOA structural gene that resulted in a severe deficiency of enzyme activity that in turn led to disturbed biogenic amine metabolism. Although this process is intriguing, it is not known whether the defective MAOA gene directly influences aggression or whether it results in the mild retardation that in turn is associated with behavior disturbance (see Chapter 28, this volume). Since aggression and antisocial behavior in humans do not show an X-linked pattern of inheritance it is unlikely that this particular genetic defect accounts for a substantial amount of antisocial behavior (Virkkunen et al., 1996).

Recently the gene for tryptophan hydroxylase (TH) has been examined in impulse control disorders (Nielsen et al., 1994). The TH gene has a U and an L allele, with the U allele the more rare of the two. TH is the rate-limiting enzyme in the synthesis of 5-HT. In the impulsive offender group the UU genotype had the highest CSF 5-HIAA concentration and the LL groups had the lowest. (Recall that the impulsive offenders overall had lower CSF 5-HIAA.) There was no relationship of TH genotype to CSF 5-HIAA in nonimpulsive offenders or controls. There was no relationship of TH genotype to psychiatric diagnosis (APD, IED, nonimpulsive offender, or controls) but among violent offenders (impulsive or nonim-

pulsive), having the L allele was associated with a greater number of suicide attempts. No definite findings have emerged but linkage studies are currently under way to determine whether mutations of the 5-HT2C or 5-HT1D receptors are linked to violent or antisocial behavior (Virkkunen et al., 1996).

5-HT Studies in Children

A number of studies have examined 5-HT function in children and adolescents. The methodological and ethical issues are much more profound in using techniques such as lumbar puncture and neuroendocrine stimulation tests in this age group. The seriousness of the condition under study clearly justifies these procedures in the clinical group, but it is often difficult to interpret the results in the absence of a normal control group. These procedures are not dangerous, but they are invasive, and even if approved for pediatric controls the investigator will rarely find parents eager to volunteer their child for a spinal tap or multiple venipunctures. If the parent wishes their normal child to volunteer, the child himself may still refuse, and it would not be ethical for the child to be forced to participate. Early studies obtained CSF from other populations undergoing lumbar puncture for a medical identification (i.e., follow-up of childhood leukemia, headache workup) (Shaywitz, Cohen, & Bowers, 1977; Shetty & Chase, 1976) but it is not clear whether such children represent adequate controls given that there is at least a suspicion of CNS dysfunction. Aside from this it is difficult from a practical standpoint for an investigator to be "at the ready" to collect CSF whenever a pediatric lumbar tap happens to be performed in the clinic.

Kruesi and colleagues (1990) first examined CSF monoamine metabolites in children with Disruptive Behavior Disorders (DBD). The 29 children with DBD had at least one diagnosis of ADHD, ODD, or CD according to a structured interview. Twenty-one met criteria for ADHD at the time of the study; the other 8 had a history of ADHD in the past. Twenty-two of the subjects had either ODD or CD. All the subjects were medication free for at least 3 weeks before the lumbar puncture. The contrast group was 43 children with Obsessive-Compulsive Disorder (OCD) who were tapped under conditions identical to the DBD group. CSF 5-HIAA was significantly lower in the DBD group relative to the OCD group; all but one subject in the DBD group had levels of CSF 5-HIAA below the mean of the OCD group. Ratings of aggression against people correlated negatively with 5-HIAA in the DBD group ($r = -.40$, $p = .04$) but not in the OCD group. There were no correlations of 5-HIAA with either clinical or laboratory measures of impulsivity but 5-HIAA correlated positively with the Social Competence Scale of the Child Behavior Checklist (Achenbach & Edelbrock, 1983) ($r = .39$, $p < .005$).

The 29 children with DBD were followed up 2 years later (Kruesi *et al.*, 1992). All but one of the subjects continued to meet criteria for a DBD at follow-up. 5-HIAA remained negatively correlated with overt physical aggression ($r = -.53$, $p = .006$) and contributed significantly to the prediction of poor outcome above that predicted by the clinical variables alone.

A subset of the sample ($n = 20$) were compared in terms of CSF 5-HIAA to a group of boys with primarily ADHD ($n = 29$) (Castellanos *et al.*, 1994). Castellanos and colleagues stated that their ADHD group was "more hyperactive and less aggressive" than the Kruesi and colleagues (1990) sample, but examination of Table 1 in their study shows the groups to be more similar than different. Equal numbers of subjects had a diagnosis of CD, for instance. The aggression ratings were higher and the inattention ratings were lower in the Kruesi and colleagues sample relative to the ADHD sample. Child Behavior Checklist (Achenbach & Edelbrock, 1983) ratings did not differ between the groups for any of the subscales, including Aggression, Hyperactivity, and Delinquency. CSF 5-HIAA did not differ between the two groups and in the ADHD group there was an unexpected positive correlation of 5-HIAA with aggression ratings. It is possible that indices of 5-HT function correlate negatively with aggression only in groups of children specifically selected for aggression as in the Kruesi and colleagues sample. Recall that CSF 5-HIAA also did not correlate with aggression in the OCD sample. All of the adult work has also been done with populations selected for aggressive behavior.

Fenfluramine was found to increase prolactin in children and adolescents and such responses were stable over time (Stoff, Pasatiempo, Yeung, Bridger, & Rabinovich, 1992). Next, 15 prepubertal children with DBD were administered fenfluramine and serial prolactin and cortisol levels were obtained (Stoff, Pasatiempo, Yeung, Cooper, *et al.*, 1992). There were no prepubertal controls. Fenfluramine clearly induced prolactin and cortisol responses, but there was no correlation between peak prolactin or cortisol levels and any measure of aggressivity. As part of the same study, 8 adolescents with DBD were compared to 8 age-matched controls on the same measures; no differences in prolactin or cortisol response to fenfluramine between the groups were found. Again, no correlation of peak prolactin or cortisol response was found with aggression ratings in the adolescent sample.

Halperin and colleagues (1994) divided a sample of 25 ADHD boys aged 7 to 11 into those with and without significant aggression. Children were classified as aggressive by three investigators who reviewed all the history, rating scales, and psychiatric interview data for the presence or absence of clinically significant aggression. The aggressive ADHD children were found to have an augmented prolactin response to fenfluramine, findings opposite from adult work. Halperin, Newcorn, Schwartz, and colleagues (1997) then attempted to replicate this finding in a second, independent sample of 25 ADHD boys. This time, they found no differences between the aggressive and nonaggressive ADHD boys in prolactin response to fenfluramine. In an attempt to reconcile the discrepant findings, Halperin, Newcorn, Schwartz, and colleagues compared the first and second samples and noted that the second sample was significantly older than the first (9.5 years vs. 8.5 years). The second sample was closer in age to the prepubertal sample of Stoff,

Pasatiempo, Yeung, Cooper, and colleagues (1992) (mean age = 10.2 years). They combined the samples and found significant main effects of age (greater prolactin response in older children), no effect of aggression, but a significant age by aggression interaction. That is, in children under age 9, nonaggressive ADHD subjects had a blunted prolactin response to fenfluramine relative to aggressive ADHD children. In children over age 9, the nonaggressive ADHD children had nonsignificantly higher prolactin response than the aggressive children. Examination of their Figure 2 shows that the aggressive ADHD subjects had a similar prolactin response regardless of age, whereas the nonaggressive ADHD subjects showed developmental changes. Prolactin responses were lower in nonaggressive younger children and nearly doubled in the older nonaggressive children. This finding is consistent with the hypothesis that the 5-HT system responds differently in aggressive versus nonaggressive groups.

In an elegant series of studies, Halperin and his colleagues elucidated other factors that may affect the fenfluramine prolactin stimulation test in children (see Table 2). Forty-one ADHD boys were subdivided into those who had (n = 16) and those who did not have (n = 25) a parent with aggressive behavior (Halperin, Newcorn, Kopstein, et al., 1997). Each child was then classified as either aggressive or nonaggressive based on a best-estimate procedure using data from multiple sources. Aggressive children with a family history of aggression had a blunted prolactin response relative to those without such a family history. The nonaggressive children had prolactin responses intermediate between the two aggressive groups. Interestingly, this suggests that an enhanced prolactin response may be found in aggressive children without a family history of aggression, but this was not confirmed in a more recent study.

The fenfluramine prolactin test was performed on 34 African American and Hispanic boys with a mean age of 10 (Pine et al., 1997). Thirteen had comorbid ADHD and ODD/CD, 5 had ADHD alone, and 16 had other psychiatric diagnoses or no diagnosis. The prolactin response correlated positively with Child Behavior Checklist (Achenbach & Edelbrock, 1983) ratings of Aggression and Delinquency. Boys with ODD/CD had significantly enhanced prolactin response relative to boys with ADHD alone or those without an externalizing diagnosis. An enhanced prolactin response was also associated with a negative home environment. The results point out that young CD children may differ significantly from adult

TABLE 2. Effects of Multiple Factors: The Fenfluramine Prolactin and Cortisol Stimulation Tests in ADHD Children and Adolescents

Factor	Study	Result
Age	Halperin, Newcorn, Schwartz, et al. (1997)	Young (< 9 years) aggressive ADHD children have enhanced prolactin response. No difference in prolactin response between ADHD aggressive and nonaggressive boys in older (>9 years) age subjects.
Family history of aggression	Halperin, Newcorn, Kopstein, et al. (1997)	Aggressive ADHD child with aggressive parent had blunted prolactin response. Aggressive ADHD children without aggressive parent had an enhanced prolactin response.
Family history of alcoholism	Schulz et al. (1996)	ADHD children with an alcoholic father had enhanced cortisol response. Prolactin response in ADHD children does not vary as a function of family history of alcoholism.
Ratings of affective ability	Newcorn et al. (1996)	Low prolactin response in aggressive ADHD children with high ratings of irritability, no relationship of irritability ratings to prolactin response in nonaggressive group.
Pervasiveness of aggression	McKay et al. (1996)	Pervasively aggressive boys had low prolactin response relative to situationally aggressive boys.

antisocial persons in the nature of any dysfunction in the 5-HT system.

The relationship of the prolactin secretion in response to fenfluramine is complex. Table 2 indicates that there is a subgroup of aggressive children (most of whom also have ADHD) who have a family history of aggression, are affectively labile, and have pervasive aggression who show a blunted prolactin response to fenfluramine. There are clear effects of age. Thus any study that compares an unselected group of aggressive children to a control group on the prolactin stimulation test will most likely yield negative findings.

Studies of Peripheral Serotonin Measures

A number of measures of 5-HT functioning in the platelet have been studied in normal controls and aggressive subjects. These include platelet 5-HT content, platelet 5-HT2 receptor density and affinity, and binding of imipramine or paroxetine to the 5-HT reuptake site. 5-HT functioning can also be affected in some cases by manipulating dietary tryptophan. However, the relationship of these measures to central 5-HT functioning is not clear (Mann, McBride, Brown, et al., 1992; Pliszka, Rogeness, Renner, Sherman, & Broussard, 1988). Platelets do not synthesize 5-HT; instead, tryptophan is taken up from the gut and converted to 5-HT by the enterochromaffin cells. Newly synthesized platelets have storage granules and transport mechanisms but do not contain 5-HT until they reach the gut, where 5-HT is taken up from the enterochromaffin cells. 5-HT in the platelets participates in the aggregation process when blood vessels are injured.

Mann, McBride, Brown, and colleagues (1992) studied the relationship of platelet 5-HT2 receptor functioning to both CSF 5-HIAA and the prolactin response to fenfluramine in a sample of adult depressed patients. There was no relationship of CSF 5-HIAA to either number of platelet 5-HT2 receptors or to any measure of receptor functioning. In patients older than 30 years, the number of platelet 5-HT2 receptors correlated positively ($r = .59$, $p = .02$) with the peak prolactin response to fenfluramine. This relationship was not found in younger patients. Platelet content of 5-HT has been found to correlate negatively with the fenfluramine prolactin response in young adult autistic men (McBride et al., 1989). Despite the unclear nature of the relationship of platelet 5-HT functioning to central 5-HT measures, the ease of these measures has led to their use in studies with both children and adults with behavior disorders.

Platelet 5-HT was higher in hospitalized aggressive CD boys relative to boys without CD (Rogeness, Hernandez, Macedo, & Mitchell, 1982). Pliszka, Rogeness, Renner, and colleagues (1988) measured platelet 5-HT in 16 nonviolent juvenile offenders, 11 violent juvenile offenders, and 17 adolescents with internalizing disorders. Platelet 5-HT was significantly higher in the violent group; there was a positive correlation between clinician ratings of CD symptoms and platelet 5-HT content ($r = .53$, $p < .01$). ADHD/CD boys were more likely to show hyperserotonemia (platelet 5-HT > 270 ng/ml) than ADHD boys without CD (Cook, Stein, Ellison, Unis, & Leventhal, 1995). Platelet 5-HT was also found to be highly familial, with strong positive correlations between mother and child 5-HT levels. The authors pointed out a possible confound in 5-HT platelet studies in that African Americans have higher whole blood 5-HT than European Americans. Given that African Americans are more likely to be diagnosed with CD because of social factors, race must be carefully controlled in such studies. Mann, McBride, Anderson, and Mieczkowski (1992) found a positive correlation between platelet 5-HT content and both current hostility ratings ($r = .44$) and lifetime aggression history ($r = .41$) in adult patients with major depression. Incarcerated teenagers with childhood-onset CD had higher platelet 5-HT than inmates with adolescent-onset CD and platelet 5-HT correlated negatively with staff ratings of social skills (Unis et al., 1997). In contrast, Stoff, Cook, and Perry (1991) and Stoff, Ieni, and colleagues (1991) found no difference between 5-HT platelet content in boys with DBD and controls; they also found no relationship of platelet 5-HT to any measure of aggression. Nonetheless, if high platelet 5-HT content is correlated with a low prolactin response (McBride et al., 1989), then is it reasonable to speculate that 5-HT is not available for release in antisocial individuals? This would explain both the blunted prolactin response and the low 5-HIAA found in adult antisocials.

Findings have been inconsistent with other measures of platelet 5-HT functioning. The number of 5-HT transporter sites labeled by paroxetine was found to be inversely related to aggression ratings in adult personality disorders (Coccaro, Kavoussi, Sheline, Lish, & Csernansky, 1996). Pine and colleagues (1996) measured the number of 5-HT2A receptors in the platelets of boys at risk for CD because they had an older brother who had been convicted of a crime. The number of 5-HT2A receptors was decreased in those boys whose parents had a history of substance abuse or incarceration. Boys who experienced a high degree of physical punishment also had reduced 5-HT2A receptors, suggesting a role for stress in modulating 5-HT platelet function. Stoff, Cook and Perry (1991) and Stoff, Ieni, and colleagues (1991) measured a wide range of peripheral 5-HT markers in boys with DBD and controls, including free-total tryptophan, platelet 5-HT2 binding and 5-HT uptake. There were no differences between the groups on any of these measures. Only imipramine binding to the platelet 5-HT reuptake site was found to be reduced in CD boys relative to controls (Stoff, Pollock, Vitiello, Behar, & Bridger, 1987). The meaning of this finding is unclear in view of the fact that CD boys showed a normal 5-HT reuptake rate.

Lower plasma tryptophan reduced brain 5-HT release in animals (Schaechter & Wurtman, 1990) and reducing dietary tryptophan increased aggression in the vervet monkey (Chamberlain, Ervin, Pihl, & Young, 1987). Recently it was found that plasma tryptophan can be dramatically decreased by a drink containing a special mixture of amino acids; remitted depressed patients who consumed this drink showed a rapid return of their depressive symptoms (Delgado et al., 1990). It has been hypothesized that administering this trypto-

phan-lowering drink might increase aggressive behavior in humans. Normal controls, however, do not show an increase in aggression when plasma tryptophan is lowered (Smith, Pihl, Young, & Ervin, 1986), unless the subjects consume alcohol first (Pihl et al., 1995). Fourteen nondepressed adults with IED also did not show an increase in aggression when administered a tryptophan-depleted drink (Salomon, Mazure, Delgado, Mendia, & Charney, 1994). Thus, whatever 5-HT dysfunction may exist in aggressive patients, it is apparently not affected by levels of plasma tryptophan. This does not suggest that administering 5-HT or tryptophan would have therapeutic effects in aggressive behavior. (See Chapter 21, this volume.)

THE ANS AND ANTISOCIAL BEHAVIOR

The autonomic nervous system (ANS), through its sympathetic and parasympathetic branches, regulates critical life functions on a moment-to-moment basis and governs the "fight or flight" reaction. The vagal nerve (parasympathetic) primarily governs heart rate (HR). Sympathetic nerves originating in the IMC of the spinal cord project first to the sympathetic ganglia and then to the blood vessels, organs, and skin. NE is released into the bloodstream and epinephrine is released from the adrenal medulla. The relationship of the ANS to the central noradrenergic system has been reviewed elsewhere (Pliszka, McCracken, & Maas, 1996). The ANS governs such factors as HR and skin conductance (SC); both of these measures have been found to be related to CD behavior.

Fourteen studies have shown the resting HR of CD children is lower relative to controls, with an effect size averaging 0.84 (Raine, 1996). Psychophysiological variables were obtained on a community sample of 101 15-year-old males in Great Britain (Raine, Venables, & Williams, 1990). All socioeconomic classes were represented. Ten years later, police records were examined for criminal convictions. HR levels of those who would become criminals were significantly lower than those who were never convicted. Criminals-to-be also showed fewer nonspecific SC fluctuations during a rest period than noncriminals, but SC level did not distinguish the groups. Criminals-to-be also showed more delta and theta power on their EEGs. A discriminant function analysis using all four variables correctly classified 75% of the subjects into criminal or noncriminal categories. A recent reanalysis of this data shows that the lowest HRs were found in those adolescents who would ultimately be convicted of violent crime (Raine, 1996). Autonomic factors were also found to be related to protective factors against developing crime in this sample (Raine, Venables, & Williams, 1995). A group of adolescents were identified who were already engaging in antisocial behavior at age 15 but who desisted and never obtained a criminal conviction. They were compared to the criminals-to-be and to normals. The desistors showed even higher resting HRs and more nonspecific SC than the normal controls. EEG power did not distinguish the groups.

Brennan, Raine, and Mednick (1994) obtained HR and SC data in 50 men at risk for crime because they had a criminal father. About half of these men became criminals themselves. They were compared to a group of criminals who had no family history of crime and to a control group (neither father nor son were criminal). Strikingly higher SC and HR were found in the men who did not commit crimes in spite of having a criminal father. In contrast, the lowest HR and SC are found in adolescents who commited crimes despite coming from intact homes in higher social classes (Maliphant, Hume, & Furnham, 1990; Raine, 1996).

Decreased ANS arousal may translate to decreased fearfulness and a disinhibited temperament. Gray (1982) has long emphasized the role of the septohippocampal system as part of a Behavioral Inhibition System (BIS). The hippocampus has output to the hypothalamus, which plays a major role in controlling output of the ANS. Reviewing studies of SC in anxiety-provoking situations or individuals with anxiety disorders, Fowles (1980, 1988) suggested that SC activity indexes the BIS. When there is no "social push" to crime (poverty, family dysfunction) ANS underarousal must be particularly strong to result in criminal behavior. In contrast, when a person is exposed to these social factors, high autonomic arousal may be a protective factor. High anxiety, better inhibitory control, or a tendency to withdraw from stimulation may lead a vulnerable child away from antisocial behavior (Raine, 1996).

THE DOPAMINE SYSTEM

A large body of evidence from animal studies implicates the DA system of the brain in the mediation of reward-driven behaviors (Wise, 1988; Wise & Bozarth, 1987). The pathway from the ventral tegmental area (VTA) to the nucleus accumbens has been particularly implicated, as animals will work either to self-stimulate these pathways or to inject DA agonists such as cocaine or amphetamine into the nucleus accumbens. Thus increased activity in this system is hypothesized to lead the organism to seek out pleasurable stimuli; the system is also hypothesized to be highly responsive to signals in the environment that indicate the presence of reward (Gray, 1982; Quay, 1988, 1993). Solanto (1984) reviewed animal studies in which DA or apomorphine (a DA agonist) was applied iontophoretically in the substantia nigra or nucleus accumbens. Low doses of DA agonist were found to stimulate the presynaptic autoreceptor preferentially, whereas higher doses were necessary to stimulate postsynaptic DA receptors (Skirboll, Grace, & Bunney, 1979). Solanto suggested that stimulants in low doses might stimulate DA autoreceptors, leading to decreased DA release. Indeed, low doses of apomorphine decreased activity in rodents (Strombom, 1976). Solanto hypothesized that stimulants exert their therapeutic effects in ADHD by the stimulation of DA autoreceptors to reduce the activity of the DA system.

In an experimental test of this hypothesis, Solanto (1986) performed a double-blind placebo-controlled trial of a very low dose of methylphenidate (0.1 mg/kg dose). Such low doses are more likely to stimulate only DA autoreceptors as in the animal studies previously mentioned. These low doses were effective in reducing activity level in ADHD children but did not improve attention as measured by a laboratory task. Solanto (1984, 1986) suggested that hyperactivity might be related to a hyperdopaminergic state. This is similar to Quay's (1988, 1993) hypothesis that CD (but not ADHD) children relentlessly seek out exciting potentially rewarding and novel situations because of overly active DA-mediated reward systems.

Studies in humans have focused on the role of the DA system in alcoholism and sensation seeking. A genetic marker related to the DA D2 receptor was hypothesized to be linked to alcoholism (Blum *et al.*, 1990) but this has not been replicated in most studies (Gelernter, Goldman, & Risch, 1993). A variant of the D4 DA receptor was found to be related to the trait of novelty seeking in normal adults (Benjamin *et al.*, 1996; Ebstein *et al.*, 1996) but this variant was not found to be overrepresented in type II alcoholics and it does not have any relationship to CSF 5-HIAA (Adamson *et al.*, 1995).

Studies of CSF HVA have been highly inconsistent in aggressive child and adult subjects. Two studies (Linnoila *et al.*, 1983; Virkkunen *et al.*, 1994) showed decreased CSF HVA in impulsive offenders relative to controls, but other studies of antisocial adults have not found any relationship of CSF HVA to aggression or antisocial behavior (Brown *et al.*, 1979; Lidberg *et al.*, 1985; Virkkunen *et al.*, 1987). Kruesi and colleagues (1990) did not find any relationship of CSF HVA to aggression or impulsivity in children with either DBD or OCD; HVA also did not predict aggressive behavior at 2-year follow-up (Kruesi *et al.*, 1992). Boys with primarily ADHD did not differ from the aggressive Kruesi and colleagues (1990) sample in terms of CSF HVA, but HVA correlated positively with aggression in the ADHD group (Castellanos *et al.*, 1994).

Peripheral measures of the DA system are difficult to come by. Urinary HVA is derived from plasma and its relationship to central DA is unclear. Blink rate has been assessed a putative measure of DA function (Zametkin, Stevens, & Pittman, 1979) but blink rate did not differentiate children with CD from those without CD (Daugherty, Quay, & Ramos, 1993). However, across all the subjects, teacher ratings of CD behaviors and eye blinks correlated .25, just missing convential statistical significance ($p = .06$). Examination of the DA–excessive reward hypothesis of CD must await the emergence of imaging technology that can assess dopaminergic functioning in the human limbic areas.

HORMONES

The evidence relating testosterone to human aggression has been extensively reviewed (Archer, 1991; Virkkunen *et al.*, 1994) with a number of key findings: (1) plasma free or salivary testosterone correlates better with aggression than plasma total testosterone and (2) early-onset aggression and aggression under the influence of alcohol is associated with elevated testosterone levels. In adults, elevated testosterone levels in CSF, plasma, and saliva have been linked to antisocial behavior and violent crime (Dabbs & Morris, 1990; Dabbs, Frady, Carr, & Besch, 1987; Ehrenkranz, Bliss, & Sheard, 1974; Virkkunen *et al.*, 1994). Testosterone levels in older adolescents (ages 17–18) also has been found to be higher in those convicted of violent crimes (Dabbs, Jurkovic, & Frady, 1991). High-testosterone subjects in this study also broke more prison rules and were less likely to be paroled. A study of younger adolescents did not find a relationship between aggression and testosterone (Susman *et al.*, 1997).

Two studies in children yielded different results. Constantino and colleagues (1993) collected serum testosterone in 18 prepubertal aggressive children and compared them to age- and race-matched controls. No differences in serum testosterone were found. Scerbo and Kolko (1994) examined salivary testosterone in 40 children with DBD aged 7–14 years who attended a day treatment program. They found a significant positive correlation between salivary testosterone and staff ($r = .47$) and teacher ($r = .45$) ratings of aggression. Parent ratings of aggression did not correlate with the hormone. Subjects were not examined for Tanner Stage, which rates the development of secondary sexual characteristics and indicates how far puberty has progressed. The subjects were, however, more likely to be postpubertal in this study, which may account for the positive results relative to those of Constantino and colleagues. It is quite likely that the testosterone–aggression relationship does not emerge until after puberty.

Dabbs and colleagues (1991) found an interaction between testosterone and cortisol. The effect of testosterone on aggression was most pronounced in offenders who had low salivary cortisol. CD children with comorbid anxiety disorders have lower rates of aggression, fewer police contacts, and fewer school suspensions than CD boys without anxiety disorders (Walker et al., 1991). Anxious CD boys have significantly higher salivary cortisol levels than nonanxious CD boys or children with anxiety disorders alone (McBurnett et al., 1991). Scerbo and Kolko (1994) found that salivary cortisol correlated positively with internalizing symptoms but had no relationship to aggression. They did not find an interaction between cortisol and testosterone. Twenty-four-hour urine free cortisol did not differentiate boys with DBD from controls (Kruesi, Schmidt, Donnelly, Hibbs, & Hamburger, 1989). Cortisol may have more of relationship to anxiety than to CD: The high cortisol is the result of higher arousal associated with internalizing disorders. In some cases, comorbid internalizing disorders may attenuate aggressive symptoms in a child with DBD. In fact, comorbid anxiety has been shown to attenuate perseverative responding for reward found in CD children (Ewell, 1994; O'Brien & Frick, 1996). These findings support the hypothesis that activity in Gray's (1982) BIS (subjectively experienced as anxiety) serves to mitigate at least some aspects of CD behavior.

THE NOREPINEPHRINE SYSTEM

Like CSF HVA, studies of CSF MHPG in antisocial behavior have been highly inconsistent. Brown and colleagues (1979) initially found a positive correlation between CSF MHPG and aggression ($r = .64$) but other studies in adults have found no relationship of CSF MHPG to aggression or antisocial behavior (Lidberg et al., 1985; Linnoila et al., 1983; Roy et al., 1986; Virkkunen et al., 1994). One study found decreased CSF MHPG in arsonists and violent offenders relative to controls (Virkkunen et al., 1987). Kruesi and colleagues (1990, 1992) found no differences between children with DBD and OCD on CSF MHPG and no correlation with measures of impulsivity or aggression. CSF MHPG was decreased in the Kruesi and colleagues (1990) sample relative to a group of boys with ADHD; MHPG was positively correlated with aggression in the ADHD group (Castellanos et al., 1994). CSF MHPG may be too "static" a measure to assess the central noradrenergic system, which constantly changes in response to demands in the environment (Pliszka et al., 1996).

Dopamine beta hydroxylase (DBH) is the enzyme that converts DA to NE. It is coreleased with NE from sympathetic nerve terminals and although interindividual variability is extremely high, it is stable within an individual, with genetic factors playing a major role (Weinshilbaum, Raymond, Elveback, & Weidman, 1973). Rogeness, Hernandez, Macedo, Amrung, and Hoppe (1986) found an association between very low levels of DBH activity and undersocialized CD. This finding was replicated in one study (Bowden, Deutsch, & Swanson, 1988) but not in others (Pliszka, Rogeness, & Medrano, 1988; Pliszka, Rogeness, Renner, et al., 1988). In particular, Pliszka, Rogeness, Renner, and colleagues (1988) did not find that DBH levels differentiated incarcerated violent juvenile offenders from non-CD psychiatric outpatients. Rogeness, Javors, Maas, and Macedo (1990) obtained 24-hr urines for catecholamines in 31 boys with DBH activity below 6 (mole/min/L) and 33 boys with DBH activity greater than 15 (mole/min/L). All the subjects were patients in a psychiatric hospital; there was no control group. Low-DBH boys had fewer anxiety and depressive diagnoses. No differences were found in NE or its metabolites in the two groups, although the sum of NE and its metabolites were decreased in the low-DBH group. The authors interpreted this as suggesting decreased NE release in the low-DBH group. A recent study of DBH in boys at a residential treatment center for DBD boys was flawed by poor design, lack of control groups, and use of multiple correlations without correcting for the number of tests (Gabel, Stadler, Bjorn, Shindledecker, & Bowden, 1993). It remains unclear whether low DBH activity is in fact associated with aggressive or antisocial behavior.

IMAGING STUDIES

Positron emission tomography (PET) has been used to assess global and regional brain glucose metabolism in violent and personality disordered subjects (Goyer et al., 1994; Raine, Buchsbaum, et al., 1995; Volkow et al., 1995). All three studies have showed decreased glucose metabolism in violent patients relative to controls, particularly in the prefrontal cortex. Curiously, in monkeys, low CSF 5-HIAA is associated with higher glucose metabolism in the orbital frontal cortex, the opposite of the expected finding (Doudet et al., 1995). It remains to be seen whether CSF 5-HIAA is related to human brain glucose metabolism. To date, no PET or other imaging studies have been performed in aggressive or CD children.

CONCLUSIONS

Figure 1 summarizes the suggested role of the 5-HT and autonomic systems in aggressive and antisocial behavior. The 5-HT system may act on four brain areas: frontal cortex, caudate, accumbens, and suprachiasmaticus to modulate cognition, motor control, response to reward,

and physiology, respectively. The 5-HT system may do this directly or by inhibiting DA inputs to these areas (Spoont, 1992). The precise nature of the 5-HT deficit remains to be elucidated. There may be deficient release of 5-HT or a defect in one of its receptors that renders the individual less responsive to 5-HT. Also, one of the many enzymes regulating 5-HT could be dysfunctional. Elevated testosterone or a deficient response of the ANS may be an alternative pathway to antisocial behavior, or they may increase the ill effects of a dysfunctional 5-HT system.

Future research should combine methods from several fields. Children at risk for antisocial behavior could be assessed for specific DA- or 5-HT–related genes, peripheral 5-HT measures, ANS measures and CSF 5-HIAA, urinary catecholamines, and neuroendocrine stimulation tests. Large samples will be needed to stratify the subjects by sex, age, race, family environment, family history, and psychosocial stressors. Studies should also examine the relationship between the genetic and neuroimaging variables and performance on laboratory measures of disinhibition (see Chapters 4 and 5, this volume) or tasks measuring perseverative responding for reward. Only then will we be able to unravel the complex gene by environment interactions that surely underlie the development of antisocial behavior.

REFERENCES

Achenback, T. M., & Edelbrock, C. (1983). *Manual for the Child Behavior Checklist and Revised Behavior Profile.* Burlington, VT: Queen City Printers.

Adamson, M. D., Kennedy, J., Petronis, A., Dean, M., Virkkunen, M., Linnoila, M., & Goldman, D. (1995). DRD4 dopamine receptor genotype and CSF monoamine metabolites in Finnish alcoholics and controls. *American Journal of Medical Genetics, 60,* 199–205.

Agren, H., Mefford, I. N., Rudorfer, M. V., Linnoila, M., & Potter, W. Z. (1986). Interacting neurotransmitter systems: A non-experimental approach to the 5-HIAA–HVA correlation in human CSF. *Journal of Psychiatric Research, 20,* 175–193.

American Psychiatric Association. (1994). *Diagnostic and statistical manual of mental disorders* (4th ed.). Washington, DC: Author.

Archer, J. (1991). The influence of testosterone on human aggression. *British Journal of Psychology, 82,* 1–28.

August, G. J., & Stewart, M. A. (1983). Familial subtypes of childhood hyperactivity. *Journal of Nervous and Mental Diseases, 171,* 362–368.

Benjamin, J., Li, L., Patterson, C., Greenberg, B. D., Murphy, D. L., & Harner, D. H. (1996). Population and familial association between the D4 dopamine receptor gene and measures of novelty seeking. *Nature Genetics, 12,* 81–84.

Biederman, J., Munir, K., & Knee, D. (1987). Conduct and oppositional disorder in clinically referred children with attention deficit disorder: A controlled family study. *Journal of the American Academy of Child and Adolescent Psychiatry, 26,* 724–727.

Biederman, J., Faraone, S. V., Keenan, K., Benjamin, J., Krifcher, B., Moore, C., Sprich-Buckminster, S., Ugaglia, K., Jellinek, M. S., & Steingard, R. (1992). Further evidence for family-genetic risk factors in attention deficit hyperactivity disorder: Patterns of comorbidity in probands and relatives psychiatrically and pediatrically referred samples. *Archives of General Psychiatry, 49,* 728–738.

Blum, K., Noble, E. P., Sheridan, P., Montgomery, A., Ritchie, T., Jagadecswaren, P., Nogami, H., Briggs, A. H., & Cohn, J. B. (1990). Allelic association of human dopamine D2 receptor gene in alcoholism. *Journal of the American Medical Association, 263,* 2055–2060.

Bohman, M. (1978). Some genetic aspects of alcoholism and criminality. *Archives of General Psychiatry, 35,* 269–276.

Bowden, C. L., Deutsch, C. K., & Swanson, J. M. (1988). Plasma dopamine-beta-hydroxylase and platelet monoamine oxidase in attention deficit disorder and conduct disorder. *Journal of the American Academy of Child and Adolescent Psychiatry, 27,* 171–174.

Brennan, P., Raine, A., & Mednick, S. A. (1994). Psychophysiological protective factors for children at high-risk for antisocial outcome. *Psychophysiology, 31* (Suppl. 1), S30.

Brewerton, T. D., Berrettini, W. H., Nurnberger, J. I., & Linnoila, M. (1987). Analysis of seasonal fluctuations of CSF monoamine metabolites and neuropeptides in normal controls: Findings with 5HIAA and HVA. *Psychiatry Research, 23,* 257–265.

Brown, G. L., Goodwin, F. K., Ballenger, J., Goyer, P., & Major, L. (1979). Aggression in humans correlates with cerebrospinal fluid metabolites. *Psychiatry Research, 1,* 131–135.

Brown, G. L., Ebert, M. H., Goyer, P., Jimerson, D., Klein, W., Bunney, W. E., & Goodwin, F. K. (1982). Aggression, suicide, and serotonin: Relationship to CSF amine metabolites. *American Journal of Psychiatry, 139,* 741–746.

Brunner, H. G., Nelen, M., Breakfield, X. O., Ropers, H. H., & van Oost, B. A. (1993). Abnormal behavior associated with a point mutation in the structural gene for monoamine oxidase A. *Science, 262,* 578–580.

Brunner, H. G., Nelen, M. R., van Zandvoort, P., Abeling, N. G. G. M., van Gennip, A. H., Wolters, E. C., Kuiper, M. A., Ropers, H. H., & van Oost, B. A. (1993). X-Linked borderline mental retardation with prominent behavioral disturbance: Phenotype, genetic localization, and evidence for disturbed monoamine metabolism. *American Journal of Human Genetics, 52,* 1032–1039.

Cadoret, R. J., & Cain, C. (1980). Sex differences in predictors of antisocial behavior in adoptees. *Archives of General Psychiatry, 37,* 1171–1175.

Cadoret, R. J., Yates, W. R., Troughton, E., Woodworth, G., & Stewart, M. A. (1995a). Adoption study demonstrating two genetic pathways to drug abuse. *Archives of General Psychiatry, 52,* 42–52.

Cadoret, R. J., Yates, W. R., Troughton, E., Woodworth, G., & Stewart, M. A. (1995b). Genetic–environmental interaction in the genesis of aggressivity and conduct disorders. *Archives of General Psychiatry, 52,* 916–924.

Cases, O., Seif, I., Grimsby, J., Gaspar, P., Chen, K., Pournin, S., Muller, U., Aguet, M., Babinet, C., & Shih, J. C. (1995). Aggressive behavior and altered amounts of brain serotonin and norepinephrine in mice lacking MAOA. *Science, 268*(5218), 1763–1766.

Castellanos, F. X., Elia, J., Kruesi, M. J. P., Gulotta, C. S., Mefford, I. N., Potter, W. Z., Ritchie, G. F., & Rapoport, J. L. (1994). Cerebrospinal fluid monoamine metabolites in boys with attention deficit hyperactivity disorder. *Psychiatry Research, 52,* 305–316.

Centerwall, B. S., & Robinette, C. D. (1989). Twin concordance for dishonorable discharge from the military: With a review of the genetics of antisocial behavior. *Comprehensive Psychiatry, 30,* 442–446.

Chamberlain, B., Ervin, F. R., Pihl, R. O., & Young, S. N. (1987). The effect of raising or lowering tryptophan levels on aggression in vervet monkeys. *Pharmacology, Biochemistry and Behavior, 28,* 503–510.

Christiansen, K. O. (1977). A preliminary study of criminality among twins. In S. Mednick & K. O. Christiansen (Eds.), *Biosocial bases of criminal behavior* (pp. 89–108). New York: Gardner.

Clarke, A. S., Kammerer, C., George, K., Kupfer, D., McKinney, W. T., Spence, A., & Kraemer, G. W. (1995). Evidence of heritability of norepinephrine, HVA, and 5HIAA values in cerebrospinal fluid of rhesus monkeys. *Biological Psychiatry, 38,* 572–577.

Cloninger, C. R. (1989). Neurogenetic adaptive mechanisms in alcoholism. In K. L. Kelner & D. E. Koshland (Eds.), *Molecules to models* (pp. 375–387). Washington, DC: American Association for the Advancement of Science.

Coccaro, E. F., Siever, L. J., Klar, H. M., Maurer, G., Cochrane, K., Cooper, T. B., Mochs, R. C., & Davis, K. L. (1989). Serotonergic studies in patients with affective and personality disorders. *Archives of General Psychiatry, 46,* 587–599.

Coccaro, E. F., Gabriel, S., & Siever, L. J. (1990). Buspirone challenge: Preliminary evidence for a role for central 5-

HT1a receptor function in impulsive aggressive behavior in humans. *Psychopharmacology Bulletin, 26,* 393–405.

Coccaro, E. F., Kavoussi, R. J., & Hauger, R. L. (1995). Physiological responses to d-fenfluramine and ipsapirone challenge correlate with indices of aggression in males with personality disorder. *International Clinical Psychopharmacology, 10,* 177–179.

Coccaro, E. F., Kavoussi, R. J., Sheline, Y. I., Lish, J. D., & Csernansky, J. G. (1996). Impulsive aggression in personality disorder correlates with tritiated paroxetine binding in the platelet. *Archives of General Psychiatry, 53,* 531–536.

Constantino, J. N., Grosz, D., Saenger, P., Chandler, D. W., Nandi, R., & Earls, F. J. (1993). Testosterone and aggression in children. *Journal of the American Academy of Child and Adolescent Psychiatry, 32,* 1217–1222.

Cook, E. H., Stein, M. A., Ellison, T., Unis, A. S., & Leventhal, B. L. (1995). Attention deficit hyperactivity disorder and whole-blood serotonin levels: Effects of comorbidity. *Psychiatry Research, 57,* 13–20.

Crowe, R. R. (1978). Genetic studies of antisocial personalities and related disorders. In R. L. Spitzer & D. F. Klein (Eds.), *Critical issues in psychiatric diagnosis* (pp. 193–202). New York: Raven.

Dabbs, J. M., & Morris, R. (1990). Testosterone, social class, and antisocial behavior in a sample of 4,462 men. *Psychological Science, 1,* 209–211.

Dabbs, J. M., Frady, R. L., Carr, T. S., & Besch, N. F. (1987). Saliva testosterone and criminal violence in young adult prison inmates. *Psychosomatic Medicine, 49,* 174–182.

Dabbs, J. M., Jurkovic, G. J., & Frady, R. L. (1991). Salivary testosterone and cortisol among late adolescent offenders. *Journal of Abnormal Child Psychology, 19,* 469–478.

Daugherty, T. K., Quay, H. C., & Ramos, L. (1993). Response perseveration, inhibitory control, and central dopaminergic activity in childhood behavior disorders. *Journal of Genetic Psychology, 154,* 177–188.

Delgado, P. L., Charney, D. S., Price, L. H., Aghajanian, G. K., Landis, H., & Heninger, G. R. (1990). Serotonin function and the mechanism of antidepressant action. *Archives of General Psychiatry, 47,* 411–418.

DiLalla, L. F., & Gottesman, I. I. (1989). Heterogeneity of causes for delinquency and criminality: Lifespan perspectives. *Development and Psychopathology, 1,* 339–349.

Dolan, M. (1994). Psychopathy—A neurobiological perspective. *British Journal of Psychiatry, 165,* 151–159.

Doudet, D., Hommer, D., Higley, J. D., Andreason, P. J., Moneman, R., Suomi, S. J., & Linnoila, M. (1995). Cerebral glucose metabolism, CSF 5-HIAA levels, and aggressive behavior in rhesus monkeys. *American Journal of Psychiatry, 152,* 1782–1787.

Ebstein, R. P., Novick, O., Umansky, R., Priol, B., Osher, Y., Blaine, D., Bennett, E. R., Nemanov, L., Katz, M., & Bolmaker, R. H. (1996). Dopamine D4 receptor (D4DR) exon III polymorphism associated with the human personality trait of novelty seeking. *Nature Genetics, 12,* 78–88.

Ehrenkranz, J., Bliss, E., & Sheard, M. H. (1974). Plasma testosterone: Correlation with aggressive behavior and social dominance in man. *Psychosomatic Medicine, 36,* 469–475.

Ewell, K. K. (1994). *Response perseveration and conduct and anxiety symptoms in clinic referred children.* Unpublished doctoral dissertation, University of Miami, Coral Gables, FL.

Faraone, S. V., Biederman, J., Keenan, K., & Tsuang, M. T. (1991). Separation of DSM-III attention deficit disorder and conduct disorder: Evidence from a family-genetic study of American child psychiatric patients. *Psychological Medicine, 21,* 109–121.

Fishbein, D. H., Lozovsky, D., & Jaffe, J. H. (1989). Impulsivity, aggression, and neuroendocrine responses to serotonergic stimulation in substance abusers. *Biological Psychiatry, 25,* 1049–1066.

Fontenot, M. B., Kaplan, J. R., Shively, C. A., Manuck, S. B., & Mann, J. J. (1996). Cholesterol, serotonin, and behavior in young monkeys. *Annals of the New York Academy of Sciences, 794,* 352–354.

Fowles, D. C. (1980). The three arousal model: Implications of Gray's two factor learning theory for heart rate, electrodermal activity and psychopathy. *Psychophysiology, 17,* 87–104.

Fowles, D. C. (1988). Psychophysiology and psychopathy: A motivational approach. *Psychophysiology, 25,* 373–391.

Gabel, S., Stadler, J., Bjorn, J., Shindledecker, R., & Bowden, C. (1993). Dopamine-beta-hydroxylase in behaviorally disturbed youth: Relationship between teacher and parent ratings. *Biological Psychiatry, 34,* 434–442.

Gately, P. F., Poon, S. L., Segal, D. S., & Geyer, M. A. (1985). Depletion of brain serotonin by 5, 7-dihydroxytryptamine alters the response to amphetamine and the habituation of locomotor activity in rats. *Psychopharmacology, 87,* 400–405.

Gelernter, J., Goldman, D., & Risch, N. (1993). The A1 allele at the D2 dopamine receptor gene and alcoholism: A reappraisal. *Journal of the American Medical Association, 269,* 1673–1677.

Gerson, S. C., & Baldessarini, R. J. (1980). Motor effects of serotonin in the central nervous system. *Life Science, 27,* 1435–1451.

Gottesman, I. I., & Goldsmith, H. H. (1994). Developmental psychopathology of antisocial behavior: Inserting genes into its ontogenesis and epigenesis. In C. A. Nelson (Ed.), *Threats to optimal development: Integrating biological, psychological, and social risk factors* (pp. 69–104). Hillsdale, NJ: Erlbaum.

Goyer, P. F., Andreason, P. J., Semple, W. E., Clayton, A. H., King, A. C., Compton-Toth, B. A., Schulz, S. C., & Cohen, R. M. (1994). Positron-emission tomography and personality disorders. *Neuropsychopharmacology, 10,* 21–28.

Gray, J. A. (1982). *The neuropsychology of anxiety: An enquiry into the functions of the septo-hippocampal system.* New York: Oxford University Press.

Grove, W. M., Elke, E. D., Heston, L., Bouchard, T. J., Segal, N., & Lykken, D. T. (1990). Heritability of substance abuse and antisocial behavior: A study of monozygotic twins reared apart. *Biological Psychiatry, 27,* 1293–1304.

Halperin, J. M., Sharma, V., Siever, L. J., Schwartz, S. T., Matier, K., Wornell, G., & Newcorn, J. H. (1994). Serotonergic function in aggressive and non-aggressive boys with attention deficit hyperactivity disorder. *American Journal of Psychiatry, 151,* 243–248.

Halperin, J. M., Newcorn, J. H., Kopstein, I., McKay, K. E., Schwartz, S. T., Siever, L. J., & Sharma, V. (1997). Serotonin, aggression, and parental psychopathology in children with attention deficit hyperactivity disorder. *Journal of the American Academy of Child and Adolescent Psychiatry, 36,* 1391–1398.

Halperin, J. M., Newcorn, J. H., Schwartz, S. T., Sharma, V., Siever, L. J., Koda, V. H., & Gabriel, S. (1997). Age-related changes in the association between serotonergic function and aggression in boys with ADHD. *Biological Psychiatry, 41,* 682–689.

Handelsman, L., Holloway, K., Shiekh, I., Sturiano, C., & Bernstein, D. (1993). Serotonergic challenges in cocaine addicts and alcoholics. *New Research Abstracts (NR 433), 146th meeting of the American Psychiatric Association,* San Francisco.

Hetey, L., Kudrin, V. S., Shemanow, A. Y., Rayevsky, K. S., & Oelssner, W. (1985). Presynaptic dopamine and serotonin receptors modulating tyrosine hydroxylase activity in synaptosomes of the nucleus accumbens of rats. *European Journal of Pharmacology, 113,* 1–10.

Higley, J. D., Suomi, S. J., & Linnoila, M. (1991). CSF monoamine metabolite concentrations vary according to age, rearing, and sex, and are influenced by the stressor of social separation in rhesus monkeys. *Psychopharmacology, 103,* 551–556.

Higley, J. D., Mehlman, P. T., Taub, D. M., Higley, S. B., Suomi, S. J., Vickers, J. H., & Linnoila, M. (1992). Cerebrospinal fluid monoamine and adrenal correlates of aggression in free-ranging rhesus monkeys. *Archives of General Psychiatry, 49,* 436–441.

Higley, J. D., Suomi, S. J., & Linnoila, M. (1992). A longitudinal study of CSF monoamine metabolite and plasma cortisol concentrations in young rhesus monkeys: Effects of early experience, age, sex, and stress on continuity of individual differences. *Biological Psychiatry, 32,* 127–145.

Higley, J. D., Thompson, W. W., Champoux, M., Goldman, D., Hasert, M. F., Kraemer, G. W., Scanlan, J. M., Suomi, S. J., & Linnoila, M. (1993). Paternal and maternal genetic and enviromental contributions to cerebrospinal fluid monoamine metabolites in rhesus monkeys (*macaca mulatta*). *Archives of General Psychiatry, 50,* 615–623.

Higley, J. D., King, S. T., Hasert, M. F., Champoux, M., Suomi, S. J., & Linnoila, M. (1996). Stability of interindividual differences in serotonin function and its relationship to severe aggression and competent social behavior in rhesus macaque females. *Neuropsychopharmacology, 14,* 67–76.

Higley, J. D., Mehlman, P. T., Higley, S. B., Fernald, B., Vickers, J., Lindell, S. G., Taub, D. M., Suomi, S. J., & Linnoila, M. (1996). Excessive mortality in young free-ranging male nonhuman primates with low cerebrospinal fluid 5-hydroxyindoleacetic acid concentrations. *Archives of General Psychiatry, 53,* 537–543.

Higley, J. D., Suomi, S. J., & Linnoila, M. (1996a). A nonhuman primate model of Type II excessive alcohol consumption? Part 1. Low cerebrospinal fluid 5-hydroxyindoleacetic acid concentrations and diminished social competence correlate with excessive alcohol consumption. *Alcoholism, Clinical and Experimental Research, 20,* 629–642.

Higley, J. D., Suomi, S. J., & Linnoila, M. (1996b). A nonhuman primate model of Type II alcoholism? Part 2. Diminished social competence and excessive aggression correlates with low cerebrospinal fluid 5-hydroxyindoleacetic acid concentrations. *Alcoholism, Clinical and Experimental Research, 20,* 643–650.

Hutchings, B., & Mednick, S. A. (1974). Registered criminality in the adoptive and biological parents of registered male adoptees. In S. A. Mednick, F. Schulsinger, J. Higgins, & B. Bell (Eds.), *Genetics, environment and psychopathology* (pp. 215–227). Amsterdam: North-Holland.

Kaplan, J. R., Shively, C. A., Fontenot, M. B., Morgan, T. M., Howell, S. M., Manuck, S. B., Muldoon, M. F., & Mann, J. J. (1994). Demonstration of an association among dietary cholesterol, central serotonergic activity, and social behavior in monkeys. *Psychosomatic Medicine, 56,* 479–484.

Kapur, S., & Remington, G. (1996). Serotonin–dopamine interaction and its relevance to schizophrenia. *American Journal of Psychiatry, 153,* 466–476.

Kelland, M. D., Freeman, A. S., & Chiodo, L. A. (1990). Serotonergic afferent regulation of the basic physiology and pharmacological responsiveness of nigrostriatal dopamine neurons. *Journal of Pharmacology and Experimental Therapeutics, 253,* 803–811.

Kraemer, G. W., & Clarke, A. S. (1996). Social attachment, brain function, and aggression. *Annals of the New York Academy of Sciences, 794,* 121–135.

Kraemer, G. W., Ebert, M. H., Schmidt, D. E., & McKinney, W. T. (1989). A longitudinal study of the effect of different social rearing conditions on cerebrospinal fluid norepinephrine and biogenic amine metabolites in rhesus monkeys. *Neuropsychopharmacology, 2,* 175–189.

Kruesi, M. J., Schmidt, M. E., Donnelly, M., Hibbs, E. D., & Hamburger, S. D. (1989). Urinary free cortisol output and disruptive behavior in children. *Journal of the American Academy of Child and Adolescent Psychiatry, 28,* 441–443.

Kruesi, M. J., Rapoport, J. L., Hamburger, S., Hibbs, E. D., Potter, W. Z., Lenane, M., & Brown, G. L. (1990). Cerebrospinal fluid monoamine metabolites, aggression, and impulsivity in disruptive behavior of children and adolescents. *Archives of General Psychiatry, 47,* 419–426.

Kruesi, M. J., Hibbs, E. D., Zahn, T. P., Keysor, C. S., Hamburger, S. D., Bartko, J. J., & Rapoport, J. L. (1992). A 2-year prospective follow-up study of children and adolescents with disruptive behavior disorders: Prediction by cerebrospinal fluid 5-hydroxyindoleacetic acid, homovanillic acid, and autonomic measures? *Archives of General Psychiatry, 49*, 429–435.

Kyes, R. C., Botchin, M. B., Kaplan, J. R., Manuck, S. B., & Mann, J. J. (1995). Aggression and brain serotonergic responsivity: Response to slides in male macaques. *Physiology and Behavior, 57*, 205–208.

Lahey, B. B., Piacentini, J. C., McBurnett, K., Stone, P., Hartdagen, S., & Hynd, G. (1988). Psychopathology in the parents of children with conduct disorder and hyperactivity. *Journal of the American Academy of Child and Adolescent Psychiatry, 27*, 163–170.

Lidberg, L., Tuck, J., Asberg, M., Scalia-Tomba, G., & Bertilsson, L. (1985). Homoicide, suicide and CSF 5-HIAA. *Acta Psychiatrica Scandinavica, 71*, 230–236.

Linnoila, V. M., & Virkkunen, M. (1992). Aggression, suicidality, and serotonin. *Journal of Clinical Psychiatry, 53*(10, Suppl.), 46–51.

Linnoila, M., Virkkunen, M., Scheinin, M., Nuutila, A., Rimon, R., & Goodwin, F. K. (1983). Low cerebrospinal fluid 5-hydroxyindoleacetic acid concentration differentiates impulsive from non-impulsive violent behavior. *Life Science, 33*, 2609–2614.

Linnoila, M., Delong, J., & Virkkunen, M. (1989). Monoamines, glucose metabolism, and impulse control. *Psychopharmacology Bulletin, 25*, 404–406.

Lyons, M. J., True, W. R., Eisen, S. A., Goldberg, J., Meyer, J. M., Faraone, S. V., Eaves, L. J., & Tsuang, M. T. (1995). Differential heritability of adult and juvenile antisocial traits. *Archives of General Psychiatry, 52*, 906–915.

Maliphant, R., Hume, F., & Furnham, A. (1990). Autonomic nervous system (ANS) activity, personality characteristics and disruptive behaviour in girls. *Journal of Child Psychology and Psychiatry, 31*, 619–628.

Mann, J. J., McBride, P. A., Anderson, G. M., & Mieczkowski, T. A. (1992). Platelet and whole blood serotonin content in depressed inpatients: Correlations with acute and life-time psychopathology. *Biological Psychiatry, 32*, 243–257.

Mann, J. J., McBride, P. A., Brown, R. P., Linnoila, M., Leon, A. C., DeMeo, M., Mieczkowski, T., Myers, J. E., & Stanley, M. (1992). Relationship between central and peripheral serotonin indexes in depressed and suicidal psychiatric inpatients. *Archives of General Psychiatry, 49*, 442–446.

Mannuzza, S., Klein, R. G., Konig, P. H., & Giampino, T. L. (1989). Hyperactive boys almost grown up: IV. Criminality and its relationship to psychiatric status. *Archives of General Psychiatry, 46*, 1073–1079.

Mannuzza, S., Klein, R. G., Bonagura, N., Malloy, P., Giampino, T. L., & Addalli, K. A. (1991). Hyperactive boys almost grown up: V. Replication of psychiatric status. *Archives of General Psychiatry, 48*, 77–83.

Mansour, A., Chalmers, D. T., Fox, C. A., Meador-Woodruff, J. H., & Watson, S. J. (1996). Biochemical anatomy: Insights into the cell biology and pharmacology of the neurotransmitter systems in the brain. In A. F. Schatzberg & C. B. Nemeroff (Eds.), *The American Psychiatric Press textbook of psychopharmacology* (pp. 45–63). Washington, DC: American Psychiatric Press.

McBride, P. A., Anderson, G. M., Hertzig, M. E., Sweeney, J. A., Kream, J., Cohen, D. J., & Mann, J. J. (1989). Serotonergic responsivity in male young adults with autistic disorder. *Archives of General Psychiatry, 46*, 213–221.

McBurnett, K., Lahey, B. B., Frick, P. J., Risch, C., Loeber, R., Hart, E. L., Christ, M. A., & Hanson, K. S. (1991). Anxiety, inhibition, and conduct disorder in children: II. Relation to salivary cortisol. *Journal of the American Academy of Child and Adolescent Psychiatry, 30*, 192–196.

McGee, R., Williams, S., & Silva, P. A. (1984a). Background characteristics of aggressive, hyperactive, and aggressive-hyperactive boys. *Journal of the American Academy of Child Psychiatry, 23*, 280–284.

McGee, R., Williams, S., & Silva, P. A. (1984b). Behavioral and developmental characteristics of aggressive, hyperactive, and aggressive-hyperactive boys. *Journal of the American Academy of Child and Adolescent Psychiatry, 23*, 270–279.

McGuffin, P., & Gottesman, I. I. (1985). Genetic influences on normal and abnormal development. In M. Rutter & L. Hersov (Eds.), *Child and adolescent psychiatry: Modern approaches* (pp. 17–33). Boston: Blackwell.

McKay, K. E., Newcorn, J. H., & Halperin, J. M. (1996, October). *Situationally vs. pervasively aggressive boys: Behavioral, cognitive, and neurochemical differences.* Paper and poster presented at the 43rd annual meeting of the American Academy of Child and Adolescent Psychiatry, Philadelphia.

Mehlman, P. T., Higley, J. D., Faucher, I., Lilly, A. A., Taub, D. M., Vickers, J., Suomi, S. J., & Linnoila, M. (1994). Low CSF 5-HIAA concentrations and severe aggression and impaired impulse control in nonhuman primates. *American Journal of Psychiatry, 151*, 1485–1491.

Mehlman, P. T., Higley, J. D., Faucher, I., Lilly, A., Taub, D. M., Vickers, J., Suomi, S. J., & Linnoila, M. (1995). Correlation of CSF 5-HIAA concentration with sociality and the timing of emigration in free-ranging primates. *American Journal of Psychiatry, 152*, 907–913.

Moffitt, T. E. (1990). Juvenile delinquency and attention deficit disorder: Boys' developmental trajectories from age 3 to age 15. *Child Development, 61*, 893–910.

Moss, H. B., Yao, Y. K., & Panzak, G. L. (1990). Serotonergic responsivity and behavioral dimensions in antisocial personality disorder with substance abuse. *Biological Psychiatry, 28*, 325–328.

Muldoon, M. F., Manuck, S. B., & Matthews, K. A. (1990). Lowering cholesterol concentrations and mortality: A quantitative review of primary prevention trials. *British Medical Journal, 301,* 309–314.

Newcorn, J. H., McKay, K. E., Loeber, R., Bonfina, M., Sharma, V., & Halperin, J. M. (1996, October). *Emotionality and serotonergic function in aggressive and non-aggressive ADHD children.* Paper presented at the 43rd annual meeting of the American Academy of Child and Adolescent Psychiatry, Philadelphia.

Nielsen, D. A., Goldman, D., Virkkunen, M., Tokola, R., Rawlings, R., & Linnoila, M. (1994). Suicidality and 5-hydroxyindoleacetic acid concentration associated with a tryptophan hydroxylase polymorphism. *Archives of General Psychiatry, 51,* 34–38.

Nieuwenhuys, R. (1985). *Chemoarchitecture of the brain.* New York: Springer-Verlag.

O'Brien, B. S., & Frick, P. J. (1996). Reward dominance: Associations with anxiety, conduct problems and psychopathy in children. *Journal of Abnormal Child Psychology, 24,* 223–240.

O'Keane, V., Moloney, E., O'Neill, H., O'Connor, A., Smith, C., & Dinan, T. G. (1992). Blunted prolactin responses to d-fenfluramine in sociopathy: Evidence for subsensitivity of central serotonergic function. *British Journal of Psychiatry, 160,* 643–646.

Pihl, R. O., Young, S. N., Harden, P., Plotnick, S., Chamberlain, B., & Ervin, F. R. (1995). Acute effect of altered tryptophan levels and alcohol on aggression in normal human males. *Psychopharmacology, 119,* 353–360.

Pine, D. S., Wasserman, G. A., Coplan, J., Fried, J. A., Huang, Y. Y., Kassir, S., Greenhill, L., Shaffer, D., & Parsons, B. (1996). Platelet serotonin 2A (5-HT2A) receptor characteristics and parenting factors for boys at risk for delinquency: A preliminary report. *American Journal of Psychiatry, 153,* 538–544.

Pine, D. S., Coplan, J. D., Wasserman, G. A., Miller, L. S., Fried, J. E., Davies, M., Cooper, T. B., Greenhill, L., Shaffer, D., & Parsons, B. (1997). Neuroendocrine response to fenfluramine challenge in boys. *Archives of General Psychiatry, 54,* 839–846.

Pliszka, S. R., Rogeness, G. A., & Medrano, M. A. (1988). DBH, MHPG, and MAO in children with depressive, anxiety, and conduct disorders: Relationship to diagnosis and symptom ratings. *Psychiatry Research, 24,* 35–44.

Pliszka, S. R., Rogeness, G. A., Renner, P., Sherman, J., & Broussard, T. (1988). Plasma neurochemistry in juvenile offenders. *Journal of the American Academy of Child and Adolescent Psychiatry, 27,* 588–594.

Pliszka, S. R., McCracken, J. T., & Maas, J. W. (1996). Catecholamines in attention deficit hyperactivity disorder: Current perspectives. *Journal of the American Academy of Child and Adolescent Psychiatry, 35,* 264–272.

Quay, H. C. (1987). Patterns of delinquent behavior. In H. C. Quay (Ed.), *Handbook of juvenile delinquency* (pp. 118–138). New York: Wiley.

Quay, H. C. (1988). The behavioral reward and inhibition systems in childhood behavior disorders. In L. M. Bloomingdale (Ed.), *Attention Deficit Disorder* (Vol. 3, pp. 176–186). Oxford, England: Pergamon.

Quay, H. C. (1993). The psychobiology of undersocialized aggressive conduct disorder: A theoretical perspective. *Development and Psychopathology, 5,* 165–180.

Raine, A. (1996). Autonomic nervous system factors underlying disinhibited, antisocial, and violent behavior. *Annals of the New York Academy of Sciences, 794,* 46–59.

Raine, A., Venables, P. H., & Williams, M. (1990). Relationships between central and autonomic measures of arousal at age 15 years and criminality at age 24 years. *Archives of General Psychiatry, 47,* 1003–1007.

Raine, A., Buchsbaum, M. S., Stanley, J., Lottenberg, S., Abel, L., & Stoddard, J. (1995). Selective reduction in prefrontal glucose metabolism in murderers. *Biological Psychiatry, 38,* 342–343.

Raine, A., Venables, P. H., & Williams, M. (1995). High autonomic arousal and electrodermal orienting at age 15 years as protective factors against criminal behavior at age 29 years. *American Journal of Psychiatry, 152,* 1595–1600.

Raleigh, M. J., & McGuire, M. T. (1994). Serotonin, aggression, and violence in vervet monkeys. In M. D. Masters & M. T. McGuire (Eds.), *The neurotransmitter revolution* (pp. 129–145). Carbondale: Southern Illinois University Press.

Raleigh, M. J., Brammer, G. L., Ritvo, E. R., Geller, E., McGuire, M. T., & Yuwiler, A. (1986). Effects of chronic fenfluramine on blood serotonin, cerebrospinal fluid metabolites, and behavior in monkeys. *Psychopharmacology, 90,* 503–508.

Reeves, J. C., Werry, J. S., Elkind, G. S., & Zametkin, A. (1987). Attention deficit, conduct, oppositional, and anxiety disorders in children: II. Clinical characteristics. *Journal of the American Academy of Child and Adolescent Psychiatry, 26,* 144–155.

Rogeness, G. A., Hernandez, J. M., Macedo, C. A., & Mitchell, E. L. (1982). Biochemical differences in children with conduct disorder socialized and undersocialized. *American Journal of Psychiatry, 139,* 307–311.

Rogeness, G. A., Hernandez, J. M., Macedo, C. A., Amrung, S. A., & Hoppe, S. K. (1986). Near-zero plasma dopamine-beta-hydroxylase and conduct disorder in emotionally disturbed boys. *Journal of the American Academy of Child Psychiatry, 25,* 521–527.

Rogeness, G. A., Javors, M. A., Maas, J. W., & Macedo, C. A. (1990). Catecholamines and diagnoses in children. *Journal of the American Academy of Child and Adolescent Psychiatry, 29,* 234–241.

Rowe, D. C. (1983). A biometrical analysis of perceptions of family environment: A study of twin and singleton sibling kinships. *Child Development, 54,* 416–423.

Rowe, D. C., & Osgood, D. W. (1984). Sociological theories of delinquency and heredity: A reconsideration. *American Sociological Review, 49,* 526–540.

Roy, A., Adinoff, B., & Linnoila, M. (1986). Acting out hostility in normal volunteers: Negative correlations with CSF 5-HIAA. *Psychiatry Research, 24,* 187–194.

Rutter, M. & Giller, H. (1983). *Juvenile delinquency: Trends and perspectives.* New York: Guilford.

Salomon, R. M., Mazure, C. M., Delgado, P. L., Mendia, P., & Charney, D. S. (1994). Serotonin function in aggression: The effect of acute plasma tryptophan depletion in aggressive patients. *Biological Psychiatry, 35,* 570–572.

Scerbo, A. S., & Kolko, D. J. (1994). Salivary testosterone and cortisol in disruptive children: Relationship to aggressive, hyperactive, and internalizing behaviors. *Journal of the American Academy of Child and Adolescent Psychiatry, 33,* 1174–1184.

Schaechter, J. D., & Wurtman, R. J. (1990). Serotonin release varies with brain tryptophan levels. *Brain Research, 532,* 203–210.

Schulsinger, F. (1972). Psychopathy: Heredity and environment. *International Journal of Mental Health, 1,* 190–206.

Schulz, K. P., McKay, K. E., Newcorn, J. H., Sharma, V., and Halperin, J. M. (1996, October) *Serotonin and risk for alcoholism in boys with ADHD.* Paper presented at the 43rd annual meeting of the American Academy of Child and Adolescent Psychiatry, Philadelphia.

Shaywitz, B. A., Cohen, D. J., & Bowers, M. B. (1977). CSF monoamine metabolites in children with minimal brain dysfunction: Evidence for alteration of brain dopamine. *Journal of Pediatrics, 90,* 67–71.

Shetty, T., & Chase, T. N. (1976). Central monoamines and hyperkinesis of childhood. *Neurology, 26,* 1000–1002.

Skirboll, L. R., Grace, A. A., & Bunney, B. S. (1979). Dopamine auto- and postsynaptic receptors: Electrophysiological evidence for differential sensitivity to dopamine agonists. *Science, 206,* 80–82.

Slutske, W. S., Health, A. C., Dinwiddie, S. H., Madden, P. A. F., Bucholz, K. K., Dunne, M. P., Statham, D. J., & Martin, N. G. (1997). Modeling genetic and environmental influences in the etiology of conduct disorder: A study of 2,682 adult twins. *Journal of Abnormal Psychology, 106,* 266–279.

Smith, S. E., Pihl, R. O., Young, S. N., & Ervin, F. R. (1986). Elevation and reduction of plasma tryptophan and their effects on aggression and perceptual sensitivity in normal males. *Aggressive Behavior, 12,* 393–407.

Solanto, M. V. (1984). Neuropharmacological basis of stimulant drug action in attention deficit disorder with hyperactivity: A review and synthesis. *Psychological Bulletin, 95,* 387–409.

Solanto, M. V. (1986). Behavioral effects of low dose methylphenidate in chilhood attention deficit disorder: Implications for a mechanism of stimulant drug action. *Journal of the American Academy of Child Psychiatry, 25,* 96–101.

Soubrie, P. (1986). Reconciling the role of central serotonin neurons in human and animal behavior. *Behavioral and Brain Sciences, 9,* 319–364.

Spoont, M. R. (1992). Modulatory role of serotonin in neural information processing: Implications for human psychopathology. *Psychological Bulletin, 112,* 330–350.

Stoff, D. M., Pollock, L., Vitiello, B., Behar, D., & Bridger, W. (1987). Reduction of 3H-imipramine binding sites on platelets of conduct-disordered children. *Neuropsychopharmacology, 1,* 55–62.

Stoff, D. M., Cook, E., & Perry, B. (1991). Blood serotonin (5HT) indices in children. *Biological Psychiatry, 29*(Suppl. 12), 523.

Stoff, D. M., Ieni, J., Friedman, E., Bridger, W. H., Pollock, L., & Vitiello, B. (1991). Platelet 3 H-imipramine binding, serotonin uptake, and plasma alpha 1 acid glycoprotein in disruptive behavior disorders. *Biological Psychiatry, 29,* 494–498.

Stoff, D. M., Pasatiempo, A. P., Yeung, J. H., Bridger, W. H., & Rabinovich, H. (1992). Test–retest reliability of the prolactin and cortisol responses to d,l-fenfluramine challenge in disruptive behavior disorders. *Psychiatry Research, 42,* 65–72.

Stoff, D. M., Pasatiempo, A. P., Yeung, J., Cooper, T. B., Bridger, W. H., & Rabinovich, H. (1992). Neuroendocrine responses to challenge with d,l-fenfluramine and aggression in disruptive behavior disorders of children and adolescents. *Psychiatry Research, 43,* 263–276.

Strombom, U. (1976). Catecholamine receptor agonists: Effects on motor activity and rate of tyrosine hydroxylation in mouse brain. *Naunyn Schmiedeberg's Archives of Pharmacology, 292,* 167–176.

Susman, E. J., Inoff-Germain, G., Nottleman, E. D., Loriaux, D. L., Cutler, G. B., & Chrousos, G. P. (1997). Hormones, emotional disposition, and aggressive attributes in young adolescents. *Child Development, 58,* 1114–1134.

Swedo, S. E., Kruesi, M. J., Leonard, H. L., Hamburger, S. D., Cheslow, D. L., Stipetic, M., & Potter, W. Z. (1989). Lack of seasonal variation in pediatric lumbar cerebrospinal fluid neurotransmitter metabolite concentrations. *Acta Psychiatrica Scandinavica, 80,* 644–649.

Unis, A. S., Cook, E. H., Vincent, J. G., Gjerde, D. K., Perry, B. D., Mason, C., & Mitchell, J. (1997). Platelet serotonin measures in adolescents with conduct disorder. *Biological Psychiatry, 42,* 553–559.

Virkkunen, M., & Linnoila, M. (1993). Brain serotonin, type II alcoholism and impulsive violence. *Journal of Studies on Alcohol* (Suppl. 11), 163–169.

Virkkunen, M., Nuutila, A., Goodwin, F. K., & Linnoila, M. (1987). Cerebrospinal fluid monoamine metabolite levels in male arsonists. *Archives of General Psychiatry, 44,* 241–247.

Virkkunen, M., Rawlings, R., Tokola, R., Poland, R. E., Guidotti, A., Nemeroff, C., Bissette, G., Kalogeras, K., Karonen, S. L., & Linnoila, M. (1994). CSF biochemistries, glucose metabolism, and diurnal activity rhythms in alcoholic, violent offenders, fire setters, and healthy volunteers. *Archives of General Psychiatry, 51,* 20–27.

Virkkunen, M., Goldman, D., & Linnoila, M. (1996). Serotonin in alcoholic violent offenders. In G. R. Bock &

J. A. Goode (Eds.), *Genetics of criminal and antisocial behaviour* (pp. 168–182). Chichester, England: Wiley.

Volkow, N. D., Tancredi, L. R., Grant, C., Gillespie, H., Valentine, A., Mullani, N., Wang, C. J., & Hollister, L. (1995). Brain glucose metabolism in violent psychiatric patients. *Psychiatry Research, 61,* 243–253.

Waldmier, P. C., & Delini-Stula, A. A. (1979). Serotonin–dopamine interactions in the nigrostriatal system. *European Journal of Pharmacology, 55,* 363–373.

Walker, J. L., Lahey, B. B., Russo, M. F., Frick, P. J., Christ, M. A., McBurnett, K., Loeber, R., Stouthamer-Loeber, M., & Green, S. M. (1991). Anxiety, inhibition, and conduct disorder in children: I. Relations to social impairment. *Journal of the American Academy of Child and Adolescent Psychiatry, 30,* 187–191.

Weinshilbaum, R. M., Raymond, F. A., Elveback, L., & Weidman, W. H. (1973). Serum DBH activity: Sibling:sibling correlation. *Science, 181,* 943–945.

Wise, R. A. (1988). The neurobiology of craving: Implications for the understanding and treatment of addiction. *Journal of Abnormal Psychology, 97,* 118–132.

Wise, R. A., & Bozarth, M. A. (1987). A psychomotor stimulant theory of addiction. *Psychological Review, 94,* 469–492.

Yodyingyuad, U., De La Riva, C., Abbott, D. H., Herbert, J., & Keverne, E. B. (1985). Relationship between dominance hierarchy, cerebrospinal fluid levels of amine transmitter metabolites (5-hydroxyindole acetic acid and homovanillic acid) and plasma cortisol in monkeys. *Neuroscience, 16,* 851–858.

Zametkin, A. J., Stevens, J. R., & Pittman, R. (1979). Ontogeny of spontaneous blinking and of habituation of the blink reflex. *Annals of Neurology, 5,* 453–457.

18

Temperament and Behavioral Precursors to Oppositional Defiant Disorder and Conduct Disorder

ANN SANSON and MARGOT PRIOR

INTRODUCTION

In this chapter we discuss the role played by early temperament and behavioral characteristics of the child in the development of Disruptive Behavior Disorders (DBD), in the context of current models of developmental psychopathology. We begin with a discussion of definitional, conceptual, and theoretical issues before examining current literature. We attempt to review the most relevant literature; we also draw extensively on the data emerging from the Australian Temperament Project (ATP), in which almost 2000 children have been followed from infancy to (currently) 14 years of age. We then discuss evidence of gender-specific pathways from early temperament and behavior to Oppositional Defiant Disorder (ODD) and Conduct Disorder (CD). Finally, the implications of findings for theoretical models of causative influences on DBD and for prevention and early intervention are explored.

ANN SANSON and MARGOT PRIOR • Department of Psychology, University of Melbourne, Parkville, Victoria 3052, Australia

Handbook of Disruptive Behavior Disorders, edited by Quay and Hogan. Kluwer Academic/Plenum Publishers, New York, 1999.

CONCEPTUAL AND METHODOLOGICAL ISSUES

What Is Temperament?

Temperament refers to constitutionally based individual differences in behavioral style that are visible from early childhood. The term *style* draws attention to the "how" of behavior rather than its specific content or the "what" of behavior. It can be regarded as individual differences in reactivity to internal and external stimulation and in patterns of motor and attentional self-regulation (Prior, 1992; Sanson & Rothbart, 1995); it thus comprises the emotional, motivational, and attentional bases of later personality.

Ideas about temperament go back to the ancient Greco-Roman notion that the balance of the four bodily humors determined temperament type (Diamond, 1974; Sanson & Rothbart, 1995) and to ancient Chinese and Indian traditions (Needham, 1973). In the first half of the 20th century, a school of temperament research emerged in Eastern Europe and the Soviet Union and continues today, building on the work of Pavlov on strength of neural activation (Strelau, 1983). However, the modern Western interest in temperament dates particularly to the pioneering work of Thomas and

Chess in the New York Longitudinal Study beginning in the mid-1950s (Thomas, Chess, Birch, Hertzig, & Korn, 1963). In reaction to the prevailing environmentalism of the time, they drew attention to the measurable individual differences in temperament, apparent from infancy, that have a substantial impact on psychosocial development, beyond the influence of parenting and other environmental factors. Another major impetus to recognition of children's contributions to their own psychosocial development came from Bell's (1968, 1974) reconceptualization of socialization as a mutually interactive process in which child and parent modify each other's behavior.

Although a broad conceptualization of temperament as behavioral style would receive general support among researchers and clinicians, a more specific definition has posed more problems. Researchers have derived their own lists of temperament dimensions and have varied in requiring evidence of a genetic contribution, stability over time and across situations, and in the narrowness or breadth of content. Thomas and Chess (1977) identified nine dimensions of temperament that have been widely accepted, especially in clinical settings (namely, Approach, Adaptability, Mood, Threshold, Rhythmicity, Intensity, Activity, Distractibility, and Persistence). However, in recent years consensus has been emerging that a smaller number of dimensions more adequately reflects the structure of temperament, and these show substantial commonality across research samples (Martin, Wisenbaker, & Huttenen, 1994). In broad terms, three aspects of temperament that emerge relatively consistently are positive affect and approaching tendencies, negative emotionality, and effortful control or self-regulation. For example, in a second-order factor analysis of data on a large sample of toddlers in the ATP, one factor principally reflected Approach or Sociability; a second (negative reactivity) tapped Cooperation-Manageability, Irritability, Intensity-Activity, and Reactivity; and the third (self-regulation) tapped Persistence and Distractibility (Prior, Sanson, & Oberklaid, 1989; Sanson & Rothbart, 1995). Other narrow-band factors reflecting rhythmicity of biological func-

tioning and activity level also emerge in some studies. The three broad factors show strong similarities to adult personality factors (e.g., Goldberg, 1993; John, Caspi, Robins, Moffitt, & Stouthamer-Loeber, 1994), with positive affect–approach being mapped onto the broad adult dimension of extroversion or surgency, negative emotionality onto neuroticism, and effortful control onto conscientiousness (see Ahadi & Rothbart, 1994).

Temperament is viewed as a biologically based construct. It is beyond the scope of this chapter to review the growing evidence for biological underpinnings of temperament and the reader is referred to Bates and Wachs (1994) and Rothbart and Bates (1998) for reviews. In brief, there is some evidence of the heritability of temperament, stronger for some dimensions than others. For example, Matheny (1995, cited in Rothbart & Bates, 1998), using parent reports of the nine Thomas and Chess dimensions for twins from 1 to 9 years, concluded that there were consistent heritable effects for activity and approach–withdrawal, with low to negative correlations for DZ twins; persistence, adaptability, and threshold also showed heritability but with more substantial DZ correlations; and genetic effects were absent for mood and distractibility and mixed for rhythmicity and intensity. Models from neuroscience, including those of Eysenck (1970), Cloninger (1987), and Gray (1981), are being explored for their applicability to temperament research (see Rothbart & Bates, 1998). Some specific psychobiological variables are also being examined. For example, right frontal asymmetry appears to be associated with fearfulness and inhibition (Fox, Calkins, & Bell, 1994) and vagal tone, an index of parasympathetic function, has been found to be associated with irritability, positive affect, and attention (Fox, 1989). Much more research is needed to specify how developing biological mechanisms interact with environmental events to result in differences in observed temperament but our understanding of its biological underpinnings is growing.

The argument that temperament may have a biological basis does not imply that it is not subject to modification through interaction with the environment. A child's experience with the environment may magnify or reduce initial individual differences. If a child approaches a stranger easily and positively, this is likely to lead to a positive interaction between them which will encourage further approaching behaviors, whereas fearful avoidance may reinforce such avoidance in future. However, carefully modulated exposure to strangers may help the child moderate an initially fearful response. "Niche-picking" may also occur, meaning that the child will seek environments in which temperamental proclivities can find expression. Thus, a shy, withdrawing child might engage in computer games, while an active, outgoing child might join sports clubs; in both cases, temperament characteristics are likely to be maintained. These postulated processes are reminiscent of Scarr and McCartney's (1983) passive, active, and evocative genotype–environment interactions.

In general, modest to moderate stability of temperament has been found across ages (Hubert, Wachs, Peters-Martin, & Gandour, 1982; Prior et al., 1989; Rothbart, 1989; Slabach, Morrow, & Wachs, 1991). Some apparent instability is likely due to measurement error. When Pedlow, Sanson, Prior, and Oberklaid (1993) used structural equation modeling (which corrects for attenuation of correlations due to measurement error) to assess stability in the ATP sample from infancy to 7–8 years, stability coefficients were considerably higher than those reported previously; they were mostly in the .7–.8 range. Even so, it is clear that stability is far from absolute, and the norm is for individuals to change somewhat (but not greatly) in temperament characteristics over time.

Much past research has used the concept of "difficult" temperament, originating as one of the four clusters in Thomas and Chess's work, along with "easy," "average," and "slow to warm up." Difficult temperament was characterized as negative mood, withdrawal, low adaptability, high intensity, and low rhythmicity (Thomas et al., 1963). Later empirical research has found that these dimensions do not cluster together (e.g., Bates, 1989). As a result,

different researchers have tended to use their own clusters of temperament dimensions to define "difficult," creating problems in comparing research findings (Sanson & Rothbart, 1995). The "difficult" construct also ignores the fact that any temperament characteristic can be easy or difficult, depending on the requirements of the situation, and the term clearly carries strong value-laden overtones. Further, it precludes investigation of whether there is specificity in the predictive role of particular temperament dimensions for emerging emotional and behavioral disorders.

How Temperament Works

As noted, most theorists agree that child characteristics do not operate in isolation but are part of a process of interaction with parents and the social environment. Thomas, Chess, and Birch (1968) first emphasized the goodness of fit model in which behavior problems were seen to result from the interaction of the child's temperament and the parents' responses to that temperament. Thus they argued that irritable, intense, and nonadaptable temperament only led to maladjustment when parents responded maladaptively with forceful confrontation or surrender. According to this model, interaction effects between temperament and parenting are expected. Such a model is accepted by many researchers as representing the process underlying much of social development, although it has proved difficult to operationalize goodness of fit (Lerner & Lerner, 1994) and empirical demonstrations of the posited interaction effects have been few, with even fewer replicated interactions (Bates, Bayles, Bennett, Ridge, & Brown, 1991).

One explanation for links between early child characteristics and later outcome is simple stability of problematic behaviors manifested differently at different ages. Although there is a worrisome level of stability of aggressive behavior from childhood to adulthood, for example (Loeber, 1990; Robins, 1978; West & Farrington, 1973; see also Chapter 24, this volume), it is far from absolute. Thus, our explanatory paradigms need to be more complex.

Rothbart and Bates (1998) refer to four categories of theoretically plausible ways in which temperament could be related to psychopathology: (1) direct linear effects, (2) indirect linear effects, (3) temperament by temperament interaction effects, and (4) temperament by environment interaction effects.

The simplest of these is direct linear effects, whereby an extreme on a temperament dimension either is synonymous with disorder (e.g., low manageability with ODD, low approach tendencies with shyness and social phobia, poor attentional control with Attention-Deficit/Hyperactivity Disorder [ADHD]) or leads to or affects the symptomatology of a closely related condition. The broad temperament factor with the clearest conceptual links to later DBD is negative emotionality: Its inflexible and reactive components may be linked with "reactive" CD; a negative, irritable temperament style may lead to "proactive" (trouble-seeking) CD (see Chapter 1, this volume); and negative emotionality is implicated in priming or readiness for outbursts of angry and aggressive behaviors (Cairns & Cairns, 1991; Ledingham, 1991).

Indirect linear effects include those where a child's temperament negatively affects the environment, thus increasing the risk of psychopathology (e.g., a highly irritable child elicits coercive parenting which in turn increases the risk of aggressive behavior; an impersistent child receives negative feedback from school leading to poor school motivation and school failure). Temperament by temperament interaction effects include the possibility that self-regulatory aspects of temperament could change the expression of other facets, so a combination of high approach and activity with good self-regulation might lead to a competent outcome, whereas without good self-regulation it may lead to ADHD.

Temperament by environment interactions refer to temperament as a risk (or vulnerability) or protective (resilience) factor; a child high in negative emotionality and reactivity may respond more poorly to stressors, while one high on adaptability and positive affect may be buffered against stress. Lytton (1990),

in reviewing the literature on the development of CD among boys, concluded that this model best fits the data. He contrasted theories positing three different factors as the major influence on CD: the parental environment, the child's own characteristics (e.g., temperament), and reciprocal effects from the interaction of parental and child factors. Among child factors, Lytton included not only temperament but biological and genetic factors, which may or may not be reflected in temperament differences. He concluded that the child's own contribution had primacy over parental contributions, but this was embedded in a reciprocal parent–child interactive system. He argued that, at times, what look like parental effects may in fact be determined in an important way by child factors. Child difficultness may provoke or exacerbate parental rejection and lack of supervision and involvement, factors that have been found to predict later antisocial behavior (e.g., Loeber & Stouthamer-Loeber, 1986). Lytton concluded that the data reviewed best fit a vulnerability-stress model, where some boys had a biologically based predisposition to CD, and the liability to actually develop this disorder was increased by stressors in the family environment and poor parenting, or reduced by protective factors such as maternal affection.

The notion of temperament by environment interactions is also compatible with a cumulative risk model. There is good evidence that outcome deteriorates as the number of risk factors increases (Rutter, 1978; Sameroff, Seifer, Barocas, Zax, & Greenspan, 1987; see also Chapter 19, this volume). Most researchers have focused on environmental and familial risk factors in such research but when temperament has been included (e.g., Sanson, Oberklaid, Pedlow, & Prior, 1991; Werner & Smith, 1982), it is clear that both temperament characteristics such as irritability and inflexibility, along with early behavior problems (BP), can be conceptualized as risks operating in cumulative fashion. The limitation with using cumulative risk as an explanatory model, though, is its failure to show *how* particular child characteristics interact with other (positive or negative) characteristics of the environment to affect outcome. Recent trends in developmental psychopathology have been toward greater efforts to understand developmental processes (Richters & Cicchetti, 1993). A cumulative risk perspective only offers the explanation of overload of risk somehow overwhelming coping processes, although the nature of that overload may vary from one individual to another. A transactional model offers greater potential for understanding how the presence of a risk factor affects developmental processes such that the individual is vulnerable to poor outcome. This implies that the contribution of both an active individual (with temperament, behavioral, and cognitive individuality) and an active environment (comprising parents, families, communities, and social norms) need to be considered, and that it is the continuous interaction between these that determines developmental outcome. Such a model also raises the concept of resilience, the processes by which an individual overcomes risk status to achieve good developmental outcome (i.e., manages to "play a bad hand well") (Garmezy, 1985; Smith & Prior, 1995).

From a transactional perspective, partitioning the contributors to ODD and CD into various individual and environmental influences is somewhat arbitrary. However, since there is communicative value to making such separations, we will focus on child characteristics but point out when their influence needs to be understood in a broader context.

Most models of the development of DBD specify a temperament component as one of the primary influences on the development of these disorders (e.g., Cairns & Cairns, 1991; Patterson, Reid, & Dishion, 1992). Hence there is general acceptance of the theoretical links between temperament and BP, and a number of reports of these associations in younger children. However, there are very few specific studies of temperament precursors of CD and ODD. Because these categorizations have limited relevance to early childhood, we will say little about the many studies that have examined only the first few years of life.

As noted earlier, there is considerable variation within the child psychopathology literature in the way temperament is described and in the weight and complexity of proposed influences of temperament characteristics. Relatively few studies of the antecedents of *clinically identified* DBD actually define and measure specific factors such as "reactivity" or "irritability." For example, Patterson and colleagues (1992) acknowledged the likelihood that temperament is an early influence in the cascade of factors and effects that culminate in serious antisocial behavior, but they did not measure temperament in any of their studies. Campbell and colleagues (see Campbell, 1994), on the other hand, in following up preschoolers at risk for the development of DBD in middle childhood, were interested in the effects of an early-appearing factor they term "hard to manage." This descriptor is not part of the set of terms usually used to describe temperament characteristics but has clear conceptual and behavioral links to them. Others, such as Bates (1989), Earls and Jung (1987), Sanson and colleagues (1991), and Shaw and Bell (1993) have proposed models of the development of behavior disorders which are clearly driven by traditional temperament theory and previous research. Whether or not specific temperament concepts and measures are used, all these writers ascribe important influences to temperamentlike factors in pathways to adjustment and maladjustment in early childhood; they acknowledge these as part of a complex mix of intrinsic and extrinsic influences that converge in the developmental pathways leading to DBD.

General Methodology

To identify temperament and behavioral predictors of DBD, longitudinal methodology is essential. Evidence of concurrent linkages can be suggestive but causal inferences must be cautious at best. Even in longitudinal studies, of course, direct causal linkages cannot be assumed from empirical associations between early and late variables. We focus our review on longitudinal studies, but include experimental and observational studies where appropriate. There are few studies covering the entire period from infancy through later childhood or early adolescence, that is, the stage at which diagnoses of DBD are more likely than in early childhood. We therefore follow our general review with a more detailed review of data from the ATP, which is arguably the largest study of a representative sample of children followed from infancy to adolescence that has had temperament as a consistent core focus. Here we also discuss the evidence for gender-specific paths to DBD.

A further methodological point concerns statistical approaches used to examine temperament–behavior connections. A substantial proportion of findings from published studies is based on the use of regression statistics and path analyses, where continuously distributed levels of disruptive behavior are predicted from selected prior variables. Alternative methods can also be found, such as comparisons of extreme groups, whether by temperament classification or clinical status (e.g., Maziade *et al.,* 1990; Sanson, Smart, Prior, & Oberklaid, 1993), and discriminant function analytic approaches (e.g., Prior, Smart, Sanson, & Oberklaid, 1998). The latter approaches are more suited to examining relationships between temperament and diagnosable DBD.

Dimensional and Diagnostic Approaches to Precursors of DBD

Research investigating the behavioral precursors of DBD in early childhood has tended to focus on specific problematic behaviors such as noncompliant and aggressive behaviors, usually assessed via rating scales. Such behaviors are often themselves symptoms of diagnosable disorders such as ODD. However, very few young children receive formal diagnoses of ODD and CD, and most research has adopted a dimensional rather than categorical or diagnostic approach to behavioral precursors, using scores on rating scales, or sometimes observational data, as predictors.

Similarly, few studies have used diagnosed ODD and CD disorders as outcome variables. This is particularly true of studies investigating temperament precursors and their effects. This is probably in part because the temperament

literature predominantly relates to early development; by late childhood and adolescence, personality factors are more likely to be the focus (see, e.g., Tremblay, 1992). Outcome variables have more commonly been behavioral symptoms or signs of disorders of the disruptive type (Campbell, 1994; Prior, Smart, Sanson, & Oberklaid, 1993; Prior, Sanson, Smart, & Oberklaid, 1997; Shaw, Keenan, & Vondra, 1994) or aggressive behavior (Kingston & Prior, 1995; Sanson, Smart, *et al.,* 1993; Tremblay, Pihl, Vitaro, & Dobkin, 1994), often using rating scale cutoffs to approximate clinical groups. In the research we review, therefore, outcomes may range from formal DBD diagnoses to extreme scores on aggression or externalizing behavior problem (EBP)* scales on parent and/or teacher questionnaires. Both in the assessment of behavioral precursors and in the identification of disordered behavioral outcome, the issue of comorbidity poses central questions that are explored further in the following sections.

The Temperament–Behavior Confound

Temperament has typically been viewed as referring to behavioral *style* whereas behavior refers to discrete actions or behavioral *content.* This distinction, however, may give a misleadingly straightforward impression. In fact, the two constructs have been rather difficult to discriminate in operational terms, a fact that often has been noted but rarely investigated. In a study where child development experts were asked to rate items from commonly used temperament and BP scales as to whether they were temperament or BP items (Sanson, Prior, & Kyrios, 1990), items supposedly assessing internalizing BP (IBP; e.g., anxiety, shyness) were commonly viewed as temperament items. Thus, an item tapping a child's reactions to strangers can equally be seen as assessing the temperament trait of approach–withdrawal or as a symptom of IBP. Items tapping active, intense,

*The term *externalizing behavior problems* (EBP) subsumes symptoms of ODD, CD, and ADHD, but does not imply that formal diagnostic criteria for any of these disorders have been met.

and irritable temperament characteristics (quick to react, impulsive) were often seen as tapping both IBP and EBP. EBP items, on the other hand, were rarely viewed as measures of temperament. Since all types of BP are assumed to arise through an interaction of intrinsic child factors such as temperament with environmental (e.g., parental) factors, it is not surprising that the dividing line between the two at times may be blurred. Often researchers have used the terms almost interchangeably or have used observations of behavior to identify temperament characteristics without specifying how they are making the distinction (e.g., Caspi, Henry, McGee, Moffitt, & Silva, 1995), or have used behavioral descriptors that are conceptually very close to temperament (e.g., Campbell's [1994] focus on "hard-to-manage" children).

For all these reasons, empirically demonstrated relationships between temperament and behavior at one time may be artefactual, especially if the temperament and behavioral data are given by the same informant. When predictions from early temperament to later behavior are found, it cannot be concluded that temperament caused the behavior but at least the opposite interpretation is precluded. These issues are important from a theoretical perspective but in pragmatic terms they do not need to cause great concern here, because the research we review is predominantly longitudinal and both temperament and behavioral contributors to later DBD are considered.

Comorbidity Issues

An additional challenge in seeking temperament and DBD associations comes from the common finding of a substantial level of comorbidity not only within externalizing disorders such as ODD and ADHD but between EBP and IBP (Bird, Gould, & Staghezza, 1993; Sanson, Oberklaid, Prior, Amos, & Smart, 1996). For example, Prior, Sanson, Smart, and Oberklaid (1998) found 44% comorbidity of diagnosed disorders at 12 years of age in the large community ATP sample. Dunedin Multidisciplinary Health and Development Study Christchurch Child Development Study reported 55% diagnosed co-

morbidity at 11 years using the DISC (Anderson, Williams, McGee, & Silva, 1987); the Christchurch Child Development Study reported that 41% of problem adolescents had two or more diagnosed disorders at 15 years of age (Fergusson, Horwood, & Lynskey, 1993). Although comorbidity within DBD, with ODD and ADHD being the prime exemplar, is always higher than across EBP and IBP categories, even the latter comorbidity is substantial (e.g., 15% in the Prior et al., 1998 study of 12-year-olds, and up to 21% in Bird et al., 1993).

RESEARCH STUDIES

Temperament Predictors of EBP

Bates and colleagues have reported a series of studies using data from the Bloomington Longitudinal Study, in which they have derived an "infant difficultness" factor from temperament measured in infancy and toddlerhood. This factor incorporated frequent and intense negative affect and attention-demanding characteristics, and predicted later EBP and IBP problems as seen in conflict in the mother–child relationship, from preschool to middle childhood periods (Bates & Bayles, 1988; Bates, Maslin, & Frankel, 1985; Bates et al., 1991; Lee & Bates, 1985). For boys in these studies, the major antecedents to DBD involved resistance to control and low manageability.

In these studies, the temperament factors were relatively weak predictors of disorder, suggesting their importance as precursors that need other "setting conditions" to affect the development and entrenchment of DBD. In discussing various influences on antisocial behavior, Bates and colleagues (1991) noted that the tendency to a demanding or coercive type of behavioral disposition is not only an intrinsic temperament precursor but will impact parental practices which can then potentiate effects. For example, a temperament cluster of difficultness that comprised negative emotionality, unadaptability to the new, and resistance to control was associated with negative management interactions and conflict with parents at 2 years of age and predicted hostile and aggressive behavior at preschool and middle-school age, especially for boys. Thus, the mechanism of effects is likely to be through the enhanced likelihood of setting up coercive interchanges in families with specific vulnerabilities or risks, operating through parental personal characteristics such as depression, and in parenting styles that are not conducive to reasoned negotiation of conflicts. Resistance to control and low manageability are reminiscent of characteristics identified by Patterson and colleagues (1992) as theoretically salient in setting up coercive cycles of negative interactions between mother and child in their antisocial boys (although, as noted previously, here they predicted both IBP and EBP). Van den Boom (1994) noted how innate child characteristics interact with the qualities of caregiving to produce different social-developmental outcomes among very young children.

In a recent 10-year longitudinal study of the relationships between temperament (assessed at 1 year of age) and BP ratings from parents and teachers of children ages 3–12 (Guerin, Gottfried, & Thomas, 1997), the temperament difficultness factor correlated consistently with parent reports of BP across all ages, more strongly for EBP than IBP problems, and with teacher report of EBP at 6–8 years. Those at the extreme of the difficultness factor were more likely to be above clinical cutoffs on aggression (by parent report) and attention and thought problems (by both parent and teacher report) at each age grouping. Although they did not report data on parenting or other contextual factors, the authors argued that the relationships found are likely to reflect goodness and poorness of fit with such contextual factors.

A French Canadian study by Maziade and his colleagues (e.g., Maziade, 1989; Maziade *et al.*, 1990) also assessed the contribution of temperament in a prospective longitudinal design. Children who were nonadaptable, withdrawing, emotionally intense, and negative in mood at 7 years of age, for example, were significantly more likely to have diagnosed clinical disorders at 12 years of age. However, clinical status at age 12 and also at age 16 was much better pre-dicted when aspects of family functioning were taken into account along with the temperament precursors. In the 1990 study, the relationship between extremely difficult temperament and diagnosis was assessed in a *clinical sample* comprising two groups of children aged 3–7 and 8–12 years. Among the younger age group, 24% of diagnosed children had an extremely difficult temperament; by contrast, 9% of a normative sample were at this extreme. The contrast was less in the older group (16% clinical vs. 7% normative) but still significant. The children with DBD were more likely to have high scores on a temperament factor very similar to Thomas and Chess's difficult temperament, comprising low adaptability, distractibility, and approach, high intensity, and negative mood. Temperament difficultness as measured in these studies seemed more strongly related to EBP than IBP. Maziade and colleagues (1990) argued that the consistency of the findings across normative and clinical samples supports the generalizability and clinical significance of these relationships between temperament and behavior problems.

So-called temperament ratings derived from observational measures aggregated across 3 to 5 years were predictive of parent- and teacher-rated EBP and IBP in late childhood and early adolescence, in Caspi and colleagues' (1995) analysis of the Dunedin longitudinal study of a community sample of almost 1000 children. Lack of control, with irritability and distractibility (similar to Bates's resistance to control factor noted previously) were predictive of EBP for both boys and girls. By comparison, lack of positive affect, passivity, wariness, and withdrawal from novelty predicted both IBP and EBP for girls but not for boys. As discussed in more depth later in this chapter, sex differences are a common feature of the temperament–behavior association literature, possibly particularly so for DBD. In the same Dunedin study, the precursors to criminal convictions by age 18 years were examined by Henry, Caspi, Moffitt, and Silva (1996). They reported that lack of control (not measured specifically as temperament but clearly a temperamentlike factor) had a direct effect on the propensity for violent crime. This interacted with family status (single parenthood) at 13 years, implicating additional social regulation factors in the association.

Temperament factors that have been described under more encompassing terms such as emotionality and impulsivity feature in a number of studies. Hagekull (1994) found that impulsivity, activity, and negative emotionality in toddlerhood predicted EBP at 4 years, although the emotionality factor was connected with *both* IBP and EBP. Cairns and Cairns (1991) and Ledingham (1991) saw such characteristics as negative emotionality functioning as readiness or priming factors for outbursts of angry and aggressive behavior. Coon, Carey, Corley, and Fulker (1992) used the Colorado Adoption Project sample to investigate temperament–behavior associations in a small (N = 15) sample of "poor conduct" boys considered at risk for DBD on the basis of parent and teacher ratings of EBP, low attention, high activity, and low achievement at 4–7 years of age and also at 8–9 years of age. Early histories showed that children with poor conduct had been rated by mothers as having more difficult temperament at 2 years of age and were more active according to observer ratings.

In a review of CD research, Robins (1991) noted that although CD is seldom diagnosed early in life, parents of older children with this diagnosis often report earlier characteristics of uncooperativeness and irritability; such data, although marred by retrospectivity, converge with the prospective studies reported previously.

There are also a number of studies examining *concurrent* rather than predictive associations. For example, McClowry and colleagues (1994) found 44% of the variance in concurrent EBP in 8- to 11-year-old children was accounted for by negative reactivity, 4% by nonpersistence, and 7% by maternal hassles. Concurrent associations between a child-reported delinquency measure and the maternal-reported temperament factors of persistence, activity, and approach, come from the ATP sample at 14 years of age. Twelve percent of the variance in delinquency was explained by temperament factors, with most of this (9.8%) being related to nonpersistence.

Wertlieb, Weigel, Springer, and Feldstein (1987) in another cross-sectional study reported results similar to those seen in longitudinal research, with negative mood characteristics correlating with both IBP and EBP, and manageability factors (nonadaptability, activity, intensity) and self-regulation factors (nonpersistence, irregularity) more closely associated with EBP (see Teglasi & McMahon, 1990, for similar findings).

Temperament factors can be conceptualized as risk factors but at least one aspect of temperament can be regarded as protective against the development of DBD, namely, approach–withdrawal or inhibition, which reflects discomfort and withdrawal in new situations and with new people. In the ATP data set, boys who at 11–12 years of age had EBP were significantly *less* likely to have been withdrawing at 3–4 years (Sanson, Oberklaid, *et al.*, 1996), although a small relationship in the reverse direction held for girls and early withdrawal predicted IBP for both boys and girls. Similarly, Schwartz, Snidman, and Kagan (1996) found that children who at 21 months had been classified as inhibited received lower scores on parent-rated externalizing, delinquent, and aggressive scales at 13 years than a group who had been classed as uninhibited. Similar findings emerged for boys (but not girls) identified as inhibited versus uninhibited at 31 months. Other research also documents the potential for temperament characteristics to create resilience against adverse outcome even in the context of other risks. Werner and Smith (1982) found that resilient individuals in their Kauai study tended to have been affectionate, responsive, and moderately active as infants. In a study of high-risk families in Australia (Smith & Prior, 1995), the resilient children tended to show low emotional reactivity and high social engagement. Individual dispositional characteristics such as these form one cluster in Garmezy's (1985) triad of protective factors.

In summary, both cross-sectional and longitudinal studies amply document associations between particular temperament features and DBD-type behaviors. The most prominent temperament factors that emerge as significant predictors are negative emotionality, characteristics involving intense and highly reactive responses in a variety of situations, and inflexibility, which encompasses resistance to control, unmanageability, and nonadaptability. Inflexibility features in a number of studies often with different but clearly related descriptors (e.g., Barron & Earls, 1984; Prior et al., 1993; Thomas & Chess, 1977). However, as noted earlier it can be difficult to distinguish between temperament and BP, with many terms used interchangeably and independently of particular measurement approaches (e.g., temperament scales vs. behavior problem scales). The next section illustrates some of these boundary problems.

Behavioral Predictors of EBP

The best predictors of DBD and related problems are almost invariably previous EBP (Bates et al., 1991; Prior et al., 1993; Prior, Smart, et al., 1998; see also Chapter 19, this volume). Their significance stands no matter what kinds of statistical approaches are used to assess predictive power and is evidence for the substantial stability of EBP once established. Despite the incontrovertibility of this finding, it is important to seek more specific behavioral predictors of DBD and to identify at what ages and under what conditions early BP are predictive of later adjustment.

McGee, Feehan, and Williams (1996) found that children who were hard to manage and showing hyperactive-type behaviors at age 3 were highly likely to show BP at one or more of ensuing ages (7, 9, 11, and 13 years). This association also included consistent links with poor academic performance and impaired early language skills. Findings applied to both boys and girls. The same sample provided the data for the Caspi and colleagues (1995) research previously cited in which DBPs in adolescence were predicted by undercontrolled behavior at preschool age. White, Moffitt, Earls, Robins, and Silva (1990), again drawing on the same data set, found consistent relationships between aggressive and disobedient behavior at age 3

and CD in childhood; the associations continued to police arrest in adolescence (Moffitt, 1990). The histories of children deemed to have antisocial problems in middle childhood and adolescence indicated that they had had a range of behavioral and cognitive problems (often with comorbid ADHD), had shown high rates of EBP, and had been hard to manage during the preschool years. A consistent theme in these Dunedin study findings, however, is the moderating effect of family adversity variables such as socioeconomic disadvantage, poor family relationships including parental separation, and poor maternal mental health on such relationships (Anderson et al., 1987).

In a series of studies focusing on the behavioral outcome of hard to manage preschool boys, Campbell and colleagues (Campbell, 1994, 1995) provide a prime example of the overlapping of constructs noted previously. Their work focuses on preschool behaviors described as active, inattentive, impulsive, hard to manage, and the like (in other words, temperamentlike constructs) and their effects on later adjustment in young boys. Problems with manageability and self-regulation as assessed in home, laboratory, and preschool settings were related (in combination with adverse family factors) to later self-regulation problems and oppositional BP in the children (Campbell, 1994). The boys in the studies were not categorized as having DBD but a smaller subgroup of the sample assessed as having more extreme and pervasive problems with disruptive, high intensity, noncompliant, and irritable behaviors (Campbell, Pierce, March, Ewing, & Szumowski, 1994) showed the most disorganized and noncompliant behavior in middle childhood. Campbell and Pierce (1996) reported that approximately 30% of problem boys who were living in dysfunctional families showed diagnosable disorders by 9 years of age, again illustrating the transactional effects already noted. Similarly, Richman, Stevenson, and Graham (1982), following up British children from 3 to 8 years of age, found that EBP and attention problems, along with sibling conflict, were characteristic of those children with persisting difficulties.

Campbell (1995), in reviewing studies of BP development in young children, concluded that children identified as hard to manage at 3 or 4 years of age had an approximately 50% chance of continuing maladjustment in middle childhood and adolescence, and that the data applied consistently across different populations, measures, and information sources.

Perhaps the most consistent and robust behavioral precursor to many forms of antisocial behavior is aggression, which appears to develop very early and in at least half of cases to remain a stable problem, particularly for boys (but see gender differences section later). The literature on this topic is substantial and covers many different populations. It includes studies of aggression and bullying by Olweus (1979); of aggression and proneness to watch violent TV programs, with prediction from age 8 to adulthood (Huesmann, Eron, Lefkowitz, & Walder, 1984); the Ensminger, Kellam, and Rubin (1983) Woodlawn study in which teacher-rated aggression in first grade predicted self-reported delinquency 10 years later; reports from Farrington (1991) and Loeber, Stouthamer-Loeber and Green (1991) of relationships between childhood aggression and violent offending; and the work of Robins (1978, 1986, 1991) documenting the life histories of identified offenders in adult life.

An additional generally agreed behavioral (or perhaps temperament) precursor to DBD is impulsivity (Farrington, 1989; Robins, 1991). In a review outlining temperament and personality antecedents to delinquent behavior, including impulsivity, Tremblay (1992) theorized how the biological and social learning influences combine to produce antisocial behavior, suggesting that consideration of models of personality such as those of Eysenck (1970), Gray (1981), and Cloninger (1987) helps to systematize and explain the links between childhood behaviors and antisocial outcomes (see Quay, 1993, for an extrapolation of Gray's work to CD). Given the role of impulsivity in DBD, a further link with hyperactivity (or ADHD symptoms) may be made, with evidence suggesting that ADHD may itself constitute a set of precursor behaviors to later

ODD and CD. Like Robins (1991), some suggest ADHD symptoms as the early pattern, with these being followed developmentally by ODD symptoms, then CD behaviors. Within the CD category there is an age-related progression of behaviors in terms of seriousness as judged by the reports of parents and teachers (see also Chapter 1, this volume). However, as described in more detail later, analyses of data from the ATP (Sanson, Smart, *et al.*, 1993) support the view that noncompliant, hostile behavior emerges early in the lives of children who develop aggressive BP, whereas ADHD symptoms emerge later and only for a subset of these aggressive children as well as for some children who do not have aggressive problems. In any case, aggression and impulsivity feature strongly and consistently as major behavioral precursors to DBDs and to legally defined delinquency.

Generally, behavioral precursors of DBDs may be best described as being less elaborated, more developmentally consistent forms of behaviors that will, in adverse family, parenting, and community contexts, blossom into DBD of a serious kind. The combination of aggression and impulsivity, especially if co-occurring with deficient problem-solving skills (see Chapter 14, this volume), poses a particularly high risk.

The Australian Temperament Project

The ATP is a large-scale, prospective longitudinal study of children's development from infancy onward that began in 1983. It is unique in that it contains detailed information from infancy to adolescence on temperament, as well as other individual and contextual data. Several analyses of this data set speak to the issue of temperament and behavioral precursors of DBD, although analyses to date mostly concern the children only up to 11–12 years and use EBP of various kinds as outcome. We therefore review selected findings from this study in more detail to flesh out those reported previously from other researchers.

The initial sample comprised 2443 infants from urban and rural areas of the state of Victoria, Australia. Sampling details are given in Sanson, Prior, and Oberklaid (1985). In brief, a stratified sample of municipalities in the state of Victoria was obtained with the assistance of the Australian Bureau of Statistics. Then, all families with an infant 4 to 8 months of age who attended a Maternal and Child Health (MCH) Centre in one of these municipalities over a specified 2-week period in 1983 were enrolled in the study. The MCH service achieved contact with 94% of live births at that time. Analyses showed that the participating families were representative of the population on parental age, ethnic background, and socioeconomic status. In 10 waves of data collection, parents, MCH nurses, teachers, and in recent years the children themselves have provided information on temperament, BP, mother–child relationship, health, school achievement and adjustment, social skills, peer relationships, parenting practices, stressful life events, and sociodemographic background. As noted, the influence of temperament on adjustment has been a unique, consistent and central focus throughout the study. About two thirds of the original cohort was still enrolled in the study at 11–12 years of age.

The pathways to DBD from infancy to 8 years of age were investigated by Sanson, Smart, and colleagues (1993). Four groups of children from the ATP were selected at 8 years of age on the basis of ratings at both 5–6 and 7–8 years on hyperactive-distractible and hostile-aggressive scales—a "pure" ADHD group, pure aggressive, comorbid, and a problem-free comparison group. Even in infancy, these groups differed significantly on the temperament factors of cooperation-manageability, activity-reactivity, and irritability, with the comorbid group showing the most negative characteristics and the pure ADHD group generally indistinguishable from the comparison group. At 2–3 years of age, a similar pattern of differences was apparent. At 3–4 and 5–6 years, inflexible and impersistent temperament characteristics were associated with aggressive behavior, with the comorbid group still retaining the highest risk levels. By these ages the pure ADHD group was higher than the comparison group on these temperament char-

acteristics, but still lower than the aggressive groups. Thus, some specificity of temperament predictors for these disorders was apparent at least in the early years.

These temperament differences were accompanied by a range of other risk variables. Overall, the groups with aggressive behaviors were perceived most negatively by their parents from infancy onward. These families also tended to have more environmental disadvantage, larger family size, more negative life events, and poorer perceived coping skills. The relative influence of temperament and family variables was not assessed in this study, but results could be interpreted to support direct linear effects for aggression, from irritability and inflexibility to aggressive behavior but in the context of a transactional model whereby the difficult temperament characteristics interacted with a poor mother–child relationship and environmental stress and disadvantage to lead to the development of aggressive behavior problems. Since identifiable temperamental precursors of pure ADHD did not emerge clearly until 3–4 years of age, it may be the mismatch between the child's characteristics and environmental demands of preschool and school that plays a major role.

Kingston and Prior (1995) also studied ATP children up to the age of 8 years, this time with a focus on stable, transient, and school-age-onset aggressive behavior. Approximately 3% of the sample (with a ratio of 3.5 boys to 1 girl) had been rated as aggressive (more than 1 SD above the mean) at each sampling point from 3 years of age. This stable aggressive group could be distinguished from the transient and late-onset groups and from nonaggressive children by difficult temperament characteristics at every measurement point from 2–3 years on, poor mother–child relationship (mother's overall rating of the child as difficult), higher levels of sibling hostility, harsher parenting practices, lower reading achievement and task orientation in school, and overall higher levels of aggressive behavior. It appears, then, that temperament and various contextual factors were combining to create a situation in which aggressive behavior was maintained in this group.

The extent to which EBP, IBP, or both at 11–12 years could be predicted from risk factors assessed in five previous waves, from infancy to 9–10 years, was investigated by Sanson, Oberklaid, and colleagues (1996) and Sanson, Smart, Prior, Oberklaid, and Amos (1996). Here BP groups were selected on the basis of agreement by at least two of three informants (parents, teachers, and the children themselves). From infancy, the children who had developed problems by 11–12 years had considerably more risk factors present than problem-free comparison groups. EBP boys were more irritable or inflexible in temperament than the comparison group at 3 time points; between 27% and 36% of EBP boys were at an extreme on irritability (toddler years) and inflexibility (from 3 years on), compared to 10% or less of the comparison group. These factors also predicted IBP. Thus, these temperament factors, reflecting aspects of emotional self-regulation and reactivity to frustration and control efforts, appeared to be a moderately strong risk for both types of disorders for boys, reminiscent of Bates's findings for his difficultness factor. The results for girls on these factors were less consistent and less strong. Low persistence (i.e., inability to stay on task) was related to EBP (but not IBP) for both boys and girls. Among boys, about a third with later EBP were nonpersistent at 3–4 and 5–6 years and half were so by teacher report at 5–6 years; among girls, about 20% with EBP had early signs of nonpersistence. At 9–10 years, boys who later had EBP were more likely to be very active.

As at 7–8 years, a range of other variables besides these temperament predictors discriminated between groups. A poorer mother–child relationship was characteristic of EBP boys and girls from infancy, and interestingly was a much stronger predictor for EBP than IBP problems. EBP groups also tended to have lower SES. Early-emerging BP in toddlerhood had predictive power for both boys and girls. Similar differences, and of strengthening magnitude, were revealed in data from later time points. Accuracy of classification, based on logistic regression analyses, ranged from 65% to 80%. However, no one risk was necessary or sufficient for a problem outcome, and each particular risk was present only in a minority of the problem group. Using categorical analyses made it easier for this fact to emerge: The highly significant results that emerge from correlational analyses with these data can make it tempting to overemphasize the strength of relationships. Again, a transactional model of interacting intrinsic and extrinsic factors appears to fit the data.

About one third of EBP children had comorbid IBP. Comorbid girls did not differ greatly from EBP-only girls in their early risk factors until 9–10 years, when they were higher on negative emotionality. In contrast, comorbid boys clearly had more risk factors present in early childhood than pure EBP boys, in particular higher irritability, lower cooperation-manageability, and poorer mother–child relationship in the first 2 years of life, but had higher SES than the pure EBP group. Thus temperament appeared to be implicated for boys in developmental pathways to comorbid conditions.

Recent analyses (Prior et al., 1997) focused on the 93 most aggressive children (66 boys, 27 girls) in the sample at 12–13 years, representing the top 7% of the sample and including 43 children in the 11- to 12-year EBP sample reported previously. Among these 93 children, 73% were comorbid with other types of problems, most often with ADHD (50%), indicating that aggression is most commonly part of a constellation of problems. As with the EBP groups at 11–12 years, the aggressive group showed differences from a randomly selected comparison group on temperament and other measures from infancy onward, showing consistent problems across family, school, and peer domains for many years. Aggressive BP from preschool age onward was highly predictive of 12- to 13-year aggression (odds ratio of 9.8).

In general, the ATP data confirm and extend the conclusions drawn from the research on samples reported earlier. Negative emotionality and inflexibility again appear to be generalized vulnerability factors for disorder. Poor self-regulation, as reflected in nonpersistence, has been assessed by relatively few other researchers, but it appears to have a growing influence as the children develop, specifically for EBP. The ATP focuses especially on intrinsic child characteristics but the consistent appearance of environmental and relationship variables as discriminators between problem and no-problem groups reinforces the need to interpret temperament differences in the context of a transactional model. Finally, the ATP data demonstrate clearly the impact of temperament from very early in life in affecting developmental pathways, as well as the predictive role of early-emerging aggressive behavior problems for later DBD. Both these findings argue for early intervention.

Gender-Specific Predictors

Analyses with the ATP data set have also addressed the issue of gender-specific paths to EBP (Prior *et al.*, 1993; Sanson, Prior, Smart, & Oberklaid, 1993; Sanson, Smart, *et al.*, 1996). We found that gender differences were minimal in infancy, but emerged and increased with age. Boys showed more negative temperament characteristics (e.g., on irritability, intensity, and cooperation-manageability) from toddlerhood and substantially lower persistence from 5 years on (see Kohnstamm, 1989, for a review of findings regarding sex differences in temperament). Maternal ratings revealed more problems with adaptive behavior and social competence, and more hyperactive and aggressive BP from toddlerhood. Gender differences for aggression were large and consistent but there were no gender differences on IBP by parent or teacher report. Teachers rated boys as having more academic problems and BP in their first 3 years of school, and lower school readiness at 5–6 years. We suggested that girls' faster development during early childhood may partially account for the differences on aggression: Faster language development and better self-regulation skills may result in parents' finding girls easier to manage, promoting a more positive parent–child relationship and thus fewer BP (Sanson, Prior, *et al.*, 1993).

Path analyses of 112 boys and 115 girls followed from 3 to 8 years were used to predict behavioral maladjustment separately by sex (Prior *et al.*, 1993). (Here our outcome measure combined symptoms of EBP and IBP.) Our predictors included the temperament factors of inflexibility and persistence; additional child measures included social maturity, intelligence, and reading achievement. Maternal variables included psychological adjustment, marital adjustment, social support, life stresses, and the child-rearing variables of child centeredness and use of punishment. Temperament inflexibility was the best predictor for both boys' and girls' BP, but in other ways the paths differed substantially. For boys at most ages, inflexibility and persistence had direct links to BP and inflexibility was the only direct predictor of boys' BP at 7–8 years. Maternal variables generally exerted their influence only indirectly, through the use of punishment. A more complex picture emerged for girls, with BP consistently related to a range of child, maternal, and interactional factors. Persistence contributed to the prediction for girls only at 6–7 years, whereas child rearing was more important: Punishment contributed at every age, and child centeredness had both direct and indirect influences. Neither IQ nor reading achievement were predictive for either sex. Overall, our results suggested greater sensitivity to family influences among girls.

The later analyses of predictors of EBP and IBP at 11–12 years described previously (Sanson, Smart, *et al.*, 1996) also revealed somewhat different predictors for boys and girls. From infancy, boys with problems tended to have a higher number of risks present than did girls with problems, suggesting greater male vulnerability. Low approach and high anxiety (which could be considered early indicators of IBP) were at some ages predictors of EBP for girls, but never for boys, whereas inflexibility and irritability were stronger predictors for boys' EBP than for girls'. This latter finding in particular is consistent with Prior and colleagues' (1993) findings at 7–8 years.

Others have also found evidence of gender-specific pathways, typically with more complex pathways for girls. Most of these also involve young children, so extrapolation is needed to draw implications for adolescence. The study by Bates and colleagues (1991) predicting IBP and EBP at 8 years from data collected from 6 months, had results similar to ours. While their difficultness measure had similar predictive value for boys and girls, it appeared that resistance to control (measured at 13 months) was a stronger predictor for boys; girls' EBP were more closely associated with the absence of positive parental involvement, discordant parent–child relationships, and poor joint problem solving.

Using participants from the longitudinal Colorado Adoption Project, Rende (1993) examined the associations between temperament assessed in infancy and early childhood and disorder at 7 years of age, focusing on parent-rated anxiety-depression, attention problems, and delinquent behavior. Sex differences were a notable feature of the findings. Only one weak (but significant) relationship with delinquency emerged, that being with high emotionality in early childhood for boys only. Emotionality was also moderately associated with an attention problems scale for boys. High emotionality in infancy and early childhood was associated with high scores on an anxiety-depression scale for boys, whereas both high emotionality and low sociability were the correlates for girls.

In contrast to our findings, Keenan and Shaw (1994) found that family variables predicted boys' aggression more reliably than girls'. Fagot (1995) followed toddlers to 5 years of age and concluded that, if they had studied boys only, the findings would have been a strong confirmation of Patterson's coercion model of antisocial behavior in older boys. Two-year-old boys' observed negative peer interactions, along with family and maternal variables, predicted teacher ratings of behavior problems at 5 years. However, no such predictive relationships held for girls. The complexity of prediction for girls was confirmed by Caspi, Lynam, Moffitt, and Silva (1993), where prediction of girls' delinquency involved complicated relations among family history, age of menarche, and school setting. Finally, while aggression, once established, predicts later aggressive tendencies for girls as well as for boys (Cairns, Cairns, Nederman, Ferguson, & Gariepy, 1989; Pulkkinnen, 1987), aggressive girls are more likely than boys to exhibit comorbidity with depression in adolescence (Loeber & Keenan, 1994).

The exploration of gender-specific temperament and behavioral contributors to DBD is complicated by three facts. First, the incidence of EBP is lower for girls than boys. Zoccolillo (1993), while noting the paucity of studies of girls' CD, reported that about half of epidemiological studies showed no sex differences in CD after puberty, and these were mostly in relation to aggressive CD; however, there were consistent differences in childhood. About 2%–9% of girls, versus 6%–16% of boys, were likely to meet criteria for CD (DSM-IV, American Psychiatric Association, 1994; see also Chapter 2, this volume). Second, EBP appear to be expressed differently by boys and girls. Boys' physical aggression often develops out of rough-and-tumble play, whereas indirect or relational aggression, which often takes the form of alienation, ostracism, character defamation, and collusion directed at relational bonds between "friends" is reported to be more common among girls (Cairns et al., 1989; Crick & Grotpeter, 1995; Zahn-Waxler, 1993). Third, the available assessment instruments are much more tuned to male-type EBP. Although DSM-IV acknowledges that girls' presenting problems may be different, diagnostic criteria for CD have not been validated with females, so researchers may not accurately assess the nature of CD in girls (Zoccolillo, 1993). This has resulted in a call for gender-specific assessments and normative data regarding EBP (Keenan & Shaw, 1994; Zoccolillo, 1993), an issue still subject to debate (Zahn-Waxler, 1993). Of the few predictive investigations of adolescence that have included girls in their samples *and* have analyzed for sex differences (e.g., Caspi *et al.*, 1993; Keenan & Shaw, 1994; Robins, 1986), even fewer have explored temperament as a predictor (Maziade *et al.*, 1990; Sanson, Smart, *et al.*, 1996). Thus, we are left with some suggestive evidence of differential paths but no organized picture, and the need for further research on the influence of gender on the role of temperament in the etiology of BP.

CONCLUSIONS

The research reviewed demonstrates that it is possible to identify children at risk for DBD from quite early in life, on the basis of a confluence of child characteristics and parent, family, and environment characteristics. Intrinsic child characteristics undoubtedly contribute to risk. The consistency of findings of the salience of temperament and behavioral precursors, despite variations in methodology (e.g., longitudinal and cross-sectional studies, clinical and unselected samples) is notable. Negative emotionality seems to be a ubiquitous predictor of many kinds of problems; resistance to control (low manageability), poor self-regulation (low persistence), and impulsivity appear more salient as precursors to EBP or embryonic DBD problems. We conclude that the literature supports direct linkages, with specific temperament dimensions relating in a differentiated way to EBP. As noted, too little research has focused on diagnosable DBD to make strong claims here, but the level of continuity of aggressive behavior in particular (Loeber, 1990; Robins, 1978) supports the validity of generalization to diagnosed DBD from the symptom-level outcomes in childhood and adolescence that are considered in most of the available research. The data generally favor regarding temperament characteristics such as emotionality as constituting a vulnerability or predisposition to disorder (although low approach, at least for boys, may be protective against DBD). This is consistent with a transactional model in which a predisposition does not become actualized unless other potentiating factors (such as poor parent–child relationships, stress) co-occur. This is also consistent with the notion that temperament in itself does not constitute a negative versus positive adjustment, but that temperament impacts the developmental process that determines adjustment (Rothbart & Bates, 1998).

One implication of finding such early intrinsic child (and extrinsic environmental) predictors of later DBD is of course the advisability of early intervention. Early intervention is argued to be more effective than later (e.g., Feehan, McGee, Williams, & Nada-Raja, 1995; Loeber, 1990; Sanders, 1995; see also Chapter 25, this volume), and the body of research reviewed gives indications as to where such intervention should be focused. Temperament in itself is not immutable, especially as developing capacities for self-regulation give the child the ability to modify the expression of temperament traits. More fundamentally, we have argued that temperament has its effects within a transactional system, and thus the response of parents and teachers to difficult or poorly fitting temperament traits is a critical focus for intervention. The task of parenting is harder with some children than others, and parents need education and support (Sanson & Rothbart, 1995). Van den Boom (1989, 1994) has shown how parental training for mothers of highly irritable babies can be effective in improving parent–child relationships and preventing the development of problems. The literature also supports intervention focused as much on an individual's context as on individuals themselves.

A second conclusion emerging from this review relates to stability and change. Although lawful associations can be found between early status and later outcome, there is plasticity and openness in developmental paths at all times; a difficult child is not absolutely doomed to a path toward ODD and/or CD. On the other hand, odds ratios for ongoing DBD, given the early appearance of EBP, are often very high; for example, in the ATP, the odds ratio for aggressive and antisocial behavior at 12 years from aggression at 5 years is 9.8 (Prior *et al.,* 1997). Thus, the combination of problematic temperament traits and adverse circumstances is a potent predictor of poor outcome and, without intervention, substantial stability of problem behavior can be expected.

Our review of gender differences in pathways toward DBD revealed first the paucity of relevant studies. As Zoccolillo (1993) noted, there has been a remarkable failure by researchers to attend to the DBD of girls. However, from the extant literature there are strong pointers to the need to investigate the precursors of DBD separately for boys and girls. Our own studies suggest that young boys are more strongly influenced by temperament characteristics such as inflexibility and impersistence, whereas family factors may have more influence on girls. Others have found that boys are more influenced by family stress (e.g., Keenan & Shaw, 1994). Sample differences are probably part of the answer to these inconsistencies, but the data may also be interpretable as greater male vulnerability to risks (at least up to adolescence), whether intrinsic or extrinsic (see Werner & Smith, 1982). In terms of DBD, another part of the answer is also likely to lie in cultural factors. The evidence that boys and girls do not differ in temperament in infancy and that differences increasingly emerge with age suggests (but of course cannot prove) the impact of environmental factors in that emergence. Since boys are less condemned, and sometimes rewarded, for displaying aggressive behavior, it may take less risk to actualize whatever predispositions they may have. Despite cultural change in sex role expectations in the past decades, it remains the case that boys have available a range of models of male aggression, ranging from sports through television and other media to politics (Sanson, Prior, *et al.*, 1993) and that parents and teachers respond to child behavior differentially depending on whether it is exhibited by boys or girls. Hinde and Stevenson-Hinde (1988), for instance, reported that parents warmly accepted girls' shyness, whereas boys' shyness was disapproved of; in contrast, boys' aggression was more accepted than girls'. Until and unless the early experiences of boys, in their homes, schools, and general environment, give clear messages about the unacceptability of DBD, the higher prevalence rate for boys is likely to remain.

Although the evidence we have presented does support the case that a large proportion of those who develop DBD have embarked upon developmental pathways leading them in that direction very early in life, and that the individual's early temperament and behavior are an important part of this story, we conclude by reiterating that the evidence best fits a transactional model, whereby temperament may constitute a vulnerability factor that is actualized only in the context of other suboptimal environmental situations. It may often be that these extrinsic factors are more amenable to change.

ACKNOWLEDGMENT. The authors would like to thank Diana Smart for her help with analyses and in the preparation of this chapter.

REFERENCES

Ahadi, S. A., & Rothbart, M. K. (1994). Temperament, development and the Big Five. In C. F. Halverson, G. A. Kohnstamm, & R. P. Martin (Eds.), *The developing structure of temperament and personality from infancy to adulthood* (pp. 189–207). Hillsdale, NJ: Erlbaum.

American Psychiatric Association. (1994). *Diagnostic and statistical manual of mental disorders* (4th ed.). Washington, DC: Author.

Anderson, J. C., Williams, S., McGee, R., & Silva, A. (1987). DSM-III disorders in preadolescent children: Prevalence in a large sample from the general population. *Archives of General Psychiatry, 44,* 69–76.

Barron, A. P., & Earls, F. (1984). The relation of temperament and social factors to behavior problems in three year old children. *Journal of Child Psychology and Psychiatry, 25,* 23–33.

Bates, J. E. (1989). Concepts and measures of temperament. In G. A. Kohnstamm, J. E. Bates, & M. K. Rothbart (Eds.), *Temperament in childhood* (pp. 3–26). Chichester, England: Wiley.

Bates, J. E., & Bayles, K. (1988). The role of attachment in the development of behavior problems. In J. Belsky & T. Nezworski (Eds.), *Clinical implications of attachment* (pp. 253–299). Hillsdale, NJ: Erlbaum.

Bates, J. E., & Wachs, T. D. (1994). *Temperament: Individual differences at the interface of biology and behavior.* Washington, DC: American Psychological Association.

Bates, J. E., Maslin, C. A., & Frankel, K. A. (1985). Attachment security mother–infant interaction and temperament as predictors of behavior problem ratings at age three years. In I. Bretherton & E. Waters (Eds.), *Growing points of attachment theory and research* (Monographs of the Society for Research in Child Development, Serial No. 209, pp. 167–193).

Bates, J. E., Bayles, K., Bennett, D. S., Ridge, B., & Brown, M. M. (1991). Origins of externalizing behavior problems at eight years of age. In D. J. Pepler & H. Rubin (Eds.), *The development and treatment of childhood aggression* (pp. 93–121). Hillsdale, NJ: Erlbaum.

Bell, R. Q. (1968). A reinterpretation of the direction of effects in studies of socialization. *Psychological Review,* 75, 81–95.

Bell, R. Q. (1974). Contributions of human infants to caregiving and social interactions. In M. Lewis & L. A. Rosenblum (Eds.), *The effect of the infant on its caregiver* (pp. 1–19). New York: Wiley.

Bird, H. R., Gould, M. S., & Staghezza, B. M. (1993). Patterns of diagnostic comorbidity in a community sample of children aged 9 through 16 years. *Journal of the American Academy of Child and Adolescent Psychiatry,* 32, 361–378.

Boom, D. C. Van Den. (1989). Neonatal irritability and the development of attachment. In G. A. Kohnstamm, J. E. Bates, & M. K. Rothbart (Eds.), *Temperament in childhood* (pp. 299–318). Chichester, England: Wiley.

Boom, D. C. Van Den. (1994). The influence of temperament and mothering on attachment and exploration: An experimental manipulation of sensitive responsiveness among lower-class mothers with irritable infants. *Child Development,* 65, 1457–1477.

Cairns, R. B., & Cairns, B. D. (1991). Social cognition and social networks: A developmental perspective. In D. J. Pepler & H. Rubin (Eds.), *The development and treatment of childhood aggression* (pp. 249–278). Hillsdale, NJ: Erlbaum.

Cairns, R. B., Cairns, B. S., Nederman, H. J., Ferguson, L. L., & Gariepy, J. L. (1989). Growth and aggression: I. Childhood to early adolescence. *Developmental Psychology,* 25, 320–330.

Campbell, S. B. (1994). Hard-to-manage preschool boys: Externalizing behavior, social competence, and family context at two-year followup. *Journal of Abnormal Child Psychology,* 22, 147–166.

Campbell, S. B. (1995). Behavior problems in preschool children: A review of recent research. *Journal of Child Psychology and Psychiatry,* 36, 113–149.

Campbell, S. B., & Pierce, E. W. (1996, August). *Hard-to-manage preschool boys in middle childhood: Mother–child conflict and family dysfunction as predictors of externalizing problems.* Paper presented at the International Society for the Study of Behavioral Development conference, Quebec City, Quebec, Canada.

Campbell, S. B., Pierce, E. W., March, C. L., Ewing, L. J., & Szumowski, E. K. (1994). Hard-to-manage preschool boys: Symptomatic behavior across contexts and time. *Child Development,* 65, 836–851.

Caspi, A., Lynam, D., Moffitt, T. E., & Silva, P. A. (1993). Unravelling girls' delinquency: Biological, dispositional and contextual contributions to adolescent misbehavior. *Developmental Psychology,* 29, 19–30.

Caspi, A., Henry, B., McGee, R. O., Moffitt, T. E., & Silva, P. A. (1995). Temperamental origins of child and adolescent behavior problems: From age three to age fifteen. *Child Development,* 66, 55–68.

Cloninger, C. R. (1987). A systematic method for clinical description and classification of personality variants. *Archives of General Psychiatry,* 44, 573–588.

Coon, H., Carey, G., Corley, R., & Fulker, D. W. (1992). Identifying children in the Colorado Adoption Project at risk for conduct disorder. *Journal of the American Academy of Child and Adolescent Psychiatry,* 31, 503–511.

Crick, N. R., & Grotpeter, J. K. (1995). Relational aggression, gender and social-psychological adjustment. *Child Development,* 66, 710–722.

Diamond, S. (1974). *The roots of psychology.* New York: Basic Books.

Earls, F., & Jung, K. G. (1987). Temperament and home environment characteristics as causal factors in the early development of childhood psychopathology. *Journal of the American Academy of Child and Adolescent Psychiatry,* 26, 491–498.

Ensminger, M. E., Kellam, S. G., & Rubin, B. B. (1983). School and family origins of delinquency: Comparisons by sex. In K. T. Van Dusen & S. A. Mednick (Eds.), *Prospective studies of crime and delinquency* (pp. 73–97). Boston: Kluwer-Nijhoff.

Eysenck, H. J. (1970). *The structure of human personality* (3rd ed.). London: Methuen.

Fagot, B. I. (1995). Parenting of boys and girls. In M. Bornstein (Ed.), *Handbook on parenting* (Vol. 4, pp. 163–183). Hillsdale, NJ: Erlbaum.

Farrington, D. P. (1989). Later adult life outcomes of offenders and non-offenders. In M. Bambring, F. Losel, & H. Skowronek (Eds.), *Children at risk: Assessment and longitudinal research* (pp. 220–244). Berlin, Germany: De Gruyter.

Farrington, D. P. (1991). Childhood aggression and adult violence: Early precursors and later-life outcomes. In D. J. Pepler & H. Rubin (Eds.), *The development and treatment of childhood aggression* (pp. 5–28), Hillsdale, NJ: Erlbaum.

Feehan, M., McGee, R., Williams, S. M., & Nada-Raja, S. (1995). Models of adolescent psychopathology: Childhood risk and the transition to adulthood. *Journal of the American Academy of Child and Adolescent Psychiatry,* 34, 670–679.

Fergusson, D. M., Horwood, L. J., & Lynskey, M. T. (1993). Prevalence and comorbidity of DSM-III-R diagnoses in a birth cohort of 15 year olds. *Journal of the American Academy of Child and Adolescent Psychiatry,* 32, 1127–1134.

Fox, N. A. (1989). Psychophysical correlates of emotional reactivity during the first year of life. *Developmental Psychology,* 25, 364–372.

Fox, N. A., Calkins, S. D., & Bell, M. A. (1994). Neural plasticity and development in the first two years of life: Evidence from cognitive and socioemotional domains of research. *Development and Psychopathology,* 6, 677–696.

Garmezy, N. (1985). Stress-resistant children: The search for protective factors. In J. E. Stevenson (Ed.), *Recent research in developmental psychopathology* (Book suppl. 4 to *Journal of Child Psychology and Psychiatry,* pp. 213–220). Oxford, England: Pergamon.

Goldberg, L. R. (1993). The structure of phenotypic personality traits. *American Psychologist,* 48, 26–34.

Gray, J. A. (1981). A critique of Eysenck's theory of personality. In H. J. Eysenck (Ed.), *A model for personality* (pp. 246–276). New York: Springer.

Guerin, D. W., Gottfried, A. W., & Thomas, C. W. (1997). Difficult temperament and behavior problems: A longitudinal study from 1. 5 to 12 years. *International Journal of Behavioral Development, 21,* 71–90.

Hagekull, B. (1994). Infant temperament and early childhood functioning: Possible relations to the five-factor model. In C. F. Halverson, G. A. Kohnstamm, & R. P. Martin (Eds.), *The developing structure of temperament and personality from infancy to adulthood* (pp. 227–240). Hillsdale, NJ: Erlbaum.

Henry, B., Caspi, A., Moffitt, T. E., & Silva, P. A. (1996). Temperamental and familial predictors of violent and nonviolent criminal convictions: Age 3 to age 18. *Developmental Psychology, 32,* 614–623.

Hinde, R. A., & Stevenson-Hinde, J. (1988). Epilogue. In R. A. Hinde & J. Stevenson-Hinde (Eds.), *Relationships within families: Mutual influences* (pp. 365–385). Oxford, England: Clarendon.

Hubert, N. C., Wachs, T. D., Peters-Martin, P., & Gandour, M. J. (1982). The study of early temperament: Measurement and conceptual issues. *Child Development, 53,* 571–600.

Huesmann, L. R., Eron, I. D., Lefkowitz, M. M., & Walder, I. O. (1984). Stability of aggression over time and over generations. *Developmental Psychology, 20,* 1120–1134.

John, O. P., Caspi, A., Robins, R. W., Moffitt, T. E., & Stouthamer-Loeber, M. (1994). The "Little Five": Exploring the nomological network of the Five-Factor Model of personality in adolescent boys. *Child Development, 65,* 335–344.

Keenan, K., & Shaw, D. S. (1994). The development of aggression in toddlers: A study of low-income families. *Journal of Abnormal Child Psychology, 22,* 53–77.

Kingston, L., & Prior, M. (1995). The development of patterns of stable, transient and school-age onset aggressive behavior in young children. *Journal of the American Academy of Child and Adolescent Psychiatry, 34,* 348–358.

Kohnstamm, G. (1989). Temperament in childhood: Cross-cultural and sex differences. In G. A. Kohnstamm, J. E. Bates, & M. K. Rothbart (Eds.), *Temperament in childhood* (pp. 483–508). Chichester, England: Wiley.

Ledingham, J. E. (1991). Social cognition and aggression. In D. J. Pepler & H. Rubin (Eds.), *The development and treatment of childhood aggression* (pp. 279–286). Hillsdale, NJ: Erlbaum.

Lee, C., & Bates, J. E. (1985). Mother–child interaction at age two years and perceived difficult temperament. *Child Development, 56,* 1314–1326.

Lerner, J. V., & Lerner, R. M. (1994). Explorations of the goodness of fit model in early adolescence. In W. B. Carey & S. C. McDevitt (Eds.), *Individual differences as risk factors for the mental health of children: A Festschrift for Stella Chess and Alexander Thomas* (pp. 161–169). New York: Brunner/Mazel.

Loeber, R. (1990). Development and risk factors for juvenile antisocial behavior and delinquency. *Clinical Psychology Review, 10,* 1–41.

Loeber, R., & Keenan, K. (1994). Interaction between conduct disorder and its comorbid conditions: Effects of age & gender. *Clinical Psychology Review, 14,* 497–523.

Loeber, R., & Stouthamer-Loeber, M. (1986). Family factors as correlates and predictors of juvenile conduct problems and delinquency. In N. Morris & M. Tonry (Eds.), *Crime and justice: An annual review of research* (Vol. 7, pp. 29–149). Chicago: University of Chicago Press.

Loeber, R., Stouthamer-Loeber, M., & Green, S. M. (1991). Age of onset of problem behavior in boys, and later disruptive and delinquent behaviors. *Criminal Behavior and Mental Health, 1,* 229–246.

Lytton, H. (1990). Child and parent effects in boys' conduct disorder: A reinterpretation. *Developmental Psychology, 26,* 683–697.

Martin, R. P., Wisenbaker, J., & Huttenen, M. (1994). Review of factor analytic studies of temperament measures based on the Chess–Thomas structural model: Implications for the Big Five. In C. F. Halverson., G. A. Kohnstamm, & R. P. Martin (Eds.), *The developing structure of temperament and personality from infancy to adulthood* (pp. 157–172). Hillsdale, NJ: Erlbaum.

Matheny, A. P., Jr. (1995, June–July). *Temperamental stability and genetic influences for questionnaires from infancy to 9 years.* Paper presented at the 13th meeting of the International Society for the Study of Behavioral Development, Amsterdam.

Maziade, M. (1989). Should adverse temperament matter to the clinician? An empirically based answer. In G. A. Kohnstamm, J. E. Bates, & M. K. Rothbart (Eds.), *Temperament in childhood* (pp. 421–435). Chichester, England: Wiley.

Maziade, M., Caron, C., Cote, R., Merette, C., Bernier, H., Laplante, B., Boutin, P., & Thivierge, J. (1990). Psychiatric status of adolescents who had extreme temperaments at age seven. *American Journal of Psychiatry, 147,* 1531–1536.

McClowry, S. G., Giangrade, S. K., Tommasini, N. R., Clinton, W., Foreman, N. S., Lynch, K., & Ferketich, S. (1994). The effects of child temperament, maternal characteristics, and family circumstances on the maladjustment of school-age children. *Research in Nursing and Health, 17,* 25–35.

McGee, R., Feehan, M., & Williams, S. (1996). Mental health. In P. A. Silva & W. R. Stanton (Eds.), *From child to adult: The Dunedin Multidisciplinary Health and Development Study* (pp. 150–162). Auckland, New Zealand: Oxford University Press.

Moffitt, T. E. (1990). Juvenile delinquency and attention-deficit disorder: Developmental trajectories from age three to fifteen. *Child Development, 61,* 893–910.

Needham, J. (1973). *Chinese science.* Cambridge, MA: MIT Press.

Olweus, D. (1979). Stability of aggressive reaction patterns in males: A review. *Psychological Bulletin, 86,* 852–875.

Patterson, G. R., Reid, J. B., & Dishion, T. J. (1992). *Antisocial boys.* Eugene, OR: Castalia.

Pedlow, R., Sanson, A. V., Prior, M., & Oberklaid, F. (1993). The stability of maternally reported temperament from infancy to eight years. *Developmental Psychology, 29,* 998–1007.

Prior, M. (1992). Temperament: A review. *Journal of Child Psychology and Psychiatry, 33,* 249–279.

Prior, M., Sanson, A., & Oberklaid, F. (1989). The Australian Temperament Project. In G. A. Kohnstamm, J. E. Bates, & M. K. Rothbart (Eds.), *Temperament in childhood* (pp. 537–554). Chichester, England: Wiley.

Prior, M., Smart, D. F., Sanson, A. V., & Oberklaid, F. (1993). Sex differences in psychological adjustment from infancy to eight years. *Journal of the American Academy of Child and Adolescent Psychiatry, 32,* 291–304.

Prior, M., Sanson, A., Smart, D., & Oberklaid, F. (1997, April). *Longitudinal trajectories in aggressive behavior: Infancy to adolescence.* Paper presented at the Society for Research in Child Development, Washington, DC.

Prior, M., Sanson, A., Smart, D., & Oberklaid, F. (in press). *Psychological disorders and their correlates in an Australian community sample of pre-adolescent children. Journal of Child Psychology and Psychiatry.*

Prior, M., Smart, D., Sanson, A., & Oberklaid, F. (1998). *Longitudinal predictors of behavioural adjustment in pre-adolescent children.* Manuscript submitted for publication.

Pulkkinnen, L. (1987). Offensive and defensive aggression in humans: A longitudinal perspective. *Aggressive Behavior, 13,* 197–212.

Quay, H. C. (1993). The psychobiology of undersocialized aggressive conduct disorder. *Development and Psychopathology, 5,* 165–180.

Rende, R. D. (1993). Longitudinal relations between temperament traits and behavioral syndromes in middle childhood. *Journal of the American Academy of Child and Adolescent Psychiatry, 32,* 287–290.

Richman, N., Stevenson, J., & Graham, P. J. (1982). *From pre-school to school: A behavioral study.* London: Academic Press.

Richters, J. E., & Cicchetti, D. (1993). Mark Twain meets DSM III-R: Conduct disorder, development and the concept of harmful dysfunction [Special Issue: *Towards a developmental perspective on Conduct Disorder,* pp. 5–29]. *Development and Psychopathology, 5.*

Robins, L. N. (1978). Sturdy childhood predictors of adult antisocial behavior: Replications from longitudinal studies. *Psychological Medicine, 8,* 611–622.

Robins, L. N. (1986). Changes in conduct disorder over time. In D. C. Farran & J. D. McKinney (Eds.), *Risk in intellectual and psychosocial development* (pp. 227–259). New York: Academic Press.

Robins, L. N. (1991). Conduct disorder. *Journal of Child Psychology and Psychiatry, 32,* 193–212.

Rothbart, M. K. (1989). Temperament and development. In G. A. Kohnstamm, J. E. Bates & M. K. Rothbart (Eds.), *Temperament in childhood* (pp. 187–248). Chichester, England: Wiley.

Rothbart, M. K., & Bates, J. E. (1998). Temperament. In W. Damon (Ed.), *Handbook of child psychology: Vol. 3. Social, emotional and personality development* (5th ed., pp. 105–176). New York: Wiley.

Rutter, M. (1978). Family, area and school influences in the genesis of conduct disorders. In L. A. Hersov & D. Shaffer (Eds.), *Aggression and antisocial behavior in childhood and adolescence* (pp. 95–114). Oxford, England: Pergamon.

Sameroff, A. J., Seifer, R., Barocas, R., Zax, M., & Greenspan, S. (1987). Intelligence quotient scores of 4-year-old children: Social-environmental risk factors. *Pediatrics, 79,* 343–350.

Sanders, M. (1995). *Healthy families, healthy nation: Strategies for promoting family mental health in Australia.* Brisbane, Australia: Australian Academic Press.

Sanson, A., & Rothbart, M. K. (1995). Child temperament and parenting. In M. Bornstein (Ed.), *Handbook of parenting* (Vol. 4, pp. 299–321). Hillsdale, NJ: Erlbaum.

Sanson, A., Prior, M., & Oberklaid, F. (1985). Normative data on temperament in Australian infants. *Australian Journal of Psychology, 37,* 185–195.

Sanson, A., Prior, M., & Kyrios, M. (1990). Contamination of measures in temperament research. *Merrill-Palmer Quarterly, 36,* 179–192.

Sanson, A., Oberklaid, F., Pedlow, R., & Prior, M. (1991). Risk indicators: Assessment of infancy predictors of preschool behavioural maladjustment. *Journal of Child Psychology and Psychiatry, 32,* 609–626.

Sanson, A., Prior, M., Smart, D., & Oberklaid, F. (1993). Gender differences in aggression in childhood: Implications for a peaceful world. *Australian Psychologist, 28,* 86–92.

Sanson, A., Smart, D., Prior, M., & Oberklaid, F. (1993). Precursors of hyperactivity and aggression. *Journal of the American Academy of Child and Adolescent Psychiatry, 32,* 1207–1216.

Sanson, A., Oberklaid, F., Prior, M., Amos, D., & Smart, D. (1996, August). *Risk factors for 11–12 years olds' internalising and externalising behaviour problems.* Paper presented at the International Society for the Study of Behavioral Development conference, Quebec City, Quebec, Canada.

Sanson, A., Smart, D., Prior, M., Oberklaid, F., & Amos, D. (1996, October). *Temperamental precursors of externalising and internalising behavior problems at 11–12 years.* Paper presented at the 11th Occasional Temperament conference, Eugene, OR.

Scarr, S., & McCartney, K. (1983). How people make their own environments: A theory of genotype–environment effects. *Child Development, 54,* 424–435.

Schwartz, C. E., Snidman, N., & Kagan, J. (1996). Early childhood temperament as a determinant of externalizing behavior in adolescence. *Development and Psychopathology, 8,* 527–537.

Shaw, D. S., & Bell, R. C. (1993). Developmental theories of parental contributions to antisocial behavior. *Journal of Abnormal Child Psychology, 21,* 493–518.

Shaw, D. S., Keenan, K., & Vondra, J. I. (1994). Developmental precursors of externalizing behavior: Ages 1 to 3. *Developmental Psychology, 30,* 355–364.

Slabach, E. H., Morrow, J., & Wachs, T. D. (1991). Questionnaire measurement of infant and child temperament: Current status and future directions. In J. Strelau & A. Angleitner (Eds.), *Explorations in temperament: International perspectives on theory and measurement* (pp. 205–234). New York: Plenum.

Smith, J., & Prior, M. (1995). Temperament and stress resilience in school-age children: A within-families study. *Journal of the American Academy of Child and Adolescent Psychiatry, 34,* 168–179.

Strelau, J. (1983). *Temperament personality activity.* New York: Academic Press.

Teglasi, H., & McMahon, B. V. (1990). Temperament and common problem behaviors of children. *Journal of Applied Developmental Psychology, 11,* 331–349.

Thomas, A., & Chess, S. (1977). *Temperament and development.* New York: Brunner/Mazel.

Thomas, A., Chess, S., Birch, H. G., Hertzig, M. E., & Korn, S. (1963). *Behavioral individuality in early childhood.* New York: New York University Press.

Thomas, A., Chess, S., & Birch, H. G. (1968). *Temperament and behavior disorders in children.* New York: New York University Press.

Tremblay, R. E. (1992). The prediction of delinquent behavior from childhood behavior: Personality theory revisited. In J. McCord (Ed.), *Facts, frameworks and forecasts* (pp. 193–230). New Brunswick, NY: Transaction.

Tremblay, R. E., Pihl, R. O., Vitaro, F., & Dobkin, P. L. (1994). Predicting early onset of male antisocial behavior from preschool behavior. *Archives of General Psychiatry, 51,* 732–739.

Werner, E. E., & Smith, R. S. (1982). *Vulnerable but invincible: A study of resilient children.* New York: McGraw-Hill.

Wertlieb, D., Weigel, C., Springer, T., & Feldstein, M. (1987). Temperament as a moderator of children's stressful experiences. *American Journal of Orthopsychiatry, 57,* 234–245.

West, D. J., & Farrington, D. P. (1973). *Who becomes delinquent?* London: Heinemann.

White, J., Moffitt, T. E., Earls, F., Robins, L. N., & Silva, P. A. (1990). How early can we tell? Predictors of childhood conduct disorder and adolescent delinquency. *Criminology, 28,* 507–533.

Zahn-Waxler, C. (1993). Warriors and worriers: Gender and psychopathology. *Development and Psychopathology, 5,* 79–89.

Zoccolillo, M. (1993). Gender and the development of conduct disorder. *Development and Psychopathology, 5,* 65–78.

19

Environmental Risk Factors in Oppositional-Defiant Disorder and Conduct Disorder

ROB McGEE and SHEILA WILLIAMS

INTRODUCTION

More than 10 years ago, Farrington (1986) concluded his review of the sociocultural context of childhood disorders by stating that there was a clear correlation between the sociocultural environment in which children are raised and antisocial behavior such as delinquency and Conduct Disorder (CD). Farrington focused on social class, ethnic background, the peer group, and the neighborhood, but other social and familial factors might equally have been included. Many if not most psychosocial environmental risk factors for antisocial behavior have been identified for some time. As Farrington pointed out, what remains to be described are the causal relationships among these risk factors and outcomes to address the question "What leads to what?" This endeavor is no less relevant today.

This chapter reviews the recent literature on psychosocial environmental risk factors for CD and Oppositional Defiant Disorder (ODD). Several fine reviews already exist detailing as-

pects of risk factors for CD, delinquency, and antisocial behavior (e.g., Loeber & Hay, 1997; Rothbaum & Weisz, 1994). In this chapter, then, we have tried to avoid going over ground covered elsewhere. Rather, we hope to illustrate the directions in which research on risk factors for CD/ODD has been going, and future directions that such research might profitably take. The answer to questions concerning which risk factors lead to which particular outcome will come best from longitudinal studies where it is known that the risk in question precedes the outcome (Kraemer et al., 1997). Interventions to modify risk factors provide another way of addressing this question and these are discussed elsewhere in this handbook. In this chapter, therefore, emphasis will be placed on findings of longitudinal research; indeed, models of risk are inherently longitudinal. The chapter begins with a brief overview of measurement issues relating to the identification of environmental risk factors, followed by a discussion of more general models of environmental risk. Here we present some findings from a reanalysis of data on environmental risk factors for CD/ODD from the Dunedin Multidisciplinary Health and Development Study (DMHDS) to inform the direction such models might profitably move, at least at the individual level. The subtyping CD and the relationship between CD

ROB McGEE and SHEILA WILLIAMS • Department of Preventive and Social Medicine, University of Otago Medical School, Dunedin, New Zealand.

Handbook of Disruptive Behavior Disorders, edited by Quay and Hogan. Kluwer Academic/Plenum Publishers, New York, 1999.

and ODD are discussed next, with an emphasis on identifying possible risk factors that might move individuals along particular developmental paths. The remainder of the chapter examines environmental risk factors at different levels of analysis, from the family to the neighborhood and to the community or societal level. The main theme arising from this discussion is the future challenge provided in attempting to integrate analyses of antisocial behavior across these domains.

MEASUREMENT MODELS OF CD/ODD AND ENVIRONMENTAL RISK

The identification of environmental risk factors for CD/ODD, at least in part, is dependent on the measurement models used to identify disorder. Risk factors might differ according to the nature of the informant, whether CD and ODD are conceptualized as categorical or dimensional in nature, and the degree of comorbidity between these and other disorders; in this section we briefly discuss approaches to addressing these issues. Although information is often obtained from multiple informants, there does not appear to be any clear consensus on how best to represent this information as outcomes in models of CD and ODD. Typically, information obtained from different sources is not highly correlated, so that risk factors identified using separate analyses by informant may well differ. For example, Offord, Boyle, and Racine (1989) reported that family dysfunction, parental mental health (for boys), parent arrest, and the child's chronic medical illness predicted CD identified by parent report; in contrast, of these four variables only family dysfunction predicted CD identified by teacher or youth self-report. Pooling of information from different sources is common (we have been guilty of this in the past) but doing so potentially ignores situationally specific risk factors. A recent approach to this problem was reported by Fitzmaurice, Laird, Zahner, and Daskalakis (1995) who proposed testing simultaneous logistic regressions in a single

analysis for categorical outcomes using multiple informants. An advantage of this approach is the identification of risk factor effects common to informants as well as risk factor–informant interactions. The authors tested their model on parent and teacher reports of externalizing and internalizing behavior problems from two large mental health surveys of 6- to 11-year-olds in Connecticut. Common environmental factors for parent and teacher externalizing reports included effects for social class and family stress. Area of residence showed an effect for teacher but not for parent report but maternal distress showed an effect for parent report only. This form of analysis has the advantage of examining the extent to which risk factors and outcomes vary among informants.

Dimensional approaches to the measurement of antisocial behavior are largely concerned with identifying what holds for the majority and are the preserve of those interested mainly in antisocial behavior as a broad spectrum within the community. Categorical approaches, on the other hand, reflect a concern with what is happening at the extremes of the distribution and are the preserve of those primarily interested in clinical models of CD/ODD. As noted in Chapter 1 (this volume), Fergusson and Horwood (1995) examined this question from the basis of the predictive validity of the categorical and dimensional positions. CD and ODD symptom scores, together with respective DSM-III-R diagnoses based on the same data, were formed for self- and parent report at age 15. The dimensional and categorical approaches were used to predict related adverse outcomes 1 year later; these included smoking, alcohol problems, cannabis use, criminal offending, and early school leaving. The findings showed strong evidence for linear dose–response relations between the dimensional measures and each outcome. Furthermore, in all cases, dimensions were more strongly predictive of outcome than categories. It is likely that because of the increased variability associated with dimensions as opposed to categories a similar finding would hold for the relationships between disruptive disorder outcomes and sources of environmental risk.

The past 10 years of psychiatric epidemiological research have shown the extent to which different disorders coexist in the same individuals (see Chapter 2, this volume). Comorbidity has important implications when identifying environmental risk factors. Epidemiological research has shown that CD and ODD are frequently comorbid with ADHD, anxiety, and affective disorders particularly in early childhood and preadolescence (McConaughy & Achenbach, 1994). More recently, we have argued that comorbidity needs to be considered from a developmental perspective to account for the significant shifts in comorbidity from childhood to adulthood (McGee & Williams, 1997). The implication of comorbidities for studies of risk factors for CD/ODD, particularly in the preadolescent years, is for the identification of unique risk factors. Fergusson, Lynskey, and Horwood (1996), for example, have shown that the risk factors that increase the adolescent's vulnerability to CD overlap substantially with those that increase vulnerability to depression. Common environmental risk factors included troubled parent–child relationships, family conflict, and parental criminal offending; these common causal factors explained a substantial amount of the shared variance between the two types of disorder. In the past, analyses have proceeded on a disorder by disorder basis; the nature of comorbidity forces researchers to identify both common and unique predictors for CD/ODD.

MODELS OF ENVIRONMENTAL RISK FACTORS FOR CD/ODD

Farrington and Loeber (in press) described the key risk factors experienced during childhood (ages 8–10 years) that predict court appearances for delinquency over the ensuing 7 years in two large longitudinal studies, the Cambridge Study in Delinquent Development and the Pittsburgh Youth study. They identified factors associated with socioeconomic disadvantage (e.g., low SES, mother as single parent), parental background (e.g., parental mental health, criminality) and child-rearing

(e.g., parental conflict, poor supervision) as showing consistent predictive relationships with later appearance in juvenile court for delinquency. By and large, the factors identified from these two longitudinal studies agree with those identified in psychiatric epidemiological studies as being associated with CD and to a lesser extent ODD. These studies include the Isle of Wight (Rutter, 1989) and Inner London studies (Rutter, Cox, Tupling, Berger, & Yule, 1975); the Newcastle Thousand Family study (Kolvin, Miller, Fleeting, & Kolvin, 1988); the Ontario Child Health study (Offord et al., 1989); the New York Child Longitudinal study (Velez, Johnson, & Cohen, 1989); the Puerto Rican Child study (Bird, Gould, Yager, Staghezza, & Canino, 1989); the Pittsburgh Health Maintenance Study (Costello, 1989); the Christchurch Child Development Study (Fergusson, Horwood, & Lynskey, 1994); and the DMHDS (McGee, Feehan, & Williams, 1996). The findings reflect consistency across place and time. Characteristics of the child's immediate environment reflecting socioeconomic disadvantage, poor family climate, and troubled parent–child interaction have been found to be associated with CD and ODD.

In Table 1, following Farrington and Loeber (in press), we have used data ($N = 927$) from the DMHDS to illustrate the strength of the relationship between some of these characteristics of the social environment identified during the early school years (ages 3–9 years) and receiving a diagnosis of CD, ODD, or some other disorder at some time from preadolescence to adolescence (ages 11–15 years). Identification of disorder was based on confirmation by at least two informant sources (typically the child self-report with confirmation by parent or teacher report) at ages 11, 13, or 15 years (McGee et al., 1996). The category of "Other" disorder was included to show the extent to which these factors might represent unique predictors of CD and ODD, or predictors of disorders in general. For the most part, this category represents those with anxiety or depressive disorders or both. By combining these ages, 75 sample members were identified with CD representing 8.1% of the sample, 23 with

TABLE 1.   Environmental Predictors (Ages 3–9 Years) of CD, ODD, and Other Disorders (Ages 11–15 Years) in the DMHDS

Predictor	CD (N = 75)	ODD (N = 23)	Other (N = 87)
Socioeconomic disadvantage			
low SES	1.8 (1.0–3.1)[a]	1.4 (0.5–3.7)	1.5 (0.9–2.5)
baby < 21 years	1.8 (1.1–2.9)[a]	0.8 (0.3–2.1)	1.1 (0.7–1.8)
lower maternal education	2.8 (1.5–5.1)[a]	2.3 (0.8–6.2)	1.2 (0.7–1.8)
solo parent	3.2 (1.7–5.8)[a]	1.1 (0.2–4.6)	2.1 (1.1–3.9)[a]
Family climate			
parental separation	2.3 (1.3–4.0)[a]	1.4 (0.5–4.1)	1.9 (1.1–3.2)[a]
low intrafamily social support	1.7 (1.0–2.9)[a]	2.4 (1.0–5.7)[a]	1.2 (0.7–2.0)
maternal depression	2.9 (1.7–5.0)[a]	1.5 (0.5–4.4)	2.8 (1.7–4.7)[a]
Parent–child interaction			
maternal rejection	1.3 (0.6–2.6)	2.3 (0.8–6.3)	1.2 (0.6–2.4)
low egalitarianism	1.4 (0.7–2.5)	2.9 (1.2–7.0)[a]	0.8 (0.4–1.5)
high authoritarianism	2.2 (1.3–3.7)[a]	0.6 (0.2–2.2)	1.2 (0.7–2.0)
lax-inconsistent discipline	1.9 (0.9–4.0)	3.3 (1.2–9.1)[a]	1.5 (0.7–3.1)

Figures shown are Odds Ratios and 95% confidence intervals.
[a]OR significant, $p < 0.05$.

ODD (2.5%), and 87 with Other disorders (9.4%). There were slightly more males in the three groups with disorder, but the gender differences were not significant. If an individual had ODD at one age and CD at another, they were placed in the CD group; some of those with CD/ODD had other comorbid disorders, so these are not pure diagnostic categories. The variables representing the child's social environment were chosen on the basis of the previous literature and experience from the DMHDS.

The findings in Table 1 are shown as odds ratios (OR) adjusted for gender, and were estimated using the STATA procedure mlogit for multiple logistic regression (StataCorp, 1997). The OR is a measure of association that can be interpreted as how much more likely an outcome is to be present among those having a particular risk factor in comparison with those not having that risk factor. For example, Table 1 indicates that those children experiencing low SES were nearly twice as likely (OR = 1.8) to be identified with later CD than those children from higher SES backgrounds; single parenting was associated with a greater than

threefold increase in the later risk of CD (OR = 3.2). The interactions between gender and risk factor were not significant, indicating associations between specific risk factors and outcome to be similar for boys and girls. Inspection of the patterns of findings suggests that a wider variety of environmental risk factors were predictive of CD than was the case with ODD or Other disorder. ODD in the absence of CD was significantly associated with few sources of environmental risk and with different sources of risk, although this may partially reflect the fewer cases of ODD in the sample and consequent lower power to detect associations. Other disorder was similar to CD in the significance of single parenting, parental separations, and maternal depression. This analysis relies on a univariate approach to the relationship between risk factors and outcome but it is now clear that such risk factors should not be considered in isolation. Rather, complex patterns among various forms of risk are causally related to childhood and adolescent psychopathology. Such a view includes notions of family adversity (Rutter, 1978) and cumulative risk (Cichetti, 1994). Also implicit in these models is the idea that the number of risk factors may assert a more important influence on child development than the exact nature of the risk factors, and that risk factors operating in isolation may not be as important as the cumulative effect of risk.

To illustrate these ideas, the risk factors identified in Table 1 have been grouped into domains of risk following the approach of Farrington and Loeber (in press) to represent socioeconomic disadvantage, family climate, and parent–child interaction. By summing the number of adverse factors in each block experienced by the child it was possible to look at the association between cumulative environmental risk within a domain and later adverse outcome in the preadolescent to adolescent years. Table 2 shows the association between each domain of risk and type of disorder; OR are shown both unadjusted and adjusted for the other domains of risk. Further modeling of the data indicated that different domains were associated with different patterns of disorder. Family climate was a significant predictor of all three types of disorder, suggesting that it may operate as a rather general risk factor for psychopathology. The domain of parent–child interaction was predictive of both CD and ODD, suggesting that it may operate as a general risk factor for disruptive and antisocial behavior. Socioeconomic disadvantage, on the other hand, was particularly predictive of CD. This model also suggests that

the association between socioeconomic disadvantage and CD is not entirely mediated by effects associated with either family climate or parent–child interaction, at least as measured in the Dunedin study. A further finding of interest was that summing across all three domains to produce a single index of risk actually led to less predictive power in the model. This suggests that these three domains of risk represented a more powerful description of the child's early environment than did a global index.

A related issue in modeling environmental risk concerns the extent to which environmental risk factors might enhance or attenuate the effects of other sources of risk; in other words, developing models that acknowledge multiple and possibly interacting sources of risk. As Cichetti (1994) argued, "it is likely that a multitude of rather general factors across the broad domains of biology, psychology and sociology will be at least indirectly related to psychopathological outcomes, such as conduct disorder, because they represent the gamut of potential determinants of individual adaptation" (p. 292). In a similar vein, Campbell (1990) proposed that "some combination of child characteristics and parenting behaviors are seen as the primary determinants of problem outcomes, with family and social context effects exacerbating and/or maintaining them" (p. 24). Both writers reflect a general view that there are multiple paths to disorder, resulting

TABLE 2. Domains of Environmental Risk (Ages 3–9 Years) and CD, ODD, and Other Disorders (Ages 11–15 Years) in the DMHDS

Predictor	CD (N = 75)	ODD (N = 23)	Other (N = 87)
Socioeconomic disadvantage			
Unadjusted OR	1.81	1.18	1.24
Adjusted OR[a]	1.52 (1.17–1.99)	0.99 (0.62–1.59)	1.09 (0.86–1.40)
Family climate			
Unadjusted OR	1.97	1.58	1.67
Adjusted OR	1.53 (1.10–2.12)	1.47 (0.82–2.64)	1.60 (1.18–2.17)
Parent–child interaction			
Unadjusted OR	1.61	1.69	1.12
Adjusted OR	1.37 (1.01–1.85)	1.61 (0.98–2.63)	1.03 (0.76–1.40)

[a]Adjusted odds ratio (OR) refers to OR and 95% confidence interval adjusted for other risk domains in the model.

from various additive and possibly interactive effects among risk factors both in the same developmental domain and between domains. At the same time, sources of resilience or protection residing in the child and his or her environment may operate to counterbalance risk.

An early example of a developmental model of the effects of different domains of risk comes from the Kauai longitudinal study, in which Werner and Smith (1979) found evidence for an interaction between early biological stress and early family instability. Biological vulnerability in the form of perinatal stress placed the child at risk of adverse mental health outcomes only in the presence of environmental risk. This finding was partially replicated in the DMHDS where the risk of showing significant problem behavior during the early school years, associated with being small for gestational age, was higher among such children from adverse family backgrounds compared with those children who were similarly small for gestational age, but who came from more advantaged backgrounds (McGee, Silva, & Williams, 1984). Similarly, Raine, Breenan, and Mednick (1994) examined evidence for an interaction between biological and environmental risk in explaining violent behavior. They found a significant interaction between birth complications and early child rejection, and violent criminal offending among 17- to 19-year-old males in a longitudinal cohort born in Denmark. Among those young men with both of these risk factors, nearly 10% had committed violent crimes compared with about 3% of those men with one or no risk factors. This interaction was not observed for nonviolent offending. Furthermore, it was specific to early parental rejection; poor social circumstances, while predicting later offending, did not interact with perinatal risk. Nevertheless, it should be noted that 90% of men experiencing both biological risk and parental rejection had not committed violent offenses, suggesting that the combination of risk factors for most men was offset by other constitutional, developmental, or experiential factors.

The idea of individual vulnerabilities colliding with psychosocial circumstances to

heighten risk of CD and ODD has been applied similarly to the combined effects of individual temperament and parental separation (Kasen, Cohen, Brook, & Hartmark, 1996). In a longitudinal study of families studied pre- and postdivorce, it was found that while temperament variables directly predicted later antisocial behavior, these effects were moderated by the characteristics of the family after the divorce. Thus, among youth initially high on immaturity, those in stepfamilies postdivorce had over twice the risk of ODD compared with those in intact or single-mother families. Similarly, those with affective problems predivorce were at higher risk of ODD if they were in stepfamilies later. Among the boys, the combination of predivorce immaturity and later stepfamily was strongly predictive of CD. These findings suggest that pathways to antisocial behavior reflect combinations of sources of risk or resilience, with environmental risk factors enhancing or attenuating preexisting vulnerabilities.

SUBTYPES OF CD AND ENVIRONMENTAL RISK

As discussed in Chapter 1 (this volume), much research effort continues to be expended in developing valid subtypes of antisocial behavior. What are the implications of subtyping for the identification of environmental risk factors? We begin with Moffitt's (1993) proposed distinction between two types of delinquency. The first, called "life course persistent," is identified with that small group of males who show early onset of antisocial behavior that continues into adolescence and adulthood. In the DMHDS, for example, Moffitt and Harrington (1996) identified 7% of boys at age 15 who showed a history of aggressive, hyperactive, impulsive, and inattentive behavior dating from their preschool years. In contrast, "adolescence-limited" delinquency reflects antisocial behavior showing onset in adolescence and it is also relatively common; in the Dunedin study, 36% of boys showed this pattern of rapid-onset delinquency from age 11 to 13 years. As a group, these boys showed no history of antisocial behavior before that age. This pattern of late onset is predominant among girls with antisocial behavior in adolescence. Mc-Gee, Feehan, Williams, and Anderson (1992) reported a marked increase in nonaggressive (late-onset) CD among both sexes but particularly among girls at age 15 compared with age 11; the prevalence of aggressive (early-onset) CD showed no such change over time.

The distinction between these two subtypes appears to be a useful one. There has long been a clear distinction between aggressive and nonaggressive types of CD. Similarly, age of onset has been identified as an important predictor of later outcome. Moffitt's subtyping captures both of these dimensions in describing the development of antisocial behavior. The distinction may also be important in identifying environmental risk factors. In the Dunedin study, boys showing life-course persistent antisocial behaviors tended to come from adverse family backgrounds characterized by conflict and lower SES in childhood; boys with later onset did not show the same early background adversity. Other research has suggested that psychosocial environmental factors such as SES, parental unemployment, family functioning, and parental separations best predict early-rather than late-onset delinquency (Capaldi & Patterson, 1994; Tolan, 1987), but tend not to discriminate to the same extent between aggressive and nonaggressive offending (Farrington, 1978; Henry, Caspi, Moffitt, & Silva, 1996). Henry and colleagues proposed that family instability as indicated by a childhood history of parental separations, single parenting, and frequent changes in residence acts as a general risk factor for both types of offending. It is the combination of individual temperament factors such as lack of control and family instability that best predicts early onset of frequent violent offending. However, it is clear that not all aggression later in life is committed by those who were aggressive earlier in life, so that the distinction between life-course persistent and adolescence-limited antisocial behavior is not synonymous with the distinction between aggressive and nonaggressive behavior (Loeber & Hay, 1997).

What of the distinction between ODD and CD? Table 1 indicates that a small proportion of children show later ODD that does not seem to have progressed to CD. While undoubtedly a problem for the relationships between the individual and other adults, ODD in adolescence does not place the individual at risk for later disorder in early adulthood (Feehan, McGee, & Williams, 1994). The significance of ODD perhaps more clearly is as a childhood risk factor for later disorder in adolescence. In examining early oppositional behavior for this chapter, we used combined parent and teacher ratings of disobedience and irritability at ages 5 and 7 years to identify those children with persistently high levels of oppositional behavior. The latter were at higher risk of CD (OR = 3.6; 95% CI: 2.1–6.1), ODD (OR = 3.9; 95% CI: 1.6–9.4) and other disorder (OR = 2.4; 95% CI: 1.4–4.0), suggesting that early oppositional behavior acts as a general risk factor for later psychiatric disorder. In contrast, high levels of antisocial behavior appearing from 5 to 7 years (parent and teacher ratings of destructiveness, fighting, lying, and bullying) predicted only later CD (OR = 2.9; 95% CI: 1.7–4.9), not later ODD or Other disorder. Modeling of early oppositional and antisocial behavior indicated that their effects were additive; children who showed high levels of both from 5 to 7 years were at high risk of later CD (OR = 10.4).

Are there environmental risk factors that might enhance the progression from ODD to CD? Biederman and colleagues (1996) partially addressed this question in a longitudinal study of progression from ODD to CD among children with ADHD. Nearly all those with CD had comorbid ODD, with ODD preceding CD by several years. Sociodemographic characteristics did not discriminate between children with ODD who progressed to CD and those with ODD who did not progress, although there was an increased risk of familial antisocial disorders among the former group. This finding should be treated with some caution, however, as all the children had comorbid ADHD.

Table 1 and accompanying analyses suggest that there are differences primarily relating

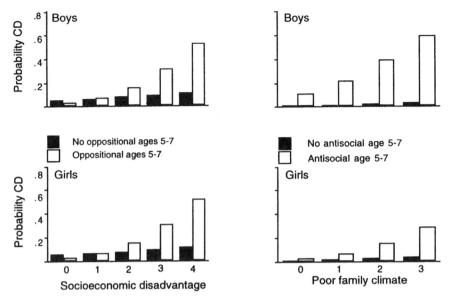

FIGURE 1. Interactions between domains of socioeconomic disadvantage and family climate, and early oppositional and antisocial behavior. Upper graphs show findings for boys.

to socioeconomic disadvantage between CD and ODD that does not progress to CD. We addressed this question of the effects of environmental risk on the progression of early behavior to later CD with the data from the DMHDS. Using the oppositional and antisocial behavior ratings from 5 to 7 years, we examined whether the predictive significance of these varied across levels of socioeconomic disadvantage, family climate, or parent–child interaction. Models that included interaction effects between these domains of variables were considered. Significant interaction effects were found for early oppositional behavior and socioeconomic disadvantage, and for early antisocial behavior and family climate. Neither of the interaction effects between early behavior and parent–child interaction was significant. The nature of these significant interactions are shown in Figure 1; these findings are shown separately for boys and girls. The figure shows the probability of developing CD across the four levels of socioeconomic disadvantage for those with and without early oppositional behavior. There was no predictive association between socioeconomic disadvantage and later CD in the absence of oppositional behavior from 5 to 7 years. For

children showing such behavior, increasing levels of disadvantage increased the probability of later CD. In contrast, the effects of family climate were related to early antisocial behavior. Again, family climate appeared to have no predictive significance for later CD in the absence of early antisocial behavior. When antisocial behavior was present, increasing levels of poor family climate predicted increased probability of later CD. Overall, these results suggest that different domains of disadvantage interact with different early behaviors to predict later CD. Environmental risk appears to hasten the progression from early oppositional and antisocial behavior to CD; by itself, such risk does not predict the development of the disorder.

ENVIRONMENTAL RISK FACTORS AT THE FAMILY LEVEL

In the following sections we examine recent developments in research involving selected environmental risk factors for CD/ODD. These particular risk factors have been chosen on the basis of the literature; they represent those factors frequently identified and studied or factors beginning to assume some importance in the etiology of antisocial disorders. We begin with risk factors identified at the family level and then discuss risk factors at the neighborhood or community level. We finish with a discussion of changes in risk factors at the societal level and how these might account for changes in levels of antisocial behaviors over time.

Socioeconomic Disadvantage

As noted, previous evidence from epidemiological studies suggests an association between indicators of socioeconomic disadvantage and both CD and ODD, although our findings from the DMHDS indicate that this association is more evident in the case of CD. More recent longitudinal studies have continued to identify socioeconomic disadvantage experienced during childhood as a risk factor for antisocial behavior in adolescence (Kratzer & Hodgins, 1997) and in early adulthood (Pakiz, Reinherz, & Giaconia, 1997). Perhaps this is not surprising given the consistent patterning of various health indicators by social position (Adler *et al.,* 1994). Some recent evidence, however, suggests that the mental health inequalities associated with socioeconomic disadvantage are not invariant over the life course. Modeling mental health data from the DMHDS from childhood to early adulthood indicates that the effects of early disadvantage are evident in childhood but disappear in adolescence only to reappear in early adulthood (Feehan, McGee, Williams, & Nada-Raja, 1995). Reappearance in early adulthood constitutes a direct effect of early childhood disadvantage on adult mental health, independent of intervening mental health and adolescent-to-adult transition events. Others have argued that variables such as social class are antecedents of antisocial behavior in childhood and it is this early antisocial behavior that places the individual at risk of future delinquent behavior; social class per se is not directly related to later delinquency in adolescence (Roff & Wirt, 1984). This is consistent with age-specific associations between low income and CD reported in other epidemiological studies (e.g., Offord *et al.,* 1989) and

with the distinction made between life-course persistent and adolescent-limited delinquency. It should be recognised, however, that this patterning of effects associated with social disadvantage across developmental stages is not limited to antisocial behavior; it is also apparent in medical mortality, acute and chronic illness, and injury (West, 1997). The effects of socioeconomic disadvantage on the lives of children are particularly salient; youth is characterized by relative equality in physical and mental health. This relative equality in health may occur when age-based experiences such as social mixing, coupled with the increasing influence of the high school, peer group, and youth culture, may attenuate the effects of disadvantage (West, 1997). Reemergence of childhood disadvantage as a risk factor for disorder in early adulthood, as observed in the DMHDS, may reflect effects of early disadvantage on aspects of the transition from education to work, and family life to life outside the family, limiting rather than enhancing opportunities in these domains.

A second feature of socioeconomic deprivation and poverty as environmental risk factors for CD/ODD concerns the "snow-balling" nature of such disadvantage. From a longitudinal perspective, the cumulative nature of risk suggests that earlier exposure to risk increases the chance of exposure to later risk factors. In a study of the mothers of the children in the DMHDS, Williams, McGee, Olaman, and Knight (1997) found that a pattern of being young at the birth of their first child and having poor educational achievement placed these women and their children in an ongoing pattern of deprivation and disadvantage. The two factors of early childbirth and poor education appeared to operate in an additive fashion. Women with both of these risk factors experienced higher levels of chronic depression over a 20-year follow-up period. Their families were more likely to experience socioeconomic disadvantage, high conflict, and family breakup, all risk factors for CD as shown in Table 1. Unfortunately, we do not know to what extent childhood and adolescent psychopathology among these women contributed to their low educational attainment and early pregnancy in the first place. However, data from their daughters suggest that adolescent disorder does predict low educational achievement, leaving home early, and acquiring a family role at an earlier age among young women (Feehan *et al.*, 1995).

McLeod and Shanahan (1996) have used data from the National Longitudinal Studies of Youth to examine the dynamic relationship between children's experience of poverty and developmental trajectories for antisocial behavior and depression. The children were aged 4 to 5 years at study outset, and were followed up at 6–7 and 8–9 years of age. The findings differed for the two mental health outcomes. Early experience of poverty predicted ongoing depression in the children, irrespective of subsequent poverty experiences. By contrast, subsequent poverty experience influenced the child's trajectory for antisocial behavior. Children experiencing unremitting poverty showed higher rates of increase in antisocial behavior over time than did other children. The authors speculated that the latter finding might be attributable to any number of factors: Persistent poverty places greater stresses on the parents, interfering with their parenting skills; it may expose the children to unsafe or unhealthy environments; it may limit access to health care for the child and thereby increase the impact of ill health on school performance. Unremitting poverty might also reflect parental psychopathology and poorer educational or cognitive skills, which would interfere with the child's development. The interest in this study lies in the application of a life-course perspective to the study of the dynamic relationship between disadvantage and antisocial outcome.

Family Climate

Parental Discord and Separation

In their review of evidence for an association between marital conflict and child adjustment, Davies and Cummings (1994) proposed that marital conflict has the frequent effect of undermining the child's sense of emotional security. The most salient immediate reaction to such conflict is emotional distress, but in the longer term, repeated exposure also leads to anger and aggression; CD is clearly more common in families where there is marital discord (see Chapter 15, this volume). Temperament and family conflict may also interact to enhance levels of externalizing behaviors (Tschann, Kaiser, Chesney, Alkno, & Boyce, 1996; see also Chapter 18, this volume); as noted in Figure 1, the predictive significance of antisocial behavior at age of school entry for later CD was markedly enhanced by increasing levels of poorer family climate. The breakdown of their parents' relationship may be one of the most catastrophic events children will experience, and such breakdowns are common. In the DMHDS, for example, 35% of children had experienced parental separation by age 15 years, half of them by early adolescence. Separations between the child's parents can lead to the disruption of the emotional bonds that form the basis of a secure attachment to the parents, thereby increasing the child's vulnerability to disorder. This may be particularly so for early separations. Woodward, Belsky, McGee, and Nada-Raja (1997) examined the effects of timing of parental separations on attachment to parents in adolescence. Using data from the DMHDS, these authors found that separations during the preschool years, compared with those in middle childhood or adolescence, were most strongly associated with the adolescents' poorer perceived attachment to parents. This effect was not observed for attachment to peers.

Epidemiological evidence shows a clear association between parental separation and CD/ODD. What is the nature of this association? Rutter (1971) mapped out the future research terrain in this area through a series of elegant analyses from the Isle of Wight and other studies. He concluded that the separation itself is of little direct consequence for the development of antisocial disorder in later life. Of more importance was the social and psychological context in which separations occurred. This proposal has been examined in other longitudinal cohorts. For example, Cherlin and colleagues (1991) examined longitudinal data from the National Child Development Study in the United Kingdom and the National Survey of Children in the United States. By adjusting for preexisting differences in behavior between children from divorced and intact families, much of the effect of divorce on subsequent behavior was attenuated. The implication of these findings is that antisocial problems precede the separation and presumably reflect the child's experience of living in a poorly functioning family characterized by protracted marital conflict. However, not all recent longitudinal studies have found these preseparation behavioral difficulties among children (Kasen *et al.*, 1996; Shaw, Emery, & Tuer, 1993).

What of the consequences of separation? In the DMHDS, after separations 90% of children remained in the custody of the mother. As younger maternal age and less education are more often associated with later separation (Williams *et al.*, 1997), there is a worsening pattern of ongoing hardship for those families with children. For example, a study of Family Court clients in New Zealand showed that separation improved the income of most men but decreased the income for most women with many moving onto social welfare (Maxwell & Robertson, 1993). Psychological morale among the women was low, and many had fears for their own and their children's safety.

Many such women will also face the prospect of raising their children alone. The father's absence appears to increase the levels of antisocial behavior postseparation and these effects of single parenting seem particularly powerful for younger boys. In a longitudinal study of boys and girls from the 4th grade (U.S.), those boys living in single-mother families were over four times more likely to receive teacher reports of high levels of aggressiveness 2 years later, than boys from mother–partner families (Vaden-Kiernan, Ialongo, Pearson, & Kellam, 1995). At least part of this may derive from an overall pattern of ambivalence in the mother–son interaction. For example, in Hetherington's (1990) study of children of divorce, among those women

who remained single, interactions in the family were characterized by mothers feeling less attached or close to their sons and spending less time with them. Added to this were problems with control and coercion, with the boys becoming more independent and disengaging from the family. Nevertheless, there may well be direct effects associated with family structure that are independent of parental attachment and family stress and conflict, perhaps deriving from father absence and absence of role modeling (Paschall, Ennett, & Flewelling, 1996). In any new relationship the woman enters, stepfathers are more likely to have a disengaged style of parenting with low involvement, warmth, and supervision of the child, a pattern of parenting found among fathers predivorce (Block, Block, & Gjerde, 1988) and once again increasing the risk of CD among boys (Kasen *et al.*, 1996).

Violence between Parents

Witnessing physical violence between parents is a relatively common experience for children. Estimates suggest that anywhere from 1 in 10 to 1 in 5 children witness such aggression, and they generally witness frequent acts of aggression (Henning, Leitenberg, Coffey, Bennett, & Jankowski, 1997). Are children who witness such violence at higher risk for later antisocial behavior? The answer to that question is complicated by the fact that domestic violence often occurs in a context of poverty and disadvantage, of ongoing marital conflict, abuse, threat, and divorce, parental alcoholism or other drug dependence, and, in many instances, physical abuse of the children themselves. Children under the age of 5 seem to be at higher risk of witnessing such violence, and particularly multiple episodes of violence (Fantuzzo, Boruch, Beriama, Atkins, & Marcus, 1997; Henning *et al.*, 1997). Analysis of the potential effects of witnessing violence, then, involves teasing out such effects from the context in which they occur. As yet, prospective follow-up studies of representative samples of children witnessing violence have not appeared in the literature. What evidence there is derives from retrospective reports from adult samples (e.g., Henning *et al.*, 1997) or accounts usually obtained in refuges, from women who have endured aggression, about their children's experiences (Kolbo, Blakely, & Engleman, 1996).

In their review of the evidence from these studies, Kolbo and colleagues (1996) concluded that the findings provide some support for an association between witnessing violence and children's externalizing and internalizing behavior, particularly the findings of more recent research. The fact that witnessing violence appears to be associated with both types of behavior problems is consistent with our notion that family climate variables act as general risk factors for psychopathology. Typically, these studies have used measures of externalizing behaviors from checklists. At the same time, witnessing violence was associated with poorer social competence, school failure, and poorer language and cognitive functioning, all of which in turn might place the child at higher risk of later antisocial behavior. It is difficult to assess, however, to what extent these differences are a function of witnessing violence per se or other uncontrolled factors. In a retrospective study of young adults who had witnessed parental violence as children, Henning and colleagues (1997) reported higher externalizing as well as internalizing behavior problems among the 14% of young men and women who had witnessed at least one episode of physical aggression. Some, but not all, of the observed relationship was accounted for by background factors and, in particular, parental alcoholism and physical abuse as a child. This suggests that the effect of witnessing violence is not simply an artifact of other concurrent risk factors. There was no evidence for a dose–response relationship between frequency and severity of the observed violence and externalizing behavior, but witnessing violence toward the same-sex parent was associated with higher problem scores. Parental violence was associated with a perception of less parental caring and warmth in childhood, and this in turn explained most of the relationship between violence and exter-

nalizing behavior. Nevertheless, a small direct effect of witnessing violence was still observed.

Parent–Child Interaction

Parental Warmth and Restrictiveness

In an extensive review of the associations between parental caregiving characteristics and externalizing behavior, Rothbaum and Weisz (1994) identified six key variables that pervade the literature. These characteristics include parental approval, guidance, positive motivation, synchrony (perhaps best captured by the notions of availability for and involvement with the child), coercive control, and restrictiveness. At a higher-order level, these individual variables appear to reflect orthogonal dimensions of acceptance-responsiveness (warmth) and restrictiveness. Meta-analyses by these authors indicated that both individual variables and higher-order factors are associated with externalizing behavior, with the strength of association being particularly strong for patterns of caring involving aggregate dimensions. Associations were stronger for children who were older and male, with a critical shift occurring around the time of school entry. In Chapter 15 (this volume), Carlson, Tamm, and Hogan also conclude that the parent–child interactions of children with CD can be characterized as aversive, less warm, more disapproving, and showing more efforts at restrictive parental control. Finally, our composite measure of parent–child interaction during early childhood in the DMHDS predicted later CD and ODD.

Much of the available data come from cross-sectional studies; longitudinal research investigating the critical dimensions of parental responsiveness and restrictiveness is needed (Rothbaum & Weisz, 1994). Recent longitudinal studies have emphasized the importance of parental involvement with the child and parent–child conflict for the prediction of later conduct problems, even after controlling for preexisting behavior (e.g., Kingston & Prior, 1995; Wasserman, Miller, Pinner, & Jaramillo, 1996). An important concept in this regard is the idea of coercive interpersonal parental style proposed by Patterson and colleagues (Capaldi & Patterson, 1994) to describe how children are trained to behave antisocially by escalating coercive interchanges with their parents, combined with ineffective monitoring and discipline. A relatively recent aspect of this research is the extension of inquiry into the preschool years to identify aspects of early parenting that might predict the development of antisocial behavior. Earlier work has suggested that low parental responsivity in the first year of life was predictive of later hostility and aggression at the end of primary school (Bradley, Caldwell, & Rock, 1988). More recent longitudinal studies of preschoolers by Shaw and colleagues (1993 & 1998) provide good examples of this new direction in research. These studies have attempted to assess combinations of child and maternal characteristics through behavior observations in the first 2 years of life that might predict later externalizing problems. Results highlight the centrality of parental rejection in the etiology of later externalizing behaviors among boys and girls, but particularly among boys when occurring in combination with a high negative responsiveness indicative of maternal frustration. High responsiveness in association with low rejection characterized a warm interaction between parent and child and was predictive of the lowest level of externalizing behavior. Campbell (1994) also reported that behavior observations of parent–preschooler interactions, characterized by negativity and control, predicted ongoing ODD behavior and poor impulse control 2 years later. These findings point to the usefulness of finer grained measures of parent–child interaction in predicting later antisocial behavior.

Physical and Sexual Abuse

If warmth lies at one extreme of the continuum of parent–child interaction, abuse lies at the other. As was the case with witnessing violence, the experience of physical and sexual abuse is quite common among the young. In community samples, about 1 in every 10 men and women report physical abuse as a child or adolescent that exceeded slapping or spanking, and about 1 in 10 women and 1 in 25 men report sexual abuse (Harrison, Fulkerson, & Beebe, 1997; MacMillan *et al.,* 1997). Recent longitudinal analyses indicate that a history of abuse in childhood is strongly predictive of antisocial behavior in adolescence and adulthood. Widom and Maxfield (1996) reported a 25-year follow-up of 908 children aged 11 years and younger, identified from court records as experiencing abuse, neglect, or both. In comparison with matched controls, these children were more likely to be arrested as a juveniles and as adults, a finding that held for both men and women. Physical abuse and neglect were particularly associated with arrest for violent offending; sexual abuse, predominantly experienced by girls, did not predict later violence. In the Christchurch Child Development Study, Fergusson, Horwood, and Lynskey (1996) were able to use prospectively collected information to examine the influence of childhood sexual abuse prior to age 16, on psychiatric disorder from 16 to 18 years. The importance of this study lies in the wealth of childhood and family factors that could be examined as confounders of observed relationships. These included measures of family socioeconomic disadvantage, family stability, parent–child relationships, and parental psychiatric disorder and offending. There was clear evidence for an increased risk of later CD associated with earlier sexual abuse; those experiencing such abuse were 12 times more likely to be diagnosed with CD even after adjustment for background factors.

What Predicts Characteristics of Parent–Child Interactions?

Menaghan, Kowaleski-Jones, and Mott (1997) used longitudinal data from the National Longitudinal Survey of Youth to examine the effects of family composition and employment stressors on the quality of family interaction (parent-reported warmth, involvement, and intellectual stimulation) and ultimately the child's academic progress and behavior. The findings indicated that higher levels of positive family interactions were associated with lower interparental conflict, committed as opposed to informal parent relationships, childbearing at a later age, spousal employment, and quality of the mother's occupation (if employed). This last effect of better working conditions also attenuated the influence of single mothering on family interactions. These family interaction patterns, in turn, were predictive of lower levels of behavior problems in early adolescence, including aggressive and undercontrolled behavior. These effects appeared to be independent of prior behavior problems among the children, and prior characteristics of the mother, such as self-esteem, which might be expected to influence each woman's current economic and family circumstances. These findings are consistent with other models suggesting that the effects of economic and social disadvantage on antisocial behavior are mediated, at least to some extent, through variables reflecting parental warmth, attachment, and discipline (Capaldi & Patterson, 1994; Kendler, Sham, & MacLean, 1997). However, the caveat of "to some extent" may be important given our findings from the DMHDS that the effect of socioeconomic disadvantage on the progression from oppositional behavior to CD was *independent* of family climate and parent–child interactions. The impact of the family environment in the etiology of CD is thus a function of the individual's history of early antisocial behavior and family processes embedded in a larger matrix of contextual variables that in turn are embedded in wider economic and social processes at the neighborhood and societal level. It is to these processes we now turn.

ENVIRONMENTAL RISK FACTORS AT THE NEIGHBORHOOD LEVEL

Socioeconomic Disadvantage

In his review of the association between neighborhood context and juvenile delinquency, Farrington (1986) concluded that delinquency rates have shown stronger associations with the social class of neighborhoods than with the social class of families. Recent studies have examined further the association between the socioeconomic characteristics of the neighborhood in which the child lives and antisocial behavior. Most of the studies fall into two groups: those analyzed using an ecological approach and those that included variables measuring characteristics of the neighborhood in addition to variables measuring the socioeconomic climate of the home. Ecological studies are sometimes used to explore the associations among routinely collected data. For example, LeClair and Innes (1997) examined mental health referrals for conduct-, mood-, and stress-related concerns in the light of two neighborhood factors, one measuring housing quality and the other social status and mobility. The results indicated that the spatial distribution of such referrals was not even across the city of Windsor (Canada); rather, such referrals were concentrated in areas of the city characterized by higher-density, older rental accommodation. Loeber and Wikstrom (1993) examined self-reported aggressive (overt) and nonaggressive (covert) pathways to crime in different neighborhoods in Pittsburgh. Neighborhoods were classified on dimensions of socioeconomic disadvantage and residential stability. The findings suggested that neighborhood socioeconomic disadvantage but not residential stability was associated with both aggressive and nonaggressive pathways, particularly among younger boys. Results from ecological studies such as these need to be treated with some caution, however, because they are subject to the ecological fallacy in part because it is necessary to adjust for confounding variables at the level of the individual. Consequently, ecological studies should be treated as generating hypotheses rather than as tests of hypotheses.

A more powerful form of analysis involves the measurement of both neighborhood characteristics and individual family characteristics, with the most appropriate analytic strategy being to examine effects of neighborhood characteristics after controlling for family characteristics. Aber (1994), for example, using data from the Adolescent Pathways Project, examined the influences of family poverty and neighborhood poverty on adolescent antisocial behavior. The analysis showed that these two sources of poverty were interrelated and both were correlated with the adolescent's experience of negative life events which in turn was more directly predictive of antisocial behavior. Poverty at either level did not have effects over and above the adolescent's experience of adverse life events. As Aber pointed out, however, even this approach to analysis is not the most appropriate; it ignores the hierarchical nature of the data collected and the interdependence among the data introduced by sampling related individuals from particular census tracts. The most appropriate approach to modeling such data is the use of multilevel analysis. In this type of analysis, data are hierarchically organized so that adjustments are made for individual characteristics at the lowest level and for neighborhood characteristics at a higher level. It also has the advantage of being able to adjust for the interdependence that might be found among individuals from the same school or district. Consequently, the multilevel model accounts for variation within individuals, variation among individuals in the same neighborhoods, and variation between neighborhoods. Sampson, Raudenbush, and Earls (1997) have recently reported an excellent example of a multilevel analysis of neighborhood characteristics and crime in the city of Chicago, based on a survey of more than 8000 residents in more than 300 neighborhoods. These characteristics included socioeconomic disadvantage, residential stability, and immigration patterns. The first two neighborhood characteristics were shown to be related to violent crime, although the effects of these variables were largely accounted for by the extent of neighborhood social cohesion and informal social control. (We return to this important paper in our discussion of the association between social cohesion and antisocial behavior.)

Ethnicity

Much early research used the notions of race and ethnicity interchangeably. However, this ignores the difficulty in actually measuring race, particularly if it is considered as a biological marker; indeed, a case can be made that the notion of race as a biological marker has been discredited (Senior & Bhopal, 1994). Ethnicity as a socially constructed phenomenon measuring the extent of access to and identification with a particular cultural tradition appears to be a more useful concept. Early evidence suggested significant differences among ethnic groups in antisocial behavior but much of this research relied on officially adjudicated delinquency, which raises the issue of differential treatment of ethnic groups in the police and justice systems (Farrington, 1986). More recent study indicates that at least as far as the United States is concerned, ethnic differences in adjudicated delinquency between African Americans and other Americans reflect differences in delinquent behavior overall (Farrington, Loeber, Stouthamer-Loeber, Van Kammen, & Schmidt, 1996). Typically, such differences in antisocial behavior have been explained in terms of the correlation between ethnic differences and socioeconomic disadvantage, although this is not always so (Herrnstein & Murray, 1994).

The danger with an exclusive focus on ethnicity as an explanatory variable is that it may draw attention away from other environmental risk factors. For example, Lillie-Blanton, Anthony, and Schuster (1993) pointed out that differences among ethnic groups in the United States relating to crack cocaine use, reported widely from the 1988 National Household Survey on Drug Abuse, disappeared after controlling for socially shared environmental conditions at the community level. The latter included availability of drugs, neighborhood income and educational levels, and age distribution. It may also be the case that ethnic differences are not fully accounted for by economic disadvantage. Muntaner, Nieto, and O'Campo (1996) have argued that many ethnic groups are exposed to sources of discrimination of an economic, political, and cultural nature that might operate as cumulative exposures over a lifetime. These authors made a plea for considering a broad range of such social determinants in examining ethnic inequalities in health outcome. In New Zealand, for example, Durie

(1996) argued that measures of poverty that depend exclusively on a socioeconomic perspective are inadequate in assessing the wealth or poverty experienced by Maori children (Maori are the indigenous people of New Zealand). In addition to access to traditional economic resources (land and fisheries), he argued that Maori children need access to *whanau* (extended family), *marae* (traditional meeting places), *te reo* (Maori language), and Maori culture to construct a meaningful identity. What evidence there is suggests that such cultural identity and cultural values may be a protective factor against antisocial behavior (Staub, 1996). Research on the association between ethnicity and antisocial behavior may well be extended by considering these wider meanings of ethnicity.

Exposure to Violence

Many young people are exposed to crime and violence in their neighborhood. This is particularly so among those from disadvantaged backgrounds. In the United States, studies of predominantly African American youth, both boys and girls from preschool age onward, indicate that at least 1 in every 2 have witnessed violence such as beatings, stabbings, or shootings (Sheehan, DiCara, LeBailly, & Christoffel, 1997), although in some samples the rates approach 9 in every 10 (Farrell & Bruce, 1997). Many have had violence inflicted on them or been threatened with violence; many do not feel safe in particular environments, such as schools and playgrounds. Violence may be seen as an acceptable response to a wide range of perceived threats (Sheehan *et al.,* 1997) and many young people predict their own death will be violent (Hinton-Nelson, Roberts, & Snyder, 1996), suggesting that exposure to violence desensities the child toward future violence and increases its acceptability. To what extent does witnessing such mayhem in their communities predict violent behavior on the part of the adolescent? Fitzpatrick (1997) examined predictors of fighting among youth in three nationally representative samples from the United States, and found that exposure to violence in the form of victimization or threats

with a weapon was consistently associated with fighting. Adolescents' perception of their neighborhood as dangerous, a characteristic of more socioeconomically disadvantaged neighborhoods, is predictive of self-reported CD and ODD (Aneshensel & Sucoff, 1996). This finding suggests the importance of the "experienced neighborhood," in addition to its more objective characteristics. These findings come from cross-sectional studies so it is difficult to disentangle the nature of predictive relationships. Farrell and Bruce (1997) recently tested a longitudinal model examining the effect of exposure to violence on subsequent violent behavior among 11- to 15-year-old boys and girls. Among boys, self-reported exposure to violence and frequency of violent behavior were significantly related at study outset, but such exposure did not predict subsequent violence. Among girls, higher initial exposure to violence predicted subsequent violent behavior, which in turn predicted greater exposure to violence. Further longitudinal study is needed to examine the extent to which the traumatic effects of childhood exposure to community violence are played out in later perpetration of violence by its witnesses.

SOCIETAL LEVEL ANALYSES

In reviewing the evidence for changes in the crime rate over the past 50 years, Smith (1995) concluded that there have been significant increases in crime in industrialized nations since World War II, and that an explanation in terms of changes in environmental risk factors must be invoked to account for these increases. However, some caution is needed in discussing these trends, particularly given differences between countries in offending and in access to firearms. With respect to the United States, some commentators have suggested that the magnitude of increase in violent offending is not as great as many believe; even so, the proportion of violent acts committed by adolescents has been steadily increasing over the past quarter century (Stanton, Baldwin, & Rachuba, 1997). Evidence from epidemiological studies of behavior problems also suggests that children's behavior, including antisocial behavior, is getting worse, although the changes are relatively small (Achenbach & Howell, 1993). Nevertheless, small changes spread uniformly across a population can amplify into increases in the prevalence of serious problems (Rose, 1985). What might account for these changes in antisocial behavior?

Major changes in divorce and parental separations over time, with the attendant consequences for effective parenting, might account for some of this change. Further, changes in the meaning of adolescence and increases in the tension between continued economic dependence of youth but earlier psychological independence may be a factor (Rutter & Smith, 1995). An additional factor may be the increasing influence of youth culture (West, 1997). Staub (1996) has argued that societal processes must be considered in accounting for the widespread youth violence that exists in the United States particularly; such an explanation also seems necessary to account for any increases in antisocial behavior among the young. Staub identified potential influences including an increase in difficult life conditions associated with changes in societal norms, greater opportunities for modeling of violence by children, and continuing economic problems, especially for minorities.

Putnam (1995), among others, writing of the United States, identified the enormous increases over the past 30 or so years in the civic and social disengagement of Americans from politics and government, community organizations and associations, and indeed from the extended and nuclear family. This has coincided with decreases in community feelings of "neighborliness" and "trust of others" as measured in ongoing surveys. Putnam argued that the overall effect has been the erosion of social connectedness and a decline in social capital. The latter refers to the accumulated ongoing goodwill and mutual trust between people. The importance of social integration for health is certainly not a new idea but the idea of social capital provides the opportunity to extend ideas about social connectedness and health to

an analysis at the neighborhood and societal (macrosocial) level. This is particularly so in examining the other societal processes that might impact social capital. At the individual level, alienation and low social closeness are among those personality characteristics most closely associated with offending (Caspi *et al.,* 1995). It is reasonable to hypothesize that societal processes that decrease the amount of social cohesiveness in the general community, as seems to have been happening over the past generation, might also result in significant shifts of whole groups of people along a dimension of behavior toward the antisocial end. This model of community social disorganization appears to be relevant to crime and delinquency. In an ecological analysis, Sampson and Groves (1989) examined data from a large sample of British residents in some 300 localities. Both criminal victimization and offending were related to the extent of social disorganization in a given community, where social disorganization reflected the degree of friendship networks, local participation in formal and voluntary organizations, and unsupervised youth peer groups in the community. Sampson and colleagues (1997) in their multilevel analysis of neighborhoods and crime (discussed previously) found that "collective efficacy" reflecting community cohesion, trust, and shared social values was negatively associated with variations in violence when individual level characteristics, measurement error, and prior violence had been taken into account.

Why has social cohesion declined? There is emerging evidence from both cross-sectional and longitudinal research that a major factor determining the health of communities is the distribution of economic resources in the population, not simply the absolute level of wealth in the community, at least as far as industrialized nations are concerned. The extent of income inequality, popularly characterized as the gap between rich and poor has been shown to be associated with life expectancy (Wilkinson, 1992); infant mortality (Wennemo, 1993); total mortality, coronary heart disease, and cancer (Kennedy, Kawachi, & Prothrow-Stith, 1996); and most interestingly in terms of the current discussion, both homicide and violent crime, as well as educational outcome (Kaplan, Pamuk, Lynch, Cohen, & Balfour, 1996; Kennedy *et al.,* 1996). The Kaplan and colleagues and Kennedy and colleagues analyses involved comparisons among states in the United States. Where income inequalities were higher, health indicators were poorer, as was social capital assessed by membership in voluntary groups and levels of social trust (Kawachi, Kennedy, Lochner, & Prothrow-Stith, 1997). Unfortunately, this kind of analysis does not appear to have been extended to juvenile crime, but it might be expected that the same patterning of antisocial behavior would occur with differences in income inequalities. Overall, the lesson seems to be that economic policies that influence the distribution of wealth within a country will also influence adversely the health of that country, and this could include the level of antisocial behavior among its youth; the mechanism linking increased income inequality and adverse outcome may well be the decline in social capital that Putnam (1995) described.

CONCLUDING COMMENTS

Most psychosocial environmental risk factors for antisocial behavior have been identified and researched for some time, although variations on existing risk factors are being identified. For example, the recognition of homelessness as a significant health issue for children has occurred relatively recently (Breakey, 1997), as has the impact of income distribution just reviewed. Much seems to be known about environmental risk factors at the individual or family level, although it can be argued that the legacy from cross-sectional studies of risk is often a static view of the relationships between risk and outcome and a passive view of the individual in relation to risk. Increasingly, the discourse in developmental psychopathology has turned toward different levels or domains of risk and the additive or interactive effects of these domains on outcome. The research we have reviewed suggests that the notion of environmental risk is gradually

being placed into a more dynamic developmental framework to examine the influence of risk at different developmental stages of the individual, how patterns of risk evolve over time, and the reciprocal relationship between risk and the individual.

That less is known about how environmental risks operate at levels of analysis beyond the individual and family may be due at least in part to the preoccupation of psychology and psychiatry with a categorical approach to the identification of antisocial disorder, thereby identifying who should be treated. We are clearly not immune to this as is evident from Table 1! The danger is that we may be led to believe that there is no such thing as society, only individuals and their families. McKinlay (1993) discussed the notion of "level of cause" to distinguish between upstream and downstream causal factors associated with health outcome; the former refers to those processes at progressively more macro levels of analysis and the latter refers to those processes revealed at the more micro level. The former cannot be simply reduced to the latter, at least as far as the recognition of preventable environmental risk and where to intervene is concerned (Aber, 1994). For example, it is now apparent that homelessness is not rare and while it may reflect the consequences of individual factors such as mental illness, unemployment, and domestic violence, broader societal processes including housing shortages, inadequate welfare support, and deinstitutionalization probably play a more significant role in determining the levels of homelessness in the community. Cross-sectional research on the effects of homelessness on children are beginning to appear in the literature, no doubt to be followed, if at all possible, by longitudinal studies of homeless children. However, to analyze the effects of homelessness on children only at the individual and family level misses the whole story. We believe this is true for many of the risk factors we have discussed in this chapter. Their analysis needs to take place at several levels, particularly to identify how upstream causes impact the more immediate downstream ones, and to identify the extent to which upstream variables have direct influences on outcome. The trick is, as Aber pointed out, to effectively integrate analyses to describe relationships between these different levels.

ACKNOWLEDGMENTS. The program of mental health research in the DMHDS has been supported by the Health Research Council of New Zealand and the Antisocial and Violent Behavior Branch of the National Institute of Mental Health (United States). We wish to acknowledge the contributions of many people to this research program over the years. Thanks to Dr. Richie Poulton and Dr. Phil Silva for their critical comments on this chapter. Finally, our special thanks to those many individuals enrolled in the DMHDS and to their parents for their long-term commitment to this research effort.

REFERENCES

Aber, J. L. (1994). Poverty, violence and child development: Untangling family and community level effects. In C. A. Nelson (Ed.), *Threats to optimal child development: The Minnesota Symposia on Child Psychology* (Vol. 27, pp. 229–272). Hillsdale, NJ: Erlbaum.

Achenbach, T. M., & Howell, C. T. (1993). Are American children's problems getting worse? A thirteen year comparison. *Journal of the American Academy of Child and Adolescent Psychiatry, 32,* 1145–1154.

Adler, N. E., Boyce, T., Chesney, M. A., Cohen, S., Folkman, S., Kahn, R. L., & Syme, S. L. (1994). Socioeconomic status and health: The challenge of the gradient. *American Psychologist, 49,* 15–24.

Aneshensel, C. S., & Sucoff, C. A. (1996). The neighborhood context of adolescent mental health. *Journal of Health and Social Behavior, 37,* 293–310.

Biederman, J., Faraone, S. V., Milberger, S., Jetton, J. G., Chen, L., Mick, E., Greene, R. W., & Russell, R. L. (1996). Is childhood oppositional defiant disorder a precursor to adolescent conduct disorder? Findings for a four-year follow-up study of children with ADHD. *Journal of the American Academy of Child and Adolescent Psychiatry, 35,* 1193–1204.

Bird, H., Gould, M. S., Yager, T., Staghezza, B., & Canino, G. (1989). Risk factors for maladjustment in Puerto Rican Children. *Journal of the American Academy of Child and Adolescent Psychiatry, 28,* 847–850.

Block, J. H., Block, J., & Gjerde, P. F. (1988). Parental functioning and the home environment in families of divorce: Prospective and concurrent analyses. *Journal of the American Academy of Child and Adolescent Psychiatry, 27,* 207–213.

Bradley, R. H., Caldwell, B. M., & Rock, S. L. (1988). Home environment and school performance: A ten year follow-up and examination of three models of environmental action. *Child Development, 59,* 852–867.

Breakey, W. R. (1997). It's time for the public health community to declare war on homelessness [Editorial]. *American Journal of Public Health, 87,* 153–155.

Campbell, S. B. (1990). *Behavior problems in preschool children.* New York: Guilford.

Campbell, S. B. (1994). Hard-to-manage preschool boys: Externalizing behavior, social competence, and family context at two-year follow-up. *Journal of Abnormal Child Psychology, 22,* 147–166.

Capaldi, D. M., & Patterson, G. R. (1994). Interrelated influences of contextual factors on antisocial behavior in childhood and adolescence for males. In D. C. Fowles, P. Sutker & S. H. Goodman (Eds.), *Progress in experimental personality and psychopathology research* (pp. 165–198). New York: Springer.

Caspi, A., Begg, D., Dickson, N., Langley, J., Moffitt, T. E., McGee, R., & Silva, P. A. (1995). Identification of personality types at risk for poor health and injury in late adolescence. *Criminal Behaviour and Mental Health, 5,* 330–350.

Cherlin, A. J., Furstenberg, F. F., Chase-Lansdale, L., Kiernan, K. E., Robins, P. K., Morrison, D. R., & Teitler, J. O. (1991). Longitudinal studies of effects of divorce on children in Great Britain and the United States. *Science, 252,* 1386–1389.

Cichetti, D. (1994). Integrating developmental risk factors: Perspectives from developmental psychopathology. In C. A. Nelson (Ed.), *Threats to optimal child development: The Minnesota Symposia on Child Psychology* (Vol. 27, pp. 285–325). Hillsdale, NJ: Erlbaum.

Costello, E. J. (1989). Child psychiatric disorders and their correlates: A primary care pediatric sample. *Journal of the American Academy of Child and Adolescent Psychiatry, 28,* 851–855.

Davies, P., & Cummings, M. (1994). Marital conflict and child adjustment: An emotional security hypothesis. *Psychological Bulletin, 116,* 387–411.

Durie, M. H. (1996). *The right of Maori rangatahi to be Maori.* Hamilton, New Zealand: Massey University, Department of Maori Studies.

Fantuzzo, J., Boruch, R., Beriama, A., Atkins, M., & Marcus, S. (1997). Domestic violence and children: Prevalence and risk in five major US cities. *Journal of the American Academy of Child and Adolescent Psychiatry, 36,* 116–122.

Farrell, A. D., & Bruce, S. E. (1997). Impact of exposure to community violence on violent behavior and emotional distress among urban adolescents. *Journal of Clinical Child Psychology, 26,* 2–14.

Farrington, D. P. (1978). The family background of aggressive youths. In L. A. Hersov, M. Berger, & D. Shaffer (Eds.), *Aggression and antisocial behaviour in childhood and adolescence* (pp. 73–93). Oxford, England: Pergamon.

Farrington, D. P. (1986). The sociocultural context of childhood disorders. In H. C. Quay & J. S. Werry (Eds.), *Psychopathological disorders of childhood* (3rd ed., pp. 391–422). New York: Wiley.

Farrington, D. P., & Loeber, R. (in press). Transatlantic replicability of risk factors in the development of delinquency. In P. Cohen, C. Slomkowski, & L. N. Robins (Eds.), *Where and when: The influence of history and geography on aspects of psychopathology.* Mahwah, NJ: Erlbaum.

Farrington, D. P., Loeber, R., Stouthamer-Loeber, M., Van Kammen, W. B., & Schmidt, L. (1996). Self-reported delinquency and a combined delinquency seriousness scale based on boys, mothers and teachers: Concurrent and predictive validity for African-Americans and Caucasians. *Criminology, 34,* 501–525.

Feehan, M., McGee, R., & Williams, S. (1994). Mental health disorders from age 15 to age 18 years. *Journal of the American Academy of Child and Adolescent Psychiatry, 32,* 1118–1126.

Feehan, M., McGee, R., Williams, S., & Nada-Raja, S. (1995). Models of adolescent psychopathology: Childhood risk and the transition to adulthood. *Journal of the American Academy of Child and Adolescent Psychiatry, 34,* 670–679.

Fergusson, D. M., & Horwood, L. J. (1995). Predictive validity of categorically and dimensionally scored measures of disruptive childhood behaviors. *Journal of the American Academy of Child and Adolescent Psychiatry, 34,* 477–485.

Fergusson, D. M., Horwood, L. J., & Lynskey, M. (1994). The childhoods of multiple problem adolescents: A fifteen year longitudinal study. *Journal of Child Psychology and Psychiatry, 35,* 1123–1140.

Fergusson, D. M., Horwood, L. J., & Lynskey, M. (1996). Childhood sexual abuse and psychiatric disorder in young adulthood: II. Psychiatric outcomes of childhood sexual abuse. *Journal of the American Academy of Child and Adolescent Psychiatry, 35,* 1365–1374.

Fergusson, D. M., Lynskey, M. T., & Horwood, L. J. (1996). Origins of comorbidity between conduct and affective disorders. *Journal of the American Academy of Child and Adolescent Psychiatry, 35,* 451–460.

Fitzmaurice, G. M., Laird, N. M., Zahner, G. E. P., & Daskalakis, C. (1995). Bivariate logistic regression of childhood psychopathology ratings using multiple informants. *American Journal of Epidemiology, 142,* 1194–1203.

Fitzpatrick, K. M. (1997). Fighting among America's youth: A risk and protective factors approach. *Journal of Health and Social Behavior, 38,* 131–148.

Harrison, P. A., Fulkerson, J. A., & Beebe, T. J. (1997). Multiple substance use among adolescent physical and sexual abuse victims. *Child Abuse & Neglect, 21,* 529–539.

Henning, K., Leitenberg, H., Coffey, P., Bennett, T., & Jankowski, M. K. (1997). Long-term psychological adjustment to witnessing interparental physical conflict during childhood. *Child Abuse & Neglect, 21,* 501–515.

Henry, B., Caspi, A., Moffitt, T. E., & Silva, P. A. (1996). Temperamental and familial predictors of violent and nonviolent criminal convictions: Age 3 to age 18. *Developmental Psychology, 32,* 614–623.

Herrnstein, R. J., & Murray, C. (1994). *The bell curve: Intelligence and class structure in American life.* New York: Free Press.

Hetherington, E. M. (1990). Parents, children and siblings: Six years after divorce. In R. A. Hinde & J. Stevenson-Hinde (Eds.), *Relationships within families: Mutual influences* (pp. 311–331). Oxford, England: Clarendon.

Hinton-Nelson, M. D., Roberts, M. C., & Snyder, C. R. (1996). Early adolescents exposed to violence: Hope and vulnerability to victimization. *American Journal of Orthopsychiatry, 66,* 346–353.

Kaplan, G. A., Pamuk, E. R., Lynch, J. W., Cohen, R. D., & Balfour, J. L. (1996). Inequality in income and mortality in the United States: Analysis of mortality and potential pathways. *British Medical Journal, 312,* 999–1003.

Kasen, S., Cohen, P., Brook, J. S., & Hartmark, C. (1996). A multiple-risk interaction model: Effects of temperament and divorce on psychiatric disorders in children. *Journal of Abnormal Child Psychology, 24,* 121–150.

Kawachi, I., Kennedy, B. P. Lochner, K., & Prothrow-Stith, D. (1997). Social capital, income inequality, and mortality. *American Journal of Public Health, 87,* 1491–1498.

Kendler, K. S., Sham, P. C., & MacLean, C. J. (1997). The determinants of parenting: An epidemiological multi-informant, retrospective study. *Psychological Medicine, 27,* 549–563.

Kennedy, B. P., Kawachi, I., & Prothrow-Stith, D. (1996). Income distribution and mortality: Cross sectional ecological study of the Robin Hood index in the United States. *British Medical Journal, 312,* 1004–1007.

Kingston, L., & Prior, M. (1995). The development of stable patterns of stable, transient, and school-age onset aggressive behavior in young children. *Journal of the American Academy of Child and Adolescent Psychiatry, 34,* 348–358.

Kolbo, J. R., Blakely, E. H., & Engleman, D. (1996). Children who witness domestic violence: A review of empirical literature. *Journal of Interpersonal Violence, 11,* 281–293.

Kolvin, I., Miller, F. J. W., Fleeting, M., & Kolvin, P. A. (1988). Social and parenting factors affecting criminal offence rates: Findings from the Newcastle Thousand Families study (1947–1980). *British Journal of Psychiatry, 152,* 80–90.

Kraemer, H. C., Kazdin, A. E., Offord, D. R., Kessler, R. C., Jensen, P. S., & Kupfer, D. J. (1997). Coming to terms with the terms of risk. *Archives of General Psychiatry, 54,* 337–343.

Kratzer, L., & Hodgins, S. (1997). Adult outcomes of child conduct problems: A cohort study. *Journal of Abnormal Child Psychology, 25,* 65–81.

LeClair, J. A., & Innes, F. C. (1997). Urban ecological structure and perceived child and adolescent psychological disorder. *Social Science & Medicine, 44,* 1649–1659.

Lillie-Blanton, M., Anthony, J. C., & Schuster, C. R. (1993). Probing the meaning of racial/ethnic differences in crack cocaine smoking. *Journal of the American Medical Association, 269,* 993–997.

Loeber, R., & Hay, D. (1997). Key issues in the development of aggression and violence from childhood to early adulthood. *Annual Review of Psychology, 48,* 371–410.

Loeber, R., & Wikstrom, P. H. (1993). Individual pathways to crime in different types of neighborhoods. In D. P. Farrington, R. J. Sampson, & P. H. Wikstrom (Eds.), *Integrating individual and ecological aspects of crime* (pp. 169–204). Stockholm: Liber-Verlag.

MacMillan, H. L., Fleming, J. E., Trocme, N., Boyle, M. H., Wong, M., Racine, Y. A., Beardslee, W. R., & Offord, D. R. (1997). Prevalence of child physical and sexual abuse in the community: Results from the Ontario health supplement. *Journal of the American Medical Association, 278,* 131–135.

Maxwell, G. M., & Robertson, J. P. (1993). *Moving apart: A study of the role of family court counselling services.* Wellington: New Zealand Department of Justice.

McConaughy, S. H., & Achenbach, T. M. (1994). Comorbidity of empirically based syndromes in matched general population and clinical samples. *Journal of Child Psychology and Psychiatry, 35,* 1141–1157.

McGee, R., & Williams, S. (1997). *Developmental changes in comorbidity among dimensions of disorder.* Paper in preparation.

McGee, R., Silva, P. A., & Williams, S. (1984). Perinatal, neurological, environmental and developmental characteristics of seven year old children with stable behaviour problems. *Journal of Child Psychology and Psychiatry, 25,* 573–586.

McGee, R., Feehan, M., Williams, S., & Anderson, J. (1992). DSM-III disorders from age 11 to age 15. *Journal of the American Academy of Child and Adolescent Psychiatry, 31,* 50–59.

McGee, R., Feehan, M., & Williams, S. (1996). Mental health. In P. A. Silva & W. R. Stanton (Eds.), *From child to adult: The Dunedin Multidisciplinary Health and Development Study* (pp. 150–162). Auckland, New Zealand: Oxford University Press.

McKinlay, J. B. (1993). The promotion of health through planned sociopolitical change: Challenges for research and policy. *Social Science & Medicine, 36,* 109–117.

McLeod, J. D., & Shanahan, M. J. (1996). Trajectories of poverty and children's mental health. *Journal of Health and Social Behavior, 37,* 207–220.

Menaghan, E. G., Kowaleski-Jones, L., & Mott, F. L. (1997). The intergenerational costs of parental social stressors: Academic and social difficulties in early adolescence for children of young mothers. *Journal of Health and Social Behavior, 38,* 72–86.

Moffitt, T. E. (1993). Adolescence-limited and life-course-persistent antisocial behavior: A developmental taxonomy. *Psychological Review, 100,* 674–701.

Moffitt, T. E., & Harrington, H. L. (1996). Delinquency: The natural history of antisocial behaviour. In P. A. Silva & W. R. Stanton (Eds.), *From child to adult: The Dunedin Multidisciplinary Health and Development Study* (pp. 163–185). Auckland, New Zealand: Oxford University Press.

Muntaner, C., Nieto, F. J., & O'Campo, P. (1996). The bell curve: On race, social class, and epidemiological research. *American Journal of Epidemiology, 144,* 531–536.

Offord, D. R., Boyle, M. H., & Racine, Y. (1989). Ontario child health study: Correlates of disorder. *Journal of the American Academy of Child and Adolescent Psychiatry, 28,* 856–860.

Pakiz, B., Reinherz, H. Z., & Giaconia, R. M. (1997). Early risk factors for serious antisocial behavior at age 21: A longitudinal community study. *American Journal of Orthopsychiatry, 67,* 92–101.

Paschall, M. J., Ennett, S. T., & Flewelling, R. L. (1996). Relationships among family characteristics and violent behavior by black and white male adolescents. *Journal of Youth and Adolescence, 25,* 177–197.

Putnam, R. D. (1995). Bowling alone: America's declining social capital. *Journal of Democracy, 6,* 65–78.

Raine, A., Breenan, P., & Mednick, S. A. (1994). Birth complications combined with early maternal rejection at age 1 predispose to violent crime at age 18 years. *Archives of General Psychiatry, 51,* 984–988.

Roff, J. D., & Wirt, R. D. (1984). Childhood aggression and social adjustment as antecedents of delinquency. *Journal of Abnormal Child Psychology, 12,* 111–126.

Rose, G. (1985). Sick individuals and sick populations. *International Journal of Epidemiology, 14,* 32–38.

Rothbaum, F., & Weisz, J. R. (1994). Parental caregiving and child externalizing behavior in nonclinical samples: A meta-analysis. *Psychological Bulletin, 116,* 55–74.

Rutter, M. (1971). Parent–child separation: Psychological effects on the children. *Journal of Child Psychology and Psychiatry, 12,* 233–260.

Rutter, M. (1978). Family, area and school influences in the genesis of conduct disorders. In L. A. Hersov, M. Berger, & D. Shaffer (Eds.), *Aggression and anti-social behaviour in childhood and adolescence* (pp. 95–133). Oxford, England: Pergamon.

Rutter, M. (1989). Isle of Wight revisited: Twenty-five years of child psychiatric epidemiology. *Journal of the American Academy of Child and Adolescent Psychiatry, 28,* 633–653.

Rutter, M., & Smith, D. J. (Eds.). (1995). *Psychosocial disorders in young people: Time trends and their causes.* Chichester, England: Wiley.

Rutter, M., Cox, A., Tupling, C., Berger, M., & Yule, W. (1975). Attainment and adjustment in two geographical areas: I. The prevalence of psychiatric disorder. *British Journal of Psychiatry, 125,* 493–509.

Sampson, R. J., & Groves, W. B. (1989). Community structure and crime: Testing social disorganization theory. *American Journal of Sociology, 94,* 774–802.

Sampson, R. J., Raudenbush, S. W., & Earls, F. (1997). Neighborhoods and violent crime: A multilevel study of collective efficacy. *Science, 277,* 918–924.

Senior, P. A., & Bhopal, R. (1994). Ethnicity as a variable in epidemiological research. *British Medical Journal, 309,* 327–330.

Shaw, D. S., Emery, R. E., & Tuer, M. D. (1993). Parental functioning and children's adjustment in families of divorce: A prospective study. *Journal of Abnormal Child Psychology, 21,* 119–134.

Shaw, D. S., Winslow, E. B., Owens, E. B., Vondra, J. I., Cohn, J. F., & Bell, R. Q. (1998). The development of early externalizing problems among children from low-income families: A transformational perspective. *Journal of Abnormal Child Psychology, 26,* 95–107.

Sheehan, K., DiCara, J. A., LeBailly, S., & Christoffel, K. K. (1997). Children's exposure to violence in an urban setting. *Archives of Pediatric and Adolescent Medicine, 151,* 502–504.

Smith, D. J. (1995). Youth crime and conduct disorders: Trends, patterns and causal explanations. In M. Rutter & D. J. Smith (Eds.), *Psychosocial disorders in young people: Time trends and their causes* (pp. 389–489). Chichester, England: Wiley.

Stanton, B., Baldwin, R. M., & Rachuba, L. (1997). A quarter century of violence in the United States: An epidemiologic assessment. *Psychiatric Clinics of North America, 20,* 269–282.

StataCorp. (1997). *Stata statistical software: Release 5.0.* College Station, TX: Stata Corp.

Staub, E. (1996). Cultural-societal roots of violence: The examples of genocidal violence and of contemporary youth violence in the United States. *American Psychologist, 51,* 117–132.

Tolan, P. H. (1987). Implications of age of onset for delinquency risk. *Journal of Abnormal Child Psychology, 15,* 47–65.

Tschann, J. M., Kaiser, P., Chesney, M. A., Alkno, A., & Boyce, W. T. (1996). Resilience and vulnerability among preschool children: Family functioning, temperament, and behavior problems. *Journal of the American Academy of Child and Adolescent Psychiatry, 28,* 861–864.

Vaden-Kiernan, N., Ialongo, N. S., Pearson, J., & Kellam, S. (1995). Household family structure and children's aggressive behavior: A longitudinal study of urban elementary school children. *Journal of Abnormal Child Psychology, 23,* 553–568.

Velez, C. N., Johnson, J., & Cohen, P. (1989). A longitudinal analysis of selected risk factors for child psychopathology. *Journal of the American Academy of Child and Adolescent Psychiatry, 28,* 861–864.

Wasserman, G. A., Miller, L. S., Pinner, E., & Jaramillo, B. (1996). Parenting predictors of early conduct problems in urban, high-risk boys. *Journal of the American Academy of Child and Adolescent Psychiatry, 35,* 1227–1236.

Wennemo, I. (1993). Infant mortality, public policy and inequality—A comparison of 18 industrialised countries 1950–85. *Sociology of Health and Illness, 15,* 429–446.

Werner, E. E., & Smith, R. S. (1979). An epidemiologic perspective on some antecedents and consequences of childhood mental health problems and learning disabilities. *Journal of the American Academy of Child Psychiatry, 8,* 292–306.

West, P. (1997). Health inequalities in the early years: Is there equalisation in youth? *Social Science & Medicine, 44,* 833–858.

Widom, C. S., & Maxfield, M. G. (1996). A prospective examination of risk for violence among abused and neglected children. *Annals of the New York Academy of Sciences, 794,* 224–237.

Wilkinson, R. G. (1992). Income distribution and life expectancy. *British Medical Journal, 304,* 165–168.

Williams, S., McGee, R., Olaman, S., & Knight, R. G. (1997). Level of education, age of bearing children and mental health of women. *Social Science & Medicine, 45,* 827–836.

Woodward, L., Belsky, J., McGee, R., & Nada-Raja, S. (1997, July). *Parental separation and attachment to parents and peers in adolescence.* Paper presented at the 10th Australasian Human Development conference, Adelaide, South Australia, Australia.

20

Interventions for Oppositional Defiant Disorder and Conduct Disorder in the Schools

KENNETH A. KAVALE, STEVEN R. FORNESS, and HILL M. WALKER

INTRODUCTION

The clinical categories of Oppositional Defiant Disorder (ODD) and Conduct Disorder (CD) are of relatively minor importance to educators who see a significant increase in the number of students, with and without formal diagnoses, who are exhibiting Disruptive Behavior Disorders (DBD) in the schools.* In general, DBD is

*Attention-Deficit/Hyperactivity Disorder (ADHD) is not a disorder that qualifies a student for special education services in most school districts. However, since there is considerable comorbidity with Learning Disabilities, many students are served under this label. ADHD students may also be served under the SED label when ADHD is comorbid with a qualifying disorder (e.g., Anxiety Disorder, Depression).

   In this chapter, we use the terms *disruptive* and *aggressive* to encompass the types of behavior symptomatic of CD and ODD.

KENNETH A. KAVALE • Department of Special Education, The University of Iowa, Iowa City, Iowa 52242-1529.   STEVEN R. FORNESS • Department of Special Education, University of California, Los Angeles, Los Angeles, California 90095-1759.   HILL M. WALKER • Department of Special Education, University of Oregon, Eugene, Oregon 97403-1215.

Handbook of Disruptive Behavior Disorders, edited by Quay and Hogan. Kluwer Academic/Plenum Publishers, New York, 1999.

marked by aggression, hostility, rule breaking, defiance of authority, and violation of social norms. (See Chapter 1, this volume, for an extended discussion.)

   In a school context, DBD have commonly been referred to as Social Maladjustment and, although historically excluded from the federal Serious Emotional Disturbance (SED) category, are now being proposed as part of a new definition of emotional and behavior disorder for education (Forness & Knitzer, 1992).

   With prevalence ranging from 2% to 6%, CD is considerably more frequent than SED (<1%) and appears to be increasing to an extent that severely constrains the ability of schools to educate all students effectively (Walker, 1993). Walker, McConnell, and Clarke (1985) described two types of critical social-behavior adjustments required of school children: teacher-related and peer-related. Patterns of disruptive behavior place children at risk for failure in both adjustment areas. Because of aggressive behavior, social rejection by peers is probable. If noncompliant with teacher directives, then teacher rejection is a real possibility.

   Disruptive behavior is aversive to others and often leads to rejection and social avoidance (Dodge, Pettit, McClaskey, & Brown, 1986;

Patterson, DeBaryshe, & Ramsey, 1989). In the classroom, aggressive behavior is considered inappropriate and unacceptable and on the playground, it often results in negative social behaviors (e.g., bullying, fighting) (Walker, Shinn, O'Neill, & Ramsey, 1987). As might be expected, DBD are often associated with academic skill deficits and low achievement (Hinshaw, 1992; see Chapters 14 & 16, this volume). Finally, DBD are frequently associated with low self-esteem and depression (Kovacs, Paulauskas, Gatsonis, & Richards, 1988; Walker, Stieber, Ramsey, O'Neill, & Eisert, 1994). The consequences of disruptive behavior include higher rates of high school dropout, drug abuse, delinquency, and incarceration (Walker & Reid, 1997).

Disruptive behavior is not only negative and destructive but also highly stable and difficult to manage. Early educational intervention is necessary and should be directed at three settings and social agents: home and parents, playground and peers, and classroom and teachers. The difficulty, however, is that many interventions have not been validated, yet they are claimed to be "cures" for the difficult and enduring problems associated with disruptive behavior. There are no "magic bullets," and it is necessary to judge the effectiveness of an intervention with respect to its intensity, length, comprehensiveness, and fidelity (Kazdin, 1985; Reid, 1993). In addition, the goals and methods of intervention may change over time and roughly fall into four developmental phases emphasizing necessary services and interventions (Bullis & Walker, 1994).

Prevention needs to be attempted in the preschool to grade 3 age range with a comprehensive, multisetting approach applied consistently and with a high level of treatment fidelity. The goal is to divert the at-risk child. From grades 4 to 6, *active remediation* is attempted, and although cure per se is unlikely, specific associated deficits may be ameliorated (e.g., social skills, self-control, peer relations). By grades 7 and 8, the goal becomes one of *attenuating* negative effects on the student, family, peers, and the society at large. The emphasis is on buffering these negative effects through teaching coping and survival skills. Finally, in grades 9 to 12, the emphasis is on *accommodation* that implies a degree of acceptance brought on through the understanding that the disruptive behavior is not likely to change significantly. The goal is to maintain school attendance and prepare the student for transition from school to work and adult life.

EARLY IDENTIFICATION OF DBD

Early identification and intervention appears decisive. Zigler, Taussig, and Black (1992) found that, although prevention of delinquency was often difficult and disappointing, intervention directed at reducing or preventing precursors to delinquency (e.g., DBD) hold promise along with efforts targeting socializing agents (e.g., Hawkins, VonCleve, & Catalano, 1991; see also Chapter 25, this volume).

What must precede intervention is the early identification of children at risk. It has been demonstrated that the social behavior of preschool children is sufficiently well differentiated for patterns of disruptive behavior to be identified (Hinshaw, Han, Erhardt, & Huber, 1992). To identify young children at risk, a number of screening measures have been suggested, for example, the Student Risk Screening Scale developed by Drummond (1993). Another procedure was developed by Walker, Severson, and Feil (1994) in the Early Screening Project that is a downward extension of the Systematic Screening for Behavior Disorders (Walker & Severson, 1990). It is a multiple-gating, screening-identification procedure for children 3–5 years of age. Other approaches and instruments for assessing disruptive behavior, as described in Chapter 3 (this volume), are also used in the schools.

INTERVENTIONS FOR DBD

Once a child is deemed at risk, intervention is necessary. It is abundantly clear that a single intervention is insufficient to deal with the complex and multidimensional nature of disruptive behavior (Bullis & Walker, 1994). The primary goal of intervention is to teach replacement behaviors that are adaptive and functional. A comprehensive program is required that includes strategies for both reducing disruptive behavior and enhancing prosocial behavior.

Intervention begins with providing a classroom structure where events in the classroom become as predictable as possible (Paine, Radicchi, Rosellini, Deutchman, & Darch, 1983). Classroom structure helps provide the stability necessary for controlling behavior and setting the stage for effective learning. It includes physical arrangements in the classroom, operating procedures (e.g., classroom rules, daily schedule), teacher expectations, and information on the kinds of academic and behavioral responses required for efficient learning (Cangelosi, 1992). An optimally structured classroom should be combined with "best practice" to ensure the delivery of effective teaching strategies where the primary goal is to provide high levels of academic-engaged time. In this context, teachers need to be prepared to deal with problem behavior during instruction. Recommendations for avoiding such problem behavior may be found in Walker, Colvin, and Ramsey (1995).

Teaching Adaptive Behavior

Even under optimal circumstances, disruptive behavior is likely to be manifested. Increasingly, managing problem behavior has emphasized the direct teaching of adaptive behavior patterns (Colvin & Sugai, 1988; Evertson, Emmer, Clements, Sanford, & Worsham, 1984; Sprick, 1994). The underlying assumption is that students have not learned the essential competencies required for school success (see Hersh & Walker, 1983), and the teaching of these adaptive forms of behavior are conceptualized in an eight-step process (see Walker *et al.*, 1995, for details).

Even the most effective strategies are sometimes unsuccessful but often attempts to ameliorate the situation are made only after

problems have occurred. Kameenui and Simmons (1990) have suggested "precorrection" whereby a teacher anticipates problems and adjustments are made before a student has the opportunity to respond inappropriately. This strategy is recommended for reducing the likelihood that the teacher will respond to inappropriate behavior only after the fact rather than acting preemptively.

Disruptive behavior is not solely a classroom problem but is also likely to be encountered in a larger environment. It is, therefore, necessary to take a broader view and examine ways to reduce it by developing and implementing a schoolwide discipline plan. In addition, emphasis must be placed on reducing aggressive behavior in the situation where adult supervision and monitoring is weakest—the playground.

Schoolwide Discipline Plans

To ensure a strong, positive climate to support learning, schools should develop plans to institute structures and strategies for establishing desirable behaviors across *all* students (Clapp, 1989).

Schoolwide discipline plans need to be based on validated practices and include the following components:

1. Discipline is viewed as a means to achieve primary goals such as academic achievement and social development (Knitzer, Steinberg, & Fleisch, 1990).
2. Emphasis should be on positive and constructive problem-solving approaches that can serve prevention goals as opposed to reactive or punitive approaches that focus on controlling behavior (Gettinger, 1988).
3. Supportive leadership from the principal is necessary.
4. All school staff need to be involved in order to establish a consistent and predictable school environment (Smylie, 1988).
5. When expectations are high, teachers are likely to assume greater responsibility for effecting behavior change, students perform better, and discipline problems are reduced (Wong, Kauffman, & Lloyd, 1991).

6. Roles and responsibilities must be clearly articulated with respect to who does what, when, and how (Sprick, 1994).
7. School staff persons should increase efforts to establish relationships with other service agencies (e.g., mental health services, courts, parent support agencies, children's protective services).
8. To provide accountability, the discipline plan should include a systematic data-management and evaluation plan.

The initial step in establishing a schoolwide discipline plan is to write a mission statement and statement of purpose. The mission statement is designed to capture the broad-based direction and values of the school, staff, and students; the statement of purpose communicates the need to establish and maintain student behavior that permits school goals to be attained.

The next step defines expected behaviors in positive terms that illustrate an acceptable range of behaviors such as (1) providing a safe and supportive environment for learning, (2) managing oneself, and (3) respecting the rights and property of others.

The process continues with the establishment of behavioral expectations for specific settings such as the cafeteria, hallways, and playground.

With expected behaviors specified, attention is directed at teaching these schoolwide behavioral expectations. The most effective means for establishing appropriate behavior is to systematically and directly teach the specific behaviors that support each behavioral expectation (Walker et al., 1995).

An important component is to develop ways to reward positive behavior which may include, for example, trophies for exemplary leadership, citizenship awards presented at school assemblies, and "caught-in-the-act" coupons distributed to those students following school rules.

Discipline and Interventions

A comprehensive discipline plan should include procedures for correcting problem behavior. A first step is to define and categorize problem behavior in the school setting. For ex-

ample, some school infractions may be relatively minor but nevertheless disruptive (e.g., talking too loudly, being tardy for class, truancy), and may escalate into more serious problems. Serious school violations represent substantial breaches of school rules and social norms that seriously disrupt school functioning (e.g., verbal abuse toward staff, vandalism, sustained noncompliance and defiance). Illegal behavior involves violation of law (e.g., theft, assault, possession of weapons or controlled substances).

Minor school infractions are usually managed by a teacher who should possess a range of procedures that strike a balance between positive reinforcement for promoting expected behavior and delivering negative consequences, as appropriate. For serious school violations, an office referral is typical and an administrative staff person takes primary responsibility. The consequences for serious violations should be stated in school policy and consequences delivered automatically and consistently. Consequences include parent conferences, after-school detention, in-school suspension, out-of-school suspension, and expulsion. For illegal behavior, a police referral is also a consequence.

On the Playground

Aggressive behavior is very likely to be manifested on the playground. In general, aggressive students require structure to manage and control the aversive features of their behavior, but the relatively unstructured nature of the playground, combined with low levels of adult supervision, make peer conflict highly likely. Consequently, for an aggressive student, the playground is an especially difficult setting in which to demonstrate self-control, cooperation, and positive social behavior (Pepler & Rubin, 1991).

Playground Behavior. Dodge, Coie, and Brakke (1982) demonstrated that aggressive children have difficulties in several social situations with peers and adults. Specifically, aggressive students tend to be unskilled in joining ongoing peer groups, in responding to teasing and provocation without intense anger accompanied by threats, and in following the requests and commands from teachers and peers. The problems posed by joining peer groups and compliance with requests and commands have been well studied; the investigation of teasing and provocation has been less extensive. From the available literature, it is possible to glean a list of "do's" and "don'ts" for children in these contexts (i.e., peer entry, teasing, and provocation) (see Walker *et al.*, 1995, for details on specific suggestions).

Bullying. One of the most prominent features of aggressive behavior is bullying. The prevalence of bullying in U.S. schools is particularly high in comparison to European schools (Hoover & Juul, 1993). This behavior is often a precursor to more overt violence and thus demands attention. Gagnon (1991) suggested that interventions for bullying must directly involve all parties (i.e., students, teachers, parents, and community). Olweus (1991) has developed intervention techniques for reducing bullying emphasizing monitoring by adults with appropriate use of sanctions.

Remediating Aggressive Behavior on the Playground. A number of strategies are available for preventing aggressive behavior on the playground. One such strategy is the teaching of normative standards; disruptive students often possess standards governing peer relations that are divergent from those of their peers. Walker, Hops, and Greenwood (1984) developed a procedure that employs direct instruction to teach awareness and understanding of playground rules and normative standards governing peer relations. The training is followed by a behavior-management system on the playground and has generally proved an effective means for aggressive students to acquire more adaptive and prosocial behavior.

A second strategy involves teaching adaptive strategies for specific social situations (e.g., joining peer group). Dodge (1996) proposed a model to teach the skills necessary for improving aggressive behavior; the model provides structured instruction-intervention efforts. For example, three different situations are provided to teach discrimination between interruptive and noninterruptive ways of approaching and seeking to join a peer group. Similar scenarios are used to teach strategies for coping with teasing and provocation or complying with teacher and peer directives.

A third strategy targets problematic playground behaviors by teaching anger-management skills and conflict-resolution procedures. The goals of anger management and control are to teach aggressive students (1) to recognize when they are angry and experience the emotional arousal associated with anger, (2) to identify the events that appear to trigger anger, (3) to recognize the unpleasant consequences that may result from the expression of anger, and (4) to learn appropriate methods for expressing anger. Coie, Underwood, and Lochman (1991) described a comprehensive program for improving social relations and reducing aggressive behavior that includes social problem-solving skills, positive-play training, group-entry skill training, and dealing with negative feelings.

Perhaps the most comprehensive program for reducing aggressive behavior that may translate to the playground is Reprogramming Environmental Contingencies for Effective Social Skills (RECESS) (Walker, Hops, & Greenwood, 1993). This program, targeted for grades K–3, includes four major components: (1) systematic training in cooperative, positive social behavior using prepared scripts, discussions, and role playing for the aggressive child and other class members, (2) a response–cost point system in which points are subtracted for inappropriate social behavior and rule infractions, (3) praise for positive, cooperative, and interactive behavior, and (4) concurrent group and individual reinforcement contingencies with group activity rewards available at school and individual rewards available at home. The RECESS program has proved to be successful (see Walker *et al.*, 1993, for details).

DISRUPTIVE BEHAVIOR IN THE CLASSROOM

Disruptive behavior in the classroom is difficult to manage and is likely to escalate from agitation to defiance and noncompliance and, finally, to verbal and physical abuse of others. A major dilemma is the discovery by teachers that management practices that have been successful in the past are not effective with disruptive students and may, in fact, exacerbate the problem.

Colvin (1993) described a seven-phase cycle illustrating how disruptive behavior escalates and de-escalates over the course of an incident. Space does not permit a discussion of these seven phases and the suggested interventions for each phase (see Colvin, 1993, for details).

INTERVENTION STRATEGIES

Most teacher interventions to manage disruptive behavior are based on social learning theory and applied behavior analysis (Baer, Wolf, & Risley, 1987; Bandura, 1973). It is assumed that disruptive behaviors are learned, and prosocial behaviors can be taught in their place. Two types may be used: behavior enhancement and behavior reduction strategies.

Interventions to Increase Desired Behavior

A number of strategies exist for enhancing behavior. A time-tested method is the use of *tangible reinforcement* in which material items that have reinforcing value are delivered immediately following desired behavior. Rhode, Jenson, and Reavis (1993) suggested that tangible reinforcement tends to be more effective with younger students who may not respond initially to teachers' social reinforcement.

The *opportunity to engage in desired behavior* as a reinforcer was first described by Premack (1959). The aggressive behavior of a 10-year-old student was reduced by making after-school activities contingent on progressively lower rates of disruptive behavior on the bus (e.g., pushing, hitting, name calling) (Jackson, Salzberg, Pacholl, & Dorsey, 1981).

In *token reinforcement* systems, earned tokens are exchanged for desired activities (Kazdin, 1982). For example, aggressive behavior was reduced when a 7-year-old student received stars exchangeable for time on the playground for every 2-min period during which no aggressive behaviors were exhibited (Deitz *et al.,* 1978).

In *contingency contracting,* a formal contract is negotiated between a student and teacher, parent, peer, or other person. The contract specifies the behavior to be increased or decreased, and the consequences associated with attaining or not attaining the goals (see Rutherford, 1975). Results have generally been found to be positive and a major contributor to behavior change (Rutherford & Polsgrove, 1981).

Modeling occurs when students observe adult or peer models performing and being reinforced for demonstrating prosocial behaviors. When students then initiate these behaviors, they are reinforced; reinforcement involves vicarious reinforcement when the model is being reinforced and direct reinforcement when the student performs the same behavior. Modeling is particularly useful for teaching complex prosocial behaviors and is typically implemented with other behavioral procedures.

Social reinforcement uses positive verbal and physical feedback, attention, and approval for desired student behaviors usually delivered by the teacher. In combination with other behavioral procedures, it is effective in increasing prosocial behaviors (Rutherford, Chipman, Di-Gangi, & Anderson, 1992). Walker and colleageus (1995) indicated that behavior-specific adult praise is a powerful form of attention that communicates approval and positive regard. Although students may not be responsive initially to adult praise because of a history of negative adult interactions, social reinforcement paired with other behavior-enhancement methods will eventually increase the value of praise.

Interventions to Decrease Disruptive Behavior

Disruptive behavior may be so well entrenched, aversive, and resistant to change that behavior-enhancement procedures used in isolation may not be effective and may need to be combined with behavior-reduction techniques. The use of *differential reinforcement* includes four strategies (see Deitz & Repp, 1983). Differential reinforcement of incompatible behavior (DRI) and differential reinforcement of alternative behavior (DRA) involve reinforcing behaviors that are incompatible with or that are alternatives to problem behaviors. Differential reinforcement of low rates of behavior (DRL) provides reinforcement when problem behavior occurs less than a specified amount during a period of time. Finally, differential reinforcement of the omission of behavior (DRO) requires the suppression of problem behavior for an entire time interval.

Both DRI and DRA increase behaviors that are incompatible with or alternative to aggressive behaviors, thus replacing the unwanted behavior. The DRL procedure is most effective in reducing minor misbehavior or in eliminating, in a stepwise process, a limited number of aggressive responses that may have been tolerated initially (e.g., Epstein, Repp, & Cullinan, 1978; Trice & Parker, 1983). For more severe behavior problems, DRO usually in combination with other techniques has been shown to be effective (e.g., Stainback, Stainback, & Dedrick, 1979).

The removal of reinforcers following the occurrence of undesired target behaviors (Response Cost) has been shown to be a powerful procedure for suppressing disruptive behaviors (Walker, 1983). Response cost most often involves either the removal of the opportunity to participate in specified activities or the removal of tokens representing "fines" in a token economy system following inappropriate behavior.

Response-contingent time-out or *time-out from positive reinforcement* is a procedure in which access to reinforcement is removed for a period of time following the occurrence of disruptive behavior. Time-out may be implemented at several levels (e.g., planned ignoring to seclusion) and is influenced by a number of factors (e.g., how it is applied, administration schedule, procedures for removing student from time-out). For disruptive behavior in young children, evidence supports the use of planned ignoring, time-out plus social reinforcement, (e.g., Pinkston, Reese, LeBlanc; & Baer, 1973), contingent observation time-out plus social reinforcement (e.g., Porterfield, Herbert-Jackson, & Risley,

1976), time-out to reduce stimuli plus group free time (e.g., Devine & Tomlinson, 1976), exclusion time-out plus social reinforcement (e.g., Firestone, 1976), and seclusion time-out plus social reinforcement (e.g., Walker, Hops, & Fiegenbaum, 1976).

In contrast, a number of behavior-reduction techniques have *not* proven to be effective in reducing disruptive behavior. These procedures include (1) *extinction* (Polsgrove & Reith, 1983), (2) *verbal reprimands* (Rutherford, 1983), (3) *physical punishment* (not often used in public school settings), and (4) *overcorrection* (Axelrod, Brantner, & Meddock, 1978).

DIRECT TEACHING OF PROSOCIAL BEHAVIOR

The behavioral procedures outlined in the preceding discussion are effective for managing disruptive behavior but must be supplemented by techniques that offer the possibility of teaching disruptive students new and appropriate behaviors, some of which have been discussed earlier (e.g., modeling). Two additional interventions have been used to reduce disruptive behavior and teach prosocial behavior.

Anger Management

Although behavioral approaches are effective in reducing overt aggressive behavior, disruptive students often have high levels of anger that are displayed in out-of-school interactions with adults and peers. Therefore, the direct treatment of high anger arousal, an antecedent of impulsive and explosive behavior, is an important strategy in managing aggressive behavior (Fendler & Ecton, 1986).

A number of anger-control programs have been developed. These include (1) Managing Anger Skills Training (Eggert, 1994), (2) Helping Kids Handle Anger: Teaching Self-Control (Huggins, 1992), (3) Stress Inoculation Training (Maag, Parks, & Rutherford, 1988; Meichenbaum, 1985), (4) "Think-Aloud" cognitive-behavioral approach (Camp, Blum, Hebert, & Van Doornick, 1977), (5) Adolescent Anger Control (Feindler & Ecton, 1986), (6) Aggression Replacement Training (Goldstein & Glick, 1987), and (7) comprehensive program for reducing aggressive behavior (Coie *et al.*, 1991). Each of these programs is a comprehensive intervention that attempts to aid students in identifying and controlling anger before it escalates into more overt aggressive and impulsive behavior.

Social Skills

Among the most often used strategies, and one that has received a great deal of attention over the past 10 years, is the direct teaching of social skills to promote prosocial behavior. The goal is to aid students in acquiring social skills needed to avoid interpersonal rejection and gain acceptance by adults and peers who often identify disruptive students as undesirable classmates and playmates (Dodge *et al.*, 1982). Similarly, teachers believe that disruptive students lack social skills and are more likely to violate social norms (Walker *et al.*, 1987).

Aggressive students also tend to misinterpret neutral situations as hostile or negative (e.g., Dodge & Frame, 1982; see also Chapter 14, this volume), to associate primarily with other antisocial students (Walker, Stieber, Ramsey, & O'Neill, 1990), and to realize that acting aggressively comes easily (i.e., aggressive impulses are difficult to inhibit and aggressive acts usually get them what they want) (Perry, Perry, & Rasmussen, 1986). Social skill deficits seem to underlie many of the problems experienced by aggressive students (Kazdin, 1995).

Classroom teachers tend to be intolerant of the behavior of disruptive students (e.g., Gersten, Walker, & Darch, 1988); this sometimes interferes with access to school-based support services and is a reason why a large percentage of aggressive students are excluded from school (Walker, Block-Pedego, Todis, & Severson, 1991).

Defining Social Skills

Social skills are difficult to define in either theoretical or practical terms. Van Hasselt, Hersen, Whitehill, and Bellack (1979) suggested that social skills are learned, situation-specific skills that lead to interpersonal effectiveness. Subsequently, social skill definitions became more differentiated. McFall (1982) distinguished between social competence and social skills. Social competence is evaluated on the basis of whether a social task has been performed competently. Social skills, on the other hand, represent *specific* behaviors exhibited in situations requiring competent performance on social tasks. For example, Walker and colleagues (1995) defined social skills as behaviors that (1) allow an individual to initiate and maintain positive social relationships, (2) contribute to peer acceptance and satisfactory school adjustment, and (3) allow an individual to cope effectively and adaptively with the larger social environment. The effectiveness of these skills in producing positive social outcomes (e.g., teacher and peer acceptance) is the basis for making judgments about social competence.

A further distinction was made by Gresham (1986b). For the case of social skill deficits, students do not possess the necessary skills to perform in a socially competent manner (e.g., not knowing how to make friends). A *skill* deficit exists when the student either does not know how to execute the skill or has never previously demonstrated the skill. A *performance* deficit exists when a student possesses the requisite social skill but does not perform it or does not do so at acceptable levels.

In addition to problems in defining social skill deficits, there are also measurement problems (Gresham, 1986a). Maag (1989) described how most measures assess only gross levels of performance and may not be associated with desired outcomes such as positive peer relationships. Thus, measurement problems that limit precision are contributors to difficulties in defining social skills.

Although problematic, social skill deficits need to be assessed formally in order to avoid subjectivity in decision making about what needs to be taught. A number of social skill rating scales are available. The most comprehensive assessments are found in the Social Skills Rating System (Gresham & Elliott, 1990) and the Walker–McConnell Scale of Social Competence and School Adjustment (Walker & McConnell, 1988). In these approaches, information is generated by teacher ratings that can pinpoint specific problem areas that can then be used to guide the content and direction of the intervention.

Social Skills Training

Two major approaches can be identified: social skills training and interpersonal cognitive problem solving (social problem solving). The former is skills based and the latter is strategy based. Social skills training assumes that key behaviors underlie social competence and that these behaviors can be systematically taught. In contrast, social problem solving emphasizes the teaching of generic strategies for responding to social situations. Skills-based approaches tend to rely on direct instruction and use techniques such as coaching, modeling, behavioral rehearsal, feedback, reinforcement, role playing, and discussion (Zaragoza, Vaughn, & McIntosh, 1991). Strategy-based approaches focus on developing improved cognitive awareness of social situations and adaptive ways of responding to them; the actual procedures may include social problem solving, modeling, and self-instruction (Ager & Cole, 1991).

A number of social skills training programs have been developed to promote social competence in aggressive students. Alberg, Petry, and Eller (1994) developed a resource manual for selecting and guiding social skills training (see also Walker *et al.,* 1985). Two examples of widely used programs are provided by the Walker Social Skills Curriculum: ACCESS and ACEPTS (Walker *et al.,* 1983; Walker, Todis, Holmes, & Horton, 1988).

Meta-Analytic Evaluation of Social Skills Training

Kavale, Mathur, Forness, Rutherford, and Quinn (1997) investigated the effectiveness of social skills training using methods of meta-analysis (see Glass, McGaw, & Smith, 1981). From an initial pool of 133 studies, 34 were eliminated, primarily for lack of usable data,

leaving 99 as the database. The 99 studies included both group design and single-subject studies necessitating different procedures for calculating the Effect Size (ES) statistic. For group designs, the ES is the outcome variable represented by the mean of the treatment group minus the mean of the control group divided by the standard deviation of the control group. For single-subject studies, the ES equivalent is the percentage of nonoverlapping data (PND) between the treatment and the immediately preceding baseline phase (Scruggs, Mastropieri, & Casto, 1987).

The ES may be interpreted as a z-score and shows the level of improvement associated with social skills training. An ES of +1.00 indicates a one standard deviation superiority of the treatment group, which means that 84% of subjects receiving social skills training were better off than untreated (comparison) subjects. The PND may be interpreted directly: the larger the better. If PND = 100%, then the treatment would be deemed highly effective; PND = 0% represents no treatment efficacy. Within the context of applied behavior analysis, a PND of 75% or better indicates a useful treatment and a PND of 50% or below indicates a questionable intervention since in at least half the instances treatment produces an effect no better than that demonstrated during baseline.

Group Designs. The 35 group studies investigating the efficacy of social skills training produced a total of 328 ES measurements. The average ES ($\overline{ES}$) across all ES measurements was .199 with standard deviation (*SD*) of .541. The range of ES was −1.321 to +2.136 with a median of .161 suggesting a modest positive skew. However, 27% of ES were negative suggesting that, in better than one in four instances, better outcomes were found for students receiving no training.

The average disruptive student gained about eight percentile ranks on the outcome assessment; a modest gain that in Cohen's (1988) classification of ES magnitude would be termed "small." Thus, it would be difficult to endorse the inclusion of social skills training in a DBD intervention program.

Sixty-three percent of studies used training programs that were specifically designed for research purposes. The remaining 37% used either commercially available social skills training programs or programs already described in the literature. The experimental programs produced an $\overline{ES}$ of .194 (SD = .593) and established programs produced an $\overline{ES}$ of .203 (SD = .499). These $\overline{ES}$ approximate the overall $\overline{ES}$ (.199) and suggest that the nature of the program (experimental vs. established) had limited influence on outcomes.

Treatment efficacy was not influenced by either age of subjects or length of the training. The average training program lasted about 12 weeks with students receiving about $2\frac{1}{2}$ hr of training per week. When aggregated into two groupings representing more or less than the average 12 weeks of training, no differences were found.

Ratings of the quality (high, medium, low) of the research studies included were based primarily on criteria provided by Campbell and Stanley (1966) and those suggested by Lytton and Romney (1991). Sixty-five percent came from the medium research quality category and produced an $\overline{ES}$ (.194) that closely approximated the overall $\overline{ES}$ (.199). Although the high category produced the lowest $\overline{ES}$ (.179) and the low category the highest $\overline{ES}$ (.232), there were no significant differences among the $\overline{ES}$ associated with research quality.

Single-Subject Designs. The 64 single-subject studies produced a total of 463 graphs from which a PND could be calculated. The majority of studies used multiple baseline designs across subjects (34%), across behaviors (17%), or across settings (6%). The most often used method was a reversal design (ABAB).

The mean PND was 62% with an SD of 33% with 10% (n = 47) showing 0% and 22% (n = 103) showing 100% PND. The mean PND (62%) indicates only modest efficacy as it falls between the 50% (moderate) and 75% (good) figures. The correlation between PND and number of data points in the intervention phase was not significant (r = .086, p < .10)

suggesting no relationship between outcome and length of training.

The smallest PND (55%) was found at the preschool level, indicating limited effectiveness. The PND were similar at the elementary and secondary levels with both approximating the overall PND (62%). In both cases, the effects of social skills training was modest.

Overall Evaluation of Social Skills Training

Since social skill deficits are a very frequent accompaniment of DBD, much effort has been directed at ameliorating those deficits with social skills training. Our findings (i.e., Kavale *et al.,* 1997) suggest that such efforts have met with limited success and cannot be interpreted as an endorsement for interventions to enhance social skills.

In the context of special education, social skills training as a "special" intervention has the same modest effects associated with other special practices (e.g., perceptual-motor training [$\overline{ES}$ = .081], modality instruction [$\overline{ES}$ = .15], psycholinguistic training [$\overline{ES}$ = .391]) (see Kavale & Forness, 1998). Part of the difficulty of social skills training is that it deals with unobservable constructs that result in a variety of conceptual and definitional issues (e.g., Gresham, 1986a; McFall, 1982; Walker *et al.,* 1995) as well as a variety of measurement problems (e.g., Hughes & Sullivan, 1988; Maag, 1989).

A number of factors may contribute to the modest effects found for social skills training. A majority of studies used training programs specifically designed for research purposes; these were found to be of limited status as determined from the descriptions provided. Consequently, it was difficult to determine what was actually happening during training.

The length of training may also have limited outcomes. Recall that the average training program lasted about 12 weeks with only about $2\frac{1}{2}$ hr per week devoted to training. Although no differences were found between programs above or below this average, it may be that even with the longer programs, the time allocated to modify social functioning was insufficient. Future efforts should direct attention to determining whether more training results in larger effects. We repeat, however, that the literature examined did not offer compelling evidence about the efficacy of social skills training, particularly with DBD students.

CONCLUSIONS

Disruptive behavior is becoming more problematic in the schools. Children and youth are involved in aggressive and disruptive behavior at ever younger ages (American Psychological Association, 1993). Schools are thus facing complex challenges but are often not prepared to cope with such extensive and involved problems. Traditionally, schools have employed such strategies as control, containment, punishment, and exclusion to deal with disruptive students. Fortunately, recent research has identified antecedents of DBD and has led to the development of new and better strategies for reducing it.

It has become evident that proactive strategies, in which new skills are taught systematically, offer an advantage over reactive strategies (e.g., punishment) primarily because prevention approaches are not dependent on the (unwanted) occurrence of the disruptive behavior. Because the disruptive behavior is likely to occur at low rates, although it may be of high intensity, proactive strategies have the further advantage of permitting positive instruction to be delivered far more frequently. Finally, proactive strategies tend to be less intrusive and more effective than interventions applied after the behavior has occurred.

Most important, the techniques outlined in this chapter represent best practice and not magical cures. Disruptive behavior tends to become ingrained quite early and is often highly resistant to change. Therefore, interventions must be applied comprehensively and systematically to be useful and must also be monitored carefully so practitioners can adjust and adapt interventions to enhance effectiveness. It is only under these circumstances that the established patterns of disruptive behavior can be modified and replaced with more prosocial behavior.

REFERENCES

Ager, C., & Cole, C. (1991). A review of cognitive-behavioral interventions for children and adolescents with behavioral disorders. *Behavioral Disorders. 16,* 276–287.

Alberg, J., Petry, C., & Eller, A. (1994). *A resource guide for social skills instruction.* Longmont, CO: Sopris West.

American Psychological Association. (1993). *Violence and youth: Psychology's response.* Washington, DC: Author.

Axelrod, S., Brantner, J. P., & Meddock, T. D. (1978). Overcorrection: A review and critical analysis. *Journal of Special Education, 12,* 367–391.

Baer, D. M., Wolf, M. M., & Risley, T. R. (1987). Some still current dimensions of applied behavior analysis. *Journal of Applied Behavior Analysis, 20,* 313–328.

Bandura, A. (1973). *Aggression: A social learning analysis.* Englewood Cliffs, NJ: Prentice Hall.

Bullis, M., & Walker, H. M. (1994). *Comprehensive school-based systems for troubled youth.* Eugene: University of Oregon, Center on Human Development.

Camp, B. W., Blum, G., Hebert, F., & Van Doornick, W. (1977). "Think-Aloud": A program for developing self-control in aggressive young boys. *Journal of Abnormal Child Psychology, 5,* 152–169.

Campbell, D. T., & Stanley, J. C. (1966). *Experimental and quasi-experimental designs for research.* Chicago: Rand McNally.

Cangelosi, J. S. (1992). *Systematic teaching strategies.* New York: Longman.

Clapp, B. (1989). The discipline challenge. *Instructor, 99,* 32–34.

Cohen, J. (1988). *Statistical power analysis for the behavioral sciences* (2nd ed.). Hillsdale, NJ: Erlbaum.

Coie, J., Underwood, M., & Lochman, J. (1991). Programmatic intervention with aggressive children in the school setting. In D. Pepler & K. Rubin (Eds.), *The development and treatment of childhood aggression* (pp. 389–407). Hillsdale, NJ: Erlbaum.

Colvin, G. (1993). *Managing acting-out behavior.* Eugene, OR: Behavior Associates.

Colvin, G. T., & Sugai, G. M. (1988). Proactive strategies for managing social behavior problems: An instructional approach. *Education and Treatment of Children, 11,* 341–348.

Deitz, D. E., & Repp, A. C. (1983). Reducing behavior through reinforcement. *Exceptional Education Quarterly, 3,* 34–46.

Deitz, S. M., Slack, D. J., Schwarzmueller, E. G., Wilander, A. P., Weatherly, T. J., & Hilliard, G. (1978). Reducing inappropriate behavior in special classrooms by reinforcing average interresponse times: Interval DRL. *Behavior Therapy, 9,* 37–46.

Devine, V. T., & Tomlinson, J. R. (1976). The "workclock": An alternative to token economies in the management of classroom behaviors. *Psychology in the Schools, 13,* 163–170.

Dodge, K. (1996). Social information processing variables in the development of aggression and altruism in children. In C. Zahn-Waxler, E. M. Cummings, & R. Ianotti (Eds.), *Altruism and aggression: Biological and social origins* (pp. 280–302). New York: Cambridge University Press.

Dodge, K., & Frame, C. L. (1982). Social cognitive biases and deficits in aggressive boys. *Child Development, 53,* 620–635.

Dodge, K., Coie, J., & Brakke, N. (1982). Behavior patterns of socially rejected and neglected adolescents: The roles of social approach and aggression. *Journal of Abnormal Child Psychology, 10,* 389–410.

Dodge, K., Pettit, G., McClaskey, C., & Brown, M. (1986). *Social competence in children* (Monographs of the Society for Research in Child Development, 51 [2, Serial No. 213]).

Drummond, T. (1993). *The Student Risk Screening Scale (SRSS).* Grants Pass, OR: Josephine County Mental Health Program.

Eggert, D. L. (1994). *Anger management for youth: Stemming aggression and violence.* Bloomington, IN: National Educational Service.

Epstein, M. H., Repp, A. C., & Cullinan, D. (1978). Decreasing "obscene" language of behaviorally disordered children through the use of a DRL schedule. *Psychology in the Schools, 15,* 419–423.

Evertson, C. M., Emmer, E. T., Clements, B. S., Sanford, J. P., & Worsham, M. E. (1984). *Classroom management for elementary teachers.* Englewood Cliffs, NJ: Prentice-Hall.

Feindler, E. L., & Ecton, R. B. (1986). *Adolescent anger control: Cognitive-behavioral techniques.* New York: Pergamon.

Firestone, P. (1976). The effects and side effects of time-out on an aggressive nursery school child. *Journal of Behavior Therapy and Experimental Psychiatry, 6,* 79–81.

Forness, S. R., & Knitzer, J. (1992). A new proposed definition and terminology to replace "seriously emotional disturbance" in the Individuals with Disabilities Education Act. *School Psychology Review, 21,* 12–20.

Gagnon, C. (1991). School based interventions for aggressive children: Possibilities, limitations and future directions. In D. Pepler & K. Rubin (Eds.), *The development and treatment of childhood aggression* (pp. 449–450). Hillsdale, NJ: Erlbaum.

Gersten, R., Walker, H. M., & Darch, C. (1988). Relationships between teachers' effectiveness and their tolerance for handicapped students. *Exceptional Children, 54,* 433–438.

Gettinger, M. (1988). Methods of pro-active classroom management. *School Psychology Review, 17,* 227–242.

Glass, G. V., McGaw, B., & Smith, M. L. (1981). *Meta-analysis in social research.* Beverly Hills, CA: Sage.

Goldstein, A. P., & Glick, B. (1987). *Aggression replacement training.* Champaign, IL: Research Press.

Gresham, F. M. (1986a). Conceptual and definitional issues in the assessment of social skills: Implications for classification and training. *Journal of Clinical Child Psychology, 15,* 16–25.

Gresham, F. M. (1986b). Conceptual issues in the assessment of social competence in children. In P. S. Strain, M. J. Guralnick, & H. M. Walker (Eds.), *Children's social behavior: Development, assessment, and modification* (pp. 143–179). New York: Academic Press.

Gresham, F. M., & Elliott, S. (1990). *The social skills rating system (SSRS).* Circle Pines, MN: American Guidance.

Hawkins, J. D., VonCleve, E., & Catalano, R. F., Jr. (1991). Reducing early childhood aggression: Results of a primary prevention program. *Journal of the American Academy of Child and Adolescent Psychiatry, 30,* 208–217.

Hersh, R. H., & Walker, H. M. (1983). Great expectations: Making schools effective for all students. *Policy Studies Review, 2* (Special No. 1), 147–188.

Hinshaw, S. (1992). Externalizing behavior problems and academic underachievement in childhood and adolescence: Causal relationships and underlying mechanisms. *Psychological Bulletin, 111,* 127–155.

Hinshaw, S., Han, S., Erhardt, D., & Huber, A. (1992). Internalizing and externalizing behavior problems in preschool children: Correspondence among parent and teacher ratings and behavior observations. *Journal of Clinical Child Psychology, 21,* 143–150.

Hoover, J., & Juul, K. (1993). Bullying in Europe and the U.S. *Journal of Emotional and Behavioral Problems, 2,* 25–29.

Huggins, P. (1992). *Helping kids handle anger: Teaching self-control.* Longmont, CO: Sopris West.

Hughes, J. N., & Sullivan, K. A. (1988). Outcome assessment in social skills training with children. *Journal of School Psychology, 26,* 167–183.

Jackson, A. T., Salzberg, C. L., Pacholl, B., & Dorsey, D. S. (1981). The comprehensive rehabilitation of a behavior problem child in his home and community. *Education and Treatment of Children, 4,* 195–215.

Kameenui, E. J., & Simmons, D. C. (1990). *Designing instructional strategies: The prevention of academic and learning problems.* Columbus, OH: Merrill.

Kavale, K. A., & Forness, S. R. (1998). *Efficacy of special education and related services.* Washington, DC: American Association on Mental Retardation.

Kavale, K. A., Mathur, S. R., Forness, S. R., Rutherford, R. G., & Quinn, M. M. (1997). The effectiveness of social skills training for students with emotional or behavioral disorders: A meta-analysis. In T. E. Scruggs & M. A. Mastropieri (Eds.), *Advances in learning and behavioral disabilities* (Vol. 11, pp. 1–26). Greenwich, CT: JAI.

Kazdin, A. E. (1982). The token economy: A decade later. *Journal of Applied Behavior Analysis, 15,* 431–445.

Kazdin, A. E. (Ed.). (1985). *Treatment of antisocial behavior in children and adolescents.* Pacific Grove, CA: Brooks/Cole.

Kazdin, A. E. (1995). *Conduct disorders in childhood and adolescence* (2nd ed.). Thousand Oaks, CA: Sage.

Knitzer, J., Steinberg, Z., & Fleisch, B. (1990). *At the school house door: An examination of programs and policies for children with behavioral and emotional problems.* New York: Bank Street College of Education.

Kovacs, M., Paulauskas, S., Gatsonis, C., & Richards, C. (1988). Depressive disorders in childhood: A longitudinal study of comorbidity with and risk for conduct disorders. *Journal of Affective Disorders, 15,* 205–217.

Lytton, H., & Romney, D. (1991). Parents' differential socialization of boys and girls: A meta-analysis. *Psychological Bulletin, 190,* 267–296.

Maag, J. W. (1989). Assessment in social skills training: Methodological and conceptual issues for research and practice. *Remedial and Special Education, 10,* 6–17.

Maag, J. W., Parks, B. T., & Rutherford, R. B. (1988). Generalization and behavior covariation of aggression in children receiving stress inoculation therapy. *Child and Family Behavior Therapy, 10,* 29–47.

McFall, R. (1982). A review and reformulation of the concept of social skills. *Behavioral Assessment, 4,* 1–33.

Meichenbaum, D. (1985). *Stress inoculation training.* New York: Pergamon.

Olweus, D. (1991). Bully/victim problems among school children: Basic facts and effects of a school-based intervention program. In D. Pepler & K. Rubin (Eds.), *The development and treatment of childhood aggression* (pp. 411–446). Hillsdale, NJ: Erlbaum.

Paine, S. C., Radicchi, J., Rosellini, L. C., Deutchman, L., & Darch, C. B. (1983). *Structuring your classroom for academic success.* Champaign, IL: Research Press.

Patterson, G. R., DeBaryshe, B. D., & Ramsey, E. (1989). A developmental perspective on antisocial behavior. *American Psychologist, 44,* 329–335.

Pepler, D., & Rubin, D. (1991). *The development and treatment of childhood aggression.* Hillsdale, NJ: Erlbaum.

Perry, D. G., Perry, L. C., & Rasmussen, P. (1986). Cognitive social learning mediators of aggression. *Child Development, 57,* 700–711.

Pinkston, E. M., Reese, N. M., LeBlanc, J. M., & Baer, D. M. (1973). Independent control of a preschool child's aggression and peer interaction by contingent teacher attention. *Journal of Applied Behavior Analysis, 6,* 115–124.

Polsgrove, L. J., & Reith, H. (1983). Procedures for reducing children's inappropriate behavior in special education settings. *Exceptional Education Quarterly, 3,* 20–33.

Porterfield, J. K., Herbert-Jackson, E., & Risley, T. R. (1976). Contingent observation: An effective and acceptable procedure for reducing disruptive behavior of young children in a group setting. *Journal of Applied Behavior Analysis, 9,* 55–64.

Premack, D. (1959). Toward empirical behavior laws: I. Positive reinforcement. *Psychological Review, 66,* 219–233.

Reid, J. (1993). Prevention of conduct disorder before and after school entry: Relating interventions to developmental findings. *Development and Psychopathology, 5,* 243–262.

Rhode, G., Jenson, W. R., & Reavis, H. K. (1993). *The tough kid book: Practical classroom management strategies.* Longmont, CO: Sopris West.

Rutherford, R. B. (1975). Establishing behavioral contracts with delinquent adolescents. *Federal Probation, 34,* 28–32.

Rutherford, R. B. (1983). Theory and research on the use of aversive procedures in the education of moderately behaviorally disordered and emotionally disturbed children and youth. In F. H. Wood & K. C. Lakin (Eds.), *Punishment and aversive stimulation in special education* (pp. 41–64). Reston, VA: Council for Exceptional Children.

Rutherford, R. B., & Polsgrove, L. J. (1981). Behavioral contracting with behaviorally disordered and delinquent children and youth: An analysis of the clinical and experimental literature. In R. B. Rutherford, A. G. Prieto, & J. E. McGlothlin (Eds.), *Severe behavior disorders of children and youth* (Vol. 4, pp. 49–69). Reston, VA: Council for Children with Behavioral Disorders.

Rutherford, R. B., Chipman, J., DiGangi, S. A., & Anderson, K. (1992). *Teaching social skills: A practical instructional approach.* Ann Arbor, MI: Exceptional Innovations.

Scruggs, T. E., Mastropieri, M. A., & Casto, G. (1987). The quantitative synthesis of single-subject research: Methodology and validation. *Remedial and Special Education, 8,* 24–33.

Smylie, M. A. (1988). The enhancement function of staff development: Organizational and psychological antecedents to individual teacher change. *American Educational Research, 25,* 1–30.

Sprick, R. (1994). School-wide discipline policies: An instructional classroom management approach. In E. Kameenui & C. Darch (Eds.), *Instructional classroom management* (pp. 179–200). White Plains, NY: Longman.

Stainback, W., Stainback, S., & Dedrick, C. (1979). Controlling severe maladaptive behaviors. *Behavioral Disorders, 4,* 99–115.

Trice, A. D., & Parker, F. C. (1983). Decreasing adolescent swearing in an instructional setting. *Education and Treatment of Children, 6,* 29–35.

Van Hasselt, V., Hersen, M., Whitehill, M., & Bellack, A. (1979). Social skill assessment and training for children: An evaluative review. *Behavior Research and Therapy, 17,* 413–437.

Walker, H. M. (1983). Applications of response cost in school settings: Outcomes, issues and recommendations. *Exceptional Education Quarterly, 3,* 47–55.

Walker, H. M. (1993). Antisocial behavior in school. *Journal of Emotional and Behavior Problems, 2,* 20–24.

Walker, H. M., & McConnell, S. R. (1988). *The Walker–McConnell scale of social competence and school adjustment.* Austin, TX: PRO-ED.

Walker, H. M., & Reid, J. (1997). *Long-term follow-up of antisocial and at-risk boys: Stability, change and group differences over a decade.* Unpublished report, Institute on

Violence and Destructive Behavior, University of Oregon, Eugene.

Walker, H. M., & Severson, H. H. (1990). *Systematic screening for behavior disorders (SSBD): User's guide and technical manual.* Longmont, CO: Sopris West.

Walker, H. M., Hops, H., & Fiegenbaum, E. (1976). Deviant classroom behavior as a function of combinations of social and token reinforcement and cost contingency. *Behavior Therapy, 7,* 76–88.

Walker, H. M., McConnell, S. R., Holmes, D., Todis, B., Walker, J., & Golden, N. (1983). *The Walker social skills curriculum: The ACCEPTS program (a curriculum for children's effective peer and teacher skills).* Austin, TX: PRO-ED.

Walker, H. M., Hops, H., .& Greenwood, C. R. (1984). The CORBEH research and development model: Programmatic issues and strategies. In S. Paine, G. T. Bellamy, & B. Wilcox (Eds.), *Human services that work* (pp. 57–78). Baltimore: Brookes.

Walker, H. M., McConnell, S. R., & Clarke, J. Y. (1985). Social skills training in school settings: A model for the social integration of handicapped children into less restrictive settings. In R. McMahon & R. D. Peters (Eds.), *Childhood disorders: Behavioral-developmental approaches* (pp. 140–168). New York: Brunner/Mazel.

Walker, H. M., Shinn, M. R., O'Neill, R. E., & Ramsey, E. (1987). A longitudinal assessment of the development of antisocial behavior in boys: Rationale, methodology and first year results. *Remedial and Special Education, 8,* 7–16, 27.

Walker, H. M., Todis, B., Holmes, D., & Horton, G. (1988). *The Walker social skills curriculum: The ACCESS program (adolescent curriculum for communication and effective social skills).* Austin, TX: PRO-ED.

Walker, H. M., Stieber, S., Ramsey, E., & O'Neill, R. E. (1990). School behavioral profiles of arrested versus nonarrested adolescents. *Exceptionality, 1,* 249–265.

Walker, H. M., Block-Pedego, A., Todis, B., & Severson, H. (1991). *School archival records search (SARS): User's guide and technical manual.* Longmont, CO: Sopris West.

Walker, H. M., Hops, H., & Greenwood, C. (1993). *RECESS: A program for reducing negative-aggressive behavior.* Seattle, WA: Educational Achievement Systems.

Walker, H. M., Severson, H. H., & Feil, E. G. (1994). *The Early Screening Project: A proven child-find process.* Longmont, CO: Sopris West.

Walker, H. M., Stieber, S., Ramsey, E., O'Neill, R. E., & Eisert, D. (1994). *Psychosocial correlates of at-risk status among adolescent boys: Static and dynamic relationships.* Unpublished report, Institute on Violence and Destructive Behavior, University of Oregon, Eugene.

Walker, H. M., Colvin, G., & Ramsey, E. (1995). *Antisocial behavior in school: Strategies and best practices.* Pacific Grove, CA: Brooks/Cole.

Wong, K., Kauffman, J., & Lloyd, J. W. (1991). Choices for integration: Selecting teachers for mainstreamed students with emotional or behavioral disorders. *Intervention in School and Clinic, 27,* 108–115.

Zaragoza, N., Vaughn, S., & McIntosh, R. (1991). Social skills interventions and children with behavior problems: A review. *Behavioral Disorders, 16,* 260–275.

Zigler, E., Taussig, C., & Black, K. (1992). Early childhood intervention: A promising preventative for juvenile delinquency. *American Psychologist, 47,* 997–1006.

21

Pharmacotherapy and Toxicology of Oppositional Defiant Disorder and Conduct Disorder

BRUCE WASLICK, JOHN S. WERRY,
and LAURENCE L. GREENHILL

INTRODUCTION

The development of specific treatments for the symptoms of Oppositional Defiant Disorder (ODD) and Conduct Disorder (CD) is a priority area for child and adolescent mental health. Antisocial behavior committed by children and adolescents has been on the rise and has been likened to an epidemic (Whitman, Benbow, & Good, 1996). Violence and criminal behavior attributed to adolescents continue to lead to substantial personal and social costs (Yoshikawa, 1994). However, as of yet there are few if any psychosocial treatments that have been clearly shown to reduce the personal and social impacts of juvenile antisocial behavior in a durable and reliable way (see Chapters 22 & 23, this volume). In some areas of child and adolescent psychopathology, pharmacotherapy offers a powerful approach in the treatment of mental disorders, and it is therefore important to look at the value of drug treatment in children with CD.

Psychopharmacologic intervention is predicated on the idea that certain forms of Disruptive Behavior Disorders (DBD) are at least partly attributable to and maintained by underlying patterns of or disturbances in brain function, represented by neurochemical, anatomical, or neurocircuitry changes in some functional area of the brain. These changes can be pathologically based or learned. As is seen later in this chapter, medications primarily have been used in CD to reduce levels of aggressive behavior or the emotional arousal and reactivity preceding aggressive action.

Animal models of aggression offer a means of testing hypotheses about the biological basis of aggressive behavior and provide an arena for the preclinical testing of drugs. Promising preclinical strategies of reducing aggressive behavior in animals have begun to be applied to human subjects with, as of yet, mixed results. In addition, medications developed or used for other indications distinct from DBD, whether discovered by serendipity or through rational drug-selection strategies, have been tested as therapeutic antiaggression agents. The purpose of this chapter is to briefly

BRUCE WASLICK and LAURENCE L. GREENHILL • Division of Child Psychiatry, New York State Psychiatric Institute/Columbia University, New York, New York 10032.   JOHN S. WERRY • Department of Psychiatry, University of Auckland, Auckland, New Zealand.

Handbook of Disruptive Behavior Disorders, edited by Quay and Hogan. Kluwer Academic/Plenum Publishers, New York, 1999.

discuss a theoretical basis for pharmacologic strategies targeting the reduction of aggressive behavior and other key behaviors present in CD and to summarize preclinical and clinical studies that have applied these strategies to aggressive children and adolescents. Because of the strong association of CD with alcohol and drug abuse, discussion of the pharmacology of these substances is included.

SUMMARY OF NODAL SYMPTOMS AND BEHAVIORS OF ODD AND CD

Overview

Verbal and physical aggression is one of the key features of children and adolescents with DBD. As was discussed in Chapter 1 (this volume), in the DSM-IV (American Psychiatric Association, 1994) aggression to people and animals is one of the four subcategories of behavior problems that has been highlighted as a feature of CD, and includes behavior such as bullying and threatening, fighting, weapon usage, physical cruelty, face-to-face robbery, and forcible sexual activity. These are overtly aggressive and potentially harmful actions that are directly perpetrated on others. They are distinguished from what can be thought of as more covert or rule-breaking symptoms that have the potential for less direct harm to other individuals, or behaviors that are meant to be destructive of property and not directly harmful to people. In the past this distinction between symptom clusters had been the basis of subtyping CD. As discussed in Chapter 1 (this volume), the DSM-IV (American Psychiatric Association, 1994) subtyping, now based on age of onset, nevertheless remains closely associated with the aggressive versus nonaggressive symptom clusters.

In children with ODD, overt aggression and violation of the safety or rights of others is a less prominent feature, but certain symptoms contain the seeds of aggressive responding. Loss of temper, frequent arguing, defiance of adult requests, deliberate annoyance of others, and spitefulness or vindictiveness all imply the potential for aggressive behavior. These symptoms have been thought to be, at least in some children, precursors of escalating antisocial and directly violent behavior, and indeed a high percentage of individuals who proceed to early-onset CD pass through a phase of predominantly ODD behavior patterns (see Chapter 1, this volume).

It appears that, at least to some extent, aggressive behavior has been conserved in the evolution of modern animal species. Animals display different types of aggression that may be common to many species or may be specific to a single particular species. There have been many attempts to describe and categorize patterns of animal aggression. Building on Moyer's (1968) classification of aggression into predatory, intermale, fear-induced, territorial, irritable, sex-related, maternal, and instrumental forms, Reis (1971, 1974) distinguished two major subtypes of aggression: (1) affective and (2) predatory. Affective aggression in animals is characterized by hyperarousal and increased sympathetic activity, and can further be divided into offensive and defensive subcategories (Mann, 1995). Predatory aggression, often occurring between animal species as opposed to within a single species (as is more characteristic of affective aggression), generally occurs with low levels of arousal (Eichelman, 1992). Vitiello, Behar, Hunt, Stoff, and Ricciuti (1990) have investigated and hypothesized about the distinction between affective and predatory aggression in children and adolescents with DBD and found the distinction to be useful in approaching therapeutic interventions for child psychiatric patients. Similar distinctions between types of aggression in children have been proposed as a way of subtyping CD (see Chapter 1, this volume).

Thus, it appears logical to postulate that the appropriate candidates for pharmacological alleviation of aggressive behavior manifest a primarily emotionally or affectively based form of aggressive responding to provoking stimuli (Campbell, Gonzalez, & Silva, 1992). This is because the power of current psychopharmacological agents to reduce arousal is greater than their capacity to change instrumental or specific behavior. Highly planned, goal-directed rule-breaking or criminal activity may be more learning-based than emotional-based and may be less "hard-wired" in neuropathological lesions or circuitry aberrations (Vitiello *et al.,* 1990). The individual who responds aggressively in a more impulse-driven manner, reacting with fear or anger toward provocative stimuli and performing acts of aggression in a state of affective arousal, is contrasted with the low levels of emotional and physiological arousal of individuals manifesting highly planned antisocial behavior.

Theoretical Foundations

The precise neurobiological mechanisms that lead to aggressive, antisocial responding in humans are not yet determined. However, psychobiological models exist that contribute to our understanding of aggressive behavior and, at least in part, provide explanation of the mechanism for some of our current pharmacologic intervention strategies. Chapters 8 and 17 (this volume) provide information on the biological bases of ODD and CD and these are not reiterated here. However, two general psychobiological models that provide broad theoretical foundations for antisocial behavior are briefly summarized, and the interested reader is directed to the cited references for more detailed discussions.

The first model of relevance is that of Gray (1982a, 1982b, 1987a, 1987b), advanced in a series of works (reviewed in Quay, 1993) summarizing models of brain function in animals and humans. He postulates three distinct but functionally interrelated brain systems that regulate organism functioning, particularly instrumental learning and emotion. The Behavioral Inhibition System (BIS), which is represented in the brain primarily by noradrenergic (NE) projections from the locus ceruleus and serotonergic (5-HT) projections from the brainstem raphe nuclei to diverse areas of the lower brain and higher cortical centers, reduces the frequency of a response, especially when the organism senses that punishment is likely or that little chance of reward is present. Gray postu-

lates that the primary emotional experiences that result from activity in this system are anxiety and frustration.

The Reward System (REW), primarily linked to dopaminergic (DA) projections, controls behavior that is motivated by the prospect of reward and the escape from or avoidance of punishment. This system directs behavior to approach or actively avoid or escape stimuli, based in part on the likelihood of experiencing reward or relief from punishment. Emotional representations of this system correspond to hope and relief. According to Gray this system underlies most types of predatory aggression.

The third system is the Fight/Flight System (F/F), which is primarily activated during times of perceived threats to the organism, resulting in defensive actions or flight behavior. Aggressive behavior can therefore result from enhanced or diminished function in these three systems: (1) A poorly functioning BIS (perhaps a hyposerotonergic state) can lead to uninhibited, impulsive behavior, (2) a hyperfunctioning (hyperdopaminergic state) REW can lead to enhanced levels of predatory aggression, or (3) a supersensitive F/F can lead to exaggerated defensive reaction (fight or flight) to minimal provocative stimuli.

Gray's model has some similarities with a model of psychobiological brain function of Cloninger, advanced primarily in his theoretical papers (Cloninger, Svrakic, & Przybeck, 1993) dealing with personality characteristics and underlying temperament. Cloninger's original tridimensional model of human temperament diathesis consisted of three factors: (1) "novelty seeking," a characteristic primarily driven by DA functioning, which drives the individual to seek out new sources of stimulation and avoidance of monotony and punishment; (2) "harm avoidance," presumably a 5-HT-mediated factor, which leads to inhibition of behavior that direct the individual toward strongly perceived, aversive experience; and (3) "reward dependence," an NE-derived trait which relates to how strongly the individual maintains behaving in a particular way based on past or present experiences of reward. A fourth temperament factor has more recently been added and is referred to as "persistence," which relates to the individual's capacity to persevere in the face of fatigue or frustrated efforts. Harm avoidance correlates well with the BIS of Gray, with the characteristic of inhibition of behavior that leads to punishment being a feature of intactness of the biological (5-HT) system moderating it. The REW system of Gray has features in common with both novelty seeking and reward dependence of Cloninger and the F/F system of Gray has no direct correlate in Cloninger's model except for some features of the harm avoidance factor. Predatory aggression in Cloninger's model may result from excess novelty seeking traits, low harm avoidance concerns, or exaggerated reward dependence for previously rewarded aggressive experiences.

Neither of these models was specifically generated to address the range of aggressive behavior seen in humans or animals, and the models are not based on empirical studies of DBD children. However, the psychobiological premises advanced by these theories have been extended to many types of disordered behavior. Particularly attractive to psychobiological models of human aggression is the fact that the theories postulate long-standing, for all practical purposes temperament, biologically mediated traits that relate well to the chronic disease that is CD in children and adolescents. The models also have been used to attempt to explain the biological effects of various pharmacological interventions in human aggression. Gray's (1982a) model in particular has led to a variety of behavioral studies of both CD and Attention-Deficit/Hyperactivity Disorder (ADHD) children (see Quay, 1993, 1997).

NEUROLEPTICS

History and Classification

Because these drugs have figured so prominently historically and are still in widespread use in the management of CD, they are discussed in more detail than most other drugs except stimulants. Most of what follows here

unreferenced is a synopsis of authoritative pharmacological texts (e.g. Reiss & Aman, 1998; Rall, Nies, & Taylor, 1991; Werry & Aman, in press) and reviews (Campbell & Cueva, 1995a, 1995b; Ernst et al., in press; Schroeder, 1988; Stoewe, Kruesi, & Lelio, 1995; Werry, 1994; Whitaker & Rao, 1992) where more detail and supporting studies can be obtained.

Neuroleptics were among the first of the modern psychiatric drugs to be discovered with the advent of chlorpromazine in 1950. The original name for this class of drug given by the French discoverers was neuroleptic or "lowering of neurological tension," but in keeping with other pharmacological trends that emphasize the therapeutic action of drugs, these drugs are now equally often referred to as antipsychotics. This is in keeping with their main and most strikingly effective use, but it does little credit to the wide range of other uses particularly in child psychopathology. Chlorpromazine was quickly followed by a large number of analogs such as thioridazine and haloperidol, but it was not until the past decade that there was any substantial change or innovation in this class of drug with the advent into clinical use of the "atypical" antipsychotics such as clozapine and respirodone, the number of which is now growing rapidly. One way or another, the neuroleptics have been used over the past 50 years in millions of patients including children and adolescents, often in high doses and for many years. They are among the best studied drugs in medicine. Although they were discovered serendipitously and their use initially was empirical, efforts to discover how they produced their therapeutic effects have rendered them major tools in the study of brain function in health and disease.

Neuroleptics can be grouped usefully into three main classes: (1) atropinic or low potency, (2) high potency, and (3) atypical. The term *potency* is somewhat misleading since it suggests that the low-potency drugs are not as effective as the high. This is true only in terms of milligram dose required to achieve the same effect (mostly in ratios of 50:1) but if the proper dose is used for each drug, the quality of therapeutic effects is the same. Though these drugs have common actions, these three divisions are indicative of the main differences in pharmacological profile. One benefit of this classification is that it defines the predominant non-core side effects (atropinic versus extrapyramidal).

Clinical Effects

As the name neuroleptic suggests, these drugs have the capacity to reduce the level of activation in the central nervous system and this effect is most relevant to CD since the active, externalized behavior is the cause of concern in that disorder. The earliest and most characteristic manifestation of neurolepsis is a special type of sedation, called ataraxis, in which the patient can be readily aroused with sufficiently strong stimulation and which blandness of affect and lack of interest in the environment is more prominent than sleep. However, the most important feature of this type of sedation compared with the true sedatives such as alcohol, barbiturates, or benzodiazepines is that the neuroleptics do not produce a pleasurable mood and thus are seldom abused or produce dependence. It also means, however, that patients on the whole do not like the sensation produced by these drugs and they may complain that it makes them feel heavy, slow, and uninterested. Such unwelcome effects are dose dependent. Doses of neuroleptics used in schizophrenia and for the control of DBD in the past often have been unnecessarily high (see Ernst *et al.,* 1998; Reiss & Aman, in press).

Unwanted Effects

Most of these effects are predictable consequences of the pharmacological profiles of action of the drug concerned. Occasionally there may be idiosyncratic effects that are probably related to some individual sensitivity to the drug. The most notable of these is the bone marrow depression that can occur with clozapine.

The most important side effects of this group of drugs lie in the four main areas discussed in the following sections.

Autonomic

These include increased heart rate which is of no significance but may cause undue alarm, lowered blood pressure especially on standing which may case faintness, dry mouth which is common in minor but annoying degrees, blurred vision, constipation, and initial oversedation.

Acute Extrapyramidal

These side effects are seen mostly with high-potency drugs and are dose dependent. Neuroleptics act by blocking DA in the key nigrostriatal tract; they cause down-regulation of the extrapyramidal system and thus a pharmacologically induced but reversible type of Parkinson's disease (increased tone and slow, rhythmic, 8 Hertz tremor; slowed and impaired motor movement, facial expression, gait, and posture). Young persons are particularly prone to acute dystonic reactions in which muscles of the head and neck may suddenly go into spasm; these reactions may be mistaken for tetanus or epilepsy. They tend to occur in the first few days after starting medication or increasing dosage and their cause is rather obscure but seems to be related primarily to DA function. They occur mainly at higher doses and above those that are indicated in CD, though some children are especially sensitive. Parkinsonism and dystonic reaction are easily treated and prevented by anticholinergic drugs such as benztropine or antihistamines such as diphenhydramine.

Probably the most important extrapyramidal side effect, however, is *akathisia,* which is a state of inner tension felt especially in the legs; it can be dispelled only by motor movement. Unfortunately, although antiparkinson and even adrenolytic (reduction of NE function) medications such as propanolol (discussed later) have been tried, there is usually no effective treatment for akathisia other than dosage reduction or a change of drug to a low-potency type.

There are a number of other much less common side effects appearing primarily as muscle spasms and spontaneous muscle movements (including tics) of which any prescriber of medication must be aware.

Late-Appearing (Tardive) Side Effects

Most of these affect the motor system and probably originate in the extrapyramidal system. Chronic blockade of DA receptors is thought in some cases to result in increased numbers or activity in those that remain. After some months or years of neuroleptic medication this can result in the appearance of *tardive dyskinesias*—spontaneous muscle movements affecting the face often in the form of chewing- or tongue-protruding-type movements. Unlike parkinsonian side effects they are slow and irregular and are most likely to be seen after dose reduction or cessation of medication because neuroleptics, though causing these, mute their appearance somewhat.

Less commonly, these dyskinesias may take the form of dystoniclike torsions of the head, neck, or trunk and appearance of Tourettelike syndrome has also been described.

In children and young persons, these tardive dyskinesias and dystonias are most commonly described as occurring after cessation of medication or as "withdrawal dyskinesis" which are neither severe nor conspicuous. There is dispute about whether or not tardive dyskinesias are permanent, but it now seems that in the majority of cases there is, as a minimum, considerable diminution in their severity with time in the absence of continued neuroleptic administration. They are thought to be more likely to occur in older persons and with longer term administration of medication. Only the atypical antipsychotics have a reputation for being less likely to cause tardive dyskinesias but that may well be a function of their recency since they do appear to be able to produce them (Ernst *et al.*, 1998).

Cognitive Dulling

There has been a great deal of concern in view of their ataractic sedative properties that neuroleptics could depress cognitive function and thus impair the most critical developmental function of learning, both academic and social. With the discovery of the critical role of acetylcholine in memory and the strong anticholinergic properties of the low-potency neuroleptics most commonly used in CD, this concern has increased. In fact, the various reviewers cited (most notably Ernst *et al.*, 1998; Schroeder, 1988; Whitaker & Rao, 1992) have all concluded first, that especially in CD, there has been insufficient study; second, that there is some evidence that in high doses, depression of cognitive function may occur; third, the balance of evidence so far does not support the idea that low-dose (less than 100-mg chlorpromazine equivalents) neuroleptic therapy depresses cognition (indeed, a few studies suggest facilitation); and fourth, that it makes best theoretical sense to use high-potency neuroleptics to minimize anticholinergic disruptions. It seems, then, that the key to avoiding any possible depression of cognition lies in minimal dosage with well-spaced intervals between dosage increments to allow dissipation of anticholinergic effects and where appropriate to use high-potency drugs such as haloperidol preferentially.

Other

There is a group of less frequent side effects such as skin sensitivities, obesity, menstrual disturbances, spontaneous lactation (galactorrhea), and seizures which occur occasionally and can be quite distressing. Most remit when medication is stopped or changed or the dose is lowered, and these side effects are infrequent.

Use in CD and ODD

In the absence of definite evidence that CD and ODD are distinct disorders rather than positions of severity (see Chapter 1, this volume), they are treated in this discussion as if they are the same except where there is specific evidence relating to ODD.

Ideally, as with any medication, clinical use would follow logically from a clear idea of what the underlying neurologic disturbances are. However, clinical use of the neuroleptics has developed out of empirical attempts to control undesirable behavior of CD; the outstanding target has been aggressive, violent behavior. With the rise of modern theorizing about CD discussed elsewhere in this handbook and summarized in the beginning of this chapter, it is possible to speculate that neuroleptics might have a nonspecific effect by, for example, lowering general motivation, that is, depressing the amount of behavior in general. This is basically a form of sedation and since all neuroleptics can produce ataratic sedation, there might be a useful role in CD where there is quantitatively a clear excess of behavior. However, this could result in reduction of prosocial behavior as well. Thus, use of medication in this way is more likely justifiable as a short-lived intervention in a crisis or at the start of a behavioral management program. It is also theoretically possible that by lowering the tone of the brain, the threshold of emotional arousal may be raised. As was discussed earlier in the chapter, reactive (stimulus-elicited) or emotive aggression might be reduced in frequency especially if medication were to be combined with social learning of alternative behaviors.

On the other hand, neuroleptics that block 5-HT, such as clozapine, might diminish inhibition of behavior and thus increase aggression. Since all neuroleptics have multiple effects, the outcome would depend on the predominant effect.

DA systems have been posited to be involved in the reward dominance that has been reported to be a problem in CD (see Quay, 1993). Thus, neuroleptics that block DA might reduce the amount of unacceptable behavior that represents perseverative-for-reward behavior. However, studies have not shown an excess of DA metabolites in CD or ODD (see Chapter 17, this volume). Another system that may be involved in aggression (probably both types, emotive *and* predatory or instrumental) is the adrenergic system. The low-potency neuroleptics have varying but sometimes quite strong adrenolytic actions and so might be useful in countering aggression.

Unfortunately, studies of the clinical use of neuroleptics are seldom designed to unscramble the hypothetically possible effects. To do so would require the use of assessment methods that clearly separated the target behaviors in line with the theoretical formulations. The most striking thing about studies of neuroleptics in CD is their paucity and poor quality. Most were done many years ago before the advent of proper diagnosis and clinical trial methodology. There seems to have been little recent interest in assessing neuroleptics in CD or ODD despite their considerable theoretical interest.

Summarizing such studies as there are, there is evidence to support the usefulness of the neuroleptics in low dosage in reduction of aggression, hostility, hyperactivity, and social unresponsiveness (Ernst *et al.,* 1998). However, effects are small and data limited. It is also not possible to separate out the posited greater effect on reactive or emotive aggression from predatory or instrumental aggression. The array of behaviors, however, suggests that the main effect of neuroleptics seen clinically is probably a nonspecific lowering of the tone of the nervous system (i.e., ataractic). The greatest, and in some ways best-documented use of neuroleptics in children and adolescents is in those who are developmentally disabled (although the quality of most of the older studies leaves much to be desired). Some of this arises from court orders in the 1970s and 1980s enforcing drug cessation in institutions in the United States (Schroeder, 1988). There seems to be general agreement that low-dose neuroleptics may be useful in reducing unwanted externalizing behaviors such as aggression. The implications for CD/ODD in those with developmental disabilities, however, can be only tenuously extrapolated (see Chapter 26, this volume).

Summary

Considering how serious and common CD is, and the evidence suggesting that neuroleptics may be of value in treating reactive aggression, impulsivity, and hyperactivity, there is a need to research this issue in greater detail, paying attention not only to proper diagnosis, but to modern neurological and theoretical formulations of psychopathology. The attitude in the United States that this should not be done because of the risk of tardive neurological syndromes pays little attention to the actual risks (which are low) as opposed to the costs to themselves, and to society, that children and young people with CD present. If the initial reputation of some of the atypical antipsychotics such a respiridone for producing fewer extrapyramidal side effects is sustained, this would be the ideal group of drugs to study. Trials of neuroleptics in children with ODD, however, are less defensible because although this disorder is troublesome it scarcely has the social valence of CD. In the meantime, there seems little objection to cautious, low-dosage use of neuroleptics in young persons with CD where emotive aggression is a problem. There seems little to choose among the various neuroleptics as far as efficacy is concerned but there is merit in trying low-potency drugs such as haloperidol first. It is hoped that clinical trials will show that respiridone offers not only equal efficacy but lower frequency of side effects than either high- or low-potency neuroleptics.

STIMULANTS

For a more detailed description of the pharmacology and mechanism of action of psychostimulants, see Chapter 10 (this volume). This material is not reviewed here; rather, the focus of this section is the use of stimulants specifically in modifying symptoms of CD and aggressive behavior.

Psychostimulants are thought to exert their primary neuropharmacologic effects by facilitating the release of norepinephrine (NE) and DA (reviewed in Hunt, Mandl, Lau, & Hughes, 1991). This release produces a wide variety of behaviors in humans and animals, but the bulk of data in animal models of aggression suggests that increases in NE and DA neurotransmission are positively correlated with levels of aggression (Mann, 1995). It therefore seems paradoxical that stimulants

have been shown to decrease aggressive behavior in some groups of children and adolescents. For the most part, psychostimulants have been determined to be effective in the reduction of aggressive behavior primarily in individuals who have ADHD in association with their aggressive behavior. Stimulants decrease motor activity level and reduce disinhibited behavior, both of which are cardinal features of ADHD, and this overall therapeutic effect may translate to reductions in aggression. Outside of the subgroup of individuals who have ADHD, there is little evidence that stimulants decrease aggressive behavior, although preliminary studies suggest that this class of drugs may be worthy of continued clinical investigation.

Stimulants have been used in attempts to decrease aggression in animal models of aggressive behavior. In mice and rat models, the psychostimulant amphetamine appears to have a dose-related effect on aggressive behavior, where low doses of amphetamine appear to stimulate aggressive behavior and moderate to high doses suppress it (Kulkarni & Plotnikoff, 1978). Methylphenidate (MPH) has been less well studied than amphetamine but appears to suppress aggressive behavior in mice (Miczek & O'Donnell 1978).

Stimulants have been demonstrated to reduce aggressive behavior in children with ADHD. Typical studies of children with ADHD involve separating the group into aggressive and nonaggressive subtypes and comparing treatment response between the groups. MPH decreases overall aggression in both aggressive and nonaggressive children with ADHD, demonstrating that the effects of the medication are not necessarily specific to aggressive children. Gadow, Nolan, Sverd, Sprafkin, and Paolicelli (1990) demonstrated that MPH can decrease the level of peer-directed aggression committed by children with ADHD in the classroom and on the playground. Hinshaw, Henker, Whalen, Erhardt, and Dunnington (1989) demonstrated that the aggression of ADHD boys can be reduced to levels indistinguishable from a group of normal controls in a dose-dependent manner, although the medication had no effects on increasing prosocial behaviors. A laboratory model of aggression called the Point Subtraction Aggression Paradigm (PSAP) was used as an analog of aggressive behavior to measure the effects of MPH on aggressive responding in children in a study by Casat, Pearson, Van Davelaar, and Cherek (1995) and MPH was found to decrease aggressive responding in a dose-related fashion.

There have been few studies of the use of stimulants in the treatment of the symptoms of CD or ODD without comorbid ADHD. One recent positive study conducted by Klein and colleagues (1997) studied the effects of MPH in a double-blind comparison with placebo in a group of outpatient CD youth with and without comorbid ADHD and found that MPH had a significant effect on reducing aggression and improving the symptoms of antisocial behavior when compared to placebo. Kaplan, Busner, Kupietz, Wassermann, and Segal (1990) reported on a small sample of 9 adolescents with "aggressive CD," 3 who were treated in open fashion and 6 who were treated in a placebo-controlled trial. They reported significant effects of MPH on the reduction of one measure of aggression, and a nonsignificant tendency for improvement using another. Stringer and Josef (1983) reported on 2 inpatients with Antisocial Personality Disorder (both of whom had childhood histories of ADHD) who became less aggressive during an open trial of MPH.

In summary, it appears that psychostimulants, in a dose-dependent manner, reduce aggressive responding in animal models and have clear effects on aggressive behavior in children with ADHD. The study by Klein and colleagues (1997) provides the first substantive evidence that stimulants can be used in CD children (many of whom also have ADHD) with any degree of confidence to reduce the aggressive symptoms of the disorder. Given the long history of safety of these medications in the application to childhood disorders, stimulants are a good initial choice for the aggressive child with underlying ADHD. They may prove to be useful as well for aggressive children with ODD and CD without underlying ADHD. The potential for abuse may be a cause for concern in adolescents with any significant degree of antisocial behavior.

ANTIDEPRESSANTS

A full review of the pharmacological dosing regimens, actions, and side effects of all the different antidepressant agents available for clinical usage is beyond the scope of this chapter. Reference is made to the major classes of antidepressants in Chapter 10 (this volume). The reader is directed to other reviews of the use of antidepressants in pediatric psychopharmacology for further information on this topic (see Werry & Aman, 1998). This chapter concentrates instead on the available information that suggests the potential use of these agents in aggression and antisocial behavior.

Tricyclic antidepressants have been used as pharmacologic probes in animal models of aggression. Although some conflicting reports are available in this literature, the majority of studies support the idea that tricyclics, especially those with a significant degree of NE-enhancing activity, tend to enhance aggressive responding in animals. Desipramine and imipramine, for example, have been studied extensively by one group and found to enhance the duration of aggressive responding in one model of mouse aggression (Matsumoto, Cai, Satoh, Ohta, & Watanabe, 1991). It should be noted that, in this study, the tricyclics enhanced aggression only in a group of already aggressive animals; it did not increase aggressive responding in nonaggressive mice. Chronic administration of tricyclics also appear to enhance or potentiate the aggression-inducing effects of other pharmacological agents, such as clonidine (Maj, Mogilnicka, & Kordecka-Magiera, 1980) and apomorphine (Maj, Mogilnicka, & Kordecka-Magiera, 1979), in mice and rats. The aggression-enhancing effects of tricyclics may result from the NE effects; at least one study suggests that pretreatment of mice with a noradrenergic neurotoxin significantly interfered with the ability of desipramine to enhance aggressive behavior (Matsumoto, Ojima, & Watanabe, 1995). The extent to which these findings translate to human effects is unknown. Occasional reactions of increased agitation and behavioral dyscontrol have been noted in humans during treatment with tricyclics, but this is not a common response to this class of medications.

Serotonin-specific reuptake inhibitors (SSRIs) also have been studied in animal models of aggression based on the extensively replicated finding that decreased central nervous system (CNS) 5-HT function is associated with increased aggression in many different species. A review of the wide body of literature demonstrating the association of aggression with alterations in 5-HT function in animals and humans is beyond the scope of this chapter but the reader is directed to recent reviews of this subject (Mann, 1995; Olivier, Mos, van Oorschot, & Hen, 1995; Chapter 17, this volume). Fluoxetine, a prototypical SSRI, has been studied in a variety of animal models and has been shown to be a modulator of intraspecies aggression in dogs (Dodman *et al.*, 1996), lizards (Deckal, 1996), rats (Datla, Mitra, & Bhattacharya, 1991), and monkeys (Raleigh, McGuire, Brammer, Pollack, & Yuwiler, 1991). Fluoxetine also appears to inhibit mouse-killing behavior by rats (Kostowski, Valzelli, Kozak, & Bernasconi, 1984).

The use of tricyclic antidepressants or other types of antidepressants in the therapy of human aggression has not been directly studied. Translation of the antiaggressive effects of 5-HT agents in animal models to human therapy has been proposed but remains experimental. Suggestions that fluoxetine reduces anger and hostility in subgroups of affectively disordered individuals are promising but unproven (Fava *et al.*, 1993). In fact, in one open trial with aggressive adults suffering concurrently from mental retardation and epilepsy, fluoxetine treatment was associated with an increase in aggressive responding in 9 out of 19 patients (Troisi, Vicario, Nuccetelli, Ciani, & Pasini, 1995). This contrasts with a report of decreased aggressive behavior and self-injury associated with fluoxetine treatment in a sample of 21 developmentally disabled patients (Markowitz, 1992).

The use of antidepressants in children with ODD or CD is being investigated. There are few FDA-approved indications for the use of tricyclics, SSRIs, or any other antidepressant medications in children. Controlled studies support the use of tricyclic agents (primarily desipramine and imipramine) in the treatment of children with ADHD who do not respond to or tolerate treatment with stimulants (see Chapter 10, this volume). However, no specific studies of the use of tricyclics for aggressive children are currently available. The use of fluoxetine in the subgroup of DBD with a concurrent major depression may be feasible, but the single controlled trial demonstrating the effectiveness of fluoxetine in child and adolescent depression specifically excluded CD children from the trial (Emslie, 1996).

MOOD STABILIZERS

The mood-stabilizing medications, consisting of lithium, carbamazepine, and valproic acid have been studied as potential pharmacological interventions for aggression. Each of these three medications has demonstrated effectiveness in the reduction of behavioral dyscontrol and manic excitement in the presence of bipolar disorder, the disorder for which they are most commonly prescribed. These medications have also been studied for use in aggressive patients without a diagnosis of underlying bipolar disorder, and in some studies have been found to be effective.

Lithium

Lithium has been demonstrated to reduce aggression in several animal models. Lithium inhibits mouse-killing behavior in rats (Broderick & Lynch, 1982) and decreases fighting behavior in mice reared in isolation (Malick, 1978). Lithium has also been studied as an antiaggression therapy in adults with a variety of conditions that lead to outward-directed or self-directed aggressive behavior. In a chart review of a sample of 38 mentally retarded individuals who were institutionalized for DBD and treated with lithium carbonate, Spreat, Behar, Reneski, and Miazzo (1989) determined that lithium treatment was associated with a reduction of aggressive behavior in 63% of cases. A placebo-controlled, double-blind study of lithium in a similar population by Craft and colleagues (1987) supported the safety and effectiveness of lithium in reducing episodes of aggression in this population. Seven of 10 patients with aggressive behavior or affective instability resulting from serious head injury responded positively to lithium carbonate when used in the context of a physical rehabilitation program (Glenn *et al.,* 1989). Sheard, Marini, Bridges, and Wagner (1976) performed a placebo-controlled, double-blind study of lithium in 66 subjects with a history of chronic impulsive violence who were in a medium security penal institution for a variety of offenses, and found that the lithium-treated group had significantly less violent infractions during the 3-month trial.

Lithium has been studied as an anti-aggression intervention in children with CD. Campbell and colleagues (1984) compared haloperidol and lithium carbonate to placebo in a double-blind study of children aged 5–13 who were institutionalized with treatment-resistant, aggressive CD. This important study found that both lithium and haloperidol were superior to placebo in reducing aggressive behavior and that lithium had fewer untoward side effects. There was no statistically significant difference between haloperidol and lithium. The superiority of lithium to placebo in reducing aggressive behavior in a similar population was replicated by this group (Campbell *et al.,* 1995) in a two-arm, lithium versus placebo design. Again the children studied were mostly prepubertal and had a diagnosis of CD. Malone, Luebbert, Pena-Ariet, Biesecker, and Delaney (1994) conducted an open study of lithium in children and adolescents with aggressive CD and found a decrease in ratings of aggression over time.

Anticonvulsants

The theoretical basis for the potential of anticonvulsant medications to reduce impulsive types of aggression is the finding that a subset of individuals who manifest violence have abnormal EEG tracings (Barratt, 1993). For example, in an open trial of valproic acid in the mentally retarded, a history of epilepsy or suspected seizure activity was strongly associated with a good response of the behavioral symptoms to anticonvulsant treatment (Kastner, Finesmith, & Walsh, 1993). There have been case reports (e.g., Rapport, Sonis, Fialkov, Matson, & Kazdin, 1983; Yassa & Dupont, 1983, Yatham & McHale, 1988) and open label studies (ie., Kafantaris *et al.,* 1992; Patterson, 1988) of carbamazepine in patients with a variety of conditions underlying their aggressive tendencies that suggest the therapeutic benefits of this medication. Addition of carbamazepine to a neuroleptic regimen in a placebo-controlled combination medication trial led to modest improvements in the experimental group in a study with schizophrenic patients who had a history of aggressive behavior or excited mental states (Okuma *et al.,* 1989). The only controlled study of the use of carbamazepine in children with CD found no superiority to active medication over placebo in a group of prepubertal children who were hospitalized and treatment resistant (Cueva *et al.,* 1996). Donovan and colleagues (1997) found that valproic acid was beneficial in decreasing mood lability and impulsive behavior in a group of adolescents who were at risk for substance abuse. There are no available controlled studies of valproic acid for the treatment of aggression or CD in children and adolescents.

In summary, there is some support for the use of lithium as a therapeutic option in prepubertal children with aggressive CD, and in general it appears to be safe when used for this indication. Anticonvulsant therapy must be considered experimental at this time and has no support from controlled trials in children or adolescents.

ADRENOLYTIC DRUGS

These drugs act to lower the level of activity in the NE system. While the functions of this system are complex and widespread both in the brain and autonomic nervous system (ANS), the basic function is concerned with fight or flight. In the brain, one important mechanism by which this is achieved is through a nonspecific setting of basal "tone" of neurons mediated largely through fibers that run in and are part of the reticular activating systems. Thus, adrenolysis that affects the brain often results in a kind of sedation. However, there are also more specific functions particularly in those parts of the brain that are important in the execution of the fight or flight response, such as the amygdala which coordinates the motor and autonomic components of the rage response. Thus, in theory, adrenolytic drugs might help mute aggressive behaviors that are part of an alarm response (reactive or emotive aggression) by a general lowering of activation (sedation) or by muting the execution of the aggressive response, or both. Conversely, in theory adrenergic drugs such as some of the stimulants should increase aggression but with the exception of cocaine most do not. Thus, this model of adrenergic function oversimplifies its role in that it is involved in day-to-day brain function but not alarm states. It also ignores the fact that there are two major kinds of NE receptors (alpha [α] and beta [β]) and thus two different NE systems; in contrast to the peripheral autonomic systems, the role of each in the brain is poorly differentiated. It is usual to classify adrenergic-adrenolytic drugs according to which receptor they affect.

Clonidine and α-Adrenergic Drugs

These drugs are discussed in detail in Chapter 10 (this volume). Basically, they are adrenolytic drugs that act by stimulating presynaptic autoreceptors that control the synthesis and storage of neurotransmitters. This blocking action is most pronounced in low dosage and, if too much is given, postsynaptic (enhancing) adrenergic effects may appear. There are two main drugs in current clinical use: clonidine and guanfacine, both of which are used primarily as antihypertensive drugs and have thus been in general medical use for many years, although their use in child and adolescent psychopharmacology is quite recent.

There have been some good reviews of these drugs and their use in pediatric psychopharmacology (Chapter 10, this volume; Horrigan & Barnhill, 1995; Hunt, Capper, & O'Connell, 1990; Hunt, Arnsten, & Asbell, 1995; Werry & Aman, 1998). Clonidine, the most popular of the two, is very short acting (about 2–4 hr) and the slow-release patches (introduced to solve this problem) may produce local allergic reactions. Guanfacine has a longer action and is thus potentially more attractive. It is only beginning to be studied; its action seems much the same as clonidine although there are minor differences in its cellular action. There can be serious interactions between these drugs and β-adrenergic blockers discussed later.

The most conspicuous effect is sedation. Extrapolations from theory and uncontrolled or anecdotal clinical reports suggest that these drugs have the power to inhibit hyperaroused states including anger and aggression (see Werry & Aman, 1998). This seems largely to be rumor rather than evidence-based medicine; there are good theoretical reasons to study these drugs in aggression and CD, but at this point, there is no evidence for or against their use in CD. Proper studies are urgently needed.

Propranolol and β-Adrenergic Blockers

Like α-adrenergic blockers just discussed, the β-blockers are used primarily in cardiovascular medicine. In psychiatry, their main use has been in the peripheral sympathetic psychophysiological symptoms of anxiety such as palpitations, panics, and sweating, but evidential support is surprisingly sparse. Like clonidine, they tend to have short duration of action, although there are longer-acting forms such as nadolol. Like clonidine, they have acquired a reputation for usefulness in explosive rage and aggression. A review (Arnold & Aman, 1991) of propranolol in DBD in young persons or those with developmental disabilities found 11 studies, none of which was properly controlled or used proper measures. More than three quarters of subjects in these studies were reported as improved in such symptoms as rage, aggression, agitation, and frustration tolerance. Stoewe and colleagues (1995) found much the same although they seemed more impressed by the gap between clinical enthusiasm and supporting data. Recently, Werry and Aman (1998) updated the data on β-blockers and found little change in the intervening 5 years or so.

In summary, the role of β-blockers in CD and its symptoms is very similar to that of the α-blockers: There are theoretical reasons and anecdotal clinical reports to suggest that these drugs may have a role to play but properly controlled and measured evaluation is needed. This paucity of studies probably suggests that the researchers are less impressed than their clinical colleagues about the efficacy of this class of medications.

Extreme care is needed with β-blockers in patients with cardiovascular disease and especially with asthma since it can provoke serious attacks. This is important because asthma is by far the most common chronic disorder in children and adolescents. There may also be pharmacokinetic interactions with neuroleptics and other psychotropic drugs though these are of less consequence.

CNS DEPRESSANTS

Since, as will be seen, these substances have no therapeutic role in CD, the extended discussion that follows may seem prolix and irrelevant but, for reasons which will become clear, it is most germane.

Pharmacology and Clinical Effects

The collation of substances may seem rather strange but it is pharmacologically sound (Werry & Aman, 1998) in that all these substances have a common core of effects on the brain: a progressive, dose-dependent, general depressant effect on all or most neuronal excitability. Most succinctly stated, the progressive effect on the brain gradually transforms humans from alert, sentient, considerate, social and esthetic beings to less and less complex mechanisms until finally, just before death they are no more than a heart–lung machine. Although many substances cause "sedation" (e.g. antihistamines, anticholinergics, adrenolytics, neuroleptics) only what are known pharmacologically as the CNS depressants cause this kind of systematic, general, widespread depression of function (hence their name).

The mode by which this depression of excitability is achieved varies, but in the end it is by altering ionic flows (mostly chloride) across cellular membranes, thus making it less probable that neuronal and axonal transmission will occur. Not surprisingly, those parts of the brain that are concerned with the most recently acquired and complex functions are first affected but, in the end, paralysis of most brain function occurs so that first drunken sleep, then coma, then death occur. The paradigm for this kind of effect is seen with alcohol. Too often this process of reversible brain dysfunction is portrayed as sophisticated, grown-up, or as an excuse for the kind of social behavior that ordinarily is kept under control by self-control, the group, and society.

In psychopharmacotherapy, the main use of these drugs is for anxiolysis and now only the benzodiazepines and analogs are so used. The basis of the anxiety-relieving effect is unclear but it is probably partly simply an early stage of sedation that reduces awareness, including of painful things, and partly some specific effect on posited "anxiety" receptors. It seems a part of the spectrum of clinical activity of all depressants including alcohol.

This process of progressive general brain depression can be achieved by an astoundingly large number of chemical substances, mostly lipid soluble organic substances such as alcohols, industrial gases and solvents, gasoline, general anesthetic agents, old-fashioned hypnotics (sleep-inducing agents) such as barbiturates, and the so-called minor tranquilizers such as benzodiazepines like diazepam and analogs like zopiclone. The speed with which intoxication occurs depends on the route of administration; inhalation of gases or volatile substances such as solvents is rapid, and other routes such as oral are much slower. Inhalation leads to rapid intoxication through a bolus of substance entering the brain circulation but since these substances are highly lipid soluble, they are rapidly distributed through all fatty tissues and so the effect dissipates—at first. This is highly valuable in anethesiology and in solvent sniffing, making it safer than drinking alcohol. However, if the dosage of the inhaled substances is continued and sufficient to induce intoxication, the fatty tissues become saturated and the state of brain depression continues for some time. Most persons who use these substances socially are saved from death because dosage ceases with the onset of drowsiness, sleep, or unconsciousness; in the case of some substances such as alcohol and ether, vomiting is induced by gastric irritation; in other cases, detectors in the chemo-receptor center in the brain limit further absorption of the substance.

This model of alcohol intoxication–sedation–anesthesia is of course somewhat simplistic since it is unlikely that all substances produce exactly the same effects, especially those that extend beyond what is observable with the "naked eye." Also, although basically correct for the anxiolytics (formerly known as minor tranquilizers), the model is only partially so, because the process stops at deep sleep and does not ordinarily proceed to coma and death. This is because the action of these drugs is indirect through GABA (γ-aminobutyric acid), a widely but selectively distributed inhibitory neurotransmitter that does not act directly on membranes themselves but through special receptors in the membrane wall. Presumably, these receptors become saturated and increasing doses produce few further effects or they are less numerous in vital centers of the brain that control life-sustaining processes such as respiration. Up to the point of deep sleep, however, the alcohol model seems quite valid clinically.

One further mystery about all these substances is that they can cause abuse and dependence. At a psychological level this is because in most individuals they cause a spurious sense of well-being and a sense of empowerment and diminish existential angst and self-doubt. True dependence, however, usually also involves altered physiological processes, which are poorly understood but in which genetic factors may play a role, making some individuals more vulnerable than others.

The other factors that cause different effects of substances are the potency of the substance and hence potential for serious overdose (anesthetic substances and most solvents are highly potent; diazepam is not) and other toxicities of the substance. For example, halogenated hydrocarbons, like chloroform or fire-extinguishing chemicals, make the heart more susceptible to fatal arrhythmias; acetone can cause irritative pulmonary edema; and the most toxic of them all, alcohol, attacks a wide variety of tissues causing acute and, more important, long-term toxic effects on liver, stomach, cardiovascular, brain, and other systems. Unlike tobacco, which principally affects the health of the smoker, alcohol is often involved in health problems (e.g., motor vehicle accidents, homicide, violence) with widespread misery to innocent bystanders and enormous economic cost to society.

CNS Depressants and CD

In order to understand the clinical implications of these substances for CD, it is necessary to have a grasp of the essential features and common correlates of the disorder, what the neurobiological bases might be, the pharmacological actions of the substance, the extent to which those with CD encounter them, and societal attitudes and canons.

For diverse reasons set out elsewhere in this handbook, those with CD are, in general, unsuccessful, socially gauche, educationally impaired and disadvantaged individuals; many grow up loveless in violent, drug and alcohol environments. By virtue of poor affectional bonding, distorted perceptions of others, and limited social, recreational, and educational opportunities, CD children or adolescents often do not have the behaviors, skills, motivations, or knowledge of the rules by which to succeed in normal society. Their repertoire of behavior is limited and in it, disinhibited, poorly thought-through, egocentric, exciting, reward-seeking, intimidating, and violent solutions figure large. The veneer of civilization, as it were, is thin and incomplete.

What, then, will be the effect of alcohol and other CNS depressant drugs in CD given that they produce euphoria, spurious empowerment, and generally diminish the quintessentially humanness of behavior? First, it is not surprising that many with CD will be exposed to these substances early in life, abuse them, and become dependent on them because of subjective pharmacological effects. Second, they will be at greater risk of suffering their health consequences such as death from overdose and accidents (and suicide) because of greater use. Third, what skills they do have to interact prosocially with the world will be diminished and more disinhibited and primitive behaviors will emerge. Little wonder then that alcohol is a major factor in most countries in crime and violence, both domestic and beyond. Youth have fewer and less well-learned social skills and lower tolerance through fewer years of exposure to these substances and we can but speculate just how much these substances add to the disability of CD and its adverse consequences.

The pharmacotherapeutic implications are that these substances should not be used in CD because of the risks of causing disinhibition and possible abuse and dependence. In addition, there are no studies that support their value (Werry & Aman, 1998). However, a problem may arise when CD is comorbid with the very few disorders in which temporary or crisis use of these substances (e.g., benzodiazepines) may be indicated (e.g., in manic episodes, acute psychotic states, and panic disorder). Any such use would have to balance the prospect of violent behavior against the gravity of the comorbid disorder and no simple rules can be given.

Summary

It is surely unnecessary to belabor the point that these substances present a serious threat and complication in CD and that every effort in therapy must be directed toward moderate and sensible use. No program to deal with CD can ignore these substances, the need for evaluation of their role in each affected individual, and the need for preventive social action.

MISCELLANEOUS SEDATIVES

Antihistamines

These drugs have been widely used in the past in infants and toddlers with ODD symptoms but there is almost no evidence to support their value (Werry & Aman, 1998) and nothing recent. It is unclear whether their undoubted mild sedating power is due to their anticholinergic action or their antihistamine action or both. They have no established role in ODD or CD.

Atypical Anxiolytics

A novel and interesting drug is buspirone which is classified as an atypical anxiolytic or sedative. Though said to be anxiolytic, it is quite unlike the CNS depressants and causes no euphoria, disinhibition, or dependence. Initially it was welcomed as the ideal anxiolytic but it has failed to live up to early enthusiasm. Even so, there is clinical anecdotal evidence to suggest that this drug may mute explosive aggression (Werry & Aman, 1998) and if so, it surely warrants proper study in CD in view of its lack of deleterious actions.

DRUGS OF ABUSE

Substance abuse has been associated with violence and aggression in many different settings and clinical situations. The effects of various recreational drugs on the risk for aggressive action is complicated and often depends on the specific drug as well as the phase of abuse (i.e., acute intoxication, chronic dependence, or withdrawal). There appears to be little doubt that illicit substance abuse is associated with a substantial amount of antisocial behavior, as well as outwardly directed and self-directed aggression. We focus here primarily on marijuana and cocaine; a full review of all the different substances is beyond the scope of the chapter. We highlight the ways in which these particular substances interact psychologically and neurobiologically with the individual organism to increase the risk of aggressive responding. It should be understood that substances that are pharmacologically similar (e.g., cocaine and psychostimulants) may have similar effects on aggression in humans through similar pharmacologic mechanisms of action. However, substances with different mechanisms of biological activity (e.g., opiates, phencyclidine [PCP]) may have effects on behavior that are vastly different from the substances highlighted here.

Nicotine

Experts have postulated that smoking cigarettes in some individuals may be a strategy to help regulate affective states and minimize negative emotions (reviewed in Ockene & Kristeller, 1994). The biological mechanism by which this occurs is unclear but it is clear that after repeated use physiological dependence follows, so that a withdrawal reaction will occur on cessation of smoking or begin during a prolonged abstinence. There is no evidence to suggest that nicotine itself would increase the likelihood of an individual engaging in antisocial acts or aggression. Its central nervous system effects are probably mild and may help decrease levels of agitation or anxiety in some individuals. Physiological withdrawal is at times associated with irritability and mild impulsive behavior. However, smoking behavior and nicotine dependence is fairly common in CD youth and smoking often is a prelude to use and abuse of illicit substances (Yamaguchi & Kandel, 1984).

Cannabis

The primary psychoactive substance in marijuana is delta-9-tetrahydrocannabinol (THC). Intoxication with this substance produces substantial psychological, physiological, and behavioral effects (for review, see Millman & Beeder, 1994). Psychological reactions include altered perceptual sensitivity, euphoria, anxiety, depression, relief of boredom, and supposed facilitation of creative or abstract thinking. Physiological effects include tachycardia, conjunctival injection, decrease in salivation, and increase of appetite. Behavioral changes include acute social withdrawal, increased talkativeness, drowsiness, silliness, or hyperactivity. Striking adverse reactions to intoxication that can be associated with agitation or increase risk of violence include (1) a well-described induction of severe anxiety states or panic attacks that can induce severe fear and hysterical upset and (2) a cannabis-induced psychotic reaction. The anxiety state often responds to maintaining a safe environment for the patient and talking in a calm, supportive manner, often in combination with a small-to-moderate dosage of a sedating benzodiazepine. The psychotic reaction can be associated with anxiety, emotional lability, persecutory delusions, and, rarely, hallucinations. These reactions are usually self-limited as the body is able to metabolize and clear the offending intoxicant. Frank delirium is possible when very high doses of the drug are ingested, and has been associated with violent behavior.

In the animal laboratory, delta-9-THC has had mixed results on aggressive behavior in different animal models. Some studies support the idea that in rats delta-9-THC leads to a reduced tendency to respond aggressively to various provocation stimuli (e.g., Cutler & Mackintosh, 1984, Miczek & Barry, 1977) but the same compound has also been demonstrated to increase fighting behavior in a different strain of rats (Fujiwara, Kataoka, Hori, & Ueki, 1984). Pigeons displayed some evidence of tolerance to the aggression-reducing effects of acute THC administration, where with repeated dosing, the measures of aggressive behavior returned to pre-exposure levels (Cherek, Thompson, & Kelly, 1980).

Dose-dependent effects of THC on human behavior have been demonstrated. In one study, acute administration of THC (in varying doses) to 30 normal volunteers found that individuals administered a low-dose condition were more likely to respond aggressively to "intense provocation" than were individuals administered either a moderate or high dose (Myerscough & Taylor, 1985).

With chronic cannabis use, a syndrome of apathy, low motivation, withdrawal, and personality deterioration has been noted. Acute cessation of the drug has been associated with some symptoms of withdrawal in some animal and human studies and can be associated with irritability and restlessness, but the association of withdrawal with aggressive or violent behavior is not common.

Cocaine

Similar to the model based on cannabis just described, cocaine and other stimulant drugs that have been abused can, at various phases of use and abuse, contribute to antisocial and aggressive behavior (see review in Gawin, Khalsa, & Ellinwood, 1994). Acute intoxication produces various behavioral and psychological consequences, including euphoria, increased behavioral activity, disinhibition, increased sexual desire, and acute feelings of increased competence and self-esteem. Unusual intoxication reactions based on some underlying predisposition in the individual or due to pharmacological dosing effect can result in impulsive behavior, agitation, or violence. Loss of judgment can result in risk-taking behavior that may be dangerous to the self or others. At times a delirium can result that resembles paniclike levels of anxiety or a paranoid psychosis. In this delirious state, agitation and aggression can ensue.

Prolonged stimulant binges or chronic abuse can lead to more severe levels of psychotic thought content, and delusional psychoses can result. Often the delusional content is paranoid in quality and rarely may lead to violence or homicide. Periods of prolonged or intense use can lead to "crash" periods, where cessation of use leads to intense feelings of psychological dysphoria that may resemble depressive disorders. At times these crashes can be of sufficient severity to stimulate suicidal ideation or behavior. Preparations of smokable stimulants such as "crack" can lead to greatly

enhanced physiological and psychological experience of the reinforcing qualities of stimulant use, and may contribute to the relatively early phase of high-intensity abuse associated with these preparations.

REFERENCES

American Psychiatric Association. (1994). *Diagnostic and statistical manual of mental disorders* (4th ed.). Washington, DC: Author.

Arnold, L. E., & Aman, M. G. (1991). Beta blockers in mental retardation and developmental disorders. *Journal of Child and Adolescent Psychopharmacology, 1,* 361–373.

Barratt, E. S. (1993). The use of anticonvulsants in aggression and violence. *Psychopharmacology Bulletin, 29,* 75–81.

Broderick, P., & Lynch, V. (1982). Behavioral and biochemical changes induced by lithium and L-tryptophan in muricidal rats. *Neuropharmacology, 21,* 671–679.

Campbell, M., & Cueva, J. E. (1995a). Psychopharmacology in child and adolescent psychiatry: A review of the past seven years: Part I. *Journal of the American Academy of Child and Adolescent Psychiatry, 34,* 1124–1132.

Campbell, M., & Cueva, J. E. (1995b). Psychopharmacology in child and adolescent psychiatry: A review of the past seven years: Part II. *Journal of the American Academy of Child and Adolescent Psychiatry, 34,* 1262–1272.

Campbell, M., Small, A. M., Green, W. H., Jennings, S. J., Perry, R., Bennett, W. G., & Anderson, L. (1984). Behavioral efficacy of haloperidol and lithium carbonate: A comparison in hospitalized aggressive children with conduct disorder. *Archives of General Psychiatry, 41,* 650–656.

Campbell, M., Gonzalez, N. M., & Silva, R. R. (1992). The pharmacologic treatment of conduct disorders and rage outbursts. *Psychiatric Clinics of North America, 15,* 69–85.

Campbell, M., Adams, P. B., Small, A. M., Kafantaris, V., Silva, R. R., Shell, J., Perry, R., & Overall, J. E. (1995). Lithium in hospitalized aggressive children with conduct disorder: A double-blind and placebo-controlled study. *Journal of the American Academy of Child and Adolescent Psychiatry, 34,* 445–453.

Casat, C. D., Pearson, D. A., Van Davelaar, M. J., & Cherek, D. R. (1995). Methylphenidate effects on a laboratory aggression measure in children with ADHD. *Psychopharmacology Bulletin, 31,* 353–356.

Cherek, D. R., Thompson, T., & Kelly, T. (1980). Chronic delta 9-tetrahydrocannabinol administration and schedule-induced aggression. *Pharmacology, Biochemistry and Behavior, 12,* 305–309.

Cloninger, C. R., Svrakic, D. M., & Przybeck, T. R. (1993). A psychobiological model of temperament and character. *Archives of General Psychiatry, 50,* 975–990.

Craft, M., Ismail, I. A., Krishnamurti, D., Mathews, J., Regan, A., Seth, R. V., & North, P. M. (1987). Lithium in the treatment of aggression in mentally handicapped patients: A double-blind trial. *British Journal of Psychiatry, 150,* 685–689.

Cueva, J. E., Overall, J. E., Small, A. M., Armenteros, J. L., Perry, R., & Campbell, M. (1996). Carbamazepine in aggressive children with conduct disorder: A double-blind and placebo-controlled study. *Journal of the American Academy of Child and Adolescent Psychiatry, 35,* 480–490.

Cutler, M. G., & Mackintosh, J. H. (1984). Cannabis and delta-9-tetrahydrocannabinol. Effects on elements of social behaviour in mice. *Neuropharmacology, 23,* 1091–1097.

Datla, K. P., Mitra, S. K., & Bhattacharya, S. K. (1991). Serotonergic modulation of footshock induced aggression in paired rats. *Indian Journal of Experimental Biology, 29,* 631–635.

Deckel, A. W. (1996). Behavioral changes in Anolis carolinensis following injection with fluoxetine. *Behavioural Brain Research, 78,* 175–182.

Dodman, N. H., Donnelly, R., Shuster, L., Mertens, P., Rand, W., & Miczek, K. (1996). Use of fluoxetine to treat dominance aggression in dogs. *Journal of the American Veterinary Medical Association, 209,* 1585–1587.

Donovan, S. J., Susser, E. S., Nunes, E. V., Stewart, J. W., Quitkin, F. M., & Klein, D. F. (1997). Divalproex treatment of disruptive adolescents: A report of 10 cases. *Journal of Clinical Psychiatry, 58,* 12–15.

Eichelman, B. (1992). Aggressive behavior: From laboratory to clinic—Quo vadit? *Archives of General Psychiatry, 49,* 488–492.

Emslie G. J. (1996, October). *Pharmacological treatment of early onset major depressive disorder.* Paper presented at the scientific proceedings of the annual meeting of the American Academy of Child and Adolescent Psychiatry, Philadelphia.

Ernst, M., Malone, R. P., Rowan, A. B., George, R., Gonzalez, N. M., & Silva, R. R. (1998). Antipsychotics (neuroleptics). In J. S. Werry & M. G. Aman (Eds.), *A practitioner's guide to psychoactive drugs for children and adolescents* (2nd ed, pp. 297–328). New York: Plenum.

Fava, M., Rosenbaum, J. F., Pava, J. A., McCarthy, M. K., Steingard, R. J., & Bouffides, E. (1993). Anger attacks in unipolar depression: Part 1. Clinical correlates and response to fluoxetine treatment. *American Journal of Psychiatry, 150,* 1158–1163.

Fujiwara, M., Kataoka, Y., Hori, Y., & Ueki, S. (1984). Irritable aggression induced by delta 9-tetrahydrocannabinol in rats pretreated with 6-hydroxydopamine. *Pharmacology, Biochemistry and Behavior, 20,* 457–462.

Gadow, K. D., Nolan, E. E., Sverd, J., Sprafkin, J., & Paolicelli, L. (1990). Methylphenidate in aggressive-hyperactive boys: I. Effects on peer aggression in public school settings. *Journal of the American Academy of Child and Adolescent Psychiatry, 29,* 710–718.

Gawin, F. H., Khalsa, M. E., & Ellinwood, E. (1994). Stimulants. In M. Galanter & H. D. Kleber (Eds.), *Textbook of substance abuse treatment* (pp. 111–140). Washington, DC: American Psychiatric Press.

Glenn, M. B., Wroblewski, B., Parziale, J., Levine, L., Whyte, J., & Rosenthal, M. (1989). Lithium carbonate for aggressive behavior or affective instability in ten brain-injured patients. *American Journal of Physical Medicine and Rehabilitation, 68,* 221–226.

Gray, J. A. (1982a). *The neuropsychology of anxiety: An inquiry into the function of the septo-hippocampal system.* New York: Oxford University Press.

Gray, J. A. (1982b). The neuropsychology of anxiety: An inquiry into the functions of the septo-hippocampal system. *Behavioral and Brain Sciences, 5,* 469–534.

Gray, J. A. (1987a). Perspectives on anxiety and impulsivity: A commentary. *Journal of Research in Personality, 21,* 493–509.

Gray, J. A. (1987b). *The psychology of fear and stress.* New York: Cambridge University Press.

Hinshaw, S. P., Henker, B., Whalen, C. K., Erhardt, D., & Dunnington, R. E., Jr. (1989). Aggressive, prosocial, and nonsocial behavior in hyperactive boys: Dose effects of methylphenidate in naturalistic settings. *Journal of Consulting and Clinical Psychology, 57,* 636–643.

Horrigan, J. P., & Barnhill, L. J. (1995). Guanfacine for treatment of Attention Deficit Hyperactivity Disorder. *Journal of Child and Adolescent Psychopharmacology, 5,* 215–223.

Hunt, R. D., Capper, L., & O'Connell, P. (1990). Clonidine in child and adolescent psychiatry. *Journal of Child and Adolescent Psychopharmacology, 1,* 87–102.

Hunt, R. D., Mandl, L., Lau, S., & Hughes, M. (1991). Neurobiological theories of ADHD and ritalin. In L. L. Greenhill & B. Osman (Eds.), *Ritalin: Theory and patient management* (pp. 267–288). New York: Liebert.

Hunt, R. D., Arnsten., A., & Asbell, M. D. (1995). An open trial of guanfacine in the treatment of attention deficit hyperactivity disorder in boys. *Journal of the American Academy of Child and Adolescent Psychiatry, 34,* 50–54.

Kafantaris, V., Campbell, M., Padron-Gayol, M. V., Small, A. M., Locascio, J. J., & Rosenberg, C. R. (1992). Carbamazepine in hospitalized aggressive conduct disorder children: An open pilot study. *Psychopharmacology Bulletin, 28,* 193–199.

Kaplan, S. L., Busner, J., Kupietz, S., Wassermann, E., & Segal, B. (1990). Effects of methylphenidate on adolescents with aggressive conduct disorder and ADDH: A preliminary report. *Journal of the American Academy of Child and Adolescent Psychiatry, 29,* 719–723.

Kastner, T., Finesmith, R., & Walsh, K. (1993). Long-term administration of valproic acid in the treatment of affective symptoms in people with mental retardation. *Journal of Clinical Psychopharmacology, 13,* 448–451.

Klein, R. G., Abikoff, H., Klass, E., Ganeles, D., Seese, L. M., & Pollack, S. (1997). Clinical efficacy of methylphenidate in conduct disorder with and without ADHD. *Archives of General Psychiatry, 54,* 1073–1080.

Kostowski W., Valzelli, L., Kozak, W., & Bernasconi, S. (1984) Activity of desipramine, fluoxetine and nomifensine on spontaneous and p-CPA-induced muricidal aggression. *Pharmacological Research Communications, 16,* 265–271.

Kulkarni, A. S., & Plotnikoff, N. P. (1978). Effects of stimulants on aggressive behavior. *Modern Problems of Pharmacopsychiatry, 13,* 69–81.

Maj, J., Mogilnicka, E., & Kordecka-Magiera, A. (1979). Chronic treatment with antidepressant drugs: Potentiation of apomorphine-induced aggressive behaviour in rats. *Neuroscience Letters, 13,* 337–341.

Maj, J., Mogilnicka, E., & Kordecka-Magiera, A. (1980). Effects of chronic administration of antidepressant drugs on aggressive behavior induced by clonidine in mice. *Pharmacology, Biochemistry and Behavior, 13,* 153–154.

Malick, J. G. (1978). Inhibition of fighting in isolated mice following repeated administration of lithium chloride. *Pharmacology, Biochemistry and Behavior, 8,* 579–581.

Malone, R. P., Luebbert, J., Pena-Ariet, M., Biesecker, K., & Delaney, M. A. (1994). The Overt Aggression Scale in a study of lithium in aggressive conduct disorder. *Psychopharmacology Bulletin, 30,* 215–218.

Mann, J. J. (1995). Violence and aggression. In F. E. Bloom & D. Kupfer (Eds.), *Psychopharmacology: The fourth generation of progress* (pp. 1919–1928). New York: Raven.

Markowitz, P. I. (1992). Effect of fluoxetine on self-injurious behavior in the developmentally disabled: A preliminary study. *Journal of Clinical Psychopharmacology, 2,* 27–31.

Matsumoto, K., Cai, B., Satoh, T., Ohta, H., & Watanabe, H. (1991). Desipramine enhances isolation-induced aggressive behavior in mice. *Pharmacology, Biochemistry and Behavior, 39,* 167–170.

Matsumoto, K., Ojima, K., & Watanabe, H. (1995) Noradrenergic denervation attenuates desipramine enhancement of aggressive behavior in isolated mice. *Pharmacology, Biochemistry and Behavior, 50,* 481–484.

Miczek, K. A., & Barry, H. (1977). Comparison of the effects of alcohol, chlordiazepoxide, and delta 9-tetrahydrocannabinol on intraspecies aggression in rats. *Advances in Experimental Medicine and Biology, 85B,* 251–264.

Miczek, K. A., & O'Donnell, J. M. (1978). Intruder-evoked aggression in isolated and nonisolated mice: Effects of psychomotor stimulants and L-dopa. *Psychopharmacology, 57,* 47–55.

Millman, R. B., & Beeder, A. B. (1994). Cannabis. In M. Galanter & H. D. Kleber (Eds.). *Textbook of substance abuse treatment* (pp. 99–110). Washington, DC: American Psychiatric Press.

Moyer, K. E. (1968). Kinds of aggression and their physiological basis. *Communications in Behavioral Biology, 2,* 65–87.

Myerscough, R., & Taylor, S. (1985). The effects of marijuana on human physical aggression. *Journal of Personality and Social Psychology, 49,* 1541–1546.

Ockene, J. K., & Kristeller, J. L. (1994). Tobacco. In M. Galanter & H. D. Kleber (Eds.), *Textbook of substance abuse treatment* (pp. 157–178). Washington, DC: American Psychiatric Press.

Okuma, T., Yamashita, I., Takahashi, R., Itoh, H., Otsuki, S., Watanabe, S., Sarai, K., Hazama, H., & Inanaga, K. (1989). A double-blind study of adjunctive carbamazepine versus placebo on excited states of schizophrenic and schizoaffective disorders. *Acta Psychiatrica Scandinavica, 80,* 250–259.

Olivier, B., Mos, J., van Oorschot, R., & Hen, R. (1995). Serotonin receptors and animal models of aggressive behavior. *Pharmacopsychiatry, 28* (Suppl. 2), 80–90.

Patterson, J. F. (1988). A preliminary study of carbamazepine in the treatment of assaultive patients with dementia. *Journal of Geriatric Psychiatry and Neurology, 1,* 21–23.

Quay, H. C. (1993). The psychobiology of undersocialized aggressive conduct disorder: A theoretical perspective. *Development and Psychopathology, 5,* 165–180.

Quay, H. C. (1997). Inhibition and Attention Deficit Hyperactivity Disorder. *Journal of Abnormal Child Psychology, 25,* 7–13.

Raleigh, M. J., McGuire, M. T., Brammer, G. L., Pollack, D. B., & Yuwiler, A. (1991). Serotonergic mechanisms promote dominance acquisition in adult male vervet monkeys. *Brain Research, 559,* 181–190.

Rall, T. W., Nies, A. S., & Taylor, P. (1991). *Goodman and Gilman's The pharmacological basis of therapeutics* (8th ed.). New York: Maxwell McMillan.

Rapport, M. D., Sonis, W. A., Fialkov, M. J., Matson, J. L., & Kazdin, A. E. (1983). Carbamazepine and behavior therapy for aggressive behavior: Treatment of a mentally retarded, postencephalitic adolescent with seizure disorder. *Behavior Modification, 7,* 255–265.

Reis, D. (1971). Brain monoamines in aggression and sleep. *Clinical Neurosurgery, 18,* 471–502.

Reis, D. (1974). Central neurotransmitters in aggression. *Research Publications of the Association for Research in Nervous and Mental Disease, 52,* 119–148.

Reiss, S., & Aman, M. G. (Eds.). (1998). *Psychotropic drugs and developmental disabilities: The international consensus handbook.* Columbus, OH: Nisonger Center.

Schroeder, S. R. (1988). Neuroleptic drugs for persons with developmental disabilities. In M. G. Aman & N. N. Singh (Eds.), *Psychopharmacology of the developmental disabilities* (pp. 82–100). New York: Springer-Verlag.

Sheard, M. H., Marini, J. L., Bridges, C. I., & Wagner, E. (1976). The effect of lithium on impulsive aggressive behavior in man. *American Journal of Psychiatry, 133,* 1409–1413.

Spreat, S., Behar, D., Reneski, B., & Miazzo, P. (1989). Lithium carbonate for aggression in mentally retarded persons. *Comprehensive Psychiatry, 30,* 505–511.

Stoewe, J. K., Kruesi, M. J. P., & Lelio, D. F. (1995). Pharmacotherapy of aggressive states and features of conduct disorder. *Child and Adolescent Psychiatric Clinics of North America, 4,* 359–380.

Stringer, A. Y., & Josef, N. C. (1983). Methylphenidate in the treatment of aggression in two patients with antisocial personality disorder. *American Journal of Psychiatry, 140,* 1365–1366.

Troisi, A., Vicario, E., Nuccetelli, F., Ciani, N., & Pasini, A. (1995). Effects of fluoxetine on aggressive behavior of adult inpatients with mental retardation and epilepsy. *Pharmacopsychiatry, 28,* 73–76.

Vitiello, B., Behar, D., Hunt, J., Stoff, D., & Ricciuti, A. (1990). Subtyping aggression in children and adolescents. *Journal of Neuropsychiatry, 2,* 189–192.

Werry, J. S. (1994). Pharmacotherapy of disruptive behavior disorders. *Child and Adolescent Psychiatric Clinics of North America, 3,* 321–342.

Werry, J. S., & Aman, M. G. (1998). Anxiolytic and miscellaneous drugs. In J. S. Werry & M. G. Aman (Eds.), *A practitioner's guide to psychoactive drugs for children and adolescents* (2nd ed., pp. 433–470). New York: Plenum.

Whitaker, A., & Rao, U. (1992). Neuroleptics in pediatric psychiatry. *Psychiatric Clinics of North America, 15,* 243–276.

Whitman, S., Benbow, N., & Good, G. (1996). The epidemiology of homicide in Chicago. *Journal of the National Medical Association, 88,* 781–787.

Yamaguchi, K., & Kandel, D. B. (1984). Patterns of drug use from adolescence to young adulthood: II. Sequences of progression. *American Journal of Public Health, 74,* 668–672.

Yassa, R., & Dupont, D. (1983). Carbamazepine in the treatment of aggressive behavior in schizophrenic patients: A case report. *Canadian Journal of Psychiatry, 28,* 566–568.

Yatham, L. N., & McHale, P. A. (1988). Carbamazepine in the treatment of aggression: A case report and a review of the literature. *Acta Psychiatrica Scandinavica, 78,* 188–190.

Yoshikawa, H. (1994). Prevention as cumulative protection: Effects of early family support and education on chronic delinquency and its risks. *Psychological Bulletin, 115,* 28–54.

22

Treatment of Oppositional Defiant Disorder and Conduct Disorder in Home and Community Settings

SONJA K. SCHOENWALD and SCOTT W. HENGGELER

INTRODUCTION

Youth with serious and persistent conduct problems receive treatment in primary care and mental health clinics, foster group homes, residential treatment centers, foster family homes (see Chapter 23, this volume), family homes, and the public schools. Such settings are often operated or funded through public agencies legally mandated to treat (mental health), rehabilitate (juvenile justice), educate (special education), or protect (social services) youth. Irrespective of the service system (e.g., mental health, juvenile justice) or setting (clinic, foster home) in which youth presenting with Conduct Disorder (CD)* receive treatment, psy-

---

*We will use *conduct disorder* as a term that encompasses children and adolescents with serious disruptive and often antisocial behavior irrespective of whether a formal diagnosis has been made. The vast majority of clients of the treatment programs described would very likely meet criteria for conduct disorder had they been assessed for that purpose.

SONJA K. SCHOENWALD and SCOTT W. HENGGELER • Department of Psychiatry and Behavioral Sciences, Medical University of South Carolina, Charleston, South Carolina 29425-0742.

Handbook of Disruptive Behavior Disorders, edited by Quay and Hogan. Kluwer Academic/Plenum Publishers, New York, 1999.

chotherapy of some type generally bears the burden of producing change (Kazdin, 1994).

Unfortunately, the knowledge base regarding the nature and effectiveness of psychotherapies rendered in community settings is both slim and discouraging. Surveys of community-based mental health practitioners suggest that the predominant treatment is general counseling of the child and parent in accordance with psychodynamic or eclectic theoretical orientations (Kazdin, Siegel, & Bass, 1990) and that the nature of treatment is determined by what clinicians know and philosophically prefer rather than by the nature of the presenting problem and circumstances of the family (Kruesi & Tolan, in press). In addition, the majority of treatment approaches have never been evaluated, and little evidence supports the effectiveness of predominant treatment models that have been tested with CD youth (Kazdin, 1987, 1994). Moreover, meta-analyses indicate that, in contrast with treatments as delivered in university-based research protocols, treatments delivered in community clinic settings are not effective (Hoagwood, Hibbs, Brent, & Jensen, 1995; Kazdin, 1997; Weisz, Han, & Valeri, 1997). Documented differences between "clinic" and "research" treatments include greater severity and heterogeneity of problems presented by clinic cases, higher caseloads of community-based clinicians, and a relative lack of training of clinicians in specific treatment protocols and monitoring of treatment adherence in community settings (Weisz, Donenberg, Han, & Kauneckis, 1995; Weisz, Donenberg, Han, & Weiss, 1995). Finally, reviews of ambitious service system initiatives designed to develop and coordinate service sectors' organization and financing of innovative community-based models of mental health service delivery, such as individualized or "wrap-around" treatment, intensive case management, family preservation services, and family support services, have yielded disappointing child outcomes. Reviewers have suggested that inattention to the nature of clinical interventions deployed in the service system initiatives is one likely explanation for the disappointing findings (Henggeler, Schoenwald, & Munger, 1996; Oswald & Singh, 1996; Rosenblatt, 1996; Weisz *et al.*, 1997).

Given the heterogeneity of service systems, settings, and treatment practices likely to be encountered by a treatment-seeking parent, youth, or referring agent (e.g., school counselor, probation officer, pediatrician, judge) and the significant differences between clinic versus research treatment, it is not surprising that few community-based treatments for youth with persistent CD have been empirically validated. The purpose of this chapter is to describe treatment approaches deployed in community-based settings that have demonstrated promise in controlled evaluations with clinically representative samples (e.g., inclusive of youth and families from diverse racial backgrounds, experiencing low SES status, and living in a variety of family structures). By community-based, we mean treatment that is delivered to youth and their caregivers (generally parents or relatives; in some cases, foster parents) in their indigenous communities, in the home or another service setting likely to be available in most communities. Treatments validated primarily with samples of volunteers who have no agency involvement or with youth presenting nonclinical levels of disruptive behavior are not described. We begin with a brief overview of the interfaces between community service systems and youth with CD.

YOUTH WITH CD IN THE CONTEXT OF COMMUNITY SERVICE SYSTEMS

Mental health, juvenile justice, child welfare and social services, and special education agencies mandate, finance, and provide (or contract with others to provide) treatment for the majority of youth with serious and persistent antisocial behavior. Youth with such behavior consume the majority of mental health resources and generate significant and costly responses across multiple service systems (e.g., arrest, incarceration, residential placement, hospitalization) (Cohen, Miller, & Rossman, 1994). Several legal terms are used to describe youth whose repetitive and persistent patterns of antisocial behavior prompt contact with mental health or juvenile justice systems. In the juvenile justice system, youths who are arrested for engaging in illegal antisocial activities are designated as delinquent. Milder or less serious forms of delinquent behavior include those activities referred to as status offenses (e.g., alcohol use, not attending school, truancy, staying out late, running away, incorrigibility); such activities are illegal for youths only and would not be considered offenses if the youths were adults. In contrast to status offenses, index offenses (e.g., murder or nonnegligent manslaughter, forcible rape, robbery, aggravated assault, burglary, larceny-theft, motor vehicle theft, arson) reflect a less common and more serious form of criminal behavior among youths. Other delinquent activities (e.g., damaging property, petty larceny, buying stolen goods, breaking and entering, joyriding) fall somewhere between status offenses and index offenses in terms of their seriousness and effects on others.

Many youths arrested for delinquent behavior meet diagnostic criteria for CD or Oppositional Defiant Disorder (ODD), and the treatment needs of youths in the juvenile justice system (i.e., delinquent youths) and mental health system (i.e., diagnosed with CD) are largely the same (Melton & Pagliocca, 1992). As noted previously, treatment for CD youth provided in community mental health settings appear not to be effective. Similarly, meta-analyses of treatments for juvenile delinquents (Lipsey, 1992) indicate community-based counseling, special school classes, and tutoring programs had no effects; deterrence-based programs such as boot camps and shock incarceration had negative effects; and well-specified multimodal behavioral treatment programs that led to involvement with prosocial peers reduced recidivism an average of 10% (though the effect size varied greatly across studies; see also Chapter 23, this volume).

TREATMENTS AVAILABLE IN COMMUNITY-BASED SETTINGS

Behavioral Parent Training Approaches

Behavioral parent training (BPT) protocols are the most widely researched therapeutic interventions for children with ODD and CD (Forehand & Kotchick, 1996) and a recent review asserts that mental health, social service, and juvenile justice agencies across the nation offer (or require, in the case of juvenile justice) some form of such training for parents (Serketich & Dumas, 1996).

Many investigators have contributed to the behavioral parent training literature, but the most influential architects of these treatment approaches are Gerald Patterson and colleagues at the Oregon Social Learning Center (OSLC), Alan Kazdin and colleagues at Yale University, and Rex Forehand and colleagues at the University of Georgia. Treatment protocols vary somewhat across investigators and studies, but most share the following core characteristics.

- They have a theoretical foundation in social learning and cognitive theory.
- The parent, rather than the therapist, changes the child's behavior.
- Behaviors and parent–child interactions targeted for intervention are known family correlates of CD (e.g., coercive interchanges, harsh and inconsistent discipline, parental monitoring; see previous chapters, this volume).
- Parents are taught to use rewards, consequences, and nonattending techniques to increase positive and decrease negative child behavior.
- Between-session homework to be completed by parents with their children is assigned.
- Treatment staff often contact parents by phone between sessions to monitor parent and child behavior changes.
- Treatment is time-limited.

Tools commonly used to teach parents behavioral parenting practices include within-session modeling of desired behavior by the therapist and role-played practice, though some protocols have used live parent models effectively (O'Dell, 1985) and others have relied more heavily on verbal methods such as lectures, discussion, and use of reading materials.

Narrative (Kazdin, 1994; Wierson & Forehand, 1994) and meta-analytic reviews (Serketich & Dumas, 1996) of controlled evaluations of BPT have generally affirmed its short-term effectiveness with children ages 6 to 12 years. The reviews also note, however, that the effectiveness of BPT is seriously limited by other family variables such as marital distress, single-parent status, and parental depressive mood, and by contextual variables such as adverse SES circumstances and lack of social support (Forehand & Kotchick, 1996; Kazdin, 1996; Sanders, 1996; Serketich & Dumas, 1996; Wierson & Forehand, 1994). These variables are particularly likely to characterize youth referred by or receiving services through public agencies with mandated responsibility for the treatment and safety of youth with CD. For example, a disproportionate number of legally delinquent youth live in poverty (Fraser, 1996; Tolan, 1996), and SES disadvantage contributes independently to the likelihood that a child will be identified by school systems or other state agencies as having a Serious Emotional Disturbance (Costello *et al.*, 1996). Similarly, parent training studies conducted with samples of young and school-aged children referred by community agencies reveal high rates of marital distress, single parenthood, clinical levels of parental depression, or a combination of these in the samples (for reviews of this work, see Patterson & Chamberlain, 1988,

1994; Webster-Stratton, 1996). Moreover, parent training protocols have generally not been effective with adolescents (Wierson & Forehand, 1994) or juvenile delinquents (for reviews, see Dodge, 1993; Jensen, Hoagwood, & Petti, 1996; Kazdin, 1996; Mulvey, Arthur, & Reppucci, 1993; Tolan, Guerra, & Kendall, 1995). Finally, and importantly, it is not known whether BPT as practiced in treatment studies resembles BPT as implemented by community-based practitioners. Treatment at the OSLC, for example, is implemented by well-trained therapists averaging 1 to 10 years experience with the treatment protocol (Patterson & Chamberlain, 1988), whereas BPT procedures in community settings are likely to be implemented by staff with an eclectic treatment orientation who receive no specialized training or adherence monitoring in BPT (Kazdin, 1994, 1997). Thus, little evidence supports the effectiveness of BPT with the types of children, adolescents, and families that most often come to the attention of public mental health, juvenile justice, and social welfare authorities.

Multicomponent Behavioral Treatments

Videotape Modeling Programs for Families of Young Children

The programmatic research of Caroline Webster-Stratton and her colleagues focuses on the development and evaluation of "widely applicable" (Webster-Stratton, 1996, p. 435) clinically and cost-effective early intervention programs for families with young children exhibiting ODD and CD (see Webster-Stratton, 1996, for a review of this research). Although validated in the context of a university-affiliated parenting clinic, the treatment components were designed expressly with mass dissemination and cost-effectiveness in mind, and a treatment manual and videotapes are available for purchase (Webster-Stratton & Herbert, 1994). In contrast to approaches that use live therapist or parent models, videotaped intervention was based on the hypothesis (supported by Bandura's [1977] modeling theory of

learning) that parents could develop parenting skills by watching and modeling videotape examples of other parents interacting with children in ways that promoted prosocial and decreased disruptive behaviors. To enhance the relevance of the models and exposure to a variety of target situations and to more and less effective parent interventions, videotaped models were parents of differing ages, cultures, SES backgrounds, and temperaments; these parents interacted (unrehearsed) with their own children in a variety of settings—home, school, grocery stores, with other adults and children, and so on.

The original program, called BASIC, consists of three components: videotape modeling, group support and discussion, and therapist development of a collaborative context intended to support and empower parents (Webster-Stratton & Herbert, 1993, 1994). The therapist's role is to teach, lead, reframe, predict, and support participants in the context of discussion about parents' reactions to videotapes and about ideas and problem-solving strategies of group members. The group context was designed to serve several functions: increase cost effectiveness, reduce family isolation, reduce family sense of stigmatization associated with having a child with CD or ODD, and model parental social support networks. Duration of the BASIC parent training program is 26 hours, distributed over 13–14 weekly sessions, during which 10 videotape programs of modeled parenting skills exemplifying behavioral principles are viewed and discussed by groups of 8–12 parents and a therapist. Details of therapeutic processes are described in a treatment guide for clinicians (Webster-Stratton & Herbert, 1994).

Data from randomized trials comparing BASIC with no-treatment controls and other treatments support its efficacy in changing parent attitudes and behavior and child behavior at 1-year follow-up (Webster-Stratton, 1982). A deconstruction study comparing the effects of the components of BASIC—videotape with no group or therapist discussion, videotape with group-only discussion, videotape with therapist-only discussion—indicated that the combined videotape with group and therapist discussion protocol sustained the best improvements at 3-year follow-up (Webster-Stratton, 1990). Consistent with the results of BPT programs implemented with school-aged children, however, treatment efficacy was consistently moderated by marital distress, single-parent status, low SES, high levels of negative life stressors, substance (alcohol, drugs) use, and spousal abuse. Of these factors, single-parent status and marital adjustment were the strongest predictors of child outcomes (i.e., deviant behavior) measured during home observations.

In response to these findings, a 14-session videotape program targeting marital communication and problem-solving skills, personal self-control, and cultivation of social support and self-care was developed. This program, called ADVANCE, was offered following completion of BASIC. The scope of interventions in this program included marital distress, maternal depression, and parental anger. As with the BASIC program, a group format utilizing therapist leadership was used. To evaluate the effects of this enhancement, families were randomly assigned to receive the ADVANCE program or no additional treatment following the completion of BASIC. At 1- and 2-year follow-up, significant improvements in child adjustment and behavior problems, parent–child interactions, and parent distress were maintained in both groups. Children in the AD-VANCE group, however, demonstrated greater nonaggressive problem-solving skills, and the parents in this group demonstrated significant improvements in marital communication, problem solving, and collaboration skills relative to parents in the BASIC group. The improved marital communication skills, in turn, were related to reductions in fathers' criticisms of their children and to improvements in the children's prosocial skills. Finally, consumer satisfaction was significantly greater in the ADVANCE group (Webster-Stratton, 1994).

In response to family requests for assistance with children's homework and with school–family interactions around management of children in school settings, a 6- to 8-week intervention targeting communication and problem solving with individuals in the school and other systems was developed. This program is called PARTNERS, and it is currently being evaluated. Across all programs—BASIC, ADVANCE, and PARTNERS—a combination of videotape modeling, role playing, homework, and therapist-led group discussion occurs. In addition, Webster-Stratton and colleagues (Webster-Stratton & Spitzer, 1996) are conducting qualitative research which suggests that the parent's subjective experiences of the child and family, negative responses and stigmatization from teachers and other members of the community, and ability to maintain a sense of competence despite relapses and stigmatization may moderate engagement and progress in treatment and should inform treatment improvements.

The programmatic research of Webster-Stratton and her colleagues is noteworthy in its consistent and ongoing commitment to enhancing outcomes. In an iterative process, innovations in the treatment model are based on previously identified barriers to achieving favorable outcomes. Moreover, each new treatment component developed by Webster-Stratton's group has incrementally shifted the conceptualization of the etiology and treatment of ODD and CD in young children from a nearly exclusive focus on parent deficits in behavioral techniques to a model that hypothesizes "that the child's eventual outcome will be dependent on the interrelationships among children, parents, teachers, and peers" (Webster-Stratton, 1996, p. 468)—a model that emphasizes the social-ecological nature of behavior (Bronfenbrenner, 1979).

Combined Parent Management Training (PMT) and Problem-Solving Skills Training (PSST)

The programmatic research of Alan Kazdin and his colleagues at Yale University focuses on the individual and combined effects of parent training and child cognitive-behavioral interventions on youth ages 7–13 years with ODD and CD (for treatment details and research review, see Kazdin, 1996). The child-focused intervention, Problem Solving Skills

Training (PSST), and parent-focused intervention, Parent Management Training (PMT) had been tested as single-component interventions in previous studies (for a review of these studies, see Kazdin, 1994). In the combined protocol, PMT and PSST procedures are individualized to take into account the structure of a particular family (e.g., single- or dual-parent status, divorced parents with joint custody), incentives readily available for the parent, and parameters that influence a parent's ability to implement and monitor the interventions (e.g., number of children in the home, parent's work schedule, financial situation). The elements of the PMT protocol are consistent with the shared characteristics of BPT enumerated earlier (e.g., parent as change agent, clearly defined target behaviors, role-play rehearsal of parent behavior, homework, monitoring). Behavior contracts between parents and children are crafted in sessions and carried out at home, where a token reinforcement system is established by the parent. The contract also involves home-based reinforcement for behavior that occurs in school. The PSST protocol is implemented in the context of therapist–child sessions, with collateral parent involvement to reinforce the child's efforts at more effective problem solving. As with most problem-solving approaches for youth, PSST uses situations the child actually encounters to model, role-play, coach, and help the child practice the development of more effective social problem-solving skills.

Although conducted in the context of a university-based clinic, Kazdin's study samples included significant proportions of families of diverse racial backgrounds and lower to lower-middle SES. Results of a series of studies indicate that PSST, when delivered alone or in conjunction with PMT over the course of 8–12 months, produced reliable and significant reductions in CD and increases in prosocial behavior at home, at school, and in the community as long as 1 year following treatment (Kazdin, Siegel, & Bass, 1992). As with BPT programs, however, family (e.g., marital discord, single-parent families), parent (e.g., depression, stress, psychopathology), and SES variables were associated with premature termination from treatment and with decreased magnitude and duration of treatment gains. Also, treatment was less effective with CD of greater severity and with families of color. In discussing these findings, Kazdin has suggested that advances in the development of more effective treatment for youth with CD require a deeper understanding of the multiple contexts in which families of such youth are embedded (Kazdin, 1996, 1997) and specification of intervention models that effectively address contextual barriers to favorable outcomes.

Family Therapies

Controlled evaluations of certain pragmatic (vs. aesthetic; cf. Henggeler, Borduin, & Mann, 1993) forms of family therapy have demonstrated their promise in the treatment of adolescent CD and drug use problems (for reviews, see Alexander, Holtzworth-Munroe, & Jameson, 1994; Henggeler, Borduin, & Mann, 1993; Kazdin, 1987; Liddle & Dakof, 1995). The treatment approaches are Functional Family Therapy (FFT), developed by James Alexander and his colleagues (Alexander & Parsons, 1982); multidimensional family therapy (MDFT), developed by Howard Liddle and colleagues (Liddle & Dakof, 1995; Liddle, Dakof, & Diamond, 1991); a structural family therapy (SFT) approach for families from culturally diverse backgrounds developed by Jose Szapocznik and colleagues (for a review, see Kurtines & Szapocznik, 1996); and Multisystemic Therapy, developed by Scott Henggeler and colleagues (MST; Henggeler & Borduin, 1990; Henggeler, Schoenwald, Borduin, Rowland, & Cunningham, 1998). Although the SFT and MDFT models have focused on drug use rather than CD, evidence regarding the covariation of drug use and CD and of etiologic factors common to both (for a review, see Henggeler, 1997), and findings regarding tandem reductions in drug use and CD following treatment (Liddle & Dakof, 1995; Szapocznik, Santisteban, Rio, Perez-Vidal, & Kurtines, 1989) suggest that these models are also effective in reducing conduct problems in adolescents.

Functional Family Therapy

Functional Family Therapy (FFT; Alexander & Parsons, 1982), introduced originally as a behavioral-systems approach to family therapy (Alexander & Parsons, 1973), was among the first family therapies to combine social learning and family systems interventions and to target delinquent youth. Initial outcome studies demonstrated the efficacy of FFT in reducing status offenses in a target population of first-time status offenders largely from middle-class Mormon families (see Alexander & Parsons, 1982). Subsequent tests of its efficacy with youth engaged in delinquent (as opposed to status) offenses were conducted in the context of three quasi-experimental studies characterized by differing methodologies (e.g., single group design, post hoc comparison of FFT and standard services as delivered by probation workers, planned comparison of FFT and behavioral group home treatment) (Barton, Alexander, Waldron, Turner, & Warburton, 1985). Archival data regarding recidivism were favorable, though standardized assessments were not conducted and variations in design rigor limited the conclusiveness of study results.

Subsequent to these studies, Gordon and colleagues (Gordon, Arbuthnot, Gustafson, & McGreen, 1988) compared FFT and a no-treatment control condition in a quasi-experimental study involving 56 white juveniles most of whom had committed only status offenses (57% of offenses), some of whom had committed misdemeanors (30% of offenses), and felonies (13% of offenses). The FFT group consisted of 15 male and 12 female youth, and the comparison group was composed of 23 male and 4 female youth randomly selected from a population of delinquents adjudicated during the same period as the FFT group. This project was the first to deliver FFT in families' homes, which were located in a rural and lower-SES community. Clinicians were relatively inexperienced but well-trained graduate students. Family sessions, each lasting approximately 1.5 hr, extended over an average of 5.5 months, and the average number of sessions was 16 (range 7–38). Archival data available for 83% of the sample 2.8 years after the original follow-up period, when participants were 20–22 years of age, showed significant differences favoring the treatment group with respect to misdemeanor, but not felony, recidivism rates.

These findings suggest that FFT delivered in the home is a promising home- and community-based treatment for youth engaged in status offenses, and, potentially, for youth engaged in criminal activity. The treatment model may also be cost-effective, particularly if paraprofessionals can deliver it effectively (see Gordon & Arbuthnot, 1988). However, the lack of a single randomized trial with predominantly delinquent (as opposed to status-offending) populations limits the confidence with which the efficacy of FFT with serious antisocial behavior can be presumed. Thus, although the investigators have recommended that home-based FFT be disseminated widely (Gordon, Graves, & Arbuthnot, 1995) and have done the laudable service of developing a training and consultation format that can be delivered to paraprofessionals, more rigorous evaluations of FFT with delinquent youth should be undertaken to identify the target populations potential practitioners can be expected to treat effectively with the model.

Multidimensional Family Therapy (MDFT)

Multidimensional family therapy (MDFT; Liddle, 1995; Liddle *et al.*, 1991) is a new, empirically derived, multicomponent intervention developed for the treatment of adolescent substance abuse. Results of a controlled trial comparing MDFT with adolescent group therapy and multifamily educational interventions indicated that MDFT was more effective in reducing drug use posttreatment and in maintaining reductions in use at 1-year follow-up (Liddle & Dakof, 1995; Liddle *et al.*, 1995). Youth receiving MDFT also evidenced more improvement in school performance relative to youth in the other two treatment conditions.

MDFT targets four domains for intervention, and each of these has several dimensions. The domains are (1) the adolescent's intrapersonal and interpersonal (family, peers) functioning, (2) the parents' intrapersonal and interpersonal functioning (e.g., parenting practices, functioning as an adult apart from the parenting role), (3) parent–adolescent interactions as observed in sessions and reported by parent and adolescent, and (4) family interactions with extrafamilal sources of influence (e.g., school and child welfare personnel, probation officers) (Schmidt, Liddle, & Dakof, 1996). Specific modules guide assessment and intervention in each of these domains and coordination of interventions across domains, although these modules are still being refined and tested (see Liddle, 1995).

As with all pragmatic family interventions, a basic tenet of MDFT is that change in the behavior of an individual results from change in the family system. A recent study conducted with a subsample of 29 families who had completed 16 sessions of MDFT provides evidence to support the link between changes in parental subsystem functioning and reductions in adolescent substance use and problem behaviors (Schmidt *et al.,* 1996). Significant improvement in parenting, as evidenced by decreased negative practices and affect and increased positive practices and affect was observed in 69% of parents. Although most parents and adolescents improved in tandem, change patterns varied, with 21% of families experiencing adolescent change in the absence of parent change and 10% experiencing parent change but no adolescent change. In exploring hypotheses to explain these patterns, the authors suggested that an advantage of MDFT is its access to alternative domains (e.g., the adolescent) if interventions with a primary target (e.g., the parental subsystem) fail. They also raised the possibility, however, that for some problems, such as chronic delinquency and serious adolescent drug use, "intervention simply may have come too late to reverse these powerful, already well-established, detrimental influences" (pp. 20-21). Although future research may support this position, an alternative hypothesis—that interventions can be effective if they focus intensely on the interfaces between these "detrimental influences" and the family, in the natural environment—is supported by

the outcomes of multisystemic therapy (MST) with violent and chronic delinquents (described later in this chapter).

Structural Family Therapy in Diverse Cultural Contexts

For over two decades, Jose Szapocznik and his colleagues have conducted programmatic research on the use of structural family therapy (SFT) with adolescent youth engaged in drug use and CD. The hallmark of this programmatic research is its focus on families of diverse cultural contexts and communities. To this end, the group has moved beyond monolithic constructions of culture and its implications for behavior and treatment to a conceptualization that honors variations among individuals who share a similar cultural heritage that arise as a function of cohort (e.g., recent Cuban immigrants vs. Cuban-born American citizens vs. Cuban Americans), community context (largely monocultural vs. increasingly diverse), and the values and experiences of a particular family within a culture and community. Reviews of this work chronicle the group's development of specialized applications for recent Hispanic immigrant families, Hispanic American families, African American families living in largely Hispanic communities, and non-Cuban Hispanic families (Kurtines & Szapocznik, 1996; Szapocznik, Kurtines, Santisteban, & Rio, 1990).

The bedrock of the group's treatment is Minuchin's structural family therapy approach (Minuchin, 1974; Minuchin & Fishman, 1981). The structural approach embodies the systems view that interdependence between parts of a system can be understood in terms of repetitive patterns of interactions between the parts. Three putative change mechanisms associated with structural family therapy, and specific techniques subsumed within them form the basis of the therapeutic process examined across several of the group's studies. These mechanisms are joining, the techniques used by the therapist to enter the system, diagnosing or identifying maladaptive interactions, and restructuring or changing maladaptive interactions that are demonstrably related to the particular symptoms (behavior problems) exhibited in the family. Techniques used to accomplish one or more phases of treatment vary as a function of the family's cultural context. Thus, for example, inasmuch as white Americans have come to value individuation and separation more than Hispanics (Kurtines & Szapocznik, 1996), a therapist may view interaction patterns that signal enmeshment in a white American family as normative for a Hispanic family. Alternatively, if the interactions that signal enmeshment are clearly associated with a referral problem, even in a Hispanic family, the treatment would target the interactions with structural interventions.

The group's early studies established the efficacy of SFT in reducing drug use among adolescents on treatment termination (Szapocznik, Santisteban, et al., 1986; Szapocznik et al., 1989) and of one-person (i.e., structural techniques are used to change family interactions through one person) and conjoint family therapy (Szapocznik, Kurtines, Foote, Perez-Vidal, & Hervis, 1986) in sustaining reductions in adolescent drug use and behavior problems and improved family functioning 6–12 months following termination (albeit with small sample sizes). A second series of studies focused on engaging adolescents and families in treatment and compared Strategic Structural Systems Engagement (SSSE; Szapocznik & Kurtines, 1989; see also Santisteban et al., 1996), designed to join, diagnose, and restructure the family on first contact, with traditional engagement strategies (i.e., expression of polite concern, interviewing about problems and well-being of family members). Three engagement strategies comprised the experimental condition, and the highest level included making out-of-office visits to family members and engaging significant others to help. Findings indicated that the specialized engagement strategy was more effective in engaging and retaining adolescent drug users and their families in treatment: Of the 93% successfully engaged in the SSSE condition, 75% completed treatment; of the 42% successfully engaged in the control condition, only 25% completed treatment. A subsequent study indicated, however, that the SSSE strategy was more successful in engaging non-Cuban Hispanic families than with Cuban Hispanic families, who wanted hospitalization or individual therapy for their drug-using adolescents and were willing to work with formal service systems to obtain it. The authors hypothesized that the greater adoption of mainstream American orientations and behaviors of Cuban Hispanic families might account for the differential effects of the engagement strategies.

Most recently, Szapocznik and colleagues have expanded intervention targets beyond within-family interactions. The emerging model, called a Structural Ecological Theory (SET; Szapocznik et al., 1997) views interactions between systems as (1) contributing to the maintenance of adolescent problem behavior, and (2) amenable to structural interventions. This theory draws on the social ecological theory of Bronfenbrenner (1979), the drug abuse prevention models of Hawkins and Weis (1985), and Multisystemic Therapy (MST) (Henggeler & Borduin, 1990; Henggeler et al., 1998). SET-informed intervention programs currently being examined in experimental studies include a neighborhood-based, parent-focused approach designed to enhance interactions in parent–peer and parent–community mesosystems and exosystems through such interventions as parent organization of youth field trips and sports teams and parent involvement in social support networks in the community. A second intervention program seeks to reduce drug use among African American and Hispanic adolescents through the application of the structural techniques of joining, diagnosing, and restructuring maladaptive interaction patterns not only within the family system but between the family, school, and peer systems.

Multisystemic Therapy

Multisystemic Therapy (MST; Henggeler & Borduin, 1990; Henggeler et al., 1998) is an intensive, time-limited (3- to 5-month) treatment approach predicated on social-ecological (Bronfenbrenner, 1979) and pragmatic family systems models of behavior (Haley, 1976;

Minuchin, 1974) and informed by findings from multivariate studies that implicate a combination of family (inadequate parental monitoring of youth whereabouts, high conflict, low warmth, inconsistent or harsh discipline practices, and parental problems), peer (association with deviant peers), school (low family–school bonding, problems with academic and social performance), and neighborhood (transience, disorganization, criminal subculture) factors in the development of delinquency and drug use (Elliott, 1994; Thornberry, Huizinga, & Loeber, 1995; Tolan & Guerra, 1994). Thus, MST views individuals as being nested in a complex of interconnected systems that encompass individual (e.g., biological, cognitive), family, and extrafamilial (peer, school, neighborhood) factors, and behavior problems as maintained by problematic transactions within and between any one or combination of the systems. Targets of MST intervention therefore include interactions within the family and between the family and other systems in the natural (e.g., peers, neighborhood, workplace) and service (e.g., mental health, juvenile justice, education, child welfare) ecologies (Schoenwald, Borduin, & Henggeler, 1998). Nine treatment principles (see Table 1) guide the development and implementation of MST interventions, the overarching goal of which is to empower parents with the skills and resources needed to address the inevitable difficulties that arise in rearing adolescents and to empower youth to cope with family, peer, school, and neighborhood problems. Although implemented within a broad social-ecological clinical paradigm, MST interventions are both individualized and consistent with those (i.e., behavioral, cognitive-behavioral, pragmatic family systems) evidencing the largest effect sizes in the meta-analytic literature (Lipsey, 1992; Weisz & Weiss, 1993). Treatment sessions are active, highly focused, and held as often as every day early in treatment, and as infrequently as once a week later in treatment. A clinically oriented volume introduced MST to the field of family therapy (Henggeler & Borduin, 1990) and a manual for practitioners details the ongoing and interrelated assessment and intervention

practices that characterize MST (Henggeler *et al.*, 1998).

Throughout the development and validation of MST, considerable attention has been devoted to issues of external validity and ecological validity—the applicability of the treatment model to real-world clinical populations seen in community settings by public sector mental health professionals. Thus, MST as delivered in community-based clinical trials and in subsequent community-initiated programs around the country has been provided in a family preservation or home-based model of service delivery (described in the next section of this chapter). As such, MST is (1) provided in the home, school, neighborhood, and community setting; (2) intense (2–15 hours of service provided per family per week); (3) flexible (clinicians are available 24 hours per day, 7 days a week); (4) time-limited (4–6 months); and (5) characterized by low caseloads (4–6 families per clinician).

TABLE 1.   MST Treatment Principles

Principle 1 The primary purpose of assessment is to understand the fit between the identified problems and their broader systemic context

Principle 2 Therapeutic contacts should emphasize the positive and should use systemic strengths as levers for change

Principle 3 Interventions should be designed to promote responsible behavior and decrease irresponsible behavior among family members

Principle 4 Interventions should be present-focused and action-oriented, targeting specific and well-defined problems

Principle 5 Interventions should target sequences of behavior within and between multiple systems that maintain the identified problems

Principle 6 Interventions should be developmentally appropriate and fit the developmental needs of the youth

Principle 7 Interventions should be designed to require daily or weekly effort by family members

Principle 8 Intervention efficacy is evaluated continuously from multiple perspectives with providers assuming accountability for overcoming barriers to successful outcomes

Principle 9 Interventions should be designed to promote treatment generalization and long-term maintenance of therapeutic change by empowering caregivers to address family members' needs across multiple systemic contexts

MST was originally developed in a university research setting, with early clinical trials supporting its short-term efficacy in treating delinquent inner-city adolescents (Henggeler et al., 1986), maltreating families (Brunk, Henggeler, & Whelan, 1987), and a small sample of juvenile sex offenders (Borduin, Henggeler, Blaske, & Stein, 1990). In these early clinical trials, clinicians were doctoral-level students in clinical psychology. Treatment fidelity was monitored through weekly clinical group supervision and review of treatment logs. Posttreatment measures of youth behavior problems (Henggeler et al., 1986), family functioning, and reoccurrence of offending (Borduin et al., 1990) indicated that MST was significantly more effective as compared with usual community treatments (Henggeler et al., 1986), behavioral parent training (Brunk et al., 1987), and individual outpatient counseling (Borduin et al., 1990).

Subsequent studies demonstrating the longer-term efficacy of MST were conducted under the auspices of university (Borduin et al., 1995) and public service sector (Henggeler, Melton, & Smith, 1992; Henggeler, Melton, Smith, Schoenwald, & Hanley, 1993) settings. These studies were characterized by similarities in design (randomized, two groups, pre- and posttest, follow-up for recidivism), participants (serious juvenile offenders and their families), treatment intensity, clinical supervisory practices, treatment fidelity, and favorable outcome (see Henggeler, Schoenwald, & Pickrel, 1995). In the university-based study, MST clinicians were doctoral students. In the community-based study, MST clinicians were master's level counselors with an average of 2 years experience employed by a public community mental health agency. In these studies, MST sustained reductions in criminal behavior 2.4 years (Henggeler et al., 1992; Henggeler, Melton, et al., 1993) and 4 years (Borduin et al., 1995) following treatment. The relative efficacy of MST was moderated neither by demographic characteristics (race, age, social class, gender, arrest and incarceration history) nor by psychosocial variables (family relations, peer relations, social competence, behavior problems, and parental

symptomatology). Thus, MST was equally effective with youth and families of divergent backgrounds. In addition, reductions in substance use and arrests for substance-related crimes were achieved (Henggeler et al., 1991), as were improvements in family functioning. Finally, a comparison of cost indicated that the cost per client for treatment in the MST group was about $3,500, which compares favorably with the average cost of institutional placement in South Carolina of $17,769 per offender; such placement was significantly greater for youth in the usual services condition.

The success of MST with serious juvenile offenders and their families has led to evaluations of the effectiveness of MST with other populations presenting serious problems. For example, data from an ongoing randomized trial with 118 substance abusing or dependent adolescent offenders suggest that MST is effective in reducing soft-drug and hard-drug use at posttreatment and incarceration and out-of-home placement at 1-year postreferral (Henggeler, Pickrel, & Brondino, 1998). Moreover, cost analyses have shown that the costs of MST were nearly offset by savings accrued as a result of reductions in days of out-of-home placement (hospitalization, residential treatment) in the MST condition, relative to the usual services condition, 1 year following referral (Schoenwald, Ward, Henggeler, Pickrel, & Patel, 1996). Finally, the MST engagement and alliance process resulted in a 98% completion rate (Henggeler, Pickrel, Brondino, & Crouch, 1996).

As a second example of the extension of MST to other challenging clinical populations, MST is being evaluated as an alternative to hospitalization of youths presenting psychiatric emergencies (i.e., suicidal, homicidal, psychotic) in a randomized trial. Data from the pilot study portion of the trial suggest that MST is a more effective and less costly strategy than psychiatric hospitalization for addressing the mental health emergencies of adolescents with severe emotional disturbances (Henggeler, Rowland, et al., 1997). This study will eventually include 252 youth and families and both clinical (e.g., symptomatology, adaptive functioning) and service-level (utilization, cost-effectiveness) outcomes will be examined. Clinical trials evaluating the effectiveness of MST as an alternative to incarceration, out-of-state residential placement, and community-based treatments for youth engaged in serious antisocial behavior are also being conducted by investigators in Ohio (Timmons-Mitchell, 1997), Texas (Thomas, 1994), Delaware (Miller, 1997), and Ontario, Canada (Lescheid, 1997).

Newly funded projects further expand the target populations, intervention components, and service system parameters (e.g., location of services; cross-agency and grassroots collaboration in service design and delivery) to be addressed using MST. All projects were designed in collaboration with public agencies (e.g., mental health, substance abuse, juvenile justice, education). Projects already under way include a federally funded quasi-experimental study of the effectiveness of MST blended with the Community Reinforcement Approach (Higgins & Budney, 1993) in the treatment of substance-abusing parents or guardians of young children, and a qualitative and quantitative evaluation of a program of integrated substance abuse, mental health, primary care, and educational–vocational services for pregnant adolescents and adolescent parents. This study is embedded in a national evaluation of Head Start for children of teen parents. Two recently funded projects focus on developing ecologically based services for settings characterized by high prevalence of mental health problems: (1) a neighborhood with extremely high rates of adult and juvenile crime, abuse or neglect, infant mortality, and poverty; and (2) an inner-city middle school in a low SES neighborhood that has very high rates of violence, drug use, and dropout. Both projects are funded by the South Carolina Department of Health and Human Services. In the first, an assessment of needs in a neighborhood characterized by high rates of adult and juvenile crime, child abuse and neglect, infant mortality, and poverty will form the basis for the development of a neighborhood–research center collaborative that will design and implement an empirically informed array of neighborhood-based services. In the second, ecologically based prevention and intervention strategies (including MST) will be developed, implemented, and evaluated in collaboration with school personnel, neighborhood residents, and staff from state agencies.

Alternative Models of Treatment Delivery for CD Youth

Family Preservation Services

Family preservation services (FPS) increasingly have been recommended by clinical child psychology (Culbertson, 1993; Roberts, 1994) and mental health services researchers (Burns & Friedman, 1990; Stroul & Friedman, 1994) as desirable alternatives to the use of restrictive and expensive placements for youth with serious behavioral and emotional problems. Family preservation is a model of service delivery through which a variety of counseling and concrete service interventions are implemented in the homes and communities of referred families. A basic assumption underlying most programs is that children are better off being reared in their natural families than in surrogate families or institutions (Nelson & Landsman, 1992). Thus, the family is seen as a source of strengths, even when serious and multiple needs are evident, and a common objective is to empower families to meet, and garner resources to meet, their needs in the future.

In the past decade, family preservation programs have proliferated, distinct practice models have emerged, and target populations have diversified to include youth and families referred by juvenile justice and mental health agencies (Nelson & Landsman, 1992; Wells & Biegel, 1991). Dimensions on which programs vary include service delivery characteristics (e.g., caseload, duration of service), type of clinical interventions deployed, and relative emphasis on the provision of clinical as opposed to concrete services (e.g., transportation to medical appointments, cleaning house). Discussion of the common and distinctive elements of various programs and of research on their effectiveness with different target populations is beyond the scope of this chapter and appears elsewhere (see Fraser, Nelson, & Rivard, 1997; Kutash & Rivera, 1996; Nelson & Landsman, 1992; Schoenwald & Henggeler, 1997). In general, however, crisis-based models developed initially for use with abuse and neglect referrals last 4–6 weeks and combine a package of concrete services with skills-building techniques (e.g., parent–child conflict resolution, parent behavior management); home-based and family treatment models are of longer duration (3–5 months), incorporate family systems theory in their conceptualization of referral problems, use behavioral interventions such as parent training only as needed, and attend to family interactions with the community more directly than is the case with crisis-intervention models.

Studies indicate that failure rates among family preservation programs are high (Feldman, 1991; Fraser, Pecora, & Haapala, 1991; Nelson, 1990; Nelson & Landsman, 1992; Yuan, McDonald, Wheeler, Struckman-Johnson, & Rivest, 1990). A recent meta-analytic review (Fraser et al., 1997) of their effects on child welfare, juvenile justice, and mental health populations suggests, however, that they may be relatively more successful with older children referred for CD or ODD than with child abuse referrals. It should be noted, however, that clinical trials of MST comprised the majority of the controlled studies in the juvenile justice category. Thus, with the exception of MST, little evidence supports the effectiveness of family preservation services with youth engaged in antisocial behavior and data regarding its effectiveness with children at risk of abuse and neglect are discouraging.

Despite scant evidence of their effectiveness, various models of family preservation have been implemented by child-serving agencies seeking alternatives to out-of-home placement. As a result, child welfare, juvenile justice, and mental health agencies in many communities seek to avert placement by referring youth and families to family preservation services (typically the 4- to 6-week crisis-oriented model) which are no more likely to be effective in achieving desired outcomes (e.g., reductions in abuse or neglect, delinquency) than are community-based practices delivered

in clinic settings. A cadre of practitioners (social workers, therapists, psychologists) are delivering home-based services to youth referred for antisocial behavior who are perceived (by the referring agent) to be at imminent risk for removal from the home but these practitioners have very little, if any, knowledge and skill in the identification and treatment of the proximal processes within and outside of the family system associated with CD. Thus, reviewers have suggested (Fraser et al., 1997; Oswald & Singh, 1996; Rosenblatt, 1996), and we concur, that the FPS model of service delivery is not likely to become more effective until interventions delivered to target populations (e.g., children at risk of abuse and neglect, youth with ODD and CD, delinquent youth) address the known correlates of the referral problem (child abuse and neglect, ODD or CD, delinquency) with evidence-based interventions (for further discussion, see Schoenwald & Henggeler, 1997).

Therapeutic Foster Care

Although the treatments described thus far focus on the youth's natural environment, the fact remains that many youth whose CD has attracted service system attention are ordered to institutional and residential placements for treatment. A promising alternative to institutionalization being evaluated in clinical trials is therapeutic foster care. Therapeutic foster care programs have proliferated in recent years, although controlled evaluation of their effectiveness is rare (for reviews, see Kutash & Rivera, 1996; Reddy & Pfeiffer, 1997). Foster family and group home care are two prevalent service models, and both have been implemented with juvenile delinquents. In the group home model, several delinquents reside with professionally trained foster parents and both the foster parents and the other delinquents are believed to facilitate treatment. Perhaps the most widely disseminated of the group home model is the Teaching Family Model, which demonstrated promise in early studies but fell short of expectations in subsequent investigations (for a review, see Wolf,

Kirigin, Fixsen, & Blase, 1995). Given recent findings (Dishion & Andrews, 1995) supporting the hypothesis that increased contact with problem peers in treatment settings can exacerbate problem behavior and the fact that youth return to unchanged ecologies (i.e., family, peer group, school, neighborhood) following discharge, the failure of the Teaching Family Model to obtain lasting results might have been expected.

In the foster family model, individual youths are placed with foster families in which the parents are seen as critical change agents. The advantages of this model include the nonrestrictiveness of placement, increased exposure to prosocial peers, and lower costs (Chamberlain, 1990). Patricia Chamberlain and her colleagues at the OSLC have developed and tested a Treatment Foster Care (TFC) treatment protocol with two adolescent populations: those with chronic delinquency and CD and those with serious emotional disturbances. Descriptions of the program elements are available in a manual (Chamberlain, 1994) and in a recent review of research on the model (Chamberlain, 1996). This treatment approach is described in detail in Chapter 23 (this volume) and need not be discussed further here.

TOWARD MORE EFFECTIVE COMMUNITY-BASED TREATMENT

Several chapters in this volume, and research cited in this chapter attest to the multidetermined nature of CD and ODD and to more serious antisocial behaviors such as delinquent acts and drug abuse often committed by youth carrying such a diagnosis. Leading researchers have suggested that it may be necessary to address a comprehensive range of the proximal processes that contribute to the disorder (Dodge, 1993; Henggeler, 1997; Tolan, 1996) if favorable clinical outcomes are to be achieved. The accumulating longitudinal database on the etiologic pathways to CD, delinquency, and adolescent drug abuse have given rise to an ecological-developmental framework that suggests that the nature and number of

proximal processes may change at different points of development (Fraser, 1996; Kazdin, 1997; Liddle, 1996; Tolan et al., 1995). The most promising treatments reviewed in this chapter can be conceptualized as addressing aspects of the youth's ecology implicated by multivariate models of the behavior problem at a particular stage in the child or adolescent's development. Thus, for example, Webster-Stratton's program focused initially on the parenting variables associated with ODD in young children (e.g., coercive parent–child cycles that reinforce aggressive behavior, harsh and inconsistent discipline practices); subsequent iterations targeted additional intrafamilial (marital, single-parent stresses) and extrafamilial factors (relations with school, social support) that moderated treatment effects and became more relevant as children began attending school. By virtue of their systemic (as opposed to behavioral) perspective and focus on older youth, Szapocznik and colleagues focused from the outset on a broader range of within-family processes and more recently have targeted interactions between the family and the known correlates of adolescent drug use and problem behavior in other systems (peers, neighborhood, school) for structural intervention. MST has, from its inception, targeted the variables known to directly or indirectly predict delinquency, has been delivered in the family's indigenous environment, and has produced the largest effect sizes of any treatment delivered in a family preservation model of service with juvenile justice populations (Fraser et al., 1997).

To significantly impact the availability and effectiveness of community-based treatments for youth with persistent and serious CD, however, interventions with demonstrated effectiveness must be integrated into extant service systems. Accomplishing this objective is likely to require the development of effective dissemination strategies that address service system, fiscal, organizational, and professional factors that sustain current practices (see Brown, 1995; Schoenwald & Henggeler, in press; Weisz, Donenberg, Han, & Weiss, 1995), as well as expansions in the conceptualizations of treatment (along ecological-developmental lines) and methods of testing their efficacy (see Hoagwood *et al.*, 1995; Kazdin, 1997; Weisz *et al.*, 1997) to better reflect the real-world conditions under which families and community-based practitioners jointly seek to change the behavior of CD youth.

ACKNOWLEDGMENTS. Preparation of this manuscript was supported in part by National Institute of Mental Health Grants MH-51852 and R01-MH51852, National Institute on Drug Abuse Grant RO1 DA10079-01A1, The Center for Mental Health Services, Substance Abuse and Mental Health Services Administration, Administration for Children and Families, DHHS, 90FYF0012/01, and the Annie E. Casey Foundation.

REFERENCES

Alexander, J. F., & Parsons, B. V. (1973). Short-term behavioral intervention with delinquent families: Impact on family process and recidivism. *Journal of Abnormal Psychology, 81,* 219–225.

Alexander, J. F., & Parsons, B. V. (1982). *Functional family therapy.* Monterey, CA: Brooks/Cole.

Alexander, J. F., Holtzworth-Munroe, A., & Jameson, P. (1994). The process and outcome of marital and family therapy: Research review and evaluation. In A. E. Bergin & S. L. Garfield (Eds.), *Handbook of psychotherapy and behavior change* (pp. 595–630). New York: Wiley.

Bandura, A. (1977). *Social learning theory.* Englewood Cliffs, NJ: Prentice Hall.

Barton, C., Alexander, J. F., Waldron, H., Turner, C. W., & Warburton, J. (1985). Generalizing treatment effects of functional family therapy: Three replications. *American Journal of Family Therapy, 13,* 16–26.

Borduin, C. M., Henggeler, S. W., Blaske, D. M., & Stein, R. (1990). Multisystemic treatment of adolescent sexual offenders. *International Journal of Offender Therapy and Comparative Criminology, 34,* 105–113.

Borduin, C. M., Mann, B. J., Cone, L. T., Henggeler, S. W., Fucci, B. R., Blaske, D. M., & Williams, R. A. (1995). Multisystemic treatment of serious juvenile offenders: Long-term prevention of criminality and violence. *Journal of Consulting and Clinical Psychology, 63,* 569–578.

Bronfenbrenner, U. (1979). *The ecology of human development: Experiments by nature and design.* Cambridge, MA: Harvard University Press.

Brown, B. S. (1995). Reducing impediments to technology transfer in drug abuse programming. *Reviewing the behavioral science knowledge base on technology transfer*

(NIDA Monograph No. 155, pp. 169–185). Rockville, MD: National Institute on Drug Abuse.

Brunk, M., Henggeler, S. W., & Whelan, J. P. (1987). A comparison of multisystemic therapy and parent training in the brief treatment of child abuse and neglect. *Journal of Consulting and Clinical Psychology, 55,* 311–318.

Burns, B. J., & Friedman, R. M. (1990). Examining the research base for child mental health services and policy. *Journal of Mental Health Administration, 17,* 87–97.

Chamberlain, P. (1990). Comparative evaluation of specialized foster care for seriously delinquent youths: A first step. *Community Alternatives: International Journal of Family Care, 2,* 21–36.

Chamberlain, P. (1994). *Family connections* (Vol. 5). Eugene, OR: Castalia.

Chamberlain, P. (1996). Intensified foster care: Multi-level treatment for adolescents with conduct disorders in out-of-home care. In E. D. Hibbs & P. S. Jensen (Eds.), *Psychosocial treatments for child and adolescent disorders: Empirically based strategies for clinical practice* (pp. 475–490). Washington, DC: American Psychological Association.

Cohen, M. A., Miller, T. R., & Rossman, S. B. (1994). The costs and consequences of violent behavior in the United States. In A. J. Reiss, Jr., & J. A. Roth (Eds.), *Understanding and preventing violence* (pp. 67–166). Washington, DC: National Research Council, National Academy Press.

Costello, E. J., Angold, A., Burns, B. J., Erkanli, A., Stangle, D. K., & Tweed, D. L. (1996). The Great Smoky Mountains Study of Youth: Functional impairment and serious emotional disturbance. *Archives of General Psychiatry, 53,* 1137–1143.

Culbertson, J. (1993). Clinical child psychology: Broadening our scope. *Journal of Clinical Child Psychology, 22,* 116–122.

Dishion, T. J., & Andrews, D. W. (1995). Preventing escalation in problem behaviors with high-risk young adolescents: Immediate and 1-year outcomes. *Journal of Consulting and Clinical Psychology, 63,* 538–548.

Dodge, K. A. (1993). The future of research on the treatment of conduct disorder. *Development and Psychopathology, 5,* 311–319.

Elliott, D. S. (1994). *Youth violence: An overview.* Boulder: University of Colorado, Center for the Study and Prevention of Violence, Institute for Behavioral Sciences.

Feldman, L. H. (1991). Evaluating the impact of intensive family preservation services in New Jersey. In K. Wells & D. E. Biegel (Eds.), *Family preservation services: Research and evaluation* (pp. 33–47). Newbury Park, CA: Sage.

Forehand, R., & Kotchick, B. A. (1996). Cultural diversity: A wake-up call for parent training. *Behavior Therapy, 27,* 187–206.

Fraser, M. W. (1996). Aggressive behavior in childhood and early adolescence: An ecological-developmental perspective on youth violence. *Social Work, 41,* 347–361.

Fraser, M. W., Pecora, P. J., & Haapala, D. A. (1991). *Families in crisis: The impact of intensive family preservation services.* New York: Aldine de Gruyter.

Fraser, M. W., Nelson, K. E., & Rivard, J. C. (1997). The effectiveness of family preservation services. *Social Work Research, 21,* 138–153.

Gordon, D. A., & Arbuthnot, J. (1988). The use of paraprofessionals to deliver home-based family therapy to juvenile delinquents. *Criminal Justice and Behavior, 15,* 364–378.

Gordon, D. A., Arbuthnot, J., Gustafson, K., & McGreen, P. (1988). Home-based behavioral-systems family therapy with disadvantaged juvenile delinquents. *American Journal of Family Therapy, 16,* 243–255.

Gordon, D. A., Graves, K., & Arbuthnot, J. (1995). The effect of functional family therapy for delinquents on adult criminal behavior. *Criminal Justice and Behavior, 22,* 60–73.

Haley, J. (1976). *Problem solving therapy.* San Francisco: Jossey-Bass.

Hawkins, J. D., & Weis, J. G. (1985). The social development model: An integrated approach to delinquency prevention. *Journal of Primary Prevention, 6,* 73–97.

Henggeler, S. W. (1997). The development of effective drug abuse services for youth. In J. A. Egertson, D. M. Fox, & A. I. Leshner (Eds.), *Treating drug abusers effectively* (pp. 253–279). A copublication with the Milbank Memorial Fund. New York: Blackwell.

Henggeler, S. W., & Borduin, C. M. (1990). *Family therapy and beyond: A multisystemic approach to treating the behavior problems of children and adolescents.* Pacific Grove, CA: Brooks/Cole.

Henggeler, S. W., Rodick, J. D., Borduin, C. M., Hanson, C. L., Watson, S. M., & Urey, J. R. (1986). Multisystemic treatment of juvenile offenders: Effects on adolescent behavior and family interaction. *Developmental Psychology, 22,* 132–141.

Henggeler, S. W., Borduin, C. M., Melton, G. B., Mann, B. J., Smith, L. A., Hall, J. A., Cone, L., & Fucci, B. R. (1991). Effects of multisystemic therapy on drug use and abuse in serious juvenile offenders: A progress report from two outcome studies. *Family Dynamics of Addiction Quarterly, 1,* 40–51.

Henggeler, S. W., Melton, G. B., & Smith, L. A. (1992). Family preservation using multisystemic therapy: An effective alternative to incarcerating serious juvenile offenders. *Journal of Consulting and Clinical Psychology, 60,* 953–961.

Henggeler, S. W., Borduin, C. M., & Mann, B. J. (1993). Advances in family therapy: Empirical foundations. In T. H. Ollendick & R. J. Prinz (Eds.). *Advances in clinical child psychology* (Vol. 15, pp. 207–241). New York: Plenum.

Henggeler, S. W., Melton, G. B., Smith, L. A., Schoenwald, S. K., & Hanley, J. (1993). Family preservation using multisystemic therapy: Long-term follow-up to a clinical trial with serious juvenile offenders. *Journal of Child and Family Studies, 2,* 283–293.

Henggeler, S. W., Schoenwald, S. K., & Pickrel, S. G. (1995). Multisystemic therapy: Bridging the gap between university- and community-based treatment. *Journal of Consulting and Clinical Psychology, 63,* 709–717.

Henggeler, S. W., Pickrel, S. G., Brondino, M. J., & Crouch, J. L. (1996). Eliminating (almost) treatment dropout of substance abusing or dependent delinquents through home-based multisystemic therapy. *American Journal of Psychiatry, 153,* 427–428.

Henggeler, S. W., Schoenwald, S. K., & Munger, R. L. (1996). Families and therapists achieve clinical outcomes, systems of care mediate the process. *Journal of Child and Family Studies, 5,* 177–183.

Henggeler, S. W., Rowland, M. D., Pickrel, S. G., Miller, S. L., Cunningham, P. B., Santos, A. B., Schoenwald, S. K., Randall, J., & Edwards, J. E. (1997). Investigating family-based alternatives to institution-based mental health services for youth: Lessons learned from the pilot study of a randomized field trial. *Journal of Clinical Child Psychology, 26,* 226–233.

Henggeler, S. W., Pickrel, S. G., & Brondino, M. J. (1998). *Multisystemic treatment of substance abusing and dependent delinquents: Outcomes, treatment fidelity, and transportability.* Manuscript submitted for publication.

Henggeler, S. W., Schoenwald, S. K., Borduin, C. M., Rowland, M. D., & Cunningham, P. B. (1998). *Multisystemic treatment for antisocial behavior in children and adolescents.* New York: Guilford.

Higgins, S. T., & Budney, A. J. (1993). Treatment of cocaine dependence through the principles of behavior analysis and behavioral pharmacology. In L. S. Onken, J. D. Blaine, & J. J. Boren (Eds.), *Behavioral treatments for drug abuse and dependence* (NIH Publication No. 93-3684; NIDA Research Monograph No. 137, pp. 97–122). Rockville, MD: National Institute on Drug Abuse.

Hoagwood, K., Hibbs, E., Brent, D., & Jensen, P. (1995). Introduction to the special section: Efficacy and effectiveness in studies of child and adolescent psychotherapy. *Journal of Consulting and Clinical Psychology, 63,* 683–687.

Jensen, P. S., Hoagwood, K., & Petti, T. (1996). Outcomes of mental health care for children and adolescents: II. Literature review and application of a comprehensive model. *Journal of the American Academy of Child and Adolescent Psychiatry, 35,* 1064–1077.

Kazdin, A. E. (1987). Treatment of antisocial behavior in children: Current status and future directions. *Psychological Bulletin, 102,* 187–203.

Kazdin, A. E. (1994). Psychotherapy for children and adolescents. In A. E. Bergin & S. L. Garfield (Eds.), *Handbook of psychotherapy and behavior change* (pp. 543–594). New York: Wiley.

Kazdin, A. E. (1996). Problem solving and parent management in treating aggressive and antisocial behavior. In E. D. Hibbs & P. S. Jensen (Eds.), *Psychosocial treatments for child and adolescent disorders: Empirically based strategies for clinical practice* (pp. 377–408). Washington, DC: American Psychological Association.

Kazdin, A. E. (1997). A model for developing effective treatments: Progression and interplay of theory, research, and practice. *Journal of Clinical Child Psychology, 26,* 114–129.

Kazdin, A. E., Siegel, T. C., & Bass, D. (1990). Drawing upon clinical practice to inform research on child and adolescent psychotherapy: A survey of practitioners. *Professional Psychology: Research and Practice, 21,* 189–198.

Kazdin, A. E., Siegel, T. C., & Bass, D. (1992). Cognitive problem-solving skills training and parent management training in the treatment of antisocial behavior in children. *Journal of Consulting and Clinical Psychology, 60,* 737–747.

Kruesi, M. J. P., & Tolan, P. H. (in press). Disruptive disorders. In J. Nospitz (Ed.), *Basic handbook of child psychiatry* (2nd ed.). New York: Basic Books.

Kurtines, W. M., & Szapocznik, J. (1996). Family interaction patterns: Structural family therapy within contexts of cultural diversity. In E. D. Hibbs & P. S. Jensen (Eds.), *Psychosocial treatments for child and adolescent disorders: Empirically based strategies for clinical practice* (pp. 671–697). Washington, DC: American Psychological Association.

Kutash, K., & Rivera, V. R. (1996). *What works in children's mental health services? Uncovering answers to critical questions.* Baltimore: Brooks.

Lescheid, A. W. (1997). *Evaluation of clinical trials of multisystemic therapy targeting high-risk young offenders.* London, Ontario, Canada: Author.

Liddle, H. A. (1995). Conceptual and clinical dimensions of a multidimensional, multisystemic engagement strategy in family-based adolescent treatment. *Psychotherapy, 32,* 39–58.

Liddle, H. A. (1996). Family-based treatment for adolescent problem behaviors: Overview of contemporary developments and introduction to the special section. *Journal of Family Psychology, 10,* 3–11.

Liddle, H. A., & Dakof, G. A. (1995). Efficacy of family therapy for drug abuse: Promising but not definitive. *Journal of Marital and Family Therapy, 21,* 511–543.

Liddle, H. A., Dakof, G. A., & Diamond, G. (1991). Adolescent substance abuse: Multidimensional family therapy in action. In E. Kaufman & P. Kaufman (Eds.), *Family therapy with drug and alcohol abuse* (pp. 120–171). Boston: Allyn & Bacon.

Liddle, H. A., Dakof, G. A., Parker, K., Barrett, K., Diamond, G. S., Garcia, R. G., & Palmer, R. B. (1995). *Multidimensional family therapy for treating adolescent substance abuse: A controlled clinical trial.* Manuscript submitted for publication.

Lipsey, M. W. (1992). Juvenile delinquency treatment: A meta-analytic inquiry into the variability of effects. In T. D. Cook, H. Cooper, D. S. Cordray, H. Hartman, L. V. Hedges, R. J. Light, T. A. Louis, & F. Mosteller (Eds.), *Meta-analysis for explanation: A casebook* (pp. 83–127). New York: Russell Sage Foundation.

Melton, G. B., & Pagliocca, P. M. (1992). Treatment in the juvenile justice system: Directions for policy and practice. In J. J. Cocozza (Ed.), *Responding to the mental health needs of youth in the juvenile justice system* (pp. 107–139). Seattle, WA: National Coalition for the Mentally Ill in the Criminal Justice System.

Miller, M. L. (1997). *The multisystemic therapy pilot program: Fifth quarter status report.* Wilmington: Delaware Department of Services to Children, Youth, and Their Families.

Minuchin, S. (1974). *Families and family therapy.* Cambridge, MA: Harvard University Press.

Minuchin, S., & Fishman, H. C. (1981). *Family therapy techniques.* Cambridge, MA: Harvard University Press.

Mulvey, E. P., Arthur, M. W., & Reppucci, N. D. (1993). The prevention and treatment of juvenile delinquency: A review of the research. *Clinical Psychology Review 13,* 133–167.

Nelson, K. E. (1990). Family based services for juvenile offenders. *Children and Youth Services Review, 12*(3), 193–212.

Nelson, K. E., & Landsman, M. J. (1992). *Alternative models of family preservation: Family-based services in context.* Springfield, IL: Thomas.

O'Dell, S. L. (1985). Progress in parent training. *Progress in Behavior Modification, 19,* 57–108.

Oswald, D. P., & Singh, N. N. (1996). Emerging trends in child and adolescent mental healthservices. In T. H Ollendick & R. J Prinz (Eds.), *Advances in clinical child psychology* (Vol. 18, pp. 331–365). New York: Plenum.

Patterson, G. R., & Chamberlain, P. (1988). Treatment process: A problem at three levels. In L. C. Wynne (Ed.), *The state of the art in family therapy research: Controversies and recommendations* (pp. 189–233). New York: Family Process Press.

Patterson, G. R., & Chamberlain, P. (1994). A functional analysis of resistance during parent training therapy. *Clinical Psychology: Science and Practice, 1,* 53–70.

Reddy, L. A., & Pfeiffer, S. I. (1997). Effectiveness of treatment foster care with children and adolescents: A review of outcome studies. *Journal of the American Academy of Child and Adolescent Psychiatry, 36,* 581–588.

Roberts, M. S. (1994). Models for service delivery in children's mental health: Common characteristics. *Journal of Clinical Child Psychology, 23,* 212–219.

Rosenblatt, A. (1996). Bows and ribbons, tape and twine: Wrapping the wraparound process for children with multi-system needs. *Journal of Child and Family Studies, 5,* 101–116.

Sanders, M. R. (1996). New directions in behavioral family intervention with children. In T. H. Ollendick & R. J. Prinz (Eds.), *Advances in clinical child psychology* (Vol. 18, pp. 293–330). New York: Plenum.

Santisteban, D. A., Szapocznik, J., Perez-Vidal, A., Kurtines, W. M., Murray, W. J., & LaPerriere, A. (1996). Engaging behavior problem drug abusing youth and their families into treatment: An investigation of the efficacy of specialized engagement interventions and factors that contribute to differential effectiveness. *Journal of Family Psychology, 10,* 35–44.

Schmidt, S. E., Liddle, H. A., & Dakof, G. A. (1996). Changes in parenting practices and adolescent drug abuse during multidimensional family therapy. *Journal of Family Psychology, 10,* 12–27.

Schoenwald, S. K., & Henggeler, S. W. (1997). Combining effective treatment strategies with family preservation models of service delivery: A challenge for mental health. In R. J. Illback, H. Joseph, Jr., & C. Cobb (Eds.), *Integrated services for children and families: Opportunities for psychological practice* (pp. 121–136). Washington, DC: American Psychological Association.

Schoenwald, S. K., & Henggeler, S. W. (in press). Services research and family based treatment. In H. Liddle, G. Diamond, R. Levant, J. Bray, & D. Santisteban (Eds.), *Family psychology intervention science.* Washington, DC: American Psychological Association.

Schoenwald, S. K., Ward, D. M., Henggeler, S. W., Pickrel, S. G., & Patel, H. (1996). MST treatment of substance abusing or dependent adolescent offenders: Costs of reducing incarceration, inpatient, and residential placement. *Journal of Child and Family Studies, 4,* 431–444.

Schoenwald, S. K., Borduin, C. M., & Henggeler, S. W. (1998). Changing the natural and service ecologies of adolescents and their families. In M. H. Epstein, K. Kutash, & A. Duchnowski (Eds.), *Community based programming for children with serious emotional disturbance and their families: Research and evaluations* (pp. 485–511). Austin, TX: PRO-Ed.

Serketich, W. J., & Dumas, J. E. (1996). The effectiveness of behavioral parent training to modify antisocial behavior in children: A meta-analysis. *Behavior Therapy, 27,* 171–186.

Stroul, B. A., & Friedman, R. M. (1994). *A system of care for children and youth with severe emotional disturbance.* Washington, DC: Georgetown University Child Development Center.

Szapocznik, J., & Kurtines, W. M. (1989). *Breakthroughs in family therapy with drug-abusing and problem youth.* New York: Springer.

Szapocznik, J., Kurtines, W. M., Foote, E., Perez-Vidal, A., & Hervis, O. E. (1986). Conjoint versus one-person family therapy: Further evidence for the effectiveness of conducting family therapy through one person. *Journal of Consulting and Clinical Psychology, 54,* 395–397.

Szapocznik, J., Santisteban, D., Rio, A. T., Perez-Vidal, A., Kurtines, W. M., & Hervis, O. E. (1986). Bicultural effectiveness training: An experimental test of an intervention modality for families experiencing intergenerational/intercultural conflict. *Hispanic Journal of Behavioral Sciences, 8,* 303–330.

Szapocznik, J., Santisteban, D., Rio, A. T., Perez-Vidal, A., & Kurtines, W. M. (1989). Family effectiveness training: An intervention to prevent problem behaviors in Hispanic adolescents. *Hispanic Journal of Behavioral Sciences, 11,* 4–27.

Szapocznik, J., Kurtines, W. M., Santisteban, D. A., & Rio, A. T. (1990). Interplay of advances between theory, research, and application in treatment interventions aimed at behavior problem children and adolescents. *Journal of Consulting and Clinical Psychology, 58,* 696–703.

Szapocznik, J., Kurtines, W. M., Santisteban, D. A, Pantin, H., Scopetta, M., Mancilla, Y., Aisenberg, S., McIntosh, S., & Coatsworth, J. D. (1997). The evolution of structural ecosystemic theory for working with Latino families. In J. Garcia & M. C. Zea (Eds.), *Psychological interventions and research with Latino populations* (pp. 166–190). Boston: Allyn & Bacon.

Thomas, C. R. (1994). *Island youth programs.* Galveston: University of Texas Medical Branch, Galveston.

Thornberry, T. P., Huizinga, D., & Loeber, R. (1995). The prevention of serious delinquency and violence: Implications from the program of research on the causes and correlates of delinquency. In J. C. Howell, B. Krisberg, J. D. Hawkins, & J. J. Wilson (Eds.), *A sourcebook: Serious, violent, & chronic juvenile offenders* (pp. 213–237). Newbury Park, CA: Sage.

Timmons-Mitchell, J. (1997). *Multisystemic therapy (MST) Replication,* Cuyahoga and Lorain Counties, Ohio. Cleveland, OH: Author.

Tolan, P. H. (1996). Characteristics shared by exemplary child clinical interventions for indicated populations. In M. C. Roberts (Ed.), *Model programs in child and family mental health* (pp. 91–107). Mahwah, NJ: Erlbaum.

Tolan, P. H., & Guerra, N. C. (1994). *What works in reducing adolescent violence: An empirical review of the field.* Boulder: University of Colorado, Center for the Study and Prevention of Violence, Institute for Behavioral Sciences.

Tolan, P. H., Guerra, N. C., & Kendall, P. (1995). A developmental-ecological perspective on antisocial behavior in children and adolescent: Towards a unified risk and intervention framework. *Journal of Consulting and Clinical Psychology, 63,* 579–584.

Webster-Stratton, C. (1982). The long term effects of a videotape modeling parent training program: Comparison of immediate and one year follow-up results. *Behavior Therapy, 13,* 702–714.

Webster-Stratton, C. (1990). Long-term follow-up of families with young conduct problem children: From preschool to grade school. *Journal of Clinical Child Psychology, 19,* 144–149.

Webster-Stratton, C. (1994). Advancing videotape parent training: A comparison study. *Journal of Consulting and Clinical Psychology, 62,* 583–593.

Webster-Stratton, C. (1996). Early intervention with videotape modeling: Programs for families of children with oppositional defiant disorder or conduct disorder. In E. D. Hibbs & P. S. Jensen (Eds.), *Psychosocial treatments for child and adolescent disorders: Empirically based strategies for clinical practice* (pp. 435–474). Washington, DC: American Psychological Association.

Webster-Stratton, C., & Herbert, M. (1993). What really happens in parent training? *Behavior Modification, 17,* 407–456.

Webster-Stratton, C., & Herbert, M. (1994). *Troubled families—Problem children. Working with parents: A collaborative process.* New York: Wiley.

Webster-Stratton, C., & Spitzer, A. (1996). Parenting a young child with conduct problems. New insights using qualitative methods. In T. H. Ollendick & R. J. Prinz (Eds.), *Advances in clinical child psychology* (Vol. 18, pp. 1–63). New York: Plenum.

Weisz, J. R., & Weiss, B. (1993). *Effects of psychotherapy with children and adolescents.* New York: Sage.

Weisz, J. R., Donenberg, G. R., Han, S. S., & Kauneckis, D. (1995). Child and adolescent psychotherapy outcomes in experiments versus clinics: Why the disparity? *Journal of Abnormal Child Psychology, 23,* 83–106.

Weisz, J. R., Donenberg, G. R., Han, S. S., & Weiss, B. (1995). Bridging the gap between laboratory and clinic in child and adolescent psychotherapy. *Journal of Consulting and Clinical Psychology, 63,* 688–701.

Weisz, J. R., Han, S. S., & Valeri, S. M. (1997). More of what? Issues raised by the Fort Bragg study. *American Psychologist, 52,* 541–545.

Wells, K., & Biegel, D. E. (Eds.). (1991). *Family preservation services research and evaluation.* Newbury Park, CA: Sage.

Wierson, M., & Forehand, R. (1994). Parent behavioral training for child noncompliance: Rationale, concepts, and effectiveness. *Current Directions in Psychological Science, 3,* 146–150.

Wolf, M., Kirigin, K. A., Fixsen, D. L., & Blase, K. A. (1995). The teaching-family model: A case study in data-based program development and refinement (and dragon-wrestling). *Journal of Organizational Behavior Management, 15,* 11–68.

Yuan, Y. Y., McDonald, W. R., Wheeler, C. E., Struckman-Johnson, D., & Rivest, M. (1990). *Evaluation of AB1562 in-home care demonstration projects: Final report* (Vols. 1 & 2). Sacramento, CA: McDonald.

23

Residential Care for Children and Adolescents with Oppositional Defiant Disorder and Conduct Disorder

PATRICIA CHAMBERLAIN

BACKGROUND AND OVERVIEW

The practice of placing children and adolescents with severe conduct problems (e.g., Oppositional Defiant Disorder [ODD] and Conduct Disorder [CD]) in residential settings is expanding. In 1983, estimates were that more than 19,000 such youngsters were in residential care. By 1986, the number had increased 32% to more than 25,000 (Select Committee on Children, Youth, and Families, 1990). These data are surely an underestimate in that they exclude those placed in for-profit residential treatment centers. The American Public Welfare Association estimated that approximately 70% of the total funding for children's mental health services was used for residential services. Yet little research exists on either the short-term effectiveness or long-term benefits of these placements (Burns & Freidman, 1990). In commenting on the effectiveness of various components of the system of care for children and adolescents, Burns, Hoagwood, and Maultsby (1998) noted that "A dominant observation is that the least evidence of effectiveness exists for residential services, where the vast majority of dollars are spent" (p. 690). Moreover, there is some indication in the literature that children and adolescents who have disruptive behavior problems with antisocial and aggressive symptoms are among the most difficult population to treat in residential settings and that they tend to benefit the least when compared to their nonantisocial counterparts in care (Zoccolillo & Rogers, 1991).

Contemporary approaches to residential care are characterized by a range of placement types (Wells, 1991); the most prevalent of these include community-based family-style group homes, cottages in larger institutional settings, large group living situations with shift staff, and, more recently, treatment or therapeutic foster care with one or two youths placed in family homes in the community. The theoretical foundations that underpin these program types vary as widely as their physical characteristics. Commonly used treatment modalities include psychoanalytic (Bettleheim, 1982), psychoeducational (Hobbs, 1982), behavioral

PATRICIA CHAMBERLAIN • Oregon Social Learning Center, Eugene, Oregon 97401.

Handbook of Disruptive Behavior Disorders, edited by Quay and Hogan. Kluwer Academic/Plenum Publishers, New York, 1999.

(Fixsen *et al.,* 1978), and peer cultural (Vorrath & Brendtro, 1985). However, there are few systematic studies that examine the application of various theories using well-controlled designs.

The empirical gap in research on residential care is difficult to explain, especially for children and adolescents with severe and antisocial problems, given the well-developed body of research on the development and treatment of these problems. Considering the growing use of residential placements and the proportion of mental health dollars spent on this form of care, increased emphasis is long overdue on studies devoted to examination of effectiveness and on studies that bridge the gap between empirical work on child and adolescent CD treatments and their applications to residential care.

In this chapter, research on the effectiveness of residential care, descriptive data on factors that predict successful outcomes in residential treatment, and issues and controversies related to treating children and adolescents with CD in residential settings are discussed. In addition, directions for future research are suggested.

RESEARCH ON THE EFFECTIVENESS OF RESIDENTIAL TREATMENT

Although it would be desirable to restrict studies reviewed to those that had well-controlled research designs, the lack of systematic work in this area precludes this approach. Instead, studies reviewed are those with research designs of sufficient rigor to allow for meaningful conclusions on effectiveness or to identify key processes relating to program effectiveness. Several reviews of the state of research on residential treatment have identified promising program models (e.g., Curry, 1991; Quay, 1986; Whittaker & Pecora, 1984). This chapter is not intended to reexamine programs and studies that have been previously reviewed but rather to review more recently published studies and to attempt to identify implications for practice and for future research. Two types of studies are the focus: (1) those with single samples and

without comparison or control groups (these represent the majority of studies conducted); and (2) studies that compared residential treatment to no treatment, that compared residential treatment to other forms of treatment, or that compared different forms of residential treatment.

Studies without Control or Comparison Groups: Predictors of Good Outcomes

Two major earlier reviews have examined factors that predicted positive outcomes in residential care. Blotcky, Dimperio, and Gossett (1984), in a subjective narrative review, found that in 24 studies conducted from 1936 to 1982, the following child factors predicted relatively successful outcomes: (1) higher intelligence, (2) nonpsychotic diagnosis, (3) no neurological dysfunction, (4) absence of antisocial behavior, (5) healthy family functioning, (6) adequate time in the program, and (7) adequate aftercare services.

Pfeiffer and Strzelecki (1990) summarized results from studies on residential treatment and hospitalization from the period 1975–1990. Because only 2 of the 34 studies that they examined reported means and standard deviations for outcome scores, they devised a system of rating program effects as negative, neutral, or positive and then adjusted this value according to sample size. In their analysis, less severe dysfunction (in both child and family), the presence of a specialized treatment regime, and availability of aftercare services were all related to positive outcomes. Higher child or adolescent intelligence and length of stay were moderately related to positive outcomes; age and gender were unrelated to outcomes.

Both of these reviews called for more scientific rigor in the design and conduct of future studies. For example, Pfeiffer and Strzelecki (1990) suggested four conceptual and methodological advances: (1) identification of the necessary and sufficient dimensions of the treatment to be examined, (2) use of multiple measures and perspectives to define success or adjustment, (3) use of statistical techniques and experimental designs to test specific hypotheses, and (4) use of both micro- (e.g., small, observable behaviors) and macro-level indicators (e.g., broad-based traits) of outcomes.

Other studies have been published since the two reviews just described. A study reviewed by Dalton, Muller, and Forman (1989) found that for 26 children with CD there was no significant change in behavior at 3 months follow-up from discharge from an inpatient unit. Curry (1991) reviewed three studies of residential treatment that found that 71% of the youngsters were functioning "adequately" at follow-up but that progress in treatment was not predictive of good adjustment in follow-up. He and others (e.g., Durkin & Durkin, 1975; Quay, 1979; Whittaker & Pecora, 1984) concluded that several key factors are important in determining positive postdischarge adjustment. These include the degree of support provided to the child in aftercare, the need to work with the child's family, and the need to include in residential programming opportunities for learning that can be generalized to the community environment to which the child will return.

In three Swedish studies that used an adaptation of the Teaching Family Group Home model with samples of antisocial boys, Slot, Jagers, and Dangel (1992) found that boys improved significantly from pre- to postresidential treatment on occurrences of problems and on abilities for relationships but not on rates of drinking. They also improved on rates of arrest from pre- to posttreatment and residential care was only one fourth as costly as care in a Swedish institution, which was the logical alternative placement for the boys studied. Treatment consisted of placing boys with an adult couple who emphasized teaching social competency skills, educational problem solving, vocational skills, and interpersonal interaction skills.

Day, Pal, and Goldberg (1994) examined the postdischarge functioning of CD children treated in a residential setting that emphasized family involvement and treatment. Parents participated in mealtime and bedtime activities and attended weekly family therapy sessions and parent training groups. At 6 months post-discharge, improvements were found on Child Behavior Checklist scores (Achenbach & Edlebrock, 1983) with significantly fewer children being in the clinical range at 6 months postdischarge than they had been at admission on both externalizing and internalizing scales. Children who had the most severe symptoms of CD at admission had the poorest adjustment at follow-up.

Hoagwood and Cunningham (1992) examined outcomes for 114 children and adolescents who had been placed in residential care by school districts in a large southwestern state. All subjects had been identified as Seriously Emotionally Disturbed (SED),* and their average length of stay in residential care was 18.2 months. In 63% of the cases, subjects were rated as having made either no or minimal progress at the time of discharge. Positive outcomes were associated with shorter lengths of stay. However, subjects with positive outcomes and shorter lengths of stay were not less disturbed than their less successful counterparts according to preplacement ratings of severity of problems. In fact, they were rated as being significantly more disturbed on the severity of impairment of functioning measure used. The availability of community-based services during the transition from residential care to home was the single most likely reason reported for positive discharge. The services that were mentioned as being important included family support, respite care, crisis intervention, and day treatment.

Treatment Foster Care (TFC) is currently one of the most widely used forms of out-of-home placement for children and adolescents with severe emotional and behavioral disorders and is considered the least restrictive form of residential care (Kutash & Rivera, 1996; Stroul, 1989). TFC differs from most Group Care (GC) settings in several important ways: community families are recruited, trained, and supported to provide placements; children generally attend public schools; no more than two youngsters are placed in a home; and most TFC

*SED is an educational label that does not correspond to any particular psychiatric diagnosis.

programs include a family therapy component with the biological parent or parents (or relatives or other aftercare resource). These components are thought to predict positive outcomes. TFC is significantly less costly than GC. Single sample studies of TFC were reviewed by Meadowcroft, Thomlinson, and Chamberlain (1994) and included surveys describing the components and clinical orientations of TFC programs, descriptions of the children served, and descriptions of TFC parents. In addition, four outcome studies were reviewed that did not involve comparison or control groups (Fanshel, Finch, & Grundy, 1990; Hazel, 1989; Larson, Allison, & Johnston, 1978; Smith, 1986). In summary, these studies found that the majority of placements were completed as planned, that participants improved on behavioral indicators of adjustment, and that 60% to 89% of the children and adolescents were discharged to less restrictive living settings.

Outcome studies, even without control groups, can provide documentation of clinical progress or lack thereof, but do not compare the effectiveness of the treatment or program examined with that of alternative or no treatments. As noted by Curry (1991), such studies can illuminate the nature of the treatment process. In the studies reviewed here, treatments that included components that attempted to strengthen the child's postresidential environment (e.g., increased family skills and support and community support) and that included family treatment seemed to be more likely to have positive outcomes.

Studies with Control or Comparison Groups

A few studies have been conducted in the 1990s that have looked at the components or key factors in daily life in residential care of different types. Other studies have focused on outcomes in residential care in comparison to other alternatives. Some studies have used quasi-experimental designs with matched comparison groups; others have used more powerful random assignment designs.

Studies on Daily Life

Friman and colleagues (1996) compared measures of quality of life in residential care using the Teaching Family (TF) model at Boys' Town to "treatments as usual" for youngsters referred to Boys' Town but not admitted due to lack of a program opening or to quicker availability of a placement in another program. The two groups were comparable on age, gender, and ethnicity at baseline. Participants were assessed every 3 months for up to 4 years. The variables studied were (1) delivery of helpful treatment, (2) satisfaction with supervising adults, (3) isolation from family, and (4) sense of personal control. Several differences favoring the TF model of treatment were found. There was a greater increase in participant ratings of the amount of helpful treatment delivered after admission to the TF program compared to controls. Youngsters in TF reported being more satisfied with supervising adults than those in the comparison condition. Furthermore, that high level of satisfaction with adults generalized to their postplacement settings. Feelings of isolation from family and friends decreased from baseline to a greater extent for the TF group than for the comparison group. No reliable differences were found between groups for sense of personal control but a trend favored participants in the TF condition. This was a carefully conducted study that challenged some of the negative beliefs about residential care and documented the fact that substantial variability exists in the quality of daily life in residential care.

In another study examining the characteristics of daily life in care, Chamberlain, Ray, and Moore (1996) examined program assumptions and daily practices in GC and TFC settings. Participants were male adolescents referred by the juvenile court for severe and chronic delinquent behavior. They were randomly assigned to TFC or GC conditions. As part of a larger study (outcomes are reported later in this chapter), four key variables that were identified in the literature as being instrumental in the prediction of continued delinquency were measured during treatment. These variables were hypothesized to influence treatment success or failure regardless of the condition (GC or TFC) in which the boy was placed. The variables examined were the intensity of the supervision youngsters received, the consistency and perceived fairness of the discipline received, the quality of the relationship with caretaking adults, and relationships and associations with delinquent peers. These four variables were examined using data from multiple perspectives (caretakers and boys). Prior to the boys' placement, caretakers in each setting were interviewed about what they considered to be the key elements of their treatment programs.

After boys had been residents for 3 months, boys and caretakers were interviewed about characteristics of daily life. At the preplacement interviews with caretakers, several differences were found between the two models in caretakers' perceptions of the key treatment elements for their respective models. For example, in GC, peers were thought to play a more influential role in program operations. Peers were thought to contribute to a boy's success in the program and they helped decide what was appropriate discipline and for what events boys should be disciplined. In TFC, adults were thought to be more influential; adults decided on discipline and were more instrumental in setting house rules.

After 3 months of placement, in addition to interviewing boys and caretakers, three data collection telephone calls were made to each site asking about occurrences of behaviors during the previous day. Caretakers in both GC and TFC reported that boys engaged in approximately the same numbers of problem behaviors per day; however, boys in the two programs differed in their accounts. Boys in GC reported engaging in twice the number of problem behaviors as did boys in TFC. In TFC, boys and caretakers both reported that given the occurrence of a problem behavior, boys were disciplined twice as often as were boys in GC. In TFC, boys spent less time unsupervised with peers and more time one-on-one with caretakers. Boys in TFC reported that they were influenced less by peers than did boys in GC.

These two studies highlight the differences in living experiences to which youngsters in residential care are exposed. How these and other differences in program structure and treatment processes affect outcomes is an obvious avenue for future research.

Outcome Studies

Thompson and colleagues (1996) examined the short- and long-term educational outcomes for adolescents who had participated in TF homes at Boys' Town compared to a group of youngsters who had been admitted to that program but never attended. The comparison group was similar to the Boys' Town group in terms of demographic characteristics. Participants in the comparison group received treatment in alternative settings. The study followed youngsters after admission for up to 4 years. There was an initial increase in academic grade point average after the initial interview for the TF but not for the comparison group. Although the grade point average for the TF group decreased at 6 months after discharge, it was still higher than that obtained for the comparison group after discharge.

The TF group completed years of school at a faster rate than those in the comparison group. Eighty-three percent of the TF group and 69% of the comparison group completed high school; this difference was statistically significant. Participants in the TF group rated the importance of college as being higher in assessments conducted after the initial interview than did those in the comparison group. Although this score decreased after discharge, the TF group reported that they believed college was important more than did participants in the comparison group at follow-up. Finally, the amount of help the child was given with homework was assessed during residential placement and after discharge. As with the other measures, the TF group reported a significantly greater amount of help with homework than did comparison cases during their placements. This score decreased for both groups after discharge, but the TF group mean remained statistically higher than the mean for the comparison group. It was unclear from the report on this study if there was more parental involvement in the homes of TF graduates, or if TF graduates sought out more help from parents, or both.

This study demonstrated a carryover of positive treatment effects into follow-up; an unfortunately rare finding for outcome studies on residential care. The TF program model specifically targets school achievement during placement and apparently produces lasting gains that are evident once the placement is ended. More research needs to be conducted on such interventions that can facilitate turning points that are likely to have a positive effect on the trajectory of the teenager's adjustment in the community postplacement.

Three studies on the effectiveness of TFC using comparison or control groups have been conducted at the Oregon Social Learning Center. In the first, Chamberlain (1990) matched adolescents referred for delinquency and treated in TFC on age, sex, and date of commitment to the state training school with adolescents served in GC programs. Subjects did not differ on a set of child and family characteristics examined at baseline (e.g., age, number of prior out-of-home placements, parents with criminal histories, child drug and alcohol use). Rates of incarceration for the TFC youngsters were lower at 1- and 2-year follow-up, program completion rates for the TFC group were higher, and the number of days in treatment was correlated with subsequent lower incarceration rates for subjects in the TFC group but not for those in the GC group. Limitations of this study were that the sample size was small (32, 16 in each group), arrest rates were not examined, and a matched comparison design rather than random assignment of subjects to groups was used.

A second study improved on some of these limitations. Chamberlain and Reid (1991) randomly assigned youngsters ages 9–18 leaving the state hospital to TFC or "treatment as usual" in the community. Over a 7-month period, participants were assessed on rates of daily problem behaviors, rehospitalization rates, restrictiveness of living situation, and presence or absence of symptoms. TFC youngsters spent more time living in family-based settings (and therefore spent fewer days living in a hospital setting) and had fewer daily problem behaviors. No differences were observed between the groups on self-reports of symptoms. This study was also conducted with a small sample ($n = 20$).

The third and largest Oregon study on the effectiveness of TFC began in 1990 and involved the random assignment of 79 boys referred because of chronic and serious delinquency to TFC or GC programs. In addition to examining outcomes, investigators studied four key variables thought to mediate the effectiveness of treatment (as reported earlier in this chapter in Chamberlain et al., 1996). Key outcomes examined included official and self-reported delinquency rates, drug use, school attendance and performance, and mental health status. Data were reported on delinquency outcomes (Chamberlain, 1997; Chamberlain & Reid, 1997).

Participating boys were an average of 14 years old and had been arrested more than 13 times prior to entering the study. They averaged 1.4 previous out-of-home placements, excluding detention stays, and had spent an average of 80 days in detention during the previous year. Fifteen percent had been charged with a sex offense and 18% had been arrested for fire-setting.

The TFC program consisted of placing boys (usually one per home) in a trained and supported community family where they underwent a structured daily program including the use of point and level systems. Boys also participated in weekly individual therapy that was skill focused and their parents (or other aftercare resource) participated in family treatment.* Frequent contact between boys and

*Parents were told that participation in family therapy was a requirement of the program prior to their son's admission. Nevertheless, some parents were reluctant to participate in the family therapy once the placement was made. Program staff worked to remove barriers to parents' participation by providing funds for transportation, meeting in family homes, and being flexible about times for meetings. As a result, all of the parents in the experimental group participated in the family therapy to some extent.

parents or relatives was promoted as were weekly home visits where parents were taught to use a management system that was parallel to the one used in the TFC home. Psychiatric consultation and medication management was used on an "as needed" basis. The TFC placements lasted an average of 6.8 months. Detailed descriptions of the program model are given in Chamberlain (1994) and Chamberlain and Moore (1998).

In GC programs, boys lived with from 6 to 15 other boys in family-style group homes, in stand-alone group homes, or in cottages on the grounds of larger institutions. In GC, most boys participated in daily group therapy. Most programs used variations of the Positive Peer Culture model (Vorrath & Brendtro, 1985) where peers were expected to participate in daily governance and decision making. Boys' families participated in family therapy in 40% of the cases, and boys participated in individual therapy in 53% of the cases. Eleven group homes located throughout the state participated in the study.

Data on official arrest rates at 1 year postdischarge showed that boys in TFC had significantly fewer arrests (TFC mean = 2.6 arrests; GC mean = 5.4 arrests). Postdischarge self-reports of delinquent activities also showed that TFC boys reported engaging in significantly fewer delinquent activities including serious and person crimes (TFC mean = 12.8 self-reported criminal activities; GC mean = 28.9 self-reported criminal activities). TFC boys also spent fewer days incarcerated than did boys in the GC group (means = 53 vs. 129 days, respectively) and they ran away from their placements less often (means = 18 days vs. 36 days, respectively). In addition, TFC boys at follow-up reported using hard drugs less frequently.

Analyses are now under way to examine the effect of mediating variables on outcomes. For example, we hypothesized that boys' rates of contact with delinquent peers during placement would predict criminal behavior in follow-up. In addition, we hypothesized that supervision and consistent discipline during treatment would be protective factors in terms of subsequent criminality as would having a quality relationship with a prosocial adult. These analyses will begin to identify what factors or practices are active or key ingredients in successful versus unsuccessful treatment as measured by boys' desistance or continuance in criminal activities.

CONTROVERSIAL ISSUES IN RESIDENTIAL CARE

What components of residential care are necessary and sufficient for children and adolescents with CD? Are such children and adolescents effectively served in residential placements and, if so, what are the characteristics of those placements that relate to successful outcomes? Do youngsters with CD disrupt residential settings to the extent that they damage treatment opportunities for other residents and, if so, how should programs be structured to prevent or minimize this problem? What should be the criteria for discharge and for elements of follow-up care? These are all questions that could be addressed in the context of well-designed clinical trials. There are a few "leads" from the existing literature that may be of relevance.

Necessary and Sufficient Components: Should Families Be Included in Residential Treatment?

Whether family treatment should be a routine part of residential care is controversial in the residential care field. As many providers of residential services point out, logistical barriers interfere with including families in treatment; however, given the contextual nature of most severe conduct problems, it is not reasonable to expect that in-placement changes in child behavior will be maintained postplacement without consistent adult support. Ideally, parents or aftercare parent substitutes can be helped to provide consistent daily structure and support for youngsters that is similar to that which they received in the residential care setting. This would include similar levels of supervision, discipline, expectations, and encouragement for academic and work skills.

Failure to include parents in youngsters' treatment may be the single largest barrier to generalization of treatment effects from residential care to living at home. Children and adolescents with CD are likely to gravitate toward like peers when they return to their home communities. Parents or other community caregivers need the resources and skills to prevent this drift, which has been shown to be a key part of the progression toward delinquency and drug use (e.g., Elliott, Huizinga, & Ageton, 1985). For youths whose parents or relatives are not available to provide support and guidance, communities may find that efforts to establish alternative surrogate parental relationships are worthwhile and cost-effective in terms of producing positive outcomes for youngsters and for society in general.

There is some evidence that family therapy has a positive influence on posttreatment adjustment. Garrett (1985), in a meta-analysis on components of treatments in residential care for juvenile offenders, found that while individual and group therapies had no impact on recidivism, family therapy appeared to be more effective. Borduin and colleagues (1995) found that recidivism for institutionalized delinquents after release was significantly less for those who received family therapy than for those in a control group (60% vs. 93%).

Provision of Appropriate Treatment

During the past decade a number of promising treatments have been developed for children and adolescents with CD. These approaches have largely relied on parents to implement daily behavioral programs aimed at changing the oppositional behavior of their child. Parent Management Training (Miller & Prinz, 1990; Patterson, 1982; Patterson, Dishion, & Chamberlain, 1993) is a well-researched therapy for treatment of ODD and CD youngsters. Treatment effects have been demonstrated for a number of related problems such as compliance, attention-deficit and hyperactivity problems, destructiveness, and rates of aggression toward adults and other children at home and on the playground. Treatment effects

are evident for up to 3 years following treatment and in one program for from 10 to 14 years following treatment (Long, Forehand, Wierson, & Morgan, 1994). Yet these methods have not been generally accepted for use in residential settings. In most residential placements for adolescents, peer-mediated treatments are used extensively. Exceptions are the application of social learning principles and methods of parent management training in TFC and to residential populations in the TF model. Numerous studies have demonstrated robust in-program behavior changes using TF (Braukmann & Wolf, 1987; Phillips, Phillips, Fixsen, & Wolf, 1974). Studies on long-term outcomes have been fewer in number and less promising.

Are Children and Adolescents with CD Good Candidates for Participation in Residential Treatment?

In 1991, the staff from six residential care centers for emotionally and behaviorally disturbed youth in the state of Washington convened a conference on the treatment of children with CD (Colyar, 1991). The conference focused on three issues: (1) the impact of CD children on the program and staff, (2) methods that had been successful or unsuccessful in their treatment, and (3) recommendations to program directors regarding policy and personnel changes. Among the most salient problems identified in serving this population were staff members' having to deal with frequent episodes of aggression and violence, high levels of staff fear, frequent sexual concerns, CD youths dominating and controlling the agenda for group meetings, negative peer leadership, and staff focus on negative behaviors. The staff identified several factors that disrupted treatment or were countertherapeutic that were associated with serving CD youth. These included staff's avoiding confrontations when negative behavior occurred so as to avoid negative outbursts, staff's using the majority of their energy on crises, high staff turnover and feelings of frustration and powerlessness, and staff's emotional problems developing from work-associated stress.

Successful treatment strategies included use of highly structured level systems as a behavioral management tool, immediate feedback to youngsters about positive and negative behaviors, having the program (rather than individual staff) dictate the consequences of behavior, de-emotionalizing negative consequences, consequences that can be applied quickly and over short periods of time, rewards and consequences that are individualized, and programming the maximum amount of structure and predictability possible.

Colyar's (1991) thoughtful summary of the conference proceedings lays out relevant issues in dealing with CD youngsters in residential settings. There appears to be a negative emotional cost to staff and other residents associated with treatment of these youngsters, especially if the residential unit is not prepared to engage in specialized programming to address the challenges of managing the therapeutic environment. The literature on residential care is peppered with references to the fact that inclusion of children and adolescents with CD has a negative impact on the therapeutic milieu, yet these youngsters comprise a growing, and probably the largest, group of children referred for residential services. Clearly, studies are needed that test models of intervention for this population.

Contamination Effects

A number of longitudinal and survey studies have identified deviant peer associations as a strong predictor of delinquency. For example, the National Youth Survey (Elliott *et al.,* 1985) sampled more than 1000 adolescents using a longitudinal design. They found that association with delinquent peers strongly contributed to continued and escalated patterns of criminal behavior. Without the variable of association with delinquent peers, the growth in delinquency over time was virtually nonexistent. These investigators commented that given the negative effects of becoming involved in a delinquent subculture, it is ironic that most delinquency treatment and prevention programs aggregate high-risk adolescents to implement their programs.

Dishion and Andrews (1995) found iatrogenic effects of group work in their study aimed at the prevention of conduct problems and substance use. They compared the effectiveness of five conditions (parent groups, adolescent groups, parents and adolescents combined, and two control groups). Participants were 158 families with young adolescents. The parent-only group was superior to all of the others in producing reduced family conflict, teacher ratings of reduced externalizing behaviors, and reduced tobacco use. Conversely, teachers reported significantly higher externalizing scores for those in the adolescent-only group than for youth in any other condition. These findings suggest that strategies that aggregate high-risk youth in intervention conditions should be reassessed, as in this study the group treatments produced the highest escalation in tobacco use and problem behaviors in school beginning at termination and persisting during the 1-year follow-up period. Other studies also reported iatrogenic effects for association with negative peers (Chamberlain & Reid, 1997; McCord, 1997).

IMPLICATIONS FOR A RESEARCH AGENDA IN RESIDENTIAL CARE

In their forward-looking article summarizing future directions in research on residential care, Whittaker and Pfeiffer (1994) made several recommendations for establishing a research agenda on residential care, including (1) the incorporation of new knowledge and research findings into residential care practice, (2) the conduct of research training staff, (3) the investigation of what subgroups of children might be best served in residential care, (4) the investigation of mechanisms for improving coordination of residential care and community programs, (5) the examination of characteristics of successful transitions and maintenance of treatment gains, (6) the conduct of systems-level research on the role of residential placements in the overall system of care, (7) the investigation of innovative models of residential care, (8) the examination of the role of family involvement, and (9) the carrying out of longitudinal studies on outcomes.

These suggestions are all relevant to bridging the gap between practice and research, in terms of both incorporating findings from existing studies and initiating programmatic work on the efficacy of residential care and on the role of residential care in the system of care. Given the amount of resources committed to residential care and the increasing emphasis on accountability and program efficacy, those providing funds should be motivated to promote the development of such studies. Although there are well-known barriers to implementing research in community-based treatment settings, there are indications that residential care providers are open to conducting studies. For example, Pfeiffer, Burd, and Wright (1992) reported that a national sample of clinicians involved in residential treatment said they had favorable attitudes toward research. Eighty-eight percent said that integration of research and practice was important and more than half reported that they would be willing to do research in their settings. The top three obstacles identified to conducting research were insufficient time, that research was not formally part of the job, and the lack of financial support for research; these barriers could be removed in the context of a funded research study.

The need for and the problems inherent in designing meaningful research studies in real-world contexts have been the focus of much recent attention in the literature (e.g., Burns 1994; Clarke, 1995). This new attention has been at least in part prompted by the disturbing findings of Weisz, Weiss, and Donenberg (1992) that the positive findings of the effectiveness of psychotherapy for children that were found in research studies were not found in clinic-based studies. Incorporation of a rigorous research design and appropriate measurement strategies into community-based mental health service settings requires melding the agendas of the practitioner and the researcher. It is probably no more satisfactory to try to impose a research design on an existing program with established procedures than it is to have re-

search goals dictate program operations. Most practitioners are not in a good position in terms of training or other resources to design and initiate studies, and researchers might lack the practical knowledge of day-to-day practice and local funding issues to implement community programs. An ideal scenario for integration of research and practice might be to establish and support partnerships between experienced researchers and practitioners.

ACKNOWLEDGMENTS. Support for this project was provided by Grant No. R01 MH47458 from the Center for Studies of Violent Behavior and Traumatic Stress, NIMH, U.S. PHS and Grant No. P50 MH46690 from the Prevention Research Branch, NIMH, U.S. PHS.

REFERENCES

Achenbach, T. M., & Edelbrock, C. S. (1983). *Manual for the Child Behavior Checklist and Revised Child Behavior Profile.* Burlington, VT: Queen City Printers.

Bettleheim, B. (1982). The necessity and value of residential treatment for severely disturbed children. *Family and Mental Health Journal, 8*(1&2), 55–61.

Blotcky, M. J., Dimperio, T. L., & Gossett, J. T. (1984). Follow-up of children treated in psychiatric hospitals: A review of studies. *American Journal of Psychiatry, 141,* 1499–1507.

Borduin, C. M., Mann, B. J., Cone, L. T., Henggeler, S. W., Fucci, B. R., Blaske, D. M., & Williams, R. A. (1995). Multisystemic treatment of serious juvenile offenders: Long-term prevention of criminality and violence. *Journal of Consulting and Clinical Psychology, 63,* 569–578.

Braukmann, C. J., & Wolf, M. M. (1987). Behaviorally based group homes for juvenile offenders. In E. K. Morris & C. J. Braukmann (Eds.), *Behavioral approaches to crime and delinquency* (pp. 135–155). New York: Plenum.

Burns, B. J. (1994). The challenge of child mental health services research. *Journal of Emotional and Behavioral Disorders, 2,* 254–259.

Burns, B. J., & Freidman, R. M. (1990). Examining the research base for children's mental health services and policy. *Journal of Mental Health Administration, 17,* 87–99.

Burns, B. J., Hoagwood, K., & Maultsby, L. T. (1998). Improving outcomes for children and adolescents with serious emotional and behavioral disorders: Current and future directions. In M. H. Epstein, K. Kutash, & A. Duchnowski (Eds.), *Community-based programming for children with serious emotional disturbance and their families: Research and evaluations* (pp. 685–707). Austin, TX: Pro-Ed.

Chamberlain, P. (1990). Comparative evaluation of specialized foster care for seriously delinquent youths: A first step. *Community Alternatives: International Journal of Family Care, 2,* 21–36.

Chamberlain, P. (1994). *Family connections: Treatment foster care for adolescents with delinquency.* Eugene, OR: Castalia.

Chamberlain, P. (1997, April). *The effectiveness of group versus family treatment settings for adolescent juvenile offenders.* Paper presented at the meeting of the Society for Research on Child Development, Washington, DC.

Chamberlain, P., & Moore, K. (1998). Models of community treatment for serious juvenile offenders. In J. Crane (Ed.), *Social programs that really work* (pp. 258–276). New York: Russell Sage.

Chamberlain, P., & Reid, J. B. (1991). Using a specialized foster care community treatment model for children and adolescents leaving the state mental hospital. *Journal of Community Psychology, 19,* 266–276.

Chamberlain, P., & Reid, J. B. (1997). *Comparison of two community alternatives to incarceration for chronic juvenile offenders.* Manuscript submitted for publication.

Chamberlain, P., Ray, J., & Moore, K. J. (1996). Characteristics of residential care for adolescent offenders: A comparison of assumptions and practices in two models. *Journal of Child and Family Studies, 5,* 259–271.

Clarke, G. N. (1995). Improving the transition from basic efficacy research to effectiveness studies: Methodological issues and procedures. *Journal of Consulting and Clinical Psychology, 63,* 718–725.

Colyar, D. E. (1991). Residential care and treatment of youths with conduct disorders: Conclusions of a conference of child care workers. *Child and Youth Care Forum, 20,* 195–201.

Curry, J. F. (1991). Outcome research on residential treatment: Implications and suggested directions. *American Journal of Orthopsychiatry, 61,* 348–357.

Dalton, R., Muller, B., & Forman, M. (1989). The psychiatric hospitalization of children: An overview. *Child Psychiatry and Human Development, 19,* 231–244.

Day, D. M., Pal, A., & Goldberg, K. (1994). Assessing the post-residential functioning of latency-aged conduct disordered children. *Residential Treatment for Children and Youth, 11,* 45–52.

Dishion, T. J., & Andrews, D. W. (1995). Preventing escalation in problem behaviors with high risk young adolescents: Immediate and 1-year outcomes. *Journal of Consulting and Clinical Psychology, 63,* 538–548.

Durkin, R. P., & Durkin, A. B. (1975). Evaluating residential treatment programs for disturbed children. In M. Guttentag & E. L. Streuning (Eds.), *Handbook of evaluation research* (Vol. 2, pp. 275–339). Beverly Hills, CA: Sage.

Elliott, D. S., Huizinga, D., & Ageton, S. S. (1985). *Explaining delinquency and drug use.* Beverly Hills, CA: Sage.

Fanshel, D., Finch, S. J., & Grundy, J. F. (1990). *Foster children in life course perspective.* New York: Columbia University Press.

Fixsen, D. L., Phillips, E. L., Baron, R. L., Coughlin, D. D., Daly, D. L., & Daly, R. B. (1978, November). The Boys' Town revolution. *Human Nature,* 54–61.

Friman, P. C., Osgood, D. W., Shanahan, D., Thompson, R. W., Larzelere, R., & Daly, D. L. (1996). A longitudinal evaluation of prevalent negative beliefs about residential placement for troubled adolescents. *Journal of Abnormal Child Psychology, 24,* 299–324.

Garrett, C. J. (1985). Effects of residential treatment on adjudicate delinquents: A meta-analysis. *Journal of Research in Crime and Delinquency, 22,* 287–308.

Hazel, N. (1989). Adolescent fostering as a community resource. *Community Alternatives: International Journal of Family Care, 1,* 47–52.

Hoagwood, K., & Cunningham, M. (1992). Outcomes of children with emotional disturbance in residential treatment for educational purposes. *Journal of Child and Family Studies, 1,* 129–140.

Hobbs, N. (1982). *The troubled and troubling child.* San Francisco: Jossey-Bass.

Kutash, K., & Rivera, V. R. (1996). *What works in children's mental health services?* Baltimore: Brookes.

Larson, G., Allison, J., & Johnston, E. (1978). Alberta Parent Counselors: A community treatment program for disturbed youth. *Child Welfare, 57,* 47–52.

Long, P., Forehand, R., Wierson, M., & Morgan, A. (1994). Does parent training with young noncompliant children have long-term effects? *Behaviour Research and Therapy, 32,* 101–107.

McCord, J. (1997, April). *Some unanticipated consequences of summer camps.* Paper presented at the meeting of the Society for Research on Child Development, Washington, DC.

Meadowcroft, P., Thomlinson, B., & Chamberlain, P. (1994). Treatment foster care services: A research agenda for child welfare. *Child Welfare, 33,* 565–581.

Miller, G. E., & Prinz, R. J. (1990). Enhancement of social learning family interventions for childhood conduct disorder. *Psychological Bulletin, 108,* 291–307.

Patterson, G. R. (1982). *Coercive family process.* Eugene, OR: Castalia.

Patterson, G. R., Dishion, T. J., & Chamberlain, P. (1993). Outcomes and methodological issues relating to treatment of antisocial children. In T. R. Giles (Ed.), *Handbook of effective psychotherapy* (pp. 43–88). New York: Plenum.

Pfeiffer, S. I., & Strzelecki, S. C. (1990). Inpatient psychiatric treatment of children and adolescents: A review of outcome studies. *Journal of the American Academy of Child and Adolescent Psychiatry, 29,* 847–853.

Pfeiffer, S. I., Burd, S., & Wright, A. (1992). Clinicians and research: Recurring obstacles and some possible solutions. *Journal of Clinical Psychology, 48,* 140–145.

Phillips, E. L., Phillips, E. A., Fixsen, D. L., & Wolf, M. M. (1974). *The teaching-family handbook* (Rev. ed.).

Lawrence: The University of Kansas, Bureau of Child Research.

Quay, H. C. (1979). Residential treatment. In H. C. Quay & J. S. Werry (Eds.), *Psychopathological disorders of childhood* (2nd ed., pp. 387–410). New York: Wiley.

Quay, H. C. (1986). Residential treatment. In H. C. Quay & J. S. Werry (Eds.), *Psychopathological disorders of childhood* (3rd ed., pp. 558–582). New York: Wiley.

Select Committee on Children, Youth, and Families, U.S. House of Representatives. (1990). *No place to call home: Discarded children in America.* Washington, DC: U.S. Government Printing Office.

Slot, N. W., Jagers, H, D., & Dangel, R. F. (1992). Cross-cultural replication and evaluation of the Teaching Family Model of community-based residential treatment. *Behavioral Residential Treatment, 7,* 341–354.

Smith, P. (1986). Evaluation of Kent placements. *Adoption and Fostering, 10,* 22–33.

Stroul, B. (1989). *Community-based services for children and adolescents who are severely emotionally disturbed: Therapeutic foster care.* Washington, DC: CASSP Technical Assistance Center, Georgetown University Child Development Center.

Thompson, R. W., Smith, G. L., Osgood, D. W., Dowd, T. P., Friman, P. C., & Daly, D. (1996). Residential care: A study of short- and long-term effects. *Children and Youth Services Review, 18,* 139–162.

Vorrath, H., & Brendtro, L. K. (1985). *Positive peer culture.* Chicago: Aldine.

Weisz, J. R., Weiss, B., & Donenberg, G. R. (1992). The lab versus the clinic: Effects of child and adolescent psychotherapy. *American Psychologist, 47,* 1578–1585.

Wells, K. W. (1991). Placement of emotionally disturbed children in residential treatment: A review of placement criteria. *American Journal of Orthopsychiatry, 61,* 339–347.

Whittaker, J. K., & Pecora, P. J. (1984). A research agenda for residential care. In T. Philpot (Ed.), *Group care practice: The challenge of the next decade* (pp. 71–86). Surrey, England: Community Care/Business Press International.

Whittaker, J. K., & Pfeiffer, S. I. (1994). Research priorities for residential group care. *Child Welfare, 73,* 583–592.

Zoccolillo, M., & Rogers, K. (1991). Characteristics and outcome of hospitalized adolescent girls with conduct disorder. *Journal of the American Academy of Child and Adolescent Psychiatry, 30,* 973–981.

24

Outcomes of Children and Adolescents with Oppositional Defiant Disorder and Conduct Disorder

PAUL J. FRICK and BRYAN R. LONEY

INTRODUCTION

Children and adolescents with severe conduct problems, such as those diagnosed with conduct disorders (CD), by definition have significant impairments in their social, emotional, and educational functioning (Frick & O'Brien, 1995; Lahey *et al.*, 1994). In addition, their behavior is highly costly to society (e.g., costs of incarceration) and to the victims of their antisocial and aggressive acts. Perhaps the greatest cause for concern for children and adolescents with CD, however, is the fact that their behavior is often quite stable and persistent. In fact, it is one of the most persistent forms of childhood psychopathology (Offord *et al.*, 1992). Given the impairment, cost, and stability of CD, it is not surprising that a great deal of research has focused on understanding the developmental course of youth with this disorder.

Before focusing on the specific findings, we consider several general issues that provide a context for understanding this area of research. The first of these relates to the widely varying definitions of CD that have been used in research. As was discussed in Chapter 1 (this volume), the most recent terms are Oppositional Defiant Disorder (ODD) and Conduct Disorder (American Psychiatric Association, 1994). However, limiting our discussion only to those studies that have employed the current diagnostic criteria for defining CD would have severely limited the available research on which to base conclusions. Therefore, studies that have used definitions of CD derived from behavior rating scales and other psychometric measures, or that have used legal definitions of norm violating behavior (e.g., delinquency), or that have focused on a specific type of conduct problem (e.g., aggression) are considered as well. We believe that including research that has used these various operational definitions of CD is justified because they seem to be significantly intercorrelated and, with some notable exceptions discussed in later sections, the conclusions on stability and outcome are quite similar across them.*

PAUL J. FRICK and BRYAN R. LONEY • Department of Psychology, University of Alabama, Tuscaloosa, Alabama 35487.

Handbook of Disruptive Behavior Disorders, edited by Quay and Hogan. Kluwer Academic/Plenum Publishers, New York, 1999.

*We use CD as the generic term that subsumes the various operational definitions of severe and impairing patterns of antisocial and aggressive behavior except when it is important to specify an exact condition (e.g., delinquency).

A second important issue in understanding the outcomes of children with CD is the developmental and hierarchical relation between the behaviors associated with ODD (e.g., negative, noncompliant, angry, and defiant behaviors) and the behaviors associated with CD (e.g., norm-breaking behaviors and violations of the rights of others). The relation between these two behavioral domains is *developmental* in that longitudinal studies of preadolescent children have documented a typical progression from the less severe ODD behaviors to the more severe symptoms of CD. For example, in a 4-year longitudinal study of clinic-referred boys (initially ages 6-13), 82% of the boys who developed CD in the third and fourth years of the study had shown ODD in prior years (Lahey & Loeber, 1994; Lahey *et al.,* 1995). In this progression from a less severe to a more severe disorder, the boys did not change the types of behavior that they exhibited but seemed instead to add the more serious symptoms to their behavioral repertoire (see also Patterson, 1993). In addition to being developmental, this relation between ODD and CD symptoms seems to be *hierarchical* in nature. For example, whereas Lahey and Loeber (1994) reported that the majority of preadolescent boys who developed CD had ODD in previous years, they also reported that only about half (47%) of all the boys diagnosed with ODD progressed to CD over the 4-year course of the study.

This developmental and hierarchical association between ODD and CD has been consistently replicated in samples of preadolescent children (Hinshaw, Lahey, & Hart, 1993). However, this pattern has not been consistently found in youth who first show CD in adolescence (Moffitt, Caspi, Dickson, Silva, & Stanton, 1996). Despite the fact that it may not be typical of all youth who develop CD, this common progression from ODD to CD has some important implications. For example, because treatment success for older children with CD is somewhat limited, successful intervention strategies need to focus on intervening with children at high risk for developing CD (e.g., Conduct Problems Prevention Research Group, 1992; see also Chapter 25, this volume). Clearly,

the presence of ODD can be considered a marker for children at high risk for developing CD. It is also important to note that little is known about the outcomes of children with ODD who do not go on to show the more severe CD in childhood or adolescence. Much of the literature that is discussed in this chapter focuses on children or adolescents who have been diagnosed with CD or who show the antisocial and aggressive symptoms that characterize this disorder.

A third issue that is important in interpreting research on the outcomes of children with CD is the type of research design that is used. Specifically, "retrospective" studies look backward into the childhood histories of adults with antisocial behavior to determine the extent of CD in their childhood. "Prospective" studies follow children with CD into adulthood to determine the persistence and stability of their behavior over time. In retrospective studies of the life-span course of antisocial behavior, research has consistently found that most adults who show severe patterns of antisocial behavior have childhood histories of CD (Robins, Tipp, & Pryzbeck, 1991). When viewed prospectively, research has also documented a fairly substantial degree of stability in antisocial behavior across the life span. However, the level of stability is not nearly as high as that found in retrospective studies, because a substantial number of children and adolescents with CD do not go on to show severe patterns of antisocial behavior in adulthood. Given the substantial differences in results between these two research methods, we decided to focus only on prospective studies in an attempt to accomplish two main goals. Our first goal was to quantify the degree of stability associated with CD throughout the life span and our second goal was to explain some of the variability in outcomes in children with CD.

THE STABILITY OF CONDUCT DISORDER

The results of early prospective longitudinal studies were summarized by Olweus (1979) who reviewed 16 longitudinal studies involving predominantly male children ages 2 to 18, ranging in the length of time between the initial and follow-up assessments from 6 months to 21 years. Across the studies, there was an average stability coefficient of about .55 between measures of CD symptoms obtained at two assessment times. Two factors seemed to affect the size of the stability estimates. First, as would be expected, the stability coefficients were inversely related to the length of time between measurement periods; studies with longer intervals between measurement periods tended to produce smaller stability coefficients. Second, the age of the sample at the initial assessment time was related to stability; older children tended to exhibit more stable patterns of behavior.

Since this seminal article, numerous studies have provided additional estimates of the stability of CD. The findings from these studies, as well as three early studies not included in Olweus's (1979) review, are summarized in Tables 1 and 2. The studies are divided into those in which the sample was followed over relatively short periods of time (8 months to 5 years—Table 1) and those with longer follow-up intervals (6 to 30 years—Table 2). It is evident from both Tables 1 and 2 that (1) a number of different definitions of CD were used, (2) many different informants or informant combinations were used to assess CD, and (3) several types of stability estimates were calculated. It is also evident that the vast majority of these studies estimated the stability of CD in nonreferred samples of children or adolescents.

Despite the substantial heterogeneity across studies, there was substantial consistency in the estimates of stability. In studies using relatively short follow-up periods (Table 1), the majority of the correlations between initial and follow-up assessments fell between .42 and .64. These stability estimates are consistent with Olweus's (1979) findings and support the notion that there is substantial stability in measures of CD symptoms over relatively short periods of time. These studies employing correlation coefficients provide estimates of stability across the entire range of symptom severity. Three studies in Table 1 estimated the stability

of a diagnosis of CD and thereby focused exclusively on stability in children showing a more severe symptom pattern. Cohen, Cohen, & Brook (1993), in a community sample of children and adolescents (ages 9–18 at initial assessment), estimated the 2-year stability of CD defined by DSM-III criteria (American Psychiatric Association, 1980). They reported kappa coefficients ranging from .34 to .40 between diagnoses of CD at the initial assessment and 2-year follow-up. Given that the coefficient kappa is a fairly conservative estimate of stability, these estimates represent substantial levels of stability. Lahey and colleagues (1995) reported a similar stability estimate (kappa = .33) for a diagnosis of CD over a 4-year study period in a clinic-referred sample of boys (ages 6–13 at initial assessment). In this study, DSM-III-R criteria were used to diagnose CD (American Psychiatric Association, 1987). Approximately 51% of the boys diagnosed with CD at the initial assessment were rediagnosed with CD at the 4-year follow-up assessment. This percentage of children rediagnosed at follow-up is very similar to the estimate provided by Offord and colleagues (1992) who found that in a community sample of children (ages 4–12 at initial assessment) diagnosed with CD by DSM-III criteria, 45% were rediagnosed at the 4-year follow-up assessment.

Another source of consistency that is evident from Table 1 is the fact that the estimates did not vary greatly across different sources of the assessment information (e.g., parent, teacher, child self-report, or peer nominations) or across the type of CD symptoms assessed. Furthermore, a number of studies provided separate stability estimates for boys and girls and there was little difference in the stability of CD due to sex. This finding is consistent with two previous reviews of this literature. Olweus (1984) reported average stability coefficients of .44 and .50 for measures of conduct problems in boys and girls, respectively. Zumkley (1994) reported correlations of .44 and .56 in samples of boys and girls.

Table 2 summarizes data on the stability of CD over longer time intervals (i.e., > 6 years). As would be expected, the stability esti-

TABLE 1. Short-Term Stability of Conduct Problems (< 6 Years)

Article	Sample size/type (% male)	Age of sample	Length of follow-up	Informant(s)	Description of conduct problems	Stability estimate
Cohen, Cohen, & Brook (1993)	734 (Co)	9–18	2½ years	Parent & child	DSM-III CD	Kappa = .34 (mild) Kappa = .40 (mod.) Kappa = .39 (severe)
Dumas, Neese, Prinz, & Blechman (1996)	478 (Co) (49%)	6–8	8 months	Teacher	Oppositional/ aggressive behavior	r = .66
Fergusson & Horwood (1993)	783 (Co)	8	4 years	Parent Teacher	Conduct/oppositional behavior	r = .63 (parent) r = .48 (teacher)
Gersten et al. (1976)	732 (Co)	6–18	5 years	Parent	Delinquent behavior	r = .44
Jessor & Jessor (1977)	432 (Co) (44%)	13–15	3 years	Child	General deviancy	r = .45 (boys) r = .53 (girls)
Lahey et al. (1995)	174 (Cl) (100%)	7–12	4 years	Parent, teacher, & child	DSM-III-R CD	Kappa = .33
Loeber et al. (1991)	1517 (Co) (100%)	6–12	2 years	Parent, teacher, & child	Classified delinquent	Percent reclassified = 31% to 52%
McConaughy, Stanger, & Achenbach (1992)	2466 (Co)	4–16	3 years	Parent	Opposition/Aggression Antisocial	r = .58 (opp/agg) r = .44 (anti.)
Moskowitz, Schwartzman, & Ledingham (1985)	377 (Co) (49%)	6–12	3 years	Peers	Aggression	r = .42–.64 (boys) r = .43–.64 (girls)
Offord et al. (1992)	881 (Co) (50%)	4–12	4 years	Parent & teacher	DSM-III CD	Percent rediagnosed = 44.8%
Verhulst, Koot, & Berden (1990)	1200 (Co) (48%)	4–12	4 years	Parent	Opposition/aggression Antisocial	r = .67 (opp/agg) r = .31 (anti.)
Verhulst & Van Der Ende (1991)	797 (Co) (46%)	4–12	4 years	Teacher	Opposition/aggression	r = .34 (boys) r = .52 (girls)

Note. Sample type: Co = nonreferred community; Cl = clinic referrals.

TABLE 2. Long-Term Stability of Conduct Problems (> 6 Years)

Article	Sample size/type (% male)	Age of sample	Length of follow-up	Informant(s)	Description of conduct problems	Stability estimate
Huesmann et al. (1984)	402 (Co) (48%)	8	22 years	Peers (I) Self (F)	Aggression & antisocial behavior	$r = .30$ (boys) $r = .16$ (girls)
Farrington (1991)	411 (Co) (100%)	8–10	22–24 years	Teacher (I) Self (F)	Disruptive (I) Aggressive/ criminal (F)	Percent of most disruptive (I) rated as most aggressive (F) = 49% or with any criminal offense (F) = 57%
Fergusson, Lynskey, & Horwood (1996)	901 (Co)	7–9	7 years	Parent & teacher (I) Parent & self (F)	Conduct problems (I) ODD/CD (F)	Percent in upper 10% (I) Diagnosed (F) = 58%
Kratzer & Hodgins (1997)	12,717 (Co) (51%)	12–16	16 years	Teacher (I) Record review (F)	Conduct problems (I) Criminality (F)	Percent with conduct problems (I) who committed crime (F) 64% (boys) 17% (girls)
Lefkowitz et al. (1977)	427 (Co) (49%)	8	10 years	Peer (I) Peer & self (F)	Aggression (I) Aggression & antisocial (F)	$r = .38$ (boys—peer/peer) $r = .21$ (boys—peer/self) $r = .47$ (girls—peer/peer) $r = .13$ (girls—peer/self)
Moffitt (1990, 1993a)	435 (Co)	5	8 years	Teacher	Antisocial	$r = .28$
Robins (1966)	314 (Cl) (74%)	6–17	30 years	Parent (I) Self & record review (F)	Conduct problems (I) Sociopathic personality (F)	Percent referred for conduct problems (I) Diagnosed (F) = 31% (boys) 17% (girls)
Stattin & Magnusson (1991)	709 (Co) (100%)	15	14 years	Record review (I&F)	Criminality	$r = .34$
Tremblay et al. (1992)	147 (Co) (46%)	7	7 years	Peer (I) Self (F)	Disruptive behavior (I) Delinquency (F)	$r = .46$ (boys) $r = .11$ (girls)

Note. Sample type: Co = nonreferred community; Cl = clinic referrals. (I) = initial assessment; (F) = follow-up assessment.

mates presented in these studies are somewhat lower than those reported in Table 1. However, they still show substantial stability, especially relative to the stability in measures of other psychological traits over extended time periods (e.g., Huessman, Eron, Lefkowitz, & Walder, 1984). Specifically, the correlation coefficients for the long-term follow-up studies generally fell between .20 and .40. Several studies provided estimates of stability in samples of youth with severe patterns of behavior who were likely to meet formal diagnostic criteria for CD. However, the degree of stability was somewhat variable across studies. This variability seemed partly related to the choice of outcome measure. For example, Kratzer and Hodgins (1997) found that about 64% of boys and 17% of girls (ages 12–16) with CD had committed a crime during a 16-year follow-up period. In contrast, Robins (1966) reported that 31% of boys and 17% of girls referred to a mental health clinic for CD symptoms were diagnosed with sociopathic personality disorder as adults. The definition of sociopathic personality disorder was similar to the DSM-IV criteria for Antisocial Personality Disorder (APD; American Psychiatric Association, 1994) which requires a more severe, varied, and chronic pattern of antisocial behavior than the commission of a single criminal offense. In fact, when Robins estimated the percentage of children with CD who had criminal histories over the 30-year follow-up period, she found that 43% of the boys and 12% of girls who had been referred for CD symptoms had been imprisoned at least once as an adult. While these percentages still do not approach the high figures reported by Kratzer and Hodgins for boys, they do suggest that at least some of the variability in stability estimates may be attributed to the choice of outcome measure.

A second source of variability that is evident in these long-term outcome studies is that boys had greater stability of CD into adulthood than girls. As mentioned previously, there was no evidence of sex differences in stability from the short-term outcome studies summarized in Table 1. Therefore, there seem to be no sex differences in the stability of CD over short time periods, whereas boys with CD seem to show a more stable disorder over long periods of time than girls with CD, especially when studies include follow-up assessments into adulthood. The outcomes that were the focus of Table 2 were antisocial outcomes (e.g., criminal histories, diagnosis of an antisocial disorder). There is evidence that girls with CD may have substantially impaired adult outcomes but the impairment may not be as specific to antisocial behavior as is the case for the adult outcome of boys with CD. For example, girls with CD seem to be at high risk for (1) showing somatization disorders and other emotional disorders, (2) making suicide attempts, and (3) having severe impairments in their occupational and social adjustment (see Robins *et al.,* 1991; Silverthorn & Frick, in press; Zoccolillo, 1993).

METHODOLOGICAL FACTORS AFFECTING STABILITY ESTIMATES

These prospective studies suggest that there is a substantial degree of stability in CD over both short and long follow-up periods. However, there is reason to believe that many of these studies may even have *underestimated* the stability of CD because of several methodological factors. One possible reason for such underestimation is that the stability estimates were typically based on outcome assessed at a single point (e.g., at a 4-year follow-up). Estimates of stability based on only one follow-up assessment do not take into account the substantial waxing and waning of symptom severity that occurs over time. For example, Lahey and colleagues (1995) reported on a 4-year longitudinal study of 171 clinic-referred boys; they found that about 50% of the boys diagnosed with CD at the start of the study were rediagnosed at the 4-year follow-up, which led to the kappa of .33 reported in Table 1. However, 88% of the boys were rediagnosed with CD at any one of the yearly follow-up assessments across the 4-year study.

The estimates of stability reported in Tables 1 and 2 can also be attenuated by the use of measures that are insensitive to the changing manifestations of CD over the course of development (Patterson, 1993). Numerous longitudinal studies have shown that the types of CD symptoms shown by children of different ages vary, with very young children showing more oppositional and argumentative behaviors, followed by an increase in physical aggression in later childhood, and followed even later by "delinquent" behaviors (e.g., vandalism, stealing) (Lahey & Loeber, 1994; Patterson, 1993). As mentioned previously, this process is often one of the subjects' adding more severe behaviors to their repertoire (Lahey & Loeber, 1994). However, there can also be qualitative changes in the types of behavior shown by children of different ages, such as a decrease in the level of interpersonal aggression that is exhibited by a child as he or she approaches adolescence and a corresponding increase in nonaggressive illegal behaviors (e.g., substance abuse, shoplifting, truancy, vandalism) (Patterson, 1993). Patterson has described these age-related variations as illustrating the stability of an antisocial "trait" that may take on developmentally distinct forms. The implication of this issue for interpreting stability estimates is that many studies have used measures of only one aspect of the antisocial trait (e.g., interpersonal aggression). Therefore, they potentially underestimated the stability of the trait by not adequately capturing developmental changes in how the trait is expressed.

A third reason that the estimates provided in Tables 1 and 2 may underestimate the actual stability of CD is that most estimates were based on a single assessment method at both the initial assessment point and at follow-up. Any single assessment method is associated with some degree of measurement error. The imperfections in measurement techniques are compounded in longitudinal studies when they are used in multiple administrations to estimate stability. The resulting estimate of stability is affected by measurement error occurring at multiple administrations (Fergusson, Horwood, & Lynskey, 1995). To illustrate the effects of measurement error in estimating stability, Fergusson and colleagues provided data on a subset (81%) of a birth cohort of New Zealand children ($n = 905$) studied between the ages of 7 and 15. Using an estimate of stability that did not control for measurement error, these authors found that 50% of the children with CD were not rediagnosed 2 years later, estimates quite similar to the ones reported in Table 1. However, using a second approach to estimating stability, one that controlled for measurement error using latent variable analysis, these authors found that only 14% of children with CD showed a remission in behavior over a 2-year period. These authors have reported similar changes in stability estimates when continuous measures of CD symptoms were used and measurement error was controlled using latent variable models. Specifically, without controlling for measurement error, CD symptoms were correlated at approximately .39 across 2 to 4 years. However, the same correlations across time were estimated as being approximately .90 when latent variable models were used to control for measurement error (Fergusson & Horwood, 1993).

PREDICTORS OF STABILITY

Because of these methodological factors, it is quite possible that the stability estimates provided in Tables 1 and 2 underestimate the actual stability of CD. However, even when these methodological factors are taken into account, there still seems to be important and systematic sources of variability in the stability of CD. This variability is dramatically illustrated by the fact that the most persistent 5% to 6% of youthful offenders account for about 50% of reported crimes (Farrington, Ohlin, & Wilson, 1986). Similarly, estimates of stability such as those reported in Tables 1 and 2 are dramatically reduced when the most persistent 5% of boys with CD are excluded from the estimates (Moffitt, 1993a). Therefore, an important focus of longitudinal research has been to identify variables that predict the stability of CD.

One important issue in this research on predictors of persistence is the need to disentangle factors that are related to the *development* of CD with factors that are related to the *persistence* of CD. Although some factors may be related to both the cause and the stability of CD, Lahey and colleagues (1995) outlined three reasons for their differing. First, some causal variables may be related only to the development of relatively transient forms of CD and therefore may only weakly predict persistence. Second, some variables may play a role only in the maintenance of CD and not in the initial etiology. As a result, these variables predict only persistence. Third, some variables may be so strongly associated with the development of CD that they are nearly ubiquitous among children with CD and therefore there is little variance in the prediction of persistence for which these variables could account.

A good illustration of this third point is the association between having a delinquent peer group and CD. It is well documented that children and adolescents with CD are more likely to associate with peers who also show CD symptoms (Elliott, Huizinga, & Ageton, 1985; Keenan, Loeber, Zhang, Stouthamer-Loeber, & Van Kammen, 1995). The importance of this association with an antisocial peer group for the development of CD is the subject of great debate. For some, delinquent peers provide the single most critical environmental influence on the development of antisocial behavior (Elliott *et al.,* 1985). For others, the association with delinquent peers is secondary to other factors associated with CD, such as rejection from a prosocial peer group and poor monitoring and supervision from parents (Patterson, Reid, & Dishion, 1992; see also Chapter 16, this volume). However, the important point is that there has been no clear evidence to date to link the association with delinquent peers to greater *stability* of CD. This failure to clearly predict persistence seems to be due to the ubiquitous nature of having delinquent peers in children with CD. For example, Moffitt and colleagues (1996) compared the level of involvement with delinquent peers between two groups of boys with CD. The first group were boys who had shown a chronic pattern of CD through childhood and into adolescence and therefore were at high risk for continuing antisocial behavior

into adulthood. The second group were boys who had an adolescent-onset CD and therefore were at lower risk for continuing antisocial behavior into adulthood. Both groups of boys with CD reported having more peers who engaged in delinquent activities than did children without CD, with all three groups being matched on various demographic characteristics (see Fergusson, Lynskey, & Horwood, 1996, for similar results).

This example illustrates the distinction between factors that may be critical in the etiology of CD but may not be useful in the prediction of stability. Since the focus of this chapter is primarily the stability of CD, the following discussion focuses on factors that longitudinal research has documented as playing a role in predicting the stability of CD, irrespective of their role in the initial development of the disorder. However, many studies have not used a methodology that allows one to clearly disentangle causal factors from predictors of persistence. For example, many prospective studies have followed cohorts of children longitudinally; these children are often selected because they are at high risk for CD and have documented background factors (e.g., family dysfunction) that predict adult antisocial behavior (e.g., McCord, 1979). However, this design does not control for the association of these background predictors with childhood CD. As a result, many "predictors" of adult outcome may be related to the development of CD in childhood or adolescence and thus predict adult antisocial outcomes only because of the stability of CD over time. Although we tried to focus on factors that seemed to predict persistence independent of their association with the development of CD, in some instances this distinction was not often clear because of the methodology of the studies reviewed.

Severity of Conduct Problems

One of the more consistent predictors of poor outcome for children with CD is the severity of the initial disorder (Loeber, 1982, 1991). This fact may sound intuitively obvious but it is important to illustrate that even in children who cross a formal diagnostic threshold there remain substantial variations in severity. Research has documented certain aspects of these variations in severity that seem to be most predictive of persistence. The frequency and intensity of the behavior exhibited, the variety of types of symptoms displayed, and the presence of symptoms in more than one setting have all been related to a more severe and persistent form of CD (see Loeber, 1982, 1991). For example, Robins (1966) found that in a sample of 314 children referred to a child mental health clinic for CD symptoms, the risk for being diagnosed with an antisocial disorder as an adult was a linear function of the number of symptoms exhibited in childhood. Specifically, of the children with 3 to 5 symptoms in childhood, 15% were rediagnosed with an antisocial disorder as an adult, in comparison to 25% of children with 6 or 7 symptoms, 29% of children with 8 or 9 symptoms, and 43% of children with greater than 10 symptoms. Related to the cross-setting aspect of severity, Mitchell and Rosa (1981) found that boys rated by both parents and teachers as stealing or lying were two to six times more likely to show chronic criminal behavior as adults than boys rated by only one of these informants as showing these symptoms. And finally, Stattin and Magnusson (1991) reported on criminal activity of males followed from childhood (before age 14) through early adulthood (ages 21–30) and found that the more diversified the offending pattern (i.e., involvement in multiple types of offenses) in adolescence, the more varied and severe the person's criminal activity tended to be in early adulthood.

Early Age of Onset

Another consistent finding in this literature is that children who begin showing CD symptoms early in childhood are more likely to show a chronic and stable pattern of behavior than children who start showing CD symptoms in adolescence (e.g., Farrington, Gallagher, Morley, St. Ledger, & West, 1988; Moffitt et al., 1996; Patterson, 1993; Robins, 1966). For example, Farrington and colleagues found that

boys who were arrested before age 12 showed almost twice as many convictions at two later times (between the ages of 16 and 18 and between the ages of 22 and 24). Similarly, Robins found that boys referred to a mental health clinic for antisocial behavior before age 11 were twice as likely to receive a diagnosis of an antisocial disorder as an adult, as compared to boys who began showing antisocial behavior after age 11.

The strong and consistent association between the age of onset of CD symptoms and outcome was a major factor in the adoption of the current subtyping approach to CD which distinguishes between childhood-onset and adolescent-onset subtypes, as discussed in Chapter 1 (this volume). The differences in prognosis between the childhood- and adolescent-onset patterns of CD also correspond to a number of differences in the symptom presentation and clinical correlates of the two subtypes (see Moffitt, 1993a; Patterson, 1993; see also Chapter 1, this volume). These differences in both prognosis and correlates led Moffitt to propose a theoretical model that outlines two distinct causal pathways through which children develop CD. According to Moffitt, the childhood-onset pathway typically involves a child with temperament and cognitive vulnerabilities, such as impulsivity and lower intelligence. In addition, the child often has parents who have difficulty in using effective socialization strategies. This "juxtaposition of a vulnerable and difficult child with an adverse rearing context" (Moffitt, 1993a, p. 682) initiates a transactional process that evokes a chain of failed and aversive parent–child interactions that prevents the child from developing prosocial patterns of behavior, especially in interpersonal relations (see also Patterson et al., 1992). The adolescent-onset CD pathway is conceptualized as an exaggeration of a normative pattern of rebellion associated with the maturity gap that occurs in most industrialized society. This maturity gap refers to the period between reaching biological and cognitive maturity and attaining societally accepted adult status. Moffitt proposed that this maturity gap, combined with the influence of delinquent peers and a personality type that rejects traditional status hierarchies, leads persons in the adolescent-onset group to engage in antisocial behavior as a misguided attempt to gain a sense of maturity.

A thorough evaluation of Moffitt's theory in terms of causal predictions is beyond the scope of this chapter. However, this model provides a theoretical rationale for the differences in outcome between the two groups of children with CD. Specifically, when the adolescent-onset group achieves adult status, the primary motivation for the antisocial behavior (e.g., achieving adult status) is removed. In contrast, the temperament and cognitive vulnerabilities associated with the childhood-onset pattern, vulnerabilities that result from a combination of biological factors (see Chapter 17, this volume) and early learning experiences, likely place a person at risk for continued antisocial behavior throughout the life span. Consistent with this notion, persons with childhood-onset CD show greater problems in a number of areas of occupational and psychosocial adjustment as adults than persons with adolescent-onset CD, in addition to showing more severe antisocial behavior in adulthood (Nagin, Farrington, & Moffitt, 1995).

Both the differences in correlates and differences in outcome for the childhood- and adolescent-onset CD have been well supported in research on boys with CD (see Moffitt, 1993a). However, the findings are less clear for girls. Girls with CD are much more likely to have an adolescent-onset antisocial behavior than boys and, despite this later onset, the correlates (e.g., poor impulse control, adverse family backgrounds) are similar to the correlates found in studies of childhood-onset boys (Silverthorn & Frick, in press). More important, however, is the fact that, despite the later onset of their antisocial behavior, girls with CD seem to have poor adult outcomes. For example, Zoccolillo and Rogers (1991) presented outcome data for a sample of girls (ages 13–16) diagnosed with CD and admitted to a psychiatric hospital. Two to 4 years later, 50% had been arrested or placed on probation, 41% had dropped out of school permanently, and 22% had attempted suicide. Similarly, Lewis and colleagues (1991) reported

a 7-year follow-up of delinquent girls (age 14 years 9 months at initial assessment) and found that 71% of the girls had been arrested as an adult with a mean of 3.8 adult arrests. Furthermore, 71% had serious drug problems and 90% had attempted suicide. The literature on the outcome of girls with CD is quite limited and fraught with numerous methodological problems, the most apparent being the lack of adequate comparison groups with which to compare the outcomes of girls with CD (Silverthorn & Frick, in press). However, the literature that is available suggests that an adolescent-onset of CD does not predict a more positive outcome for girls with CD, as it does for boys.

Comorbid Attention-Deficit/Hyperactivity Disorder

Another factor that seems to play an important role in determining the outcome of children with ODD or CD is the presence of Attention-Deficit/Hyperactivity Disorder (ADHD). ADHD may be one of the most common co-occurring problems in adjustment experienced by children with CD, affecting between 65% and 90% of clinic-referred boys with CD (Abikoff & Klein, 1992; Stewart, Cummings, Singer, & deBlois, 1981; see also Chapter 3, this volume). The presence of ADHD seems to predict certain aspects of poor outcome for children with CD. For example, Loeber, Brinthaupt, and Green (1990) reported data on boys in grades 4, 7, and 10 who were followed over a 5-year period. Boys with CD, with or without ADHD, were highly likely to have police contacts over the follow-up period (54% of the group with ADHD and 48% of the group without ADHD). However, the group with ADHD were more likely to be multiple offenders (31% vs. 21%) and were more likely to self-report a variety of delinquent acts (62% vs. 21%). Similar findings were reported by Moffitt (1990) in a longitudinal study of 435 boys followed prospectively from age 3. When these boys were divided at age 13 into (1) those who self-reported delinquent behaviors and who were diagnosed with ADHD and (2) those who reported delinquent acts but who did not show ADHD, both delinquent groups were found to have high rates of self-reported delinquent acts at age 15. However, the ADHD group reported significantly more aggression than the non-ADHD group. Finally, Klinteberg, Andersson, Magnusson, and Stattin (1993) reported that boys (age 13) who had CD and who showed motor hyperactivity were more likely to be convicted of violent offenses (18%) between the ages of 15 and 25 than boys who had CD but who were not hyperactive (7%).

These data suggest that children with CD, either with or without ADHD, are at increased risk for antisocial outcomes. However, children with both ADHD and CD seem to show a greater variety of delinquent acts in adolescence (Loeber et al., 1990), a greater number of aggressive acts in adolescence (Moffitt, 1993a), and more violent offending in adulthood (Klinteberg et al., 1993). It is not clear, however, whether this risk is independent of other factors that predict antisocial outcomes. For example, children with both ADHD and CD tend to show an earlier age of onset of CD, a greater number of symptoms, and more aggressive symptoms in childhood (Moffitt, 1990; Walker, Lahey, Hynd, & Frame, 1987), all of which predict poor outcome. Therefore, it is unclear whether the influence of ADHD on the outcome of children with CD is a result of its influence on the severity and onset of CD in childhood or whether it contributes independently to the prediction of outcome in later adolescence and adulthood.

Another issue in this research is the debate over what aspects of ADHD contribute to the poor outcome for children with both ADHD and CD. For many authors, it is the impulsivity associated with ADHD that leads to the poor outcome (Moffitt, 1993a). Moffitt has proposed that the impulsivity associated with ADHD can lead a child with CD to have difficulty anticipating the consequences of his or her behavior, thus contributing directly to a more severe and stable pattern of CD. Alternatively, Moffitt proposed that impulsivity could have an indirect effect on the stability of CD by disrupting a child's school performance which

further limits his or her options for adopting a prosocial lifestyle. In another conceptualization of the influence of ADHD on the stability of CD, Lynam (1996) proposed that children with ADHD and CD represent a unique and qualitatively distinct subtype of CD that more closely corresponds to adult conceptualizations of psychopathy. Lynam proposed that children with ADHD and CD show a specific deficit in response inhibition, one that prevents these children from inhibiting goal-directed behaviors in the face of changing environmental contingencies. This pattern of deficient response modulation has been associated with psychopathy in adults (Newman & Wallace, 1993).

Low Intellectual Ability

There is a large body of research linking low intelligence, especially lower verbal intelligence, to CD (Moffitt, 1993b; see also Chapter 14, this volume). Furthermore, several studies have found that the most persistent offenders from childhood to adolescence (Fergusson et al., 1996; Moffitt, 1990) or from childhood to adulthood (Farrington, 1991) tend to have lower scores on measures of intelligence. Also, Robins (1966) found that low intelligence predicted which children with antisocial behaviors were at greatest risk for receiving a diagnosis of an antisocial disorder as an adult. Despite these generally positive findings, the literature linking low intelligence to the persistence of CD has not always been consistent. For example, Huesmann, Eron, and Yarmel (1987) reported on a 22-year prospective study of 600 subjects assessed from age 8 to age 30. These authors reported that, whereas intelligence was related to the onset of aggression at age 8, it did not influence the stability of aggression into adulthood.

One possible explanation for these inconsistent findings is that intelligence may influence stability in persons with severe CD but not the persistence of less severe symptoms. Another explanation for this inconsistency comes from Lahey and colleagues' (1995) longitudinal study in which intelligence scores did not predict persistence in boys with CD in isolation from other variables. However, it did interact with the presence of a family history of APD in predicting stability. Specifically, higher intelligence was predictive of less persistence in children with CD *only* if they did not have a family history of APD. In contrast, CD children with high intelligence and a family history of APD showed a highly stable pattern of symptoms. These results suggest that intelligence may be differentially related to the persistence of conduct problems depending on the presence of other variables. In a later section we provide a theoretical context that might explain this interactive effect of intelligence in predicting persistence in children with CD.

Predictors in the Child's Social Ecology

The predictors of persistence that have been reviewed thus far have largely focused on factors in the child that might predict a more chronic pattern of antisocial behavior. There are several factors in a child's social ecology that might also predict the persistence of CD throughout the life span. For example, McCord (1979) reported on a longitudinal study of 253 boys (age 5 to 13) who were enrolled in a treatment program designed to prevent delinquency. When these participants were evaluated 30 years later, several factors from their childhood home environment were predictive of later criminality. The one aspect of family functioning that predicted both property crimes and crimes against persons was the quality of supervision that the child's parent provided. Parental conflict and parental aggression predicted later crimes against persons and low maternal affection and low maternal self-confidence in parenting ability predicted property crimes. Farrington (1991) also identified factors in the early home environment that predicted chronic and violent antisocial behavior in adolescence and adulthood such as harsh parental discipline and parental conflict. In addition, Farrington found that several indicators of economic hardship in childhood, such as low family income, poor paternal employment history, and large family size, predicted adult antisocial behavior.

Although the findings from both Farrington (1991) and McCord (1979) suggest that certain aspects of a child's social ecology predict adult antisocial behavior, these studies did not control for the association of these background factors with the initial development of CD to see whether they predicted adult outcome independent of their association with childhood behavior. There are two pieces of evidence that relate to this issue. First, Moffitt (1990) differentiated children at age 13 who reported delinquent behaviors but who either did or did not have a diagnosis of ADHD. The subgroup with ADHD, who had a more continuous childhood history of CD, scored higher on a family adversity index than the delinquent group who did not have ADHD. The family adversity index was a composite of parental education, parental occupation, parental income, maternal mental health, and family social climate. This study provides the first clear evidence that measures of family dysfunction and other stressors in the child's background may be specifically associated with stability in children with CD. However, this stable group of CD children also exhibited ADHD, so it is unclear how much the environmental stressors as opposed to ADHD contributed to stability. In fact, the effect may be interactive in that children with ADHD may be more susceptible to the influence of less than optimal rearing environments (see Colder, Lochman, & Wells, 1997). Second, Lahey and colleagues (1995) reported that low socioeconomic status (SES) was clearly associated with the onset of CD but did not contribute to the prediction of the persistence of CD over the 4-year study. This latter finding illustrates that, although factors in the child's family and the broader social ecology may be associated with the development of CD (see Frick, 1994), their role in predicting the stability of CD is less clear.

SUMMARY AND FUTURE DIRECTIONS

It is evident that there have been a number of prospective longitudinal studies documenting both the short- and long-term stability of

CD in children and adolescents. From these studies, there is evidence for substantial stability across many types of samples, using many different definitions of CD, and using many different methods for estimating stability. There is also evidence that these stability estimates may even underestimate the true level of stability due to a number methodological factors, such as a failure to use measures that capture varying manifestations of CD across development, reliance on single follow-up assessments that do not capture the fluctuating severity of symptoms over time, and a failure to control for measurement error in the estimates of stability.

The literature is also important in uncovering several variables that fairly consistently predict poor outcome in children with CD. For example, children with CD who show a large number and multiple types of CD symptoms in multiple settings, who develop CD symptoms at an early age (before adolescence), and who have comorbid problems of disinhibition associated with ADHD seem to show a more chronic disorder. The literature also suggests that under certain conditions low intelligence might be a predictor of poor outcome but its effects may be best understood in the context of other variables. Environmental stressors, such as a dysfunctional family environment and low SES, may also play a role in predicting poor outcome. However, the current database on the role of these factors is limited and does not allow for a clear conclusion about their role in predicting persistence independent of their role in the initial development of CD.

This review has also uncovered a number of problems that must be addressed in future research. The first is the need for future studies to control for factors that can attenuate stability estimates in longitudinal studies. Future research needs to use methodology that recognizes the changing symptoms of CD over the course of development, that takes into account the fluctuating severity of symptoms over time, and that controls for the influence of measurement error on estimates of stability. The second problem is that of differentiating factors that are involved in the onset of CD and factors that are involved in its persistence. We have high-

lighted a number of reasons that these two processes may involve different variables, yet much of the research to date has failed to use a methodology that clearly differentiates variables involved in the two processes. This failure to disentangle causal factors from predictors of persistence has been especially problematic for determining the influence of the child's social ecology on persistence.

A third limitation in the existing research is the minimal information available on the outcome of at least two groups of children with severe conduct problems: girls with CD and children with ODD who do not go on to show CD. The outcome of girls with CD has not been studied systematically and the limited data that are available suggest that at least some of the predictors of poor outcome (e.g., early onset) for boys may not operate in the same manner for girls. Furthermore, there is virtually no information on the lifelong course of children with ODD who do not go on to develop CD, despite that fact that this is a sizable proportion of children who have clinically significant conduct problems (Lahey *et al.,* 1994).

A fourth problem documented by this review relates to the predominant focus in outcome research on the predictors of *poor* outcome. There is an assumption that predictors of *good* outcome are simply the absence of predictors of poor outcome. However, there is a growing literature on protective factors in children (e.g., Garmezy, 1993) suggesting that some variables, both in the child and in the child's social ecology, may act primarily through moderating the negative effects of certain risk factors. That is, they may not have detrimental effects on the child's outcome if they are absent but, when present, serve to buffer or protect a child from the negative effects of risk factors. This approach to research has not been systematically applied to the study of the outcome of children with CD. Such studies could provide tremendously important data on factors that could be enhanced through treatment programs designed to alter the negative outcome of children and adolescents with CD.

A fifth need not yet met by the existing longitudinal research is that for more theory-driven research into the mechanisms that might affect the stability of CD in children and adolescents. It is fairly well accepted that advances in our understanding of the causes of CD will largely come from theory-driven research that attempts to go beyond simply describing correlates of CD to actually attempting to understand the mechanisms involved in the development of this disorder (Richters & Cicchetti, 1993). A similar case has been made in developing innovative prevention and treatment programs. That is, advances in treatment typically are based on sound theoretical foundations and specifically attempt to alter mechanisms involved in the development of CD (Dodge, 1993; see also Chapter 25, this volume). This focus on sound theoretical models has been absent in much of the longitudinal research on the outcomes of children with CD. There has been an implicit assumption in much of the research that the best approach is an atheoretical or actuarial approach in which one studies as many variables as possible and simply charts those that seem predictive of poor outcome. This approach leads to a list of predictors that can be dependent on the sample in which they are studied and a list that is quite limited in advancing our understanding of how the predictors might lead to poor outcomes.

One notable exception to this atheoretical trend is the approach taken by Moffitt (1993a) in defining distinct mechanisms to explain the development and differential stability of childhood-onset and adolescent-onset subtypes of CD. As an illustration of the importance of embedding predictors of stability in a theoretical framework, Silverthorn and Frick (in press) used Moffitt's model to explain why an early onset of CD as a predictor of poor outcome may be sample specific. These authors proposed that age of onset may not predict poor outcome for girls with CD because girls with CD generally have a later onset of their antisocial behavior yet they often have the dispositional and environmental characteristics that are similar to childhood-onset boys (e.g., poor impulse control, familial dysfunction). Therefore, despite the later age of onset of CD in girls, the devel-

opment of CD may involve the same processes that enhance the stability of CD in the childhood-onset boys. This extension of Moffitt's model illustrates how a focus on the processes that enhance stability (e.g., specific dispositional vulnerabilities), rather than simply documenting markers of persistence (e.g., age of onset), can help explain why some predictors of persistence may be sample dependent (e.g., apply mainly to boys).

One final problem in the current outcome research is the need to move away from sole reliance on variable-centered approaches to predicting outcome and to include more person-centered approaches to prediction (see also Magnusson & Bergman, 1990). Much of the outcome research to date has attempted to find *variables* (e.g., intelligence, low SES) that predict poor outcome. In contrast, person-centered approaches attempt to isolate *persons* with certain constellations of variables or profiles of variables that are at high risk for having a poor long-term outcome. The two approaches to studying outcome can lead to different predictors of persistence if a variable is predictive of poor outcome only when it occurs in combination with another variable or variables, as illustrated previously in the findings of Lahey and colleagues (1995) in which low intelligence and parental APD interacted to predict the persistence of CD. This recommendation for more person-centered approaches to research should be considered in conjunction with the recommendation for more theory-driven research. Specifically, the testing of particular constellations of characteristics that might designate a person at high risk for a stable pattern of CD should be guided by a theoretical framework that explains why these characteristics tend to form distinct profiles that predict poor outcome.

As an example of this person-centered approach, we have been developing an approach to subtyping children with CD based on the presence of callous-unemotional traits (Christian, Frick, Hill, Tyler, & Frazer, 1997). We have proposed that children who show both CD and a callous and unemotional interpersonal style develop their disorder through a unique set of causal factors, one related to a deficit in fearful inhibition (Frick, 1998). This deficit in fearful inhibition places these children at risk for developing callous and unemotional (CU) traits (Frick, 1998; Kochanska, 1993). In turn the cold and callous interpersonal style makes them more likely to violate the rights of others and disregard societal norms; this leads to an especially severe and aggressive pattern of antisocial behavior (Christian *et al.,* 1997). This multiple pathway model assumes that children with CD who also show CU traits, because they develop CD through a unique causal pathway, would show a pattern of correlates different from CD children who do not show these traits. For example, we have found that CD children with these CU traits show a preference for thrill- and adventure-seeking activities (Frick, O'Brien, Wootton, & McBurnett, 1994) and a decreased sensitivity to punishment relative to rewards (O'Brien & Frick, 1996), both of which are consistent with the proposed temperament deficit in low fearful inhibition. In contrast, children with CD who do not show these traits have been shown to be more likely than CD children with CU traits to evidence intellectual deficits (Christian *et al.,* 1997) and to be more likely to come from homes in which parents used ineffective socialization strategies (Wootton, Frick, Shelton, & Silverthorn, 1997).

The predictive utility of this model has not yet been tested in longitudinal research. However, Christian and colleagues (1997) found that children with ODD or CD who also exhibited CU traits showed a number of markers of poor outcome, such as a greater number and variety of CD symptoms, an earlier arrest history, and a family history of APD. However, this group of children did not show low intelligence. As a result, this person-centered approach could explain the interaction between intellectual ability and a family history of APD found in previous research (Lahey *et al.,* 1995). The combination of a family history of APD and high intelligence in CD children may have designated a group with a large number of children with CU traits which contributed to the high degree of stability in this group. Clearly this model utilizing the presence of CU traits to designate a unique subgroup of chil-

dren with CD has not been adequately tested to determine its usefulness in predicting outcome. It is presented here to illustrate the *potential* utility of person-centered approaches to research, that are embedded within a clear theoretical framework, for enhancing our understanding of the differential outcomes of children with CD.

In conclusion, we have attempted to summarize an important body of research showing substantial stability in CD over both short and long periods. We have also attempted to highlight some of the inadequacies in this research to date, inadequacies that point the way to some important goals in the next generation of outcome studies. These goals focus on enhancing our understanding of the children who are at greatest risk for poor outcomes and developing a better understanding of the mechanisms involved in creating and moderating this risk. As the field attempts to develop intensive yet cost-effective prevention approaches to alter the mechanisms involved in this poor outcome (Dodge, 1993), these goals are quite important. When we identify those children at greatest risk for poor outcome, we can begin to focus the most intensive treatment on them. By developing a better understanding of the mechanisms involved in the poor outcome for many children with CD, we can begin to design treatments that specifically target changes in these mechanisms so that we can become more effective in altering the negative life-course followed by many children and adolescents with CD.

REFERENCES

Abikoff, H., & Klein, R. G. (1992). Attention-deficit hyperactivity disorder and conduct disorder: Comorbidity and implications for treatment. *Journal of Consulting and Clinical Psychology, 60,* 881–892.

American Psychiatric Association. (1980). *Diagnostic and statistical manual of mental disorders* (3rd ed.). Washington, DC: Author.

American Psychiatric Association. (1987). *Diagnostic and statistical manual of mental disorders* (3rd ed., rev.). Washington, DC: Author.

American Psychiatric Association. (1994). *Diagnostic and statistical manual of mental disorders* (4th ed.). Washington, DC: Author.

Christian, R., Frick, P. J., Hill, N., Tyler, L. A., & Frazer, D. (1997). Psychopathy and conduct problems in children: II. Subtyping children with conduct problems based on their interpersonal and affective style. *Journal of the American Academy of Child and Adolescent Psychiatry, 36,* 233–241.

Cohen, P., Cohen, J., & Brook, J. (1993). An epidemiological study of disorders in late childhood and adolescence: II. Persistence of disorders. *Journal of Child Psychology and Psychiatry, 34,* 869–877.

Colder, C. R., Lochman, J. E., & Wells, K. C. (1997). The moderating effects of children's fear and activity level on relations between parenting practices and childhood symptomology. *Journal of Abnormal Child Psychology, 25,* 251–263.

Conduct Problems Prevention Research Group. (1992). A developmental and clinical model for the prevention of conduct disorder: The FAST Track Program. *Development and Psychopathology, 4,* 509–527.

Dodge, K. A. (1993). The future of research on the treatment of conduct disorder. *Development and Psychopathology, 5,* 311–320.

Dumas, J., Neese, D., Prinz, R., & Blechman, E. (1996). Short-term stability of aggression, peer rejection, and depressive symptoms in middle childhood. *Journal of Abnormal Child Psychology, 24,* 105–119.

Elliott, D. S., Huizinga, D., & Ageton, S. S. (1985). *Explaining delinquency and drug use.* Beverly Hills, CA: Sage.

Farrington, D. P. (1991). Childhood aggression and adult violence: Early precursors and later-life outcomes. In D. J. Pepler & K. H. Rubin (Eds.), *The development and treatment of childhood aggression* (pp. 5–19). Hillsdale, NJ: Erlbaum.

Farrington, D. P., Ohlin, L., & Wilson, J. Q. (1986). *Understanding and controlling crime.* New York: Springer-Verlag.

Farrington, D. P., Gallagher, B., Morley, L., St. Ledger, R. J., & West, D. J. (1988). A 24-year follow-up of men from vulnerable backgrounds. In R. L. Jenkins & W. K. Brown (Eds.), *The abandonment of delinquent behavior: Promoting the turnaround* (pp. 155–173). New York: Praeger.

Fergusson, D. M, & Horwood, L. J. (1993). The structure, stability and correlations of the trait components of conduct disorder, attention deficit and anxiety/withdrawal reports. *Journal of Child Psychology and Psychiatry, 34,* 749–766.

Fergusson, D. M., Horwood, L. J., & Lynskey, M. T. (1995). The stability of disruptive childhood behaviors. *Journal of Abnormal Child Psychology, 23,* 379–396.

Fergusson, D. M., Lynskey, M. T., & Horwood, L. J. (1996). Factors associated with continuity and changes in disruptive behavior patterns between childhood and adolescence. *Journal of Abnormal Child Psychology, 24,* 533–553.

Frick, P. J. (1994). Family dysfunction and the disruptive behavior disorders: A review of recent empirical findings. In T. H. Ollendick & R. J. Prinz (Eds.), *Advances in clinical child psychology* (Vol. 17, pp. 203–226). New York: Plenum.

Frick, P. J. (1998). Callous-unemotional traits and conduct problems: A two-factor model of psychopathy in children. In D. J. Cooke, A. Forth, & R. D. Hare (Eds.), *Psychopathy: Theory, research, and implications for society* (pp. 161–187). Dordrecht, The Netherlands: Kluwer.

Frick, P. J., & O'Brien, B. S. (1995). Conduct disorder. In R. T. Ammerman & M. Hersen (Eds.), *Handbook of child behavior therapy in the psychiatric setting* (pp. 199–216). New York: Wiley.

Frick, P. J., O'Brien, B. S., Wootton, J. M., & McBurnett, K. (1994). Psychopathy and conduct problems in children. *Journal of Abnormal Psychology, 103,* 700–707.

Garmezy, N. (1993). Vulnerability and resilience. In D. C. Funder, R. D. Parke, C. Tomlinson-Keasey, & K. Widaman (Eds.), *Studying lives through time: Personality and development* (pp. 377–398). Washington, DC: American Psychological Association.

Gersten, J., Langner, T., Eisenberg, J., Simcha-Fagan, O., & McCarthy, E. (1976). Stability and change in types of behavioral disturbance of children and adolescents. *Journal of Abnormal Child Psychology, 4,* 111–127.

Hinshaw, S. P., Lahey, B. B., & Hart, E. L. (1993). Issues of taxonomy and co-morbidity in the development of conduct disorder. *Development and Psychopathology, 5,* 31–50.

Huesmann, L., Eron, L., Lefkowitz, M., & Walder, L. (1984). Stability of aggression over time and generations. *Developmental Psychology, 20,* 1120–1134.

Huesmann, L. R., Eron, L. D., & Yarmel, P. W. (1987). Intellectual functioning and aggression. *Journal of Personality and Social Psychology, 52,* 232–240.

Jessor, R., & Jessor, S. (1977). *Problem behavior and psychosocial development.* New York: Academic Press.

Keenan, K., Loeber, R., Zhang, Q., Stouthamer-Loeber, M., & Van Kammen, W. B. (1995). The influence of deviant peers on the development of boys' disruptive and delinquent behavior: A temporal analysis. *Development and Psychopathology, 7,* 715–726.

Klinteberg, B. A., Andersson, T., Magnusson, D., & Stattin, H. (1993). Hyperactive behavior in childhood as related to subsequent alcohol problems and violent offending: A longitudinal study of male subjects. *Personality and Individual Differences, 15,* 381–388.

Kochanska, G. (1993). Toward a synthesis of parental socialization and child temperament in early development of conscience. *Child Development, 64,* 325–347.

Kratzer, L., & Hodgins, S. (1997). Adult outcomes of child conduct problems: A cohort study. *Journal of Abnormal Child Psychology, 25,* 65–81.

Lahey, B. B., & Loeber, R. (1994). Framework for a developmental model of oppositional defiant disorder and conduct disorder. In D. K. Routh (Ed.), *Disruptive behavior disorders in childhood* (pp. 139–180). New York: Plenum.

Lahey, B. B., Applegate, B., Barkley, R. A., Garfinkel, B., McBurnett, K., Kerdyk, L., Greenhill, L., Hyne, G. W., Frick, P. J., Newcorn, J., Biederman, J., Ollendick, T., Hart, E. L., Perez, D., Waldman, I., & Shaffer, D. (1994). DSM-IV field trials for oppositional defiant disorder and conduct disorder in children and adolescents. *Journal of the American Academy of Child and Adolescent Psychiatry, 151*, 1163–1171.

Lahey, B., Loeber, R., Hart, E., Frick, P., Applegate, B., Zhang, Q., Green, S., & Russo, M. (1995). Four-year longitudinal study of conduct disorder in boys: Patterns and predictors of persistence. *Journal of Abnormal Psychology, 104*, 83–93.

Lefkowitz, M., Eron, L., Walder, L., & Huesmann, L. (1977). *Growing up to be violent: A longitudinal study of the development of aggression.* New York: Pergamon.

Lewis, D. O., Yeager, C. A., Cobham-Portorreal, C. S., Klein, N., Showalter, C., & Anthony, A. (1991). A follow-up of female delinquents: Maternal contributions to the perpetuation of deviance. *Journal of the American Academy of Child and Adolescent Psychiatry, 30*, 197–201.

Loeber, R. (1982). The stability of antisocial and delinquent child behavior: A review. *Child Development, 53*, 1431–1446.

Loeber, R. (1991). Antisocial behavior: More enduring than changeable? *Journal of the American Academy of Child and Adolescent Psychiatry, 30*, 393–397.

Loeber, R., Brinthaupt, V. P., & Green, S. M. (1990). Attention deficits, impulsivity, and hyperactivity with or without conduct problems: Relationships to delinquency and unique contextual factors. In R. J. McMahon & R. DeV. Peteres (Eds.), *Behavior disorders of adolescence: Research, intervention, and policy in clinical and school setting* (pp. 39–61). New York: Plenum.

Loeber, R., Stouthamer-Loeber, M., Van Kammen, W., & Farrington, D. (1991). Initiation, escalation and desistance in juvenile offending and their correlates. *Journal of Criminal Law and Criminology, 82*, 36–82.

Lynam, D. R. (1996). Early identification of chronic offenders: Who is the fledgling psychopath? *Psychological Bulletin, 120*, 209–234.

Magnusson, D., & Bergman, L. R. (1990). A pattern approach to the study of pathways from childhood to adulthood. In L. N. Robins & M. Rutter (Eds.), *Straight and devious pathways from childhood to adulthood* (pp. 101–115). Cambridge, England: Cambridge University Press.

McConaughy, S., Stanger, C., & Achenbach, T. (1992). Three-year course of behavioral/emotional problems in a national sample of 4- to 16- year-olds: I. Agreement among informants. *Journal of the American Academy of Child and Adolescent Psychiatry, 31*, 932–940.

McCord, J. (1979). Some child-rearing antecedents of criminal behavior in adult men. *Journal of Personality and Social Psychology, 37*, 1477–1486.

Mitchell, S., & Rosa, P. (1981). Boyhood behavior problems as precursors of criminality: A fifteen year follow-up study. *Journal of Child Psychology and Psychiatry, 22*, 19–33.

Moffitt, T. E. (1990). Juvenile delinquency and attention deficit disorder: Boys' developmental trajectories from age 3 to age 15. *Child Development, 61*, 893–910.

Moffitt, T. E. (1993a). Adolescence-limited and life-course persistent antisocial behavior: A developmental taxonomy. *Psychological Review, 100*, 674–701.

Moffitt, T. E. (1993b). The neuropsychology of conduct disorder. *Development and Psychopathology, 5*, 135–152.

Moffitt, T. E., Caspi, A., Dickson, N., Silva, P., & Stanton, W. (1996). Childhood-onset versus adolescent-onset antisocial conduct problems in males: Natural history from ages 3 to 18 years. *Development and Psychopathology, 8*, 399–424.

Moskowitz, D., Schwartzman, A., & Ledingham, J. (1985). Stability and change in aggression and withdrawal in middle childhood and early adolescence. *Journal of Abnormal Psychology, 94*, 30–41.

Nagin, D. S., Farrington, D. P., & Moffitt, T. E. (1995). Life-course trajectories of different types of offenders. *Criminology, 33*, 111–139.

Newman, J. P., & Wallace, J. F. (1993). Diverse pathways to deficient self-regulation: Implications for disinhibitory psychopathology in children. *Clinical Psychology Review, 13*, 699–720.

O'Brien, B. S., & Frick, P. J. (1996). Reward dominance: Associations with anxiety, conduct problems, and psychopathy in children. *Journal of Abnormal Child Psychology, 24*, 223–240.

Offord, D., Boyle, M., Racine, Y., Fleming, J., Cadman, D., Blum, H., Byrne, C., Links, P., Lipman, E., MacMillan, H., Grant, N., Sanford, M., Szatmari, P., Thomas, H., & Woodward, C. (1992). Outcome, prognosis, and risk in a longitudinal follow-up study. *Journal of the American Academy of Child and Adolescent Psychiatry, 31*, 916–923.

Olweus, D. (1979). Stability of aggression reaction patterns in males: A review. *Psychological Bulletin, 86*, 852–875.

Olweus, D. (1984). Stability in aggressive and withdrawn, inhibited behavior patterns. In R. Kaplan, V. Konecni, & R. Novaco (Eds.), *Aggression in children and youth* (pp. 104–137). The Hague, The Netherlands: Nijhoff.

Patterson, G. R. (1993). Orderly change in a stable world: The antisocial trait as a chimera. *Journal of Consulting and Clinical Psychology, 61*, 911–919.

Patterson, G. R., Reid, J. B., & Dishion, T. J. (1992). *Antisocial boys.* Eugene, OR: Castalia.

Richters, J. E., & Cicchetti,. D. (1993). Toward a developmental perspective on conduct disorder. *Development and Psychopathology, 5*, 1–4.

Robins, L. N. (1966). *Deviant children grown up.* Baltimore: Williams and Wilkins.

Robins, L. N., Tipp, J., & Pryzbeck, T. (1991). Antisocial personality. In L. N. Robins & D. A. Regier (Eds.), *Psychiatric disorders in America* (pp. 224–271). New York: Free Press.

Silverthorn, P., & Frick, P. J. (in press). Developmental pathways to antisocial behavior: The delayed-onset pathway in girls. *Development and Psychopathology.*

Stattin, H., & Magnusson, D. (1991). Stability and change in criminal behaviour up to age 30. *British Journal of Criminology, 31*, 327–346.

Stewart, M. A., Cummings, C., Singer, S., & deBlois, C. S. (1981). The overlap between hyperactive and unsocialized aggressive children. *Journal of Child Psychology and Psychiatry, 22,* 35–45.

Tremblay, R., Masse, B., Perron, D., Leblanc, M., Schwartzman, A., & Ledingham, J. (1992). Early disruptive behavior, poor school achievement, delinquent behavior, and delinquent personality: Longitudinal analyses. *Journal of Consulting and Clinical Psychology, 60,* 64–72.

Verhulst, F., & Van Der Ende, J. (1991). Four-year follow-up of teacher-reported problem behaviours. *Psychological Medicine, 21,* 965–977.

Verhulst, F., Koot, H., & Berden, G. (1990). Four-year follow-up of an epidemiological sample. *Journal of the American Academy of Child and Adolescent Psychiatry, 29,* 440–448.

Walker, J. L., Lahey, B. B., Hynd, G. W., & Frame, C. L. (1987). Comparison of specific patterns of antisocial behavior in children with conduct disorder with and without coexisting hyperactivity. *Journal of Consulting and Clinical Psychology, 55,* 910–913.

Wootton, J. M., Frick, P. J., Shelton, K. K., & Silverthorn, P. (1997). Ineffective parenting and childhood conduct problems: The moderating role of callous-unemotional traits. *Journal of Consulting and Clinical Psychology, 65,* 301–308.

Zoccolillo, M. (1993). Gender and the development of conduct disorder. *Development and Psychopathology, 5,* 65–78.

Zoccolillo, M., & Rogers, K. (1991). Characteristics and outcomes of hospitalized adolescent girls with Conduct Disorder. *Journal of the American Academy of Child and Adolescent Psychiatry, 30,* 97.

Zumkley, H. (1994). The stability of aggressive behavior: A meta-analysis. *German Journal of Psychology, 18,* 273–281.

25

The Prevention of Oppositional Defiant Disorder and Conduct Disorder

RICHARD E. TREMBLAY, DAVID LeMARQUAND,
and FRANK VITARO

INTRODUCTION

The aim of this chapter is to review preventive experiments for Oppositional Defiant (ODD) or Conduct (CD) Disorders and evaluate their efficacy. To our surprise, we found no preventive interventions that met our selection criteria (see later discussion) and used DSM-III-R or DSM-IV (American Psychiatric Association, 1987, 1994) categories of ODD and CD as outcomes. We thus broadened the scope and selected studies with outcome measures related to CD/ODD symptoms, including court-recorded or self-reported delinquency, self-, parent-, or teacher-rated measures of aggressive-externalizing behavior, and observer-rated measures of aversive behavior in the classroom. We generally refer to these outcomes using the term Disruptive Behavior Disorders (DBD).

Only studies employing random assignment or quasi-experimental (pre- and post measures in intervention and adequate control

RICHARD E. TREMBLAY, DAVID LeMARQUAND, and FRANK VITARO • Research Unit on Children's Psychosocial Maladjustment, University of Montreal, Montreal, Quebec, Canada H3T 1J7.

Handbook of Disruptive Behavior Disorders, edited by Quay and Hogan. Kluwer Academic/Plenum Publishers, New York, 1999.

groups) designs were included. The review was also limited to those studies using nonreferred children ages 12 and under to ensure that the interventions were preventive in nature (i.e., not studies with children referred for treatment) and that the focus was on interventions designed to alter developing DBD tendencies in childhood. The differences in behavioral characteristics between nonreferred subjects in a prevention experiment and referred subjects in a clinical experiment are often tenuous. Inclusion of studies was limited to those studies with follow-up periods of at least 1 year, congruent with the idea that effective preventive interventions have relatively long-term outcomes. We would have preferred to set the limit at 3 years of follow-up at least; however, not enough studies met that criterion. The fact that none of the studies used DSM criteria for outcome and very few studies have at least a year of follow-up after the end of the intervention tells us much concerning the state of research on the prevention of ODD and CD. Only 20 studies met our criteria and only 11 were originally designed to specifically prevent DBD (numbers 1, 2 in Figure 1; number 3 in Figure 2; numbers 11, 12, 13, 14, 15, 16, 17, 18 in Figure 3). The nine other studies were designed to foster children's development more generally and eventually assessed DBD. A visual summary of these studies is presented in Figures 1, 2, and 3, and descriptive statistics of

some of the studies' characteristics are presented in Table 1.

To obtain a uniform measure of treatment effects we calculated Hedges and Olkin's (1985)

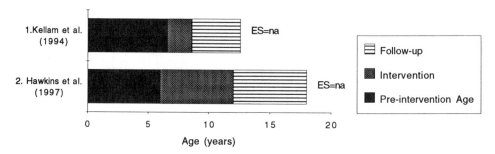

FIGURE 1. Preintervention ages, length of interventions, and length of follow-up periods for the 2 universal prevention studies for disruptive behavior. Effect size (ES) at the most recent follow-up is included: na = not available.

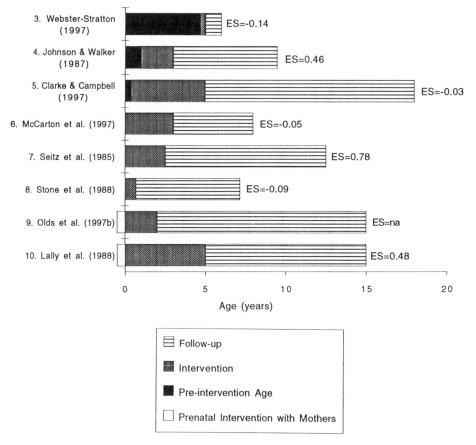

FIGURE 2. Preintervention ages, length of interventions, and length of follow-up periods for the 8 selective prevention studies for disruptive behavior included in the review. Studies are ordered by decreasing age of start of intervention. Effect size (ES) at the most recent follow-up is included: na = not available.

effect size (ES) *d* statistic. When possible the comparisons between intervention and control groups were expressed by the standard ES where the mean of the control group is subtracted from the mean of the intervention group and divided by the pooled within-group standard deviation (Hedges & Olkin, 1985). ESs were calculated so that positive scores reflected improvement in the intervention group relative to the controls. Thus, an ES of 0.50 indicates that the mean of the intervention group was one-half of one standard deviation better on the outcome measure than the mean of the control group. An effect size of 0.2 can be considered to be small, 0.5 medium, and 0.8 large (Cohen, 1977).

ESs were calculated for all disruptive behavior outcomes, then averaged to obtain an overall study ES. Disruptive behavior outcomes included (1) externalizing behavior (including mother, father, peer and/or teacher-rated disruptive behavior), (2) aversive behavior (observer-rated disruptive behavior in the classroom), and (3) delinquency (self-reported or court-recorded delinquent behavior). ESs were calculated for the most recent follow-up period. For studies that had more than one intervention group, ESs were calculated for each intervention–control group comparison separately.

Of the 20 studies, 16 provided enough information to calculate ESs. There were 29 experimental groups in the 20 studies. Seventeen

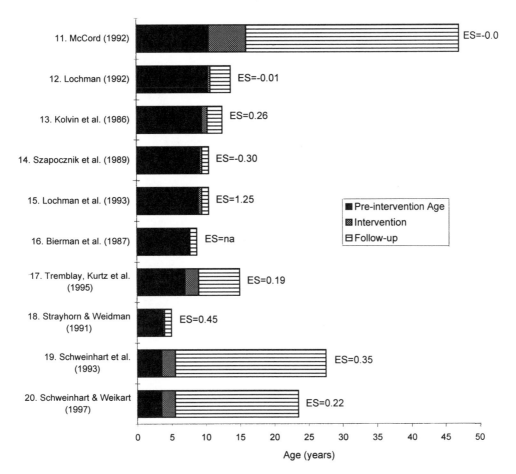

FIGURE 3. Preintervention ages, length of interventions, and length of follow-up periods for the 10 indicated prevention studies for disruptive behavior included in the review. Studies are ordered by decreasing age of start of intervention. Effect size (ES) at the most recent follow-up is included: na = not available.

TABLE 1.   Descriptive Statistics for the 20 Preventive Intervention Studies
for Disruptive Behavior Included in the Meta-Analysis

Variable	n	Mean	SD	Range
Total number of participants (preintervention)	20	314.7	274	32–985
Mean age (preintervention)	20	4.6	3.9	0–10.5
Percent male[a]	18	64.5	23.1	42.9–100
Length of intervention (months)	20	24.5	22.1	2–72
Length of follow-up (years)	20	8.1	8.0	1–31

[a]Number of males and females could not be determined in 2 studies.

studies employed random assignment to intervention and control conditions. ESs in 8 of the studies were calculated using means and *SDs*; in 6 studies ESs were estimated using *F, t,* or chi-square statistics, or proportions. In 2 studies, ESs were provided in the reports.

PREVENTION: A RAPIDLY EVOLVING PARADIGM?

In child psychopathology, "prevention" still sounds as if it were a new area of practice and research. Although in recent years much emphasis has been put on prevention, calls for a preventive approach have been made for a long time.

Plato made it clear in his *Republic* that the future of the state depended on the quality of early education. Following a conference on the care of dependent children, Theodore Roosevelt (1909) wrote to the Senate and House of Representatives: "Each of these children represents either a potential addition to the productive capacity and the enlightened citizenship of the nation, or, if allowed to suffer from neglect, a potential addition to the destructive forces of the community. The ranks of criminals and other enemies of society are recruited in an altogether undue proportion from children bereft of their natural homes and left without sufficient care" (p. 5).

Most prevention specialists have not realized that the first two monographs published by the World Health Organization after its creation in 1948 concerned children's mental health. The second monograph has been widely cited. It was written by John Bowlby (1951)

and titled *Maternal Care and Mental Health*. The first monograph has generally been forgotten, probably because its author, Lucien Bovet, died in a car accident soon after the publication of the monograph.

Bovet created the child psychiatry unit at Lausanne University in Switzerland. The World Health Organization commissioned him to write a report on the psychiatric aspects of the etiology, prevention, and treatment of juvenile delinquency (Bovet, 1951). Many of his conclusions still read as if they were an agenda for the next century. He concluded that the best approach to delinquency was a mental health campaign to prevent children's behavioral disorders. He even suggested that "[t]reatment of the non-delinquent little girl or teen-age girl might perhaps have been the most efficacious prophylaxis for the delinquency which a few years later will break out in her sons" (p. 46).

Prevention has appeared to be the logical next step for at least the past 2400 years probably because corrective interventions are simply not very effective. If treatment of DBD were effective, it would be simpler to treat those who have the disorder than to try to help all those who could have it, unless, of course, there was an easy and inexpensive way of preventing the disorder.

The developmental trajectory of CD is another reason that many people have proposed early prevention. Most students of human behavior have realized the importance of early childhood. However, the developmental paths that lead from early childhood problems to serious antisocial behavior have only started to be explored.

Our knowledge of the developmental paths to disruptive and serious antisocial behavior has been greatly advanced by longitudinal studies that have followed subjects from childhood to adolescence and adulthood (see Chapters 18 and 19, this volume). One would expect that the age at which the subjects were first assessed would reveal the investigators' best approximation concerning the age at which the building blocks of later disorder are put in place.

When reviewing longitudinal studies that were specifically designed to study the development of DBD from childhood to adolescence, one is struck by the fact that most started with subjects who were in elementary school. This appears to indicate that investigators trying to understand the development of DBD and ready to embark on a long-term enterprise believed that the origins could be found between 6 and 10 years of age. For example, after having studied the development of aggression for 30 years, Eron (1990) concluded that an aggressive tendency crystallized around 8 years of age.

Some have suggested that a limited set of underlying behavioral–psychobiological–personality dimensions underlie DBD and adult antisocial behavior (Cloninger, 1987; Eysenck & Gudjonsson, 1989; Gray, 1990; Newman, 1987; Quay, 1993). Others have proposed a cumulative effect model (Coie, Lochman, Terry, & Hyman, 1992; Yoshikawa, 1994) where individual and environmental characteristics interact and create different developmental paths (Loeber, 1991), becoming, over time, more and more difficult to deflect.

Because the origins of DBD appear during early childhood (Moffitt, 1993; Patterson, DeBaryshe, & Ramsey, 1989; Yoshikawa, 1994) and are related to the parents' own history of antisocial behavior (Lahey et al., 1988; Lahey, Russo, Walker, & Piacentini, 1989; Rowe & Farrington, 1997), the lack of repeated measurements on key variables from early in life to school entry constitutes a serious handicap to the identification of the early development of DBD. This lack also handicaps the identification of means to prevent this early deviant development.

Longitudinal studies have shown that there are long-term consequences of DBD for the disordered individual, his family, his friends, his community, and the following generation (Farrington, 1994; Huesmann, Eron, Lefkowitz, & Walder, 1984; Serbin, Peters, & Schwartzman, 1996). Investment in early preventive efforts could reduce the burden of suffering and the financial costs related to the development of DBD (Carnegie Task Force, 1994; Keating & Mustard, 1996; National Crime Prevention Council, 1996).

Finally, over the past 40 years, intervention specialists have developed an array of technologies to promote the development of behaviors and conditions incompatible with DBD. Training programs have been developed for pregnant women to foster the development of their fetus, for mothers to provide adequate care of their infants, for toddlers to enhance their cognitive development, for parents to learn disciplining skills, for kindergarten children to learn prosocial skills, and for families to solve problems. At the same time, school specialists have developed new ways of helping children who have learning problems and community specialists have developed ways to help communities help the most disadvantaged. It appears that everything is ready for making the first century of the next millennium "the prevention century."

WHAT POPULATIONS SHOULD BE THE TARGET OF PREVENTIVE INTERVENTIONS?

Offord, Chmura Kraemer, Kazdin, Jensen, and Harrington (1998) recently published an excellent summary of the advantages and disadvantages of universal versus targeted preventive strategies. Universal preventive interventions aim at all children in a geographic area or setting without any further selection criteria. Targeted preventive interventions focus on children at risk because of socio-familial and environmental factors or personal characteristics. Targeting children on the basis of socio-familial risk factors is referred to as *selective* preventive intervention; targeting children on the basis of personal risk factors is referred to as *indicated* preventive intervention (Mrazek & Haggerty, 1994). Although universal and targeted preventive interventions differ with respect to their "clientele," they share one important feature: Children who participate in either type of program are not initially referred for treatment. They are identified from the general population (after a screening process for targeted preventive programs).

Offord and colleagues (1998) concluded that the optimal preventive strategy includes successive steps. The first step is to put in place effective universal programs to promote all children's competencies. These programs should focus on the implementation of protective factors. Two recent large-scale preventive experiments are examples of a universal component in a multistep strategy. In both the multisite Fast Track Program (Conduct Problems Prevention Research Group, 1992) and the Chicago Metropolitan Area Child Study (Metropolitan Area Child Study Research Group, 1997), a curriculum was applied in all participating classrooms, irrespective of the children's characteristics.

For children with multiple (personal or socio-familial) risk factors, a second step is to implement more intensive interventions targeting the children, their families, or their community. Without such additional interventions, these children and their families would still be at risk because the universal component of the global preventive strategy is not sufficient to eliminate all the risk factors or promote sufficient protective factors.

The screening of the at-risk children who would participate in a targeted preventive intervention should be inexpensive, easy to administer, and nonstigmatizing. In addition, threshold criteria for inclusion should be low to ensure high sensitivity (i.e., all possible at-risk children, families, or communities are included), even running the risk of including cases that are not at risk. Inclusion criteria can be refined further if desired to improve specificity by eliminating false positive cases.

The multistep screening and intervention strategy is necessary to overcome the respective limitations of universal and targeted prevention strategies. However, the importance of the targeted component to prevent DBD in children must be stressed. Many if not all of the disadvantages underlined by Offord and colleagues (1998) with respect to the targeted component in a combined strategy can be overcome in the specific case of DBD.

The first obstacle is that a targeted approach might be hard to sell to the public and politicians because the actual disorder may not be impressive. Clearly, DBD have a high potential to convince everyone of the necessity to intervene early and effectively because of the costs and low effectiveness of treatment and the DBD burden on individuals and society. Epstein and colleagues (1993) estimated that the annual cost for treating an individual with serious behavioral problems in an out-of-home setting was $50,000. The predictors of DBD such as inadequate parenting or disruptiveness have already gained support as potential targets or screening criteria for preventive interventions because longitudinal studies have repeatedly shown their predictive power.

A second potential disadvantage of a targeted approach is the predictive power and costs for screening at-risk cases. For indicated prevention there are easy-to-administer, easy-to-analyze, and valid measures that can be used with caregivers to assess the child's personal risk status. As complements to behavior rating scales, there are other potentially valuable instruments but with higher costs: diagnostic interviews, sociometrics, and direct observations in natural or simulated settings (see Chapter 3, this volume).

For selective preventive interventions, broad and accessible criteria such as poverty level or rate of unemployment in a community can be used to determine the level of risk. Of course, the general and very inexpensive sources of information used for screening purposes can be crossed with other sources (e.g., school resources) to improve specificity.

The third limitation identified by Offord and colleagues (1998) refers to the stability of risk status and the difficulty of choosing an appropriate threshold. The stability issue should not represent a major obstacle for DBD since personal and socio-familial predictors of DBD are relatively stable. Globally, it has been estimated that half of the children at risk for DBD because of early behavior problems will continue to have problems during adolescence and possibly adulthood (Kazdin, Mazurick, & Bass, 1993). Tremblay, Boulerice, Pihl, Vitaro, & Zoccolillo (1996) showed that 60% of low-SES kindergarten boys who had Cloninger's (1987) antisocial personality profile according to teacher ratings had a DSM-III-R diagnosis of externalizing or internalizing disorder between 14 and 16 years of age. Disruptive youth who do not meet DSM criteria are often just below the cutoff point and at risk for other problems such as drug abuse, school dropout, early pregnancy, vocational problems, and family violence. If needed, the screening measures can be administered at two different times or include different informants to ensure temporal and situational stability.

Although relatively stable, personal and family predictive factors do not guarantee that DBD will develop because some protective factors, personal or environmental, may have been overlooked in the screening process (see Chapter 19, this volume). Some protective factors may have an impact after the screening process. Conversely, very few low-risk children (e.g., children below the median on teacher-rated disruptiveness and above median on school performance or social skills) will develop DBD (Vitaro, Tremblay, Gagnon, & Pelletier, 1994). Although some might still develop adolescence-limited CD, many will remit on their own and may need minimal intervention at some critical periods of development only.

The problem lies with the DBD children living in disorganized families or in poor neighborhoods, some of whom may develop serious CD. The adoption of rather lenient thresholds (at the first step) will maximize sensitivity even if specificity may be low. A low threshold is further supported by the possibility that preventive interventions might prove useful for children who are high but not extreme on risk factors rather than with very extreme cases. For example, high but not extreme

cases have been found to be those most at risk of being negatively influenced by deviant peers in early adolescence (Vitaro, Tremblay, Kerr, Pagani-Kurtz, & Bukowski, 1997).

The last two disadvantages raised by Offord and colleagues (1998) are not easily overcome by preventive interventions aimed at children at risk for DBD if these interventions are not embedded in a combined strategy that includes a universal component. The first of these disadvantages concerns labeling and stigmatization. One could always argue that disruptive children do not need to be targeted by a preventive intervention to be labeled by teachers and thus stigmatized by peers; that is, they are already stigmatized by their behavior. However, one way to avoid more labeling and stigmatization is to state the objectives of the preventive intervention in positive ways such as promoting social acceptance or school performance. A second strategy is to include low-risk children and their families in the prevention program. Their presence can prove beneficial to the prevention process (through, for example, modeling of appropriate behaviors). Tremblay, Kurtz, Mâsse, Vitaro, and Pihl (1995) illustrated the use of prosocial children in social skills training sessions with DBD boys.

Finally, Offord and colleagues (1998) referred to the difficulty targeted preventive interventions have in focusing on macro-social variables that might be responsible for the higher prevalence rate of DBD in one particular community. This difficulty can and should be dealt with through the universal component of the integrated global strategy; however, further research is needed on the distribution of high-risk children in high-risk areas. Although there are prevalence rate differences between communities and SES clusters, there are important prevalence rate differences within these communities and SES clusters. Tremblay, Boulerice, Harden, and colleagues (1996) have shown an SES gradient for family effects on children's physical aggression. Family effects are greater in low-SES families than in high-SES families. This suggests that community-wide interventions could be more appropriate for higher-SES communities, while targeting high-risk families would be more appropriate for lower-SES communities. It certainly suggests that community-level interventions in low-SES communities need to reach out for (target) the high-risk families.

In summary, a combination of universal and targeted strategies can prove optimal by capitalizing on the advantages and reducing the disadvantages of each strategy to an acceptable level. The reader is referred to Offord and colleagues (1998) for further advantages and disadvantages of both universal and targeted strategies.

WHEN IS THE BEST TIME TO PREVENT THE DEVELOPMENT OF DBD?

During Adolescence?

Over the past 40 years most interventions for DBD have targeted male adolescents. It is extremely difficult for any family, school, or community simply to ignore them. Consequently, families, schools, and communities have mobilized their resources to help delinquent adolescents, although the general effectiveness of the interventions is, as Lipsey (1992) concluded after a meta-analysis of 443 evaluation studies, "perilously close to zero" (p. 126).

Longitudinal studies have clearly shown that most adolescents with DBD and antisocial adults had behavior problems during childhood (Farrington, 1994; Pulkkinen & Tremblay, 1992; Robins, 1966; Tremblay, Pihl, Vitaro, & Dobkin, 1994; White, Moffitt, Earls, Robins, & Silva, 1990). Those who appear to be late starters or adolescent-onset cases (Moffitt, 1993) may be the most difficult to identify before the onset of their DBD. As their problem behavior may not persist beyond adolescence, the most economic strategy could be to give support to these individuals and their environment during their short period of disruptive activity. However, to prevent these late-onset cases, it may be useful to consider the hypothesis that DBD are unlikely to appear suddenly without any developmental antecedents. If

these late-onset cases could be identified early, one would expect that interventions before adolescence would have more of an impact than interventions just before onset.

Following this logic we decided to review only preventive interventions that targeted individuals before the start of adolescence, which we set at the end of their 13th year after birth, that is, when most children leave elementary school.

During Middle Childhood?

All but two (Strayhorn & Weidman, 1991; Webster-Stratton, 1997) of the 11 prevention experiments we selected that were clearly devised to prevent the development of DBD (nos. 1, 2 in Figure 1, no. 3 in Figure 2; nos. 11–18 in Figure 3) targeted elementary school children. This reflects the fact that the majority of longitudinal studies that attempted to understand the development of DBD started with elementary school children.

These interventions with elementary school children were considered preventive because the children were not referred for treatment. However, most of them (seven of nine; nos. 11–17 in Figure 3) targeted children who had some behavior problem. These interventions were, in fact, attempting to change the trajectory of individuals already engaged in disruptive behavior. Some cases may not have met criteria for ODD, others may have but may not have met criteria for CD, and still others may have met criteria for CD. In most cases we do not know because no DSM diagnoses were made.

There is good evidence that oppositional and physically aggressive elementary school children generally had behavior problems during the preschool years (Bates, Bayles, Bennett, Ridge, & Brown, 1991; Tremblay et al., 1995; White et al., 1990). Thus, preventive interventions during the elementary school years are generally attempts to prevent the problem from following its course to a full-blown case of CD in adolescence and adult Antisocial Personality Disorder (APD). Unfortunately, none of the prevention studies displayed in Figures 1, 2, and 3 have published follow-up assessments using DSM criteria. The long-term follow-up assessments using disruptive behavior scales show that five of the nine experiments (nos. 1, 2 in Figure 1; nos. 13, 15, 17 in Figure 3) had positive effects.

During Early Childhood?

For the purpose of our review we defined early childhood as the period from 25 months to 71 months of age. Most people are surprised, and some are outraged, when children of these ages are described as showing DBD tendencies. However, it is quite clear that the frequency of temper tantrums and physically aggressive behavior peaks around the end of the second year and the beginning of the third year (Dunn & Munn, 1985; Restoin et al., 1985; Sand, 1966; Tremblay, Boulerice, Harden, et al., 1996). It is between 18 and 30 months of age that a human is most at risk of physically aggressing or being aggressed by a peer. Every mother of a toddler understands very well the meaning of the expression "the terrible twos." At 27 months of age close to 50% of mothers from a random sample of Canadian mothers reported that their son sometimes hits, bites, or kicks other children (Tremblay, Boulerice, Harden, et al., 1996). For girls the figure was close to 40%. However, for both boys and girls, the percentage had dropped to nearly 25% by 39 months and 10% by 11 years of age.

As they grow older most children learn that physical aggression is not acceptable. Unfortunately, some do not learn. Cummings, Iannotti, and Zahn-Waxler (1989) showed that the correlation between frequency of observed aggression in a play situation with a friend at 2 and 5 years of age was .75. Although a large proportion of 2-year-olds and a much smaller proportion of 5-year-olds use physical aggression, this correlation indicates that those who use physical aggression often at age 2 are more likely to use physical aggression most often at age 5. They are also likely to follow the DBD trajectory.

Longitudinal studies have shown that we can identify these children with reasonable accuracy. They have a characteristic behavior pro-

file, and their environments also have particular characteristics (Henry, Moffitt, Robins, Earls, & Silva, 1993; Raine, Brennan, Mednick, & Mednick, 1996; Stattin & Klackenberg-Larsson, 1990; Tremblay et al., 1994; White et al., 1990). By targeting 2-year-olds, preventive interventions are close to the beginning of the DBD path, at least with regard to physical aggression. If the intervention starts at age 5, then a number of the children will be firmly caught in their DBD groove.

Only four of the prevention studies that met our criteria aimed at children between 2 and 5 years of age, and only two were specifically planned to prevent the development of DBD (Strayhorn & Weidman, 1991; Webster-Stratton, 1997). The High/Scope Perry Preschool Study (Schweinhart, Barnes, & Weikart, 1993) and the High/Scope Preschool Curriculum Study (Schweinhart & Weikart, 1997) were both *indicated studies* designed to help prepare low-SES children at risk of school failure because of their cognitive performance. These two studies did show important long-term (18 and 22 years) positive effects on DBD. The indicated study by Strayhorn and Weidman (1991) implemented a parent–child interaction training program in Pittsburgh with low-income parents who reported behavioral or emotional problems in their preschool children. Results from a short-term follow-up (1 year) also showed important positive effects on DBD. However, no significant effects were observed after a 1-year follow-up of the Seattle *selective study* (Webster-Stratton, 1997) aimed at preventing DBD in children of Head Start centers with a parent- and teacher-training program.

The two High/Scope indicated studies' aim was to foster the development of intellectual abilities by providing a high-quality preschool education for 3- and 4-year-old low-IQ children from poor families (see Berrueta-Clement, Schweinhart, Barnett, Epstein, & Weikart, 1984). Because the positive effects on DBD were observed only when self-reported and official delinquency data was obtained after the subjects were 14 years of age (Schweinhart et al., 1993), it is impossible to compare the developmental paths of DBD from the start of the intervention to midadolescence. Did the differences in DBD start early when the prevention subjects were making gains in intellectual abilities, or did they start during adolescence when the intervention subjects were staying in school while the control subjects were dropping out? Only a similar intervention with repeated measures of DBD and school achievement from preschool to high school will answer this important question. From this perspective it is difficult to decide whether the 1-year follow-up nonsignificant results of the Seattle selective study (Webster-Stratton, 1997) are an indication that it was ineffective for DBD, or that it is much too early to observe its effectiveness on DBD. The Pittsburgh indicated study (Strayhorn & Weidman, 1991) suggests that important short-term effects are possible, although it remains to be seen if they translate into long-term effects.

We are fortunate that the participants in the two High/Scope prevention studies were followed for such a long period. Most preventive interventions have relatively short follow-ups. Of the nine elementary school intervention experiments aiming to prevent DBD, only four had follow-ups of 4 years or more.

During Pregnancy and Infancy?

Preventive interventions with pregnant women and infants generally aim at fostering the physical, cognitive, and emotional development of the babies. Some of these experiments, that is, those with relatively long-term follow-ups, eventually assessed the children's behavior problems. These studies give an indication of the effectiveness of very early interventions to prevent DBD.

However, we did not find any that at the onset clearly targeted the prevention of DBD. This could be explained by the fact that few granting agencies would be willing to invest in a prevention experiment that would show results only 15 years later. But this logic does not recognize the fact that chronic disruptive behavior often starts in the first 700 days after birth (Bates et al., 1991; Cummings et al.,

1989; Dunn & Munn, 1985; Tremblay, Boulerice, Harden, et al., 1996; Yoshikawa, 1994; see also Chapter 18, this volume). Interventions with pregnant women and infants would be ideal to test the possibility of influencing early control over physical aggression, and its impact on the path toward chronic DBD.

The seven experiments that met our selection criteria were selective interventions. Five targeted low-SES teen mothers and their infants. The two other experiments targeted low-SES families with an infant. Only two studies included prenatal programs (Lally, Mangione, & Honig, 1988; Olds et al., 1997b). The length of the follow-up for each of the five studies varied from 5 to 15 years. However, the attrition rate was often high and two studies did not have random assignment.

Five of the seven studies showed some long-term (3 to 15 years) effectiveness for the prevention of DBD. The Abecedarian project showed long-term positive impacts on cognitive development (Campbell & Ramey, 1995) but not on offending in late adolescence and early adulthood (Clarke & Campbell, 1997). The Mailman Center program for low-SES adolescent mothers reported higher developmental scores for the children of the intervention group at 3 years of age, 2 years after the end of the intervention. However, when the children were between age 5 and 8 years, the assessments did not show any positive impact on a wide range of outcomes, including mother ratings of behavior problems. The Infant Health Program for low-birth-weight premature infants reported significant positive effects on mother-rated behavior problems at 3 years of age, at the end of the intervention (Infant Health and Development Program, 1990), but no positive effects on DBD were observed at the age 8 follow-up (McCarton et al., 1997).

Second Thoughts about Adolescence

We began this section by explaining that we had chosen to review preventive studies with children before age 13 because by adolescence it was generally too late to prevent the development of chronic disruptive behavior.

In the preceding subsection we described studies targeting mothers and their infants. It is important to realize that babies born to adolescent mothers with a history of behavior problems are at very high risk for many developmental problems (Serbin *et al.*, 1996). Adolescent mothers with behavior problems not only give inadequate care to their fetus and infant, they also tend to mate with males who have a history of behavior problems (Castaignede & Tremblay, 1984; Rowe & Farrington, 1997).

If adolescence is late for preventing chronic DBD for a given individual, it may not be too late to prevent the development of chronic DBD in the next generation. Many preventive interventions rely on the training of parents to forestall the development of DBD in their children. Many of these parents are adolescents or young adults with a history of DBD. Training them to be adequate parents is in fact training them to be less impulsive, less aggressive, more caring, and thus more prosocial.

If interventions do not generally work with DBD adolescents, why would they work with DBD teen parents or young adults? One reason it may be more effective to intervene when the individual has become a parent is that having a baby may for some, because of biological, psychological, and social factors, create a sensitive period that favors change (Pryce, Martin, & Skuse, 1995). It has been clear for some time that children do elicit caring behaviors from adults (Bell & Harper, 1977), and the biological mechanisms underlying this phenomenon are becoming clearer (Carter, Lederhendler, & Kirkpatrick, 1997). Having a baby also changes the way an individual perceives his role in society and the way others perceive the new parent (Musick, 1993).

As Bovet (1951) suggested, the ideal is, of course, to prevent young girls from developing behavior problems. If such a strategy were to be implemented, the risk of adolescent pregnancy would be reduced, the risk of substance use and abuse during pregnancy would be reduced, the risk of inadequate care of infants would be reduced, and even the risk of mating with a DBD male and becoming a single mother would be reduced (Castaignede & Tremblay, 1984; Robins, 1986; Schweinhart *et al.*, 1993; Tremblay, 1991). Unfortunately, society is more afraid of aggressive juvenile males than of maladjusted females at risk of being inadequate mothers. This is clear from the male–female ratio in the ten experiments specifically designed to prevent DBD. None targeted only girls, five targeted only males, and five targeted approximately an equal number of males and females.

The price we pay in terms of social, human, and monetary capital for focusing on male DBD to the exclusion of females may be very high. Let us imagine that by increasing the resources invested in the prevention of male DBD we would completely eliminate the DBD (genetics notwithstanding) in the present generation of adolescent males. What effect would this extraordinary feat have on the next generation of males if we had not managed to help the maladjusted females? Now imagine the reverse. From the intergenerational perspective, our stubborn concentration on antisocial males does appear short-sighted. If the child is the father to man, the female child is his mother.

WHO SHOULD BE THE FOCUS OF THE INTERVENTION AND WHICH TYPE OF INTERVENTION SHOULD BE USED?

As illustrated in the preceding section, the targets of preventive interventions are potentially almost unlimited. Some have argued that changing children's diet will have a significant impact on their behavior problems (Prinz, 1985), others have focused on the effects of television (Huesmann, Eron, Klein, Brio, & Fisher, 1983), many have targeted parenting abilities or children's social or academic skills, and others argue that eliminating environmental pollutants (Fergusson, Horwood, & Lynskey, 1997; Reiss & Roth, 1993) or community disorganization (Sampson, 1995) reduces the risk of DBD. Many believe that the target should be the most likely causal factors, some argue for protective factors, and still others underscore the fact that past risk and protective factors cannot be changed (Farrington, 1992; Mrazek & Haggerty, 1994; Rob-ins, 1992).

The field of preventive interventions has progressed over the past few decades from experiments that target one factor to experiments with multiple targets. We first review the prevention studies by discussing one target at a time. Table 2 presents the 20 studies we selected classified by targets and type of interventions. When it was not possible to use one of the 20 studies we selected to illustrate an important type of intervention, we referred to the best studies we could find. At the end of this section we discuss the experiments that had many targets.

The At-Risk Child as Target

If a child is at risk for developing one of the DBD, it makes intuitive sense to target him for help. Most of the 20 studies we reviewed included the child as a specific target. From Table 2 it can be seen that six studies for infants provided quality day care, seven studies with elementary school children targeted either social skills (five) and/or social-cognitive skills (three), three studies with preschool children and two with elementary school children targeted the child's academic skills, and two other studies offered psychodynamic psychotherapy.

Day Care

The cognitive, affective, and social development of children born to parents who have difficulties providing adequate parental care during early childhood can easily be compromised and quickly lead to serious DBD. Quality day care centers have been created to foster the development of these children.

The Syracuse University Family Development Research Program (Lally et al., 1988) is a good example of a major preventive effort that included quality day care from 6 to 60 months of age. The program targeted poor pregnant adolescent girls who had not completed high school. The day care center had been developed in the 1960s by Betty Caldwell in an effort to apply the latest child development knowledge to early childhood education. The staff was trained to stimulate active child and parent participation based on Piaget's work (1960), while giving responsive loving attention. Language skills acquisition was a key component of the program, and attempts were made to tailor the activities to the level of each child. The environment was based on the British Infant School philosophy, giving children freedom of choice to four areas in the day care center.

The five other selective prevention programs that targeted families of at-risk infants also included some form of day care intervention. The Mailman Center program (Stone, Bendell, & Field, 1988) offered a nursery program, the Yale Child Welfare program (Seitz, Rosenbaum, & Apfel, 1985) offered day care between birth and 30 months of age, and the Houston Parent–Child program (Johnson & Walker, 1987) offered day care when the children were 2 years of age. The Abecedarian Project (Clarke & Campbell, 1997) offered day care between birth and 5 years of age and the Infant Health and Development Program (McCarton et al., 1997) provided day care from ages 1 to 3.

The impact of day care without any other form of intervention is not known because each of the six experiments included other forms of intervention, such as parent training and medical services. To the extent that cognitive development, emotional regulation, and peer interaction underlie the development of DBD, one would expect that quality day care programs would be an essential component of preventive efforts with at-risk infants and toddlers. Long-term (5–10 years) positive results were observed for three of the most intensive programs. The teacher assessments of externalizing problems 5 to 8 years after the end of the 2-year Houston Parent–Child Development Center Project (Johnson & Walker, 1987) indicated a substantial positive impact (ES = .46). The official delinquency data collected 10 years after the end of the 5-year Syracuse University Family Development Program (Lally et al., 1988) also indicated a significant impact (ES = .48). A large ES (.78) was obtained with the teacher-assessed externalizing behavior of subjects 10 years after the end of the 2.5-year Yale Child Welfare Project (Seitz et al., 1985). No significant effect (ES =

TABLE 2.   Summary of the Types of Interventions Found in the 20 Preventive Intervention Studies for Disruptive Behavior

Type of intervention	Number of studies	Studies included	Age of participants
Day care	6	4. Johnson & Walker (1987); Houston Parent–Child Development Center Project (N = 139; I = 51, C = 88)	1
		5. Clarke & Campbell (1997); Abecedarian Project (N = 105; I = 54, C = 51)	birth
		6. McCarton et al. (1997); Infant Health and Development Program (N = 874; I = 336, C = 538)	birth
		7. Seitz et al. (1985); Yale Child Welfare Research Project (N = 36; I = 18, C = 18)	birth
		8. Stone et al. (1988); Mailman Center program (N = 61; I = 31, C = 30)	birth
		10. Lally et al. (1988); Syracuse University Family Development Research Program (N = 119; I = 65, C = 54)	pregnancy
Social skills training	5	1. Kellam et al. (1994) (N = 590)	6
		13. Kolvin et al. (1986) (N = 592)	Juniors 7–8; seniors 11–12
		15. Lochman et al. (1993) (N = 44)	9
		16. Bierman et al. (1987) (N = 29)	7 y, 7 m
		17. Tremblay, Kurtz, et al. (1995); Montréal Longitudinal Experimental Study (N = 124; I = 31, C = 93)	7
Social-cognitive skills training	3	2. Hawkins et al. (1997) (N = 598; I = 392, C = 206)	6
	1	2. Lochman (1992) (N = 145)	9–12
		15. Lochman et al. (1993)	9
Academic skills training	5	1. Kellam et al. (1994); Mastery Learning Program	6
		2. Hawkins et al. (1997)	6
		5. Clarke & Campbell (1997)	birth
		19. Schweinhart et al. (1993); High/Scope Perry Preschool Study (N = 123; I = 58, C = 65)	3–4
		20. Schweinhart & Weikart (1997); High/Scope Preschool Curriculum Study (N = 68; I = 22, C = 46)	3–4
Psychodynamic therapy	2	13. Kolvin et al. (1986) (N = 592)	Juniors 7–8; seniors 11–12
		14. Szapocznik et al. (1989) (N = 58; I = 44, C = 14)	9 y, 2 m
Parenting skills training	13	2. Hawkins et al. (1997)	6
		3. Webster-Stratton (1997) (N = 280; I = 173, C = 107)	5
		4. Johnson & Walker (1987); Houston Parent–Child Development Center Project	1
		6. McCarton et al. (1997); Infant Health and Development Program	birth
		7. Seitz et al. (1985); Yale Child Welfare Research Project	birth
		8. Stone et al. (1988); Mailman Center program	birth
		9. Olds et al. (1997b); Elmira Home Visitation Study (N = 400)	pregnancy
		10. Lally et al. (1988); Syracuse University Family Development Research Program	pregnancy
		13. Kolvin et al. (1986)	Juniors 7–8; seniors 11–12
		17. Tremblay, Kurtz, et al. (1995); Montréal Longitudinal Experimental Study	7
		18. Strayhorn & Weidman (1991) (N = 84; I = 45, C = 39)	4
		19. Schweinhart et al. (1993); High/Scope Perry Preschool Study	3–4

(continued)

TABLE 2.   *(Continued)*

Type of intervention	Number of studies	Studies included	Age of participants
Parenting skills training (continued)		20. Schweinhart & Weikart (1997); High/Scope Preschool Curriculum Study	3–4
Family therapy	1	14. Szapocznik *et al.* (1989) (*N* = 58; I = 44, C = 14)	9 y, 2 m
Peer training	1	17. Tremblay, Kurtz, *et al.* (1995); Montréal Longitudinal-Experimental Study	7
Teacher training	4	1. Kellam *et al.* (1994); Good Behavior Game	6
		2. Hawkins *et al.* (1997)	6
		3. Webster-Stratton (1997)	5
		13. Kolvin *et al.* (1986); Behavior Modification Nurture Work groups	Juniors 7–8; seniors 11–12
Social work	1	11. McCord (1992); Cambridge–Somerville Youth Study (*N* = 506; I = 253, C = 253)	10.5
School	0	None	—
Community	0	None	—

Note. Sample and group sizes are those at most recent follow-up. (*N* = total sample size; I = intervention; C = control)

−.09) was observed for mother-rated externalizing problems 5 to 8 years after the end of the less intensive (8 months) Mailman Center program for adolescent mothers (Stone *et al.*, 1988). Large effects on cognitive development were observed for the intensive Abecedarian Project (Campbell & Ramey, 1995) but the program did not have an impact on official criminality (Clarke & Campbell, 1997). The intensive Infant Health and Development Program did not show a significant impact at age 8 on mother-rated child externalizing behavior (McCarton *et al.*, 1997).

The outcomes of these six programs are difficult to compare because the assessments are from different sources of information (mothers, teachers, and official files), at different ages (6 to 18 years), and with different length of follow-up (5 to 13 years). On the whole, there is evidence for a positive impact in preventing DBD. It would be useful to have comparable assessments of disruptive behavior for all who have now reached adulthood.

Social Skills Training

Many disruptive children clearly lack social skills (see Chapter 20, this volume). Not only do they show physical and verbal aggres-

sion but they also show fewer prosocial behaviors than other children. In return, they are deprived of positive feedback from their environment, resulting in a weak bond with caregivers and conventional peers. Moreover, they become entangled in coercive and punitive exchanges with them.

The program implemented by Bierman, Miller, and Stabb (1987) with 32 rejected boys in grades 1 to 3 is a classic example of social skills training experiments. The boys were randomly allocated to four treatment conditions. The first condition attempted to promote three types of positive social behavior: questioning and inviting others, sharing and taking turns, and helping and cooperating in play. The second condition involved adult prohibitions to reduce the following behaviors when playing with peers: fighting, arguing, yelling, being mean, whining, and having bad temper. The third condition combined the first two and the fourth involved no treatment. The program in the first three conditions had 10 half-hour school play sessions. The combination of prohibitions and social skills training resulted in fewer sociometric negative nominations from training partners compared to prohibitions alone or social skills training alone. In the classroom, however, no effects were obtained at posttest or at 6-week or 1-year follow-ups.

The Bierman and colleagues (1987) study is a good example of experiments that have helped develop prevention programs but cannot be expected to show long-term impacts because of the lack of intensity of the program. The four other studies with social skills training (Kellam, Rebok, Lalongo, & Mayer, 1994; Kolvin *et al.,* 1986; Lochman, Coie, Underwood, & Terry, 1993; Tremblay, Kurtz, *et al.,* 1995) had other components and were more intensive. These four studies reported significant positive effects on antisocial behavior from 1 to 6 years after the intervention. The ES could be calculated for only two of these studies. In the Lochman and colleagues (1993) study, at 1-year follow-up, teacher-rated aggression was significantly lower in treated aggressive-rejected children relative to aggressive-rejected controls (ES = 1.25). In the Tremblay, Kurtz, and colleagues (1995) study, comparing self-reported delinquency for treated and untreated disruptive kindergarten boys across the 6 years after the end of the intervention led to an ES of 0.19.

Social-Cognitive Skills Training

Social-cognitive processes such as negative perceptions, attributions, and expectations have been linked to antisocial behavior (see Chapter 14, this volume). Social-cognitive skills training involves different procedures that attempt to change thought processes in situations that can lead to disruptive behavior. One of them, inspired by Shure and Spivak (1982), has been used by Tremblay and colleagues (Tremblay, Kurtz, *et al.,* 1995; Tremblay, Mâsse, Pagani, & Vitaro, 1996) and Vitaro and Tremblay (1994) as part of their intervention program. It consisted of training children in step-by-step fashion in a problem-solving process starting with problem clarification and ending with enactment and reinforcement of the desired solution. This training was conducted in a small-group format that involved prosocial peers. The components of problem solving were anchored to real-life situations involving conflict or frustra-

tion. Coupled with parent training, this study showed long-term prevention effects (see no. 17 in Figure 3).

Another version of problem-solving skills training is focused on emotional aspects and involves anger-management skills. A good illustration is Lochman's (1992) study of an anger-coping training program with 83 fourth- to sixth-grade aggressive-disruptive boys who were randomly allocated to a treatment (*n* = 31) or control (*n* = 52) group. Weekly group sessions over a period of 4 to 5 months included training in use of self-statements to inhibit impulsive behavior, training in generating alternative solutions in social situations, learning to link physiological arousal to anger, and learning to use problem-solving skills when angry. After 3 years, treated boys had higher levels of self-esteem and social problem-solving skills, and lower rates of drug and alcohol involvement. No significant effect was observed for classroom disruptive-aggressive behavior and self-reported delinquency.

Despite their promising features, social-cognitive skills training programs have not yielded generalized behavioral improvements unless used in combination with other procedures (Durlak, Fubrman, & Lampman, 1991; Mathur & Rutherford, 1996). Moreover, these interventions were intended to improve peer relations (i.e., improve children's social acceptance or foster establishment of friendships) which, in turn, might improve children's social behavior, but this impact on peer relations rarely has been attained even though children's behavior might have improved (see Chapter 20, this volume).

Academic Skills

Although school failure can contribute to the development of antisocial behavior (Maguin & Loeber, 1995), there is good evidence that behavior problems of most children with chronic DBD started before they entered elementary school (Moffitt, 1993; Stattin & Klackenberg-Larsson, 1990; Tremblay *et al.,* 1994; see also Chapter 16, this volume). Hence, it is likely that low school performance and DBD are correlated often because both are related to pre-school individual characteristics, such as in-attention, impulsivity, and disruptiveness.

Should prevention of disruptive behavior target these problems at the expense of cognitive deficits and school achievement? Probably not. First, there is good evidence that DBD are linked to cognitive deficits which could be malleable, especially during early childhood (Moffitt, 1993; Séguin, Pihl, Harden, Tremblay, & Boulerice, 1995; see Chapter 14, this volume). Second, school success could prevent the development of antisocial behavior for the late-onset cases.

The best example of an effective early intervention targeting school success is the Perry Preschool Project (Schweinhart et al., 1993). Three- and four-year-old children from poor families who had a low IQ were randomly allocated to a treatment and a control condition. The preschool program was aimed at stimulating cognitive development by active learning based on Piaget's (1960) work. The children attended the program for $2\frac{1}{2}$ hr on weekday mornings and teachers visited the mother and child for $1\frac{1}{2}$ hr a week in the afternoon. The program lasted 30 weeks a year over a 2-year period for those who entered at 3 years of age. The long-term follow-up (22 years) showed that the treatment group scored higher on IQ tests up to age 7, performed better in high school, and were less involved in delinquent behavior up to age 27. The ES for officially recorded lifetime arrests 22 years after the end of the intervention was 0.54. In a sister study, the High/Scope Preschool Curriculum Study, Schweinhart and Weikart (1997) replicated the Perry Preschool study results with a follow-up of children up to 23 years of age. The ES was 0.21 for officially recorded delinquency when comparing the High Scope curriculum to the two other curricula.

It is tempting to conclude from these studies that the treatment effects on delinquent behavior were mediated by the early effects on cognitive abilities and school performance. However, when Farnworth, Schweinhart, and Berrueta-Clement (1985) attempted to test this hypothesis with the Perry Preschool data they concluded that the effects on delinquency could not be explained by the effects on IQ or school achievement. Preschool interventions aimed at cognitive performance will probably need to monitor the development of cognitive and behavioral characteristics to understand how a preschool curriculum has a long-term impact on delinquency.

Good examples of later interventions to prevent DBD through school achievement can be found in two universal programs implemented with elementary school children. Hawkins, Catalano, Kosterman, Abbott, and Hill (1997) and Kellam and Rebok (1992) attempted to increase children's school performance to prevent disruptive behavior. Kellam and Rebok implemented a Mastery Learning program to increase first graders' mastery of reading. The follow-up assessment 1 year later (Dolan et al., 1993) indicated that the treatment group, especially the male low achievers, performed better than the control group on reading achievement. However, no impact on aggressive behavior could be shown.

In the Seattle Social Development Project (Hawkins et al., 1992; Hawkins et al., 1997), Hawkins and collaborators trained teachers in proactive classroom management methods, interactive teaching, and cooperative learning (i.e., teaching social and problem-solving skills to children, focusing on individual learning of academic objectives, monitoring children's learning process and sustaining it by rewards and incentives). They also trained parents in behavior management skills. This combination of procedures was applied over a 6-year period and produced proximal positive effects on self-reported delinquency, alcohol use, and attachment to school in comparison to control students. Results after a 6-year follow-up revealed positive effects on self-reported and officially recorded delinquency outcomes for students in the intervention group (Hawkins et al., 1997).

Individual and Group Psychotherapy

There is a long tradition of using psychodynamic therapy principles to help disruptive children, but few experimental preventive interventions. We found two experiments that met our criteria.

The Newcastle-upon-Tyne study (Kolvin et al., 1986) included group psychotherapy as one component of a preventive intervention with at-risk elementary school children. (The parent training is described in the next section.) With the youngest age cohort (7–8 years old), they implemented a playgroup procedure in which groups of four to five boys and girls met with a social worker for 10 sessions over a school term. The social worker was trained to establish a warm and friendly relationship, to accept the child as he is, to develop a feeling of permissiveness in the relationship, to be alert to the children's expression of feelings, and to not direct the children's actions but to set a minimum number of limits to help impulsive children.

With the oldest age group (11–12 years old), four to five same-sex children participated in 10 discussion sessions that focused on "here-and-now" interactions in the group. The social worker was trained not to direct the discussion. Follow-up assessments 1 and 2.5 years after the end of the interventions showed that both the younger and older treated groups were significantly less disruptive than the control groups according to parents' and teachers' ratings (ES = 0.26).

Szapocznik and colleagues (1989) used an individual psychodynamic therapy program as a comparative treatment in an experiment in family therapy described later in this chapter. Subjects were males, ages 6–12, a proportion of whom had DBD (e.g., 16% conduct disorders, 32% oppositional disorders) and were seen individually in a playroom. The approach focused on expression of feelings, limit setting, transference, and insight. At the end of the 6-months treatment (mean of 17.7 contact hours) and at the 1-year follow-up, treated boys had not made more progress than the controls on parent ratings of disruptive behaviors.

The Parents as Target

Parenting skills have repeatedly been associated with children's disruptive behavior (see Chapters 6 and 15, this volume), hence their inclusion in preventive efforts. But parents can be targets even before the child's birth. Women at risk of substance abuse during pregnancy can be the target of interventions to prevent negative effects on the child's brain development. Mothers and fathers at risk of abusing or neglecting their children can receive support and training during pregnancy.

Of the 20 studies reviewed, 13 targeted parents (see Table 2); 2 targeted pregnant women, 4 targeted parents of infants, 4 targeted parents of preschool children, and 3 targeted parents of elementary school children.

Interventions with Expecting Parents

There is a strong case for interventions with expectant parents. First, it is becoming clearer that brain development during the fetal period has lifelong consequences; it can be altered by chemical agents (such as alcohol, nicotine, and drugs), by mothers' behavior and health, and by environmental effects on the mother (Carnegie Task Force, 1994; Coe, in press; Cynader & Frost, in press). The first trimester appears to be a key developmental phase (Barker, 1992); unfortunately, some women have not yet realized that they are pregnant, and preventive interventions usually start during the second or third trimester.

Parents with a history of adjustment problems are most likely to maintain risky behaviors during pregnancy. From this perspective, a number of preventive interventions have targeted pregnant adolescents. These experiments can often be considered interventions with disruptive adolescents in an effort to prevent the intergenerational reproduction of DBD. However, most of the participants from these intervention studies have not been followed long enough to document their impact on the development of disruptive behavior for both the mother and the child.

The Elmira Home Visitation study (Olds et al., 1997b) is a fortunate exception. Participants were mostly low-income, unmarried, pregnant adolescents. Other pregnant women were included in the study to prevent stigmatization. Three experimental groups were created by random allocation. Women in the first group were visited weekly by a nurse for the first month after enrollment in the study, twice a month until birth, weekly for the first 6 weeks after birth, twice a month until the baby reached 21 months, and monthly until the child reached the end of the second year. Women in the second group received home visits only during pregnancy; women in the third group had a screening interview after birth and free transportation to the health clinic between the child's birth and the end of the second year. Mothers and children have been followed up to the child's 15th birthday. Fewer mothers in the first group were identified as perpetrators of child abuse and neglect. On a number of outcome measures, significant differences between the first group and controls were observed only when the comparison was limited to those women who were unmarried and had low incomes at initial enrollment. These mothers had fewer subsequent births, longer intervals between the birth of the first and second child, fewer substance abuse impairments, fewer self-report and officially recorded arrests, and were less often on Aid to Families with Dependent Children (AFDC) (Olds *et al.*, 1997a). Follow-up results on delinquency measures for the children in this study appear positive (Olds *et al.*, 1997b).

Interventions with Parents of Infants

Although interventions starting before birth are possibly preferable to ones starting after birth, one would expect that interventions with parents of infants would have a significant impact on their parenting skills, and thus on the socialization of their children (Patterson *et al.*, 1989; Shaw & Bell, 1993). It is of interest to note that all four experimental interventions that started with parents of infants also included some form of day care.

The Mailman Center program (Stone *et al.*, 1988) provides a good comparison to the Elmira Home Visitation study (Olds *et al.*, 1997a) just described. Both studies targeted poor adolescent mothers and both offered home visitation. The Elmira program, which was

shown to be most effective, offered home visitation from pregnancy to the child's second year of life. The Mailman study randomly allocated the adolescent mothers to a program that offered 6 months of home visitation starting at birth and a second concurrent program that added 6 months of work as teachers' aides in their infants' nursery program. At age 2, children from the second group had higher developmental scores and their mothers had a higher rate of return to work or school and fewer pregnancies, when compared to the first group and to a no-intervention control group (Field, Widmayer, Stringer, & Ignatoff, 1980; Field, Widmayer, Greenberg, & Stoller, 1982). However, at a later follow-up, when the children were between 5 and 8 years of age, no significant differences were observed between the groups for academic, behavioral, and socio-emotional assessments. Although the investigators assessed only half the families, no significant differences were found between the original sample and those followed up.

The authors concluded that low SES of the mothers may override the early positive effects of the intervention. From the perspective of the Elmira study (Olds *et al.*, 1997a, 1997b) which also targeted low-SES adolescent mothers, the lack of long-term effects could be due to the relatively late onset of the intervention (birth), and its short duration. This conclusion can also be reached by comparing the results of the Mailman study to the long-term effectiveness of the Syracuse University Family Development Research Program (Lally *et al.*, 1988), which was described earlier in the day care section. Again, both studies targeted low-SES pregnant adolescents and started after birth, but the Syracuse intervention lasted 5 years compared to 1 year for the Mailman study.

Interventions with Parents of Preschool Children

The High/Scope Perry Preschool and High/Scope Preschool Curriculum studies described earlier included components that targeted parents' abilities to support their preschool children's learning activities. Parenting interventions were also the focus of the Syracuse University program (Lally *et al.,* 1988) when the children were in their preschool years. More recently, Webster-Stratton (1997) administered a parent training program targeting risk factors for disruptive behavior. Head Start centers (8, with a total of 64 classes) were randomly assigned to experimental (296 children) and control conditions (130 children). The 8- to 9-week program focused on teaching effective parenting skills, positive discipline strategies, and ways to strengthen children's social skills and prosocial behaviors to parents of the 4-year-olds attending the Head Start centers. Groups of parents (8–16) met weekly for 2 hr with a trained family service worker and a professional to view videotapes of modeled parenting skills and discuss parent–child interaction. Posttest and 1-year follow-up assessments of parental competencies (mother reports and home observations) showed significant differences between the experimental and control condition parents.

However, at 1-year follow-up there was no clear evidence that the intervention had a significant effect on the children's DBD, although the posttest assessment had shown significant differences between the experimental and control groups on home observations of deviant and noncompliant behavior. It can only be hoped that the effects on parenting behavior will, in the long run, translate into effects on the children's behavior. Yet long-term positive effects of 16–18 hr of intervention with parents of 4-year-old children may be too much to hope for. On the other hand, similarly to the Elmira study (Olds *et al.,* 1997a), this intervention may have a positive impact only on the higher-risk families. This possibility was not investigated in the publication available.

Interventions with Parents of Elementary School Children

Three experiments with elementary school children included programs for parents. The Newcastle-upon-Tyne project (Kolvin *et al.,* 1986) included, among its different experiments, a parent counseling–teacher consultation program for one group of 7- to 8-year-olds and one group of 11- to 12-year-olds. Social workers were given the task of consulting with teachers to assist in planning individualized curricula, discuss the home environment of the child, and promote links between home and school. They also visited parents to help them understand how family factors influenced the child's school performance. Families were visited up to 10 times, most receiving four to six visits. Assessments 2 years after the intervention indicated no significant effects of the program on disruptive behavior for either age cohort.

The Seattle Social Development Project (Hawkins *et al.,* 1992; Hawkins *et al.,* 1997), described earlier, offered on a voluntary basis two parent-training components (in conjunction with teacher training). The first was a seven-session curriculum on monitoring, teaching expectations for behavior, and positive reinforcement that was offered to parents when their children were in first and second grade. The second was a four-session curriculum on how to help children succeed in school, offered to parents during the spring of the second grade and during the third grade. Unfortunately, only 43% of the parents attended at least one of the parenting classes. This is an important and frequent problem with parent training for children at risk of DBD. Many of the parents have a history of problem behaviors and will not easily and regularly come to group meetings at school. In most cases individual attention is needed, preferably through visits in their homes.

The Montréal Longitudinal-Experimental Study (Tremblay *et al.,* 1992; Tremblay, Kurtz, *et al.,* 1995) offered a parent-training program to the parents of a random sample of boys who had been rated as disruptive during their kindergarten year in schools in low-SES areas. The parent-training component was based on one developed by the Oregon Social Learning Center (Patterson, Reid, Jones, & Conger, 1975). However, instead of asking the parents to come to the school or to a clinic, professionals went to their homes approximately once every 3 weeks over a 2-year period. The mean number of visits was 17.4 including families that dropped out during the course of the experiment. Because a social skills program was also offered to the children at school, this study could not assess the specific effects of the parent-training program. However, the combined programs showed significant positive effects on self-reported delinquent behavior up to 6 years after the end of the intervention (ES = 0.24).

Interventions with Future Parents

Ideally, preventive interventions with parents of at-risk children should start long before they become parents. Because parents of children with DBD themselves often have a history of disruptive and antisocial behavior (Huesmann et al., 1984; Lahey et al., 1989; Rowe & Farrington, 1997) one would expect that, if successful, interventions with disruptive children in one generation would be a preventive intervention for the children of the next generation. Classrooms and neighborhoods are more disrupted by deviant males than deviant females but it is deviant females who become the pregnant adolescents abusing alcohol, drugs, and cigarettes and who lack the skills to give adequate care during the first few months after birth when the brain is more receptive to environmental influences (Cynader & Frost, in press; Serbin, Peters, McAffer, & Schwartzman, 1991; Serbin et al., 1996). We did not find one study that has assessed the disruptive behavior of the children of boys and girls who were in an intervention experiment. Most interventions that have shown long-term effects could do these assessments. The experiments that included both males and females would be especially useful in comparing the long-term benefits (for the next generation) targeting males as compared to females (in the previous generation).

The Family as Target

We considered that the family was the target if all members of a given family were involved. Family therapy has been used extensively for the treatment of different types of adult and childhood disorders (Hazelrigg, Cooper, & Borduin, 1987; Szapocznik et al.,

1989) but preventive interventions using the family therapy approach are much less common.

We did find a randomized experiment with boys recruited for behavior problems that compared the effectiveness of family therapy to psychodynamic child therapy and a recreational control condition. Through a media campaign and school counselors, Szapocznik and colleagues (1989) recruited Hispanic families who had lived in the United States for at least 3 years and had a 6- to 12-year-old son with behavior problems. The family therapy condition involved weekly sessions of up to 90 min with all the family members to modify maladaptive patterns of interaction between family members. A mean of 19.1 hr of treatment was given to these families over a 6-month period. The duration of treatment was similar in the two other conditions. Assessments of the boys' behavior problems were obtained from mothers prior to the start of the intervention, at the end of the intervention, and at 1-year follow-up. At the posttest assessment the family therapy group showed significant improvement on parent-rated externalizing behavior, compared to the two other conditions. However, the difference had disappeared by the 1-year follow-up assessment.

The Teachers as Target

The section on targeting academic skills clearly indicates that teachers should be targets or allies in preventive interventions. Teachers are "natural" allies to implement preventive interventions aimed at reducing DBD in their classroom or on the playground (see Chapter 20, this volume).

Among these prevention studies, there are several examples of inclusion of teacher-training components. Webster-Stratton (1997) provided a 2-day teacher-training workshop as a complement to the parent-training program for Head Start children described earlier. Teachers were shown the same videotapes as the parents. The training also stressed the importance of parent–teacher collaboration. The Good Behavior Game used by Kellam and colleagues (1994) with first-grade children illustrates the use of behavior management strategies that teachers can implement in the classroom. Essentially, individual and group reinforcement was provided by the teacher contingent on children's behavior in the classroom. Positive effects on boys with high baseline aggression were reported at the end of first grade and at a 6-year follow-up. Other roles for teachers such as instructors of social or problem-solving skills or as technologists of teaching and learning strategies have been exemplified in the Seattle preventive experiment (Hawkins *et al.*, 1997).

The Peer Group as Target

Peers represent an important target and possible source of change because of their influence which increases from childhood to adolescence as parental influence decreases (Furman & Robbins, 1985). Despite the potential of peers for prevention purposes (Coie & Jacobs, 1993), only one of the preventive interventions we reviewed used peers as targets. Tremblay and colleagues (Tremblay, Mâsse, *et al.*, 1995; Tremblay, Mâsse, *et al.*, 1996) included prosocial peers in their social and social-problem–solving skills training sessions in order to capitalize on a positive modeling effect and facilitate therapists' work in implementing reinforcement contingencies for appropriate behavior. The presence of prosocial peers also avoided the exclusive focus on disruptive children and possible risks for labeling and stigmatization. Finally, the presence of prosocial peers may have fostered the social acceptance of target children in their classroom (Vitaro & Tremblay, 1994).

Peers can also serve as models, reinforcement agents, or conflict mediators. For example, tutoring between same-age or cross-age children for social skills has proven beneficial for increasing these skills in children with behavior problems and improving their social interactions with classmates (Kohler & Greenwood, 1990). Older peers can also be used as mediators trained to help children solve conflicts in natural settings not easily accessible to adults (Powell, Muir-McClain, & Halasysmani, 1995). Finally, peers may empower children who are victimized by others and reduce bullying inside and outside the schools (Olweus, 1991). The results of these promising strategies have been assessed on short-term outcomes only, precluding their inclusion in our selection for this review.

The Community as Target

The observation made in 1942 by Shaw and McKay that delinquency and neighborhood disorganization in Chicago was linked, had also been made half a century earlier for London by Charles Booth (1891). The social-ecological approach to child development and disruptive behavior (Bronfenbrenner, 1979; Sampson, 1995) has developed a strong theoretical framework on a century of observations that there is more deviant behavior and more deviant development in low-SES areas (see also Chapter 19, this volume). However, we have not found experiments that have assessed the effects of the physical rehabilitation of slums on the development of DBD in children living in these areas. Neither did we find experiments that assessed the effects of stimulating community organization on the development of DBD. Most community interventions assess the impact of the intervention on community-level indicators rather than on individual development. Thus, changes in community-level statistics in delinquent behavior can be observed without actual changes in the individuals who were living in these communities. The observed changes in the community can be due to the fact that the delinquent individuals moved to another community or are committing their antisocial acts in the neighboring communities.

Targeting specific communities with high rates of crime is certainly a strategy, but there are important limits to taking only a "changing the place" strategy. The main message is that communities create criminals. Longitudinal studies have repeatedly shown that chronic offenders have a childhood history of disruptive behavior. It is difficult to understand how high-crime areas could have a direct effect on infants and toddlers, except through the fact that they attract or keep a large proportion of high-risk families. It is also clear that, except for prisons, there must be a very small number of communities on this planet where a majority of its inhabitants are criminals. There is evidence that the SES gradient in antisocial behavior is explained by the differences in family effects within SES classes; that is, the lower the SES of the family the higher the family concentration of antisocial behavior (Tremblay, Boulerice, Harden, *et al.,* 1996). This suggests that interventions that target high-risk (low-SES) areas must also target families in these areas. If high-risk areas are targeted without reaching out for high-risk families, there is a strong likelihood that the people who will most benefit from the neighborhood changes are those who are not antisocial nor at risk of becoming antisocial; those who need to change their behavior will not be touched by the intervention, because they do not come forward or they simply move (or are chased) to another community where there is less social pressure to conform.

Jones and Offord (1989) reported on a prevention experiment in a low-rent housing complex in Ottawa where changing people's behavior appeared to change places. A recreational program was offered to all the 5- to 15-year-olds ($N = 417$) in one of the city's low-rent housing complexes intended for low-income families. A second, similar complex, was used as a control site. This study was not included in the group of 20 studies we selected, mainly because outcome assessment was limited to community-level statistics which cannot indicate to what extent the intervention had an impact on individual DBD. The study did not randomize subjects or communities to the treatment and control conditions and the community-level information did not enable us to focus on the effects for the age span we selected (0–12 years).

The experimental program offered an opportunity to participate in scouting, orienting, and cooperative games that would increase subjects' recreational skills. One of the objectives was to help the children from the housing complex join the recreational activities of the surrounding community. Another objective was to reduce disruptive behavior. Nonparticipant children were "systematically and aggressively"

pursued to integrate them into the program. The experiment lasted 3 years.

In the first year 70.8% of eligible children participated in at least one course. Over the next 2 years the participation rate fell off to 60.2% and 49.0%, apparently because fewer courses were offered to reduce costs. However, even with an aggressive outreach approach in an attractive recreational community project, 30% of the targeted population did not participate. One would expect that these would include a large proportion of the most at-risk individuals.

The assessment of effects on delinquent and disruptive behavior was made by comparing the experimental and control housing complexes for the number of reports from the security officers in the housing complex, and police charges against people living in the housing complexes for three time periods: 6–12 months before the program, the 32 months during the program, and the 16 months after the program. Both security reports and police charges involving juveniles were significantly reduced from before to during the experiment for the experimental complex compared to the control complex.

However, the significant differences disappeared during the 16 months that followed the end of the intervention. This study indicates that targeting individuals (children) in a specific environment and "aggressively" reaching for them can have a beneficial impact on the security of the environment as long as the program is in place. The environment will revert to its original condition if the program is dropped before there is a permanent change in the participants.

It is likely that the temporary reduction in police charges and security reports were due to an effect on the activities of the older age group of youths (11–15 years) rather than on the younger age group (5–10 years). It makes sense to target the adolescents if the aim is a quick reduction of delinquent activities. However, to obtain a more permanent effect it may be necessary to target the younger children (birth to 10 years) so that the intervention will show long-term effects on their socialization through school achievement and integration in the broader community. It should be easier to help children to integrate into the broader community if the effort is made when they enter kindergarten (or even earlier), rather than attempting to integrate adolescents who may have been rejected since kindergarten.

The Better Beginnings, Better Futures Project (Peters & Russell, 1996) is an example of an ongoing community experiment targeting children from birth to 8 years of age. Eleven low-SES neighborhoods in Ontario were selected to prevent the development of serious emotional, behavioral, physical, and cognitive problems in young children. Each community is implementing over a 4-year period some of the following strategies: home visiting, enrichment of child care facilities, family and parent programs, classroom enrichment, and community programs. An evaluation team will follow the children until they are 20 years of age.

Multimodal Interventions

The first waves of experimental interventions with disruptive children tended to include only one mode of intervention. These experiments were useful to create and test the implementation of new types of interventions. The most recent waves of interventions tend to be multimodal. The majority of the 20 experiments we selected were at least bimodal. One of the best examples of the new generation of multimodal prevention experiments for conduct problems is the Fast Track Program (Conduct Problems Prevention Research Group, 1992). The aim of the program is to promote the competencies of children at risk for conduct disorder in four geographical areas of the United States. Kindergarten children identified by parents and teachers as having behavior problems were included in the prevention group or a control group based on random allocation of the schools they attended in first grade. The 6-year intervention involves seven components: parent training, home visiting, parent–child relationship enhancement, academic tutoring, social-cognitive skills training, emotional regulation skills training, and inter-

personal skills training. The content of these components for first and second grade can be found in Bierman, Greenberg, and Conduct Problems Research Group (1996) and McMahon, Slough, and Conduct Problems Research Group (1996). Although the long-term impact of this comprehensive intervention will not be known much before the end of the first decade of the next millennium, the continuous monitoring of the experimental and control subjects will provide some indication of its short-term and medium-term effectiveness.

If chronic disruptive behavior is already well established by 3 years of age, an intervention starting in first grade can be considered relatively late in the developmental process. However, there will always be disruptive kindergarten children who should be helped to prevent the development of CD. It is important to know how much effort is needed to achieve this goal. The Fast Track Program is possibly the maximum a society will be willing to pay to help these children. The strategy of identifying at-risk children in kindergarten is economical and may capitalize on the parents' hope that school will help their disruptive child. This was the logic used in the early 1980s to plan the Montreal Longitudinal-Experimental Study with disruptive kindergarten children (Tremblay, Kurtz, et al., 1995; Tremblay, Mâsse, et al., 1996). Although the intervention was less comprehensive and lasted only 2 years, the results appeared to be relatively long lasting. A more comprehensive and longer-lasting intervention should have a greater impact.

CONCLUSION

General Comments

When we started this review we identified more than 50 prevention experiments that could possibly be included. As we read through these studies we realized that many were treatment studies of referred children with ODD and CD, many had only a posttest, and very few had at least a 1-year follow-up. We were faced with the decision to use relaxed or stringent criteria. We were tempted to use relaxed criteria because we wanted to do a meta-analysis and thus needed a relatively large number of studies to be able to compare, for example, the effectiveness of preventive experiments with infants to those with preschoolers. Had we made this choice, we would have come to the conclusion that there is a relatively large body of prevention experiments which can guide theorists, practitioners, and policy makers. We did not make this choice because as we read through the studies we thought that the large majority of them were weak in either design, implementation, or outcome assessment. We cannot believe that a serious policy maker or developmental psychopathology theorist will be impressed by statistically significant or not significant differences at posttest (or even after a 10-month follow-up) on mother ratings between treatment and control groups totaling less than 100 subjects. We are not even certain that they should be impressed by studies that conform to the more stringent criteria we used. We now think that by using 12-month of follow-up as a lower limit we were using a relaxed criterion.

Having been involved in preventive experiments as well as treatment and longitudinal studies over the past three decades, we know that prevention experiments are extremely difficult to do, and more difficult and less rewarding for a research or clinical career than longitudinal or treatment studies. This is certainly one of the major reasons we found only 20 studies that met our criteria. However, we also know that the small-scale studies with only a posttest or a short-term follow-up are extremely useful to create and test new types of interventions. Thus, our conclusion is not that these studies should not be done or should not be published. However, we believe that when we want to assess the effectiveness of preventive interventions to decide which approach should be taken to reduce the prevalence of ODD and CD in a community or to decide whether more resources should be allocated to preventive rather than treatment efforts, we should take into account only well-designed and well-implemented studies with relatively long follow-ups. Preventive and treatment programs are expected to have relatively

long-term effects. Those with an impact that does not last may be useful for chronic cases if they can be maintained as long as the individual or the family is in need. These programs could be named "prosthesis interventions" for which some individuals and families may be in need for most of their lives. They should not be confounded with preventive or treatment interventions which implemented at a given point in time are expected to change the developmental course of an individual.

ODD and CD, with their links to school failure, delinquency, substance abuse, unemployment, and child neglect and abuse are among the most debilitating and socially disruptive disorders we encounter. It is difficult to understand and difficult to accept that there are only 20 prevention experiments meeting our criteria. Considering that Bovet's report to the World Health Organization in the late 1940s contained most of the present insights on the importance of early prevention of DBD, the slow progress of our experimental efforts since then is somewhat depressing.

Among the 20 studies we retained, only 11 were originally designed to specifically prevent disruptive behavior, and none used DSM diagnoses in the outcome assessment. Of the 10 studies designed to prevent disruptive behavior, half offered programs that lasted no more than 6 months. None of the studies used the same outcome criteria at the same time in the developmental course. All of these 10 studies were single-site studies designed and implemented by small teams of researchers. In fact, the 10 studies appear to be relatively unrelated and they exist almost by chance. Clearly, there has not been a concerted effort to match the magnitude of the challenge offered by the disruptive disorders.

A new generation of preventive studies has been started since the early 1990s. These studies are on a larger scale with reference to the number of subjects, the intensity of the intervention, the size of the research teams, and the size of the budgets. However, there are very few of these studies and they will come to maturity (if they do!) only in a decade or two. Can we accelerate and intensify the process?

We identified six preventive experiments with pregnant women or infants that were not specifically designed to prevent disruptive behavior but did provide interesting data because the participants' disruptive behavior was eventually assessed during childhood or adolescence. The subjects from these studies are now adults. It would be extremely useful to do a comprehensive assessment of the mental and physical health of these subjects, a retrospective assessment of their social adjustment (e.g., school performance, employment history, marital history), a prospective assessment of their parenting behaviors, and a prospective assessment of their children's development. If early interventions do have a long-term preventive impact because they initiate a positive cumulative effect trajectory and prevent a negative cumulative effect trajectory, these effects should be observed during adulthood for the participants who benefited from these intensive early preventive interventions. A large number of these interventions were implemented during the 1970s and the 1980s (see Tremblay & Craig, 1995). We did not review them in this chapter because they did not assess antisocial behavior. However, follow-ups could be done with comprehensive assessments of their psychosocial adjustment. Such studies would be less expensive than starting new early interventions. They would also relatively quickly make an extremely important contribution to a field of knowledge that is seriously in need of high-quality preventive experiments.

We offer the following comments as a set of issues we think must be taken in account when planning preventive experiments.

Design Issues

It is important that preventive interventions for ODD and CD be hypothesis-driven. Preventive interventions designed specifically to alter maladaptive processes uncovered by basic research have the potential to support a causal relationship between that process and the maladaptive outcome (Schwartz, Flamant, & Lellouch, 1980). In addition to choosing these hypothetical mediating variables as the foci of intervention, it is important to measure these mediating variables as well as outcomes of interest (e.g., CD) Assessment of mediating variables has the potential to demonstrate that (1) differences exist in these variables between CD and non CD individuals before intervention, and (2) improvements in outcome are correlated with changes in the mediating variables. This type of study design will provide supportive evidence for an etiological model of Conduct Disorder. Examples of this type of hypothesis-driven prevention research exist (Conduct Problems Prevention Research Group, 1992; Tremblay, Kurtz, et al., 1995).

It is also important that analyses be included to investigate the moderating effects of contextual variables on proximal outcomes at postintervention and distal outcome measures at follow-up. Using regression analyses and other related statistical procedures, subject characteristics and environmental variables present at the time of the intervention that predict positive long-term outcomes can be determined, thus providing additional information pertinent for the planning of future intervention outcomes. To this end, a focus on documenting study participant characteristics is needed. In particular, baseline sample characteristics such as the quality, quantity, and severity of conduct problems, frequency of co-occurring characteristics or disorders (e.g., Attention-Deficit/Hyperactivity Disorder), ethnic makeup, age, gender ratio, IQ, SES, marital status of parents, and family constellation need to be documented. These variables can be used to identify those individuals who may be more amenable to the effects of a particular preventive intervention.

In addition to investigating the moderating effects of contextual variables, it is also important to measure variables that affect the delivery of the intervention. Variables such as the degree to which an intervention was implemented can be correlated with outcome measures. Positive correlations would provide evidence that the intervention had a positive impact on the outcome measure.

An important issue in the design of preventive interventions is the need for random assignment to intervention and control conditions so that group differences can be attributed to the intervention and not to third variables. In lieu of (or in addition to) random assignment, preintervention measures identical to postintervention measures need to be included so that differences between treated and control samples can be controlled statistically (although this is not always possible if treatment duration is long). Some studies have employed random assignment with pretest measures to ensure that intervention and control groups are similar along a number of dimensions after randomization (Szapocznik *et al.*, 1989; Tremblay, Kurtz, *et al.*, 1995). It is expected that follow-up measures will differ from those at preintervention as the study participants pass into subsequent developmental periods.

Implementation Issues

Intervening in multiple contexts may be more effective than in single contexts. Intervening at home and in school, with the child, the parent or parents, and the teacher addresses the child's behavior problems in multiple settings, increasing the likelihood of generalization of intervention effects. Intervention duration may be important as well. Shorter interventions are less likely to be as effective as longer interventions.

Issues from the treatment outcome literature also are pertinent for preventive intervention research. The use of intervention manuals ensures that the intervention is delivered to the recipient as conceptualized, and that intervention fidelity is maintained across participants and over time. Intervention manuals facilitate the replication of effective intervention components in future trials. Also, random assignment of caseworkers to study groups is important to consider in the implementation of preventive interventions. This procedure ensures that the effects of the intervention compared to the control group are not due to specific caseworker variables but to the intervention itself. A still more sophisticated design will include the measurement of caseworker characteristics to ascertain which variables are associated with positive and negative outcomes.

Minimally, it is important that some measure of program integrity and completeness be included. For example, in a parent-skills–training program, investigators might assess the degree to which parents learned the skills and the degree to which they then implemented those skills when interacting with the focal child. Assessment of these variables allows a researcher to estimate the degree to which the intervention was actually implemented.

Outcome Issues

Outcome measures should encompass multiple perspectives. Combinations of teacher, parent and self-ratings of externalizing behavior, observer ratings of aversive behavior in multiple contexts (laboratory, home, and classroom), and self-ratings and official records of delinquent behavior should be included. This is particularly true when the intervention targets multiple contexts, to determine whether intervention in a particular context leads to change in that context or across contexts as well. Even when the intervention is implemented in a relatively specific context, it is important to assess other contexts to note any generalization of change. It is also important to assess related areas of adjustment (e.g., drug and alcohol abuse, hyperactivity and inattention, self-esteem) to note possible collateral effects of the intervention.

Methodologically, it is important at postintervention and follow-up assessments to show the equivalence of study participants who were assessed versus those who terminate, particularly in situations of differential mortality of participants across intervention and control groups. These statistical comparisons will increase confidence that beneficial intervention effects are in fact due to the intervention and not the differential loss of participants across groups.

Prevention trials should include follow-up periods that are long enough to determine the full effects of the intervention on CD symptoms. For preventive intervention studies commencing in early childhood, this will mean follow-up periods of at least two decades, with repeated measures to catch the developmental trajectories. This type of research puts intense demands on monetary resources; however, compared to longitudinal studies without interventions, the potential benefits outweigh the costs. Well-designed preventive intervention trials can alleviate the distress of the participant and those in his or her social sphere, decrease the costs of that individual for society, and provide important experimental information concerning the basic mechanisms contributing to the development of conduct-disordered behavior. This review has shown that there are very few preventive studies that have provided long-term information of their impact on ODD and CD.

ACKNOWLEDGMENTS. The authors wish to thank Anne Hogan and Herbert Quay for their extremely useful editorial work, and J. McCord, P. S. Klebanov, and J. Brooks-Gunn for contributing data toward the calculation of effect sizes. We also wish to thank D. Olds, J. D. Hawkins, D. Johnson, F. Campbell, and C. Webster-Stratton for providing preprints of their papers, and V. Seitz and G. Wasserman for their assistance in locating additional preventive intervention studies. This work was supported financially by the Molson Foundation, the Canadian Institute of Advanced Research, the Quebec FCAR fund, and the Social Sciences and Humanities Research Council of Canada.

REFERENCES

American Psychiatric Association. (1987). *Diagnostic and statistical manual of mental disorders* (3rd ed., rev.). Washington, DC: Author.

American Psychiatric Association. (1994). *Diagnostic and statistical manual of mental disorders* (4th ed.). Washington, DC: Author.

Barker, D. J. P. (1992). *Fetal and infant origins of adult disease.* London: British Medical Association.

Bates, J. E., Bayles, K., Bennett, D. S., Ridge, B., & Brown, M. M. (1991). Origins of externalizing behavior problems at eight years of age. In D. J. Pepler & K. H. Rubin (Eds.), *The development and treatment of childhood aggression* (pp. 93–120). Hillsdale, NJ: Erlbaum.

Bell, R. Q., & Harper, R. V. (1977). *Child effects on adults.* Hillsdale, NJ: Erlbaum.

Berrueta-Clement, J. R., Schweinhart, L. J., Barnett, W. S., Epstein, A. S., & Weikart, D. P. (1984). *Changed lives: The effects of the Perry Preschool Program on youths through age 19.* Ypsilanti, MI: High Scope.

Bierman, K., Miller, C., & Stabb, S. D. (1987). Improving the social behavior and peer acceptance of rejected boys: Effects of social skill training with instructions and prohibitions. *Journal of Consulting and Clinical Psychology, 55,* 194–200.

Bierman, K. L., Greenberg, M. T., & Conduct Problems Research Group. (1996). Social skills training in the Fast Track Program. In R. DeV. Peters & R. J. McMahon (Eds.), *Preventing childhood disorders, substance abuse, and delinquency* (pp. 65–89). Thousand Oaks, CA: Sage.

Booth, C. (Ed.). (1891). *Labour and life of the people.* London: Williams and Norgate.

Bovet, L. (1951). *Psychiatric aspects of juvenile delinquency.* Geneva, Switzerland: World Health Organization.

Bowlby, J. (1951). *Maternal care and mental health.* Geneva, Switzerland: World Health Organization.

Bronfenbrenner, U. (1979). *The ecology of human development.* Cambridge, MA: Harvard University Press.

Campbell, F. A., & Ramey, C. T. (1995). Cognitive and school outcomes for high-risk African-American students at middle adolescence: Positive effects of early intervention. *American Educational Research Journal, 32,* 743–772.

Carnegie Task Force. (1994). *Starting points: Meeting the needs of our youngest children.* New York: Carnegie Corporation of New York.

Carter, C. S., Lederhendler, I. I., & Kirkpatrick, B. (Eds.). (1997). *The integrative neurobiology of affiliation* (Annals of the New York Academy of Sciences, Vol. 807). New York: New York Academy of Sciences.

Castaignede, J., & Tremblay, R. E. (1984). Investissement parental et transmission de l'inadaptation sociale chez l'humain. In A. De Haro & X. Espalader (Eds.), *Processus d'acquisition précoce. Les communications* (pp. 65–69). Rennes, France: Société Française pour l'Etrude du Comportement Animal.

Clarke, S. H., & Campbell, F. A. (1997, April). *The Abecedarian Project and youth crime.* Paper presented at the biennial meeting of the Society for Research in Child Development, Washington, DC.

Cloninger, C. R. (1987). A systematic method for clinical description and classification of personality variants: A proposal. *Archives of General Psychiatry, 44,* 573–588.

Coe, C. (in press). Psyphoneuroimmunological reactions to stress. In D. Keating & C. Hertzman (Eds.) and the CIAR Human Development Program, *Developmental health: The wealth of nations in the information age.* New York: Guilford.

Cohen, J. (1977). *Statistical power analysis for the behavior sciences.* (Rev. ed.). New York: Academic Press.

Coie, J. D., & Jacobs, M. R. (1993). The role of social context in the prevention of conduct disorder. *Development and Psychopathology, 5,* 263–275.

Coie, J. D., Lochman, J. E., Terry, R., & Hyman, C. (1992). Predicting early adolescent disorder from childhood aggression and peer rejection. *Journal of Consulting and Clinical Psychology, 60,* 783–792.

Conduct Problems Prevention Research Group. (1992). A developmental and clinical model for the prevention of conduct disorder: The FAST Track Program. *Development and Psychopathology, 4,* 509–527.

Cummings, E. M., Iannotti, R. J., & Zahn-Waxler, C. (1989). Aggression between peers in early childhood: Individual continuity and developmental change. *Child Development, 60,* 887–895.

Cynader, M., & Frost, B. (in press). Mechanisms of brain development: Neuronal sculpting by the physical and social environment. In D. Keating & C Hertzman (Eds.) and the CIAR Human Development Program, *Developmental health: The wealth of nations in the information age.* New York: Guilford.

Dolan, L. J., Kellam, S. G., Brown, C. H., Werthamer-Larsson, L., Rebok, G. W., Mayer, L. S., Laudoff, J., Turkkan, J., Ford, C., & Wheeler, L. (1993). The short-term impact of two classroom based preventive interventions on aggressive and shy behaviors and poor achievement. *Journal of Applied Developmental Psychology, 14,* 317–345.

Dunn, J., & Munn, P. (1985). Becoming a family member: Family conflict and the development of social understanding in the second year. *Child Development, 56,* 480–492.

Durlak, J. A., Fuhrman, T., & Lampman, C. (1991). *Effectiveness of cognitive behavior therapy for maladapting children: A meta-analysis.* Unpublished manuscript, Loyola University, Chicago.

Epstein, M., Nelson, M., Polsgrove, L., Countinko, M, Cumblad, C., & Quinn, K. (1993). A comprehensive community-based approach to serving students with emotional and behavioral disorders. *Journal of Emotional and Behavioral Disorders, 1,* 127–133.

Eron, L. D. (1990). Understanding aggression. *Bulletin of the International Society for Research on Aggression, 12,* 5–9.

Eysenck, H. J., & Gudjonsson, G. H. (1989). *The causes and cures of criminality.* New York: Plenum.

Farnworth, M., Schweinhart, L. J., & Berrueta-Clement, J. R. (1985). Preschool intervention, school success and delinquency in a high-risk sample of youth. *American Educational Research Journal, 22,* 445–464.

Farrington, D. P. (1992). The need for longitudinal experimental research on offending and antisocial behavior. In J. McCord & R. E. Tremblay (Eds.), *Preventing antisocial behavior: Interventions from birth through adolescence* (pp. 353–376). New York: Guilford.

Farrington, D. P. (1994). Childhood, adolescent, and adult features of violent males. In L. R. Huesmann (Ed.), *Aggressive behavior: Current perspectives* (pp. 215–240). New York: Plenum.

Fergusson, D. M., Horwood, L. J., & Lynskey, M. T. (1997). Early dentine lead levels and educational outcomes at 18 years. *Journal of Child Psychology and Psychiatry, 38,* 471–478.

Field, T. M., Widmayer, S. M., Stringer, S., & Ignatoff, E. (1980). Teenage, lower-class, black mothers and their preterm infants: An intervention and developmental follow-up. *Child Development, 51,* 426–436.

Field, T., Widmayer, S., Greenberg, R., & Stoller, S. (1982). Effects of parent training on teenage mothers and their infants. *Pediatrics, 69,* 703–704.

Furman, W., & Robbins, P. (1985). What's the point? Issues in the selection in treatment objectives. In B. H. Schneider, K. H. Rubin, & J. E. Ledingham (Eds.), *Children's peer relations: Issues in assessment and intervention* (pp. 41–56). New York: Springer-Verlag.

Gray, J. A. (1990). Brain systems that mediate both emotion and cognition. *Cognition and Emotion, 4,* 269–288.

Hawkins, J. D., Catalano, R. F., Morrison, D. M., O'Donnell, J., Abbott, R. D., & Day, L. E. (1992). The Seattle social development project: Effects of the first four years on protective factors and problem behaviors. In J. McCord & R. E. Tremblay (Eds.), *Preventing antisocial behavior: Intervention from birth through adolescence* (pp. 162–195). New York: Guilford.

Hawkins, J. D., Catalano, R. F., Kosterman, R., Abbott, R. D., & Hill, K. G. (1997). *A twelve year study of academic success, violence, alcohol misuse, and teen pregnancy.* Manuscript submitted for publication.

Hazelrigg, M. D., Cooper, H. M., & Borduin, C. M. (1987). Evaluating the effectiveness of family therapies: An integrative review and analysis. *Psychological Bulletin, 101,* 428–442.

Hedges, L. V., & Olkin, I. (1985). *Statistical methods for meta-analysis.* New York: Academic Press.

Henry, B., Moffitt, T., Robins, L., Earls, F., & Silva, P. (1993). Early family predictors of child and adolescent antisocial behavior: Who are the mothers of delinquents? *Criminal Behaviour and Mental Health, 3,* 97–100.

Huesmann, L. R., Eron, L. D., Klein, R., Brio, D., & Fisher, P. (1983). Mitigating the imitation of aggressive behaviors by changing children's attitudes about media violence. *Journal of Personality and Social Psychology, 44,* 899–910.

Huesmann, L. R., Eron, L. D., Lefkowitz, M. M., & Walder, L. O. (1984). Stability of aggression over time and generations. *Developmental Psychology, 20,* 1120–1134.

Infant Health and Development Program. (1990). Enhancing the outcomes of low-birth weight, premature infants: A multisite, randomized trial. *Journal of the American Medical Association, 263,* 3035–3042.

Johnson, D. L., & Walker, T. (1987). Primary prevention of behavior problems in Mexican-American children. *American Journal of Community Psychology, 15,* 375–385.

Jones, M. B., & Offord, D. R. (1989). Reduction of antisocial behavior in poor children by nonschool skill-development. *Journal of Child Psychology and Psychiatry, 30,* 737–750.

Kazdin, A. E., Mazurick, J. L., & Bass, D. (1993). Risk for attrition in treatment of antisocial children and families. *Journal of Clinical Child Psychology, 22,* 2–16.

Keating, D., & Mustard, F. (1996). The National Longitudinal Survey of Children and Youth: An essential element for building a learning society in Canada. In Human Resources Development Canada & Statistics Canada (Ed.), *Growing up in Canada* (pp. 7–13). Ottawa, Ontario: Statistics Canada.

Kellam, S. G., & Rebok, G. W. (1992). Building developmental and etiological theory through epidemiologically based preventive intervention trials. In J. McCord & R. E. Tremblay (Eds.), *Preventing antisocial behavior: Interventions from birth to adolescence* (pp. 162–195). New York: Guilford.

Kellam, S. G., Rebok, G. W., Ialongo, N., & Mayer, L. S. (1994). The course and malleability of aggressive behavior from early first grade into middle school: Results of a developmental epidemiologically-based preventive trial. *Journal of Child Psychology and Psychiatry, 35,* 259–281.

Kohler, F. W., & Greenwood, C. R. (1990). Effects of collateral peer supportive behaviors within the classwide peer tutoring program. *Journal of Applied Behavior Analysis, 23,* 307–322.

Kolvin, I., Garside, R. F., Nicol, A. R., MacMillen, A., Wolstenhome, F., & Leitch, I. M. (1986). *Help starts here.* New York: Tavistock.

Lahey, B. B., Hartdagen, S. E., Frick, P. J., McBurnett, K., Connor, R., & Hynd, G. W. (1988). Conduct disorder: Parsing the confounded relation to parental divorce and antisocial personality. *Journal of Abnormal Psychology, 97,* 334–337.

Lahey, B. B., Russo, M. F., Walker, J. L., & Piacentini, J. C. (1989). Personality characteristics of the mothers of children with disruptive behavior disorders. *Journal of Consulting and Clinical Psychology, 57,* 512–515.

Lally, J. R., Mangione, P. L., & Honig, A. S. (1988). The Syracuse University Family Development Research Program: Long-range impact of an early intervention with low-income children and their families. In D. R. Powell (Ed.), *Advances in applied developmental psychology: Parent education as early childhood intervention: Emerging directions in theory, research, and practice* (Vol. 3, pp. 79–104). Norwood, NJ: Ablex.

Lipsey, M. W. (1992). Juvenile delinquency treatment: A meta-analytic inquiry into the variability of effects. In T. D. Cook, H. Cooper, D. S. Cordray, H. Hartman, L. V. Hedges, R. J. Light, T. A. Louis, & F. Mosteller (Eds.), *Meta-analysis for explanation* (pp. 83–127). New York: Russell Sage Foundation.

Lochman, J. E. (1992). Cognitive-behavioral intervention with aggressive boys: Three-year follow-up and preventive effects. *Journal of Consulting and Clinical Psychology, 60,* 426–432.

Lochman, J. E., Coie, J. D., Underwood, M. K., & Terry, R. (1993). Effectiveness of a social relations intervention program for aggressive and nonaggressive, rejected

children. *Journal of Consulting and Clinical Psychology, 61,* 1053–1058.

Loeber, R. (1991). Questions and advances in the study of developmental pathways. In D. Cicchetti & S. Toth (Eds.), *Models and integrations: Rochester symposium on developmental psychopathology* (Vol. 3, pp. 97–115). Rochester, NY: University of Rochester Press.

Maguin, E., & Loeber, R. (1995). Academic performance and delinquency. In M. Tonry & D. P. Farrington (Eds.), *Building a safer society: Strategic approaches to crime prevention* (pp. 145–264). Chicago: University of Chicago Press.

Mathur, S. R., & Rutherford, R. B. (1996). Is social skills training effective for students with emotional or behavioral disorders? Research issues and needs. *Behavioral Disorders, 22,* 21–28.

McCarton, C. M., Brooks-Gunn, J., Wallace, I. F., Bauer, C. R., Bennett, F. C., Bernbaum, J. C., Broyles, R. S., Casey, P. H., McCormick, M. C., Scott, D. T., Tyson, J., Tonascia, J., Meinert, C. L., & Infant Health and Development Program Research Group. (1997). Results at age 8 years of early intervention for low-birth-weight premature infants. *Journal of the American Medical Association, 277,* 126–132.

McCord, J. (1992). The Cambridge–Somerville study: A pioneering longitudinal-experimental study of delinquency prevention. In J. McCord & R. E. Tremblay (Eds.), *Preventing antisocial behavior: Interventions from birth to adolescence* (pp. 196–206). New York: Guilford.

McMahon, R. J., Slough, N. M., & Conduct Problems Research Group. (1996). Family-based intervention in the Fast Track Program. In R. DeV. Peters & R. J. McMahon (Eds.), *Preventing childhood disorders, substance abuse, and delinquency* (pp. 90–110). Thousand Oaks, CA: Sage.

Metropolitan Area Child Study Research Group. (1997). *A cognitive-ecological approach to preventing aggression in urban and inner-city settings: Preliminary outcomes.* Manuscript submitted for publication.

Moffitt, T. E. (1993). Adolescence-limited and life-course persistent antisocial behavior: A developmental taxonomy. *Psychological Review, 100,* 674–701.

Mrazek, P. J., & Haggerty, R. J. (Eds.). (1994). *Reducing risks for mental disorders: Frontiers for preventive intervention research.* Washington, DC: National Academy Press.

Musick, J. S. (1993). *Young, poor, and pregnant.* New Haven, CT: Yale University Press.

National Crime Prevention Council. (1996). *Preventing crime by investing in families.* Ottawa, Ontario, Canada: National Crime Prevention Council.

Newman, J. P. (1987). Reaction to punishment in extraverts and psychopaths: Implications for the impulsive behavior of disinhibited individuals. *Journal of Research in Personality, 21,* 464–480.

Offord, D. R., Chmura Kraemer, H., Kazdin, A. E., Jensen, P., & Harrington, R. (1998). Lowering the burden of suffering from child psychiatric disorder: Trade-offs among clinical, targeted, and universal interventions.

Journal of the American Academy of Child and Adolescent Psychiatry, 37, 686–694.

Olds, D. L., Eckenrode, J., Henderson, C. R., Jr., Kitzman, H., Powers, J., Cole, R., Sidora, K., Morris, P., Pettitt, L. M., & Luckey, D. (1997a). Long-term effects of home visitation on maternal life course, and child abuse and neglect. *Journal of the American Medical Association, 278,* 637–643.

Olds, D. L., Eckenrode, J., Henderson, C. R., Jr., Kitzman, H., Powers, J., Cole, R., Sidora, K., Morris, P., Pettitt, L. M., & Luckey, D. (1997b). *Long-term effects of home visitation on maternal life course, child abuse and neglect, and children's arrests: 15-year follow-up a randomized trial.* Unpublished manuscript, University of Colorado Health Sciences Center, Denver, CO.

Olweus, D. (1991). Bully/victim problems among schoolchildren: Basic facts and effects of a school based intervention program. In D. J. Pepler & K. H. Rubin (Eds.), *The development and treatment of childhood aggression* (pp. 411–448). Hillsdale, NJ: Erlbaum.

Patterson, G. R., Reid, J. B., Jones, R. R., & Conger, R. R. (1975). *A social learning approach to family intervention: Families with aggressive children* (Vol. 1). Eugene, OR: Castalia.

Patterson, G. R., DeBaryshe, B. D., & Ramsey, E. (1989). A developmental perspective on antisocial behavior. *American Psychologist, 44,* 329–335.

Peters, R. D., & Russell, C. C. (1996). Promoting development and preventing disorder: The Better Beginnings, Better Futures Project. In R. D. Peters & R. J. McMahon (Eds.), *Preventing childhood disorders, substance abuse, and delinquency* (pp. 19–47). Thousand Oaks, CA: Sage.

Piaget, J. (1960). *The psychology of intelligence.* Totowa, NJ: Littlefield, Adams.

Powell, K. E., Muir-McClain, L., & Halasysmani, L. (1995). A review of selected school-based conflict resolution and peer mediation projects. *Journal of School Health, 65,* 426–431.

Prinz, R. J. (1985). Diet–behavior research with children: Methodological and substantive issues. *Advances in learning and behavioral disabilities, 4,* 181–199.

Pryce, C. R., Martin, R. D., & Skuse, D. (Eds.). (1995). *Motherhood in human and nonhuman primates: Biosocial determinants.* New York: Karger.

Pulkkinen, L., & Tremblay, R. E. (1992). Patterns of boys' social adjustment in two cultures and at different ages: A longitudinal perspective. *International Journal of Behavioural Development, 15,* 527–553.

Quay, H. C. (1993). The psychobiology of undersocialized aggressive conduct disorder: A theoretical perspective. *Development and Psychopathology, 5,* 165–180.

Raine, A., Brennan, P., Mednick, B., & Mednick, S. A. (1996). High rates of violence, crime, academic problem, and behavioral problems in males with both early neuromotor deficits and unstable family environments. *Archives of General Psychiatry, 53,* 544–549.

Reiss, A. J., & Roth, J. A. (Eds.). (1993). *Understanding and preventing violence.* Washington, DC: National Academy Press.

Restoin, A., Montagner, H., Rodriguez, D., Girardot, J. J., Laurent, D., Kontar, F., Ullmann, V., Casagrande, C., & Talpain, B. (1985). Chronologie des comportements de communication et profils de comportement chez le jeune enfant. In R. E. Tremblay, M. A. Provost, & F. F. Strayer (Eds.), *Ethologie et développement de l'enfant* (pp. 93–130). Paris: Editions Stock/Laurence Pernoud.

Robins, L. N. (1966). *Deviant children grown up.* Baltimore: Williams & Wilkins.

Robins, L. N. (1986). The consequences of conduct disorder in girls. In D. Olweus, J. Block, & M. Radke-Yarrow (Eds.), *Development of antisocial and prosocial behavior* (pp. 385–414). New York: Academic Press.

Robins, L. N. (1992). The role of prevention experiments in discovering causes of children's antisocial behavior. In J. McCord & R. E. Tremblay (Eds.), *Preventing antisocial behavior: Interventions from birth to adolescence.* New York: Guilford.

Roosevelt, T. (1909). Special message to Senate and House of Representatives. In *Proceedings of the conference on the care of dependent children.* (pp. 5–8). New York: Arno Press & The New York Times (1971).

Rowe, D. C., & Farrington, D. P. (1997). The familial transmission of criminal convictions. *Criminology, 35,* 177–201.

Sampson, R. J. (1995). The community. In J. Q. Wilson & J. Petersilia (Eds.), *Crime* (pp. 196–216). San Francisco: Institute for Contemporary Studies.

Sand, E. A. (1966). *Contribution à l'étude du développement de l'enfant. Aspects médico-sociaux et psychologiques.* Brussels, Belgium: Éditions de l'Institut de sociologie de l'Université libre de Bruxelles.

Schwartz, D., Flamant, R., & Lellouch, J. (1980). *Clinical trials.* New York: Academic Press.

Schweinhart, L. L., & Weikart, D. P. (1997). *Lasting differences: The High/Scope preschool curriculum comparison study through age 23* (Monographs of the High/Scope Educational Research Foundation, No. 12). Ypsilanti, MI: High/Scope.

Schweinhart, L. L., Barnes, H. V., & Weikart, D. P. (1993). *Significant benefits. The High/Scope Perry School Study through age 27.* Ypsilanti, MI: High/Scope.

Séguin, J. R., Pihl, R. O., Harden, P. W., Tremblay, R. E., & Boulerice, B. (1995). Cognitive and neuropsychological characteristics of physically aggressive boys. *Journal of Abnormal Psychology, 104,* 614–624.

Seitz, V., Rosenbaum, L. K., & Apfel, H. (1985). Effects of family support intervention: A ten-year follow-up. *Child Development, 56,* 376–391.

Serbin, L. A., Peters, P. L., McAffer, V. J., & Schwartzman, A. E. (1991). Childhood aggression and withdrawal as predictors of adolescent pregnancy, early parenthood, and environmental risk for the next generation. *Canadian Journal of Behavioural Science, 23,* 318–331.

Serbin, L. A., Peters, P. L., & Schwartzman, A. E. (1996). Longitudinal study of early childhood injuries and acute illnesses in the offspring of adolescent mothers who were aggressive, withdrawn, or aggressive-withdrawn in childhood. *Journal of Abnormal Psychology, 105,* 500–507.

Shaw, C. R., & McKay, H. D. (1942). *Juvenile delinquency and urban areas.* Chicago: University of Chicago Press.

Shaw, D. S., & Bell, R. Q. (1993). Developmental theories of parental contributors to antisocial behavior. *Journal of Abnormal Child Psychology, 21,* 493–518.

Shure, M. B., & Spivak, G. (1982). Interpersonal problem-solving in young children: A cognitive approach to prevention. *American Journal of Community Psychology, 10,* 341–356.

Stattin, H., & Klackenberg-Larsson, I. (1990). The relationship between maternal attributes in early life of the child and the child's future criminal behavior. *Development and Psychopathology, 2,* 99–111.

Stone, W. L., Bendell, R. D., & Field, T. M. (1988). The impact of socio-economic status on teenage mothers and children who received early intervention. *Journal of Applied Developmental Psychology, 9,* 391–408.

Strayhorn, J. M., & Weidman, C. S. (1991). Follow-up one year after parent–child interaction training: Effects on behavior of preschool children. *Journal of the American Academy of Child and Adolescent Psychiatry, 30,* 138–143.

Szapocznik, J., Rio, A., Murray, E., Cohen, R., Scopetta, M., Rivas-Vazques, A., Hervis, O., Posada, V., & Kurtines, W. (1989). Structural family versus psychodynamic child therapy for problematic Hispanic boys. *Journal of Consulting and Clinical Psychology, 51,* 571–578.

Tremblay, R. E. (1991). Aggression, prosocial behavior and gender: Three magic words but no magic wand. In D. Pepler & K. Rubin (Eds.), *The development and treatment of aggression* (pp. 71–78). Hillsdale, NJ: Erlbaum.

Tremblay, R. E., & Craig, W. (1995). Developmental crime prevention. In M. Tonry & D. P. Farrington (Eds.), *Building a safer society: Strategic approaches to crime prevention* (pp. 151–236). Chicago: University of Chicago Press.

Tremblay, R. E., Vitaro, F., Bertrand, L., LeBlanc, M. Beauchesne, H., Boileau, H., & David, H. (1992). Parent and child training to prevent early onset of delinquency: The Montreal longitudinal-experimental study. In J. McCord & R. E. Tremblay (Eds.), *Preventing antisocial behavior: Interventions from birth through adolescence* (pp. 117–138). New York: Guilford.

Tremblay, R. E., Pihl, R. O., Vitaro, F., & Dobkin, P. L. (1994). Predicting early onset of male antisocial behavior from preschool behavior. *Archives of General Psychiatry, 51,* 732–738.

Tremblay, R. E., Kurtz, L., Mâsse, L. C., Vitaro, F., & Pihl, R. O. (1995). A bimodal preventive intervention for disruptive kindergarten boys: Its impact through mid-adolescence. *Journal of Consulting and Clinical Psychology, 63,* 560–568.

Tremblay, R. E., Mâsse, L. C., Vitaro, F., & Dobkin, P. L. (1995). The impact of friends' deviant behavior on early onset of delinquency: Longitudinal data from 6 to 13 years of age. *Development and Psychopathology, 7,* 649–668.

Tremblay, R. E., Boulerice, B., Harden, P. W., McDuff, P., Pérusse, D., Pihl, R. O., & Zoccolillo, M. (1996). Do children in Canada become more aggressive as they approach adolescence? In Human Resources Development Canada & Statistics Canada (Eds.), *Growing up in Canada: National Longitudinal Survey of Children and Youth/Grandir au Canada: Enquête longitudinale nationale sur les enfants et les jeunes* (pp. 127–137). Ottawa, Ontario: Statistics Canada.

Tremblay, R. E., Boulerice, B., Pihl, R. O., Vitaro, F., & Zoccolillo, M. (1996, January). *Male adolescent conduct disorder is predicted by kindergarten impulsivity, but there are moderating effects.* Paper presented at the meeting of the Society for Research in Child and Adolescent Psychiatry, Santa Monica, CA.

Tremblay, R. E., Mâsse, L. C., Pagani, L., & Vitaro, F. (1996). From childhood physical aggression to adolescent maladjustment: The Montréal Prevention Experiment. In R. D. Peters & R. J. McMahon (Eds.), *Preventing childhood disorders, substance abuse and delinquency* (pp. 268–298). Thousand Oaks, CA: Sage.

Vitaro, F., & Tremblay, R. E. (1994). Impact of a prevention program on aggressive-disruptive children's friendships and social adjustment. *Journal of Abnormal Child Psychology, 22,* 457–475.

Vitaro, F., Tremblay, R. E., Gagnon, C., & Pelletier, D. (1994). Predictive accuracy of behavioral and sociometric assessments of high-risk kindergarten children. *Journal of Clinical Child Psychology, 23,* 272–282.

Vitaro, F., Tremblay, R. E., Kerr, M., Pagani-Kurtz, L., & Bukowski, W. M. (1997). Disruptiveness, friends' characteristics, and delinquency: A test of two competing models of development. *Child Development, 68,* 676–689.

Webster-Stratton, C. (1997). *Preventing conduct problems in Head Start children: Strengthening parenting competencies.* Manuscript submitted for publication.

White, J. L., Moffitt, T. E., Earls, F., Robins, L., & Silva, P. A. (1990). How early can we tell? Predictors of childhood conduct disorder and adolescent delinquency. *Criminology, 28,* 507–533.

Yoshikawa, H. (1994). Prevention as cumulative protection: Effects of early family support and education on chronic delinquency and its risks. *Psychological Bulletin, 115,* 28–54.

IV

Special Problems and Issues

26

Disruptive Behavior Disorders in Children with Mental Retardation

BETSEY A. BENSON and MICHAEL G. AMAN

INTRODUCTION

The Multifaceted Nature of Mental Retardation

In discussing Disruptive Behavior Disorders (DBD) in mental retardation (MR), it is well to be aware that MR does not have one etiology but a nearly infinite number of etiologies. Indeed, insofar as individual genetic inheritance is a factor (and it often is) the mix of etiologies is enormous. Most workers agree that the presence of MR is the consequence of an array of factors that fall under the rubrics of biological, social, and psychological risk factors (Aman, Hammer, & Rojahn, 1993). Each of these factors may have different impacts on the various DBD. Examples of organic causes are genetic abnormalities, chromosomal abnormalities, and a multitude of congenital infections and maternal diseases that may harm the fetus. Subsequent to birth, encephalitis, meningitis, head trauma, toxemia, malnutrition, cerebrovascular accidents, and degenerative diseases are capable of causing MR. Environmental conditions, such as exposure to lead, mercury, radiation,

and a variety of licit and illicit drugs may also be toxic to either the fetus or the developing child. Finally, MR may be "psychosocially" determined. Psychosocial MR is presumed to exist when the person with MR has a family history of MR, there is no apparent organic cause, and there are impoverished circumstances such as poor housing, a general lack of healthy stimulation, chaotic living environment, inadequate medical care, and undernutrition (Aman et al., 1993).

Thus, MR is a final common pathway for a very large collection of potential causes. Its quintessential features are abnormally low IQ and inadequate adaptive behavior. The American Association on Mental Retardation has recently endorsed a more complex definition that emphasizes specific areas of deficit and society's obligation to provide the necessary supports for persons with MR (Luckasson et al., 1992).

Problems in Diagnosing Disorders in People with MR

Before discussing DBD in MR, it is important to recognize some of the impediments to establishing their presence. First, by virtue of their cognitive handicaps, many children and adolescents with MR have severe language limitations that can make it difficult or impossible to obtain information about internal states, such as feelings of worthlessness, thoughts of suicide,

BETSEY A. BENSON and MICHAEL G. AMAN • The Nisonger Center for Mental Retardation and Developmental Disabilities, The Ohio State University, Columbus, Ohio 43210-1296.

Handbook of Disruptive Behavior Disorders, edited by Quay and Hogan. Kluwer Academic/Plenum Publishers, New York, 1999.

anxiety, and the presence of delusions and hallucinations. Second, especially in child and adolescent disorders, one often has to establish whether symptoms are developmentally inappropriate. For example, body rocking or excessive motor activity might be tolerated for a longer time in children with severe developmental handicaps. One may be reluctant to assign the symptom of stealing to a child where it is unclear whether the child even has a concept of personal ownership. Third, the environmental-cultural context can complicate diagnosis. For example, children with psychosocial MR may have grossly inappropriate role models.

Fourth, there have traditionally been a shortage of appropriate norms for this population, making it more difficult to judge findings from psychometric instruments. Fifth, until recently (Einfeld & Aman, 1995) the field has not had a working definition of behavioral abnormality in children and adolescents with MR. Sixth, these children often have a variety of sensory and physical impairments that also complicate diagnosis (Tonge & Einfeld, 1991). For example, deafness may seriously affect a child's development and undiagnosed pain may result in bouts of self-injury. Finally, many professionals fail to look for or recognize mental disorders when they know that the person has MR. This failure to consider behavior problems in the presence of MR has been labeled "diagnostic overshadowing" (Reiss & Szyszko, 1983; Reiss, Levitan, & Szyszko, 1982).

Aman (1991) noted that formal diagnostic criteria (see Chapter 1, this volume) can be readily used in people with mild MR. However, as functional impairment becomes more severe, the use of standard diagnostic criteria may become increasingly problematic. For example, the expression of symptoms may be transformed with greater functional impairment. Some disorders may not be present in people with profound MR or the disorders may be so significantly transmogrified that they are not identifiable within current diagnostic schemata. Schizophrenia could be one such disorder. One expert has stated that people with mild MR present with essentially the same psychopathology as seen in the general population (Einfeld, 1992) and has argued that patients with moderate and severe MR experience behavior disorders found in the general population, although they often present with symptoms that are rare in the general population. However, those with profound MR were seen as having "insufficient behavior" to allow the development of true clinical behavior disorders.

Einfeld and Aman (1995) were unable to locate any systematic studies that assessed interrater agreement on psychiatric diagnosis in children with MR. Most reports lacked sufficient methodological details to judge degree of interdiagnoser reliability. Einfeld and Tonge (1991) noted several areas where they had considerable difficulty achieving agreement when diagnosing children and adolescents with MR: (1) distinguishing autism from pervasive developmental disorder not otherwise specified; (2) determining whether children with symptoms of Conduct Disorder (CD) were aware that they had violated the rights of others; (3) determining whether a diagnosis of organic brain syndrome should supersede more specific diagnoses, especially in those with moderate or greater MR; and (4) establishing whether Attention-Deficit/Hyperactivity Disorder (ADHD) symptoms were excessive for the child's developmental level. Einfeld and Aman (1995) noted that several epidemiological studies have found widely different prevalences of respective disorders in similar MR populations and suggested that this may indicate low interdiagnoser reliability when working with such patients.

Prevalence of Psychopathology and Behavioral Phenotypes

Workers are generally agreed that all of the disorders seen in the general population are also found in people with MR (Reiss, 1994; Stark, Menolascino, Albarelli, & Gray, 1988). However, certain disorders are seen much more commonly in those with MR than in the general population. Examples include autistic disorder, self-injury, and stereotypic behavior.

There are substantial data to indicate that children and adults with MR are at considerably increased risk for mental health problems (see Bruininks, Hill, & Morreau, 1988). By far the best of these studies in children was carried out by Rutter, Tizard, Yule, Graham, and Whitmore (1976) who found that children with MR were four to six times as likely to have a behavioral or emotional disorder as typically developing children.

Finally, certain syndromes of MR are associated with inflated rates of specific behaviors or disorders (Einfeld, 1992; Einfeld & Aman, 1995) which have been called *behavioral phenotypes*. Some examples of syndromes associated with disruptive behavior include the following: Prader–Willi syndrome (hyperphagia, inflated rates of behavior disturbance); Angleman syndrome (unprovoked laughing, hand flapping); Williams syndrome (short attention span); Fragile X syndrome (hand flapping, gaze avoidance); congenital rubella (irritability in infancy); and Lesch–Nyhan syndrome (severe self-injury). However, these behaviors do not necessarily occur at consistent rates or in all persons with these syndromes.

ADHD

Whereas thousands of studies and scholarly articles have been devoted to ADHD in children of normal IQ, relatively few studies have been conducted in children with MR. In the past, the British perspective maintained that "hyperkinesis" was an uncommon condition that was often associated with MR, brain damage, or both. Thus, we might expect to find a wealth of data on ADHD as it appears in MR and information on its treatment in the British literature, but this is not the case (Taylor, 1986). However, there are some notable exceptions. Interested readers may also wish to consult a chapter devoted solely to ADHD in children with MR (Pearson, Norton, & Farwell, 1997).

Prevalence

ADHD appears to be far more prevalent in children and adolescents with MR than in the general population. We found three epidemiological studies that estimated prevalence. Jacobson (1982) surveyed the clinical staff responsible for all 30,578 children and adults with MR served by the state of New York. The sample was divided into those with and without a recorded psychiatric disorder, and clinical staff were asked to rate the three most troublesome behavior problems for each subject. Hyperactivity was listed as a problem for 9.3% of subjects in the birth to 20-year-old cohort without a psychiatric diagnosis and for 21.0% of those with a psychiatric diagnosis (10.4% irrespective of whether a psychiatric diagnosis was used). Koller, Richardson, Katz, and McLaren (1983) assessed a 5-year birth cohort of 192 children with MR, aged 7 to 11 years, in a British city. Based on parent and child interviews, they classified 12% of the sample as having hyperactive behavior. Quine (1986) surveyed a stratified sample of 200 children aged birth to 14 years with severe MR. Based on structured interviews with parents, 21% of the sample was regarded as overactive.

Ando and Yoshimura (1978) had teachers complete a behavior checklist on 120 Japanese children with MR who were attending a special school; 9.4% were regarded as exhibiting high activity levels. Epstein, Cullinan, and Gadow (1986) surveyed children in classrooms for the educable mentally retarded (EMR) using a symptom questionnaire. In all, 18% of the sample was rated above 15, a commonly used cutoff for significant hyperactivity.

Studies of clinical populations, not surprisingly, indicate higher levels of hyperactivity. Philips and Williams (1977) reported on 100 consecutive referrals to a psychiatric clinic and reported that 19 of 62 nonpsychotic children with MR (31%) and 19 of 38 psychotic children with MR (54%) were hyperactive (DSM-II). In another clinical sample of 113 children with MR, Myers (1987) reported that 15% had primary or secondary diagnoses of ADHD.

Thus a wide range of prevalence data have been reported, from 10% to 21% for population studies. The obvious weakness in these surveys is that control groups were not included, so that we cannot be certain that the investigators were not predisposed to find high rates of ADHD symptoms. Nevertheless, the population surveys were remarkably consistent in some respects, and a reasonable estimate would be that at least 9% of children with MR have significant hyperactivity.

Presentation of ADHD in MR

The data on the clinical presentation of ADHD in MR are remarkably limited. In an early British study, Hutt and Hutt (1964) compared 8 brain-injured nonhyperkinetic children, 8 brain-injured hyperkinetic children, and 12 "normal" children referred for relatively minor behavior problems. IQs of the children were not provided, but we assume that the first two groups included significant numbers of children with MR. The children were observed in a test room as the environment was systematically enriched by the introduction of toy blocks and an interactive adult. The hyperkinetic children were consistently active, irrespective of environment, whereas the other groups became dramatically less active as the environment was enriched. Hyperkinetic children spent more time manipulating such things as light switches and door knobs than the other groups and spent substantially less time in block play.

In another British study, Tizard (1968a) compared 10 children regarded as severely overactive by their teachers with 11 judged as normoactive. All of these children, who had severe to profound MR were observed in their classrooms for locomotion and approach to teachers and other children. The overactive children were found to have more movement, to make fewer friendly approaches to others, and to receive fewer friendly approaches from other children. Typically developing ADHD children were not included in either of these studies. However, the general pattern of behavior appears to be broadly consistent with findings found with normal-IQ ADHD children in observational studies (see Barkley, 1990).

Thorley (1984) conducted a retrospective comparison of 73 children given a diagnosis of hyperkinetic syndrome with an equal number of CD children matched on age, sex, IQ, and social class ("Register General" level I to IV, plus "unemployed"). IQ ranged from less than 20 to 70+, with 51% of the subjects assigned to the 70+ bracket. Results indicated that the hyperkinetic group was rated higher on lack of emotional response, social disinhibition, disorders of articulation, repetitive movements, and duration of symptoms. The CD group was rated higher on stealing, aggression, coming from other than two-parent family units, and receiving National Assistance (welfare).

There are data indicating that children with both ADHD and MR may be characteristically less aggressive than typically developing ADHD children. Fee, Matson, Moore, and Benavidez (1993) compared (1) children with MR only, (2) children with MR plus ADHD, (3) typically developing children, and (4) typically developing children with ADHD. Subjects were allocated to clinical groups on the basis of the Conners Teacher Rating Scale (TRS) (Goyette, Conners, & Ulrich, 1978). Fee and colleagues found that Conners IOWA Inattention/Overactivity and Aggression subscales (Loney & Milich, 1982) were significantly correlated in group (4) but not in group (2). The same was true of the Hyperactivity and Asocial subscales of the TRS. Fee, Matson, and Benavidez (1994) examined these data further in a subsequent report and found that the typically developing children with ADHD had significantly higher Asocial subscale scores on the TRS than the children with MR and ADHD. In the Tizard (1968a) study mentioned earlier, teachers rated all children on distractibility, mood swings, aggression, tantrums, and lack of affection; only distractibility occurred more often in the hyperactive group. Hence, there is some reason to assume that aggression may be less in evidence in ADHD children with MR than in typically developing ADHD children. As in typically developing ADHD children, males outnumbered females among children with MR and ADHD. In their study of 192 children, Koller and colleagues (1983) found that 18.0% of the boys were hyperactive as compared with 7.4% of the girls. As noted later, this ratio (2.4:1) may be smaller than is typically found in ADHD in the normal population.

Handen, McAuliffe, Janosky, Feldman, and Breaux (1994) compared children with MR with and without ADHD in the context of a laboratory Saturday Education Program. Direct observations of on-task behavior, fidgetiness, and actometer readings differentiated the two groups, especially during periods of assigned work without direct teacher supervision. As noted by Handen and colleagues, this pattern of differences closely paralleled prior findings with typically developing ADHD children.

Pearson, Lachar, and Loveland (1995) compared 26 children with ADHD and MR with a matched group of 37 children with MR only. The children's mothers rated them on the Personality Inventory for Children—Revised edition (PIC–R) (Wirt, Lachar, Klinedinst, & Seat, 1984). Compared with the controls, the ADHD children had significantly higher scores on the Depression, Delinquency, Anxiety, Psychosis, and Social Skills (immature social development) subscales, a pattern that Pearson and colleagues argued is also characteristic of typically developing ADHD children.

Finally, a special note concerns the *developmental appropriateness* of the child's behavior when diagnosing ADHD symptoms in children with MR. Both DSM-III and DSM-IV (American Psychiatric Association, 1980, 1994) contain instructions to clinicians to take the child's mental age (MA) into account when assessing hyperactivity and its associated features. Some practitioners have tried to do this by calculating the child's MA and using corresponding chronological age (CA) norms from the general population when employing rating scale data to assess behavior. In commenting on problems they experienced in achieving interdiagnoser reliability, Einfeld and Tonge (1991) noted that it was difficult to reach agreement on whether levels of impulsivity and short attention span were abnormal in relation to a given child's cognitive development.

Although these DSM guidelines make intuitive sense, there are scant data available. To address this question, Pearson and Aman (1994) compared the relationship of several hyperactivity subscale scores to CA, IQ, and MA. Both parent and teacher ratings were available

on a general clinical sample (N = 58) and on a group with developmental disabilities (N = 54). Within the general clinical sample, parent ratings on six hyperactivity subscales and teacher ratings on five hyperactivity subscales were available from several standardized instruments and there were two IQ measures and one MA score available. For the developmental sample, parent ratings were available on six subscales measuring hyperactivity and teacher ratings were available on three similar subscales; there were three IQ and three MA measures. If the DSM guidelines are correct, one might expect to see a large number of significant negative correlations between IQ and MA on the one hand and hyperactivity scores on the other. In fact, in the general clinical sample, only 3 of 33 correlations (9%) between the cognitive measures (i.e., IQ and MA) and hyperactivity subscale scores were significant. In the developmental sample, 4 of 27 (15%) MA–hyperactivity correlations scores and 1 of 23 (4%) IQ–hyperactivity correlations were significant. All correlations between IQ or MA and hyperactivity ratings were modest. Furthermore, the MA associations ceased to be significant if the effect of CA was partialed out first. In contrast, 7 of 9 CA–hyperactivity comparisons (78%) were significant in the developmental sample. Pearson and Aman concluded that it is not necessary (or appropriate, given available data) to adjust for IQ or MA when using rating scores, but it may be appropriate to control for CA. They speculated that many raters, including parents and teachers, may make an implicit correction for developmental level when asked to do ratings.

Cognitive Functioning

We could locate only two studies in relation to cognition and ADHD in children with MR. Melnyk and Das (1992) chose 13 children each who scored high and low on an attention checklist. All subjects attended classes for EMR children and they had a mean IQ of 71. The children were tested on a sustained attention task requiring auditory detection and on a selective attention test in which pictures were identified if they matched physically or conceptually. The groups did not differ on the auditory sustained attention task but the children rated as inattentive took significantly longer to perform the selective matching task. The authors felt that this indicated significantly greater distractibility in the poor-attention group.

Pearson, Yaffee, Loveland, and Lewis (1996) compared ADHD and non-ADHD children with MR on sustained and selective attention tasks. The children in the ADHD group had a mean IQ on the Stanford Binet Intelligence Scale of 56.0, whereas those in the control group had a mean IQ of 55.7. On a continuous performance task, the ADHD children made significantly fewer correct detections and significantly more commission errors, findings that are usually interpreted as signifying poorer sustained attention and greater impulsivity, respectively. On a speeded classification task, the ADHD children made significantly more classification errors than the non-ADHD group, suggesting a deficit in selective attention.

Risk Factors

As in typically developing children, male gender is a risk factor for developing ADHD in children with MR (Eyman & Call, 1977; Koller et al., 1983). However, some workers have found quite low male-to-female ratios (ranging from 1.25:1 to 2:1) (Pearson et al., 1996; Tizard, 1968a, 1968b). The impact of gender may be weaker, because other risk factors may outweigh it. ADHD is typically associated with more severe functional handicap (Eyman & Call, 1977; Jacobson, 1982; Koller et al., 1983; Myers, 1987). Hyperactivity is often found to be more common as handicap progresses from mild through severe MR and it may actually lessen a little at profound MR.

Central nervous system (CNS) dysfunction has been posited as a risk factor. Reid (1980) noted a "tendency" for more structural brain damage among children diagnosed as hyperkinetic. However, Thorley (1984) observed no differences in CNS dysfunction between hyperkinetic children and a control group of CD children. Several authors have observed more evidence of hyperactivity among children with epilepsy (Aman, Richmond, Stewart, Bell, & Kissel, 1987; Myers, 1987; Tizard, 1968a). At least one study found higher rates of hyperactivity among younger children with MR (Eyman & Call, 1977). Other studies found lower rates of hyperactivity among patients who were less ambulatory (Myers, 1987) or who had cerebral palsy (Aman et al., 1987).

Treatment

According to Coe and Matson (1993), behavioral treatments for ADHD in this population have included antecedent exercise (Bachman & Sluyter, 1988; McGimsey & Favell, 1988), differential reinforcement of other behavior (DRO schedules) (Twardosz & Sajwaj, 1972), and physical restraint (Singh, Winton, & Ball, 1984). Antecedent exercise has resulted in both reduced overactivity and reduced off-task behavior, whereas the study of DRO found decreased activity and increased toy play. The study of physical restraint did not find it to be viable for managing hyperactivity.

Pharmacotherapy, especially with stimulants, has been a mainstay of treatment in typically developing ADHD children (see Chapter 10, this volume). Reid (1980) commented that neuroleptic drugs tended to be the more common treatment in his MR patient population, and this may characterize treatment of children with MR in the United Kingdom. There is a modicum of data indicating that neuroleptics have some effectiveness in children with ADHD and MR (Aman & Singh, 1980). Recently there has been a handful of well-controlled studies of stimulant medication in children with MR and ADHD, and stimulants are clearly effective in reducing overactivity and enhancing attention span (Aman, 1996; see also Chapter 10, this volume). A meta-analysis of the recent literature suggests that about 54% of such children respond to stimulants, which is substantially lower than in the general population (Aman, 1996). Further, there are some data suggesting that children of lower functional levels are less likely to respond to psychostimulants (Aman, 1996).

Outcome Studies

Follow-up data in ADHD in MR are limited. Koller and colleagues (1983) followed up 192 children (aged 7 to 11 years at first contact) when they were 22 years old. Prevalence of hyperactivity declined from 12% in childhood to 3% in the postschool years. Aman, Pejeau, Osborne, Rojahn, and Handen (1996) followed up 26 of 30 participants in a drug study 4 years later. As rated by their parents, the subjects showed significant decreases on subscales related to DBD but their scores were still abnormally high relative to norms. Six of the 26 subjects (23%) had symptoms consistent with CD or Oppositional Defiant Disorder (ODD), and another 8 (31%) had symptoms consistent with avoidant disorder or separation anxiety disorder. Some 65% of these children were taking psychotropic medication, but stimulants accounted for only 50% of medicines. Parents reported that 11 of these youngsters (42%) had no lasting friendships or only one or two weak friendships. Interestingly, hyperactivity subscales at initial contact failed to predict outcome, whereas the Irritability subscale on the Aberrant Behavior Checklist (Aman, Singh, Stewart, & Field, 1985) was a powerful predictor of both later DBD and internalizing behavior problems.

Handen, Janosky, and McAuliffe (1997) followed up 51 of 52 former participants in a medication study $2\frac{1}{3}$ years later. During that interval, they found that 31% of the children had been suspended from school. Some 69% were receiving psychotropic drugs and 22% had received inpatient psychiatric treatment over the interval. Some 67% of the children continued to be rated above the 98th percentile on the Conners Hyperactivity Index (Goyette et al., 1978) at follow-up.

We are not aware of any studies that have followed a group selected for ADHD into adulthood, so the picture is incomplete.

AGGRESSION AND CONDUCT PROBLEMS

Description

Aggressive behavior of youth with MR is a major cause of placement in restrictive residential programs and special educational environments (Bruininks et al., 1988). Behavioral disturbance, including aggression, has been cited as a primary reason for failure of community residential placement and return to institutions (Hill & Bruininks, 1984; Lakin, Hill, Hauber, Bruininks, & Heal, 1983). Physical safety concerns for the individual and those around him or her result in higher levels of staffing and supervision, reduced opportunities for independent functioning, and disrupted interpersonal relationships.

A lengthy list of behaviors is subsumed under the label "aggressive," including both verbal and physical acts. These clinically significant behaviors may exist as somewhat isolated behaviors or as part of a complex of symptoms associated with an identifiable syndrome. In addition to CD and ODD, aggressive behavior in persons with MR is comorbid with symptoms of other disorders, including mood disorders (Reiss & Rojahn, 1993).

Prevalence

There is a wide range of prevalence estimates of aggressive behavior and conduct problems among children and adolescents with MR. Variation in reported rates can be attributed to the subjects' levels of intellectual functioning, sampling methods used, and the definition of aggression. One difficulty cited by Harris (1993) is that traditional definitions of aggression often include the idea of *intent to harm,* a concept that is difficult to apply to individuals with more severe MR. Further, some investigations counted only severe aggression (Borthwick-Duffy, 1994) while others included milder forms of aggression in their surveys (Koller, Richardson, Katz, & McClaren, 1982).

Borthwick-Duffy (1994) presented the findings from a registry of more than 90,000 people served by the Department of Developmental Services in the state of California. Aggressive behavior (one or more violent episodes causing serious physical injury requiring immediate medical attention) in children was identified in 3.7% of the population and property destruction was reported for 14.4%. Somewhat higher rates were reported by Harris's (1993) survey of the residents of a single health district in England which included both institutional and community residences. All children with severe and profound MR were included. Using a definition of aggression that required tissue damage or management difficulty, they reported a prevalence rate of between 10% and 20%, depending on the age group. For those attending schools, the prevalence rate was 12.6%.

Higher rates of aggression and conduct problems are typically found in youth with MR in comparison to control groups. Koller and colleagues (1982) studied behavior disturbance in childhood and young adulthood among individuals with MR and control subjects. Higher rates of aggressive CD and antisocial behavior were reported among subjects with MR than controls. Likewise in school samples, children with mild MR were rated as having more conduct problems than students in the general population. Cullinan, Epstein, Matson, and Rosemier (1984) compared school behavior problems of children in special education classes to those of students in regular classes. Teacher ratings on the Behavior Problem Checklist (Quay & Peterson, 1975) indicated that students with mild MR, ages 6 to 18, scored significantly higher than regular class students on the Conduct Problem scale. No differences were found on the Immaturity or Socialized Delinquency scales. In a special education sample, males were rated higher than females on Conduct Problems (Polloway, Epstein, & Cullinan, 1985).

In clinic samples, aggression is among the most frequently referred problems (Phillips & Williams, 1975). Benson (1985) found that conduct problems accounted for 42% of the referrals of children and adolescents to a community clinic for persons with MR.

Cognitive Functioning

Most investigators report that level of intellectual functioning is associated with aggressive behavior, with higher rates of aggression at lower intellectual levels, although there are some conflicting results. Borthwick-Duffy (1994) noted a linear pattern of prevalence for aggression and property destruction with greater rates occurring with more severe MR.

The form of aggressive behavior may differ depending on the level of MR. In a report of the referrals to a crisis intervention program, Davidson and colleagues (1994) stated that aggressive individuals who destroyed property but were not aggressive toward people tended to be higher functioning. In a large-scale study, McGrew, Ittenbach, Bruininks, and Hill (1991) examined the factor structure of maladaptive behavior across the life span based on statewide surveys using the Inventory on Client and Agency Planning (ICAP) Problem Behavior Scales (Bruininks, Hill, Weatherman, & Woodcock, 1986). The sample was divided into two levels of MR, one mild to moderate and the other severe and profound. Different factor solutions were deemed most appropriate for different age groups and level of functioning. For youth up to age 12, a two-factor solution representing Internal and External dimensions was appropriate for both levels of MR. In the 13- to 19-year age group, the obtained factors varied with the level of functioning. For persons functioning in the mild to moderate range, the resulting factors were an Internal maladaptive behavior dimension and two External maladaptive behavior dimensions named Socially Disruptive and Destructive-General. For persons functioning in the severe and profound range, the three factors were Internal maladaptive, External maladaptive, and Destructive-Internal (hurts self).

Although we found no reports dealing with the issue specifically, it would seem that a DSM-IV (American Psychiatric Association, 1994) CD diagnosis would be associated with a higher level of intellectual functioning because of some of the behaviors included, such as deceitfulness. Likewise, for the diagnosis of ODD, some verbal skills would be necessary in order to blame others for one's mistakes and to argue with adults. Individuals with MR who meet these diagnostic criteria are seen in correctional settings with some frequency (Smith, Algonzzine, Schmid, & Hennly, 1990).

Risk Factors

Highly significant gender differences are typically reported for aggression and conduct problems in youth with MR, with males outnumbering females by ratios of 2:1 or more (Benson, 1985; Borthwick-Duffy, 1994). There are some data to indicate that nonverbal individuals are more likely to engage in aggressive behavior than verbal individuals (Borthwick-Duffy, 1994); this characteristic is often associated with greater cognitive impairment.

Age appears to be a factor as well. Quay and Gredler (1981) conducted a factor analysis of teacher ratings on the Behavior Problem Checklist (Quay & Peterson, 1975) for more than 200 residents of a state institution. CD was found to be related to age, with younger subjects (9–17 years) scoring higher than older subjects (18–26 years). A Socialized Aggression scale did not emerge in this sample. In large-scale surveys that include community residents, the rate of conduct problems is greater in children older than 10 years (Borthwick-Duffy, 1994), with the 15- to 19-year age range deemed particularly critical (Harris, 1993).

Studies have failed to find an association between neurological status and conduct problems among youth with MR. Davidson and colleagues' (1994) comparison of aggressive and nonaggressive individuals (both children and adults) found that the presence of a seizure disorder and EEG findings did not differentiate between the two groups. Richardson, Koller, and Katz (1985) also reported no significant difference in behavior disturbance in four categories including CD and antisocial behavior, based on the presence or absence of CNS impairment, broadly defined.

There is some evidence to suggest that family factors play a significant role in the occurrence of conduct problems in children and adolescents with MR. Richardson and colleagues (1985) examined four types of behavioral disturbance (emotional disturbance, aggressive CD, antisocial behavior, and hyperactive behavior) in individuals with mild MR and controls. They found significantly more behavioral disturbance among persons with MR as well as a significant effect of stability of upbringing, with greater behavioral disturbance associated with unstable upbringing. When conditions of upbringing were held constant, there was no difference in behavioral disturbance between groups with and without MR. The stability of upbringing data were not reported separately for the four categories; thus specific findings for aggression, CD, and antisocial behavior are not available.

Treatment

The primary approaches to treatment of aggression and conduct problems in children and adolescents with MR have been behavioral interventions and psychopharmacology. There have been a few reports of other interventions, including a cognitive-behavioral intervention (Benson, 1992; Benson, Rice, & Miranti, 1986).

Matson and Gorman-Smith (1986) reviewed behavioral treatment research for aggressive and DBD in persons with MR. There were 27 studies published between 1976 and 1983 that met their criteria for inclusion. Aggressive or disruptive behaviors that were treated included inappropriate verbalizations, aggression toward others, noncompliance, hyperactivity, and "maladaptive" behavior. The most commonly used procedures were positive reinforcement and time-out followed by aversive stimuli or punishment, overcorrection, DRO, DRL (differential reinforcement of low rate of behavior), and extinction. The most effective approaches were DRI (differential reinforcement of incompatible behavior), aversive stimuli or punishment, facial screening, and overcorrection. Most of the research was conducted with children 10 years of age or younger. The greatest improvements were noted for individuals ages 11 to 15 and for individuals functioning in the profound range who were nonambulatory, followed by children with mild MR. The authors pointed out that reinforcement was as effective as punishment for the behaviors treated.

According to Gardner and Cole (1993), the 1970s and 1980s were characterized by the use of aversive consequences to suppress aggressive behavior in persons with MR. In recent years, more emphasis has been placed on the functional analysis of behavior to identify proximal controlling variables and setting conditions (Thompson, Egli, Symons, & Delaney, 1994). Although a functional analysis of behavior is considered important, Lundervold and Bourland (1988) found that in a large number of studies that they reviewed (62%), a functional analysis was not reported nor was there a rationale provided for the choice of treatment. Sprague and Horner (1994) caution against instituting behavioral interventions for individual problem behaviors. They have found that individual behaviors are often elements of more complex response classes and that effective interventions deal with the class, not a behavior.

Aman and Singh (1991) reviewed the literature on pharmacotherapy. Many studies have examined the effects of antipsychotics on a variety of disruptive behaviors, including aggression, and the impression is that these drugs do reduce hostility in some subjects. However, it is not clear whether this is an indirect effect produced through sedation, and the majority of studies were conducted in adults. Lithium carbonate has been studied infrequently but there is some evidence that it may reduce aggressive, assaultive, or destructive behavior (Aman & Singh, 1991). The serotonin specific reuptake inhibitors (SSRIs) are becoming a common mode of therapy throughout society, and there are case reports suggesting that they may have utility in some aggressive individuals (Sovner et al., 1998). Finally, there is increasing evidence that stimulant drugs reduce aggression in addition to ADHD symptoms in typically developing children with ADHD (see Chapters 10 and

21, this volume) and this is likely the case also in children and adolescents with MR.

Outcome Studies

There are few long-term follow-up data on aggression and conduct problems in youth with MR. Eyman, Borthwick, and Miller (1981) conducted a 2-year follow-up of maladaptive behaviors, including aggression, in individuals from different residential settings and found no significant changes over that time. Among clinic-referred children, Reid (1980) followed 27 youth with CD and reported that one third showed persistent antisocial behavior several years later. All of these were functioning in the mild range of MR and 8 of the 9 were male.

In a retrospective study, Hurley and Sovner (1995) described 6 men with mild to moderate MR who were given a diagnosis of Antisocial Personality Disorder (APD). In each case, there was evidence of CD before age 15. Only 1 individual had previously received the diagnosis despite a long history, however. The authors suggested that clinicians are reluctant to make a diagnosis of APD in persons with MR because of the individual's limited cognitive skills.

SELF-INJURIOUS BEHAVIOR (SIB)

Description

Self-injury is not unique to MR, but as a problematic disruptive condition it is more common among people with developmental disabilities (i.e., MR and autistic disorder) than any other subject group. Definitions of SIB differ, but most contain the following three elements: (1) chronicity, (2) capability of causing tissue damage, and (3) repetitiveness of the action. Some definitions also specify that the self-injurious acts not be goal directed, but recent research suggests that SIB serves a communicative function for many patients. Thus, we will define SIB simply as repetitive mechanical acts capable of causing tissue damage to the person concerned and of moderate or longer duration.

Rojahn (1994) reviewed some of the largest studies of SIB and provided a listing of specific forms of SIB found in these investigations. The following seven behaviors were the most commonly observed among self-injurious individuals: (1) self-biting (34% of the samples), (2) head banging against own body (30%), (3) scratching (22%), (4) head banging with objects (20%), (5) hitting self with own body (10%), (6) pica (9%), and (7) hitting self with objects (7%). Pica is not mechanical, so this behavior actually falls outside our definition. This list highlights the diversity of forms that SIB can take as well as different perspectives in defining SIB.

DSM-IV allows for a diagnosis of self-injury under the heading of Stereotypic Movement Disorder (307.3) (American Psychiatric Association, 1994). The critical components of the diagnosis are as follows: (1) characterized by repetitive, "driven," and nonfunctional motor behavior (e.g., body rocking); (2) interferes with normal activities or results in bodily injury; (3) the behavior is of sufficient severity to warrant treatment; (4) the behavior is not better accounted for as a compulsion, tic, pervasive developmental disorder, or trichotillomania (compulsive hair pulling); (5) not caused by substances (e.g., stimulants) or an organic condition; and (6) is present for 4 weeks or longer. The criteria go on to state that Stereotypic Movement Disorder *with Self-Injurious Behavior* should be noted if the movements cause bodily damage requiring treatment or would result in damage if restraint is not used.

There are four points about this classification that warrant comment. First, criterion (1) states that the behaviors are nonfunctional. As is noted later in this chapter, many workers believe that SIB has a communicative function for the patient. Second, criterion (4) indicates that SIB cannot be diagnosed in the presence of a pervasive developmental disorder (PDD). This would make sense if all PDDs were accompanied by SIB, which is not the case. Since an additional diagnosis of SIB would provide useful clinical and research information, we believe that the DSM-IV should allow for this notation. Third, the DSM-IV subsumes SIB within

the category of movement disorder. Although many workers believe that SIB is an extreme form of stereotypic behavior, there are many who do not accept this position. Furthermore, there are very few research data to resolve the issue. Fourth, as the DSM-IV criteria couch SIB in the context of repetitive movement, this seems to exclude certain acts (e.g., aerophagy, pica) that many workers regard as forms of SIB.

Although SIB occurs predominantly in individuals with MR, PDD, and autism, it also occurs in other disorders (e.g., Schizophrenia) and in a minority of normal infants (Fee & Matson, 1992; Thompson, Axtell, & Schaal, 1993). The key difference between SIB as it occurs in the developmental disabilities and as it occurs in normal infants is the severity and often chronicity in the former that are almost always lacking in normal infants.

There have been several attempts to organize SIB into a sensible taxonomy. Rojahn (1994) carried out one of the best taxonomic empirical studies. Data from 431 self-injurious subjects were subjected to factor analysis, and five factors emerged as follows: (1) Factor 1 (self-hitting behaviors), (2) Factor 2 (inserting objects into body openings), (3) Factor 3, comprising miscellaneous behaviors (biting, scratching, pinching, hair pulling), (4) Factor 4 (teeth grinding), and (5) Factor 5 (vomiting and rumination). Although it is potentially instructive to structure SIB behaviors into seemingly rational categories, others point out that similar-appearing forms of SIB may serve different functions for the individual (Thompson *et al.,* 1993).

There are several syndromes that are frequently or always associated with SIB (see Harris, 1992). The Lesch–Nyhan syndrome is an X-linked disorder found only in males that is characterized by MR, spastic cerebral palsy, dysarthric speech, choreoathetosis, and torsion dystonia. This syndrome is associated with compulsive and severe self-biting (which may lead to the loss of fingers and tissue around the lips) and with the picking of skin with the fingers (Harris, 1992). Individuals with the syndrome sometimes request forms of physical restraint and often show great agitation if restraints are removed.

The Cornelia de Lange syndrome is a rare genetic disorder characterized by an abnormally small head, enlargement of the brows and lashes, small hands and feet, short limbs, delayed dentition, and webbing of the feet (Harris, 1992). The syndrome is often associated with face hitting, face picking, lip biting, and tantrum behavior. The Rett syndrome is a form of infantile dementia found only in females. It is characterized by a normal prenatal and perinatal period followed by social and psychomotor regression (after 18 months), loss of purposeful hand skills, the appearance of hand wringing, clapping, and/or washing stereotypies, and gait and truncal movement dysfunction (all between 1 and 4 years) (Harris, 1992).

Another disorder that is frequently associated with SIB is the Fragile X syndrome. This syndrome is an X-linked familial form of mental retardation with a prevalence as high as 1 in 1,000. Physical features include large testicles, large or prominent ears, and a narrow face (Harris, 1992). Autisticlike features, hyperactivity, or both occur in many of these youngsters, and hand biting may be seen in a majority of those with MR.

Prevalence

The prevalence of SIB is highly variable, depending on setting and type of definition used to identify the condition (Rojahn, 1994). Based on existing surveys, Aman (1993) estimated that 10% to 15% of residents in MR institutions have some form of SIB as compared with 1% to 2.5% of those residing in the community. Fee and Matson (1992) estimated that between 5% and 15% of all people with MR exhibit self-injury. Hill, Balow, and Bruininks (1985) conducted a stratified survey of people with MR in the United States. They found that 11% of those in community residences and 22% of those in institutions had SIB. SIB is also common in children with autism who, of course, often have MR. Fee and Matson (1992) estimated that between 5% and 15% of people with autism exhibit SIB; the actual figure may be even higher.

Cognitive Functioning

Several workers have noted associations between SIB on the one hand and cognitive variables (or proxy cognitive variables) and intellectual functioning on the other. In general, the prevalence of SIB increases as IQ and expressive language decline (Rojahn, 1994; Thompson et al., 1993). SIB is also much more common in institutions than in the community (Rojahn, 1994). This finding may be attributed to IQ differences across settings, behavioral factors leading to institutionalization, or unknown factors. In contrast to our experience with the literature on ADHD, we are not aware of sophisticated attempts to look for specific cognitive differences between children with and without SIB and having comparable IQs.

Risk Factors

Severity of MR and institutional placement have already been mentioned as variables strongly related to the presence of SIB. Gender has only inconsistently been found to relate to SIB, with males slightly outnumbering females. Rojahn (1994) speculated that this may be because of certain rare genetic disorders (e.g., Lesch–Nyhan syndrome) which occur solely or mainly in males. Some have suggested that outward aggression and SIB are linked to some degree, but the data are inconsistent on this point. Finally, age appears to be associated in curvilinear fashion with SIB, with the highest prevalence occurring between 20 and 25 years of age. Rates of SIB tend to fall off as ages move toward the extremes (i.e., in the very young and in the elderly; Rojahn, 1994).

As noted earlier, many workers conceptualize SIB as an extreme variant of stereotypic behavior. This is probably because of the repetitive and invariant appearance of many forms of SIB. In some factor analytically derived scales, stereotypic behavior and SIB have failed to load on the same factor (e.g. Aman et al., 1985), whereas mutual loading has been found in other factor analyses (Aman, Tassé, Rojahn, & Hammer, 1996). Most reviewers have concluded that any relation is uncertain at this time (e.g., Fee & Matson, 1992; Thompson *et al.*, 1993).

Treatment

Behavior Therapy

Behavioral and pharmacological treatments are clearly the most commonly used forms of therapy for SIB. In the past, the most effective forms of behavior therapy involved some type of punishment contingent on SIB. Examples of such suppressive procedures include skin shock, overcorrection, lemon juice in the mouth, contingent restraint, aromatic ammonia, facial screening, and time-out from positive reinforcement (Durand & Carr, 1985; Thompson *et al.*, 1993). Cataldo (1990; in Thompson *et al.*, 1993) reviewed 137 studies employing such approaches and concluded that many of the therapies led to rapid and fairly durable suppression of SIB. However, given the impaired ability of many children with MR to voice opposition to such "aversive" approaches, many workers object to their use or prefer to reserve them as a treatment of last resort.

A relatively recent development in the field is the idea that many individuals engage in SIB to "communicate" some special need. Four motivating conditions have been advanced as factors likely to maintain SIB: (1) social attention (the child receives adult attention following SIB), (2) tangible consequences (e.g., toys, food), (3) escape from aversive situations, and (4) sensory consequences (i.e., the child may engage in SIB for the sensory stimulation that accompanies the act) (see Durand & Carr, 1985).

It follows logically that, if the maintaining circumstances can be identified, then an appropriate therapy can be tailored for that child. To facilitate the identification of maintaining variables, Durand and Crimmins (1988) introduced the Motivation Assessment Scale (MAS) (see also Durand, 1988). The MAS comprises 16 items that are completed by significant figures in the life of the child, such as teachers. Four items each assess maintaining

variables in the areas of (1) social attention, (2) tangible consequences, (3) escape from aversive situations, and (4) sensory consequences. In this way, the MAS is intended to identify motivating conditions. Iwata, Dorsey, Slifer, Bauman, and Richman (1994) have developed another method for identifying environmental events leading to SIB. They exposed subjects to a series of analogue conditions in the laboratory to determine whether they influence rate of SIB. The conditions comprised the following: (1) social disapproval, contingent on SIB, (2) academic demand, (3) unstructured play, and (4) child left alone without toys or sources of stimulation. A majority of the subjects showed reliable increases in SIB in the presence of one or more of these conditions, suggesting that the condition elicited the event.

Logically, the treatment should be congruent with the "communicative intent" of the SIB. For example, Durand and colleagues (Durand & Carr, 1985; Durand & Crimmins, 1988) developed an approach that they refer to as Differential Reinforcement of Communication (DRC). Thus, if a child's hand biting is motivated by adult attention, the rational behavioral approach would be to withdraw all attention following hand-biting incidents *and* train the child to seek adult attention by other means (e.g., by verbal requests).

Psychotropic Drugs

Surveys of subjects with SIB consistently indicate high rates of psychotropic drug use. A wide variety of psychoactive agents have been studied, but none of them has proven to be universally helpful or even partially helpful in all patients. The most promising or widely used agents are as follows.

Neuroleptics. These are probably the most widely used agents to suppress SIB, but the evidence of efficacy is mixed. The existing research gives greatest support to thioridazine, whereas there are insufficient data to judge haloperidol; the evidence with chlorpromazine is largely negative (Aman, 1993). Gualtieri and

Schroeder (1989) have described a dopaminergic model of self-injury that implicates a dysfunction of the D_1 system; drugs specific to D_1 could have greater efficacy than the traditional neuroleptics.

Lithium Carbonate. Only a few studies and case reports are available and their findings are mixed (especially in the controlled studies). Aman (1993) concluded that it is premature to draw conclusions about efficacy for SIB, although clinical studies are warranted.

SSRIs. A number of clinicians have speculated that the presence of SIB may reflect an underlying depression or obsessive-compulsive disorder in the affected person (see Aman, 1993). There are also empirical data that implicate low serotonin levels in aggressive behavior and in suicide (Coccaro, 1989). All of these observations suggest the possible utility of SSRIs, such as fluoxetine, sertraline, and paroxetine. Several case reports have been positive (Aman, 1993; Sovner *et al.,* 1998), although controlled studies are nearly nonexistent. One group study observed no change in SIB with paroxetine in 15 institutionalized residents (Davanzo, Belin, Widawski, & King, 1998).

Opiate Blockers. Another theory posits that the opiate system may be dysfunctional and thus contribute to SIB in some patients. The idea is either (1) that endogenous levels or opiates are too high, thereby raising the pain threshold *or* (2) that SIB may be maintained (reinforced) in some individuals by the endogenous opioids that are released following SIB (Aman, 1993; Sandman *et al.,* 1998). Either theory, if correct, would suggest that opiate blockers may be a useful therapy. There have been numerous case reports and a few group studies with the opiate blockers naloxone and naltrexone. Most of the case reports were positive, but the group studies had mixed outcomes (Werry & Aman, 1998). Our appraisal of the literature leads us to conclude that further studies of naltrexone are warranted. If the opiate blockers are effective, the mechanism may not necessarily be related to the opiate system. For example, naltrexone also appears to cause a degree of anxiolysis, and we already know that SIB can be stress-related in some individuals.

STEREOTYPED BEHAVIOR

Description

Stereotyped behavior refers to a group of behaviors that are topographically quite distinct, including body rocking, mouthing, finger and hand movements, and object manipulation. It is classified as Stereotypic Movement Disorder in the DSM-IV, the same diagnostic category as self-injury (American Psychiatric Association, 1994). Stereotyped behavior is distinguished from both movement disorders such as Tourette's syndrome and from compulsive rituals. Most definitions include the concept that the behavior serves no apparent adaptive function, although the subjective nature of this criterion is viewed as problematic (Berkson, Gutermuth, & Baranek, 1995). Stereotyped behavior is said to interfere with learning, adaptive behavior, and community integration and is said to be stigmatizing.

Prevalence

It has been estimated that approximately 15% of young children with MR exhibit stereotyped behavior (Wehmeyer, 1994). Most develop it in the second year of life or later. Jacobson (1982) reported that 5.8% of individuals of all ages with MR served by the state of New York exhibited stereotyped behaviors. Only stereotyped behavior that interfered with independent functioning was recorded.

In Rojahn's (1986) large-scale survey of both stereotyped behavior and SIB, stereotypies were present in 65% of individuals (mostly adults) with SIB and in 62% of those without SIB. The most common was body rocking. The findings suggested that some stereotypies are more closely associated with certain SIBs than with others, for example, body rocking with head hitting and self-restraint with pinching.

Presentation of Stereotyped Behavior in MR

Many types of stereotyped behavior have been identified. Berkson and colleagues (1995) examined 54 behaviors including staring, licking and smelling objects, unusual play, picking objects apart, body rocking, hand flapping, unusual noises, hand gaze, and spinning objects. A factor analysis of data collected from a large survey identified several factors: Rigidity or Maintenance of Sameness, Auditory or Repetitive Verbal, Visual Orientation, Object Stereotypy, Focused Affection, Music-Motor, and two unnamed factors.

Stereotyped behavior also occurs in normal children during the course of development. When children with developmental delays and control children were compared, key differentiating characteristics were that the behavior of the children with developmental delays involved more gross motor movement and visual orientation than did the behavior of the control children (Smith & Van Houten, 1996). These characteristics contributed to the behavior's being more noticeable and seeming more "bizarre." Visual orientation to the stereotyped behavior would, of course, interfere with attention to and participation in ongoing activities.

Stereotyped behavior has been described as serving various functions, including regulating arousal level, providing stimulation, and providing perceptual feedback (Buyer, Berkson, Winnega, & Morton, 1987; Rojahn & Sisson, 1990). Buyer and colleagues found that stimulation and control of body rocking were separate processes and that control was more often preferred than not. Behavioral models suggest that it develops as a learned response to escape or avoid unpleasant situations, that it is maintained by external positive reinforcement, or both (Rojahn & Sisson, 1990). According to Berkson and colleagues (1995), "patterns of stereotyped behavior may be developed and maintained by different factors and are regulated from moment to moment by different events" (p. 137).

Risk Factors

Stereotyped behavior is characteristic of individuals with severe and profound MR (Rojahn & Sisson, 1990). It is also associated with certain syndromes, including Rett's syndrome, Fragile X, and autism. Stereotyped behavior is less common in young children and in older individuals (Rojahn & Sisson, 1990).

Low-stimulation environments are thought to contribute to the development of stereotyped behaviors. A study of nonhandicapped children in residential care reported that 58.5% displayed one or more stereotypes at least once a week and more than half at least once a day (Tröster, 1994). Stereotyped behavior was more frequent among children for whom child abuse was suspected and those with aggressive behavior problems.

Treatment

Rojahn and Sisson (1990) summarized the behavioral treatment of stereotyped behaviors. They noted that some treatment studies failed to indicate the rationale for treatment and that intervention may not be required for all stereotyped behaviors as some have few negative effects on the individual.

Gorman-Smith & Matson (1985) performed a meta-analysis of behavioral treatment studies of stereotyped behavior and SIB. The studies used interventions based on operant techniques, including DRO, DRL, and punishment procedures. The most frequently treated stereotyped behavior was body rocking. No gender differences in treatment effectiveness were found and the individual's level of functioning had an unclear effect on the outcome. The authors suggested that treatment effectiveness may be determined by the type of problem, the severity, the length of time of treatment, age, and cognitive level.

In a more recent meta-analysis, Wehmeyer (1995) measured treatment efficacy by evaluating studies based on the percentage of nonoverlapping data (PND) and the percentage of zero data (PZD). PND is the percentage of treatment data points that are below the lowest baseline point. The PZD index is the percentage of treatment data points that remain at a zero level after the first zero point. The studies were grouped according to the part of the body involved in the stereotyped behavior. A high average PND (81%) was found, indicating that many treatments were successful in reducing the behavior below baseline. Treatments were less successful in completely eliminating the behavior, however. Complete elimination was more likely to be obtained with older children (10 years and up). No significant effects were noted for gender or level of functioning. Stereotyped behavior involving the torso seemed to be the most difficult to treat. The findings suggest that one should be cautious when analyzing effects of treatment to avoid overgeneralizing results on stereotyped behaviors of different topographies.

Rojahn and Sisson (1990) concluded that elimination of stereotyped behavior is not achieved by reinforcement of some other behaviors alone (DRO). Further, studies indicate that time-out and extinction are ineffective treatments (Wehmeyer, 1995).

The influence of the setting events on the rate of occurrence of stereotyped behavior has been well documented (Repp, Singh, Karsh, & Deitz, 1991). Based on the results of an observational study of preschool children in which significant variation in rates were noted during different classroom activities, Baumeister, MacLean, Kelly, and Kasari (1980) stated that minimal generalization of treatment effects should be expected from one setting to another. Further, stereotyped behavior is related to the repertoire of appropriate behavior the individual has available in any situation. Thus, intervention aimed at increasing appropriate behaviors is a logical treatment goal. It has also been suggested that individuals be trained to engage in different stereotyped behaviors that are less disruptive (Smith & Van Houten, 1996) and be provided with more opportunities to control their environment (Buyer et al., 1987).

In terms of pharmacotherapy, patients are seldom treated solely for the presence of stereotypic behavior, although stereotypy frequently co-occurs with other disruptive behavior. Several well-controlled studies have shown that antipsychotic medication frequently reduces stereotypic behavior (Aman, 1997). Furthermore, Aman (1997) suggested that stereotypy may be a useful patient marker. He presented data suggesting that subjects with high rates of stereotypy may respond better to neuroleptics on *other* clinical variables than patients with low rates. Some authors have suggested that clomipramine and SSRIs may be useful for reducing ritualistic, stereotyped, and compulsive behavior in adults with MR (Lewis, Aman, Gadow, Schroeder, & Thompson, 1996). However, there is some question as to whether these are true stereotypies or whether they are a form of obsessive-compulsive disorder.

SUMMARY

Four types of DBD in youth with MR were addressed: ADHD, aggression and conduct problems, SIB, and stereotyped behavior. ADHD-type behavior appears to be much the same in youth with MR as it is in the general population. One area of distinction may be that aggression is less in evidence in ADHD children with MR than in other ADHD youth. Aggression and conduct problems are quite prevalent in children with MR. The form of the behavior seems to vary with the level of intellectual functioning. Interventions tend to focus on aggressive behavior and few treatment studies have been conducted with specific diagnostic groups.

Chronic SIB appears almost solely in the developmental disabilities. The potential for serious harm and the distressed reaction of caregivers has resulted in vigorous pharmacological and behavioral interventions. Stereotyped behavior, often co-occurring with SIB, has received less independent attention. Treatments are effective in reducing stereotypies, but are less successful at eliminating them completely.

The literature on DBD in children with MR often lacks the depth found in the study of youth in the general population. This is not surprising, although it is unfortunate, given that MR is an orphan clinical population. We need to bear in mind that MR is a relatively infrequent condition and that the disorders discussed in this chapter represent a percentage of all disorders in that select population. Further, the multifaceted nature of MR adds to the complexity of the etiology, diagnosis, and treatment process. For example, the etiologies associated with MR are extremely varied, which further complicates their systematic study.

REFERENCES

Aman, M. G. (1991). *Assessing psychopathology and behavior problems in persons with mental retardation: A review of available instruments* (DHHS Publication No. [ADM] 91-1712). Rockville, MD: U. S. Department of Health and Human Services.

Aman, M. G. (1993). Efficacy of psychotropic drugs for reducing self-injurious behavior in the developmental disabilities. *Annals of Clinical Psychiatry, 4,* 171–188.

Aman, M. G. (1996). Stimulant drugs in the developmental disabilities revisited. *Journal of Developmental and Physical Disabilities, 8,* 347–365.

Aman, M. G. (1997). Recent studies in psychopharmacology in mental retardation. In N. Bray (Ed.), *International review of research in mental retardation* (Vol. 21, pp. 113–146). San Diego, CA: Academic Press.

Aman, M. G., & Singh, N. N. (1980). The usefulness of thioridazine for treating childhood disorders—Fact or folklore? *American Journal of Mental Deficiency, 84,* 331–338.

Aman, M. G., & Singh, N. N. (1991). Pharmacological intervention. In J. L. Matson & J. A. Mulick (Eds.), *Handbook of mental retardation* (2nd ed., pp. 347–372). New York: Pergamon.

Aman, M. G., Singh, N. N., Stewart, A. W., & Field, C. J. (1985). The Aberrant Behavior Checklist. *Psychopharmacology Bulletin, 21,* 845–850.

Aman, M. G., Richmond, G., Stewart, A. W., Bell, J. C., & Kissel, R. C. (1987). The Aberrant Behavior Checklist: Factor structure and the effect of subject variables in American and New Zealand facilities. *American Journal of Mental Deficiency, 91,* 570–578.

Aman, M. G., Hammer, D., & Rojahn, J. (1993). Mental retardation. In T. H. Ollendick & M. Hersen (Eds.), *Handbook of child and adolescent assessment* (pp. 321–345). Boston: Allyn and Bacon.

Aman, M. G., Pejeau, C., Osborne, P., Rojahn, J., & Handen, B. (1996). Four-year follow-up of children with low intelligence and ADHD. *Research in Developmental Disabilities, 17,* 417–432.

Aman, M. G., Tassé, M. J., Rojahn, J., & Hammer, D. (1996). The Nisonger CBRF: A child behavior rating form for children with developmental disabilities. *Research in Developmental Disabilities, 17,* 41–57.

American Psychiatric Association. (1980). *Diagnostic and statistical manual of mental disorders* (3rd ed.). Washington, DC: Author.

American Psychiatric Association. (1994). *Diagnostic and statistical manual of mental disorders* (4th ed.). Washington, DC: Author.

Ando, I., & Yoshimura, I. (1978). Prevalence of maladaptive behavior in retarded children as a function of IQ and age. *Journal of Abnormal Child Psychology, 6,* 345–349.

Bachman, J. E., & Sluyter, D. (1988). Reducing inappropriate behaviors of developmentally disabled adults using antecedent aerobic dance exercises. *Research in Developmental Disabilities, 9,* 73–83.

Barkley, R. A. (1990). *Attention-deficit hyperactivity disorder: A handbook for diagnosis and treatment.* New York: Guilford.

Baumeister, A. A., MacLean, W. E., Kelly, J., & Kasari, C. (1980). Observational studies of retarded children with multiple stereotyped movements. *Journal of Abnormal Child Psychology, 8,* 501–521.

Benson, B. A. (1985). Behavior disorders and mental retardation: Associations with age, sex, and level of functioning in an outpatient clinic sample. *Applied Research in Mental Retardation, 6,* 79–85.

Benson, B. A. (1992). *Teaching anger management to persons with mental retardation.* Worthington, OH: IDS.

Benson, B. A., Rice, C. J., & Miranti, S. V. (1986). Effects of anger management training with mentally retarded adults in group treatment. *Journal of Consulting and Clinical Psychology, 54,* 728–729.

Berkson, G., Gutermuth, L., & Baranek, G. (1995). Relative prevalence and relations among stereotyped and similar behaviors. *American Journal on Mental Retardation, 100,* 137–145.

Borthwick-Duffy, S. (1994). Prevalence of destructive behaviors: A study of aggression, self-injury, and property destruction. In T. Thompson & D. B. Gray (Eds.), *Destructive behavior in developmental disabilities* (pp. 3–23). Thousand Oaks, CA: Sage.

Bruininks, R. H., Hill, B. K., Weatherman, R. F., & Woodcock, R. W. (1986). *Inventory for client and agency planning.* Allen, TX: DLM Teaching Resources.

Bruininks, R. H., Hill, B. K., & Morreau, L. E. (1988). Prevalence and implications of maladaptive behaviors and dual diagnosis in residential and other service programs. In J. A. Stark, F. J. Menolascino, M. H. Albarelli, & V. C. Gray (Eds.), *Mental retardation and mental health: Classification, diagnosis, treatment, services* (pp. 3–29). New York: Springer-Verlag.

Buyer, L., Berkson, G., Winnega, M. A., & Morton, L. (1987). Stimulation and control as components of stereotyped body rocking. *American Journal of Mental Retardation, 91,* 543–547.

Cataldo, M. F. (1990). *The effects of punishment and other behavior reducing procedures on the destructive behaviors of persons with developmental disabilities.* Unpublished manuscript provided to NIH Consensus Committee on Destructive Behavior, Washington, DC.

Coccaro, E. F. (1989). Central serotonin and impulsive aggression. *British Journal of Psychiatry, 155* (Suppl. 8), 52–62.

Coe, D. A., & Matson, J. L. (1993). Hyperactivity and disorders of impulse control. In J. L. Matson & R. P. Barrett (Eds.), *Psychopathology in the mentally retarded* (2nd ed., pp. 253–271). Boston: Allyn and Bacon.

Cullinan, D., Epstein, M. H., Matson, J. L., & Rosemier, R. A. (1984). Behavior problems of mentally retarded and nonretarded adolescent pupils. *School Psychology Review, 13,* 381–384.

Davanzo, P. A., Belin, R. R., Widawski, M. H., & King, B. H. (1998). Paroxetine treatment of aggression and self injury in persons with mental retardation. *American Journal on Mental Retardation, 102,* 427–437.

Davidson, P. W., Cain, N. N., Sloane-Reeves, J. E., Van Speybroech, A., Segal, J., Gutkin, J., Quijano, L. E., Kramer, B. M, Parter, B., Shoham, I., & Goldstein, E. (1994). Characteristics of community-based individuals with mental retardation and aggressive behavioral disorders. *American Journal on Mental Retardation, 98,* 704–716.

Durand, V. M. (1988). The Motivation Assessment Scale. In M. Hersen & A. S. Bellack (Eds.), *Dictionary of behavioral assessment techniques* (pp. 309–310). New York: Pergamon.

Durand, V. M., & Carr, E. G. (1985). Self-injurious behavior: Motivating conditions and guidelines for treatment. *School Psychology Review, 14,* 171–176.

Durand, V. M., & Crimmins, D. B. (1988). Identifying the variables maintaining self-injurious behavior. *Journal of Autism and Developmental Disorders, 18,* 99–117.

Einfeld, S. L. (1992). Clinical assessment of psychiatric symptoms in mentally retarded individuals. *Australian and New Zealand Journal of Psychiatry, 26,* 48–63.

Einfeld, S. L., & Aman, M. G. (1995). Issues in the taxonomy of psychopathology in children and adolescents with mental retardation. *Journal of Autism and Developmental Disorders, 25,* 143–167.

Einfeld, S. L., & Tonge, B. J. (1991). Psychometric and clinical assessment of psychopathology in developmentally disabled children. *Australia and New Zealand Journal of Developmental Disabilities, 17,* 147–154.

Epstein, M. H., Cullinan, D., & Gadow, K. D. (1986). Teacher ratings of hyperactivity in learning-disabled, emotionally disturbed, and mentally retarded children. *Journal of Special Education, 20,* 219–229.

Eyman, R. K., & Call, T. (1977). Maladaptive behavior and community placement of mentally retarded persons. *American Journal of Mental Deficiency, 82,* 137–144.

Eyman, R. K., Borthwick, S. A., & Miller, C. (1981). Trends in maladaptive behavior of mentally retarded persons placed in community and institutional settings. *American Journal of Mental Deficiency, 85,* 473–477.

Fee, V. E., & Matson, J. L. (1992). Definition, classification, and taxonomy. In J. K. Luiselli, J. L. Matson, & N. N. Singh (Eds.), *Self-injurious behavior: Analysis, assessment, and treatment* (pp. 3–20). New York: Springer-Verlag.

Fee, V. E., Matson, J. L., Moore, L. A., & Benavidez, D. A. (1993). The differential validity of hyperactivity/attention deficits and conduct problems among mentally retarded children. *Journal of Abnormal Child Psychology, 21,* 1–11.

Fee, V. E., Matson, J. L., & Benavidez, D. A. (1994). Attention deficit-hyperactivity disorder among mentally retarded children. *Research in Developmental Disabilities, 15,* 67–79.

Gardner, W. I., & Cole, C. L. (1993). Aggression and related conduct disorders: Definition, assessment, and treatment. In J. L. Matson & R. P. Barrett (Eds.), *Psychopathology in the mentally retarded* (2nd ed., pp. 213–252). Needham Heights, MA: Allyn and Bacon.

Gorman-Smith, D., & Matson, J. (1985). A review of treatment research for self-injurious and stereotyped responding. *Journal of Mental Deficiency Research, 29,* 295–308.

Goyette, C. H., Conners, C. K., & Ulrich, R. T. (1978). Normative data on revised Conners Parent and Teacher Scales. *Journal of Abnormal Child Psychology, 6,* 221–236.

Gualtieri, C. T., & Schroeder, S. R. (1989). Pharmacotherapy for self injurious behavior: Preliminary tests of the D_1 hypothesis. *Psychopharmacology Bulletin, 25,* 364–371.

Handen, B. L., Janosky, J., & McAuliffe, S. (1997). Long-term follow-up of children with mental retardation and ADHD. *Journal of Abnormal Child Psychology, 25,* 287–295.

Handen, B. L., McAuliffe, S., Janosky, J., Feldman, H., & Breaux, A. M. (1994). Classroom behavior and children with mental retardation: Comparison of children with and without ADHD. *Journal of Abnormal Child Psychology, 22,* 267–280.

Harris, J. C. (1992). Neurobiological factors in self-injurious behavior. In J. K. Luiselli, J. L. Matson, & N. N. Singh (Eds.), *Self-injurious behavior: Analysis, assessment, and treatment* (pp. 59–92). New York: Springer-Verlag.

Harris, P. (1993). The nature and extent of aggressive behaviour amongst people with learning difficulties (mental handicap) in a single health district. *Journal of Intellectual Disability Research, 37,* 221–242.

Hill, B. K., & Bruininks, R. H. (1984). Maladaptive behavior of mentally retarded individuals in residential facilities. *American Journal of Mental Deficiency, 88,* 380–387.

Hill, B. K., Balow, E. A., & Bruininks, R. H. (1985). A national study of prescribed drugs in institutions and community residential facilities for mentally retarded people. *Psychopharmacology Bulletin, 21,* 279–284.

Hurley, A. D., & Sovner, R. (1995). Six cases of patients with mental retardation who have antisocial personality disorder. *Psychiatric Services, 46,* 828–831.

Hutt, S. J., & Hutt, C. (1964). Hyperactivity in a group of epileptic (and some non-epileptic) brain-damaged children. *Epilepsia, 5,* 334–351.

Iwata, B. A., Dorsey, M. F., Slifer, J. K., Bauman, K. E., & Richman G. S. (1994). Toward a functional analysis of self-injury. *Journal of Applied Behavior Analysis, 27,* 197–209.

Jacobson, J. W. (1982). Problem behavior and psychiatric impairment within a developmentally disabled population: I. Behavior frequency. *Applied Research in Mental Retardation, 3,* 121–139.

Koller, H., Richardson, S. A., Katz, M., & McLaren, J. (1982). Behavior disturbance in childhood and the early adult years in populations who were and were not mentally retarded. *Journal of Preventive Psychiatry, 1,* 453–468.

Koller, H., Richardson, S. A., Katz, M., & McLaren, J. (1983). Behavior disturbance since childhood among a 5-year birth cohort of all mentally retarded young adults in a city. *American Journal of Mental Deficiency, 87,* 386–395.

Lakin, K. C., Hill, B. K., Hauber, F. A., Bruininks, R. H., & Heal, L. W. (1983). New admissions and readmissions to a national sample of public residential facilities. *American Journal of Mental Deficiency, 88,* 13–20.

Lewis, M. H., Aman, M. G., Gadow, K. D., Schroeder, S. R., & Thompson, T. (1996). Psychopharmacology. In J. W. Jacobson & J. A. Mulick (Eds.), *Manual of diagnosis and professional practice in mental retardation* (pp. 323–340). Washington, DC: American Psychological Association.

Loney, J., & Milich, R. (1982). Hyperactivity, inattention, and aggression in clinical practice. In M. Wolraich & D. K. Routh (Eds.), *Advances in developmental and behavioral pediatrics* (pp. 113–147). Greenwich, CT: JAI.

Luckasson, R., Coulter, D., Polloway, E., Reiss, S., Schalock, R. L., Snell, M., Spitalnik, D., & Stark, J. A. (1992). *Mental retardation: Definition, classification, and systems of supports.* Washington, DC: American Association on Mental Retardation.

Lundervold, D., & Bourland, G. (1988). Quantitative analysis of treatment of aggression, self-injury, and property destruction. *Behavior Modification, 12,* 590–617.

Matson, J. L., & Gorman-Smith, D. (1986). A review of treatment research for aggressive and disruptive behavior in the mentally retarded. *Applied Research in Mental Retardation, 7,* 95–103.

McGimsey, J. F., & Favell, J. E. (1988). The effects of increased physical exercise on disruptive behavior in retarded persons. *Journal of Autism and Developmental Disorders, 18,* 167–179.

McGrew, K. S., Ittenbach, R. F., Bruininks, R. H., & Hill, B. K. (1991). Factor structure of maladaptive behavior across the lifespan of persons with mental retardation. *Research in Developmental Disabilities, 12,* 181–199.

Melnyk, L. & Das, J. P. (1992). Measurement of attention deficit: Correspondence between rating scales and tests of sustained and selective attention. *American Journal on Mental Retardation, 96,* 599–606.

Myers, B. A. (1987). Psychiatric problems in adolescents with developmental disabilities. *Journal of the American Academy of Child and Adolescent Psychiatry, 26,* 74–79.

Pearson, D. A., & Aman, M. G. (1994). Ratings of hyperactivity and developmental indices: Should clinicians correct for developmental level? *Journal of Autism and Developmental Disorders, 24,* 395–411.

Pearson, D. A., Lachar, D., & Loveland, K. A. (1995, September). *Behavioral problems in children with mild mental retardation: A comparison of children with and without ADHD.* Paper presented to the first congress of Mental Health in Mental Retardation, Amsterdam.

Pearson, D. A., Norton, A. M., & Farwell, E. C. (1997). Attention deficit/hyperactivity disorder in mental retardation: Nature of attention deficits. In J. T. Enns & J. Burack (Eds.), *Attention, development, and psychopathology* (pp. 205–229). New York: Guilford.

Pearson, D. A., Yaffee, L. S., Loveland, K. A., & Lewis, K. R. (1996). Comparison of sustained and selective attention in children who have mental retardation with and without attention deficit hyperactivity disorder. *American Journal on Mental Retardation, 100,* 592–607.

Philips, I., & Williams, N. (1975). Psychopathology and mental retardation: A study of 100 mentally retarded children: I. Psychopathology. *American Journal of Psychiatry, 132,* 1265–1271.

Philips, I., & Williams, N. (1977). Psychopathology and mental retardation: A statistical study of 100 mentally retarded children treated at a psychiatric clinic: II. Hyperactivity. *American Journal of Psychiatry, 134,* 418–419.

Polloway, E. A., Epstein, M. H., & Cullinan, D. (1985). Prevalence of behavior problems among educable mentally retarded students. *Education and Training in Mental Retardation, 20,* 3–13.

Quay, H. C., & Gredler, Y. (1981). Dimensions of problem behavior in institutionalized retardates. *Journal of Abnormal Child Psychology, 9,* 523–528.

Quay, H. C., & Peterson, D. R. (1975). *Manual for the behavior problem checklist.* Unpublished checklist. Available from H. C. Quay, University of Miami, Coral Gables, FL.

Quine, L. (1986). Behavior problems in severely mentally handicapped children. *Psychological Medicine, 16,* 895–907.

Reid, A. H. (1980). Psychiatric disorders in mentally handicapped children: A clinical and follow-up study. *Journal of Mental Deficiency, 24,* 287–298.

Reiss, S. (1994). *Handbook of challenging behaviors: Mental health aspects of mental retardation.* Worthington, OH: IDS.

Reiss, S., & Rojahn, J. (1993). Joint occurrence of depression and aggression in children and adults with mental retardation. *Journal of Intellectual Disability Research, 37,* 287–294.

Reiss, S., & Szyszko, J. (1983). Diagnostic overshadowing and professional experience with retarded persons. *American Journal of Mental Deficiency, 87,* 396–402.

Reiss, S., Levitan, G., & McNally, R. J. (1982). Emotionally disturbed, mentally retarded people: An underserved population. *American Psychologist, 37,* 361–367.

Repp, A. C., Singh, N. N., Karsh, G. K., & Deitz, D. E. D. (1991). Ecobehavioral analysis of stereotypic and adaptive behaviors: Activities as setting events. *Journal of Mental Deficiency Research, 35,* 413–429.

Richardson, S. A., Koller, H., & Katz, M. (1985). Relationship of upbringing to later behavior disturbance of mildly mentally retarded young people. *American Journal of Mental Deficiency, 90,* 1–8.

Rojahn, J. (1986). Self-injurious and stereotypic behavior of noninstitutionalized mentally retarded people: Prevalence and classification. *American Journal of Mental Retardation, 91,* 268–276.

Rojahn, J. (1994). Epidemiology and topographic taxonomy of self-injurious behavior. In T. Thompson & D. B. Gray (Eds.), *Destructive behavior in developmental disabilities: Diagnosis and treatment* (pp. 49–67). Thousand Oaks, CA: Sage.

Rojahn, J., & Sisson, L. (1990). Stereotyped behavior. In J. Matson (Ed.), *Handbook of behavior modification with the mentally retarded* (2nd ed., pp. 181–223). New York: Plenum.

Rutter, M., Tizard, J., Yule, W., Graham, P., & Whitmore, K. (1976). Isle of Wight studies, 1964–1974. *Psychological Medicine, 6,* 313–332.

Sandman, C., Thompson, T., Barrett, R. P., Verhoeven, W., McCubbin, J. A., Schroeder, S. R., & Hetrick, W. D. (1998). Opiate blockers. In S. Reiss & M. G. Aman (Eds.), *Psychotropic medications and developmental disabilities: The international consensus handbook* (pp. 291–302). Columbus, OH: Nisonger Center UAP.

Singh, N. N., Winton, A. S., & Ball, P. M. (1984). Effects of physical restraint on the behavior of hyperactive mentally retarded persons. *American Journal on Mental Deficiency, 89,* 16–22.

Smith, C., Algonzzine, B., Schmid, R., & Hennly, T. (1990). Prison adjustment of youthful inmates with mental retardation. *Mental Retardation, 28,* 177–181.

Smith, E. A., & Van Houten, R. (1996). A comparison of the characteristics of self-stimulatory behaviors in "normal" children and children with developmental delays. *Research in Developmental Disabilities, 17,* 253–268.

Sovner, R., Pary, R. J., Dosen, A., Gedye, A., Barrera, F. J., Cantwell, D. P., & Huessy, H. R. (1998). Antidepressant drugs. In S. Reiss & M. G. Aman (Eds.), *Psychotropic medications and developmental disabilities: The international consensus handbook* (pp. 179–200). Columbus, OH: Nisonger Center UAP.

Sprague, J. R., & Horner, R. H. (1994). Covariation within functional response classes: Implications for treatment of severe problem behavior. In T. Thompson & D. B. Gray (Eds.), *Destructive behavior in developmental disabilities* (pp. 213–242). Thousand Oaks, CA: Sage.

Stark, J. A., Menolascino, F. J., Albarelli, M. H., & Gray, V.

(1988). Executive summary. In J. A. Stark, F. J. Menolascino, M. H. Albarelli, & V. C. Gray (Eds.), *Mental retardation and mental health: Classification, diagnosis, treatment, services* (pp. xi–xviii). New York: Springer-Verlag.

Taylor, E. A. (1986). Childhood hyperactivity. *British Journal of Psychiatry, 149,* 562–573.

Thompson, T., Axtell, S., & Schaal, D. (1993). Self-injurious behavior: Mechanisms and intervention. In J. L. Matson & R. P. Barrett (Eds.), *Psychopathology in the mentally retarded* (2nd ed., pp. 179–211). Boston: Allyn and Bacon.

Thompson, T., Egli, M., Symons, F., & Delaney, D. (1994). Neurobehavioral mechanisms of drug action in developmental disabilities. In T. Thompson & D. B. Gray (Eds.), *Destructive behavior in developmental disabilities* (pp. 133–180). Thousand Oaks, CA: Sage.

Thorley, G. (1984). Hyperkinetic syndrome of childhood: Clinical characteristics. *British Journal of Psychiatry, 144,* 16–24.

Tizard, B. (1968a). Observations of over-active imbecile children in controlled and uncontrolled environments: I. Classroom studies. *American Journal of Mental Deficiency, 72,* 540–547.

Tizard, B. (1968b). Observations of over-active imbecile children in controlled and uncontrolled environments: II. Experimental studies. *American Journal of Mental Deficiency, 72,* 548–553.

Tonge, B., & Einfeld, S. (1991). Intellectual disability and psychopathology in Australian children. *Australia and New Zealand Journal of Developmental Disabilities, 17,* 155–167.

Tröster, H. (1994). Prevalence and functions of stereotyped behaviors in nonhandicapped children in residential care. *Journal of Abnormal Child Psychology, 22,* 79–97.

Twardosz, S., & Sajwaj, T. (1972). Multiple effects of a procedure to increase sitting in a hyperactive, retarded boy. *Journal of Applied Behavior Analysis, 5,* 73–78.

Wehmeyer, M. L. (1994). Factors related to the expression of typical and atypical repetitive movements of young children with intellectual disability. *International Journal of Disability, Development and Education, 41,* 33–49.

Wehmeyer, M. L. (1995). Intra-individual factors influencing efficacy of interventions for stereotyped behaviours: A meta-analysis. *Journal of Intellectual Disability Research, 39,* 205–214.

Werry, J. S., & Aman, M. G. (1998). Anxiolytics, sedatives, and miscellaneous drugs. In J. S. Werry & M. G. Aman (Eds.), *Practitioner's guide to psychoactive drugs for children and adolescents* (2nd ed., pp. 433–469). New York: Plenum Medical Books.

Wirt, R. D., Lachar, D., Klinedinst, J. K., & Seat, P. D. (1984). *Multidimensional description of child personality: A manual for the Personality Inventory for Children* (Rev. ed.). Los Angeles: Western Psychological Services.

27

Ethical Issues in Research with Children and Adolescents with Disruptive Behavior Disorders

PETER S. JENSEN, CELIA B. FISHER,
and KIMBERLY HOAGWOOD

INTRODUCTION

Converging evidence suggests that all of the major mental illnesses affecting adults also afflict children (Institute of Medicine, 1989) but research on child and adolescent mental disorders has generally lagged far behind studies of adult mental illnesses. These research gaps continue to exist for a variety of reasons, including difficulties recruiting child and adolescent subjects into research studies; wariness of the pharmaceutical industry about potential liability if wide-scale child-based pharmaceutical research were supported; lack of agreement among the lay public, professions, and various research disciplines about the appropriateness of classification and diagnoses in children and adolescents; insufficient research funding; and the special ethical challenges in conducting research with children and adolescents. These

PETER S. JENSEN and KIMBERLY HOAGWOOD • Division of Mental Disorders, Behavioral Research, and AIDS, National Institute of Mental Health, Rockville, Maryland 20857-8030.   CELIA B. FISHER • Department of Psychology, Fordham University, New York, New York 10458.

Handbook of Disruptive Behavior Disorders, edited by Quay and Hogan. Kluwer Academic/Plenum Publishers, New York, 1999.

factors have together combined to limit research in this population, with the result that children have been described as "therapeutic orphans," less likely than adults to reap the benefits of new knowledge on the safety and efficacy of various treatment alternatives.

Interestingly, the research area of Attention-Deficit/Hyperactivity Disorder (ADHD) is perhaps the single greatest exception to this general rule, having survived over three decades. It constitutes the single greatest area of research activity in the NIMH children's mental disorders research portfolio for the past decade. Nonetheless, the ethical challenges that affect the implementation of research in ADHD and other Disruptive Behavior Disorders (DBD) are formidable, and investigators studying this population must address these difficulties if their research is to meet federal standards and achieve maximum benefit for the populations of children and families such research is ultimately destined to reach.

In this chapter we review the regulatory protections that apply to research with children and adolescents, identify areas of ethical challenges in the conduct of research with children, discuss the application of these guidelines based on examples drawn from studies of ADHD, and propose a reconceptualization of the relationships between investigators and families in order to address many of these challenges not just in studies of children and adults with ADHD but also in children with other mental illnesses.

REGULATORY PROTECTIONS

Just as is the case with adults, ethical justification for the conduct of research in children rests on demonstrating a favorable balance of risks to benefits for participating children. Under most circumstances, however, for research to be approvable for children and adolescents it must have the potential to benefit the participant directly or enhance knowledge of the child or adolescent's disorder or condition. The federal guidelines for allowable research with children were published in final form in 1983 (U.S. Department of Health and Human Services [DHHS], 1983), based on the work and findings of the National Commission for the Protection of Human Subjects of Biomedical and Behavioral Research (National Commission, 1977). These guidelines recognized the special vulnerability of child participants in human subjects research. Hence, they were written to ensure that children's rights and welfare are protected, particularly when the research entails more than minimal risk. These provisions, as described in the DHHS regulations 45 CFR 46 Subpart D, are described in the following sections.

Minimal-Risk Research

Research is considered minimal risk when "the probability and magnitude of harm or discomfort anticipated in the research are not greater in and of themselves than those ordinarily encountered in daily life or during the performance of routine physical or psychological examinations or tests" (DHHS 46.102[i]). Research involving venipunctures and most psychological assessments routinely fit under this category. Often, one can minimize risk even further by selecting minimum levels of experimental manipulation necessary, and "piggy-backing" onto procedures already being performed on subjects for diagnostic or treatment purposes.

Research with More Than Minimal Risk but with the Prospect of Direct Benefit to Individual Subjects

When research involves more than minimal risk, guidelines specify that investigators justify the possible risks and discomforts in terms of the expected benefits to the child or to society as a whole. For example, in research involving greater than minimal risk (e.g., side effects of an experimental drug) DHHS 45 CFR 46.405 requires the investigator to demonstrate that any risks are justified by anticipated direct benefits to the participants, that the ratio of these benefits to the risk is at least as favorable to participants as available alternatives, and that appropriate steps are taken to obtain both guardian consent and the child's assent. In general, this research is termed "therapeutic research," meaning that some new treatment or procedure that entails some risk is offered to the child, but that the procedure itself may benefit the child participant directly, and that this benefit likely outweighs any potential risk of the intervention or of the illness itself. Obviously, this also means that research greater than minimal risk cannot be done using children as normal controls, since risks are deemed acceptable to a given child participant *only* if outweighed by the potential benefits to the child himself or herself, by virtue of the possibility of amelioration of the child's illness or condition.

Research with More Than Minimal Risk, No Prospect of Direct Individual Benefit, but Likely to Yield Disorder-Relevant Knowledge

When research involving greater than minimal risk holds out no prospect of direct benefit to the child participant, an acceptable balance of risk to benefits can still be achieved if it is likely that the research will yield generalizable knowledge of *vital* importance for the understanding or amelioration of the child's condition. In addition, the increased risk must represent only a *minor* increment over minimal risk *and* the research risk must be reasonably consistent with risks inherent in situations the child would be expected to experience (e.g., biomedical tests consistent with the child's disorder or condition). Finally, adequate steps must be taken to obtain guardian consent and child assent (DHHS 46.406).

Research Not Otherwise Approvable

Under certain circumstances, when research may provide an understanding, prevention, or alleviation of a serious problem affecting the health or welfare of children, the Secretary of the Department of Health and Human Services may approve research not otherwise considered acceptable under the regulations just described.

CONTROVERSIES IN CHILDREN'S MENTAL HEALTH RESEARCH

Definition of Minimal Risk

As noted by Kopelman (1989), the exact definition of minimal risk is "pivotal." Arnold and colleagues (1996) suggested that some Institutional Review Boards (IRBs) seem to interpret minimal risk as *no* risk. Yet if minimal risk means that the risks of harm anticipated in the proposed research are not greater than those ordinarily encountered in daily life, then this might imply taking into consideration the everyday risks that parents and society routinely approve for children, such as bike riding, riding in a car, swimming, or skiing. But opinions are often divided about this. Kopelman (1989) points out that the phrase "ordinarily encountered in daily life" can be variously interpreted as "all the risks ordinary people encounter, or the risks all people ordinarily encounter, or the minimal risks all ordinary people ordinarily encounter" (p. 88–89). Because risk can be interpreted in different ways and no single viewpoint is acceptable in all cases, IRBs should avoid being too restrictive,

which could otherwise create unnecessary obstacles to children's participation in research.

One approach to refining the concept of minimal risk has been offered by Arnold and colleagues (1996), who suggested the need to differentiate between risk and aversiveness. A procedure can have associated risks without being aversive or uncomfortable; conversely, a procedure can be aversive without entailing any meaningful risks. For example, Kruesi and colleagues (1988) found that spinal taps are no more aversive to children than attending school. Castellanos and colleagues (1994) have noted that the psychological risk of aversiveness can be minimized by preliminary rehearsal and role playing. Indeed, in our experience, in well-run research protocols the psychological risk and aversiveness can be minimal. Nonetheless, judgments concerning the risk–benefit ratio when using invasive procedures in pediatric research can be difficult, particularly when such procedures are employed in studies of normal pediatric populations; in such instances, controversy and differences of opinion about the definitions of minimal risk are common, and often vary across IRBs.

Confidentiality

Research on children and adolescents with DBD often elicits sensitive information that an individual may not wish revealed to others or that could produce harm if known beyond the research setting. Once a participant or his or her guardian has agreed to share personal information with a research team, investigators are obligated to ensure that information is not divulged to others in a manner inconsistent with the original agreement. However, routine procedures for maintaining confidentiality may not be sufficient when researchers are investigating sensitive or potentially stigmatizing information such as mental disorders, drug or alcohol abuse, child abuse, or illegal behaviors. Although special provisions are available to protect the confidentiality of sensitive information, research situations may arise in which the maintenance of confidentiality cannot be guaranteed. In general, such limitations on confidentiality should be noted in the consent form.

The Certificate of Confidentiality

When individual identifiers are required during the conduct of sensitive research (i.e., therapeutic or longitudinal research), routine procedures for assuring confidentiality may not be sufficient to protect the participant from harmful disclosures. For example, data collected on violent behavior, substance abuse, or parenting behaviors of adults with mental disorders may be subject to subpoena stemming from criminal investigations or custody disputes. In these circumstances investigators can apply for a Certificate of Confidentiality under 301[d] of the Public Health Service Act.

According to the law, the Certificate provides the investigator immunity from any governmental or civil order to disclose identifying information contained in research records. Even here caution is warranted, however, since the Certificate has not been challenged in court, and it is possible that circumstances could arise where such challenges could determine that the Certificate is not inviolable (Hoagwood, 1994). The Certificate does not necessarily override state reporting laws on child abuse, so investigators should consult their own appropriate state laws (see discussion about disclosure later in this chapter). Furthermore, the Certificate does not insulate the researcher from the requirement to disclose data about minor children to their parents; such protection can only be assured through permission by the parent or guardian at the time of informed consent (Hoagwood, 1994). When an investigator is granted a Certificate, both the protections and limitations of protection should be explained to child and adolescent participants and their parents.

Disclosures

Investigators studying DBD in childhood and youth may, during the course of research, become privy to information suggesting child abuse or threats of harm or violence to the participant or identified others. For example, following the 1976 Child Abuse Prevention and Treatment Act, all 50 states have enacted statutes mandating the reporting of suspected child abuse or neglect. In all states, this law pertains to mental health professionals and in at least 13 states to researchers, as members of the general public (Liss, 1994). Other states vary as to whether researchers are included in mandated reporting. Thus, investigators should review their own state laws to determine whether they or members of their research team are obligated to report child abuse and neglect (Fisher, 1991, 1993; Liss, 1994). At present, it is not clear whether researchers are legally required to release to authorities research records pertinent to the abuse after it is reported, and case examples exist of investigators both withholding and releasing such records. However, once reporting obligations are determined, the principal investigator needs to ensure that research personnel are trained to recognize indicators of abuse and to follow appropriate procedures. Such obligations should be fully communicated to both parents and minor participants at the time of informed consent (Fisher, 1993). In some instances, investigators choose not to ask specific questions about child abuse in situations where the obligation to report such information might place the participant at greater social or physical risk.

Protecting Participants from Self-Harm

In the course of research, investigators studying DBD or other high-risk children and youth may come upon information suggesting they may be contemplating suicide. Investigators need to be prepared for such circumstances by determining specific procedures to be followed if the possibility of self-harm is suspected. Participants and their guardians should be informed about these procedures prior to gaining permission to participate, and the researcher must be prepared to override a child or adolescent's request that information not be released.

Protecting Third Parties from Harm

An issue particularly relevant to developmental scientists who study family violence or DBD, especially Conduct Disorder (CD), is whether mental health researchers share with practitioner colleagues the responsibility to protect third parties about dangers posed by patients (Fisher, 1993). At present, investigators conducting such research should examine whether their role in research might meet the duty to protect as outlined by *Tarasoff v. Regents of the University of California* (1976): (1) a "special relationship" with a participant, (2) the ability to predict that violence will occur, and (3) the ability to identify the potential victim (Appelbaum & Rosenbaum, 1989). The presenting problems of some research participants (i.e. pedophiles) require advanced planning for protecting both the rights of the participants and the welfare of the community (Monahan, Appelbaum, Mulvey, Robbins, & Lidz, 1993). In recent years there has been considerable debate over the obligation to protect identifiable third parties from potential harm caused by the unsafe sex practices of an HIV-positive research participant. Investigators should approach such a situation with exteme caution, taking into account the fact that some state laws prohibit certain licensed professionals from revealing a client's HIV status.

Consent Procedures

Parental or Guardian Consent

Consent procedures for children and adolescents require special consideration for several reasons. Children do not have the legal capacity to consent and, depending on the age of the child and the nature of the research context, may lack the cognitive capacity to comprehend the purpose, scope, or nature of the study (Fisher, 1993; Melton, Koocher, & Saks, 1983; Thompson, 1992). Children may also feel incapable of refusing participation (Fisher & Rosendahl, 1990; Koocher & Keith-Spiegel, 1990; Levine, 1986). Thus, to ensure that the rights of minors

are protected, federal regulations require that adequate provisions be made for soliciting consent of parents, legal guardians, or those who act *in loco parentis*. According to Federal Regulation 46.408[b] the permission of one parent is sufficient for minimal risk research or research involving greater than minimal risk but presenting the prospect of direct benefit to the individual subject. Permission of both parents, where feasible, must be sought for research involving greater than minimal risk with no prospect of direct benefit and for research not otherwise approvable. Determining guardianship can sometimes present practical difficulties for investigators who work with children who are in the custody of state agencies.

Child Assent

In addition to parental or guardian consent, the rights of minors are further protected through the requirement that provisions are made for soliciting the assent of the child when he or she is capable (Federal Regulation 46.408[a]). *Assent* assumes that a child with a necessary level of cognitive capacity and emotional maturity understands the nature of the research and its risks and benefits and agrees to participate. Responsibility for determination of whether a child is capable of giving assent rests with the local IRB. For research with a very young child deemed not capable of providing assent, the research may proceed with parental consent alone. However, the objection of a child of any age is binding, unless the research holds out the prospect of direct benefit that is important to the child and only achievable through the experimental procedures. In designing assent procedures investigators need to take into account the child's maturity, cognitive abilities, his or her unique strengths and vulnerabilities, and the context (i.e., parent-caretaker and child relationship) in which decision making will take place.

Informed consent procedures, as currently required by federal regulations and professional ethical codes, are designed to protect participant autonomy by ensuring that the decision to participate is informed, rational, and voluntary. "Informed" refers to the investigator's obligation to fully disclose information about all procedures that might influence an individual's willingness to participate in a study. According to 45 CFR 46.116, such information must include the following: explanation of the purpose and duration of the research and a description of the procedures; a description of any foreseeable risks or discomforts; a description of potential benefits to the participant or others; disclosure of alternative procedures or treatments that may be advantageous to the subject; a description of the extent and limits of confidentiality; for research involving more than minimal risk, information regarding compensation and availability and nature of treatment if injury occurs; a statement describing the voluntary nature of the research; and the right to refuse participation or withdraw participation at any time without penalty. Particularly pertinent for children and adolescents, a further requirement of informed consent is that the information must be presented in a manner that is appropriate to the language usage and level of comprehension of the participant, his or her guardian, or both (Office of Protection from Research Risks [OPRR], 1993, pp. 3–14).

Federal guidelines require that informed consent be documented in most cases. However, under certain circumstances this requirement may be waived (45 CFR 46.117[c][1]). This includes circumstances wherein data are gathered through administrative records and no identifying information is transmitted. An additional requirement for informed consent arises in cases where information to be gathered is "sensitive." The OPRR considers research in sensitive areas to include child abuse, illegal activities, or reportable communicable diseases. Consequently, where the need to report such information to authorities is legally mandated, subjects should be so informed before agreeing to participate in the study (OPRR, 1993, pp. 3–14).

Child Assent in the Absence of Parental Consent

Significant numbers of high-risk children and adolescents with DBD have undetermined custody, nonrelative guardians, or state guar-

dianship (Gibbs, 1990; Hendren, 1991). In addition, the adverse physical or social environments in which some children live may make obtaining parental consent difficult or dangerous for the child. Federal regulations provide guidelines for helping investigators and institutional review boards determine the conditions under which requiring parental consent does not reasonably protect the welfare of minor research participants (45 CFR 46.408[c]). For example, children from neglecting or abusing families may be included in this category. In other types of research (e.g., studies on adolescent sexual activity or substance abuse) the solicitation of parental consent may violate a teenager's privacy or even jeopardize his or her welfare. Current state laws granting adolescents the autonomy to make health decisions concerning treatment for venereal disease, drug abuse, or emotional disorders have been used as a model to determine conditions under which guardian consent may be waived (Fisher, 1993; Holder, 1981).

In other situations parental consent may be waived when the research cannot be practically carried out without the waiver. However, despite the availability of a waiver, when research risks are minimal and informed consent infeasible, respect for the importance of family involvement in children's lives dictates that (in addition to child assent procedures) parental notification be offered as both a courtesy and a mechanism for providing additional information (45 CFR 46.115[d]; Nolan, 1992).

The Voluntary Nature of Consent

Investigators studying children with DBD and other psychopathologic disorders must be sensitive to the potentially coercive nature of informed consent procedures. Families contacted while seeking services at a hospital, mental health center, or social service agency may be concerned that failure to consent will result in a loss of services for themselves or for their children (Fisher, 1991, 1993; Fisher & Rosendahl, 1990) or that they may lose custody of their children altogether (Friesen & Koroloff, 1990; Osher & Telesford, 1996). Investigators also need to guard against potential conflicts of interest that may restrict the perceived voluntary nature of participation. For example, in the United States few services are available to treat children and adolescents as well as adults with DBD. As a rule resources are sparse, and insurance companies and third-party payors have restricted full access to the range and level of mental health services thought to be necessary for adequate treatment for many conditions. In this context, parents may feel a great sense of urgency in obtaining care for their children. A university-based research program may appear to be a godsend, alleviating families' sense of urgency and concerns about helping their child. They may be subject to the "therapeutic misconception," i.e., the perception that participation with their children in the research will make active and effective treatments available. Yet, given the current lack of knowledge concerning many clinical treatments of child and adolescent disorders, placebo treatments or other alternatives are critical in most, if not all, circumstances. Thus, in the context of the child's clinical needs, families may be severely disappointed if active treatment is not included as a part of their participation in a research program.

Informed consent should be conceptualized as an ongoing educational process between the investigator and prospective participant. It should be monitored and discussed throughout the course of the study. This is particularly relevant for the conduct of longitudinal studies where the nature of the assessment instruments may be modified to fit the changing developmental status of the participants, where the child's cognitive understanding and personal autonomy are increasing, and where issues of confidentiality may shift as a child participant reaches adolescence.

Passive Consent

Difficulty in acquiring guardian consent is not in itself sufficient to waive the requirement for obtaining it, simply as a means of overcoming low rates of parental response. In general, passive consent (when guardians are sent forms asking them to respond only if they do not wish their child to participate) is not an appropriate or ethical substitute for guardian consent, since it does not meet the standards set by the principles of beneficence, respect for persons, and justice (Fisher, 1993). The use of passive consent procedures with vulnerable, poor, and disenfranchised populations poses special ethical problems because it can create an unjust situation in which such children are disproportionately deprived of the protections afforded by guardian consent when compared with their less vulnerable peers.

Participant Advocates

When parental consent is waived or when children or adolescents are wards of the state, federal regulations (45 CFR 46) require that an advocate for the minor be present to (1) verify the minor's understanding of assent procedures, (2) support his or her preferences, (3) ensure that participation is voluntary, (4) check periodically whether the youth wants to terminate participation, (5) assess reactions to planned procedures, and (6) ensure that debriefing addresses all participant questions and concerns (OPRR, 1993, pp. 6–22). The participant advocate should have no investment in the research project or role in subject recruitment (Fisher, 1993).

Incentives for Participation

Offering incentives for participation is often used as a means of recruiting subjects. The decision to offer inducements creates an ethical tension between fair compensation for the time and inconvenience of research participation and undue coercion to participate in procedures to which subjects might not otherwise consent. Investigators must be particularly cautious when deciding on appropriate inducements for impoverished persons who may be willing to assume, or have their children assume, extraordinary burdens to receive payment (Levine, 1986). Subject payments should reflect the degree of risk, inconvenience, or discomfort associated with participation (OPRR, 1993, pp. 4–21). However, there is little consensus on what constitutes due and undue incentives for research participation (Macklin, 1981).

Ensuring Fair Representation and Access to Research Benefits

Investigators working with diverse or disadvantaged populations have the responsibility to (1) ensure that minority and lower socioeconomic status (SES) populations have equal access to research benefits and (2) ensure that they are not exposed to unfair distribution of research risks because of their vulnerability in the community. This requirement may present special challenges to investigators assessing mental health services for children and adolescents, because there sometimes may be serious questions raised as to the validity of existing measures to identify DBD or other forms of psychopathology across different populations. Such situations run the risk of under- or over-diagnosing children from minority and lower SES communities. Diagnostic errors can, in turn, result in minority and lower SES children being unfairly excluded from potentially advantageous treatment studies or unfairly over-represented in research, such as drug studies, that may present greater than minimal risk. Recruitment strategies for diverse populations can be enhanced through the establishment of advisory committees made up of minority representatives from the community and the mental health professions. The accuracy of research inclusion and exclusion criteria and assessment approaches can be further enhanced by ensuring that such methods meet highest standards for ecological and cultural validity.

CASE STUDIES

Balancing Risks and Benefits

Case 1

In one study, investigators sought to determine the side effects of fenfluramine in hyperactive children with mental retardation, in view of its consideration as a potential treatment alternative to stimulant medication. The investigators sought to examine five drug conditions (methylphenidate, placebo, and three different doses of fenfluramine). Although the

researchers had good arguments for the importance of examining fenfluramine, the agent is also somewhat controversial, since some animal studies had indicated that doses given over a short period could have long-lasting effects on serotonin (5-HT) receptors in some species' midbrain structures. Such evidence did not necessarily apply to humans but the investigators appropriately drew this to the attention of the IRB. To further assist the IRB in determining the risk–benefit ratio, the investigators pointed out that the agent had been used in much higher doses in the animal studies than normally used with humans, and that not all studies had replicated the purported effects in animals. They further noted the marked intraspecies differences in response to the agent, the lack of any evidence linking the 5-HT receptor changes with behavioral correlates, and, most importantly, the fact that it had been used for two decades in adults with no reports of adverse CNS consequences. The IRB accepted these arguments, since the study could help determine possible fenfluramine benefits in children who did not respond well to traditional stimulant treatments. To protect children from potential harm, parents were fully informed about the fenfluramine controversy, and the parental informed consent further advised parents about the animal research and the possibility that the medication could cause permanent neurologic damage to children participating in the study (Fisher, Hoagwood, & Jensen, 1996).

Case 2

In this study investigators sought to determine whether differences in central nervous system dopamine production were associated with children's ADHD symptoms. To adequately test this hypothesis required a spinal tap for the extraction of cerebrospinal fluid. The investigators argued that the spinal tap procedure involved a minor increment over minimal risk, since previous studies indicated that about one fourth of children receiving a spinal tap may experience headaches for a period of up to one week. Because of the uncertainties about the neurochemical basis of ADHD children's response to stimulant treatments and their lack of complete response these treatments, the investigators concluded that the study could provide important understanding of the basis of the disorder to benefit the larger class of child citizens with ADHD. In contrast, however, the investigators concluded that the use of normal controls was not justified, in terms of increased understanding of the neurochemical basis of normal functioning, and because most unaffected children are not at risk for developing ADHD.

In order to minimize anxiety for participating children (thereby improving the risk–benefit ratio), the investigators used role playing to rehearse all aspects of the spinal tap procedure and allowed potential participants to speak to other children who had undergone the procedure. In addition, parents were invited to stay with their child during the tap, and the child was provided control over the procedure, in that they could request that it be stopped at any time. To minimize the risk for headache, children remained in a reclining position for 3 hr (watching TV or videos) while being allowed to move other parts of their body. None of the participating children developed posttap headaches, and some participants volunteered for a second spinal tap (Fisher *et al.*, 1996).

Ensuring Fair Representation and Access to Research Benefits; Minimizing Risk and Threats to Internal Validity

Case 3

Investigators were interested in determining the most effective treatments for ADHD, learning whether psychosocial treatment could improve the efficacy of medication treatments, and discovering whether psychosocial treatments alone could benefit children with ADHD. To examine this possibility, the study design specified that children be randomly assigned to one of four treatment arms: individually titrated stimulant medication, intensive psychosocial treatments, the treatment modalities in combination, and referral back to community providers. While some members of the study team were concerned that members of minority groups might be disproportionately identified as meeting criteria for ADHD, parallel concerns were raised by other team members that previous ADHD treatment research had not been conducted with minority populations, thereby excluding this population from potential research benefits and knowledge by default. Because both of these concerns had merit, the investigators concluded that both must be addressed and appropriately balanced, such that no class of citizens (e.g., minority children) would be deprived of research benefits, while simultaneously ensuring that vulnerable populations not be misdiagnosed and assigned to study treatments when other interventions might be more appropriate. To address these concerns, the investigators established a Task Force on Ethnicity, Gender, and Culture (chaired by an African American scientist), charged to develop ways to communicate with minority leaders as well as to ensure that diagnostic and assessment procedures were appropriate, rigorous, and culturally valid across ethnic communities. This task force met with minority community leaders and outside scientists expert in culture-fair assessments and recommended binding inclusion and exclusion criteria to the investigators that were incorporated into the final study protocol. These study criteria included *not* using lower-end intelligence scores as a cutoff (exclusion) criterion, instead utilizing measures of functioning that had been demonstrated to be culture free and establishing a final review of the child's entire psychosocial function and family context before randomizing to the treatment arms. These procedures were accepted by the minority consultants, agreeable to the scientific team and statistical consultants, and resulted in very few children who otherwise met all study criteria not being randomized to the study arms.

In the same clinical trial, during the design of the overall four arms, some investigators were concerned that withholding medication from any child would be unethical (given the well-established beneficial effects of stimulant treatment for the great majority of children), but other team members were similarly concerned that not all ADHD children required medication and that some children were not able to tolerate these treatments because of side effects. Furthermore, studies indicated that intensive psychosocial treatments could provide adequate behavioral control of ADHD symptoms. To address and balance these concerns, investigators developed novel procedures to minimize risk and maximize clinical benefits across all active study arms. First, prior to randomization, to establish the presence of ADHD caseness, all eligible study children were assessed off medication (if they had previously been on medication); this assessment was carefully coordinated with the primary care provider. The total time off medication was kept to an absolute minimum in order to avoid any untoward effects on home and school performance, while close contact was maintained between the child's study case manager and the referring primary care physician. Once the assessment was completed, and while waiting for randomization, children were returned to their normal treatment regimen.

Once randomized, for those children assigned to stimulant medication alone or to the combined treatment arm, medications were individually titrated for each child to determine that child's "best dose." For those children assigned to the psychosocial only treatment arm, the treatments were "beefed up" to make them sufficiently intense to address any likely behavior problems characteristic of ADHD. To monitor all children's clinical status, a special weekly Adjunctive Services and Attrition Prevention (ASAP) panel was established to review any emergent conditions arising for children in any treatment arm, and a "bank" of extra treatment sessions was provided to any child who showed evidence of clinical deterioration during the course of the 14-month trial. Furthermore, for any child showing persistent difficulties the ASAP recommended the child receive whatever services deemed ethically and clinically necessary, even if this recommendation constituted treatments that were not part of the original randomly assigned treatment arm. Necessary arrangements were made to track additional services received, in order to conduct any required post-hoc analyses of the number of cross-arm treatments received by subjects in each treatment arm. In this manner, the scientific integrity of the study was maintained, while also ensuring the appropriate and ethical safeguarding of each child's clinical interests (Fisher et al., 1996).

ADDITIONAL CONSIDERATIONS IN CHILD RESEARCH

Technically, most of the requirements described apply only to research supported by DHHS, but the requirements that any proposed study be reviewed by an IRB in order to receive federal funding, coupled with the application of IRB review to all research at most institutions, essentially brings all research under the purview of these regulations. The Department of Education is now revising its research regulations, proposing that all Department of Education–sponsored research meet the same criteria as DHHS-sponsored research.

Above and beyond the formal requirements established for federally supported research, two other significant issues should be considered by all parties participating in mental health research with children and adolescents. The first of these concerns the impact of stigma on IRB members' assumptions and behavior and the second concerns the need to reconceptualize the relationship between investigators and research participants as being guided not just by procedures but by an "ethical compact" between investigators and participating children and families.

The Impact of Stigma on Child and Adolescent Mental Health Research

In our view, investigators and IRBs frequently hold subtle yet stigmatizing attitudes and opinions concerning research participants who may be at risk for or are afflicted by a mental disorder. Too often, the "presumption of incompetence" seems to shape the opinions and prejudices of investigators and IRB members.

Thus, IRBs or investigators may feel the need to establish greater than usual protections for the disordered or disabled child from his or her presumably incompetent parent. This presumption of incompetence stems from the undemonstrated belief that emotional, behavioral, and developmental disorders primarily impair participants' ability to comprehend information and meaningfully evaluate the risk–benefit ratio. There is, however, no empirical support for the assumption that children suffering from psychopathologic disorders (apart from those that frequently affect cognition, e.g., pervasive developmental disorders and autism) are less able than their age-matched counterparts to evaluate and participate in the assent and consent processes in research.

The presumption of incompetence also extends to prejudices regarding the ability of parents of children with such disorders to evaluate research participation vis-à-vis the best interests of their children, such that their children require greater than usual protection (e.g., a consent auditor or parent monitor) during the course of the research. The stigmatization of parents of children with mental disorders is based in part on the same unsupported biases concerning the ability of at-risk or distressed persons to give fully informed consent and the historical assumption that parents "cause" their child's mental disorder. That parents of children with mental disorders are incompetent to provide rational and fully informed consent has not been demonstrated.

Stigma also affects investigators' and IRBs' assumptions about the kinds of questions and procedures to which children may be safely exposed in the course of research. For example, no evidence has demonstrated that asking children about suicidal feelings increases the likelihood of such feelings or gives a child passive permission to act out such suicidal impulses. Indeed, clinical experience suggests just the opposite, yet many IRBs assume that such questions may be dangerous or lead to untoward consequences. In actual fact, asking children and families such personal, highly confidential questions is regularly seen as acceptable for most participating subjects and families (Lahey et al., 1996). In our experience, ongoing education and consultation are needed to educate IRB members to allow them to render knowledgeable and sophisticated judgments concerning the balance of risks and benefits of research for child participants.

The Ethical Compact between Investigators and Research Participants

In the deepest sense, a full and consensual understanding of the nature of the research program and its potential risks and benefits must be shared between investigators and research participants. This shared understanding should form the basis of an *ethical compact* between the investigator and the participant, and the information-sharing process should be couched in candor, respect, and mutual trust. This also requires that the clinical investigator be aware of and fully communicate to prospective participants and their guardians the potential for conflicts of interest in the investigator's dual roles: the scientist embarked on a quest for knowledge versus the clinician who is bound to work solely on behalf of the patient. The clinical investigator must be aware of this conflict of interest inherent in therapeutic research and recognize that his or her actions are shaped by two competing value systems. Full awareness of this conflict of interest can form the foundation for trust between investigators and research participants. Honest communication at the initial stages of a research partnership can serve as a firm basis for a relationship built on respect. Such mutual respect can in turn enhance the ethical compact by overriding what in many instances may appear to be unequal power relationships.

This mutuality, candor, and shared participation in the research process is critical for research to proceed, and to maintain the public's trust and good will toward the goal of advancing science for the benefit of all. Clearly, this ethical compact requires more than a single consent form signed under limited or less than optimal conditions. A research partnership bound by an ethical compact begins with the initial consent procedures, continues through the duration of the research program, and ends with a thoughtful debriefing and a shared, final examination of the entire process. This process should be mutually and gladly undertaken by the investigator and the research participants. Thus, in the conduct of research, investigators should aim not just for IRB approval but for a higher standard: a plan to address human subjects issues that considers all possible ramifications of the research enterprise, embedded in ethical principles and built on systematic efforts to increase trust in the investigator–participant relationship. Although IRBs cannot fully anticipate every eventuality that may arise during the course of research, if the investigator fully grasps the essential nature of the ethical compact, he or she can make appropriate adjustments at critical points of the study, ensuring that families' confidence in the research and the researcher increase during the course of their mutual collaboration. While systematic approaches to addressing these issues have been developed (e.g., data safety, monitoring boards, ongoing reviews of side effects and treatment outcomes during the course of clinical trials), such formal mechanisms cannot replace investigators' own concern for their research participants' well-being and the active communication of these perspectives in interactions with families.

FUTURE RECOMMENDATIONS

We suggest that increased efforts are needed to strengthen the links between investigators, institutional review boards, families, and their communities. In the final analysis, the highest ethical standard will never be obtained by an elegant, well-written, explicit consent form. Although such consent procedures are to be emulated whenever possible, they fall short of an ethical standard that seeks to involve members of the larger "community of citizens" as research participants and collaborators in the goals of science and research. Although science should ultimately benefit the larger community of citizens, all too often investigators complain that their research find-

ings are not incorporated into available knowledge, nor do their findings actually change the standards of practice. On further consideration, this should not be too surprising: The terminologies used to define the research questions and the aims of the research are often very different from the policy objectives of program planners or the more personal concerns of parents and families who are dealing with the immediate effects of a member who is suffering with a disabling disorder.

To address these difficulties in research dissemination, members of the communities whom the research is intended to benefit must increasingly be part of the early definition of the research questions, research procedures, selection of domains for assessment, specific terminologies, and dissemination of research findings. This action perspective more closely joins the interests of scientists, research participants, and the larger community, and seems to us ethical in the deepest sense. Such an approach offers a more comprehensive means of strengthening collaborations between scientists and research participants, engendering trust, developing relevant research that is well received by communities, and enhancing effective research dissemination. Such partnerships between scientists and the citizenry could yield a number of important benefits, including the development of consensus on levels of acceptable risk, the cultivation of a common will to address critical research gaps (particularly in the area of children and adolescents), and the reaffirmation of the importance of science in improving the lives of all citizens.

Given concerns about difficulties in younger children's understanding of research procedures, investigators must pay greater attention to engaging participants in the research enterprise. Such engagement entails creative and sustained attention to the process of obtaining and continuing informed consent, to developmental issues, and to therapeutic comprehensiveness. For example, investigators may want to use systematic "staged consent," particularly if consent procedures are long, complex, or if the research procedures take place over a longer period of time. In the area of therapeutic research, investigators need to consider using developmentally sensitive yet scientifically sensible designs. Given the nature of children's development and their needs over time and across multiple settings and contexts, a child with a psychopathologic disorder may warrant more comprehensive treatment approaches than simple placebo-controlled, double-masked designs can offer. Studies that involve comprehensive treatment strategies are likely to be more acceptable to families, offer a better basis for trust and shared commitment to the research process, and offer sensible and generalizable findings to inform public policy and health practices.

Research with children poses special challenges in the areas of balancing risk and benefits, maintenance of appropriate confidentiality, and ensuring developmentally sensible child assent and parental consent. In part because of these challenges, children run the risk of becoming "therapeutic orphans," that is, being deprived of the benefits of medical research as a class of citizens. As a consequence, 80% of all medications approved for marketing in the United States have not been tested for safety and efficacy in children (Jensen, Vitiello, Leonard, & Laughren, 1994). In many instances, novel strategies and special arrangements can be made to enable appropriate research in children (e.g., see Hoagwood, Jensen, & Fisher, 1996). In our view, substantial progress will be possible only by increasing dialogue and more effective coalitions between families, investigators, IRBs, policy makers, and the general public. As such, research cannot and should not be the province of science and scientists alone. Science, in the public trust and on behalf of public health, is the province of us all.

REFERENCES

Applebaum, P. D., & Rosenbaum, A. (1989). Tarasoff and the researcher: Does the duty to protect apply in the research setting? *American Psychologist, 44,* 885–894.

Arnold, L., Stoff, D., Cook, E., Wright, C., Cohen, D. J., Kruesi, M., Hattab, J., Graham, P., Zametkin, A., Castellanos, F. X., MacMahon, W., & Leckman, J. (1996). Biologic procedures: Ethical issues in research with children and adolescents. In K. Hoagwood, P. S. Jensen, & C. Fisher (Eds.), *Ethical issues in mental health research with children and adolescents* (pp. 89–111). Hillsdale, NJ: Erlbaum.

Castellanos, F. X., Elia, J., Kruesi, M., Gulotta, C. S., Mefford, I. N., Potter, W. Z., Ritchie, G. F., & Rapoport, J. L. (1994). Cerebrospinal fluid monoamine metabolites in ADHD boys. *Psychiatry Research, 52,* 305–316.

Fisher, C. B. (1991). Ethical considerations for research on psychosocial interventions for high-risk infants and children. In *Psychological practice: Marketing, legal, ethical and current professional issues* (pp. 92–94). Washington, DC: National Register.

Fisher, C. B. (1993). Integrating science and ethics in research with high-risk children and youth. *Society for Research and Child Development Social Policy Report, 7*(4), 1–27.

Fisher, C. B., & Rosendahl, S. A. (1990). Emerging ethical issues in an emerging field. In C. B. Fisher & W. W. Tryon (Eds.), *Annual advances in applied developmental psychology* (Vol. 4, pp. 43–60). Norwood, NJ, Ablex.

Fisher, C. B., Hoagwood, K., & Jensen, P. (1996). Casebook on ethical issues in research with children and adolescents with mental disorders. In K. Hoagwood, C. B. Fisher, & P. Jensen (Eds.), *Ethical issues in mental health research with children and adolescents: A casebook and guide* (pp. 135–141). Hillsdale, NJ: Erlbaum.

Friesen, B. J., & Koroloff, N. M. (1990). Family-centered services: Implications for mental health administration and research. *Journal of Mental Health Administration, 17,* 13–25.

Gibbs, J. T. (1990). Mental health issues of black adolescents: Implications for policy and practice. In A. R. Stiffman & L. E. Davis (Eds.), *Ethnic issues in adolescent mental health* (pp. 21–52). Newbury Park, CA: Sage.

Hendren, R. L. (1991). Determining the need for inpatient treatment. In R. L. Hendren & I. N. Berlin (Eds.), *Psychiatric inpatient care of children and adolescents: A multi-cultural approach* (pp. 37–64). New York: Wiley.

Hoagwood, K. (1994). The Certificate of Confidentiality at NIMH: Applications and implications for service research with children. *Ethics and Behavior, 4,* 123–131.

Hoagwood, K., Jensen, P., & Fisher, C. B. (Eds.). (1996). *Ethical issues in mental health research with children and adolescents: A casebook and guide.* Hillsdale, NJ: Erlbaum.

Holder, A. R. (1981). Can teenagers participate in research without parental consent? *IRB: Review of Human Subjects Research, 3,* 5–7.

Institute of Medicine. (1989). *Research on children and adolescents with mental, behavioral, and developmental disorders* (Publication IOM-89-07). Washington, DC: National Academy Press.

Jensen, P., Vitiello, B., Leonard, H., & Laughren, T. (1994). Child and adolescent psychopharmacology: Expanding the research base. *Psychopharmacology Bulletin, 30,* 3–8.

Koocher, G. P., & Keith-Spiegel, P. C. (1990). *Children, ethics and the law: Professional issues and cases.* Lincoln: University of Nebraska Press.

Kopelman, L. M. (1989). When is the risk minimal enough for children to be research subjects? In L. M. Kopelman & J. C. Moskop (Eds.), *Children and health care: Moral and social issues* (pp. 89–99). Boston: Kluwer.

Kruesi, M. J. P., Swedo, S. E., Coffey, M. L., Hamburger, S. D., Leonard, H., & Rapoport, J. L. (1988). Objective and subjective side effects of research lumbar punctures in children and adolescents. *Psychiatry Research, 25,* 59–63.

Lahey, B., Flagg, E., Bird, H., Schwab-Stone, M., Canino, G., Dulcan, M., Leaf, P., Davies, M., Brogan, D., Bourdon, K., Horwitz, S., Rubio-Stipec, M., Freeman, D., Lichtman, J., Shaffer, D., Goodman, S., Narrow, W., Weissman, M., Kandel, D., Jensen, P., Richters, J., & Regier, D. (1996). The NIMH methods for the Epidemiology of Child and Adolescent Mental Disorders (MECA) Study: Background and methodology. *Journal of the American Academy of Child and Adolescent Psychiatry, 35,* 855–864.

Levine, R. (1986). *Ethics and regulation of clinical research* (2nd ed.). Munich, Germany: Urban & Schwarzenberg.

Liss, M. (1994). State and federal laws governing reporting for researchers. *Ethics and Behavior, 4,* 133–146.

Macklin, R. (1981). "Due" and "undue" inducements: On paying money to research subjects. *IRB: Review of Human Subjects Research, 3,* 1–6.

Melton, G. B., Koocher, G. P., & Saks, M. J. (1983). *Children's competence to consent.* New York: Plenum.

Monahan, J., Appelbaum, P. S., Mulvey, E. P., Robbins, P. C., & Lidz, C. W. (1993). Ethical and legal duties in conducting research on violence: Lessons from the MacArthur Risk Assessment Study. *Violence and Victims, 8,* 387–396.

National Commission for the Protection of Human Subjects of Biomedical and Behavioral Research Research Involving Children. (1977). *Report and recommendations* (DHEW Publication No. [OS] 77-0005). Washington, DC: U.S. Government Printing Office.

Nolan, K. (1992, Summer). Assent, consent, and behavioral research with adolescents. *AACAP Child and Adolescent Research Notes,* pp. 7–10.

Office for Protection from Research Risks, Department of Health and Human Services, National Institutes of Health. (1993). *Protecting human research subjects: Institutional review board guidebook.* Washington, DC: U.S. Government Printing Office.

Osher, T. W., & Telesford, M. (1996). Involving families to improve research. In K. Hoagwood, P. Jensen, & C. B. Fisher (Eds.), *Ethical issues in mental health research with children and familes* (pp. 29–39). Hillsdale, NJ: Erlbaum.

Thompson, R. A. (1992). Developmental changes in risk and benefit: A changing calculus of concerns. In B. L. Stanley & J. E. Sieber (Eds.), *Social research on children and adolescents: Ethical issues* (pp. 31–64). Newbury Park, CA: Sage.

U.S. Department of Health and Human Services. (1983, March). Protection of human subjects: Research involving children. *Federal Register, 48,* 9814–9820.

U.S. Department of Health and Human Services. (1991). OPRR Reports: Protection of human subjects. *Federal Register, 46* (revised June 18, 1991).

28

Research Problems and Issues

Toward a More Definitive Science of Disruptive Behavior Disorders

STEPHEN P. HINSHAW and TERON PARK

INTRODUCTION

Writing the concluding chapter for an authoritative, edited handbook on Disruptive Behavior Disorders (DBD) is both challenging and daunting. Our task, which involves appraising the status of research practices in this domain, invites a host of "big questions": Where is the field? How much substantive progress have we made in such crucial issues as understanding etiology, elucidating underlying processes, predicting long-term outcomes, or mapping the outcomes of intervention techniques? At an applied level, do our developmental trajectories, multiple-risk-factor models, and ever more sophisticated data analytic strategies stand any chance of influencing policy that might stem the rising tide of youth violence in the United States?* More basically, are we even headed in the right directions; that is, can our current research models yield predictive and explanatory success? In all, the prevalence, impairment, and destructive nature of DBD (Barkley, 1996; Hinshaw & Anderson, 1996; Stoff, Breiling, & Maser, 1997) mandate that our science carefully scrutinize its conceptual bases and practices.

Both space limitations and our lack of knowledge preclude complete answers to these essential questions. We therefore alternate between covering, at a broader level, larger-scale conceptual and philosophical concerns regarding underlying models in the field and tackling such mainstream issues as sampling methods, design, and data-analytic strategies. Our intent is to be illuminating, but we disclaim any effort to provide comprehensive solutions to the long-standing issues raised herein. We also include a section on the salient issues of culture, ethnicity, and gender—understudied variables that require far more attention in the field's subsequent research efforts.

CRITIQUES OF EXTANT RESEARCH: BOTTOM-UP OR TOP-DOWN?

Two main alternatives emerge in organizing a chapter such as this. The first would be to take a "bottom-up" perspective, systematically discussing a host of specific research issues (e.g., sample selection, assessment practices, modes of analyzing data) with the goal of

---

*National data indicate that, after years of steady and alarming increase, youth violence in the United States has finally showed declines in 1995 and 1996.

STEPHEN P. HINSHAW and TERON PARK • Department of Psychology, University of California, Berkeley, Berkeley, California 94720-1650.

Handbook of Disruptive Behavior Disorders, edited by Quay and Hogan. Kluwer Academic/Plenum Publishers, New York, 1999.

taking incremental steps toward optimal research practices. The second would be to take a larger, "top-down" view at the outset, examining more holistically the field's predominant procedures. The choice, in many respects, depends on an underlying optimism versus pessimism about the state of the art. If one's perspective is that the field is basically headed in the right direction, then such correctives as better sampling, more precise specification of diagnostic status, improved research design strategies, and clearer data analyses could each help to effect more precise findings. On the other hand, if one believes that the field is moving entirely too slowly—or, worse, may be utilizing fundamentally misguided approaches—then such an incrementalist approach would be wholly misdirected. A recent critique of the status of research in developmental psychopathology (Richters, 1997) exemplifies this latter perspective, providing a starting point for our endeavor.

Richters's Top-Down Critique

In his provocative review, Richters (1997) decried the fundamental assumptions and limited progress of current research efforts in the field, with particular content emphasis on antisocial behavior. Echoing a long tradition of deep dissatisfaction with slow progress in psychology and other social sciences (e.g., Bevan & Kessel, 1994; Lykken, 1991; Meehl, 1978), Richters contends that the field's current variable-centered research methods are predicated on paradigms borrowed from mainstream psychology which, in turn, has utilized principles from 19th-century physics. These methods were generated to investigate what are termed closed systems, that is, systems involving passive physical objects that are subject to mechanistic, general laws, instead of the open systems that characterize human functioning and interaction. Because the traditional models emphasize "the study of variables over individuals, the modeling of complex interactions among variables, and the search for invariant causal explanations to account for phenotypically similar patterns of overt functioning across individuals" (Richters, 1997, p. 199), they cannot with

validity be applied to the study of developing persons, who are characterized by adaptive, interactive, open-systems functioning and whose highly individualized natures do not yield standard or invariant responses to biological or environmental causal factors. The "catch," however, is that the field largely remains unaware of this problematic state of affairs because of the weak scientific standards employed by the dominant perspective—most notably, null-hypothesis significance testing. That is, the standards of null-hypothesis testing are so low that there is no real self-corrective function served. In all, from Richters's perspective, our current methods and paradigms are akin to the poor focus of the Hubble space telescope before the discovery and correction of the crucial lack of resolution of its main lens.

A core tenet of Richters's argument is that the field continues to assume the basic homogeneity of phenotypically similar categories. In the present context, a given category of the DBD—Oppositional Defiant Disorder (ODD), Conduct Disorder (CD), or Attention-Deficit/Hyperactivity Disorder (ADHD)—often serves as the independent variable in research studies, with the assumption that youngsters in the category are fundamentally similar in terms of their "effects" on dependent measures of interest. Alternatively, dimensional conceptions of inattentive, impulsive-hyperactive, or aggressive behavior patterns serve as dependent variables in risk-factor research.

In fact, however, these diagnoses are quite heterogeneous (e.g., Barkley, 1996; Hinshaw & Anderson, 1996; see also Chapter 1, this volume), with the implication that the field cannot assume the application of similar or invariant causal laws to all children within the taxon (or to all data points in the scatterplot of a given risk factor's association with a disruptive behavior score). Furthermore, entities in open systems are subject to both equifinality, the emergence of similar end-states from disparate developmental processes, and to multifinality, the emergence of differing developmental outcomes from similar precursors (Cicchetti & Rogosch, 1996). In both processes, any influences of causal variables differ qualitatively (as opposed to merely quantitatively) across individuals, with the clear implication that linear, static causal models are misguided. Thus, according to Richters, the field's typical research paradigms, which assume the structural homogeneity of individuals in the samples under investigation, are ill suited to the task at hand, which is the study of open-system, transactional child development. One antidote may be better understanding of truly homogeneous subgroups, particularly at the level of underlying etiology.

Implications for This Review

What is the specific pertinence of this far-reaching perspective for DBD? First, it is clearly accepted that CD and ODD, on the one hand, and ADHD, on the other, comprise distinct forms of externalizing symptomatology (Hinshaw, 1987) and result from a multitude of proclivities, background variables, and developmental pathways, thus exemplifying equifinality (Hinshaw, 1994; Loeber *et al.,* 1993; Moffitt, 1993). Second, multifinality is also pertinent: For example, such traits as impulsivity, extraversion, or sensation seeking may lead to quite different outcomes, depending on a host of interacting and transacting factors (Richters, 1997). Many current research methods, then, appear to mix disparate types of children and adolescents in a given diagnostic category—some truly disordered individuals with aberrant psychological mechanisms, other phenocopies with largely familial or neighborhood-related inducements to aggressive or attention-dysregulated behavior patterns, and still others with complex mixtures of risk factors—into the same "group" factor, with great potential for the masking of key underlying processes. To that extent, the arguments of Richters (1997) are well founded.

Authoritatively, Moffitt (1993) has made a parallel argument with respect to the study of antisocial behavior in adolescents. Her main contention is that the field has lumped together two fundamentally different types of youth, each of which displays similar behavior patterns in adolescence. One is marked by early onset of antisocial behavior, disrupted attach-

ments, verbal IQ deficits, and impulsivity (as well as other aspects of ADHD); this "life-course-persistent" group typically reveals underlying disorder or psychopathology. The other, "adolescent-limited" subtype is characterized by social mimicry, for time-limited periods, of their more persistently antisocial peers, with little sign of underlying disorder. Indeed, this latter type may, in fact, be normative in many cultures. The phenotypic similarity of their behavioral displays, however, has led to their amalgamation in most investigations, promoting considerable disinformation in the research field.* Thus, unthinking adherence to descriptive classification systems and variable-centered (as opposed to person-centered) research methods could well be slowing progress in the field.

In all, Richters's (1997) critique is erudite, lucid, and well documented, particularly with respect to his points regarding closed-system models, invariant causal factors, and the weaknesses inherent in null-hypothesis significance testing (see also Shrout, 1997). Yet groundbreaking solutions are not readily apparent. For one thing, despite the limitations of our current descriptive nosologic categories, the operational criteria of the *Diagnostic and Statistical Manual of Mental Disorders* (DSM; American Psychiatric Association, 1980, 1987, 1994) have at least established a beachhead of reliability in the field. Although empirical efforts to refine and validate the status of these conditions as actual disorders (with unifying causal mechanisms and with clear status as dysfunctions) as opposed to syndromes (constellations of covarying behaviors) must continue, the field is in better shape than it was several decades ago, when diagnostic reliability was not even established. On the other hand, reliability at the expense of validity is no virtue,

*See Chapter 1 (this volume) for elaboration of the older socialized versus undersocialized distinction among youth with antisocial behavior. Youth with early-onset and aggressive (as opposed to covert or nonaggressive) forms of antisocial activity tend to commit their actions in solitary fashion; hence, undersocialized aggressive CD is virtually synonymous with the early- or child-onset designation (Hinshaw, Lahey, & Hart, 1993).

and we see the current DSM categories as way stations, temporarily useful entities that should challenge the field to integrate operational criteria at a symptom level with the appropriate attention to causal pathways and context that must characterize future nosologies (Jensen & Hoagwood, 1997).

Second, despite the call for future nosologies to incorporate etiologic information with the aim of forming more meaningful taxa, the complex interplay of genetic, nongenetic biological, family-systemic, and sociocultural risk factors for externalizing behavioral manifestations may constrain attempts to base classification on etiologic variables. We envision the field's ability to categorize multiple-risk-factor etiologic models as an essential ingredient in this attempt; we also believe that such transactional risk models will be difficult to capture in a yes/no nosologic system.

Third, the field is still struggling with such basic assessment issues as (1) the lack of precision of most of our measurement tools (see Chapter 3, this volume), (2) the paucity of objective (as opposed to informant report) measures of the constructs of interest, and (3) the daunting problem of poor interinformant correspondence regarding the appraisal of antisocial and hyperactive behavior (see subsequent sections of this chapter). Renewed attention toward viable assessment strategies is needed to fuel progress (Hinshaw & Zupan, 1997). In summary, development of better theory, better classification systems, and better assessment devices must proceed together as we enter the next century.

Fourth, we contend that variable-centered and person-centered research models can and should provide complementary (rather than opposing) perspectives on research on DBD. As we argue later, person-centered research, which may better account for unique developmental trajectories, must still rely on strong inferences regarding the influence of risk and protective variables.

Overall, critiques like those of Richters (1997) are a necessary antidote to any naive optimism that may accrue from a cursory inspection of "progress" in the field. Clearly, the research enterprise on DBD is still in a period of relative immaturity, but easy solutions to the fundamental problems raised are not apparent. Conceptual, methodologic, and data-analytic changes (e.g, better integration of relevant theory into research, more explicit consideration of ethnicity and culture, acceptance of ethnography as well as "hard" empirical methods, employment of more explicitly falsifiable evidentiary standards) are needed to shake the existing paradigm.

We begin our specific coverage with the critical issues of (1) variable-centered versus person-centered research paradigms (also discussing the corollary issue of dimensional vs. categorical views of DBD) and (2) sample selection, with the attendant concerns of clinical versus representative samples, comorbidity, and multi-informant diagnostic methods. We then consider research design and measurement issues, data-analytic approaches, and cross-cultural perspectives before presenting a section on culture, ethnicity, and gender and making our concluding comments.

VARIABLE-CENTERED VERSUS PERSON-CENTERED RESEARCH

A longstanding tension exists in human sciences between (1) variable-centered approaches, which (in developmental psychopathology) aim to elucidate the influences of risk variables* on criterion measures of interest, and (2) person-centered research, which attempts to separate and analyze fundamentally disparate types of individuals. Indeed, from the earliest days of factor analysis, advocates of the typical "R" analyses, in which underlying dimensions are gleaned from correlation matrices of variables amalgamated across research participants have been countered by those who champion transposed "Q" analyses, in which types of persons are distinguished across measured variables.

*Kraemer and colleagues (1997) present cogent discussion about risk factors in developmental psychopathology research, discussing the concepts of variable, fixed, and causal risk factors.

Recent advocates of person-centered research strategies in the domain of DBD include, from differing perspectives and philosophies, Bergman and Magnusson (1997), Loeber and colleagues (1993), Moffitt (1993), and Stattin and Magnusson (1996). One defining feature of a person-centered approach is that persons are investigated with respect to patterns or profiles of variables. That is, "variables included in such an analysis have no meaning in themselves but as components of the pattern under analysis and interpreted in relation to all other variables simultaneously" (Bergman & Magnusson, 1997, p. 293). Unless disparate types of antisocial youth are distinguished, such investigators contend, the true influence of causal variables on developmental pathways and trajectories will be missed. An underlying assumption is that individuals in valid taxa or categories are qualitatively (as opposed to quantitatively) distinct.

Key issues with regard to person-centered paradigms include (1) the use of rational-conceptual versus statistical means of distinguishing subgroups; (2) within the statistical approach, the sheer numbers of statistical techniques that can be used to discern disparate subtypes of individuals (cf. the large variety of strategies subsumed under the rubric of cluster analysis); and (3) the dearth of viable statistical means of testing the empirical discriminability of subtypes or clusters that may emerge. The ultimate criterion for distinguishing clusters or types, however, is not statistics per se but the establishment of divergent validity through comparisons on the basis of external correlates (e.g., family history, differing biological variables, disparate developmental course, distinct response to treatments).

Variable-centered investigators, on the other hand, typically attempt to isolate the effect or effects of theoretically relevant variables, for example, socioeconomic status (SES), neuropsychological risk, accuracy of self-perception, or family history of psychopathology, on dimensions of outcome, impairment, or prognosis. Although discrete diagnostic and comparison groups are often used in such research designs, an underlying assumption is that psychopathology, as well as its predictors or precursors, is distributed dimensionally or quantitatively across the population, affording examination of linear (or, more rarely, quadratic or higher-order) patterns of influence. Person-centered research, on the other hand, presumes that psychopathology divides into qualitatively distinct categories. This long-standing dichotomy bears separate examination.

Dimensional versus Categorical Models of Disruptive Behavior

The literature on this topic is voluminous, allowing only a brief synopsis herein (for seminal reviews, see Eysenck, 1986; Quay, 1986; see also Chapter 1, this volume). Quantitative approaches assume that psychopathology is distributed continuously in the general population and that quantitative scores on such dimensions retain far more information than do arbitrary categories that might be imposed on scaled indexes. Instruments like the MMPI in adult personality and the Child Behavior Checklist (Achenbach, 1991) in child and adolescent psychopathology exemplify this tradition: Normed indicators of deviance on pertinent dimensions of interest are displayed in the form of continuous scores. Testifying to the popularity of the dimensional approach, the number of quantitative rating scales in the domain of DBD has multiplied at high rates in recent years (Hinshaw & Nigg, in press; see also Chapter 3, this volume). The dimensional perspective also has the added advantage of capturing subclinical (but potentially important) amounts of deviant functioning by retaining quantitative scores on all individuals rather than eliminating subthreshold information in a yes/no categorical system (Hinshaw, Lahey, & Hart, 1993).

Alternatively, discrete or categorical approaches rely on the assumption that distinctions between disorder and nondisorder are qualitative in nature, mandating the use of discrete types or taxa. As described in Chapter 1 (this volume), the *Diagnostic and Statistical Manual of Mental Disorders,* fourth edition (DSM-IV; American Psychiatric Association,

1994) presents discrete categories of mental disorders, with ADHD, ODD, and CD comprising the disruptive spectrum. As noted earlier, however, the DSM categories appear to reflect syndromes, which demarcate individuals only at a phenotypic or behavioral level, rather than true disorders with unified causes (Richters & Cicchetti, 1993). Renewed interest in categorical conceptions of child psychopathology is emanating from psychobiologic research on extremes of internalizing behavior: Inhibited, shy youngsters may form a temperamental category rather than simply reflecting the end of a continuum of fearful social approach (Kazdin & Kagan, 1994).

Which model is correct with regard to child psychopathology in general and the DBD in particular? As a provocative example, Rutter and colleagues (1990) discuss mental retardation, which has traditionally been defined on the basis of cutoff scores from distributions of intellectual functioning (clearly continuous in nature). Indeed, the mild to moderate range of retardation constitutes no more than the lower end of the normal distribution of IQ scores; both intellectual functioning and underlying causation appear to fall along the same continuum as normal-range scores. Yet severe and profound levels of retardation almost invariably indicate a chromosomal abnormality or other discrete biological causal factor (Rutter *et al.,* 1990). Thus, in some instances cutoffs on supposedly dimensional measures can yield categories that are etiologically distinct.

As for the subject matter at hand, strong evidence has accumulated that the relatively narrow category of adult psychopathy (marked by both a repetitive antisocial lifestyle and the presence of callous, manipulative interpersonal and emotional traits) actually captures a distinct taxon rather than simply indicating the tail of a distribution (Harris, Rice, & Quinsey, 1994). In childhood, however, the symptoms of CD may be best viewed as a dimensional (rather than categorical) indicator of antisocial behavior. For example, when Robins and McEvoy (1990) predicted adolescent and adult substance abuse from retrospectively reported symptoms of CD from the earlier DSM-III

(American Psychiatric Association, 1980), sampling from the Epidemiologic Catchment Area (ECA) study (Robins & Regier, 1991), the predictive function was entirely linear: Each additional CD symptom added incrementally to the prediction of later substance abuse, with no point at which the prediction yielded a discontinuous step function. Furthermore, recent behavior-genetic research regarding the constituent symptoms of ADHD shows strikingly high heritability coefficients for dimensional conceptions of the disorder (in this case, maternal ratings) as well as no increment of the heritability figures for any extreme grouping of the constituent behaviors (Levy, Hay, McStephen, Wood, & Waldman, 1997). The genetic liability therefore appears to relate to dimensional components of inattentive, impulsive, and hyperactive behavior patterns rather than to any distinct category.

On the other hand, with respect to CD, invoking criteria other than numbers of behavioral symptoms per se (e.g., age of onset of CD-type problems, presence of significant neuropsychological deficits, significant interpersonal violence) appears to yield subgroups of antisocial youth that do constitute discrete categories (see Moffitt, 1993). As discussed earlier, the early-onset group evidences clear psychopathology, and aberrant psychobiological findings are limited to the undersocialized, aggressive (now termed child-onset) type (Quay, 1993; see also Chapter 17, this volume). On the other hand, many if not most adolescent-onset youngsters are on a developmental trajectory that is normative, without signs of intraindividual or family-systemic disorder. In addition, Wootton, Frick, Shelton, and Silverthorn (1997) provided intriguing evidence that a constellation of callous-unemotional (CU) traits in childhood, potentially signaling precursors of subsequent psychopathy, may comprise a separable category. That is, unlike other externalizing children, whose aggressive behavior is positively correlated with inept parental discipline, the CU group shows no correspondence whatsoever between parental discipline style and levels of aggression. In other words, the type of externalizing behavior (CU vs. not) moderates the relationship between maternal discipline and severity of aggressive symptomatology. Thus, apparent dimensions with use of behavior checklists may yield discrete taxa when other conceptually relevant criteria are invoked.

In all, following the comprehensive arguments of Achenbach (1993), we contend that the dichotomy between dimensional and categorical approaches to research on child psychopathology is more apparent than real. In practice, the field would do well to view these perspectives as complementary rather than fundamentally opposed. Investigators should capture the full dimensionality of constituent symptoms, emotional indicators, degree of impairment, and related causal variables in their studies while also ascertaining and testing conceptually or empirically based subgroups, which may yield a clearer pattern of findings. An example is found in the work of Pelham and Lang (1993) regarding the tendency of parents of disruptive children to consume alcohol before an anticipated parent–child interaction. The relationship was moderated by family history of alcohol problems: Parents with a positive family history showed significantly higher levels of drinking before interacting with a disruptive child than did parents with a negative family history, an effect that was reversed preceding interactions with a nondisruptive child. Utilization of such moderator variables may be essential for accurate interpretation of results; we discuss subsequently methodologic and statistical issues regarding their detection.

In addition, invoking principles of profile or "subtype" analyses from such instruments as the MMPI, investigators can use a configural approach across multiple dimensions to capture a profile marked by a particular constellation of problems (e.g., the profile types from Achenbach's [1991] Child Behavior Checklist, or the discrete types of learning-disabled youngsters garnered from profile analysis of achievement and neuropsychological measures, advocated by Rourke [1985]). In this way, the full range of quantitative scores from well-normed instruments may yield distinct subgroups that could never be apparent from examination of any one diagnostic marker.

From the opposite perspective, those who classify children into discrete categories on the basis of structured interviews or other diagnostic instruments should maintain the underlying dimensionality of the constituent symptoms, affording quantitative and categorical examination of the same data. Jensen and colleagues (1996) have explored the relative power of dimensional and categorical approaches to child psychopathology, comparing DSM diagnoses with constituent symptom counts, discovering that each perspective provides important information. In short, neither the quantitative nor the categorical perspective has cornered the market in research on DBD; a complementarity of approaches is likely to foster the most progress.

The Variable- versus Person-Centered Debate: More Apparent than Real?

Returning to the underlying issue of variable-centered versus person-centered research, may they also be viewed as complementary rather than opposing? Despite the strong statements of Bergman and Magnusson (1997) regarding the problems inherent in variable-centered research, we contend that both approaches can offer important perspectives on the domain of DBD, so long as relevant subgroups are detected and theoretically and psychometrically sound variables are used in predictive and process-oriented research. Before exploring the influences of theoretically and conceptually driven variables on key outcomes across entire samples, investigators must be alert to the possibility of fundamentally disparate predictive patterns in important subgroups (see Richters, 1997, for an example of relating marital discord to child antisocial behavior). Creativity in examining pertinent subgroups is essential; qualitative, ethnographic methods can supplement more traditional quantitative means of discerning such typologies. However, we do not advocate casually combing a data set for possible subgroup-specific relationships, particularly on the basis of the criterion variable under investigation, an approach that is bound to yield spurious results. In all, the discovery of relevant variables is essential for identifying more precise subpopulations, in which the influence of more refined variables can be evaluated with even greater specificity.

Finally, we note that models of causation with respect to DBD, like those for many other phenomena in the social sciences, are highly likely to reflect multiple levels of analysis (from the molecular and genetic, to the cellular, progressing to individual-psychological and ultimately to ecological-systemic), with strong potential for complex causal pathways within and between levels (see Cacioppo & Berntson, 1992). For example, (1) parallel causation could occur, with either genetic or neighborhood factors separately contributing to antisocial behavior; (2) convergent causation could operate, in which environmental factors could potentiate aberrant cellular (or even genetic) processes; or (3) reciprocal causation may be salient, in which temperament factors in the child could induce negative family interactions, which, in turn, could exacerbate the child's disruptive tendencies (Patterson, Reid, & Dishion, 1992). Process-level investigations with measured variables at only one level of analysis—or static research models that do not allow interactions across levels—will be inadequate to capture the phenomena and mechanisms of interest.

SAMPLING ISSUES

Whether the investigator performs dimensional, variable-centered research, analyzes person-centered types, or utilizes a hybrid approach, a seminal issue is the composition of the sample of participants. We highlight several crucial topics in this vast area, with space limitations dictating "headline" rather than exhaustive coverage.

Clinical verus Unreferred Samples

Research on DBD includes, almost by definition, children at the extremes of such dimensions as disinhibition, aggression, or antisocial traits. Hence, most investigators select participants who have been referred for treatment or otherwise designated by caregivers or teachers as problematic. Although research on clinical samples has been and will continue to be a mainstay of the field, clinical, referred samples do not accurately represent all youngsters with mental disorders in the community. Indeed, using data from the Methodology for Epidemiology of Mental Disorders in Children and Adolescents (MECA) Study, Goodman and colleagues (1997) showed that youth referred for mental health services systematically differed from the larger group of youth with DSM-III-R (American Psychiatric Association, 1987) mental disorders. Compared to the nonreferred group, the clinically referred youngsters were more likely to be Caucasian, to show greater impairment, to have comorbid (rather than single) disorders, to have parents with both more education and a greater likelihood of having used mental health services themselves, and to have come from families with poorer parental monitoring.

The inference is clear: Investigations of underlying mechanisms of psychopathology that utilize clinically referred samples are likely to be biased in fundamental ways. Note that the same dictum need not apply to clinical intervention studies, which are likely to be intended for generalization only to other youth who have been referred for treatment (Goodman *et al.,* 1997). Investigations of general mechanisms of psychopathology, however, typically aim for wider applicability. Thus, inferences about processes and mechanisms from clinic-referred, convenience samples must be made with extreme caution. Adding to the difficulty is that mounting population-representative investigations is expensive and quite time-consuming. Even when feasible, however, epidemiologic-scale investigations are not an automatic panacea, as the instrumentation in such large studies typically begins and ends with parent (and perhaps) child informant interviews or checklists, to the exclusion of teacher measures, observational systems, peer sociometrics, laboratory measures, or other important data sources. The trade-off thus appears to be one of obtaining rich, multisource data on samples of unknown (or biased) generalizability versus gathering rather limited symptom- and impairment-based information from large, representative samples. Reconciling this troublesome state of affairs is sure to be a major item on the agendas (and budgets) of those investigating DBD in the next decades.

Comorbidity

Comorbidity is on the list of "hot topics" in contemporary research on child psychopathology. Caron and Rutter (1991) provided important theoretical discussion of the topic, making the distinction between true comorbidity (the joint presence of independent disorders in a given individual) and artifactual comorbidity (apparent overlap that may reflect inaccurate classification systems or the attribution of developmental progressions to independent disorders). At present, even in community samples, it is more likely for a child with one of the DBD to have one or more additional disorders than it is for the child to display DBD in isolation (Bird, Gould, Staghezza, & Jaramilo, 1994; see also Chapter 2, this volume). Thus, at least as currently defined, comorbidity is not an esoteric phenomenon but is quite commonplace.

The findings of Goodman and colleagues (1997) regarding an abundance of comorbid youth in clinically referred samples is reminiscent of a long-replicated finding in the fields of epidemiology and medicine: Persons with multiple conditions are quite likely to be overrepresented in clinic settings (Berkson, 1946). Crucially, extreme errors in prediction may result when comorbidity in a referred sample is attributed to the general population (Caron & Rutter, 1991). At a more basic level, we caution investigators of DBD to measure comorbid psychopathology with care and precision. Otherwise, what may be attributed to (for example) ADHD may actually pertain to the aggressive features or to the internalizing symptoms or disorders that often accompany this disorder (Hinshaw, 1987; Loney, 1987).

We reiterate this point even more explicitly: Two given children, each with identical levels of externalizing psychopathology on well-validated measures, may differ radically with respect to causal factors, correlates, course, treatment response, or some combination if one displays comorbid psychopathology and the other does not (or, alternatively, if the comorbid psychopathologies are different). Hence, assessment practices must transcend the use of narrow, syndrome-focused scales and include instruments capable of sampling broad domains of psychopathology (Hinshaw & Nigg, in press; Hinshaw & Zupan, 1997). Although the DSM practice of listing multiple comorbid diagnoses may give way, in future years, to more precise demarcation of subgroups and subtypes that are linked etiologically, there is no excuse, at present, for failing to account for diverse psychopathology and for not listing the multiple behavioral and emotional syndromes that fit the symptom picture. Indeed, neglecting comorbidity in research on the DBD is sure to lead to confusion, nonreplication of results, and stagnation in research efforts.

Conceptual issues regarding comorbidity are far from resolved. In DSM-IV (American Psychiatric Association, 1994), clinicians and investigators are encouraged to list the multiple mental disorders that a child may have, whereas the *International Classification of Diseases* (ICD-10; World Health Organization, 1993) has "comorbidities" built into the nomenclature (e.g., depressive conduct disorder; see Hinshaw & Anderson, 1996, and Chapter 1, this volume). Furthermore, as noted by Achenbach (1993), ODD may best be construed as a sensitive but nonspecific developmental precursor of early-onset, serious CD rather than a truly distinct disorder (in this regard, see also Loeber, Lahey, & Thomas, 1991, and Chapter 1, this volume). Although developmentally sensitive research will help to resolve such issues, the field cannot afford to ignore heterogeneity in our extant categories of DBD, meaning that the listing of (and, where possible, subtyping by) comorbid diagnoses should become a virtual requirement in the field. Overall, although the future may bring more clarity to the scene such that the comorbidities of today may yield to more precise specification of disordered pathways in the future, at present we must provide the most accurate depictions possible, which includes specification of multiple conditions.

Means of Establishing Diagnosis and Cross-Informant Perspectives

What are the optimal means of classifying DBD? Dimensionally, problem or symptom counts from validated and well-normed checklists appear to yield an optimal means of quantifying the domain or domains of interest; furthermore, use of cutoff scores could subsequently establish a statistically deviant group of youngsters with externalizing symptomatology. This approach has been a mainstay of obtaining samples for psychopathology and treatment investigations for many years. Yet several key problems can and often do emerge from the exclusive use of checklists or rating scales (see Hinshaw & Nigg, in press, for extended discussion). The meaning of items on checklists may be ambiguous and rater biases (e.g., "halo" effects in which a child is rated as all good or all bad depending on global impressions) may occur. Relatedly, constructs that can be differentiated clearly by objective observations may show considerable overlap with global ratings (see Hinshaw, Simmel, & Heller, 1995). Furthermore, ratings may reflect characteristics of the rater rather than of the child being appraised; a considerable literature has appeared debating the bias versus accuracy of depressed mothers' ratings (e.g., Fergusson, Lynksey, & Horwood, 1993; Richters, 1992).

For obtaining a diagnosis, rating scales are not the optimal means of appraising symptom onset, offset, and duration. Structured interviews, which typically take pains to establish timelines in order to prompt accurate temporal recall, are increasingly mandated as a means of ensuring diagnostic accuracy. Recall that dimensional symptom indexes can be obtained from the specific symptom counts of structured interviews, supplementing yes/no, categorical diagnoses per se (see Jensen *et al.*, 1996).

A key issue pertains equally to checklists and structured interviews: the differing perspectives of the various informants (usually parents, teachers, and the child himself or herself) who are sampled to yield symptom counts. The classic meta-analytic review of Achenbach, McConaughy, and Howell (1987) documents the distressingly low interinformant correspondence regarding appraisal of child psychopathology. For externalizing domains, the average intercorrelations hover around .3–.4, revealing considerable situational variability and unique informant variance in behavioral performance.

Reconciliation of disparate information across informants regarding both disruptive behavior and comorbid internalizing features is a pressing concern. Most data suggest that parents and teachers, rather than children themselves, are optimal informants for ADHD- and ODD-related behavior problems, whereas direct child report is needed for features of anxiety, depression, and thought disorder as well as for "covert" (mainly delinquent-type) conduct problems (see Hinshaw *et al.*, 1995; Loeber, Green, Lahey, & Stouthamer-Loeber, 1989). The age of the interviewed child is pertinent: Reliability figures for youth less than 10 years of age are suspect (although neglecting the child's perspective in a comprehensive evaluation can seldom be justified). Procedures for amalgamating disparate informants have focused on "either/or" algorithms: The symptom is counted as present when any informant responds positively (Bird, Gould, & Staghezza, 1992). Such "simple" algorithms have been found to outperform complex formulas that employ differential weighting (Piacentini, Cohen, & Cohen, 1992).

The ultimate validity of symptom-based diagnostic appraisal (whether quantitative or categorical) will depend on the underlying homogeneity of the dimensions or diagnoses under consideration and the expansion of purely behavioral evaluation into cognitive, neuropsychological, neurophysiological, and even genetic realms. Indeed, much of the research enterprise in the field today takes on a "bootstrapping" approach, in which reasonably reliable (but still questionably valid) diagnostic categories are examined with respect to correlates and mechanisms of interest, with the expectation (or hope) that more refined categorizations, based on processes that transcend symptom levels per se, will emerge. We thus reiterate our contention that person-centered approaches must coexist with investigations that can test, with strong inference, the effects of predictive and causal variables (see following sections).

METHODOLOGIC AND DESIGN ISSUES

Experimental versus Naturalistic Research

In a classic elaboration, four decades ago, of the two main traditions in psychological research, Cronbach (1957) described the differences between correlational (or naturalistic) investigations, on the one hand, and experimental research, on the other. Both types of research require careful observation, according to Cronbach; thus, it is inaccurate to discuss observational versus experimental paradigms. The key issue is the explicit control of extraneous variables in true experiments. The core problem for much human research, of course, is that many of the major causal or predictive variables of interest (e.g., genetic endowment, family child-rearing climate and practices, SES, neighborhood factors) are not amenable, for obvious ethical reasons, to experimental manipulation (see also Chapter 27, this volume). Viable quasi-experimental alternatives have been eloquently described (Cook & Campbell, 1979), but even these authors caution that there is no substitute for random assignment if causal inferences are to be drawn. This topic has recently received renewed interest in terms of the controversy, in treatment-related research, between "efficacy" investigations (randomized trials that typically utilize homogeneous samples and tight experimental controls with the aim of enhancing internal validity) versus "effectiveness" studies (naturalistic, broad-sample investigations that aim to promote generalizability) (see Hollon, 1996; Seligman, 1995; VandenBos, 1996).

Most of the field's research efforts directed toward understanding of causal factors are therefore correlational-predictive in nature. With (1) well-measured constructs, (2) competing causal pathways (which may include moderator and/or mediator variables; see Baron & Kenny, 1986), and (3) careful statistical means of testing such competing models, the field may be able to test relatively specific and nonambiguous predictions. Inference of "causation" must still be made with the utmost caution. Furthermore, the role of experimental treatment studies in the understanding of causal processes (beyond demonstrations of treatment effects per se) should not be underestimated. For example, Coie and Krehbiel (1984) found that improvements in academic skills produced increases in peer competence, but not vice versa, suggesting specific rather than general trajectories in achievement–peer linkages. Furthermore, the parent-training trial of Dishion, Patterson, and Kavanagh (1992) showed that changes in parental discipline style, which were associated with active behavioral intervention, accounted for (i.e., mediated) reductions in teacher-rated antisocial behavior patterns. In both of these experimental treatment studies, the effect of the independent variable of intervention type was mediated by changes in a key process variable (i.e., academic achievement, parental discipline), which in turn produced effects on outcomes of central importance (i.e., peer social status, antisocial behavior). In all, true experiments are unmatched in their ability to yield both causal inference (Hollon, 1996) and essential data on mediational processes. We turn next to consideration of moderator and mediator effects in developmental psychopathology research.

Processes, Mediators, and Moderators

In describing both experimental and correlational findings, Cook and Campbell (1979) noted that it is far easier to detect an effect of one variable on another than to explain it. Indeed, explanation, involving the uncovering of underlying processes over and above the documentation of simple predictions between predictor and criterion variables, should be the "name of the game" in most studies of biological, cognitive, psychological, familial, or environmental correlates.

As authoritatively described by Baron and Kenny (1986), a moderator is a group-level factor that changes predictive relationships between variables of interest when it is entered into the equation. For example, Robins (1978) demonstrated that only children with intermediate levels of antisocial behavior in adolescence, and not those with extremely high or low amounts, showed predictive relationships between (1) antisocial paternal histories, low socioeconomic status, or family discord and (2) adult antisociability. Thus, the level of adolescent conduct problems served to moderate the relationship between family history, impoverishment, and family interaction patterns, on the one hand, and adult antisocial outcomes, on the other. As noted earlier, Wootton and colleagues (1997) examined the presence of callous-unemotional (CU) traits in childhood as a moderator of the relationship between parenting competence and antisocial behavior patterns. In the non-CU youth with disruptive problems, the expected prediction held: Higher levels of unskilled parenting were associated with greater degrees of CD behavior. Intriguingly, however, the CU group showed a nonsignificant (and even slightly negative) predictive relationship, suggesting that children with such a temperament style may be relatively impervious to variations in parenting. In addition, Deater-Deckard and Dodge (1997) demonstrated that ethnicity moderated the relationship between harsh discipline style and subsequent aggressive behavior: In Caucasian children, authoritarian parenting predicted teacher-appraised aggression 6 years later; however, in an African American sample there was no significant predictive relationship, with a slightly negative slope.* In summary, without taking into account crucial moderator variables, predictive relationships will be masked, missed, or misunderstood.

*Note, however, that abusive parenting was strongly predictive of subsequent externalizing behavior in both ethnic groups. The findings under discussion pertain to authoritarian parenting styles but not frank abuse.

In contrast, a mediator helps to explain the process by which predictor and criterion variables are related. As articulated by Baron and Kenny (1986), the conditions for a mediational effect are as follows: First, the predictor (P) variable significantly relates to the outcome or criterion (C); second, P significantly relates to the putative mediator (M); third, M significantly predicts C; and, finally, statistically accounting for M either eliminates or significantly reduces the predictive relationship between P and C. In other words, the mediator "takes over" as the explanatory factor. In one of the experimental investigations discussed earlier, parenting discipline was the key mediator of the treatment-related impact of parent management intervention on child coercion and antisocial behavior (Dishion et al., 1992). Another example is found in Dodge, Bates, and Pettit (1990): The effects of early exposure to abuse on subsequent teacher-appraised aggression were mediated, in part, by sociocognitive information-processing measures. That is, altered perceptions of and attributions about the social world accounted for the tendency of abused youngsters to develop aggressive behavior patterns (see also Chapter 14, this volume). Overall, elucidation and analysis of psychometrically sound mediator and moderator variables is essential for explanation, over and above prediction per se. In addition, uncovering the optimal group-level variables to serve as moderators will help blend person-centered and variable-centered research strategies.

Viable Measures of Key Constructs

Our discussion of the importance of investigating processes and mechanisms is predicated, of course, on the availability of reliable and valid indicators of the constructs of interest. Indeed, Meehl (1978) pointed to the exquisite reliability and precision of measures as a key reason for the explosive progress in the 20th century in the "hard" sciences such as physics. First, issues of interinformant correspondence (see the preceding discussion) pertain just as much to predictors, outcomes, mediators, and moderators as they do to diagnostic measures. Thus, results from measures relying solely on single informants may be quite specific to such sources. Second, investigations in which predictors, mediators or moderators, and criteria all emanate from the same method, source, or both are far less persuasive than those that utilize alternative methods for different constructs. To transcend method- or source-specific findings, key constructs in predictive and explanatory research would each comprise latent variables, amalgamated from various methods and informants that include direct observation and informant report (e.g., Patterson *et al.*, 1992). Direct observations and other more objective indicators are particularly important in studies of psychosocial treatments, in which those informants (parents, teachers) who are delivering intervention cannot be expected to remain unbiased in their appraisal of child dysfunction or impairment (Hinshaw *et al.*, 1997). Although laboratory indicators of the important constructs of inattention, impulsivity, hyperactivity, aggression, or antisocial behavior cannot automatically be assumed to be more valid than informant or self-report, the objective anchoring of these constructs is an extremely desirable goal (see Teicher, Ito, Glod, & Barber, 1996). Finally, we reiterate our earlier point that although self-reports of ADHD and ODD behavior patterns do not aid appreciably in the diagnostic process, it is vital to include the child's perspective on such variables as internalizing and conduct symptoms, family relationships, community violence, and self-esteem (e.g., Coie & Lenox, 1994; Herjanic & Reich, 1982; Richters & Martinez, 1993).

Protective Factors and Resiliency

In passing, we note that the vast majority of research in the area of DBD has centered on risk factors—influences that predict increased tendencies toward externalizing features or impairment. Far less attention has been paid to those intrapersonal, familial, or environmental factors that may help to mitigate their impact (Yung & Hammond, 1997). Whereas risk factors are those variables that specifically increase the likelihood of later dysfunction, often operating on vulnerable individuals (those with predispositions that accentuate risk susceptibility), protective factors are those influences that help mitigate risk and vulnerability. In other words, a protective factor operates in the presence of a risk factor to reduce the risk; its effects are typically detected by means of statistical interactions. That is, at low levels of risk the protective factor shows little effect but at high levels of risk it enhances adaptive outcome. Such protective factors may thus help spur resiliency—the presence of optimal functioning in vulnerable or at-risk circumstances.

Investigators of developmental psychopathology are attempting to document the salient intraindividual, familial, and wider systemic influences that serve as protective factors, as well as their mechanisms of effect (for reviews, see Cicchetti & Garmezy, 1993; Masten, Best, & Garmezy, 1990). Large-scale investigations have been performed (see Werner & Smith, 1992), with encouraging findings. In terms of DBD, salient tasks would include the search for variables and processes that predict desistence from antisocial activities or that promote adaptive functioning in youth with ADHD during adolescence and adulthood. Focus on such variables and processes, that is, on the causal pathways that promote the development of amelioration of psychopathology, may well assist in the search for viable preventive intervention programs (Reid, 1993).

DATA-ANALYTIC STRATEGIES

Space limitations preclude exhaustive coverage, so we note three topics of pertinence to the field: null-hypothesis significance testing, detection of moderator and mediator effects, and longitudinal research methods.

Null-Hypothesis Significance Testing

Commentary on the standard significance-testing approach has appeared for decades, with a variety of often devastating critiques. For example, although the truth of the null hypothesis is the "standard" in this methodology—to be disconfirmed with a pattern of empirical findings—a null hypothesis of no group differences or no predictive relationship can almost never be true with any degree of precision (Hunter, 1997). Thus, significance tests are actually measures of the power of a given design; with a sufficiently large sample size, almost any null hypothesis can be rejected. Furthermore, the logic of inference from null-hypothesis testing is opposite to that of sound Bayseian inference (Loftus, 1996; Richters, 1997).

The long-standing debate over the viability of significance testing has recently intensified (e.g., Shrout, 1997). Some contend that null-hypothesis testing is actively hampering research progress (Hunter, 1997); others hold to a more conciliatory approach (Abelson, 1997; Harris, 1997). Constructively, Loftus (1996) suggested alternatives or supplements to significance tests in research reports, including inspection of plots of raw data, display of graphic figures (rather than tabular displays of means), increased use of planned comparisons, presentation of effect sizes, and greatly increased use of confidence intervals. Meehl (1978) championed more stringent criteria for the empirical backing of theoretical claims; in their innovative statistics text, Judd and McClelland (1989) advocated explicit model comparisons (rather than null-hypothesis testing) as the basis of statistical comparisons in the field. In summary, combined with promotion of more precise measures of key constructs, adoption of more stringent inferential reasoning can promote advances in our understanding of DBD.

Detection of Moderators and Mediators

Although we have emphasized the importance of explanatory research, which includes examination of moderator and mediator effects, we caution that the typical nonexperimental investigation has extremely low statistical power for their detection. Indeed, McClelland and Judd (1993) highlight the conceptual and statistical issues that make the uncovering of statistical interactions in nonrandom-assign-

ment studies problematic. One point from this incisive review is that the usual nonexperimental study does not contain enough individuals at extreme levels of both the predictor and the putative moderator to afford powerful examination of the interaction effect. This warning is particularly pertinent to those who investigate moderator variables, which by definition are those group factors that interact with predictors to yield differential patterns of influence on key outcomes. Some lessons from this problematic state of affairs are that (1) rather large samples will be needed to approach detection of interactions (but they alone do not guarantee power—see McClelland & Judd, 1993); (2) the full range of scores on predictor and moderator variables must be represented in the sample; and (3) investigators should consider, whenever possible and feasible, experimental trials, which are extremely well suited for capturing interaction effects. In the "real world," as discussed earlier, many variables of potential explanatory interest are not amenable to experimental manipulation, for logistic or ethical reasons. Nonetheless, creative investigators can and should use experimental trials, when possible, because of their considerable explanatory potential (e.g., Hollon, 1996).

Longitudinal Research Methods

Much risk and protective factor research in the field centers on the influence of causal variables on the child's development, requiring longitudinal (and ideally, prospective) research strategies. Although coverage of this topic could easily expand to book length itself, we highlight, first, the great care that must attend longitudinal investigations. Stouthamer-Loeber, Van Kammen, and Loeber (1992) and Capaldi and Patterson (1987) provided authoritative guidelines for such issues as tracking of participants, managing data files, and maintaining high retention rates.

Second, we note that increasing attention is being directed to appropriate methodologic and data-analytic procedures for handling longitudinal research designs with DBD (e.g.,

Loeber & Farrington, 1994). A key issue is that traditional statistical procedures such as repeated-measures analysis of variance have given way to random-effects regression models (Gibbons et al., 1993; Nich & Carroll, 1997) to model processes of change. These strategies allow for inclusion of all initial participants in data analyses, with imputation of missing data; for modeling of individual- (as well as group-) level trajectories of change; and for inclusion of both time-varying and "fixed" covariates. Such methods can be applied to both experimental, clinical-trials data and prospective, longitudinal investigations without random assignment. In all, new strategies for analyzing prospective, longitudinal data are quite promising and deserve the attention of investigators in the field.

Third, we point out that merely measuring the same individuals at multiple time points does not necessarily yield developmentally relevant data. Longitudinal research has great potential to uncover explanatory factors, but investigators must be aware of the assessment-related issues discussed previously, must work to amalgamate predictor and outcome variables into meaningful composites, must seek those "experiments in nature" that can help to isolate causally relevant environmental factors (Rutter et al., 1997), and must be cautious when inferring causal or explanatory processes. More sophisticated data-analytic strategies have the potential for increasing the yield from longitudinal investigations, but truly explanatory research requires considerable methodologic and conceptual efforts on the investigator's part.

CULTURE, ETHNICITY, AND GENDER

The variables of culture, ethnicity, and gender constitute areas of greatly increasing interest for developmental psychopathologists (e.g., Bird, 1996; Maccoby, 1988; Zoccolillo, 1993). The importance of these factors for thorough understanding of DBD contrasts with the limited space available for consideration of this area. Our main contention, for the issues of culture–ethnicity and gender, is that *process* investigations—those that seek to explain *how* systemic, familial, and intraindividual processes may differentially produce or maintain disruptive behavior patterns across ethnic groups or between males and females—will be more illuminating than reports that simply assert differences (or nondifferences) in rates of disruptive problems or disorders as a function of these independent variables. In other words, studies of process and explanation (including investigations of mediators and moderators) must supersede data on differential prevalence rates per se. We begin with an overview of issues pertinent to culture and ethnicity and then consider gender. For recent review chapters and articles on these topics, please refer to Arnold (1996), Dinges, Atlis, and Vincent (1997), Gaub and Carlson (1997), Giordano and Cernkovich (1997), Goodman and Kohlsdorf (1994), and Yung and Hammond (1997).

Culture and Ethnicity

The importance of recognizing culture and ethnicity in the development of DBD is apparent when one considers that culture shapes the microsocial environments (schools, families) in which behavior is defined as inattentive, impulsive, or aggressive. Indeed, one can imagine cultures or ethnic groups with greatly diverging conceptions of interpersonal boundaries, competitiveness, assertion, and/or aggression. With the ever increasing ethnic heterogeneity of American society, real progress in the field requires consideration of cultural and ethnic factors in the development, expression, maintenance, and treatment of childhood disorders. Yet a host of conceptual and methodologic problems have hampered extant research in this area, including a lack of sufficient data on ethnic groups and (particularly) ethnic subgroups, difficulties in accurate classification of ethnicity or acculturation, problems in access to immigrant or out-of-school youth, faulty instrumentation, a focus on risk factors to the exclusion of protective factors, and a lack of statistical power in data analyses (for cogent discussion, see Yung & Hammond, 1997).

Cultural and Ethnic Differences in Base Rates of Constituent Behaviors

Do prevalence rates of DBD vary as a function of cultural or ethnic status? Unfortunately, definitive data on this subject from epidemiologic samples are not plentiful. For adulthood, epidemiologic-scale investigations from the 1980s and 1990s have failed to yield consistent evidence for ethnic differences in rates of Antisocial Personality Disorder (see review in Dinges *et al.*, 1997). As for children, information from the recent MECA study, which is being analyzed at the time of the writing of this chapter, will yield better answers to this important question with respect to ODD, CD, and ADHD (see Chapter 2, this volume).

Antisocial Behavior Patterns. With existing databases, however, there are strong indications that such disenfranchised ethnic groups as African Americans display higher rates of antisocial behavior patterns and delinquency than do majority youth (see Yung & Hammond, 1997).* It is essential, however, to emphasize that nearly all African American versus white differences across multiple measures of antisocial behavior are eliminated when indicators of SES are statistically controlled (e.g., Peeples & Loeber, 1994). That is, the effects of ethnicity on rates of aggression and antisocial behavior are almost entirely explained by the substandard housing, low income, and low educational and occupational attainment that pertain to African Americans as a group (Loeber, Farrington, Stouthamer-Loeber, & Van Kammen, 1998). A comprehensive review (Hawkins, Laub, & Lauritsen, in press) demonstrates the necessity of transcending individual-level correlations between racial status and antisocial behavior by considering community or "macro" contextual factors.

*Note that samples demonstrating higher ethnic than majority representation among *incarcerated* youth may actually be indexing discriminatory policies regarding detection, sentencing, or both (Yung & Hammond, 1997).

Four additional points regarding SES as a covariate are salient. First, it appears to be income levels and poverty, rather than education and occupational status per se, that are the factors specifically related to aggression and antisocial behavior (Farrington, 1986). Second, as cogently discussed by Yung and Hammond (1997), socioeconomic variables should be expanded even further to include such ethnically relevant factors as "school quality, desegregation patterns, access to prevention resources, police/resident relationships, and other community characteristics" (p. 491). In other words, multiple levels of community and neighborhood factors may be relevant to the "disadvantage" of underrepresented minority groups. Third, as impressively demonstrated by Capaldi and Patterson (1994), effects of social systemic and socioeconomic variables on early-onset antisocial behavior are mediated almost entirely by parent–child interactions. In other words, moving from "macro" variables such as ethnic status, to associated socioeconomic disadvantage, and then further to micro-level familial processes enables the field to gain greater explanatory power. Fourth, debate continues among sociologists about the optimal means of measuring SES (e.g., Hauser, 1994), with expert opinion converging on the necessity of accounting separately for measures of income, education, neighborhood status, and occupation rather than utilizing indexes that cut across these separable factors (Entwisle & Astone, 1994).

ADHD. As for ADHD, definitive data on ethnic and cultural differences are not available. Indeed, a recent literature review revealed a paucity of pertinent studies of this topic (Samuel *et al.*, 1997). Nevertheless, several points are salient. First, to the extent that ADHD is comorbid with ODD and CD (Biederman, Newcorn, & Sprich, 1991; Hinshaw, 1987), it may also show disproportionately high rates in ethnic minority groups. An important question is whether "pure" ADHD, with aggressive and antisocial behavior controlled, is still overrepresented in either ethnic minority groups or those of lower SES. Second, in this regard, at least some risk factors for ADHD—for example, low birth weight (Breslau et al., 1996)—are associated with SES and, presumably, minority status. Indeed, as elaborated by Breslau and colleagues (1996), low birth weight is a potent and specific risk factor for later ADHD (that is, it does *not* predict later aggressive or internalizing disorders), particularly when the ADHD is accompanied by subaverage IQ. This finding holds, however, only in inner-city and not in middle-class settings (Breslau et al., 1996), suggesting strongly a multiple-risk-factor model. Alternatively, maternal intrusiveness and overstimulation early in development have also been shown to predict later ADHD (Carlson, Jacobvitz, & Sroufe, 1995). Yet, as with low birth weight, such predictions have occurred only in high-risk, low-income samples. In short, the potential for overrepresentation of ADHD among ethnic minority groups may be confounded with comorbid antisocial behavior and, if found, is likely to be part of complex causal pathways.

In addition, the push for recognition and formal diagnosis of ADHD in the 1990s may be emanating largely from middle- and upper-middle-class, suburban families who are seeking special education services and medication interventions for their offspring. Thus, SES (and ethnicity) may be interacting in disparate ways to influence prevalence of ADHD-related syndromes. In contrast to those who contend that ADHD only exists in Western, achievement-oriented societies, investigations have revealed that the symptom picture is present (and impairing) in non-Western nations (e.g., Bhatia, Nigam, Bohra, & Malik, 1991). Thus, it is not the case that only postindustrial, achievement-oriented societies foster the ADHD syndrome.

The ways in which strongly heritable temperamental characteristics (see Levy et al., 1997) such as high activity level and intensity are met with good or poor "fit" by caregivers appears to be related strongly to the cultural beliefs and expectations of families in different ethnic groups. A high priority for research on the early developmental precursors of ADHD would be to operationalize and examine the cultural influences on such family–child fit (Chess & Thomas, 1984).

Summary. In all, establishing the existence (or lack of difference) in rates of ADHD, ODD, or CD across ethnic or cultural groups is only the beginning of meaningful investigation. Understanding of the social, psychobiological, familial, and intraindividual processes that explain or "carry" any effects of culture or ethnicity is essential. At a basic level, the field must consider the cultural meaning of the risk factors for DBD. For example, do base rates of physical aggression in young children differ in different societies, cultures, or ethnic groups? How prevalent are attentional problems in agrarian societies? Furthermore, are such differences in basic behaviors related to cultural or ethnic differences in (1) expectations for appropriate behavior, (2) rater thresholds for detecting deviance, (3) child-rearing practices or parent–child "fit," or (4) schooling practices? The research agenda for investigators interested in cultural and ethnic factors is indeed large.

Relevant Processes

In a study of Anglo and Puerto Rican mothers' perceptions of temperament and attachment-related behaviors, Harwood (1992) found that although Puerto Rican parents valued calm, respectful behavior, Anglo mothers placed higher value on autonomous behavior. As another example, in Chinese families, higher parental control was viewed by adolescents as indicative of parental hostility (Lau, Lew, Hau, Cheung, & Berndt, 1990), whereas in Korean families, high parental control was associated with increased warmth and love for the child (Rohner & Pettingill, 1985). Furthermore, investigators have noted differing expectations among ethnic groups with respect to social and personal development (Pachter, Dworkin, & Bernstein, 1995). Insofar as parental expectations and parental valuation shape both behavioral displays and interactional style, ethnic or cultural differences in problem behavior and frank disorder may be likely.

As previously highlighted, important advances will not come so much from group comparison studies (that examine ethnic or gender differences in rates or levels of key behaviors) as from process or explanatory investigations, in which potential differences in underlying mechanisms within ethnic groups or gender are carefully examined. A pertinent example is the work of Deater-Deckard and Dodge (1997) discussed earlier in this chapter on the differential predictability from authoritarian parenting to subsequent child aggression in African American versus Caucasian families. To recapitulate, whereas strict, authoritarian parenting predicted later aggression in the white youth, there was no relationship (or a slightly negative association) between these variables for the African American youngsters. Thus, ethnic status moderated the relationship between parenting practices and subsequent aggression. A continuing challenge from such research is to probe further for relevant explanation. Pachter and Harwood's (1996) insightful discussion points to African American parents' perceptions of the social environment as hostile and rejecting, motivating use of strict discipline practices to prepare their offspring to survive in adverse conditions. In this context, authoritarian parenting may signify appropriate parental concern and involvement. Qualitative, ethnographic research methods may need to supplement empirical, quantitative strategies in the search for such explanations (Yung & Hammond, 1997), with focus on such variables as environmental stressors, social and political history, and parent and child perceptions of discipline practices. Research on culture and ethnicity thus necessarily incorporates a rich mix of psychological, social, and historical factors.

Methodologic and Measurement Issues

We next address a number of assessment-related and measurement issues that must be confronted in conducting research on culture and developmental psychopathology. In particular, several questions exist regarding the reliability and validity of existing measurement

tools that have been established with the majority population rather than with ethnic minority groups and the nature of sampling related to ethnic groups of interest.

Content Bias and the Meaning of Scores. As explicated by Foster and Martinez (1995), content bias may occur either when an instrument contains items that are irrelevant for a particular group or when it fails to include items important for a given subgroup. For example, Lopez, Hurwicz, Karno, and Telles (1992) found that significant differences occurred between Mexican Americans and Anglo Americans in the types of symptoms reported for schizophrenia and bipolar mood disorder, suggesting content bias in extant scales. Unless diagnostic instruments contain content relevant to diagnostic groups of interest, critical information about how psychological processes manifest in differing subcultures may be missed. The dilemma, however, is that if item content is modified to enhance culturally sensitivity and relevance, the ability to compare across majority and minority cultures is compromised. Somewhat longer scales that include sufficient items for varying subgroups may be indicated.

A related issue is whether similar scores on a given measure carry the same meaning across cultures. For example, investigations of Japanese and American mothers of preschoolers (Windle, Iwawaki, & Lerner, 1988) and adolescents (Windle, Iwawaki, & Lerner, 1987) have found that, in general, Japanese participants rate themselves less positively in such domains as self-esteem, body attractiveness, and quality of mood. These findings were not interpreted to mean that Japanese parents and youth hold less positive self-images but rather that their responses reflect the Japanese cultural value placed on reserve and modesty. Similarly, Okazaki and Sue (1995) pointed out that among middle-aged Chinese men, the endorsement of such "positive" feelings as feeling good about oneself or feeling happy about one's life may be considered immodest or frivolous.

Adult informant ratings—a cornerstone of research on DBD—have also been found to be influenced by culture. An epidemiologic study found that teachers and mothers from Puerto Rico were more likely to perceive adolescents as having externalizing behavior problems than were adults in the mainland United States (Achenbach *et al.*, 1989). Again, this difference was not interpreted to indicate that Puerto Rican adolescents are necessarily more prone to aggression than their mainland counterparts, but rather that, given the strong value in Puerto Rican society placed on calmness, rates of externalizing behavior that may be considered normative by U.S. standards could be viewed as excessive on the island (Pachter & Harwood, 1996). These results are consistent with other investigations showing that the same child behavior patterns may be rated differently by individuals from different cultural or ethnic backgrounds (Harwood, 1992).

Although the use of more objective behavior observation systems could help to mitigate such cultural "bias" in ratings and to understand "real" differences in behavior across subgroups of interest, observed behaviors may still be misinterpreted (Foster & Martinez, 1995). For example, a type of verbal dueling typical of some African American youth, termed "basing," involves the trading of insults with the understanding that there is no real harm intended. This type of behavior could easily be scored as verbally aggressive in behavior observations based on majority norms. In short, with the possibility that similar responses and behavior may carry different meaning for different ethnic or cultural groups, the issue of separate norms becomes salient.

Separate Norms? If ethnic differences in DBD exist across an item pool that is sufficiently broad, should assessment instruments provide separate norms by ethnicity? In this regard, extremely few rating scales or questionnaires pertinent to the assessment of DBD provide such differential norms (Hinshaw & Nigg, in press). Yet the utility of such norms, even if available, is a difficult question. One perspective is that, given children's need to function in the majority culture, it will be crucial for their adaptation and well-being to meet

many of the larger society's expectations. Assessment and diagnosis based on majority norms may therefore be essential for identifying those youth at risk in the mainstream culture. It would be important, however, to also consider the child's standing relative to his or her subcultural group, as such understanding may help prevent overpathologizing and inform treatment decisions.

Identifying and Categorizing Participants. In placing research participants into ethnic groups, most investigations use a classification system with broad categories such as "Native American" or "Asian American." Such categories are problematic because they group together individuals from many cultures and subcultures who differ from one another in important ways. For example, included in the category of Native American are more than 500 federally recognized tribes, known to hold markedly different practices and beliefs (Bureau of Indian Affairs, 1991; Renfry, 1992). Overly broad categories, then, may mask crucial differences between individuals, even leading to misinformation or stereotyping.

In addition, and critically, as the heterogeneity of American society increases, it becomes more difficult to characterize growing numbers of individuals with mixed ethnic heritage as belonging exclusively to one group or another. This issue is of real concern, given evidence that biracial adolescents (African American and Caucasian) differ from their monoracial counterparts (African American) in both ethnic identity and a number of indicators of family relationships (Hiraga, Cauce, Mason, & Ordonez, 1993). Coding of ethnic status is likely to become more complex in the coming years.

Some investigators believe that a more salient variable than ethnicity or race is acculturation, referring to the extent to which members of ethnic minority groups adhere to the customs and traditional practices of their culture of origin versus those of the majority culture (Berry, 1990). Level of acculturation is preferred over ethnicity per se because it is believed to be a more direct measure of cultural elements, such as values and preferences, that influence behavior

(Dinges *et al.*, 1997). Yet this construct is not without problems. For one thing, measures of acculturation vary in their content, with differential emphasis of beliefs and values across scales, resulting in ambiguity. Furthermore, whereas acculturation supposedly measures beliefs and values rather than ethnic background per se, most extant measures feature language usage and place of birth in addition to beliefs (Betancourt & Lopez, 1993). In addition, few measures of acculturation are appropriate for use with children (Foster & Martinez, 1995), an unfortunate circumstance given that acculturation level of children may well differ from that of their parents in important ways.

Differentiating Ethnicity and Culture from Social Class. Within American society, there is large confounding of the effects of ethnic background with those pertinent to social class. Careful statistical controls may be necessary to disentangle the causal or predictive effects of such correlated background variables (Yung & Hammond, 1997). In addition, individual-level and neighborhood-level analyses should not become confused or confounded (Hawkins, Laub, & Lauritsen, in press). The issues raised at the beginning of this section regarding African American youth and antisocial behavior are clearly salient here. Furthermore, as Betancourt and Lopez (1993) point out, different social classes may have their own unique cultures, and the contribution of these cultural variables needs to be differentiated from those of income level, occupational status, or education per se. To illustrate, Sobal and Stunkard (1989) posited that obesity in developing countries is attributable to both economic factors such as the availability of food supplies and cultural factors such as the valuing of larger body shapes. Clearly, complexity rather than simplicity will attend thorough investigations of culture as related to psychopathology.

Small Sample Size. Another obstacle to using culture or ethnicity as an independent variable, covariate, or moderator is that sufficiently large samples of pertinent minority groups are often difficult to obtain. For instance, the Native American population constitutes less than 1% of the U.S. population at present (Yung & Hammond, 1997). Even for ethnic minorities with larger representations, some geographical regions contain tiny percentages of important groups. As a result of the small sample sizes that may be available, investigators tend to lump individuals of diverse cultural and ethnic background together into broad categories (e.g., clustering Chinese American, Japanese American, and Korean American persons as Asian Americans; combining Mexican American and Puerto Rican individuals as Latinos-Latinas). As discussed previously, this practice is problematic to the extent that the broad categories contain significant within-group heterogeneity. Applied to the terminology of Richters (1997), assumptions of invariant causal relationships for all members of a broadly defined ethnic group may not be totally invalid. Yet sufficiently large samples of the finer-grained and more accurate classifications may be difficult, if not impossible, to identify.

Whether the investigator utilizes convenience sampling (with no stipulations regarding the final ethnic or cultural makeup of the sample) or representative sampling (ensuring that the sample reflects ethnic distributions of the larger population), assuring adequate sample sizes of ethnic groups of interest may be problematic. In particular, although ethnic group × psychological variable interactions (wherein ethnicity moderates effects of key predictors on outcomes of interest) may be instructive, the extremely low statistical power that pertains to detecting interaction terms in nonexperimental research was highlighted earlier (McClelland & Judd, 1993). To summarize, without careful attention to accurate classification of ethnic status and without samples that are sufficiently large with respect to ethnic groups of interest, the field will have difficulty uncovering explanatory processes that may diverge, in important ways, across relevant subgroups.

Gender

The majority of the literature on DBD pertains to males. Indeed, it is an almost automatic assumption that ADHD, ODD, and CD are disorders of boys and that female manifestations are atypical (Giordano & Cernkovich, 1997). Increasingly clear, however, is that ADHD, ODD, and CD are present in girls and that the understanding of gender differences and gender-related processes is necessary for progress in the field (Arnold, 1996; Eme & Kavanaugh, 1995; Goodman & Kohlsdorf, 1994).

Antisocial Behavior Patterns

A vibrant debate has unfolded, in recent years, regarding the apparently disproportionate representation of externalizing and antisocial behavior in boys (for a thorough review, see Eme & Kavanaugh, 1995). Whereas little doubt exists that base rates of acting-out behavior are higher in boys than girls before puberty, with a host of psychobiological and cultural explanations invoked to explain this difference (Goodman & Kohlsdorf, 1994), by adolescence there is considerable "catch up" by females, except in areas of interpersonal violence, where male rates remain substantially higher than those of females (Zoccolillo, 1993). The issue is greatly complicated, however, when investigators broaden the definition of antisocial activity and aggression to include such alternative manifestations as indirect, interpersonal, or relational aggression (e.g., Crick & Grotpeter, 1995; Lagerspetz & Bjorkqvist, 1994). Indeed, girls may be more likely than boys to display aggression by excluding a peer from playgroups, spreading rumors, or using social influence to retaliate; inclusion of this type of aggressive activity may render gender differences in overall aggression nonsignificant. Intriguingly, such relational aggression shows impressive predictive validity for subsequent maladjustment in female samples (Crick, 1996). Note that, like covert antisocial behavior (Hinshaw *et al.,* 1995), indirect or relational aggression is difficult to observe directly; peer sociometric ratings and nominations appear to be the gold standard for detecting such relational activity (Crick & Grotpeter, 1995). Expanded perspectives on the issue of coverage of the domain of interest is therefore essential for investigators of gender and antisocial behavior.

Because of the extremely heterogeneous nature of the symptom list for CD, which includes indicators of physical aggression, sexual assault, property destruction, status offenses, and rule violations, and because only 3 of 15 symptoms are required for diagnosis, there are a myriad of symptom configurations that can yield a diagnosis (see Chapter 1, this volume). Thus, a girl could be diagnosed with CD exclusively on the basis of covert and status behaviors, whereas a boy (with the same number of overall symptoms) may qualify on the basis of violent assault. Thus, male and female samples who supposedly have the same diagnosis of CD may diverge radically with respect to both constituent behaviors and risk factors. Investigators of gender-related aspects of CD must look to the precise symptom configurations that yield diagnosis.

Provocatively, Zoccolillo (1993) argued (1) that criteria for DBD such as CD should be gender-normed so as not to neglect clinically meaningful externalizing behavior patterns in girls and (2) that such domains as somatizing behavior, which are related familially in females to antisocial behavior patterns in male relatives, should be included in the diagnostic criteria for females. In an incisive counterpoint, Zahn-Waxler (1993) contended that separate gender norms would both water down the construct of antisocial behavior and potentially label girls with nonserious forms of aggression, thus arguing for a consistent set of behavioral criteria across genders. The debate will be furthered by the presence of data comparing levels of impairment and predictive validity for gender-specific versus gender-neutral criteria (Goodman & Kohlsdorf, 1994).

Importantly, the long-term outcomes of CD may differ for the genders. In males, CD is a sensitive (although not greatly specific) predictor of later antisocial personality disorder. For females, however, although CD does relate to antisocial outcomes, it also tends to presage depression and other internalizing disorders (Robins, 1986). The paucity of prospective, longitudinal data for sufficiently sized samples of females with aggression and conduct problems is a serious problem for the field (Giordano & Cernkovich, 1997; see also Chapter 24, this volume).

ADHD

Although boys have commonly been claimed to outnumber girls with ratios as high as 5:1 to 10:1, such figures emanate largely from referred samples, in which boys' greater propensity for comorbid antisocial behavior is presumably reflected in higher referral rates. In community samples, the ratio appears to be closer to 2:1 or 3:1 (Gaub & Carlson, 1997). Furthermore, in the field trials for DSM-IV (which utilized clinical samples), Lahey and colleagues (1994) found that although boys outnumbered girls at expected levels for the combined type of ADHD, the male:female ratio was only less than 2:1 for the inattentive type. Thus, impulsivity and hyperactivity may be the features for which males predominate, with inattention per se more equally distributed across the genders. Greater density of research on objectively measured psychological processes (attention, impulse control) in both males and females should help inform this issue.

In an incisive meta-analytic review, Gaub and Carlson (1997) examined gender differences in constituent symptoms, impairments, and correlates of ADHD. Overall, few robust differences between males and females emerged, suggesting that expression of the disorder and its common impairments does not differ appreciably with gender. On the other hand, the data of Faraone and colleagues (1995) suggest that whereas boys with ADHD evidence a host of etiological risk factors for the disorder, girls constitute a more "familial" type, with strong risk for heritable causation.

A National Institute of Mental Health conference on sex differences in ADHD (Arnold, 1996) summarized extant evidence in the field, echoing the conclusions of Gaub and Carlson (1997) that gender differences in extant samples have not been strong and providing the overall conclusion that additional research on gender-specific processes and mechanisms is clearly needed. As with ethnic minority groups, obtaining sufficient sample sizes of females is necessary if important explanatory mechanisms are to be elucidated with adequate statistical power.

CONCLUSIONS

We opened this chapter by reviewing a provocative critique of current research methods and paradigms in the field (Richters, 1997), contending that if its tenets are valid, much of the field's apparent progress is actually illusory and that substantially new approaches are necessary. We continued, however, with a set of commentaries on such issues as sampling, research design, and statistical analysis, and on the crucial topics of culture, ethnicity, and gender, that were largely framed in the predominant paradigm. Readers noting a "disconnect" between these two perspectives should be rewarded for their accuracy of perception.

How do we reconcile this disparity? As we noted at the outset, our own vision is sufficiently limited that we cannot as yet see through to what a new paradigm would entail. We therefore chose to critique what currently exists, providing commentary on the field's practices from within its prevailing methods and practices in an attempt to foster greater stringency, accuracy, and validity. Several ideas are clear: Avoiding rigid adherence to current diagnostic categories, rethinking current statistical reasoning with respect to null-hypothesis testing, and discarding assumptions of individuals' structural homogeneity should serve as partial antidotes to pursuing research that is unproductive or even misguided. Furthermore, paying greater attention to the contextual variables within which DBD develops and intensifies should pay large dividends (see Hawkins et al., in press). In all, our great respect for the many advances the field has attained is tempered by our recognition of the vast distance yet to be covered if disruptive behavior patterns are to be fully understood, treated, and prevented.

Although research on DBD is a growth industry, serious questions remain as to the importance, viability, and theoretical coherence of the many findings that have emanated from our ever increasing numbers of investigations. We close with several specific recommendations that may enhance the value of investigations in the field.

1. Investigators need to make explicit linkages with pertinent theory. Exemplary in this regard is the work of Quay (1993) regarding the neurobiological underpinnings of early-onset CD. Although careful description and documentation of developmental patterns is indeed important, understanding of causal pathways will be facilitated by linking descriptive data with developmental, personality-related, psychobiological, and cultural theory. On the other hand, overarching "theories of everything" that do not allow for the great individual and subgroup differences that exist in causal pathways, underlying mechanisms, and response to intervention are doomed to failure. That is, theories must take into account the considerable individual, developmental, and cultural differences that pertain to DBD.

2. Related to this last point, demarcation of pertinent subgroups should aid in the uncovering of causal pathways. In this regard, we have cited repeatedly the work of Moffitt (1993) and Patterson and colleagues (1992) on early- versus late-onset CD. Indeed, recent work on genetic underpinnings of reading disorders has benefited enormously from the separation of subgroups of individuals with single-word reading deficits and those with specific phonologic problems; such basic processes have not been as well specified for DBD.

3. As noted throughout the chapter, refinement of measurement tools is a priority. Objective measures are a desired aim, particularly in the areas of attentional deficits and hyperactivity (Teicher et al., 1996). Also, ecologically valid assessment in the natural environment, including the use of adult- and self-informant ratings, will continue to be a mainstay in the field.

4. Maintaining a perspective on (1) dimensional and categorical perspectives and (2) variable-centered and person-centered research strategies as complementary, rather than opposing, should facilitate more productive research enterprises.

5. Intensified focus on both ethnicity and gender will not only make research on DBD more representative and generalizable but will also help in the uncovering of basic explanatory variables. For example, over and above measur-

ing SES and ethnic status per se, investigators should consider the appraisal of exposure to neighborhood violence, patterns of school and job discrimination, acculturation of both parents and offspring, and the like.

6. Investigations of processes and mechanisms—supplementing research on diagnostic versus control group differences per se—are likely to yield the most important insights on the development of externalizing behavior patterns. We have taken pains to discuss the kinds of mediator and moderator variables that may be pertinent to development and maintenance of DBD.

7. We encourage emphasis on the potential for experimental research (in particular, clinical trials related to prevention and treatment) to answer important causal and mediational questions. Clinical trials do not automatically inform understanding of process; appropriately designed experimental investigations can yield crucial insights if measures of key mediators are included and if contrasting interventions are chosen with care. Our sense is that the explanatory potential of experimental trials is greatly underutilized in the field.

8. Attention must be paid not only to the multiple areas of concern that surround DBD—for example, molecular genetics; adequately measured temperament and parent–child "fit"; family, school, peer, and neighborhood influences; SES and wider cultural factors—but also to the transactional pathways that link these various levels. Our current methods are greatly limited in their ability to accommodate patterns of reciprocal causation and transaction; set-breaking methods and paradigms must be actively sought.

Overall, although research density in the field is increasing at high rates, we sense both a fragmentation of key findings and a distressing lack of theory-driven investigations in the field. It is indeed time for investigators of DBD to (1) actively integrate the perspectives of multiple systems (ranging from the psychobiologic to the cultural and socioeconomic) into their studies and (2) "break set" to consider alternative paradigms by adopting fresh perspectives on forming homogeneous subgroups, establishing more stringent evidentiary standards, and integrating quantitative and qualitative research methods. Certainly, the nature of the problem area and the problem populations under consideration mandates such vision and action.

ACKNOWLEDGMENTS. Work on this chapter was supported, in part, by National Institute of Mental Health Grants U01 MH50461 and R01 MH45064. We thank John Richters for his perceptive comments on drafts of this chapter.

REFERENCES

Abelson, R. P. (1997). On the surprising longevity of flogged horses: Why there is a case for the significance test. *Psychological Science, 8,* 12–15.

Achenbach, T. M. (1991). *Manual for the Child Behavior Checklist/4-18 and 1991 profile.* Burlington: University of Vermont, Department of Psychiatry.

Achenbach, T. M. (1993). Taxonomy and comorbidity of conduct problems: Evidence from empirically based approaches. *Development and Psychopathology, 5,* 51–64.

Achenbach, T. M., McConaughy, S. H., & Howell, C. T. (1987). Child/adolescent behavioral and emotional problems: Implications of cross-informant correlations for situational specificity. *Psychological Bulletin, 101,* 213–232.

Achenbach, T. M., Bird, H. R., Canino, G., Phares, V., Gould, M. S., & Rubio-Stipec, M. (1989). Epidemiological comparisons of Puerto Rican and U.S. mainland children: Parent, teacher, and self reports. *Journal of the American Academy of Child and Adolescent Psychiatry, 29,* 84–93.

American Psychiatric Association. (1980). *Diagnostic and statistical manual of mental disorders* (3rd ed.). Washington, DC: Author.

American Psychiatric Association. (1987). *Diagnostic and statistical manual of mental disorders* (3rd ed., rev.). Washington, DC: Author.

American Psychiatric Association. (1994). *Diagnostic and statistical manual of mental disorders* (4th ed.). Washington, DC: Author.

Arnold, L. E. (1996). Sex differences in ADHD: Conference summary. *Journal of Abnormal Child Psychology, 24,* 555–569.

Barkley, R. A. (1996). Attention-deficit hyperactivity disorder. In E. J. Mash & R. A. Barkley (Eds.), *Child psychopathology* (pp. 63–112). New York: Wiley.

Baron, R. M., & Kenny, D. A. (1986). The mediator–moderator distinction in social psychological research: Conceptual, strategic, and statistical considerations. *Journal of Personality and Social Psychology, 51,* 1173–1182.

Bergman, L. R., & Magnusson, D. (1997). A person-oriented approach in research on developmental psychopathology. *Development and Psychopathology, 9,* 291–319.

Berkson, J. (1946). Limitations of the application of fourfold table analysis to hospital data. *Bioethics Bulletin, 2,* 47–53.

Berry, J. (1990). Psychology of acculturation. In J. J. Berman (Ed.), *Nebraska Symposium on Motivation: Cross-cultural perspectives* (Vol. 37, pp. 201–234). Lincoln: University of Nebraska Press.

Betancourt, H., & Lopez, S. R. (1993). The study of culture, ethnicity, and race in American psychology. *American Psychologist, 48,* 629–637.

Bevan, W., & Kessel, F. (1994). Plain truths and home cooking: Thoughts on the making and remaking of psychology. *American Psychologist, 49,* 505–509.

Bhatia, M. S., Nigam, V. R., Bohra, N., & Malik, S. C. (1991). Attention deficit disorder with hyperactivity among paediatric outpatients. *Journal of Child Psychology and Psychiatry, 32,* 297–306.

Biederman, J., Newcorn, J., & Sprich, S. (1991). Comorbidity of attention deficit hyperactivity disorder with conduct, depressive, anxiety, and other disorders. *American Journal of Psychiatry, 52,* 464–470.

Bird, H. R. (1996). Epidemiology of childhood disorders in a cross-cultural context. *Journal of Child Psychology and Psychiatry, 37,* 35–49.

Bird, H. R., Gould, M. S., & Staghezza, B. (1992). Aggregating data from multiple informants in child psychiatry epidemiological research. *Journal of the American Academy of Child and Adolescent Psychiatry, 31,* 78–85.

Bird, H. R., Gould, M. S., Staghezza, B., & Jaramilo, B. M. (1994). The comorbidity of ADHD in a community sample of children aged 6 through 16 years. *Journal of Child and Family Studies, 3,* 365–378.

Breslau, N., Brown, G. G., DelDotto, J. E., Kumar, S., Ezhuthachan, S., Andreski, P., & Hufnagle, K. G. (1996). Psychiatric sequalae of low birth weight at 6 years of age. *Journal of Abnormal Child Psychology, 24,* 385–400.

Bureau of Indian Affairs. (1991). *American Indians today* (3rd ed.). Washington, DC: U.S. Department of the Interior.

Cacioppo, J., & Berntson, G. G. (1992). Social psychological contributions to the decade of the brain: Doctrine of multilevel analysis. *American Psychologist, 47,* 1019–1021.

Capaldi, D., & Patterson, G. R. (1987). An approach to the problem of recruitment and retention rates for longitudinal research. *Behavioral Assessment, 9,* 169–177.

Capaldi, D., & Patterson, G. R. (1994). Interrelated influences of contextual factors on antisocial behavior in childhood and adolescence for males. In D. C. Fowles, P. Sutker, & S. L. Goodman (Eds.), *Progress in experimental personality and psychopathology research* (Vol. 17, pp. 165–198). New York: Springer.

Carlson, E. A., Jacobvitz, D., & Sroufe, L. A. (1995). A developmental investigation of inattentiveness and hyperactivity. *Child Development, 66,* 37–54.

Caron, C., & Rutter, M. (1991). Comorbidity in child psychopathology: Concepts, issues, and research strategies. *Journal of Child Psychology and Psychiatry, 32,* 1063–1080.

Chess, S., & Thomas, A. (1984). *Origins and evolution of behavior disorders.* New York: Brunner/Mazel.

Cicchetti, D., & Garmezy, N. (1993). Prospects and promises in the study of resilience. *Development and Psychopathology, 5,* 497–502.

Cichetti, D., & Rogosch, F. (1996). Equifinality and multifinality in developmental psychopathology. *Development and Psychopathology, 8,* 597–600.

Coie, J. D., & Krebiehl, G. (1984). Effects of academic tutoring on the social status of low-achieving, socially rejected children. *Child Development, 55,* 1465–1478.

Coie, J. D., & Lenox, K. F. (1994). The development of antisocial individuals. In D. C. Fowles, P. Sutker, & S. H. Goodman (Eds.), *Progress in experimental personality and psychopathology research* (Vol. 17, pp. 45–72). New York: Springer.

Cook, T. D., & Campbell, D. T. (1979). *Quasi-experimentation: Design and analysis for field studies.* Chicago: Rand-McNally.

Crick, N. R. (1996). The role of overt aggression, relational aggression, and prosocial behavior in the prediction of children's future social adjustment. *Child Development, 67,* 2317–2327.

Crick, N. R., & Grotpeter, J. K. (1995). Relational aggression, gender, and social-psychological adjustment. *Child Development, 66,* 710–722.

Cronbach, L. J. (1957). Two disciplines of scientific psychology. *American Psychologist, 12,* 671–684.

Deater-Deckard, K., & Dodge, K. A. (1997). Externalizing behavior problems and discipline revisited: Nonlinear effects and variation by culture, context, and gender. *Psychological Inquiry, 8,* 161–175.

Dinges, N. G., Atlis, M. M., & Vincent, G. M. (1997). Cross-cultural perspectives on antisocial behavior. In D. M. Stoff, J. Breiling, & J. D. Maser (Eds.), *Handbook of antisocial behavior* (pp. 463–473). New York: Wiley.

Dishion, T. J., Patterson, G. R., & Kavanagh, K. (1992). An experimental test of the coercion model: Linking theory, measurement, and intervention. In J. McCord & R. Tremblay (Eds.), *The interaction of theory and practice: Experimental studies of interventions* (pp. 253–282). New York: Guilford.

Dodge, K. A., Bates, J., & Pettit, G. S. (1990). Mechanisms in the cycle of violence. *Science, 250,* 1678–1683.

Eme, R. F., & Kavanaugh, L. (1995). Sex differences in conduct disorder. *Journal of Clinical Child Psychology, 24,* 406–426.

Entwisle, D. R., & Astone, N. M. (1994). Some practical guidelines for measuring youth's race/ethnicity and socioeconomic status. *Child Development, 65,* 1521–1540.

Eysenck, H. J. (1986). A critique of contemporary classification and diagnosis. In T. Millon & G. L. Klerman (Eds.), *Contemporary directions in psychopathology: Toward the DSM-IV* (pp. 73–98). New York: Guilford.

Faraone, S. V., Biederman, J., Chen, W. J., Milberger, S., Warburton, R., & Tsuang, M. T. (1995). Genetic heterogeneity in attention-deficit hyperactivity disorder (ADHD): Gender, psychiatric comorbidity, and maternal ADHD. *Journal of Abnormal Psychology, 104,* 334–345.

Farrington, D. P. (1986). The sociocultural context of childhood disorders. In H. C. Quay & J. S. Werry (Eds.), *Psychopathological disorders of childhood* (3rd ed., pp. 391–422). New York: Wiley.

Fergusson, D. M., Lynskey, M. T., & Horwood, L. J. (1993). The effect of maternal depression on maternal ratings of child behavior. *Journal of Abnormal Child Psychology, 21,* 245–269.

Foster, S. L., & Martinez, C. R. (1995). Ethnicity: Conceptual and methodological issues in child clinical psychology research. *Journal of Clinical Child Psychology, 24,* 214–226.

Gaub, M., & Carlson, C. L. (1997). Gender differences in ADHD: A meta-analysis and critical review. *Journal of the American Academy of Child and Adolescent Psychiatry, 36,* 1036–1045.

Gibbons, R. D., Hedeker, D., Elkin, I., Waternaux, C., Kraemer, H. C., Greenhouse, J. B., Shea, M. T., Imber, S. D., Sotsky, S. M., & Watkins, J. T. (1993). Some conceptual and statistical issues in analysis of longitudinal psychiatric data. *Archives of General Psychiatry, 50,* 739–750.

Giordano, P. C., & Cernkovich, S. A. (1997). Gender and antisocial behavior. In D. M. Stoff, J. Breiling, & J. D. Maser (Eds.), *Handbook of antisocial behavior* (pp. 496–510). New York: Wiley.

Goodman, S. H., & Kohlsdorf, B. (1994). The developmental psychopathology of conduct problems: Gender issues. In D. C. Fowles, P. Sutker, & S. H. Goodman (Eds.), *Progress in experimental personality and psychopathology research* (pp. 121–161). New York: Springer.

Goodman, S. H., Lahey, B. B., Fielding, B., Dulcan, M., Narrow, W., & Regier, D. (1997). Representativeness of clinical samples of youths with mental disorders: A preliminary population-based study. *Journal of Abnormal Psychology, 106,* 3–14.

Harris, G. T., Rice, M. E., & Quinsey, V. L. (1994). Psychopathy as a taxon: Evidence that psychopaths are a discrete class. *Journal of Consulting and Clinical Psychology, 62,* 387–397.

Harris, R. J. (1997). Significance tests have their place. *Psychological Science, 8,* 8–11.

Harwood, R. L. (1992). The influence of culturally derived values on Anglo and Puerto Rican mothers' perceptions of attachment behavior. *Child Development, 63,* 822–839.

Hauser, R. M. (1994). Measuring socioeconomic status in studies of child development. *Child Development, 65,* 1541–1545.

Hawkins, D. F., Laub, J. H., & Lauritsen, J. L. (in press). Race, ethnicity, and serious juvenile offending. In R. Loeber & D. P. Farrington (Eds.), *Serious and violent juvenile offenders: Risk factors and successful interventions.* Thousand Oaks, CA: Sage.

Herjanic, B., & Reich, W. (1982). Development of a structured psychiatric interview for children: Agreement between child and parent on individual symptoms. *Journal of Abnormal Child Psychology, 10,* 307–324.

Hinshaw, S. P. (1987). On the distinction between attentional deficits/hyperactivity and conduct problems/aggression in child psychopathology. *Psychological Bulletin, 101,* 443–463.

Hinshaw, S. P. (1994). *Attention deficits and hyperactivity in children.* Thousand Oaks, CA: Sage.

Hinshaw, S. P., & Anderson, C. A. (1996). Conduct and oppositional defiant disorders. In E. J. Mash & R. A. Barkley (Eds.), *Child psychopathology* (pp. 108–149). New York: Guilford.

Hinshaw, S. P., & Nigg, J. T. (in press). Behavior rating scales in the assessment of disruptive behavior disorders in childhood. In D. Shaffer & J. E. Richters (Eds.), *Assessment in child and adolescent psychopathology.* New York: Guilford.

Hinshaw, S. P., & Zupan, B. A. (1997). Assessment of antisocial behavior and conduct disorder in children. In D. M. Stoff, J. Breiling, & J. D. Maser (Eds.), *Handbook of antisocial behavior* (pp. 36–50). New York: Wiley.

Hinshaw, S. P., Lahey, B. B., & Hart, E. L. (1993). Issues of taxonomy and comorbidity in the development of conduct disorder. *Development and Psychopathology, 5,* 31–49.

Hinshaw, S. P., Simmel, C., & Heller, T. L. (1995). Multimethod assessment of covert antisocial behavior in children: Laboratory observations, adult ratings, and child self-report. *Psychological Assessment, 7,* 209–219.

Hinshaw, S. P., March, J., Abikoff, H., Arnold, L. E., Cantwell, D. P., Conners, C. K., Elliott, G. R., Halperin, J., Greenhill, L. L., Hechtman, L. T., Hoza, B., Jensen, P. S., Newcorn, J. H., McBurnett, K., Pelham, W. E., Richters, J. E., Severe, J. B., Schiller, E., Swanson, J. M., Vereen, D., Wells, K., & Wigal, T. (1997). Comprehensive assessment of attention-deficit hyperactivity disorder in the context of a multisite, multimodal clinical trial. *Journal of Attention Disorders, 1,* 217–234.

Hiraga, Y., Cauce, A. M., Mason, C., & Ordonez, N. (1993, April). *Ethnic identity and social adjustment of biracial youth.* Paper presented at the meeting of the Society for Research in Child Development, New Orleans, LA.

Hollon, S. D. (1996). The efficacy and effectiveness of psychotherapy relative to medications. *American Psychologist, 51,* 1025–1030.

Hunter, J. E. (1997). Needed: A ban on the significance test. *Psychological Science, 8,* 3–7.

Jensen, P. S., & Hoagwood, K. (1997). The book of names: DSM-IV in context. *Development and Psychopathology, 9,* 231–249.

Jensen, P. S., Wantanabe, H. K., Richters, J. E., Roper, M., Hibbs, E. D., Salzberg, A. D., & Liu, S. (1996). Scales, diagnoses, and child psychopathology: II. Comparing

the CBCL and DISC against external validators. *Journal of Abnormal Child Psychology, 24,* 151–168.

Judd, C. M., & McClelland, G. H. (1989). *Data analysis: A model comparison approach.* San Diego, CA: Harcourt, Brace, Jovanovich.

Kazdin, A. E., & Kagan, J. (1994). Models of dysfunction in developmental psychopathology. *Clinical Psychology: Science and Practice, 1,* 35–52.

Kraemer, H. C., Kazdin, A. E., Offord, D. R., Kessler, R. C., Jensen, P. S., & Kupfer, D. J. (1997). Coming to terms with the terms of risk. *Archives of General Psychiatry, 54,* 337–343.

Lagerspetz, K. M. J., & Bjorkqvist, K. (1994). Indirect aggression in boys and girls. In L. R. Huesmann (Ed.), *Aggressive behavior: Current perspectives* (pp. 131–150). New York: Plenum.

Lahey, B. B., Applegate, B., McBurnett, K., Biederman, J., Greenhill, L., Hynd, G., Barkley, R. A., Newcorn, J., Jensen, P., Ricthers, J., Garfinkel, B., Kerdyk, L., Frick, P. J., Ollendick, T., Perez, D., Hart, E. L., Waldman, I., & Shaffer, D. (1994). DSM-IV field trials for attention deficit hyperactivity disorder in children and adolescents. *American Journal of Psychiatry, 151,* 1673–1685.

Lau, S., Lew, W., Hau, K., Cheung, P., & Berndt, T. (1990). Relations among perceived parental control, warmth, indulgence, and family harmony of Chinese in mainland China. *Developmental Psychology, 26,* 674–677.

Levy, F., Hay, D. A., McStephen, M., Wood, C., & Waldman, I. (1997). Attention-deficit hyperactivity disorder: A category or a continuum? Genetic analysis of a large-scale twin study. *Journal of the American Academy of Child and Adolescent Psychiatry, 36,* 737–744.

Loeber, R., & Farrington, D. P. (1994). Problems and solutions in longitudinal and experimental treatment studies of child psychopathology and delinquency. *Journal of Consulting and Clinical Psychology, 62,* 887–900.

Loeber, R., Green, S. M., Lahey, B. B., & Stouthamer-Loeber, M. (1989). Optimal informants on childhood disruptive behavior disorders. *Development and Psychopathology, 1,* 317–337.

Loeber, R., Lahey, B. B., & Thomas, C. (1991). Diagnostic conundrum of oppositional defiant disorder and conduct disorder. *Journal of Abnormal Psychology, 100,* 379–390.

Loeber, R., Wung, P., Keenan, K., Giroux, B., Stouthamer-Loeber, M., Van Kammen, W., & Maughan, B. (1993). Developmental pathways in disruptive child behavior. *Development and Psychopathology, 5,* 103–133.

Loeber, R., Farrington, D. P., Stouthamer-Loeber, M., & Van Kammen, W. B. (1998). *Antisocial behavior and mental health problems: Explanatory factors in childhood and adolescence.* Mahwah, NJ: Erlbaum.

Loftus, G. (1996). Psychology will be a much better science when we change the way we analyze data. *Current Directions in Psychological Science, 5,* 161–171.

Loney, J. (1987). Hyperactivity and aggression in the diagnosis of attention deficit disorder. In B. B. Lahey &

A. E. Kazdin (Eds.), *Advances in clinical child psychology* (Vol.10, pp. 99–135). New York: Plenum.

Lopez, S. R., Hurwicz, M., Karno, M., & Telles, C. A. (1992). *Schizophrenic and manic symptoms in a community sample: A sociocultural analysis.* Unpublished manuscript, University of California, Los Angeles.

Lykken, D. (1991). What's wrong with psychology anyway? In D. Cicchetti & W. M. Grove (Eds.), *Thinking clearly about psychology* (Vol. 1, pp. 3–39). Minneapolis: University of Minnesota Press.

Maccoby, E. E. (1988). Gender as a social category. *Developmental Psychology, 24,* 755–765.

Masten, A. S., Best, K. M., & Garmezy, N. (1990). Resilience and development: Contributions from the study of children who overcome adversity. *Development and Psychopathology, 2,* 425–444.

McClelland, G. H., & Judd, C. M. (1993). Statistical difficulties in detecting interactions and moderator effects. *Psychological Bulletin, 114,* 376–390.

Meehl, P. (1978). Theoretical risks and tabular asterisks: Sir Karl, Sir Ronald, and the slow progress of soft psychology. *Journal of Consulting and Clinical Psychology, 46,* 806–834.

Moffitt, T. E. (1993). Adolescence-limited and life-course-persistent antisocial behavior: A developmental taxonomy. *Psychological Review, 100,* 674–701.

Nich, C., & Carroll, K. (1997). Now you see it, now you don't: A comparison of traditional versus random-effects regression models in the analysis of longitudinal follow-up data from a clinical trial. *Journal of Abnormal Psychology, 65,* 252–261.

Okazaki, S., & Sue, S. (1995). Methodological issues in assessment research with ethnic minorities. *Psychological Assessment, 7,* 367–375.

Pachter, L., & Harwood, R. L. (1996). Culture and child behavior and psychosocial development. *Developmental and Behavioral Pediatrics, 17,* 191–198.

Pachter, L., Dworkin, P. H., & Bernstein, B. A. (1995). Cultural beliefs and maternal expectations regarding normal infant and child development. *Archives of Pediatrics and Adolescent Medicine, 149,* 66–78.

Patterson, G. R., Reid, J. B., & Dishion, T. J. (1992). *A social interactional approach: Vol. 4. Antisocial boys.* Eugene, OR: Castalia.

Peeples, F., & Loeber, R. (1994). Do individual factors and neighborhood context explain ethnic differences in juvenile delinquency? *Journal of Quantitative Criminology, 10,* 141–154.

Pelham, W. E., & Lang, A. R. (1993). Parental alcohol consumption and deviant child behavior: Laboratory studies of reciprocal effects. *Clinical Psychology Review, 13,* 763–784.

Piacentini, J. C., Cohen, P., & Cohen, J. (1992). Combining discrepant information from multiple sources: Are more complex algorithms better than simple ones? *Journal of Abnormal Child Psychology, 20,* 51–63.

Quay, H. C. (1986). Classification. In H. C. Quay & J. S. Werry (Eds.), *Psychopathological disorders of childhood* (3rd ed., pp. 1–34). New York: Wiley.

Quay, H. C. (1993). The psychobiology of undersocialized aggressive conduct disorder: A theoretical perspective. *Development and Psychopathology, 5,* 165–180.

Reid, J. B. (1993). Prevention of conduct disorder before and after school entry: Relating interventions to developmental findings. *Development and Psychopathology, 5,* 243–262.

Renfry, G. S. (1992). Cognitive-behavior therapy and the Native American client. *Behavior Therapy, 23,* 321–340.

Richters, J. E. (1992). Depressed mothers as informants about their children: A critical review of the evidence for distortion. *Psychological Bulletin, 112,* 485–499.

Richters, J. E. (1997). The Hubble hypothesis and the developmentalist's dilemma. *Development and Psychopathology, 9,* 193–229.

Richters, J. E., & Cicchetti, D. (1993). Mark Twain meets DSM-III-R: Conduct disorder, development, and the concept of harmful dysfunction. *Development and Psychopathology, 5,* 5–29.

Richters, J. E., & Martinez, P. E. (1993). Violent communities, family choices, and children's chances: An algorithm for improving the odds. *Development and Psychopathology, 5,* 609–627.

Robins, L. N. (1978). Aetiological implications in studies of childhood histories relating to antisocial personality. In R. D. Hare & D. Schalling (Eds.), *Psychopathic behaviour: Approaches to research* (pp. 255–271). Chichester, England: Wiley.

Robins, L. N. (1986). The consequences of conduct disorder in girls. In D. Olweus, J. Block, & M. Radke-Yarrow (Eds.), *The development of antisocial and prosocial behavior: Research, theories, and issues* (pp. 385–414). Orlando, FL: Academic Press.

Robins, L. N., & McEvoy, L. (1990). Conduct problems as predictors of substance abuse. In L. N. Robins & M. Rutter (Eds.), *Straight and devious pathways from childhood to adolescence* (pp. 182–204). Cambridge, England: Cambridge University Press.

Robins, L. N., & Regier, D. A. (1991). *Psychiatric disorders in America: The Epidemiologic Catchment Area Study.* New York: Free Press.

Rohner, R. P., & Pettingill S. M. (1985). Perceived parental acceptance–rejection and parental control among Korean adolescents. *Child Development, 56,* 524–528.

Rourke, B. P. (Ed.). (1985). *Neuropsychology of learning disabilities: Essentials of subtype analysis.* New York: Guilford.

Rutter, M., Bolton, P., Harrington, R., LeCouteur, A., Macdonald, H., & Simonoff, E. (1990). Genetic factors in child psychiatric disorders: I. A review of research strategies. *Journal of Child Psychology and Psychiatry, 31,* 3–37.

Rutter, M., Dunn, J., Plomin, R., Simonoff, E., Pickles, R., Maughan, B., Ormel, J., Meyer, J., & Eaves, L. (1997). Integrating nature and nurture: Implications of person–environment correlations and interactions for developmental psychopathology. *Development and Psychopathology, 9,* 335–364.

Samuel, V. J., Curtis, S., Thornell, A., George, P., Taylor, A., Brome, D. R., Biederman, J., & Faraone, S. V.

(1997). The unexplored void of ADHD and African-American research: A review of the literature. *Journal of Attention Disorders, 1,* 197–207.

Seligman, M. E. P. (1995). The effectiveness of psychotherapy: The Consumer Reports Study. *American Psychologist, 50,* 965–974.

Shrout, P. E. (1997). Should significance tests be banned? Introduction to a special section exploring the pros and cons. *Psychological Science, 8,* 1–2.

Sobal, J., & Stunkard, A. J. (1989). Socioeconomic status and obesity: A review of the literature. *Psychological Bulletin, 105,* 260–275.

Stattin, H., & Magnusson, D. (1996). Antisocial behavior: A holistic approach. *Development and Psychopathology, 8,* 617–645.

Stoff, D. M., Breiling, J., & Maser, J. D. (Eds.) (1997). *Handbook of antisocial behavior.* New York: Wiley.

Stouthamer-Loeber, M., Van Kammen, W., & Loeber, R. (1992). The nuts and bolts of implementing large-scale longitudinal studies. *Violence and Victims, 7,* 63–78.

Teicher, M. H., Ito, Y., Glod, C. A., & Barber, N. I. (1996). Objective measurement of hyperactivity and attentional problems in ADHD. *Journal of the American Academy of Child and Adolescent Psychiatry, 35,* 334–342.

VandenBos, G. (1996). Outcome assessment of psychotherapy. *American Psychologist, 51,* 1005–1006.

Werner, E. E., & Smith, R. S. (1992). *Overcoming the odds: High risk children from birth to adulthood.* Ithaca, NY: Cornell University Press.

Windle, M., Iwawaki, S., & Lerner, R. M. (1987). Cross-cultural comparability of temperament among Japanese and American early- and late-adolescents. *Journal of Adolescent Research, 2,* 423–446.

Windle, M., Iwawaki, S., & Lerner, R. M. (1988). Cross-cultural comparability of temperament among Japanese and American preschool children. *International Journal of Psychology, 23,* 547–567.

Wootton, J. M., Frick, P. J., Shelton, K. K., & Silverthorn, P. (1997). Ineffective parenting and childhood conduct problems: The moderating role of callous-unemotional traits. *Journal of Consulting and Clinical Psychology, 65,* 301–308.

World Health Organization. (1993). *The ICD-10 classification of mental and behavioural disorders: Diagnostic criteria for research.* Geneva, Switzerland: World Health Organization.

Yung, B. R., & Hammond, W. R. (1997). Antisocial behavior in minority groups: Epidemiological and cultural perspectives. In D. M. Stoff, J. Breiling, & J. D. Maser (Eds.), *Handbook of antisocial behavior* (pp. 474–495). New York: Wiley.

Zahn-Waxler, C. (1993). Warriors and worriers: Gender and psychopathology. *Development and Psychopathology, 5,* 79–89.

Zoccolillo, M. (1993). Gender and the development of conduct disorder. *Development and Psychopathology, 5,* 65–78.

Appendix

Note: The reader can find cited references in Chapter 2.

Handbook of Disruptive Behavior Disorders, edited by Quay and Hogan. Kluwer Academic/Plenum Publishers, New York, 1999.

TABLE A1. Methodology: Studies of Nationally Representative Samples

Key reference[a]	N[b]	Sample[c]	Age in years	Racial/ethnic background[d]	Informants	Measures
		Studies conducted in the United States				
1. Achenbach National Study Achenbach *et al.* (1991)	T1: 2600	Household sample (48 contiguous states); 3-year & 6-year follow-ups	T1: 4–16 T2: 7–19 T3: 9–22	74% White 16% Black 7% Hispanic 3% Other	Child, ages 11–19 Parent Teacher	ACQ/CBCL, TRF, YABCL, YASR, YSR
2. Adjustment Scales for Children and Adolescents Study McDermott (1993)	700 males 700 females 1400 total	School-based sample (public & private)	5–17	Not reported	Teacher	ASCA
3. Children of the National Longitudinal Survey of Youth Baker *et al.* (1993)	T1: 4971 T2: 6266 T3: 5803 T4: 6100	Children of household sample of females aged 14–21 when selected; oversampled blacks, Hispanics, low-income whites, & military (50 states); follow-ups every other year to date[e]	T1: 0–16	49% White[f] 32% Black[f] 19% Hispanic[f]	Parent	BPI
4. National Health Examination Survey Cycle II National Center for Health Statistics (1967)	3632 males 3487 females 7119 total	Household sample (50 states)	6–11	86% White 14% other	Teacher	SQ
5. National Health Interview Survey Child Health Supplement (1981) Inter-University Consortium for Political and Social Research (1985)	15,416 total	Household sample (50 states)	5–17	Not reported	Parent	BPI
6. National Health Interview Survey Child Health Supplement (1988) Inter-University Consortium for Political and Social Research (1994)	11,840 total	Household sample (50 states)	5–17	Not reported	Parent	BPI

Study	Sample size	Sample description	Age	Ethnicity	Informant	Measure
7. National Youth Survey Elliot et al. (1983)	T1: 1725 T2: 1655 T3: 1626 T4: 1543 T5: 1494	Household sample (48 contiguous states); 6 annual follow-ups	T1: 11–17 T2: 12–18 T3: 13–19 T4: 14–20 T5: 15–21 T6: 16–22	79% White 15% Black 4% Hispanic 2% Other	Child	SRD

Studies conducted outside the United States

Study	Sample size	Sample description	Age	Ethnicity	Informant	Measure
8. Child Health and Education Study Osborn et al. (1984)	T1: 16,541 T2: 13,135 T3: 14,849	Birth cohort (England, Scotland, & Wales); 5-year and 10-year follow-ups	T1: Birth T2: 5 T3: 10	Not reported	Parent	Rutter Scale A
9. National Child Development Study Pringle et al. (1966)	T1: 17,414 T2: 15,468 T3: 15,503 T4: 14,761 T5: 12,537	Birth cohort (England, Scotland, & Wales); 7-year, 11-year, 16-year, and 23-year follow-ups	T1: Birth T2: 7 T3: 11 T4: 16 T5: 23	Not reported	Parent Teacher	BSAG, Rutter Scales A & B
10. Netherlands Study Verhulst et al. (1997)	312	Screened household sample (Netherlands)	13–18	Not reported	Child Parent Teacher	CBCL, CGAS, DISC 2.3, TRF, YSR (DSM-III-R)
11. Young in Norway Study Wichstrøm et al. (1996)	5147 males 5315 females 10,462 total	School-based sample (all; Norway)	12–19[f]	Not reported	Child	SQ (DSM-III-R[g])

Abbreviations of names of measures: ACQ = Achenbach, Conners, & Quay Behavior Checklist; ASCA = Adjustment Scales for Children and Adolescents; BPI = Behavior Problem Index; BSAG = Bristol Social Adjustment Guides; CBCL = Achenbach Child Behavior Checklist; CGAS = Children's Global Assessment Scale; DISC 2.3 = Diagnostic Interview Schedule for Children, Version 2.3; SQ = structured questionnaire; SRD = Self-Reported Delinquency Scale; TRF = Achenbach Teacher Report Form; YABCL = Achenbach Young Adult Behavior Checklist; YASR = Young Adult Self-Report; YSR = Achenbach Youth Self-Report.

[a] Key publication describing the basic methodology of the study.
[b] Where not otherwise indicated, sample included both males and females, but data regarding specific gender composition were not reported. Where reported, sample sizes at follow-up are noted.
[c] Where not otherwise indicated, sample was screened for disruptive behavior problems. For school-based surveys, type of schools sampled is noted in parentheses.
[d] Where not otherwise indicated, data regarding racial or ethnic composition of the sample were not reported. For longitudinal studies, sample composition at T1 is reported. "White" = non-Hispanic white.
[e] Mothers were aged 21–29 when children were first assessed. At each follow-up, children born since the previous assessment were added to the sample.
[f] Approximate number or percentage.
[g] Behaviors indicative of conduct disorder were assessed by means of items approximating DSM-III-R criteria.

623

TABLE A2. Methodology: Studies of Locally Representative Samples

Key reference[a]	N[b]	Sample[c]	Age in years	Racial/ethnic background[d]	Informants	Measures
		Studies conducted in the United States				
12. Adolescent Depression Study Garrison *et al.* (1992)	T1: 488	Screened school-based sample (public school district; southeastern U.S.) 2 annual follow-ups	12–15	76% White 24% Black	Child Parent	CES-D, CGAS, K-SADS (DSM-III)
13. Dade County Study Warheit *et al.* (1996)	T1: 6760 males 626 females 7386 total T2: 6089 males 549 females 6638 total T3: 5370 males 554 females 5924 total	School-based sample (public; Dade County, FL)	T1: Grades 6–7 T2: Grades 7–8 T3: Grades 8–9	25% Cuban 12% American black 2% Haitian 3% Other black 41% Other[e]	Child	SQ
14. Eastern Connecticut Child Survey Zahner *et al.* (1993)	795 males 902 females 1697 total	School-based sample; (public, private, & institutional, eastern CT)	6–11	88% White[e] 5% Black[e] 3% Hispanic[e] 3% Other	Parent Teacher	CBCL, TRF
15. Great Smoky Mountains Study of Youth Costello *et al.* (1996)	T1: 1338	Screened[f] school-based sample (public & Qualla Boundary Reservation; Appalachian region of NC); annual follow-ups ongoing	T1: 9,11,13	68% White 24% Native American[g] 6% Black 2% Other	Child Parent	CAPA, CBCL (DSM-III-R, DSM-IV)

Study	Sample size	Sample type (location)	Age	Ethnicity	Informant	Measures
16. Los Angeles County Study Aneshensel & Sucoff (1996)	469 males 408 females 877 total	Household sample (Los Angeles County, CA)	12–17	38% Mexican 26% White 11% Black 11% Asian 10% Other Hispanic	Child	SBCPC
17. Methods for the Epidemiology of Child and Adolescent Disorders Study						
Lahey et al. (1996)	681 males 604 females 1285 total	Household sample; oversampled blacks and Hispanics (multiple sites[b])	9–17	51% White 28% Hispanic 15% Black 6% Other	Child Parent	CGAS, CIS, DISC 2.3 (DSM-III-R)
18. New Haven Child Survey Zahner et al. (1993)	408 males 414 females 822 total	School-based sample (public, private, & Catholic; New Haven, CT)	6–11	50% Black 30% White 18% Hispanic 2% Other	Parent Teacher	CBCL, TRF
19. New York Child Longitudinal Study/Children in the Community Project						
Cohen et al. (1993)	T1: 976	Household sample (Saratoga and Albany Counties, NY; 8-year, 10-year, and 16-year follow-ups)	T1: 1–10 T2: 9–18 T3: 11–20 T4: 17–26	Not reported	Child, T2 & T3 Parent	DISC (DSM-III-R)
20. Oregon Adolescent Depression Project Lewinsohn et al. (1993)	T1: 805 males 905 females 1710 total T2: 1508 total	School-based sample (public; west central OR); 1-year follow-up	T1: 14–18 T2: 15–19	91% White[e] 9% Other[e]	Child	K-SADS, LIFE (DSM-III-R)
21. Pittsburgh Youth Study Loeber et al. (1998)	1517 males	Screened school-based sample (public school district; Pittsburgh, PA); longitudinal follow-ups ongoing	T1: Grades 2,5,8	57% Black[j] 43% White[j]	Child Caregiver Teacher	CBCL, DISC, SRA, SRD, TRF, YSR (DSM-III-R)

(continued)

TABLE A2. (*Continued*)

Key reference[a]	N[b]	Sample[c]	Age in years	Racial/ethnic background[d]	Informants	Measures
22. Puerto Rico Child Psychiatry Epidemiologic Study						
Bird et al. (1988)	197 males 189 females 386 total	Screened household sample (Puerto Rico)	4–16	Not reported	Child Parent Teacher, ages 6–16	CBCL, CGAS, DISC, TRF (DSM-III)
23. "River City" Study						
Havighurst et al. (1962)	T1: 247 males 240 females 487 total	School-based sample (all public, selected private & special; "River City"); longitudinal follow-ups to age 20	T1: 11	Not reported	Teacher Peers	BDC, WAT
Unnamed studies						
24. Fridrich & Flannery (1995)	608 males 562 females 1170 total	School-based sample (public school district; southwestern U.S. city)	Grades 6–7	63% White 24% Hispanic 13% Other	Child	YSR-DEL
25. Reinherz et al. (1984)	T1: 774 T7: 404 T8: 386	School-based sample (public; Quincy, MA); 7 follow-ups	T1: Pre-K T2: Grade K T3: Grade 1 T4: Grade 2 T5: Grade 3 T6: Grade 4 T7: Grade 9 T8: Grade 12	Not reported	Parent Teacher	SBCL
26. Wolraich et al. (1996)	8258 total	School-based sample (public; county in TN)	Grades K–5	Majority white 7% Black	Teacher	DBD (DSM-III-R, DSM-IV)

626

Studies conducted outside the United States

27. Christchurch Health and Development Study Ferguson *et al.* (1989)	Birth cohort (Christchurch, New Zealand); initial issessment at birth, follow-ups at 4 months, 1 year, and annually to date	Not reported	T1: Birth T2: 4 months T3–T20: 1–18	Child Parent	CIDI, DISC, RBPC (DSM-III-R, DSM-IV)
	T1: 1262 T2: 1210 T3: 1180 T4: 1156 T5: 1143 T6: 1127 T7: 1123 T8: 1115 T9: 1107 T10: 1092 T11: 1079 T12: 1067 T13: 1048				
28. Dunedin Multidisciplinary Health and Development Study Silva (1990)	Birth cohort, (Queen Mary Hospital, Dunedin, New Zealand); initial assessment at birth, follow-ups at age 3, every other year to age 18, age 21	Majority European, minority Maori/ other Polynesian	T1: Birth T2: 3 T3: 5 T4: 7 T5: 9 T6: 11 T7: 13 T8: 15 T9: 18 T10: 21	Child Parent Significant other, age 18 Teacher	DIS-III-R, DISC, DYSYI, RBPC, Rutter Scales A & B (DSM-III, DSM-III-R)
	T1: 1661 T2: 1037 T3: 991 T4: 954 T5: 955 T6: 925 T7: 850 T8: 976 T9: 1008 T10: 992				
29. Hong Kong Study Leung *et al.* (1996)	Screened school-based sample (primary; British colony of Hong Kong, Southeast China)	100% Chinese	7	Parent Teacher	CRS, PACS, Rutter Scales A2 & B2, SI (DSM-III, DSM-III-R, ICD-10)
	611 males				

(*continued*)

TABLE A2. *(Continued)*

Key reference[a]	N[b]	Sample[c]	Age in years	Racial/ethnic background[d]	Informants	Measures
30. Isle of Wight/Inner London Borough Studies						
a. Rutter *et al.* (1970)	T1: 286	Screened birth cohort (Isle of Wight, England); 4-year follow-up (see 30b)	T1: 10–11	Not reported	Child Parent Teacher	Rutter Scales A & B, PI (Rutter)
b. Graham & Rutter (1973)	T2: 630	Screened birth cohort (Isle of Wight, England)	T2: 14–15	Not reported	Child Parent Teacher	Rutter Scales A & B, PI (Rutter)
c. Rutter *et al.* (1975)	211+	Screened birth cohort (Isle of Wight, England)	10	Not reported	Parent Teacher	Rutter Scale B2, PI (Rutter)
c. Rutter *et al.* (1975)	265+	Screened birth cohort (Inner borough of England)	10	Not reported	Parent Teacher	Rutter Scale B2, PI (Rutter)
31. Mannheim Study Esser *et al.* (1990)	T1: 216 T2: 191	Household sample (Mannheim, Germany); 5-year follow-up	T1: 8 T2: 13	Not reported	Child, age 13 Parent Teacher	Conners Scales, GRPI (ICD-9)
32. Ontario Child Health Study Boyle *et al.* (1987)	T1: 1329 males 1345 females 2769 total[k]	Household sample (Ontario, Canada); 4-year follow-up	T1: 4–16 T2: 8–20	Not reported	Child, ages 12–20 Parent Teacher, ages 4–11	SDI (DSM-III)
33. Ontario Study Boyle, Offord, Racine, Fleming, *et al.* (1993)	251	Screened school-based sample (public; urban area of Ontario, Canada)	6–16	Not reported	Child Parent Teacher	OCHS scales, DICA-R (DSM-III-R)
34. Young in Oslo Study Wichstrøm *et al.* (1996)	678 males	Household sample	16–19	Not reported	Child	SQ

Study	Sample (location)	Sample size	Age	Race	Informant	Measures
	(Oslo, Norway)	668 females 1346 total				(DSM-III-R[l])
Unnamed studies						
35. Al-Kuwaiti *et al.* (1995)	School-based sample (primary; Al Ain, Abu Dhabi, United Arab Emirates)	1140 males 960 females 2100 total	5–16	Not reported	Teacher	Rutter Scale B2 (Rutter)
36. Leslie (1974)	Screened household sample (public; Blackburn, England)	141	13–14	Not reported	Child Parent Teacher	BQ, GRPI, RGCI (Rutter)
37. Trites *et al.* (1979)	School-based sample (all; Ottawa–Carleton region, Ontario, Canada)	7306 males 6769 females 14,083 total	5–12	Not reported	Teacher	CTRS
38. Vikan (1985)	Screened household sample (North Troendelag County, Norway)	139	10	100% White	Child Parent Teacher Nurse	GRPI, RGCI, SCL (Rutter)
39. Wang *et al.* (1993)	Screened school-based sample (primary; Kaohsiung, Taiwan)	2181 males 2050 females 4231 total	7–12	Not reported	Parent	CTRS (DSM-III-R)

Abbreviations of names of measures: BDC = Behavior Description chart; BQ = Buckinghamshire Questionnaires; CAPA = Child and Adolescent Psychiatric Assessment; CBCL = Achenbach Child Behavior Checklist; CES-D = Center for Epidemiologic Studies Depression Scale; CGAS = Children's Global Adjustment Scale; CIDI = Composite International Diagnostic Interview; CIS = Columbia Impairment Scale; CRS = Conners Classroom Rating Scale; CTRS = Conners Teacher Rating Scale; DBD = Disruptive Behavior Disorder Rating Scale; DICA-R = Diagnostic Interview for Children and Adolescents–Revised; DIS-III-R = Diagnostic Interview Schedule, Version Three–Revised; DISC = Diagnostic Interview Schedule for Children; DISC 2.3 = Diagnostic Interview Schedule for Children, Version 2.3; DYSYI = Denver Youth Survey Youth Inventory; GRPI = Graham & Rutter Parent Interview; K-SADS = Schedule of Affective Disorders and Schizophrenia for School-Age Children; LIFE = Longitudinal Interval Follow-up Evaluation; OCHS = Ontario Child Health Study Scales; PACS = Parental Account of Childhood Symptoms; PI = psychiatric interview; RBPC = Revised Behavior Problem Checklist; RGCI = Rutter & Graham Child Interview; SBCL = Simmons Behavior Checklist; SBCPC = Stony Brook Child Psychiatric Checklist–3R; SCL = symptom checklist; SDI = Survey Diagnostic Instrument; SI = structured interview; SQ = structured questionnaire; SRA = Self-Reported Antisocial Scale; SRD = Self-Reported Delinquency Scale; TRF = Achenbach Teacher Report Form; WAT = Who Are They? Test; YSR = Achenbach Youth Self-Report; YSR-DEL = Achenbach Youth Self-Report Delinquency Subscale.

[a]Key publication describing the basic methodology of the study.

[b]Where not otherwise indicated, sample included both males and females, but data regarding specific gender composition were not reported. Where reported, sample sizes at follow-up are noted.

[c]Where noted, sample was screened for disruptive behavior problems. For school-based samples, type of schools sampled is noted (where reported) in parentheses.

[d]Where not otherwise indicated, data regarding racial or ethnic composition of the sample were not reported. For longitudinal studies, sample composition at T1 is reported. "White" = non-Hispanic white.

[e]Approximate percentage.

[f]Native American participants were not screened; interviews were attempted with all who consented to participate in the study.

[g]Majority was Cherokee.

[h]Hamden, East Haven, and West Haven, Connecticut; DeKalb, Rockdale, and Henry Counties, Georgia; Westchester County, New York; and San Juan, Puerto Rico.

[i]Authors' classification included Hispanics, Native Americans, and biracial or multiracial participants.

[j]Authors' classification included Asian American participants.

[k]Gender data missing for 5 participants.

[l]Behaviors indicative of conduct disorder were assessed by means of items approximating DSM-III-R criteria.

629

TABLE A3. Prevalence of Disruptive Disorders

Reference[a]	Diagnostic system (method)[b]	Informant[c] (method)[d]	Gender	N	Age																
					4	5	6	7	8	9	10	11	12	13	14	15	16	17	18	19	20
					Any disruptive disorder[g]																
32. Boyle, Offord, Racine, Sanford, et al. (1993)	DSM-III-R (algorithm)	C	Both	251			<———7.8———>						<———7.9———>							
		P	Both	251			<———17.4———>						<———10.8———>							
17. Shaffer et al. (1996)	DSM-III-R (algorithm; CGAS ≤ 60 or DSIC)	DSM + CGAS ≤ 60																			
		C	Both	1285					<———————3.0———————>										
		P	Both	1285					<———————3.7———————>										
		C,P (combined)	Both	1285					<———————7.2———————>										
		DSM + DSIC																			
		C	Both	1285					<———————4.7———————>										
		P	Both	1285					<———————7.6———————>										
		C,P (combined)	Both	1285					<——————11.5——————>										
20. Lewinsohn et al. (1993)	DSM-III-R (clinician)	Time 1																			
		C	Both	1710											<———1.8———>					
		C	Males	819											<———2.7———>					
		C	Females	891											<———1.0———>					
		Time 2																			
		C	Both	1508													<———0.5———>			
		C	Males	810													<———0.7———>			
		C	Females	698													<———0.2———>			
27. Fergusson et al. (1993)	DSM-III-R[f] (algorithm)	C	Both	965												8.3				
		P	Both	986												5.2				
		C,P (either)	Both	961												10.8				
		C,P (either)	Males	961												12.2				
		C,P (either)	Females	961												9.5				
		C,P (latent)	Both	961												8.1				
		C,P (latent)	Males	961												8.6				
		C,P (latent)	Females	961												7.5				

Attention Deficit Disorder

Study	Criteria	Source	Sex	N		
22. Bird et al. (1989)	DSM-III (algorithm; CGAS < 61)	C,P (combined)	Both	386	← 9.5 →	
32. Offord et al. (1987)	DSM-III (threshold score; distress or social impairment)	P,T/C^g (either)	Males	1329	← 10.1 →	← 7.3 →
		P,T/C^g (either)	Males	1329	← 8.9 →	
		P,T/C^g (either)	Females	1345	← 3.3 →	← 3.4 →
		P,T/C^g (either)	Females	1345	← 3.3 →	
32. Offord, Boyle, & Racine (1989)	DSM-III (threshold score; distress or social impairment)	P	Males	1317	← 2.1 →	← 3.1 →
		P	Females	1342	← 0.8 →	← 1.4 →
		T/C^g	Males	1317	← 7.3 →	← 4.0 →
		T/C^g	Females	1342	← 2.5 →	← 1.8 →
32. Szatmari, Offord, & Boyle (1989)	DSM-III (threshold score; distress or social impairment)	ADD + ADDH				
		P,T/C^g (either)	Males	1365	← 10.8 →	← 4.3 →
		P,T/C^g (either)	Females	1357	← 4.3 →	← 2.4 →
		ADDH				
		P,T/C^g (either)	Males	1365	← 9.4 →	← 2.9 →
		P,T/C^g (either)	Females	1357	← 2.8 →	← 1.8 →
		ADD				
		P,T/C^g (either)	Males	1365	← 1.4 →	← 1.4 →
		P,T/C^g (either)	Females	1357	← 1.3 →	← 1.0 →
29. Leung et al. (1996)	ICD-10, DSM-III, DSM-III-R (algorithm)	HKD				
		P,T (both)	Males	611	0.8	
		ADDH				
		T	Males	611	6.1	
		ADHD				
		T	Males	611	8.9	

(continued)

TABLE A3. (*Continued*)

Reference[a]	Diagnostic system (method[b])	Informant[c] (method[d])	Gender	N	Age — 8	Age — 13/14
31. Esser et al. (1990)	ICD-9 (clinician; distress or social impairment)	Time 1				
		P	Both	216	4.2[b]	
		P	Males	108	8.3[b]	
		P	Females	108	0.0[b]	
		Time 2				
		C,P (clinical)	Both	191		1.6[b]
		C,P (clinical)	Males	95		3.0[b]
		C,P (clinical	Females	96		0.0[b]
26. Wolraich et al. (1996)	DSM-III-R (threshold) score	T	Both	8258	←——7.3——→ (ages 5–10)	
		T	Males	4102	←——10.8——→	
		T	Females	3836	←——3.3——→	
	DSM-IV (threshold score; DSM-IV)	All ADHD				
		T	Both	8258	←——11.4——→	
		T	Males	4102	←——16.2——→	
		T	Females	3836	←——6.1——→	
		ADHD-AD				
		T	Both	8258	←——5.4——→	
		T	Males	4102	←——7.2——→	
		T	Females	3836	←——3.5——→	
		ADHD-HI				
		T	Both	8258	←——2.4——→	
		T	Males	4102	←——3.8——→	
		T	Females	3836	←——0.9——→	
		ADHD-CT				
		T	Both	8258	←——3.6——→	
		T	Males	4102	←——5.3——→	
		T	Females	3836	←——1.6——→	
32. Boyle, Offord, Racine, Sanford, et al. (1993)	DSM-III-R (algorithm)	Mild				
		C	Both	251	←——1.6	1.1——→ (ages 6–16)
		P	Both	251	←——2.9	0.9——→
		Moderate				
		C	Both	251	←——0.7	0.0——→
		P	Both	251	←——0.9	0.8——→

Study	Criteria	Informant	Group	N	Prevalence	Severe
33. Boyle et al. (1996)	DSM-III-R (algorithm)	C	Both	251	<——0.5——>	<——0.0——>
		P	Both	251	<——1.0——>	<——3.6——>
	DSM-III-R (clinician)	P	Both	251	<——3.9——>	>
39. Wang et al. (1993)	DSM-III-R (threshold score)	T	Both	114	<——4.2——>	
		T	Both	4231	<——9.9——>	
		T	Males	2181	<——14.9——>	
		T	Females	2050	<——4.5——>	
30a. Rutter et al. (1970)	Rutter (clinician; distress or social impairment)	C,P,T (clinical)	Both	286	<0.1[b]>	
15. Costello et al. (1996)	DSM-III-R (algorithm)	P	Both	1015	X——1.9——X[i]	
		P	Males		X——2.9——X[i]	
		P	Females		X——1.0——X[i]	
15. Costello et al. (1997)	DSM-III-R (algorithm)	P	Natives[j] Both	323	X——1.2——X[i]	
		P	Males	172	X——1.7——X[i]	
		P	Females	151	X——0.7——X[i]	
		P	Whites Both	933	X——1.9——X[i]	
		P	Males	522	X——2.9——X[i]	
		P	Females	411	X——1.0——X[i]	
28. Anderson et al. (1987)	DSM-III (algorithm)	C,P,T (combined	Both	792	6.7	
22. Bird et al. (1992)	DSM-III (algorithm)	C	Both	222	<——0.5	
		P	Both	222	<——7.0	
		C,P (optimal)	Both	222	<——7.9	
		C,P (combined)	Both	222	<——9.4	

(continued)

TABLE A3. (Continued)

Reference[a]	Diagnostic system (method)[b]	Informant[c] (method)[d]	Gender	N	Age 4	5	6	7	8	9	10	11	12	13	14	15	16	17	18	19	20
17. Shaffer et al. (1996)	DSM-III-R (algorithm; CGAS ≤ 60 or DSIC)	DSM + CGAS ≤ 60																			
		C	Both	1285						<				0.8			>				
		P	Both	1285						<				1.9			>				
		C,P (combined)	Both	1285						<				3.3			>				
		DSM + DSIC																			
		C	Both	1285						<				1.2			>				
		P	Both	1285						<				4.0			>				
		C,P (combined)	Both	1285						<				5.1			>				
30b. Graham & Rutter (1973)	Rutter (clinician; social impairment)	C,P,T (clinical)	Both	306											<0.1[b]>						
10. Verhulst et al. (1997)	DSM-III-R (algorithm; CGAS < 61)	C	Both	274									<			0.7	>				
		P	Both	274									<			1.2	>				
		C,P (either)	Both	274									<			1.6	>				
27. Fergusson et al. (1993)	DSM-III-R (algorithm)	C	Both	965												2.8					
		P	Both	986												3.0					
		C,P (either)	Males	961												4.8					
		C,P (either)	Females	961												5.7					
		C,P (either)	Both	961												2.7					
		C,P (latent)	Both	961												2.8					
		C,P (latent)	Males	961												5.0					
		C,P (latent)	Females	961												0.7					
28. McGee et al. (1990)	DSM-III[k] (algorithm)	C[l]	Both	943												2.1					
20. Lewinsohn et al. (1993)	DSM-III-R (clinician)	Time 1																			
		C	Both	1710									<			0.4	>				
		C	Males	819									<			0.5	>				
		C	Females	891									<			0.3	>				

634

Study	Criteria	Informant	Group	N	Prevalence (CI)
		C	Time 2 Both	1508	← 0.1 →
		C	Males	810	← 0.1 →
		C	Females	698	← 0.0 →
19. Velez et al. (1989)	DSM-III-R (algorithm)	Time 2 C,P (combined)	Both	776	← 16.6 → 9.9 →
		Time 3 C,P (combined)	Both	776	← 12.8 → 6.8 →
19. Cohen et al. (1993)	DSM-III-R (algorithm)	C,P (combined)	Both	749	← 17.1 → ← 11.4 → 5.8 →
		C,P (combined)	Females	746	← 8.5 → ← 6.5 → 6.2 →
Conduct Disorder					
32. Offord et al. (1987)	DSM-III (threshold score; distress or social impairment)	P,T/C^g (either)	Males	1329	← 6.5 → 10.4 →
		P,T/C^g (either)	Males	1329	← 8.1 →
		P,T/C^g (either)	Females	1345	← 1.8 → 4.1 →
		P,T/C^g (either)	Females	1345	← 2.7 →
32. Offord, Boyle, & Racine (1990)	DSM-III (threshold score; distress or social impairment)	P	Males	1317	← 1.4 → 4.0 →
		P	Females	1342	← 0.4 → 1.9 →
		T/C^g	Males	1317	← 4.9 → 7.2 →
		T/C^g	Females	1342	← 1.8 → 2.9 →
26. Wolraich et al. (1996)	DSM-IV (threshold score DSM-IV)	T	Both	8258	← 2.1 →
		T	Males	4102	← 3.1 →
		T	Females	3836	← 1.0 →
31. Esser et al. (1990)	ICD-9 (clinician; distress or social impairment)	Time 1 Pure CD P	Both	216	0.9[b]
		P	Males	108	1.9[b]
		P	Females	108	0.0[b]
		Mixed CD/ED P	Both	191	0.9[b]
		P	Males	95	1.9[b]
		P	Females	96	0.0[b]

(continued)

635

TABLE A3. *(Continued)*

Reference[a]	Diagnostic system (method)[b]	Informant[c] (method)[d]	Gender	N	4	5	6	7	8	9	10	11	12	13	14	15	16	17	18	19	20
		Time 2																			
		Pure CD																			
		C,P (clinical)	Both	216										5.8[b]							
		C,P (clinical)	Males	108										6.0[b]							
		C,P (clinical)	Females	108										5.0[b]							
		Mixed CD																			
		C, P (clinical)	Both	191										2.6[b]							
		C,P (clinical)	Males	95										3.0[b]							
		C,P (clinical)	Females	96										2.0[b]							
30c. Rutter *et al.* (1975)	Rutter (clinician; social impairment)	*Isle of Wight*																			
		C,P,T (clinical)	Both	211+							2.2[b]										
		Inner London Borough																			
		P (clinical)	Both	256+							3.5[b]										
30a. Rutter *et al.* (1970)	Rutter (clinician; distress or social impairment)	*Pure CD*																			
		P (clinical)	Both	286							<2.0[b]>										
		Mixed CD/ED																			
		C,P,T (clinical)	Both	286							<1.2[b]>										
28. Anderson *et al.* (1987)	DSM-III[m] (algorithm)	C,P,T (combined)	Both	792								3.4									
15. Costello *et al.* (1996)	DSM-III-R (algorithm)	C,P (combined)	Both	1015						X	3.3			X[i]							
		C,P (combined)	Males							X	5.4			X[i]							
		C,P (combined)	Females							X	1.1			X[i]							
32. Boyle, Offord, Racine, Sanford, *et al.* (1993)	DSM-III-R (algorithm)	*Mild*																			
		C	Both	251					<——0.0——>						0.4 ——>						
		P	Both	251					<——0.0——>						0.2 ——>						
		Moderate																			
		C	Both	251					<——0.6——>						1.4 ——>						
		P	Both	251					<——0.4——>						3.2 ——>						

Study	Diagnostic criteria	Informant/subtype	Sex	N		Severe
33. Boyle et al. (1996)	DSM-III-R (algorithm)	C	Both	251	<—0.0—>	<—0.0—>
		P	Both	251	<—0.4—>	<—0.0—>
	DSM-III-R (clinician)	P	Both	251	<——1.0——>	
		T	Both	114	<———1.6———>	
17. Shaffer et al. (1996)	DSM-III-R (algorithm; CGAS ≤ 60 or DSIC)	DSM + CGAS ≤ 60				
		C	Both	1285	<——2.1——>	
		P	Both	1285	<——0.9——>	
		C,P (combined)	Both	1285	<——3.2——>	
		DSM + DSIC				
		C	Both	1285	<——2.7——>	
		P	Both	1285	<——1.3——>	
		C,P (combined)	Both	1285	<——3.9——>	
12. Andrews et al. (1993)	DSM-III (algorithm; CGAS < 61)	C	Both	460		<——2.6[b]——>
		P	Both	460		<——2.0[b]——>
36. Leslie (1974)	Rutter (clinician)	C,P (clinical)	Both	150		2.6
30b. Graham & Rutter (1973)	Rutter (clinician; social impairment)	Pure CD				
		C,P,T (clinical)	Both	306		<2.1[b]>
		Mixed CD/ED				
		C,P,T (clinical)	Both	306		<1.9[b]>
27. Fergusson et al. (1993)	DSM-III-R (algorithm)	C	Both	965		3.2
		P	Both	986		3.3
28. McGee et al. (1990)	DSM-III (algorithm)	Aggressive CD				
		C[l]	Both	943		1.6
		Nonaggressive CD				
		C[l]	Both	943		5.7
10. Verhulst et al. (1997)	DSM-III-R (algorithm; CGAS < 61)	C	Both	274		<——1.5——>
		P	Both	274		<——1.2——>
		C,P (either)	Both	274		<——2.0——>

(continued)

TABLE A3. (*Continued*)

Reference[a]	Diagnostic system (method)[b]	Informant[c] (method)[d]	Gender	N	Age 4	5	6	7	8	9	10	11	12	13	14	15	16	17	18	19	20
28. Feehan et al. (1994)	DSM-III-R (algorithm; ad hoc impairment)	C	Both	930														5.5			
11. Wichström et al. (1996)	DSM-III-R[n] (threshold score)		Norway	10,462																	
		C	Males												←—4.9—						—→
		C	Females												←—0.8—						—→
			Oslo	1346																	
		C	Both														←—	5.6			—→
		C	Males														←—	8.0			—→
		C	Females														←—	3.1			—→
20. Lewinsohn et al. (1993)	DSM-III-R (clinician)		Time 1																		
		C	Both	1710											←—		0.1		—→			
		C	Males	819											←—		0.9		—→			
		C	Females	891											←—		0.3		—→			
			Time 2																		
		C	Both	1508											←—		0.1		—→			
		C	Males	810											←—		0.1		—→			
		C	Females	698											←—		0.1		—→			
19. Velez et al. (1989)	DSM-III-R (algorithm)	Time 2 C,P (combined)	Both	776						←—	—11.9—	—→		←—		—11.6—		—→			
		Time 3 C,P (combined)	Both	776							←—	—10.9—	—→			←—		—9.9—		—→	
19. Cohen et al. (1993)	DSM-III-R (algorithm)	C,P (combined)	Males	749							←—	—16.0—	—→	←—	—15.8—	—→	←—		—9.5—	—→	
		C,P (combined)	Females	746							←—	—3.8—	—→	←—	—9.2—	—→	←—		—7.1—	—→	

Oppositional Defiant Disorder

Study	Criteria	Source	Sex	N	Prevalence
22. Bird et al. (1989)	DSM-III (algorithm; CGAS < 61)	C,P (combined)	Both	386	<———9.9———>
26. Wolraich et al. (1996)	DSM-IV (threshold score; DSM-IV)	T	Both	8258	<—4.9—>
		T	Males	4102	<—6.8—>
		T	Females	3836	<—2.6—>
32. Boyle, Clifford, Racine, Sanford et al. (1993)	DSM-III-R (algorithm)	Mild C	Both	251	<—1.3—> <—2.6—>
		Mild P	Both	251	<—5.9—> <—2.7—>
		Moderate C	Both	251	<—0.7—> <—3.2—>
		Moderate P	Both	251	<—0.9—> <—2.2—>
		Severe C	Both	251	<—4.5—> <—0.7—>
		Severe P	Both	251	<—6.5—> <—5.5—>
28. Anderson et al. (1987)	DSM-III (algorithm)	C,P,T (combined)	Both	792	5.7
15. Costello et al. (1996)	DSM-III-R (algorithm)	C,P (combined)	Both	1015	X—2.8—X^i
		C,P (combined)	Males		X—3.2—X^i
		C,P (combined)	Females		X—2.3—X^i
15. Angold & Costello (1996)	DSM-IV (algorithm; DSM-IV)	C,P (combined)	Both	1015	X—3.0—X^i
22. Bird et al. (1992)	DSM-III (algorithm)	C	Both	222	<———7.9———>
		P	Both	222	<———24.1———>
		C,P (optimal)	Both	222	<———24.9———>
		C,P (combined)	Both	222	<———28.6———>

(continued)

TABLE A3. (Continued)

Reference[a]	Diagnostic system (method)[b]	Informant (method)[c]	Gender	N	Age (prevalence by age range)
17. Shaffer et al. (1996)	DSM-III-R (algorithm; CGAS ≤ 60 or DSIC)	DSM + CGAS ≤ 60			
		C	Both	1285	<———— 1.4 ————>
		P	Both	1285	<———— 2.7 ————>
		C,P (combined)	Both	1285	<———— 4.7 ————>
		DSM + DSIC			
		C	Both	1285	<———— 1.9 ————>
		P	Both	1285	<———— 4.4 ————>
		C,P (combined)	Both	1285	<———— 6.5 ————>
27. Fergusson et al. (1993)	DSM-III-R (algorithm)	C	Both	965	5.1 (age 15)
		P	Both	986	1.8 (age 15)
28. McGee et al. (1990)	DSM-III (algorithm)	C[f]	Both	943	1.7 (age 15)
10. Verhulst et al. (1997)	DSM-III-R (algorithm; CGAS < 61)	C	Both	274	<———— 0.6 ————>
		P	Both	274	<———— 0.6 ————>
		C,P (either)	Both	274	<———— 1.2 ————>
19. Velez et al. (1989)	DSM-III-R (algorithm)	Time 2			
		C,P (combined)	Both	776	<——15.6——> <——18.6——>
		Time 3			
		C,P (combined)	Both	776	<——22.5——> <——14.3——>
19. Cohen et al. (1993)	DSM-III-R (algorithm)	C,P (combined)	Males	749	<——14.2——> <——15.4——> <——12.2——>
		C,P (combined)	Females	746	<——10.4——> <——15.6——> <——12.5——>
20. Lewinsohn et al. (1993)	DSM-III-R (clinician)	Time 1			
		C	Both	1710	<———— 0.9 ————>
		C	Males	819	<———— 1.5 ————>
		C	Females	891	<———— 0.4 ————>
		Time 2			
		C	Both	1508	<———— 0.3 ————>
		C	Males	810	<———— 0.6 ————>
		C	Females	698	<———— 0.1 ————>

Age column headers: 4 4 6 7 8 9 10 11 12 13 14 15 16 17 18 19 20

Abbreviations: ADD = Attention-Deficit Disorder; ADDH = Attention-Deficit Disorder with Hyperactivity; ADHD = Attention-Deficit/Hyperactivity Disorder; ADHD-AD = Attention-Deficit/Hyperactivity Disorder, Inattentive type; ADHD-CT = Attention-Deficit/Hyperactivity Disorder, Combined type; ADHD-HI = Attention-Deficit/Hyperactivity Disorder, Hyperactive-Impulsive type; CD = Conduct Disorder; CGAS = Children's Global Assessment Scale; DSIC = diagnosis-specific impairment criteria; ED = Emotional Disorder; HKD = Hyperkinetic Disorder; OD = Oppositional Disorder.

[a] Number indicates the study on which the cited publication is based. Refer to Tables A1 and A2 for numbered list of studies.

[b] Method of diagnosis. Algorithm = computer algorithm. Threshold score = optimal cut scores on questionnaires set by reference to clinician diagnoses. Where diagnoses included consideration of impairment in functioning, criteria used are noted.

[c] C = child, P = parent, T = teacher.

[d] Method of combination of data from multiple informants. "Either" = diagnosis-level combination; diagnoses were made if any informant endorsed the full set of diagnostic criteria. "Combined" = symptom-level combination; diagnoses were made if the full set of diagnostic criteria was endorsed by any informant, alone or in combination with other informants. "Both" = diagnoses were made only if each informant endorsed the full set of diagnostic criteria. "Optimal" = diagnoses were made if the full set of diagnostic criteria was endorsed, each individual criterion being endorsed by the informant whose response was most predictive of disorder. "Latent" = latent class estimate. "Clinical" = clinical combination.

[e] Attention Deficit (Hyperactivity) Disorder, Conduct Disorder, or Oppositional (Defiant) Disorder.

[f] Conduct Disorder and Oppositional Defiant Disorder.

[g] Teacher for children aged 4–11, child for children aged 12–16.

[h] Unweighted percentage.

[i] Prevalence estimates were based on a sample consisting of 9-, 11-, and 13-year-old age cohorts.

[j] Native Americans.

[k] Attention-Deficit Disorder and Attention-Deficit Disorder, Residual type.

[l] Diagnosis was confirmed by parent report.

[m] Aggressive Conduct Disorder.

[n] Behaviors indicative of Conduct Disorder were assessed by means of items approximating DSM-III-R criteria.

TABLE A4. Comorbidity of Disruptive Disorders

Reference[a]	Diagnostic system (method[b])	Informant[c] (method[d])	N	Gender	Age	Diagnosis	Finding[e]
28. Anderson et al. (1987)	DSM-III (algorithm)	C,P,T (combined)	792	Both	11	ADD/ADDH CD/OD	47.2% had CD/OD* 34.7% had ADD/ADDH*
22. Bird et al. (1988)	DSM-III (clinician)	C,P (combined)	386 386	Both Both	4–16 4–16	ADD/ADDH CD/OD	53.6% had CD/OD* 44.7% had ADD/ADDH*
22. Bird et al. (1993)	DSM-III (algorithm)	C,P (combined) C,P (combined)	222 222	Both Both	9–16 9–16	ADD/ADDH CD/OD	35.7% had CD/OD* 93.0% had ADD/ADDH*
33. Boyle et al. (1996)	DSM-III-R (algorithm)	P P T T	251 251 251 251	Both Both Both Both	6–16 6–16 6–16 6–16	ADHD CD ADHD CD	2.1% had CD[f] 8.3% had ADHD[f] 21.2% had CD[f] 55.0% had ADHD[f]
27. Fergusson et al. (1993)	DSM-III-R (algorithm)	C,P (combined) C,P (latent)	961 961	Both Both	15 15	ADHD and CD/ODD ADHD and CD/ODD	OR = 26.8* OR = 23.6*
28. McGee et al. (1990)	DSM-III (algorithm)	C[g]	943	Both	15	ADD/ADDH CD	20.0% had CD[b] 4.7% had ADD/ADDH[b]
32. Offord et al. (1986)	DSM-III (threshold score)	P,T (either) P,T (either) C,P (either) C,P (either)	721 721 608 624	Males Females Males Females	4–11 4–11 12–16 12–16	CD CD CD CD	58.7% had ADD/ADDH[f] 56.3% had ADD/ADDH[f] 30.5% had ADD/ADDH[f] 37.0% had ADD/ADDH[f]
32. Offord, Boyle, Fleming et al. (1989)	DSM-III (threshold score)	P,T/C[i] (either) P,T/C[i] (either)	2687 2687	Both Both	4–16 4–16	ADD/ADDH CD	42.7% had CD[f] 42.7% had ADD/ADDH[f]
32. Szatmari, Boyle, & Offord (1989)	DSM-III (threshold score)	P,T/C[i] (either) P,T/C[i] (either) P,T (either P,T (either C,P (either) C,P (either)	2687 2687 721 721 608 624	Males Females Males Females Males Females	4–16 4–16 4–11 4–11 12–16 12–16	ADDH and CD ADDH and CD ADDH ADDH ADDH ADDH	OR = 14.7[f] OR = 40.0[f] 42.2% had CD[f] 36.0% had CD[f] 43.9% had CD[f] 50.0% had CD[f]

		N	Sample	Age		
	P,T (either)	721	Males	4–11	CD	58.7% had ADDH[f]
	P,T (either)	721	Females	4–11	CD	56.2% had ADDH[f]
	C,P (either)	608	Males	12–16	CD	30.5% had ADDH[f]
	C,P (either)	624	Females	12–16	CD	37.0% had ADDH[f]
26. Wolraich *et al.* (1996) DSM-III-R, DSM-IV (threshold score)	T	8258	Both	5–10[j]	ADHD (DSM-III-R)	22.3% had CD*
	T	8258	Both	5–10[j]	ADHD (DSM-IV)	15.6% had CD*
	T	8258	Both	5–10[j]	ADHD-AD	4.7% had CD*
	T	8258	Both	5–10[j]	ADHD-HI	19.9% had CD*
	T	8258	Both	5–10[j]	ADHD-CT	29.0% had CD*
	T	8258	Both	5–10[j]	ADHD (DSM-III-R)	44.4% had ODD*
	T	8258	Both	5–10[j]	ADHD (DSM-IV)	30.2% had ODD*
	T	8258	Both	5–10[j]	ADHD-AD	11.2% had ODD*
	T	8258	Both	5–10[j]	ADHD-HI	36.2% had ODD*
	T	8258	Both	5–10[j]	ADHD-CT	54.7% had ODD*

Abbreviations: ADD = Attention-Deficit Disorder; ADDH = Attention-Deficit Disorder with Hyperactivity; ADHD = Attention-Deficit/Hyperactivity Disorder; ADHD-AD = Attention-Deficit/Hyperactivity Disorder, Inattentive type; ADHD-CT = Attention-Deficit/Hyperactivity Disorder, Combined type; ADHD-HI = Attention-Deficit/Hyperactivity Disorder, Hyperactive-Impulsive type; CD = Conduct Disorder; OD = Oppositional Disorder; ODD = Oppositional Defiant Disorder; OR = odds ratio.

[a]Number indicates the study on which the cited publication is based. Refer to Tables A1 and A2 for numbered list of studies.

[b]Method of diagnosis. Algorithm = computer algorithm. Threshold score = optimal cut scores on questionnaires set by reference to clinician diagnoses.

[c]C = child, P = parent, T = teacher.

[d]Method of combination of data from multiple informants. "Either" = diagnosis-level combination; diagnoses were made if any informant endorsed the full set of diagnostic criteria. "Combined" = symptom-level combination; diagnoses were made if the full set of diagnostic criteria was endorsed by any informant, alone or in combination with other informants. "Latent" = latent class estimate.

[e]* = significant at $p < .001$.

[f]No significance tests were reported.

[g]Diagnoses were confirmed by parent report.

[h]Nonsignificant at $p < .05$.

[i]Teacher for children aged 4–11, child for children aged 12–16.

[j]Approximate numbers.

TABLE A5. Selected Individual-Level Correlates of Disruptive Behavior Disorders

Reference[a] (sample characteristics[b])	Definition (measure)	Informant[c] (methods[d])	Diagnosis or behavior (dependent measure[e])	Effect (control variables)
Age and diagnoses				
22. Bird et al. (1989) (Hispanic males & females; 4–16 years)	Chronological age (years, 4–5 vs. 6–11 vs. 12–16)	C,P (combined)	ADD/ADDH (PREV)	4–5 < 6–11 = 12–16 (gender)
		C,P (combined)	OD (PREV)	NS (gender)
19. Cohen et al. (1993) (white & nonwhite males & females; 10–20 years at T2 & T3)	Chronological age (years, 10–13 vs. 14–16 vs. 17–20)	C,P (combined)	ADD/ADDH (PREV)	Decreases with age
		C,P (combined)	CD (PREV)	Decreases with age for males; curvilinear for females, peak age 16 years
		C,P (combined)	OD (PREV)	Curvilinear, peak ages 13–16 years
15. Costello et al. (1996) (white & black males & females; 9, 11, 13 years at T1)	Chronological age (years, 9 vs. 11 & 13 years)	P	ADHD (PREV)	NS
		C,P (combined)	CD (PREV)	NS
		C,P (combined)	ODD (PREV)	NS
20. Lewinsohn et al. (1993) (white & nonwhite males & females; 14–18 years at T1, 15–19 years at T2)	Chronological age (years, 14–18 vs. 15–19)	C	ADHD (PREV)	NS
		C	CD (PREV)	NS
		C	ODD (PREV)	NS
32. Offord et al. (1987) (males & females; 4–16 years at T1)	Chronological age (years, 4–11 vs. 12–16)	P,T/C[f] (either)	ADD/ADDH[g] (PREV)	NS[b]
		P,T/C[f] (either)	CD[g] (PREV)	4–11 < 12–16[b]
32. Offord, Boyle, & Racine (1989) (males & females; 4–16 years at T1)	Chronological age (years, 4–11 vs. 12–16)	P	ADD/ADDH[g] (PREV)	Interaction with physical illness[i]
		P	CD[g] (PREV)	4–11 < 12–16
		T/C[f]	ADD/ADDH[g] (PREV)	12–16 < 4–11
		T/C[f]	CD[g] (PREV)	Interaction with income[i]
33. Offord et al. (1996) (males & females; 6–16 years)	Chronological age (years, 6–11 vs. 12–16)	P	CD (PREV)	NS
		P	OD (PREV)	NS
		T	CD (PREV)	NS
		T	OD (PREV)	NS
		P,T (either)	CD (PREV)	NS

(*continued*)

Study	Variable	Design	Behavior	Result
19. Velez *et al.* (1989) (white & nonwhite males & females; 11–20 years at T3)	Chronological age (years, 11–14 vs. 15–20)	P,T (either)	OD (PREV)	NS
		P,T (combined)	CD (PREV)	NS
		P,T (combined)	OD (PREV)	NS
		C,P (combined)	ADHD (PREV)	15–20 < 11–14 (gender)
		C,P (combined)	CD (PREV)	15–20 < 11–14 (gender)
		C,P (combined)	ODD (PREV)	15–20 < 11–14 (gender)

Age and behavior

Study	Variable	Design	Behavior	Result
1. Achenbach *et al.* (1991) (white, black, & other males & females 4–16 years at T1)	Chronological age (years, 4–5 vs. 6–7 vs. 8–9 vs. 10–11 vs. 12–13 vs. 14–15 vs. 16)	P	AGG (NUM)	Decreases with age [k]
		P	ATT (NUM)	Nonlinear [k]
		P	DEL (NUM)	Increases with age [k]
16. Aneshensel & Sucoff (1996) (white, black, Hispanic, Asian, & other males & females; 12–17 years)	Chronological age (years)	C	CP (NUM)	Increases with age [l]
		C	OPP (NUM)	Increases with age [l]
7. Elliott *et al.* (1983) (white, black, Hispanic, & other males & females, 12–20 years at T1–T5)	Chronological age (years)	C	DEL (PREV)[m]	Increases with age
2. McDermott (1996) (white, black, Hispanic, & other males & females; 5–17 years)	Chronological age (years, 5–8 vs. 9–11 vs. 12–14 vs. 15–17)	T	ATT/HYP (PREV)[n]	15–17 < 5–8
		T	SOL AGG/PRO (PREV)[n]	15–17 < 12–14 = 9–11 = 5–8
		T	SOL AGG/IMP (PREV)[n]	15–17 < 12–14 = 5–8
		T	OPP (PREV)[n]	NS
2. McDermott (1996) (white, black, Hispanic & other males only; 5–17 years)	Chronological age (years, 5–8 vs. 9–11 vs. 12–14 vs. 15–17)	T	ATT/HYP (PREV)[n]	NS
		T	SOL AGG/PRO (PREV)[n]	15–17 < 12–14 = 9–11 = 5–8
		T	SOL AGG/IMP (PREV)[n]	15–17 < 12–14 = 5–8
		T	OPP (PREV)[n]	NS
2. McDermott (1996) (white, black, Hispanic, & other females only; 5–17 years)	Chronological age (years, 5–8 vs. 9–11 vs. 12–14 vs. 15–17)	T	ATT/HYP (PREV)[n]	NS
		T	SOL AGG/PRO (PREV)[n]	NS
		T	SOL AGG/IMP (PREV)[n]	NS
		T	OPP (PREV)[n]	NS

TABLE A5. (*Continued*)

Reference[a] (sample characteristics)[b]	Definition (measure)	Informant[c] (methods)[d]	Diagnosis or behavior (dependent measure)[e]	Effect (control variables)
2. McDermott (1993) (white, black, Hispanic, & other, males & females; 5–17 years)	Chronological age (preadolescent vs. adolescent)	T	ATT (PREV)[o]	NS
		T	ATT/HYP (PREV)[o]	Adolescent < preadolescent
		T	SOL AGG/PRO (PREV)[o]	Adolescent < preadolescent
		T	SOL AGG/IMP (PREV)[o]	NS
		T	OPP (PREV)[o]	NS
11. Pedersen & Wichstrøm (1995) (males & females; 12–18 years)	Chronological age (years)	C	DEL (NUM)	Curvilinear; peak age 17 years for males, 16 years for females
4. Roberts & Baird (1972) (white & nonwhite males & females; 6–11 years)	Chronological age (years)	T	AGG (PREV)[m]	NS
11. Wichstrøm et al. (1996) (Norway sample; males & females; 13–19 years)	Chronological age (years)	C	CP (PREV)[p]	NS
11. Wichstrøm et al. (1996) (Oslo sample; males & females; 16–19 years)	Chronological age (years)	C	CP (PREV)[p]	NS
Gender[q] and diagnoses				
35. Al-Kuwaiti et al. (1995) (grades 1–2)	Male vs. female	T	CD (PREV)	Female < male
35. Al-Kuwaiti et al. (1995) (grades 3–4)	Male vs. female	T	CD (PREV)	Female < male
35. Al-Kuwaiti et al. (1995) (grades 5–6)	Male vs. female	T	CD (PREV)	Female < male

Study	Comparison	Type	Measure	Result
28. Anderson et al. (1987) (white, Maori, & other Polynesian; 11 years at T6)	Male vs. female	C,P,T (combined)	ADD/ADDH (PREV)	1:5.1 female:male
		C,P,T (combined)	CD^r (PREV)	1:3.2 female:male
		C,P,T (combined)	OD (PREV)	1:2.2 female:male
22. Bird et al. (1989) (Hispanic; 4–16 years)	Male vs. female	C,P (combined)	ADD/ADDH (PREV)	Female < male (age)
		C,P (combined)	OD (PREV)	NS (age)
19. Cohen et al. (1993) (white & nonwhite; 10–20 years at T2 & T3)	Male vs. female	C,P (combined)	ADD/ADDH (PREV)	Female < male
		C,P (combined)	CD (PREV)	Female < male; Effect decreases with age
		C,P (combined)	OD (PREV)	NS
28. Feehan et al. (1994) (white, Maori, & other Polynesian; 18 years at T9)	Male vs. female	C	CDSr (PREV)	Female < male
27. Fergusson et al. (1993) (Pakeha, Maori, & Pacific Island; 15 years at T17)	Male vs. female	C,P (optimal)	ADHD (PREV)	Female < male
		C,P (optimal)	CD/ODD (PREV)	NS
		C,P (latent)	ADHD (PREV)	Female < male
		C,P (latent)	CD/ODD (PREV)	NS
30b. Graham & Rutter (1973) (14–15 years at T2)	Male vs. female	C,P,T (clinical)	HKS^g (PREV)	1:1 female:male
		C,P,T (clinical)	CDS^{g,f} (PREV)	1:2.7 female:male
36. Leslie (1974) (13–14 years)	Male vs. female	C,P (clinical)	CD (PREV)	1:1.2 female:male
20. Lewinsohn et al. (1993) (white & nonwhite; 14–18 years at T1)	Male vs. female	C	ADHD (PREV)	NS
		C	CD (PREV)	NS
		C	ODD (PREV)	Female < male
20. Lewinsohn et al. (1993) (white & nonwhite; 15–19 years at T2)	Male vs. female	C	ADHD (PREV)	NS
		C	CD (PREV)	NS
		C	ODD (PREV)	NS
28. McGee et al. (1990) (white, Maori, & other Polynesian; 15 years at T8)	Male vs. female	C^t	ADD/ADDH^a (PREV)	1:2.3 female:male
		C^t	CD (PREV)	1:1 female:male
		C^t	OD (PREV)	3.1:1 female:male
32. Offord et al. (1987) (4–16 years at T1)	Male vs. female	P,T/C^g (either)	ADD/ADDH^g (PREV)	Female < male
		P,T/C^g (either)	CD^g (PREV)	Female < male

(continued)

Reference[a] (sample characteristics[b])	Definition (measure)	Informant[c] (methods[d])	Diagnosis or behavior (dependent measure[e])	Effect (control variables)
32. Offord, Boyle, & Racine (1989) (4–16 years at T1)	Male vs. female	P	ADD/ADDH[g] (PREV)	NS
		P	CD[g]	Interaction with parental psychiatric history: female < male for children with parental psychiatric history; NS for children without parental psychiatric history
		T/C[f]	ADD/ADDH[g] (PREV)	Female < male
		T/C[f]	CD[g] (PREV)	Female < male
33. Offord et al. (1996) (6–16 years)	Male vs. female	P	CD (PREV)	NS
		P	OD (PREV)	Female < male
		T	CD (PREV)	Female < male
		T	OD (PREV)	Female < male
		P,T (either)	CD (PREV)	Female < male
		P,T (either)	OD (PREV)	Female < male
		P,T (combined)	CD (PREV)	Female < male
		P,T (combined)	OD (PREV)	Female < male
30a. Rutter et al. (1970) (10–11 years at T1)	Male vs. female	C,P,T (clinical)	HKS[g] (PREV)	1:1 female:male
		C,P,T (clinical)	CD[g,s] (PREV)	1:4 female:male
19. Velez et al. (1989) (white & nonwhite; 9–12 years at T2)	Male vs. female	C,P (combined)	ADHD (PREV)	Female < male
		C,P (combined)	CD (PREV)	Female < male
		C,P (combined)	ODD (PREV)	NS
19. Velez et al. (1989) (white & nonwhite; 13–18 years at T2)	Male vs. female	C,P (combined)	ADHD (PREV)	NS
		C,P (combined)	CD (PREV)	NS
		C,P (combined)	ODD (PREV)	NS
19. Velez et al. (1989) (white & nonwhite; 11–14 years at T3)	Male vs. female	C,P (combined)	ADHD (PREV)	NS
		C,P (combined)	CD (PREV)	Female < male
		C,P (combined)	ODD (PREV)	NS
19. Velez et al. (1989) (white & nonwhite; 15–20 years at T3)	Male vs. female	C,P (combined)	ADHD (PREV)	NS
		C,P (combined)	CD (PREV)	NS
		C,P (combined)	ODD (PREV)	NS

19. Velez *et al.* (1989) (white & nonwhite; 11–20 years at T3)	Male vs. female	C,P (combined)	ADHD (PREV)	NS (age)
		C,P (combined)	CD (PREV)	Female < male (age)
		C,P (combined)	ODD (PREV)	NS (age)
10. Verhulst *et al.* (1997) (13–18 years)	Male vs. female	C,P (either)	ADHD[e] (PREV)	NS
		C,P (either)	CD[f] (PREV)	Female < male
		C,P (either)	ODD[g] (PREV)	NS
38. Vikan (1985) (white; 10 years)	Male vs. female	C,P (clinical)	CD[g] (PREV)	NS
		C,P (clinical)	HKS[g] (PREV)	NS
26. Wolraich *et al.* (1996) (white & black; grades K–5)	Male vs. female	T	DSM-III-R ADHD (PREV)	1:3.6 female:male
		T	DSM-IV ADHD[y] (PREV)	1:2.9 female:male
		T	DSM-IV ADHD-AD[y] (PREV)	1:2.2 female:male
		T	DSM-IV ADHD-HI[y] (PREV)	1:4.3 female:male
		T	DSM-IV ADHD-CT[y] (PREV)	1:3.5 female:male

Gender and behavior

1. Achenbach *et al.* (1991) (white, black, Hispanic, & other; 4–16 years at T1)	Male vs. female	P	AGG (NUM)	Female < male
		P	ATT (NUM)	Female < male
		P	DEL[i] (NUM)	Female < male
24. Anastas & Reinherz (1984) (white & nonwhite; kindergarten at T1)	Male vs. female	P	AGG (NUM)	Female < male
16. Aneshensel & Sucoff (1996) (white, black, Hispanic, Asian, & other; 12–17 years)	Male vs. female	C	CP (NUM)	NS[l]
		C	OPP (NUM)	Female < male[l]
5. Barbarin & Soler (1993) (black; 4–11 years)	Male vs. female	P	CP (NUM)	Female < male (family structure)
		P	HYP (NUM)	NS (family structure)
5. Barbarin & Soler (1993) (black; 12–17 years)	Male vs. female	P	CP (NUM)	Female < male (family structure)
		P	HYP (NUM)	Female < male (family structure)
8. Butler & Golding (1986) (white, black, Asian, & other; 5 years at T2)	Male vs. female	P	CP (NUM)	Female < male
		P	HYP (NUM)	Female < male
9. Davie *et al.* (1972) (7 years at T2)	Male vs. female	P	AGG (NUM)	Female < male
		P	HYP (NUM)	Female < male

(continued)

TABLE A5. (*Continued*)

Reference[a] (sample characteristics[b])	Definition (measure)	Informant[c] (methods[d])	Diagnosis or behavior (dependent measure[e])	Effect (control variables)
9. Davie *et al.* (1972) (7 years at T2)	Male vs. female	T	HYP (NUM)	Female < male
7. Elliott *et al.* (1983) (white, black, Hispanic, & other; 11–17 years at T1, 12–18 years at T2, 13–19 years at T3, 14–20 years at T4, 15–21 years at T5)	Male vs. female	C	DEL (PREV)	Female < male[w]
3. Luster & McAdoo (1994) (blacks; 6–9 years at T1)	Male vs. female	P	CP (NUM)	NS
2. McDermott (1996) (white, black, Hispanic, & other; 5–8 years)	Male vs. female	T T T T	ATT/HYP (PREV)[n] SOL AGG/PRO (PREV)[n] SOL AGG/IMP (PREV)[n] OPP (PREV)[n]	Female < male Female < male Female < male Female < male
2. McDermott (1996) (white, black, Hispanic, & other; 9–11 years)	Male vs. female	T T T T	ATT/HYP (PREV)[n] SOL AGG/PRO (PREV)[n] SOL AGG/IMP (PREV)[n] OPP (PREV)[n]	Female < male NS Female < male NS
2. McDermott (1996) (white, black, Hispanic, & other; 12–14 years)	Male vs. female	T T T T	ATT/HYP (PREV)[n] SOL AGG/PRO (PREV)[n] SOL AGG/IMP (PREV)[n] OPP (PREV)[n]	Female < male Female < male Female < male NS
2. McDermott (1996) (white, black, Hispanic, & other; 15–17 years)	Male vs. female	T T T T	ATT/HYP (PREV)[n] SOL AGG/PRO (PREV)[n] SOL AGG/IMP (PREV)[n] OPP (PREV)[n]	Female < male NS Female < male NS

28. McGee et al. (1984) (white, Maori, & other Polynesian; 7 years at T4)	Male vs. female	P,T (both above cutoff)	CP (PREV)[x]	1:2 female:male
28. McGee et al. (1985) (white, Maori, & other Polynesian; 7 years at T4)	Male vs. female	T T	AGG (NUM) HYP (NUM)	Female < male Female < male
11. Pedersen & Wichstrøm (1995) (12–18 years)	Male vs. female	C	DEL (NUM)	Female < male
4. Roberts & Baird (1972) (white & nonwhite; 6–11 years)	Male vs. female	T	AGG (PREV)[m]	Female < male
37. Trites et al. (1979) (5–12 years)	Male vs. female	T T T	CP (PREV)[y] ATT (PREV)[y] HYP (PREV)[y]	2.7:1 female:male 1:2.1 female:male 1:3.0 female:male
11. Wichstrøm et al. (1996) (Norway sample; 13–19 years)	Male vs. female	C	CP (PREV)[b]	Female < male
11. Wichstrøm et al. (1996) (Oslo sample; 16–19 years)	Male vs. female	C	CP (PREV)[b]	Female < male
28. Williams et al. (1990) (white, Maori, & other Polynesian; 11 years at T6)	Male vs. female	C C C C C C	ATT (NUM) CP (NUM) HYP (NUM) OPP (NUM) ATT/HYP (NUM) CP/OPP (NUM)	Female < male Female < male Female < male NS Female < male Female < male
Racial/ethnic background and diagnoses				
15. Costello et al. (1996) (males & females; 9, 11, 13 years at T1)	White vs. black	P C,P (combined) C,P (combined)	ADHD (PREV) CD (PREV) ODD (PREV)	NS NS NS
15. Costello et al. (1997) (Males & females; 9, 11, 13 years at T1)	White vs. Native American	P C,P (combined)	ADHD (PREV) CD/ODD (PREV)	NS NS
19. Velez et al. (1989) (males & females; 9–18 years at T2)	White vs. nonwhite	C,P (combined) C,P (combined) C,P (combined)	ADHD (PREV) CD (PREV) ODD (PREV)	NS (age, gender) NS (age, gender) NS (age, gender)

(continued)

TABLE A5. *(Continued)*

Reference[a] (sample characteristics)[b]	Definition (measure)	Informant[c] (methods[d])	Diagnosis or behavior (dependent measure)[e]	Effect (control variables)
19. Velez *et al.* (1989) (males & females, 11–20 years at T3)	White vs. nonwhite	C,P (combined) C,P (combined) C,P (combined)	ADHD (PREV) CD (PREV) ODD (PREV)	NS (age, gender) White < nonwhite (age, gender) NS (age, gender)
Racial/ethnic background and behavior				
1. Achenbach *et al.* (1991) (males & females; 4–16 years at T1)	White vs. nonwhite	P P P	AGG (NUM) ATT (NUM) DEL[j] (NUM)	Nonwhite < white [k] Nonwhite < white [k] NS [k]
1. Achenbach *et al.* (1991) (males & females; 4–16 years at T1)	Black vs. nonblack	P P P	AGG (NUM) ATT (NUM) DEL[j] (NUM)	NS [k] NS [k] NS [k]
16. Aneshensel & Sucoff (1996) (males & females; 12–17 years)	Black vs. nonblack	C C	CP (NUM) OPP (NUM)	NS [l] NS [l]
16. Aneshensel & Sucoff (1996) (males & females; 12–17 years)	Hispanic vs. non-Hispanic	C C	CP (NUM) OPP (NUM)	Non-Hispanic < Hispanic [l] NS [l]
7. Elliott *et al.* (1983) (males & females; 11–17 years at T1)	White vs. black[x]	C	DEL (PREV)[m]	NS
7. Elliott *et al.* (1983) (males & females; 12–18 years at T2)	White vs. black[x]	C	DEL (PREV)[m]	NS
7. Elliott *et al.* (1983) (males & females; 13–19 years at T3)	White vs. black[x]	C	DEL (PREV)[m]	NS
7. Elliott *et al.* (1983) (males & females; 14–20 years at T4)	White vs. black[x]	C	DEL (PREV)[m]	White < black

Study	Comparison	Outcome	Informant	Results
7. Elliott *et al.* (1983) (males & females; 15–21 years at T5)	White vs. black[z]	DEL (PREV)[m]	C	White < black
24. Fridrich & Flannery (1995) (males & females; grades 6–7)	White vs. Mexican American	DEL[i] (NUM)	C	White < Mexican American
7. Huizinga & Elliott (1987) (males & females; 11–17 years at T1, 12–18 years at T2, 13–19 years at T3, 14–20 years at T4, 15–21 years at T5)	White vs. black[z]	DEL (PREV)[m]	C	NS[aa]
13. Kingery (1996) (males only; grades 8–9 at T3)	White vs. American black vs. Caribbean black vs. Haitian vs. Cuban vs. non-Cuban Hispanic vs. Nicaraguan vs. other	DEL (NUM)	C	NS
21. Loeber *et al.* (1998) (males only; grade 2 at T1)	White or Asian vs. black, Hispanic, Native American, biracial, or multiracial	AGG$^{\alpha}$ (PREV)[dd]	C,T (sum)	NS
		ATT/HYP (PREV)[dd]	P	NS
		COV (PREV)[dd]	C,P,T (sum)	NS
		CP (PREV)[dd]	P	NS
		DEL (SER)	C,P,T [bb]	White or Asian < black, Hispanic, Native American, biracial, or multiracial
21. Loeber *et al.* (1998) (males only; grade 5 at T1)	White or Asian vs. black, Hispanic, Native American, biracial, or multiracial	AGG$^{\alpha}$ (PREV)[dd]	C,T (sum)	NS
		ATT/HYP (PREV)[dd]	P	NS
		COV (PREV)[dd]	C,P,T (sum)	NS
		CP (PREV)[dd]	P	NS
		DEL (SER)	C,P,T [bb]	White or Asian < black, Hispanic, Native American, biracial, or multiracial

(*continued*)

TABLE A5. (Continued)

Reference[a] (sample characteristics[b])	Definition (measure)	Informant[c] (methods[d])	Diagnosis or behavior (dependent measure[e])	Effect (control variables)
21. Loeber et al. (1998) (males only; grade 8 at T1)	White or Asian vs. black, Hispanic, Native American, biracial, or multiracial	C,T (sum)	AGG[α] (PREV)[dd]	White or Asian < black, Hispanic, Native American, biracial, or multiracial
		P	ATT/HYP (PREV)[dd]	NS
		C,P,T (sum)	COV (PREV)[dd]	NS
		P	CP (PREV)[dd]	NS
		C,P,T [bb]	DEL (SER)	White or Asian < black, Hispanic, Native American, biracial, or multiracial
2. McDermott (1996) (males & females; 5–17 years)	White vs. black vs. Hispanic vs. other	T	ATT/HYP (PREV)[n]	NS [æ]
		T	SOL AGG/PRO (PREV)[n]	NS [æ]
		T	SOL AGG/IMP (PREV)[n]	NS [æ]
		T	OPP (PREV)[n]	NS [æ]

Abbreviations: ADD = Attention-Deficit Disorder; ADDH = Attention-Deficit Disorder with Hyperactivity; ADHD = Attention-Deficit/Hyperactivity Disorder; ADHD-AD = Attention-Deficit/Hyperactivity Disorder, Inattentive type; ADHD-CT = Attention-Deficit/Hyperactivity Disorder, Combined type; ADHD-HI = Attention-Deficit/Hyperactivity Disorder, Hyperactive-Impulsive type; AGG = aggressive behavior; ATT = attention problems; CD = Conduct Disorder; COV = covert antisocial behavior; CP = conduct problems; DEL = delinquent behavior; HKS = Hyperkinetic Syndrome; HYP = hyperactive behavior; NS = nonsignificant results; OD = Oppositional Disorder; ODD = Oppositional Defiant Disorder; OPP = oppositional behavior; SOL AGG/IMP = solitary aggressive–impulsive behavior; SOL AGG/PRO = solitary aggressive–provocative behavior.

[a]Number indicates the study on which the cited publication is based. Refer to Tables A1 and A2 for numbered list of studies.
[b]Where not otherwise indicated, racial or ethnic composition of the sample was not reported. "White" = non-Hispanic white.
[c]C = child, P = parent, T = teacher.
[d]Method of combination of data from multiple informants. "Either" = diagnosis-level combination; diagnoses were made if any informant endorsed the full set of diagnostic criteria. "Combined" = symptom-level combination; diagnoses were made if the full set of diagnostic criteria was endorsed by any informant, alone or in combination with other informants. "Optimal" = diagnoses were made if the full set of diagnostic criteria was endorsed, each individual criterion being endorsed by the informant whose response was most predictive of disorder. "Latent" = latent class estimate. "Clinical" = clinical combination. "Sum" = number of symptoms or behaviors endorsed was summed across informants.
[e]PREV = prevalence. NUM = number of symptoms or behaviors endorsed. SER = seriousness of behavior.
[f]Teacher for children aged 4–11, child for children aged 12–16.
[g]Diagnosis included ad hoc impairment criterion.
[h]Separate analyses were performed for males and females. Results were the same for each gender.
[i]Nature of effect was not specified.
[j]Measure included items assessing alcohol and drug use.
[k]Multivariate analyses included age, gender, racial/ethnic background, religion, and socioeconomic status.
[l]Multivariate analyses included age, gender, racial/ethnic background, family structure, income, neighborhood type, neighborhood stability, and neighborhood quality.
[m]Prevalence threshold = one or more behaviors endorsed.
[n]Prevalence threshold = T score ≥ 60.
[o]Prevalence threshold = T score ≥ 70.
[p]Prevalence threshold = three or more behaviors endorsed.
[q]Where ratios are presented, no significance tests were reported.

654

[r]Aggressive Conduct Disorder.

[s]Includes mixed Conduct Disorder and Emotional Disorder.

[t]Diagnosis was confirmed by parent report.

[u]Includes residual type.

[v]Diagnosis included DSM-IV impairment criterion.

[w]Separate analyses were performed on each of 5 annual waves of data. Participants were 11–17 years old at Time 1 and 16–21 years old at Time 5. Results were the same for each wave.

[x]Prevalence threshold = 13 or more behaviors endorsed by parent and 9 or more behaviors endorsed by teacher.

[y]Prevalence threshold = scale score of 1.5 or greater.

[z]Racial background was interviewer-identified; participants were questioned only if the interviewer was unable to make a visual determination.

[aa]Separate analyses were performed for males and females on each of 5 annual waves of data. Participants were 11–17 years old at Time 1 and 16–21 years old at Time 5. Results were the same for each gender at each wave.

[bb]Participants were classified according to the severity of the most serious act ever committed reported by any informant.

[cc]Lifetime aggression.

[dd]Prevalence threshold = 75th percentile.

[ee]Multivariate analyses included age, gender, ethnic background, and parental education.

TABLE A6. Selected Family-Level Correlates of Disruptive Behavior Disorders

Reference[a] (sample characteristics[b])	Definition (measures)	Informant[c] (methods[d])	Diagnosis or behavior (dependent measures[e])	Effect (control variables)
		Family structure and diagnoses		
22. Bird et al. (1989) (Hispanic males & females; 4–16 years)	Single-parent household	C,P (combined)	ADD/ADDH (PREV)	NS (age, gender)
		C,P (combined)	OD (PREV)	NS (age, gender)
32. Blum et al. (1988) (males & females; 6–16 years at T1)	Head of household (two-parent vs. single parent)	P;T/C[f] (either)	ADDH[g] (PREV)	Two-parent < single
		P;T/C[f] (either)	OD[g] (PREV)	Two-parent < single
30b. Graham & Rutter (1973) (males & females; 14–15 years at T2)	Head of household (biological two-parent vs. other)	C,P,T (clinical)	CD[g] (PREV)	NS
		C,P,T (clinical)	CD/ED[g] (PREV)	Two-parent < other
32. Offord et al. (1986) (males & females; 4–16 years at T1)	Single-parent household	P;T/C[f] (either)	CD[g] (PREV)	Increases risk
33. Offord et al. (1996) (males & females; 6–16 years)	Single-parent household	P	CD (PREV)	NS
		P	OD (PREV)	NS
		T	CD (PREV)	NS
		T	OD (PREV)	Increases risk
		P,T (either)	CD (PREV)	Increases risk
		P,T (either)	OD (PREV)	NS
		P,T (combined)	CD (PREV)	Increases risk
		P,T (combined)	OD (PREV)	Increases risk
19. Velez et al. (1989) (white & nonwhite males & females; 1–10 years at T1, 9–18 years at T2)	Parents divorced at T1	C,P (combined)	ADHD at T2 (PREV)	NS (age, gender)
		C,P (combined)	CD at T2 (PREV)	Increases risk (age, gender)
		C,P (combined)	ODD at T2 (PREV)	NS (age, gender)
19. Velez et al. (1989) (white & nonwhite males & females; 9–18 years at T2, 11–20 years at T3)	Single-mother household at T2	C,P (combined)	ADHD at T3 (PREV)	NS (age, gender, SES)
		C,P (combined)	CD at T3 (PREV)	Increases risk (age, gender, SES)
		C,P (combined)	ODD at T3 (PREV)	Increases risk (age, gender, SES)
19. Velez et al. (1989) (white & nonwhite males & females; 9–18 years at T2, 11–20 years at T3)	Stepfather present at T2	C,P (combined)	ADHD at T3 (PREV)	Increases risk (age, gender, SES)
		C,P (combined)	CD at T3 (PREV)	NS (age, gender, SES)
		C,P (combined)	ODD at T3 (PREV)	NS (age, gender, SES)

Study	Variable	Informant	Measure	Result
27. Fergusson *et al.* (1994) (males & females; 15 years at T17)	Parental separation, ages 0–5	C,P (combined)	CD/ODD (PREV)	Increases risk
	Parental separation, ages 5–10	C,P (combined)	CD/ODD (PREV)	Increases risk (prior separation)
	Parental separation, ages 10–15	C,P (combined)	CD/ODD (PREV)	Increases risk (prior separation)

Family structure and behavior

Study	Variable	Informant	Measure	Result
1. Achenbach *et al.* (1995) (white, black, Hispanic, & other males & females; 4–16 years at T1, 7–19 years at T2, 9–18 years at T3)	Change in family structure between T1 and T2	C,P,T [b] C,P,T [b] C,P,T [b]	AGG at T3 (NUM) ATT at T3 (NUM) DEL[i] at T3 (NUM)	NS [j,k] NS [j,k] NS [j,k]
1. Achenbach *et al.* (1995) (white, black, Hispanic, & other males & females; 7–19 years at T2, 9–18 years at T3)	Change in family structure between T2 and T3	C,P,T [b] C,P,T [b] C,P,T [b]	AGG at T3 (NUM) ATT at T3 (NUM) DEL[i] at T3 (NUM)	NS [j,k] NS [j,k] NS [j,k]
16. Aneshensel & Sucoff (1996) (white, black, Hispanic, Asian, & other males & females; 12–17 years)	Biological two-parent household	C C	CP (NUM) OPP (NUM)	NS [l] NS [l]
16. Aneshensel & Sucoff (1996) (white, black, Hispanic, Asian, & other males & females; 12–17 years)	Single-parent household	C C	CP (NUM) OPP (NUM)	NS [l] Increases risk [l]
5. Barbarin & Soler (1993) (black males & females; 4–11 years)	Head of household biological mother vs. other single-parent vs. biological two-parent vs. other two-parent vs. three-generation)	P P	CP (NUM) HYP (NUM)	Three-generation < biological mother (gender) NS (gender)
5. Barbarin & Soler (1993) (black males & females; 12–17 years)	Head of household (biological mother vs. other single-parent vs. biological two-parent vs. other two-parent vs. three-generation)	P P	CP (NUM) HYP (NUM)	NS (gender) NS (gender)

(*continued*)

TABLE A6. *(Continued)*

Reference[a] (sample characteristics[b])	Definition (measures)	Informant[c] (methods[e])	Diagnosis or behavior (dependent measures[f])	Effect (control variables)
6. Dawson (1991) (white, black, & other males & females; 5–17 years)	Head of household (biological two-parent vs. biological mother/stepfather vs. formerly married single-mother vs. never-married single-mother)	P	CP (NUM)	Two-parent < never-married mother = formerly-married mother = mother/stepfather[m]
			OPP (NUM)	Two-parent < never-married mother = formerly-married mother = mother/stepfather[m]
			HYP (NUM)	Two-parent < never-married mother = formerly-married mother = mother/stepfather[m]
27. Fergusson & Lynskey (1993a) (males & females; 12 years at T14)	Number of changes in parenting figures prior to age 12	C,T (latent)	ATT/HYP (NUM)	Increases risk[n]
		C,T (latent)	CP/OPP (NUM)	Increases risk[n]
27. Fergusson & Lynskey (1993a) (males & females; 13 years at T15)	Number of changes in parenting figures prior to age 12	C,T (latent)	ATT/HYP (NUM)	Increases risk[n]
		C,T (latent)	CP/OPP (NUM)	Increases risk[n]
21. Loeber *et al.* (1998) (white, black, & other males only; grade 2 at T1)	Head of household (biological two-parent vs. other)	C,T (sum)	AGG[p] (PREV)[q]	Two-parent < other
		P	ATT/HYP (PREV)[q]	Two-parent < other
		C,P,T (sum)	COV (PREV)[q]	Two-parent < other
		P	CP (PREV)[q]	Two-parent < other
		C,P,T ([e])	DEL (SER)	Two-parent < other
21. Loeber *et al.* (1998) (white, black, & other males only; grade 5 at T1)	Head of household (biological two-parent vs. other)	C,T (sum)	AGG[p] (PREV)[q]	Two-parent < other
		P	ATT/HYP (PREV)[q]	Two-parent < other
		C,P,T (sum)	COV (PREV)[q]	Two-parent < other
		P	CP (PREV)[q]	Two-parent < other
		C,P,T ([e])	DEL (SER)	Two-parent < other
21. Loeber *et al.* (1998) (white, black, & other males only; grade 8 at T1)	Head of household (biological two-parent vs. other)	C,T (sum)	AGG[p] (PREV)[q]	Two-parent < other
		P	ATT/HYP (PREV)[q]	NS
		C,P,T (sum)	COV (PREV)[q]	Two-parent < other
		P	CP (PREV)[q]	Two-parent < other
		C,P,T ([e])	DEL (SER)	Two-parent < other

Study / sample	Variable		Outcome	Increases risk
3. Luster & McAdoo (1994) (black males & females; 6–9 years at T1)	Single-mother household	P	CP (NUM)	
1. Stanger et al. (1992) (white, black, Hispanic, & other males & females; 4–16 years at T1, 7–19 years at T2)	Change in family structure between T1 and T2	C	AGG at T2 (NUM)	NS (j)
		C	ATT at T2 (NUM)	NS (j)
		C	DEL[i] at T2 (NUM)	NS (j)
		P	AGG at T2 (NUM)	NS (j)
		P	ATT at T2 (NUM)	NS (j)
		P	DEL[i] at T2 (NUM)	NS (j)
		T	AGG at T2 (NUM)	NS (j)
		T	ATT at T2 (NUM)	NS (j)
		T	DEL[i] at T2 (NUM)	NS (j)
8. Wadsworth et al. (1985) (males & females; 5 years at T2)	Head of household (biological two-parent vs. biological single-parent vs. biological parent/stepparent)	P	CP (NUM)	Two-parent < single, Two-parent < step
Parental age and behavior				
27. Fergusson & Lynskey (1993b) (Pakeha, Maori, & Pacific Island males & females; 8 years at T10)	Maternal age at child's birth (years)	P,T (sum)	CP/OPP (NUM)	Inverse relationship
27. Fergusson & Lynskey (1993b) (Pakeha, Maori, & Pacific Island males & females; 10 years at T12)	Maternal age at child's birth (years)	P,T (sum)	CP/OPP (NUM)	Inverse relationship
27. Fergusson & Lynskey (1993b) (Pakeha, Maori, & Pacific Island males & females; 12 years at T14)	Maternal age at child's birth (years)	P,T (sum)	CP/OPP (NUM)	Inverse relationship
21. Loeber et al. (1998) (white, black, & other males only; grade 2 at T1)	Young maternal age at time of assessment (years; < 27)	C,T (sum)	AGG[b] (PREV)[q]	NS
		P	ATT/HYP (PREV)[q]	NS
		C,P,T (sum)	COV (PREV)[q]	NS
		P	CP (PREV)[q]	NS
		C,P,T (c)	DEL (SER)	NS

(continued)

659

TABLE A6. (*Continued*)

Reference[a] (sample characteristics)[b]	Definition (measures)	Informant[c] (methods[d])	Diagnosis or behavior (dependent measures[e])	Effect (control variables)
21. Loeber et al. (1998) (white, black, & other males only; grade 5 at T1)	Young maternal age at time of assessment (years; < 30)	C,T (sum) P C,P,T (sum) P C,P,T (?)	AGG[b] (PREV)[g] ATT/HYP (PREV)[g] COV (PREV)[g] CP (PREV)[g] DEL (SER)	NS NS NS NS Increases risk
21. Loeber et al. (1998) (white, black, & other males only; grade 8 at T1)	Young maternal age at time of assessment (years; < 33)	C,T (sum) P C,P,T (sum) P C,P,T (?)	AGG[b] (PREV)[g] ATT/HYP (PREV)[g] COV (PREV)[g] CP (PREV)[g] DEL (SER)	NS NS NS NS Increases risk
3. Luster & McAdoo (1994) (black males & females; 6–9 years at T1)	Maternal age at first childbirth (years)	P	CP (NUM)	Inverse relationship
8. Osborn et al. (1984) (white, black, Asian & other males & females; 5 years at T2)	Maternal age at child's 5th birthday (years)	P	CP (NUM)	Inverse relationship [r]
Parental psychopathology and diagnoses				
22. Bird et al. (1989) (Hispanic males & females; 4–16 years)	Maternal psychiatric history (measure not described)	C,P (combined) C,P (combined)	ADD/ADDH (PREV) OD (PREV)	NS (age, gender) NS (age, gender)
22. Bird et al. (1989) (Hispanic males & females; 4–16 years)	Paternal psychiatric history (measure not described)	C,P (combined) C,P (combined)	ADD/ADDH (PREV) OD (PREV)	NS (age, gender) NS (age, gender)
33. Boyle et al. (1996) (males & females; 6–16 years)	Parental criminal history (arrests for nontraffic violations)	P P T T	ADHD (PREV) CD (PREV) ADHD (PREV) CD (PREV)	Increases risk Increases risk Increases risk NS

Study	Predictor	Informant	Outcome	Result
30b. Graham & Rutter (1973) (males & females; 14–15 years at T2)	Maternal psychiatric disorder (PI)	C,P,T (clinical) C,P,T (clinical)	CD[g] (PREV) CD/ED[g] (PREV)	NS Increases risk
32. Offord, Boyle, & Racine (1989) (males & females; 4–16 years at T1)	Parental psychiatric history (treatment for "nerves")	P P T/C[f] T/C[f]	ADD/ADDH[g] (PREV) CD[g] (PREV) ADD/ADDH[g] (PREV) CD[g] (PREV)	NS Interaction with gender[i] NS NS
32. Offord, Boyle, & Racine (1989) (males & females; 4–16 years at T1)	Parental criminal history (arrests)	P P T/C[f] T/C[f]	ADD/ADDH[g] (PREV) CD (PREV) ADD/ADDH[g] (PREV) CD[g] (PREV)	NS Increases risk NS NS
32. Offord et al. (1991) (males & females; 4–16 years at T1)	Parental psychiatric history (treatment for "nerves")	P,T/C[f] (either)	CD[g] (PREV)	Increases risk
32. Offord et al. (1991) (males & females; 4–16 years at T1)	Parental criminal history (arrests for nontraffic violations)	P,T/C[f] (either)	CD[g] (PREV)	Increases risk
19. Velez et al. (1989) (white & nonwhite males & females; 9–18 years at T2, 11–20 years at T3)	Parental emotional problems at T2 (measure not described)	C,P (combined) C,P (combined) C,P (combined)	ADHD at T3 (PREV) CD at T3 (PREV) ODD at T3 (PREV)	NS (age, gender, SES)[f] NS (age, gender, SES)[f] NS (age, gender, SES)[f]
19. Velez et al. (1989) (white & nonwhite males & females; 1–10 years at T1, 9–18 years at T2)	Parental sociopathy at T1 (drug, alcohol, or police problem)	C,P (combined) C,P (combined) C,P (combined)	ADHD at T2 (PREV) CD at T2 (PREV) ODD at T2 (PREV)	Increases risk (age, gender, SES) Increases risk (age, gender, SES) Increases risk (age, gender, SES)
19. Velez et al. (1989) (white & nonwhite males & females; 9–18 years at T2, 11–20 years at T3)	Parental sociopathy at T2 (drug, alcohol, or police problem)	C,P (combined) C,P (combined) C,P (combined)	ADHD at T3 (PREV) CD at T3 (PREV) ODD at T3 (PREV)	Increases risk (age, gender) Increases risk (age, gender) NS (age, gender)

(continued)

Reference[a] (sample characteristics[b])	Definition (measures)	Informant[c] (methods[d])	Diagnosis or behavior (dependent measures[e])	Effect (control variables)
Parental psychopathology and behavior				
27. Fergusson & Lynskey (1993a) (males & females; 12 years at T14)	Current maternal depression (LPDI)	C	ATT/HYP (NUM)	NS (prior depression)
		C	CP/OPP (NUM)	NS (prior depression)
		T	ATT/HYP (NUM)	Increases risk (prior depression)
		T	CP/OPP (NUM)	NS (prior depression)
		C,T (latent)	ATT/HYP (NUM)	Increases risk (prior depression)
		C,T (latent)	CP/OPP (NUM)	NS (prior depression)
27. Fergusson & Lynskey (1993a) (males & females; 13 years at T15)	Current maternal depression (LPDI)	C	ATT/HYP (NUM)	NS (prior depression)
		C	CP/OPP (NUM)	NS (prior depression)
		T	ATT/HYP (NUM)	NS (prior depression)
		T	CP/OPP (NUM)	NS (prior depression)
		C,T (latent)	ATT/HYP (NUM)	NS (prior depression)
		C,T (latent)	CP/OPP (NUM)	NS (prior depression)
21. Loeber *et al.* (1998) (white, black, & other males only; grade 2 at T1)	Parental depression/anxiety (ever sought treatment)	C,T (sum)	AGG[b] (PREV)[q]	Increases risk
		P	ATT/HYP (PREV)[q]	Increases risk
		C,P,T (sum)	COV (PREV)[q]	Increases risk
		P	CP (PREV)[q]	Increases risk
		C,P,T (e)	DEL (SER)	Increases risk
21. Loeber *et al.* (1998) (white, black, & other males only; grade 5 at T1)	Parental depression/anxiety (ever sought treatment)	C,T (sum)	AGG[b] (PREV)[q]	Increases risk
		P	ATT/HYP (PREV)[q]	Increases risk
		C,P,T (sum)	COV (PREV)[q]	NS
		P	CP (PREV)[q]	Increases risk
		C,P,T (e)	DEL (SER)	Increases risk
21. Loeber *et al.* (1998) (white, black, & other males only; grade 8 at T1)	Parental depression/anxiety (ever sought treatment)	C,T (sum)	AGG[b] (PREV)[q]	NS
		P	ATT/HYP (PREV)[q]	Increases risk
		C,P,T (sum)	COV (PREV)[q]	Increases risk
		P	CP (PREV)[q]	Increases risk
		C,P,T (e)	DEL (SER)	NS

(continued)

21. Loeber *et al.* (1998) (white, black, & other males only; grade 2 at T1)	Paternal behavior problems[a] (ever sought treatment)	C,T (sum) P C,P,T (sum) P C,P,T (°)	AGG[b] (PREV)[q] ATT/HYP (PREV)[q] COV (PREV)[q] CP (PREV) DEL (SER)	Increases risk Increases risk Increases risk Increases risk NS
21. Loeber *et al.* (1998) (white, black, & other males only; grade 5 at T1)	Paternal behavior problems[a] (ever sought treatment)	C,T (sum) P C,P,T (sum) P C,P,T (°)	AGG[b] (PREV)[q] ATT/HYP (PREV)[q] COV (PREV)[q] CP (PREV)[q] DEL (SER)	Increases risk NS Increases risk Increases risk Increases risk
21. Loeber *et al.* (1998) (white, black, & other males only; grade 8 at T1)	Paternal behavior problems[a] (ever sought treatment)	C,T (sum) P C,P,T (sum) P C,P,T (°)	AGG[b] (PREV)[q] ATT/HYP (PREV)[q] COV (PREV)[q] CP (PREV)[q] DEL (SER)	NS NS NS Increases risk NS
Parental substance use and abuse and diagnoses				
27. Lynskey *et al.* (1994) (Pakeha, Maori, & Pacific Island; 15 years at T17)	Parental history of alcohol problems (SI)	C,P (either) C,P (either)	ADHD (PREV) CD/ODD (PREV)	Increases risk Increases risk
32. Offord *et al.* (1991) (males & females; 4–16 years at T1)	Excessive parental alcohol use (quantity/frequency > 3 drinks per day in 6 months)	P,T/C[f] (either)	CD[g] (PREV)	NS
Parental substance use and abuse and behavior				
21. Loeber *et al.* (1998) (white, black, & other males only; grade 2 at T1)	Parental substance abuse problems (ever sought treatment)	C,T (sum) P C,P,T (sum) P C,P,T (°)	AGG[b] (PREV)[q] ATT/HYP (PREV)[q] COV (PREV)[q] CP (PREV)[q] DEL (SER)	Increases risk Increases risk Increases risk Increases risk Increases risk

TABLE A6. (*Continued*)

Reference[a] (sample characteristics)[b]	Definition (measures)	Informant[c] (methods)[d]	Diagnosis or behavior (dependent measures)[e]	Effect (control variables)
21. Loeber et al. (1998) (white, black, & other males only; grade 5 at T1)	Parental substance abuse problems (ever sought treatment)	C,T (sum) P C,P,T (sum) P C,P,T (°)	AGG[b] (PREV)[q] ATT/HYP (PREV)[q] COV (PREV)[q] CP (PREV)[q] DEL (SER)	NS Increases risk Increases risk Increases risk Increases risk
21. Loeber et al. (1998) (white, black, & other males only; grade 8 at T1)	Parental substance abuse problems (ever sought treatment)	C,T (sum) P C,P,T (sum) P C,P,T (°)	AGG[b] (PREV)[q] ATT/HYP (PREV)[q] COV (PREV)[q] CP (PREV)[q] DEL (SER)	NS NS NS Increases risk NS
11. Wichstrøm et al. (1996) (Norway sample; males & females; 13–19 years)	Paternal alcohol use (frequency)	C	CP (PREV)[v]	Increases risk
11. Wichstrøm et al. (1996) (Norway sample; males & females; 13–19 years)	Maternal alcohol use (frequency)	C	CP (PREV)[v]	Increases risk
11. Wichstrøm et al. (1996) (Norway sample; males & females; 13–19 years)	Parental intoxication (frequency)	C	CP (PREV)[v]	Increases risk
			Family functioning and diagnoses	
22. Bird et al. (1989) (Hispanic males & females; 4–16 years)	Family dysfunction (family Apgar)	C,P (combined) C,P (combined)	ADD/ADDH (PREV) OD (PREV)	NS (age, gender) NS (age, gender)
22. Bird et al. (1989) (Hispanic males & females; 4–16 years)	Parental marital discord (measure not described)	C,P (combined) C,P (combined)	ADD/ADDH (PREV) OD (PREV)	NS (age, gender) Increases risk (age, gender)
32. Offord, Boyle, & Racine (1989) (males & females; 4–16 years at T1)	Family dysfunction (GFS)	P P	ADD/ADDH[g] (PREV) CD[g] (PREV)	Increases risk Increases risk

(continued)

		T/C[f]	ADD/ADDH[g] (PREV)	Increases risk
		T/C[f]	CD[g] (PREV)	Increases risk
32. Offord et al. (1991) (males & females; 4–16 years at T1)	Family dysfunction (GFS)	P,T/C[f] (either)	CD[g] (PREV)	Increases risk
32. Offord et al. (1991) (males & females; 4–16 years at T1)	Domestic violence (physical assault of either parent by the other)	P,T/C[f] (either)	CD[g] (PREV)	Increases risk
33. Offord et al. (1996) (males & females; 6–16 years)	Family dysfunction (GFS)	P	CD (PREV)	Increases risk
		P	OD (PREV)	Increases risk
		T	CD (PREV)	NS
		T	OD (PREV)	NS
		P,T (either)	CD (PREV)	Increases risk
		P,T (either)	OD (PREV)	Increases risk
		P,T (combined)	CD (PREV)	Increases risk
		P,T (combined)	OD (PREV)	Increases risk

Family functioning and behavior

27. Fergusson & Lynskey (1993a) (males & females; 12 years at T14)	Parental marital unhappiness (SQ)	C,T (latent)	ATT/HYP (NUM)	Increases risk [n]
		C,T (latent)	CP/OPP (NUM)	NS [n]
27. Fergusson & Lynskey (1993a) (males & females; 13 years at T15)	Parental marital unhappiness (SQ)	C,T (latent)	ATT/HYP (NUM)	NS [n]
		C,T (latent)	CP/OPP (NUM)	NS [n]
21. Loeber et al. (1998) (white, black, & other males only; grade 2 at T1)	Parental marital discord (DAS)	C,T (sum)	AGG[b] (PREV)[q]	Increases risk
		P	ATT/HYP (PREV)[q]	NS
		C,P,T (sum)	COV (PREV)[q]	NS
		P	CP (PREV)[q]	Increases risk
		C,P,T [o]	DEL (SER)	Increases risk
21. Loeber et al. (1998) (white, black, & other males only; grade 5 at T1)	Parental marital discord (DAS)	C,T (sum)	AGG[b] (PREV)[q]	Increases risk
		P	ATT/HYP (PREV)[q]	Increases risk
		C,P,T (sum)	COV (PREV)[q]	Increases risk
		P	CP (PREV)[q]	Increases risk
		C,P,T [o]	DEL (SER)	NS

TABLE A6. (*Continued*)

Reference[a] (sample characteristics[b])	Definition (measures)	Informant[c] (methods[d])	Diagnosis or behavior (dependent measures[e])	Effect (control variables)
21. Loeber *et al.* (1998) (white, black, & other males only; grade 8 at T1)	Parental marital discord (DAS)	C,T (sum) P C,P,T (sum) P C,P,T ([e])	AGG[b] (PREV)[q] ATT/HYP (PREV)[q] COV (PREV)[q] CP (PREV)[q] DEL (SER)	NS Increases risk NS NS NS
Parenting behavior				
3. Dubow & Ippolito (1994) (white, black, & Hispanic males & females; 5–8 years at T1, 9–12 years at T3)	Cognitive stimulation and emotional support at T1 and T3 (HOME-SF)	P P	CP (NUM) at T1 CP (NUM) at T3	Decreases risk Decreases risk
21. Loeber *et al.* (1998) (white, black, & other males only; grade 5 at T1)	Inconsistent discipline (DS)	C,P,T ([e])	DEL (SER)	NS
21. Loeber *et al.* (1998) (white, black, & other males only; grade 8 at T1)	Inconsistent discipline (DS)	C,P,T ([e])	DEL (SER)	Increases risk
21. Loeber *et al.* (1998) (white, black, & other males only; grade 2 at T1)	Countercontrol (CCS)	C,P,T ([e])	DEL (SER)	NS
21. Loeber *et al.* (1998) (white, black, & other males only; grade 5 at T1)	Countercontrol (CCS)	C,P,T ([e])	DEL (SER)	Increases risk
21. Loeber *et al.* (1998) (white, black, & other males only; grade 8 at T1)	Countercontrol (CCS)	C,P,T ([e])	DEL (SER)	Increases risk

21. Loeber *et al.* (1998) (white, black, & other males only; grade 2 at T1)	Physical punishment (DS)	C,T (sum) P C,P,T (sum) P C,P,T [o]	AGG[b] (PREV)[q] ATT/HYP (PREV)[q] COV (PREV)[q] CP (PREV)[q] DEL (SER)	Increases risk NS Increases risk NS Increases risk
21. Loeber *et al.* (1998) (white, black, & other males only; grade 5 at T1)	Physical punishment (DS)	C,T (sum) P C,P,T (sum) P C,P,T [o]	AGG[b] (PREV)[q] ATT/HYP (PREV)[q] COV (PREV)[q] CP (PREV)[q] DEL (SER)	Increases risk Increases risk Increases risk Increases risk Increases risk
21. Loeber *et al.* (1998) (white, black, & other males only; grade 8 at T1)	Physical punishment (DS)	C,T (sum) P C,P,T (sum) P C,P,T [o]	AGG[b] (PREV)[q] ATT/HYP (PREV)[q] COV (PREV)[q] CP (PREV)[q] DEL (SER)	Increases risk Increases risk NS Increases risk Increases risk
21. Loeber *et al.* (1998) (white, black, & other males only; grade 2 at T1)	Poor supervision (SIS)	C,T (sum) P C,P,T (sum) P C,P,T [o]	AGG[b] (PREV)[q] ATT/HYP (PREV)[q] COV (PREV)[q] CP (PREV)[q] DEL (SER)	Increases risk Increases risk NS Increases risk Increases risk
21. Loeber *et al.* (1998) (white, black, & other males only; grade 5 at T1)	Poor supervision (SIS)	C,T (sum) P C,P,T (sum) P C,P,T [o]	AGG[b] (PREV)[q] ATT/HYP (PREV)[q] COV (PREV)[q] CP (PREV)[q] DEL (SER)	Increases risk Increases risk Increases risk Increases risk Increases risk
21. Loeber *et al.* (1998) (white, black, & other males only; grade 8 at T1)	Poor supervision (SIS)	C,T (sum) P C,P,T (sum) P C,P,T [o]	AGG[b] (PREV)[q] ATT/HYP (PREV)[q] COV (PREV)[q] CP (PREV)[q] DEL (SER)	Increases risk Increases risk Increases risk Increases risk Increases risk
21. Loeber *et al.* (1998) (white, black, & other males only; grade 2 at T1)	Low reinforcement (PPS)	C,T (sum) P C,P,T (sum) P C,P,T [o]	AGG[b] (PREV)[q] ATT/HYP (PREV)[q] COV (PREV)[q] CP (PREV)[q] DEL (SER)	NS NS NS NS NS

(continued)

TABLE A6. (*Continued*)

Reference[a] (sample characteristics[b])	Definition (measures)	Informant[c] (methods[d])	Diagnosis or behavior (dependent measures[e])	Effect (control variables)
21. Loeber *et al.* (1998) (white, black, & other males only; grade 5 at T1)	Low reinforcement (PPS)	C,T (sum) P C,P,T (sum) P C,P,T ([e])	AGG[f] (PREV)[q] ATT/HYP (PREV)[q] COV (PREV)[q] CP (PREV)[q] DEL (SER)	Increases risk Increases risk Increases risk Increases risk NS
21. Loeber *et al.* (1998) (white, black, & other males only; grade 8 at T1)	Low reinforcement (PPS)	C,T (sum) P C,P,T (sum) P C,P,T ([e])	AGG[f] (PREV)[q] ATT/HYP (PREV)[q] COV (PREV)[q] CP (PREV)[q] DEL (SER)	Increases risk Increases risk Increases risk Increases risk NS
21. Loeber *et al.* (1998) (white, black, & other males only; grade 5 at T1)	Poor communication (RPACF)	C,T (sum) P C,P,T (sum) P C,P,T ([e])	AGG[f] (PREV)[q] ATT/HYP (PREV)[q] COV (PREV)[q] CP (PREV)[q] DEL (SER)	Increases risk Increases risk Increases risk Increases risk Increases risk
21. Loeber *et al.* (1998) (white, black, & other males only; grade 8 at T1)	Poor communication (RPACF)	C,T (sum) P C,P,T (sum) P C,P,T ([e])	AGG[f] (PREV)[q] ATT/HYP (PREV)[q] COV (PREV)[q] CP (PREV)[q] DEL (SER)	Increases risk Increases risk Increases risk Increases risk Increases risk
3. Luster & McAdoo (1994) (black males & females; 6–9 years at T1)	Cognitive stimulation and emotional support (HOME-SF)	P	CP (NUM)	Decreases risk
11. Wichstrøm *et al.* (1996) (Norway sample; males & females; 13–19 years)	Overprotection (PBI)	C	CP (PREV)[v]	NS
11. Wichstrøm *et al.* (1996) (Norway sample; males & females; 13–19 years)	Lack of care (PBI)	C	CP (PREV)[v]	NS

Abbreviations: ADD = Attention-Deficit Disorder; ADDH = Attention-Deficit Disorder with Hyperactivity; ADHD = Attention-Deficit/Hyperactivity Disorder; AGG = aggressive behavior; ATT = attention problems; CCS = Countercontrol Scale; CD = Conduct Disorder; COV = covert antisocial behavior; CP = conduct problems; DAS = Dyadic Adjustment Scale; DEL = delinquent behavior; DS = Discipline Scale; ED = Emotional Disorder; FHQ = Family Health Questionnaire; GFS = General Functioning subscale of McMaster Family Functioning Assessment Device; HOME-SF = Home Observation for Measurement of the Environment—Short Form; HYP = hyperactive behavior; LPDI = Levine–Pilowsky Depression Inventory; NS = nonsignificant results; OD = Oppositional Disorder; ODD = Oppositional Defiant Disorder; OPP = oppositional behavior; PBI = Parental Bonding Instrument; PI = psychiatric interview; PPS = Positive Parenting Scale; RPACF = Revised Parent–Adolescent Communication Form; SI = structured interview; SIS = Supervision/Involvement Scale; SQ = structured questionnaire.

[a]Number indicates the study on which the cited publication is based. Refer to Tables A1 and A2 for numbered list of studies.

[b]Where not otherwise indicated, racial or ethnic composition of the sample was not reported. "White" = non-Hispanic white.

[c]C = child, P = parent, T = teacher.

[d]Method of combination of data from multiple informants. "Either" = diagnosis-level combination; diagnoses were made if any informant endorsed the full set of diagnostic criteria. "Combined" = symptom-level combination; diagnoses were made if the full set of diagnostic criteria was endorsed by any informant, alone or in combination with other informants. "Latent" = latent class estimate. "Clinical" = clinical combination. "Sum" = number of symptoms or behaviors endorsed were summed across informants.

[e]PREV = prevalence. NUM = number of symptoms or behaviors endorsed. SER = seriousness of behavior.

[f]Teacher for children aged 4–11, child for children aged 12–16.

[g]Diagnosis included ad hoc impairment criterion.

[h]Three separate sets of path analyses were conducted on composite scores for participants who had (1) CBCL and TRF scores, (2) CBCL and YSR scores, and (3) CBCL, TRF, and YSR scores. Results indicate which variables were significant direct predictors in two or more sets of analyses.

[i]Measure included items assessing alcohol and drug use.

[j]Multivariate analyses included SES, poverty, family size, family structure, changes in family structure, family mental health service use, stressful life events, and other 1. Achenbach syndrome scores.

[k]Analyses were performed separately for males and females. Results were the same for each gender.

[l]Multivariate analyses included age, gender, racial/ethnic background, family structure, income, neighborhood type, neighborhood stability, and neighborhood quality.

[m]Results were generally the same for subsamples based on age, gender, race, ethnicity, number of siblings, maternal education, maternal employment, and family income.

[n]Multivariate analyses included family social position, standard of living, changes in family structure, parental marital unhappiness, current maternal depression, and maternal history of depression.

[o]Participants were classified according to the severity of the most serious act ever committed reported by any informant.

[p]Lifetime aggression.

[q]Prevalence threshold = 75th percentile.

[r]Nature of effect was not specified.

[s]Multivariate analyses included gender, family structure, family size, maternal age, maternal education, SES, and urbanization.

[t]Separate analyses were performed for maternal and paternal emotional problems. Results were also nonsignificant.

[u]"Behavior problems" was not defined

[v]Prevalence threshold = three or more behaviors endorsed.

TABLE A7. Selected Socioeconomic and Residential Correlates of Disruptive Behavior Disorders

Reference[a] (sample characteristics)[b]	Definition (measures)	Informant[c] (methods)[d]	Diagnosis or behavior (dependent measures)[e]	Effect (control variables)
Family income and diagnoses				
15. Costello et al. (1996) (white & black males & females; 9, 11, 13 years at T1)	Poverty (income below federal poverty line)	P C,P (combined) C,P (combined)	ADHD (PREV) CD (PREV) ODD (PREV)	Increases risk Increases risk Increases risk
32. Offord et al. (1986) (males & females; 4–16 years at T1)	Low income (SCLIC)	P,T/C[f] (either)	CD[g] (PREV)	Increases risk
32. Offord et al. (1986) (males & females; 4–16 years at T1)	Poverty (receipt of public assistance)	P,T/C[f] (either)	CD[g] (PREV)	Increases risk
32. Offord et al. (1986) (males & females; 4–16 years at T1)	Poverty (residence in subsidized housing)	P,T/C[f] (either)	CD[g] (PREV)	Increases risk
32. Offord, Boyle, & Racine (1989) (males & females; 4–16 years at T1)	Low income (less than $10,000 annually)	P P T/C[f] T/C[f]	ADD/ADDH[g] (PREV) CD[g] (PREV) ADD/ADDH[g] (PREV) CD[g] (PREV)	NS NS Increases risk Increases risk; effect stronger at older ages
33. Offord et al. (1996) (males & females; 6–16 years)	Low income (less than $15,000 annually)	P P T T P,T (either) P,T (either) P,T (combined)	CD (PREV) OD (PREV) CD (PREV) CD (PREV) CD (PREV) OD (PREV) CD (PREV)	NS Increases risk NS Increases risk Increases risk Increases risk Increase risk
19. Velez et al. (1989) (white & nonwhite males & females; 1–10 years at T1, 9–18 years at T2)	Low income at T1 (> 1 SD below sample mean annual income)	C,P (combined) C,P (combined) C,P (combined)	ADHD at T2 (PREV) CD at T2 (PREV) ODD at T2 (PREV)	Increases risk (age, gender) Increases risk (age, gender) Increases risk (age, gender)

Study	Variable	C,P	Outcome	Result
19. Velez *et al.* (1989) (white & nonwhite males & females; 9–18 years at T2, 11–10 years at T3)	Low income at T2 (> 1 *SD* below sample mean annual income)	C,P (combined) — C,P (combined) — C,P (combined)	ADHD at T3 (PREV) — CD at T3 (PREV) — ODD at T3 (PREV)	Increases risk (age, gender) — Increases risk (age, gender) — Increases risk (age, gender)

Family income and behavior

Study	Variable	C,P	Outcome	Result
1. Achenbach *et al.* (1995) (white, black, Hispanic, & other males & females; 4–16 years at T1, 9–18 years at T3)	Poverty at T1 (number of types of public assistance received)	C,P,T [b] — C,P,T [b] — C,P,T [b]	AGG at T3 (NUM) — ATT at T3 (NUM) — DEL[i] at T3 (NUM)	NS [j]k — NS [j]k — NS [j]k
1. Achenbach *et al.* (1995) (white, black, Hispanic, & other males & females; 7–19 years at T2, 9–18 years at T3)	Poverty at T2 (number of types of public assistance received)	C,P,T [b] — C,P,T [b] — C,P,T [b]	AGG at T3 (NUM) — ATT at T3 (NUM) — DEL[i] at T3 (NUM)	NS [j]k — NS [j]k — NS [j]k
1. Achenbach *et al.* (1995) (white, black, Hispanic, & other males & females; 9–18 years at T3)	Poverty at T3 (number of types of public assistance received)	C,P,T [b] — C,P,T [b] — C,P,T [b]	AGG at T3 (NUM) — ATT at T3 (NUM) — DEL[i] at T3 (NUM)	NS [j]k — NS [j]k — NS [j]k
16. Aneshensel & Sucoff (1996) (white, black, Hispanic, Asian, & other males & females; 12–17 years)	Income (annual)	C — C	CP (NUM) — OPP (NUM)	NS [l] — Inverse relationship [l]
3. Dubow & Ippolito (1994) (males & females; 5–8 years at T1, 9–12 years at T3)	Prior poverty (number of years prior to T1 income was below federal poverty line or received public assistance)	P — P	CP (NUM) at T1 — CP (NUM) at T3	Increases risk — Increases risk
3. Dubow & Ippolito (1994) (males & females; 5–8 years at T1, 9–12 years at T3)	Recent poverty (number of years from T1 to T3 income was below federal poverty line or received public assistance)	P — P	CP (NUM) at T1 — CP (NUM) at T3	Increases risk — Increases risk

(*continued*)

Reference (sample characteristics[b])	Definition (measures)	Informant[c] (methods[d])	Diagnosis or behavior (dependent measures[e])	Effect (control variables)
21. Loeber *et al.* (1998) (white, black, & other males only; grade 2 at T1)	Poverty (receipt of public assistance in year prior to assessment)	C,T (sum) / P	AGG[n] (PREV[o]) / ATT/HYP (PREV[o])	Increases risk / Increases risk
		C,P,T (sum) / P	COV (PREV[o]) / CP (PREV[o])	Increases risk / Increases risk
		C,P,T (m)	DEL (SER)	Increases risk
21. Loeber *et al.* (1998) (white, black, & other males only; grade 5 at T1)	Poverty (receipt of public assistance in year prior to assessment)	C,T (sum) / P	AGG[n] (PREV[o]) / ATT/HYP (PREV[o])	NS / NS
		C,P,T (sum) / P	COV (PREV[o]) / CP (PREV[o])	Increases risk / Increases risk
		C,P,T (m)	DEL (SER)	Increases risk
21. Loeber *et al.* (1998) (white, black, & other males only; grade 8 at T1)	Poverty (receipt of public assistance in year prior to assessment)	C,T (sum) / P	AGG[n] (PREV[o]) / ATT/HYP (PREV[o])	Increases risk / NS
		C,P,T (sum) / P	COV (PREV[o]) / CP (PREV[o])	Increases risk / Increases risk
		C,P,T (m)	DEL (SER)	Increases risk
3. Luster & McAdoo (1994) (black males & females 6–9 years at T1)	Income (annual)	P	CP (NUM)	Inverse relationship
3. Luster & McAdoo (1994) (black males & females; 6–9 years at T1)	Poverty (income below federal poverty line)	P	CP (NUM)	Increases risk
1. Stanger *et al.* (1992) (white, black, Hispanic, & other males & females; 4–16 years at T1, 7–19 years at T2)	Poverty at T1 (number of types of public assistance received)	C	AGG at T2 (NUM)	NS[f]
		C	ATT at T2 (NUM)	NS[f]
		C	DEL[i] at T2 (NUM)	NS[f]
		P	AGG at T2 (NUM)	NS[f]
		P	ATT at T2 (NUM)	NS[f]
		P	DEL[i] at T2 (NUM)	NS[f]
		T	AGG at T2 (NUM)	NS[f]

Study	Predictor	Outcome	Source	Result
1. Stanger et al. (1992) (white, black, Hispanic, & other males & females; 7–19 years at T2)		ATT at T2 (NUM)	T	NS[j]
		DEL at T2 (NUM)	T	NS[j]
	Poverty at T2 (number of types of public assistance received)	AGG at T2 (NUM)	C	NS[j]
		ATT at T2 (NUM)	C	NS[j]
		DEL[i] at T2 (NUM)	C	NS[j]
		AGG at T2 (NUM)	P	NS[j]
		ATT at T2 (NUM)	P	NS[j]
		DEL[i] at T2 (NUM)	P	NS[j]
		AGG at T2 (NUM)	T	NS[j]
		ATT at T2 (NUM)	T	NS[j]
		DEL[i] at T2 (NUM)	T	NS[j]
11. Wichstrøm et al. (1996) (Norway sample; males & females; 13–19 years)	Poverty (receipt of social aid)	CP (PREV)[b]	C	NS

Parental education and diagnoses

Study	Predictor	Outcome	Source	Result
32. Offord et al. (1986) (males & females; 4–16 years at T1)	Low maternal education (less than 8th grade)	CD[g] (PREV)	P,T/C[f] (either)	Increases risk
19. Velez et al. (1989) (white & nonwhite males & females; 1–10 years at T1, 9–18 years at T2)	Low maternal education at T1 (years completed; >1 SD below sample mean)	ADHD at T2 (PREV)	C,P (combined)	Increases risk (age, gender)
		CD at T2 (PREV)	C,P (combined)	Increases risk (age, gender)
		ODD at T2 (PREV)	C,P (combined)	Increases risk (age, gender)
19. Velez et al. (1989) (white & nonwhite males & females; 9–18 years at T2, 11–20 years at T2)	Low maternal education at T2 (years completed; >1 SD below sample mean)	ADHD at T3 (PREV)	C,P (combined)	Increases risk (age, gender)
		CD at T3 (PREV)	C,P (combined)	NS (age, gender)
		ODD at T3 (PREV)	C,P (combined)	Increases risk (age, gender)
19. Velez et al. (1989) (white & nonwhite males & females; 1–10 years at T1, 9–18 years at T2)	Low paternal education at T1 (years completed; >1 SD below sample mean)	ADHD at T2 (PREV)	C,P (combined)	Increases risk (age, gender)
		CD at T2 (PREV)	C,P (combined)	NS (age, gender)
		ODD at T2 (PREV)	C,P (combined)	NS (age, gender)

(continued)

TABLE A7. (Continued)

Reference[a] (sample characteristics[b])	Definition (measures)	Informant[c] (methods[d])	Diagnosis or behavior (dependent measures[e])	Effect (control variables)
19. Velez et al. (1989) (white & nonwhite males & females; 9–18 years at T2, 11–20 years at T3)	Low paternal education at T2 (years completed; >1 SD below sample mean)	C,P (combined) C,P (combined) C,P (combined)	ADHD at T3 (PREV) CD at T3 (PREV) ODD at T3 (PREV)	NS (age, gender) Increases risk (age, gender) Increases risk (age, gender)
Parental education and behavior				
27. Fergusson & Lynskey (1993b) (Pakeha, Maori, & Pacific Island males & females; 8 years at T10)	Maternal education at child's birth (highest degree obtained)	P,T (sum)	CP/OPP (NUM)	Inverse relationship
27. Fergusson & Lynskey (1993b) (Pakeha, Maori, & Pacific Island males & females; 10 years at T12)	Maternal education at child's birth (highest degree obtained)	P,T (sum)	CP/OPP (NUM)	Inverse relationship
27. Fergusson & Lynskey (1993b) (Pakeha, Maori, & Pacific Island males & females; 12 years at T14)	Maternal education at child's birth (highest degree obtained)	P,T (sum)	CP/OPP (NUM)	Inverse relationship
21. Loeber et al. (1998) (white, black, & other males only; grade 2 at T1)	Low maternal education (less than 12th grade)	C,T (sum) P C,P,T (sum) P C,P,T [m]	AGG[n] (PREV)[o] ATT/HYP (PREV)[o] COV (PREV)[o] CP (PREV)[o] DEL (SER)	NS NS NS Increases risk Increases risk
21. Loeber et al. (1998) (white, black, & other males only; grade 5 at T1)	Low maternal education (less than 12th grade)	C,T (sum) P C,P,T (sum) P C,P,T [m]	AGG[n] (PREV)[o] ATT/HYP (PREV)[o] COV (PREV)[o] CP (PREV)[o] DEL (SER)	NS NS Increases risk NS NS

Study	Variable	Method	Outcome	Result
21. Loeber *et al.* (1998) (white, black, & other males only; grade 8 at T1)	Low maternal education (less than 12th grade)	C,T (sum); P; C,P,T (sum); C,P,T [m]	AGG[n] (PREV); ATT/HYP (PREV)[o]; COV (PREV)[o]; CP (PREV)[o]; DEL (SER)	NS; NS; Increases risk; Increases risk; Increases risk
3. Luster & McAdoo (1994) (black males & females; 6–9 years at T1)	Maternal education (years completed)	P	CP (NUM)	Inverse relationship
2. McDermott (1996) (white, black, Hispanic, & other males & females; 15–17 years)	Parental education (years completed)	T; T; T; T	ATT/HYP (PREV)[q]; SOL AGG/PRO (PREV)[q]; SOL AGG/IMP (PREV)[q]; OPP (PREV)[q]	NS[r]; NS[r]; NS[r]; NS[r]
8. Osborn *et al.* (1984) (white, black, Asian, & other males & females; 5 years at T2)	Maternal education (highest degree obtained)	P	CP (NUM)	Inverse relationship[p]

Parental occupation and diagnoses

Study	Variable	Method	Outcome	Result
30b. Graham & Rutter (1973) (males & females; 14–15 years at T2)	Manual paternal employment	C,P,T (clinical); C,P,T (clinical)	CD[g] (PREV); CD/ED[g] (PREV)	NS; NS
32. Offord *et al.* (1986) (males & females; 4–16 years)	Parental unemployment	P,T/C[f] (either)	CD[g] (PREV)	Increases risk
30a. Rutter *et al.* (1970) (males & females; 10–11 years at T1)	Parental occupational status (RGCO)	C,P,T (clinical)	CD[g,t]	NS

Parental occupation and behavior

Study	Variable	Method	Outcome	Result
1. Achenbach *et al.* (1991) (white, black, Hispanic, & other; 4–16 years at T1)	Parental occupational status (Hollingshead Index)	P; P; P	AGG (NUM); ATT (NUM); DEL[i] (NUM)	Inverse relationship[p]; Inverse relationship[p]; Inverse relationship[p]
1. Achenbach *et al.* (1995) (males & females; 4–16 years at T1, 7–19 years at T2, 9–18 years at T3)	Parental occupational status at T1	C,P,T [b]; C,P,T [b]; C,P,T [b]	AGG at T3 (NUM); ATT at T3 (NUM); DEL[i] at T3 (NUM)	NS[j,k]; NS[j,k]; NS[j,k]

(continued)

TABLE A7. *(Continued)*

Reference[a] (sample characteristics[b])	Definition (measures)	Informant[c] (methods[d])	Diagnosis or behavior (dependent measures[e])	Effect (control variables)
	(Hollingshead Index)			
9. Davie *et al.* (1972) (males & females; 7 years at T2)	Paternal occupational status (RGCO, middle-class vs. working-class)	P P T	AGG (NUM) HYP (NUM) HYP (NUM)	Middle < working NS Middle < working
27. Fergusson & Lynskey (1993b) (Pakeha, Maori, & Pacific Island males & females; 8 years at T10)	Parental occupational status at time of child's birth (EII)	P,T (sum)	CP/OPP (NUM)	Inverse relationship
27. Fergusson & Lynskey (1993b) (Pakeha, Maori, & Pacific Island males & females; 10 years at T12)	Parental occupational status at time of child's birth (EII)	P,T (sum)	CP/OPP (NUM)	Inverse relationship
27. Fergusson & Lynskey (1993b) (Pakeha, Maori, & Pacific Island males & females; 12 years at T14)	Parental occupational status at time of child's birth (EII)	P,T (sum)	CP/OPP (NUM)	Inverse relationship
21. Loeber *et al.* (1998) (white, black, & other males only; grade 2 at T1)	Maternal unemployment (number of weeks in year prior to assessment)	C,T (sum) P C,P,T (sum) P C,P,T (*m*)	AGG[n] (PREV)[o] ATT/HYP (PREV)[o] COV (PREV)[o] CP (PREV)[o] DEL (SER)	NS NS Increases with weeks of unemployment Increases with weeks of unemployment NS
21. Loeber *et al.* (1998) (white, black, & other males only; grade 5 at T1)	Maternal unemployment (number of weeks in year prior to assessment)	C,T (sum) P C,P,T (sum) P C,P,T (*m*)	AGG[n] (PREV)[o] ATT/HYP (PREV)[o] COV (PREV)[o] CP (PREV)[o] DEL (SER)	NS NS NS NS Increases with weeks of unemployment

Study	Variable	Measure	Outcome	Result
21. Loeber et al. (1998) (white, black, & other males only; grade 8 at T1)	Maternal unemployment (number of weeks in year prior to assessment)	C,T (sum)	AGG[n] (PREV)[o]	Increases with weeks of unemployment
		P	ATT/HYP (PREV)[o]	NS
		C,P,T (sum)	COV (PREV)[o]	NS
		P	CP (PREV)[o]	NS
		C,P,T ([m])	DEL (SER)	NS
21. Loeber et al. (1998) (white, black, & other males only; grade 2 at T1)	Paternal unemployment (number of weeks in year prior to assessment)	C,T (sum)	AGG[n] (PREV)[o]	NS
		P	ATT/HYP (PREV)[o]	NS
		C,P,T (sum)	COV (PREV)[o]	NS
		P	CP (PREV)[o]	Increases with weeks of unemployment
		C,P,T ([m])	DEL (SER)	Increases with weeks of unemployment
21. Loeber et al. (1998) (white, black, & other males only; grade 5 at T1)	Paternal unemployment (number of weeks in year prior to assessment)	C,T (sum)	AGG[n] (PREV)[o]	NS
		P	ATT/HYP (PREV)[o]	NS
		C,P,T (sum)	COV (PREV)[o]	NS
		P	CP (PREV)[o]	NS
		C,P,T ([m])	DEL (SER)	Increases with weeks of unemployment
21. Loeber et al. (1998) (white, black, & other males only; grade 8 at T1)	Paternal unemployment (number of weeks in year prior to assessment)	C,T (sum)	AGG[n] (PREV)[o]	NS
		P	ATT/HYP (PREV)[o]	NS
		C,P,T (sum)	COV (PREV)[o]	NS
		P	CP (PREV)[o]	NS
		C,P,T ([m])	DEL (SER)	NS
28. Silva et al. (1982) (white, Maori, & other Polynesian males & females; 4 years at T3)	Parental occupational status (EII)	P	CP (NUM)	NS
		P	ATT/HYP (NUM)	Inverse relationship
		T	CP (NUM)	Inverse relationship
		T	ATT/HYP (NUM)	Inverse relationship
1. Stanger et al. (1992) (white, black, Hispanic, & other males & females; 4–16 years at T1, 7–19 years at T2)	Parental occupational status at T1 (Hollingshead Index)	C	AGG at T2 (NUM)	NS [f]
		C	ATT at T2 (NUM)	NS [f]
		C	DEL[i] at T2 (NUM)	NS [f]
		P	AGG at T2 (NUM)	NS [f]
		P	ATT at T2 (NUM)	NS [f]
		P	DEL[i] at T2 (NUM)	NS [f]
		T	AGG at T2 (NUM)	NS [f]
		T	ATT at T2 (NUM)	NS [f]
		T	DEL[i] at T2 (NUM)	NS [f]
11. Wichstrøm et al. (1996) (Norway sample; males & females; 13–19 years)	Parental occupational status (ISCO-88)	C	CP (PREV)[g]	NS

(continued)

TABLE A7. (*Continued*)

Reference[a] (sample characteristics[b])	Definition (measures)	Informant[c] (methods[d])	Diagnosis or behavior (dependent measures[e])	Effect (control variables)
		SES composite indices and diagnoses		
22. Bird *et al.* (1989) (Hispanic males & females; 4–16 years)	Parental education and occupational status (Hollingshead Index, upper vs. middle vs. lower)	C,P (combined) C,P (combined)	ADD/ADDH (PREV) OD (PREV)	Upper < middle = lower (age, gender) Upper = middle < lower (age, gender)
19. Velez *et al.* (1989) (white & nonwhite males & females; 1–10 years at T1, 11–20 years at T3)	Low SES at T1 (parental income and parental education > 1 *SD* below sample means)	C,P (combined) C,P (combined) C,P (combined)	ADHD at T3 (PREV) CD at T3 (PREV) ODD at T3 (PREV)	Increases risk (age, gender) Increases risk (age, gender) Increases risk (age, gender)
19. Velez *et al.* (1989) (white & nonwhite males & females; 9–18 years at T2, 11–20 years at T3)	Low SES at T2 (parental income and parental education > 1 *SD* below sample means)	C,P (combined) C,P (combined) C,P (combined)	ADHD at T3 (PREV) CD at T3 (PREV) ODD at T3 (PREV)	Increases risk (age, gender) Increases risk (age, gender) Increases risk (age, gender)
		SES composite indices and behavior		
7. Ageton (1983) (black & white females only; 11–17 years at T1, 12–18 years at T2, 13–19 years at T3, 14–20 years at T4, 15–21 years at T5)	Parental education and occupational status (Hollingshead Index, middle vs. working vs. lower)	C	DEL (PREV)[u]	NS[v]
8. Butler & Golding (1986) (white, black, Asian, & other males & females; 5 years at T2)	Paternal employment status, paternal occupational status (OPCS. nonmanual vs. manual)	P P	CP (NUM) HYP (NUM)	Nonmanual < manual Nonmanual < manual

7. Elliott & Huizinga (1983) (white, black, Hispanic, & other males only, 11–17 years at T1)	Parental education and occupational status (Hollingshead Index, middle vs. working vs. lower)	C	DEL (PREV)[a]	NS
7. Elliott & Huizinga (1983) (white, black, Hispanic, & other males only, 12–18 years at T2)	Parental education and occupational status (Hollingshead Index, middle vs. working vs. lower)	C	DEL (PREV)[a]	NS
7. Elliott & Huizinga (1983) (white, black, Hispanic, & other males only, 13–19 years at T3)	Parental education and occupational status (Hollingshead Index, middle vs. working vs. lower)	C	DEL (PREV)[a]	Middle < working
7. Elliott & Huizinga (1983) (white, black, Hispanic, & other males only, 14–20 years at T4)	Parental education and occupational status (Hollingshead Index, middle vs. working vs. lower)	C	DEL (PREV)[a]	Middle < working
7. Elliott & Huizinga (1983) (white, black, Hispanic, & other males only, 15–21 years at T5)	Parental education and occupational status (Hollingshead Index, middle vs. working vs. lower)	C	DEL (PREV)[a]	NS
7. Elliott & Huizinga (1983) (white, black, Hispanic, & other females, only, 11–17 years at T1, 12–18 years at T2, 13–19 years at T3,	Parental education and occupational status (Hollingshead Index, middle vs. working vs. lower)	C	DEL (PREV)[a]	NS

(continued)

679

TABLE A7. *(Continued)*

Reference[a] (sample characteristics[b])	Definition (measures)	Informant[c] (methods[d])	Diagnosis or behavior (dependent measures[e])	Effect (control variables)
14–20 years at T4, 15–21 years at T5				
23. Havighurst *et al.* (1962) (males & females, grade 9 at T4)	Family income, parental education and occupational status (ISC)	T, peers (mean)	AGG (NUM)	NS
21. Loeber *et al.* (1998) (white, black, & other males only; grade 2 at T1)	Low parental education and occupational status (Hollingshead Index)	C,T (sum) P C,P,T (sum) P C,P,T[m]	AGG[n] (PREV)[o] ATT/HYP (PREV)[o] COV (PREV)[o] CP (PREV)[o] DEL (SER)	Increases risk NS NS NS Increases risk
21. Loeber *et al.* (1998) (white, black, & other males only; grade 5 at T1)	Low parental education and occupational status (Hollingshead Index)	C,T (sum) P C,P,T (sum) P C,P,T[m]	AGG[n] (PREV)[o] ATT/HYP (PREV)[o] COV (PREV)[o] CP (PREV)[o] DEL (SER)	Increases risk Increases risk Increases risk Increases risk Increases risk
21. Loeber *et al.* (1998) (white, black, & other males only; grade 8 at T1)	Low parental education and occupational status (Hollingshead Index)	C,T (sum) P C,P,T (sum) P C,P,T[m]	AGG[n] (PREV)[o] ATT/HYP (PREV)[o] COV (PREV)[o] CP (PREV)[o] DEL (SER)	NS NS Increases risk Increases risk Increases risk
8. Osborn *et al.* (1984) (white, black, Asian, & other males & females; 5 years at T2)	Paternal occupational status (OPCS), parental education, urbanization, housing, car ownership	C,P,T[m] P	CP (NUM)	Decreases with increasing SES[i]

Neighborhood characteristics and behavior

16. Aneshensel & Sucoff (1996) (white, black, Hispanic, Asian, & other males & females; 12–17 years)	Ambient hazards (SQ; child's perceptions of safety, crime, cleanliness, etc.)	C C	CP (NUM) OPP (NUM)	Increases with hazards [f] Increases with hazards [f]
7. Elliott et al. (1983) (white, black, Hispanic, & other males & females, 11–17 years at T1)	Neighborhood crime (SQ; parental perceptions)	C	DEL (PREV)[a]	NS
7. Elliott et al. (1983) (white, black, Hispanic, & other males & females, 15–21 years at T5)	Neighborhood crime (SQ; parental perceptions)	C	DEL (PREV)[a]	Increases with crime
21. Loeber et al. (1998) (white, black, & other males only; grade 2 at T1)	Social disadvantage (census data regarding neighborhood characteristics including ethnic composition, rates of poverty, unemployment, single-mother households, out-of-wedlock births, and use of public assistance)	C,T (sum) P C,P,T (sum) P C,P,T [m]	AGG[n] (PREV)[o] ATT/HYP (PREV)[o] COV (PREV)[o] CP (PREV)[o] DEL (SER)	NS NS NS Increases risk Increases risk
21. Loeber et al. (1998) (white, black, & other males only; grade 5 at T1)	Social disadvantage (census data regarding neighborhood characteristics including ethnic composition, rates of poverty, unemployment,	C,T (sum) P C,P,T (sum) P C,P,T [m]	AGG[n] (PREV)[o] ATT/HYP (PREV)[o] COV (PREV)[o] CP (PREV)[o] DEL (SER)	NS NS NS NS Increases risk

(continued)

TABLE A7. *(Continued)*

Reference (sample characteristics[b])	Definition (measures)	Informant[c] (methods[d])	Diagnosis or behavior (dependent measures[e])	Effect (control variables[f])
	single-mother households, out-of-wedlock births, and use of public assistance)			
21. Loeber *et al.* (1998) (white, black, & other males only; grade 8 at T1)	Social disadvantage (census data regarding neighborhood characteristics including ethnic composition, rates of poverty, unemployment, single-mother households, out-of-wedlock births, and use of public assistance)	C,T (sum) P C,P,T (sum) P C,P,T [m]	AGG[n] (PREV)[g] ATT/HYP (PREV)[g] COV (PREV)[g] CP (PREV)[g] DEL (SER)	NS NS NS NS Increases risk
21. Loeber *et al.* (1998) (white, black, & other males only; grade 2 at T1)	Social disadvantage (SQ; parental perceptions of quality of housing, rates of unemployment and crime, safety, etc.)	C,T (sum) P C,P,T (sum) P C,P,T [m]	AGG[n] (PREV)[g] ATT/HYP (PREV)[g] COV (PREV)[g] CP (PREV)[g] DEL (SER)	Increases risk NS NS Increases risk Increases risk
21. Loeber *et al.* (1998) (white, black, & other males only; grade 5 at T1)	Social disadvantage (SQ; parental perceptions of quality of housing,	C,T (sum) P C,P,T (sum) P	AGG[n] (PREV)[g] ATT/HYP (PREV)[g] COV (PREV)[g] CP (PREV)[g]	NS NS Increases risk NS

	rates of unemployment and crime, safety, etc.)	C,P,T [m]	DEL (SER)	Increases risk
21. Loeber et al. (1998) (white, black, & other males only; grade 8 at T1)	Social disadvantage (SQ; parental perceptions of quality of housing, rates of unemployment and crime, safety, etc.)	C,T (sum) P C,P,T (sum) P C,P,T [m]	AGG[n] (PREV)[o] ATT/HYP (PREV)[o] COV (PREV)[o] CP (PREV)[o] DEL (SER)	Increases risk Increases risk Increases risk Increases risk Increases risk

Urbanization and diagnoses

15. Costello et al. (1996) (white & black males & females; 9, 11, 13 years at T1)	Population of geographical area of residence (urban vs. rural)	P C,P (combined) C,P (combined)	ADHD (PREV) CD (PREV) ODD (PREV)	NS (poverty) NS (poverty) NS (poverty)
32. Offord et al. (1987) (males & females; 4–16 years at T1)	Population of geographical area of residence (urban vs. rural)	P,T/C[f] (either) P,T/C[f] (either)	ADD/ADDH[g] (PREV) CD[g] (PREV)	Rural < urban NS
32. Offord, Boyle, & Racine (1989) (males & females; 4–16 years at T1)	Population of geographical area of residence (urban vs. rural)	P P T/C[f] T/C[f]	ADD/ADDH[g] (PREV) CD[g] (PREV) ADD/ADDH[g] (PREV) CD[g] (PREV)	NS NS NS NS
30c. Rutter et al. (1975) (males & females; 10 years)	Population of geographical area of residence (Inner London borough vs. Isle of Wight)	P	CD[g] (PREV)	Isle of Wight < Inner London

Urbanization and behavior

7. Ageton (1983) (black & white females only; 11–17 years at T1)	Population of geographical area of residence (urban vs. suburban vs. rural)	C	DEL (PREV)[u]	NS

(continued)

TABLE A7. *(Continued)*

Reference[a] (sample characteristics[b])	Definition (measures)	Informant[c] (methods[d])	Diagnosis or behavior (dependent measures[e])	Effect (control variables)
7. Ageton (1983) (black & white females only; 12–18 years at T2)	Population of geographical area of residence (urban vs. suburban vs. rural)	C	DEL (PREV)[u]	Rural < suburban = urban
7. Ageton (1983) (black & white females only; 13–19 years at T3)	Population of geographical area of residence (urban vs. suburban vs. rural)	C	DEL (PREV)[u]	NS
7. Ageton (1983) (black & white females only; 14–20 years at T4)	Population of geographical area of residence (urban vs. suburban vs. rural)	C	DEL (PREV)[u]	NS
7. Ageton (1983) (black & white females only; 15–21 years at T5)	Population of geographical area of residence (urban vs. suburban vs. rural)	C	DEL (PREV)[u]	Rural < suburban = urban
3. Luster & McAdoo (1994) (black males & females; 6–9 years at T1)	Population of geographical area of residence (urban vs. other)	P	CP (NUM)	NS
8. Osborn et al. (1984) (white, black, Asian, & other males & females; 5 years at T2)	Population of geographical area of residence (urban vs. rural)	P	CP (NUM)	Rural < urban (f)
11. Wichstrøm et al. (1996) (Norway sample; males & females;	Population of geographical area of	C	CP (PREV)[p]	Increases with population size

684

Study	Predictor	Behavior	Informant	Result
13–19 years)	residence (population size)			NS
14. Zahner *et al.* (1993) (white, black, Hispanic, & other males only; 6–11 years)	Population of geographical area of residence (urban vs. suburban vs. rural)	DEL[i] (PREV)[w]	P	NS
		AGG (PREV)[w]	P	NS
		HYP (PREV)[w]	P	NS
		AGG (PREV)[w]	T	NS
		ATT (PREV)[w]	T	NS
		HYP (PREV)[w]	T	NS
14. Zahner *et al.* (1993) (white, black, Hispanic, & other females only; 6–11 years)	Population of geographical area of residence (urban vs. suburban vs. rural)	DEL[i] (PREV)[w]	P	Rural/suburban < urban
		AGG (PREV)[w]	P	Rural/suburban < urban
		HYP (PREV)[w]	P	NS
		AGG (PREV)[w]	T	NS
		ATT (PREV)[w]	T	NS
		HYP (PREV)[g]	T	NS

Abbreviations: ADD = Attention-Deficit Disorder; ADDH = Attention-Deficit Disorder with Hyperactivity; ADHD = Attention-Deficit/Hyperactivity Disorder; AGG = aggressive behavior; ATT = attention problems; CD = Conduct Disorder; COV = covert antisocial behavior; CP = conduct problems; DEL = delinquent behavior; ED = Emotional Disorder; EII = Elley & Irving Index; HYP = hyperactive behavior; ISC = Index of Status Characteristics; ISCO-88 = International Standard Classification of Occupations; NS = nonsignificant results; OD = Oppositional Disorder; ODD = Oppositional Defiant Disorder; OPCS = Office of Population Censuses and Surveys' Social Class classification; OPP = oppositional behavior; RGCO = Registrar-General's Classification of Occupations; SCLIC = Statistics Canada's Low Income Cutoffs; SD = standard deviation; SES = socioeconomic status; SOL AGG/IMP = solitary aggressive–impulsive behavior; SOL AGG/PRO = solitary aggressive–provocative behavior; SQ = structured questionnaire.

[a]Number indicates the study on which the cited publication is based. Refer to Tables A1 and A2 for numbered list of studies.
[b]Where not otherwise indicated, racial or ethnic composition of the sample was not reported. "White" = non-Hispanic white.
[c]C = child, P = parent, T = teacher.
[d]Method of combination of data from multiple informants. "Either" = diagnosis-level combination; diagnoses were made if any informant endorsed the full set of diagnostic criteria. "Combined" = symptom-level combination; diagnoses were made if the full set of diagnostic criteria was endorsed by any informant, alone or in combination with other informants. "Clinical" = clinical combination. "Sum" = number of symptoms or behaviors endorsed were summed across informants. "Mean" = scale scores were averaged across informants.
[e]PREV = prevalence. NUM = number of symptoms or behaviors endorsed. SER = seriousness of behavior.
[f]Teacher for children aged 4–11, child for children aged 12–16.
[g]Diagnosis included ad hoc impairment criterion.
[h]Three separate sets of path analyses were conducted on composite scores for participants who had (1) CBCL and TRF scores, (2) CBCL and YSR scores, and (3) CBCL, TRF, and YSR scores. Results indicate which variables were significant direct predictors in two or more sets of analyses.
[i]Measure included items assessing alcohol and drug use.
[j]Multivariate analyses included SES, poverty, family size, family structure, changes in family structure, family mental health service use, stressful life events, and other 1. Achenbach syndrome scores.
[k]Analyses were performed separately for males and females. Results were the same for each gender.
[l]Multivariate analyses included age, gender, racial/ethnic background, family structure, income, neighborhood type, neighborhood stability, and neighborhood quality.
[m]Participants were classified according to the severity of the most serious act ever committed reported by any informant.
[n]Lifetime aggression.
[o]Prevalence threshold = 75th percentile.
[p]Prevalence threshold = three or more behaviors endorsed.
[q]Prevalence threshold = T score ≥ 60.
[r]Multivariate analyses included age, gender, racial/ethnic background, and parental education.
[s]Multivariate analyses included gender, family structure, family size, maternal age, maternal education, SES, and urbanization.
[t]Includes mixed Conduct Disorder and Emotional Disorder.
[u]Prevalence threshold = one or more behaviors endorsed.
[v]Separate analyses were performed on each of 5 annual waves of data. Participants were 11–17 years old at Time 1 and 16–21 years old at Time 5. Results were the same for each wave.
[w]Prevalence threshold = T score ≥ 70.

685

Index

ISBN 0-306-45974-4

90000